CLINICAL NURSING

Pathophysiological

Psychosocial
Approaches

Irene L. Beland

R.N., B.S., M.S.
Professor of Nursing, College of Nursing
Wayne State University, Detroit, Michigan

CONTRIBUTORS:

ESTHER H. READ

A.B., M.Ed., R.N.
Emeritus Professor of Nursing, College of Nursing,
Wayne State University, Detroit, Michigan;
and Visiting Professor, School of Nursing,
Universidad del Valle, Cali, Colombia

JANE FRANCES RONAN

B.S., A.M., R.N.
Assistant Professor of Nursing, College of Nursing,
Wayne State University, Detroit, Michigan

NANCY MARTIN

B.S., M.A., R.N.
Director, Nursing Department,
Rehabilitation Institute of Chicago, Chicago, Illinois

JOYCE Y. PASSOS

B.S., M.S., Ph.D., R.N.
Associate Professor and Chairman,
Department of Medical and Surgical Nursing,
College of Nursing, Wayne State University,
Detroit, Michigan

JEAN A. WERNER

M.N., R.N.
Associate Professor of Nursing, College of Nursing,
Wayne State University, Detroit, Michigan

CORINNE H. ROBINSON

M.S.
Emeritus Professor of Nutrition,
Drexel Institute of Technology, Philadelphia;
formerly Instructor of Nutrition and Diet Therapy,
Jefferson Medical College Hospital, School of Nursing, Philadelphia

ELIZABETH FORD PITORAK

B.S., M.S., R.N.
Associate Professor of Medical and Surgical Nursing,
Case Western Reserve University, Cleveland, Ohio

ROBERTA K. ADLER

B.S.N., M.S., R.N.
Instructor, College of Nursing,
Rutgers University, Newark, New Jersey

CLINICAL NURSING

Pathophysiological

&

Psychosocial
Approaches

SECOND EDITION

The Macmillan Company

Collier-Macmillan Limited/London

THE MACMILLAN COMPANY
866 Third Avenue, New York, New York 10022
COLLIER-MACMILLAN CANADA, LTD., Toronto, Ontario

Library of Congress catalog card number: 70–92079

PRINTING   8910   YEAR   3456789

PREFACE
to the First Edition

THIS book is written for the nursing student who is studying medical-surgical nursing for the first time. The approach that is used has been developed in the teaching of medical-surgical nursing over a period of many years. An attempt has been made to organize a vast quantity of material into a meaningful whole and to present the person who is ill as a total individual, not as a sick arm, leg, or heart. To further this objective the content of one chapter is related to and built upon earlier chapters and anticipates the content of later ones. Content is selected from the biological, physical, and social sciences. Emphasis is on normal as well as pathological physiology. Throughout the text the relationship of the function of one part to that of other parts of the body has been stressed. Since derangement in the function of one part is likely to affect other functions, including psychological and emoitonal functioning, these relationships are included. Further, an attempt has been made to organize all aspects of a function so that the interrelationships of different bodily functions are shown. As an example, one vital function is the maintenance of nutrition. All elements entering into the nutritional status from those affecting food supply and the ingestion, digestion, and absorption of food, to its utilization by cells, are presented. Through this approach, it is hoped that the student will have a broader base from which to evaluate the needs of each patient. A conscientious effort has been made to show how a variety of elements such as age, hereditary background, cultural background, state of nutrition, causative agent or agents, and the organs affected influence the effects of illness and the behavior manifested by the patient and his nursing requirements.

Surgery is regarded by the writer as a form of treatment. Recognition is given to the fact that the person experiencing surgical therapy has some special requirements. However, because he is a human being who has an illness, many of his needs are similar to those of other sick persons.

In the selection of content, three criteria have been given priority: first, that the information act as a basis for answering the question "Why?"; second, that it have broad rather than limited applicability; and third, that it have relevance to the practice of nursing as defined by the writer. Though nurses perform many activities, including acting as the physician's assistant, and as the protector and custodian of machines, their function in ministering to and in behalf of the patient has been emphasized.

Extensive footnoting and bibliographies have been used. It is hoped that sufficient content has been included to provide the student with a base to which she can continue to add. No effort has been made to be encyclopedic. With the rapid expansion of knowledge and techniques, it is essential that the nurse be prepared to continue her own learning. Hopefully, the content of the book will also help to prepare the student for change and to make changes. If nursing is to survive, the members of the profession must be prepared to accept and effect change. The maintenance of the *status quo* is no longer adequate.

In the development of the content a number of concepts [1] have been presented and discussed. They include:

1. Adaptation is basic to survival.
   a. The human organism is flexible and permits adaptations at all levels of activity (physiological, psychological, social).
   b. As an organism increases in complexity, specialized structures are required to facilitate adaptive functions.
   c. In health, physiological and psychological changes are regulated within limits.
   d. Some of the effects observed in disease result from the utilization of adaptive mechanisms.
   e. In disease, adaptation may be deficient, excessive, disorganized, or initiated by inappropriate stimuli.
   f. The physiological and psychological changes occurring in disease have a cause or causes, and within limits, some of them serve a useful purpose.
2. Heredity and environment interact to create individual potentials and differences.
3. Patient needs determine patient care.

[1] Many of these concepts were developed by a group of the faculty of Wayne State University College of Nursing.

v

4. Organization facilitates the utilization of resources to meet human needs.
5. Optimum health is a desirable goal.
6. The value of an observation depends on the integrity and detachment with which it is made and on its specificity.
7. Perceptions of reality vary with the perceiver.
8. The interaction of multiple factors determines the outcome of a situation.
9. Progress from disease toward health involves an increase in the capacity of the patient to cope with stress. During illness and recovery, the patient's needs shift from dependence, to independence, to interdependence.
10. Manifestations of disease and behavior during illness result from:
    a. An attempt on the part of the organism to adapt to or to compensate for disturbed function.
    b. The mobilization of defense mechanisms.
    c. The effect of injury on cells comprising a tissue or organ.
    d. The meaning that a disease and its treatment has for a person.
11. What a person does when he is ill depends on what he believes to be the cause of his illness and how he thinks it should be treated.
12. Therapy in disease includes one or more of the following: neutralizing the cause, encouraging compensatory mechanisms, and providing rest to the diseased organ so that healing can take place.
13. Respect for the rights and dignity of man is fundamental in a democratic society. This is just as essential to the sick as to the well.
14. Mutual trust is basic to the establishment of constructive nurse-patient relationships.
15. Acceptance of the patient involves considering the meaning of his behavior and recognizing that it has a cause and serves a purpose. It does not require the nurse to compromise her own system of values.
16. The behavior of a person is affected by and affects all persons and events with which he is involved.
17. Rehabilitation is a continuous process which begins with the first contact with the patient.
18. The patient has a right to participate in plans concerning his welfare.
19. The nurse has a responsibility to assist the patient and his family to utilize his resources constructively.
20. Nurses have an obligation to explore interests and aptitudes with the patient to increase his skills in living.
21. Nursing procedures can be used to facilitate communication.
22. There are limits to what can be accomplished by medical science.
23. Birth, growth, health, disease, and death are all phenomena of life.

For some readers, too much content may be provided in some areas and too little in others. Certain specialized areas of the body now included in medical-surgical nursing texts have not been included. No attempt has been made to include a wide variety of procedures. For the most part, procedures are included for the purpose of illustrating or emphasizing a point or points. Although the nurse does have a responsibility for using machines properly and for knowing whether or not they are operating properly, little attention has been given to the operation and care of machines employed in the treatment of disease. When directions provided by the manufacturer are inadequate, technicians from the factory are usually available to instruct in the use and care of complicated machines.

The writer would like to express her appreciation to the many persons who assisted in countless ways in the preparation of the manuscript. First are the students, who, over the years, asked the question, "When are you going to write a medical-surgical nursing book based on physiology?" or made statements such as, "Nursing makes more sense and is more fun when you are encouraged to seek answers to the question 'Why?'" Finally, the graduates of the class of 1962 provided concrete assistance by trying out and making constructive suggestions used in the revision of the "Guide for Assessing the Needs of Patients."

Certainly, the manuscript would have never been started or completed had it not been for the cooperation, patience, and prodding of Dean Katharine Faville of the College of Nursing of Wayne State University. Among others who provided encouragement are Miss Sylvia Peabody, R.N., Dean Mary Kelly Mullane, R.N., and Dean Rozella Schlotfeldt, R.N.

Those who read parts of the manuscript and assisted with the library research that went into its preparation and writing include the following: Mrs. Mary Ann Gray, R.N., Mrs. Joyce Passos, R.N., Miss Nancy Couture, R.N., Miss Milenca Herc, R.N. (deceased), Mrs. Lorene Fischer, R.N., Mrs. Mildred Konlande, Miss Kathlene Monahan, R.N., Mrs. Charlotte Pickering, R.N., Mrs. Claudia Watson, R.N., and Mrs. Dawn Zagornik, R.N. Special thanks go to Mr. Theodore Draves, who typed and retyped the manuscript in all of its revisions. I am greatly indebted to Dr. Gordon Doty, who, with the exception of the chapters on the special requirements of patients treated surgically and neural integration, read the entire manuscript. Dr. Raymond C. Read took time from a busy schedule to read the chapter on the special requirements of surgical patients. Dr. John Sterling Meyer read and commented on the chapter on

neural integration. My gratitude also goes to my colleagues who cheerfully assumed some of my responsibilites when the manuscript was in preparation and to those who participated in the identification of nursing concepts.

Finally, the writer wishes to express sincere appreciation to the staff of the Macmillan Company, and especially to Mr. Henry Van Swearingen, for their help and cooperation during the preparation and production of this book.

IRENE L. BELAND

PREFACE
to the Second Edition

THE objectives and approach of the second edition are similar to those of the first. In the selection of content I have tried to keep in focus Szent-Gyögyi's statement: [1]

> We, in our teaching, should place more emphasis on generalizations than on details. Of course, details and generalizations must be in proper balance: generalization can be reached only from details, while it is the generalization which gives value and interest to the detail.

and later in the same paper:

> My friend Gerard quoted Fouchet as advising us to take from the altar of knowledge the fire, not the ashes.

Changes that have been made are for the purposes of updating the content, improving the organization, deleting unnecessary repitition, and making the material easier to locate.

References, within the limits of time taken to convert the manuscript into a book, are up to date. Because of the volume of literature in some areas, not all useful articles could be included. In general, articles from nursing journals, particularly those based on nursing research or practice, and review articles were given priority.

Four contributors have been added to those who helped with the first edition. Because they are all knowledgeable in their fields, they have made a substantial contribution to this book.

Two new chapters have been added. Chapter 2 of the first edition has been divided into chapters entitled "Historical Perspectives" and "The

[1] Albert Szent-Györgyi: "Teaching and the Expanding Knowledge," *Science*, 146:1278 (Dec. 4) 1964.

Health-Illness Spectrum." "Historical Perspectives" traces the history of man's ideas about health and the causes and treatment of disease. The history of health-related legislation is reviewed. Because information about Social Security, Medicare, and Medicaid is readily available, details are not included. Chapter 3 is intended to provide a framework for understanding that health and disease are a part of life and are interrelated. The stages of health care beginning with the promotion of health, the prevention of disease, and the natural history of disease are considered.

Another new chapter, Chapter 11, is devoted to shock. Although Chapter 11 might have been placed elsewhere, it follows the chapter on transportation of material to and from cells. Much of the content presented in previous chapters is utilized and expanded, explaining the pathophysiology of shock.

To facilitate the use of this book, brief outlines have been placed at the beginning of each chapter and the number of topic headings has been increased.

The author wishes to thank all those who used the first edition and the individuals who offered constructive criticisms. Without the help of the contributors and the readers, the revision could not have been completed. The efforts of the following deserve special comment: Vainutis K. Vaitkevicius, M.D., Associate Professor and Chairman, Division of Oncology, Wayne State University School of Medicine, who read Chapter 14, commented on it, and contributed the material on chemotherapeutic agents; Robert P. Williams, Ph.D., Professor of Microbiology,

Baylor University, who read and made suggestions on Chapters 5 and 6; Robert F. Wilson, M.D., Associate Professor of Surgery, Wayne State University School of Medicine, who read and commented on Chapters 9, 11, and 17; Rubin Meyer, M.D., Professor of Pediatrics, Wayne State University School of Medicine, who read the material in Chapter 9 on acute glomerulonephritis; Robert Gruskin, Ph.D., who read Chapter 15A; and Henry C. Bock, M.D., Indiana University School of Medicine, who read Chapter 19A. Many of the improvements in these chapters follow the advice offered by these men.

The work of preparing the manuscript was greatly facilitated by Mrs. Patricia Skalski, R.N., who devoted untold hours to library research and who read each chapter. Important contributions were made by Sister Dorothy Schmidt, R.N., O.S.F., and Mrs. Leola Hogan. Sister Dorothy prepared the index and Mrs. Hogan drew some of the new figures. Special thanks also go to Miss Kathleen Monahan, R.N., Mrs. Darlene Rodgers Stewart, R.N.; Mrs. Dawn Zagornik, R.N.; Miss Edith Johnson, R.N.; Mrs. Eleanor Sheridan, R.N.; Miss Mary Patricia Endress, R.N.; Miss Fredricka Shea, R.N.; Miss Susan Beland, R.N.; Miss Wilma Geels, R.N.; Miss Katherine Marquis, R.N.; Miss Barbara Schmidt; and Mr. Theodore Draves, who typed the manuscript. Miss Ann Price also gave secretarial assistance. My brother Ralph, as well as my mother, helped in numerous ways to further the completion of the revision. I am grateful to Dean Margaret Shetland, Ed.D., R.N., College of Nursing, Wayne State University, who made it possible for me to have a leave of absence to work on the revision.

Words cannot describe my gratitude to Mrs. Barbara Johnson, chief librarian, and the other members of the Harper Hospital library staff. They were consistently helpful during the many hours Mrs. Skalski and I spent in the library.

Finally, appreciation is due Mr. Henry Van Swearingen, Mr. T. P. McConahay, and other members of the staff of The Macmillan Company for their help and encouragement.

I. L. B.

CONTENTS

1

Introduction

She opened her hands to the needy and stretched out her hands to the poor. . . . Strength and honesty are her clothing. . . . She rendered good, not evil, all the days of her life. . . . The law of clemency is on her tongue. . . . Many daughters have gathered together riches but the valiant woman has surpassed them all.

THE BOOK OF PROVERBS

THIS book, *Clinical Nursing,* is concerned with the nursing of the person whose presenting problem is primarily pathophysiological. Like many scientific terms, this one is not altogether helpful, for it tells how but not why the person is ill. Whatever its nature, illness is the consequence of the interaction of multiple factors— the susceptible host, the etiological agent(s), and the environment. Disturbances at any level of organization—biochemical, cellular, systemic, psychological, interpersonal, or social—are likely to result in disturbances at other levels. For example, Mr. Quick is angry with his wife. Not only does he feel and look angry, but also he manifests his anger by changes in behavior. On the biochemical and physiological levels, secretion of catecholamines increases. Among the changes occurring are increases in the amounts of blood glucose and cholesterol. His muscles contract, he loses his appetite, and his blood vessels constrict. On the interpersonal level he shouts at his wife, is sharp with his son, and is rude to the neighbor next door. He gets into his car and backs out of the driveway, narrowly missing a two-year-old child playing in the street. In other words, Mr. Quick is angry as a whole individual, and he manifests his anger as a unit, not as a part.

Beliefs Underlying Selection of Content

Certain beliefs underlie the selection of content for this book. The first is that every person is an individual human being with dignity and rights. A person does not, or should not, lose his dignity and rights as an individual because he is sick or well, old or young, clean or unclean, rich or poor, criminal or law abiding. Further, he has physiological, psychological, social, and spiritual needs that must be met if he is to survive, grow, and be productive. In health he is able to meet his needs through his own efforts. When he is ill he requires assistance in meeting one or more of his needs. Because of lack of specialized knowledge and skills, he may also require assistance to maintain an optimum state of health.

A second belief is that the practice of professional nursing requires a body of knowledge of facts, theories, principles, and concepts. This body of knowledge is derived from the humanities and the biological, physical, and behavioral sciences. It is necessary to the understanding of (1) the role of the nurse; (2) the needs of people; (3) the importance of the ability to adapt physiologically, emotionally, and socially to changes in the environment; and (4) the results of failure of man to adapt.

A third belief is that professional nursing has a real contribution to make in the promotion of health, in the prevention of disease, and in the care of those who are sick, those who will be cured, and those for whom cure is unlikely and/or for whom this is the last illness. The phrase "to give nursing care" has real meaning when it expresses the attitude of the nurse as she expresses her concern for the patient's welfare. She does this freely and without the expectation that he will reward her by expressing gratitude for her services. Nor will he always accept what she has to offer in ways that she expects. In fact, he may reject it. Rejection of the service should not result in the rejection of the person. In other words, care is given unconditionally. The nurse expresses her concern for the patient both by doing and by her manner of doing.

How has nursing been defined?

The attempt to define nursing is not new, for over a hundred years ago Florence Nightingale [1] wrote that nursing signified "little more than the administration of medicines and the application of poultices." She continued by saying that it ought to signify the proper use of fresh air, warmth, cleanliness, and quiet and the proper selection and administration of diet—all at the least expense of vital power to the patient. Moreover, Miss Nightingale [2] did not limit nursing to the care of the sick, for she wrote, "The same laws of health, or of nursing, for they are in reality the same, obtain among the well as among the sick."

One of the most widely quoted definitions of nursing is that of Virginia Henderson.[3]

The unique function of the nurse is to assist the individual, sick or well, in the performance of those activities contributing to health or its recovery (or to peaceful death) that he would perform unaided if he had the necessary strength, will or knowledge. And to do this in such a way as to help him gain independence as rapidly as possible. This aspect of her work, this part of her function, she

initiates and controls; of this she is master. In addition she helps the patient to carry out the therapeutic plan as initiated by the physician. She also, as a member of a medical team, helps other members, as they in turn help her, to plan and carry out the total program whether it be for the improvement of health, or the recovery from illness or support in death.

Is nursing a profession?

The question "Is nursing a profession?" raises two further questions. What are the characteristics of a professional person? And what are the characteristics of a profession? Darley [4] describes the characteristics of a professional person as follows: "the truly professional person is one, who, by virtue of intellectual capacity, education and moral outlook, is capable of the exercise of intellectual and moral judgment at a high level of responsibility." In his discussion of the professional person, Darley emphasizes the importance of judgment based on "broad knowledge, penetrating wisdom and great moral certitude."

McGlothlin [5] makes essentially the same points when he says that a professional person has four characteristics: professional competence, understanding of society, ethical behavior, and scholarly concern.

Johnson [6] states that professional practice depends on at least three elements: "(1) the knowledge, skill, and personal qualities of the practitioner; (2) an established process and methodology in decision-making; and (3) the availability of a body of knowledge relevant to the management of practical problems of considerable social significance." Johnson [7] further states that any description of professional practice must emphasize the responsibility and accountability of the practitioner. Her decisions must be skillfully and wisely made, and she must base her decisions on knowledge so that what she does is based on what she knows.

Towle [8] further defines the characteristics of a profession and professional practice by adding that "(1) a profession has attitudes toward the recipients of its service that are essential to the giving of service in ways that are helpful to the recipients, (2) a profession has something to

[1] Florence Nightingale: *Notes on Nursing: What It Is, and What It Is Not,* New Edition, revised and enlarged (London: Harrison and Sons, 1860), p. 2.

[2] *Ibid.,* p. 4.

[3] Virginia Henderson: "The Nature of Nursing," *Amer. J. Nurs.,* **64**:63 (Aug.) 1964.

[4] Ward Darley: "The Professions and Professional People," *Nurs. Forum,* **1**:83 (Winter) 1961–62.

[5] William J. McGlothlin: *The Professional Schools* (New York: Center for Applied Research in Education, Inc., 1964), pp. 22–29.

[6] Dorothy E. Johnson: "Professional Practice in Nursing" in *The Shifting Scene—Directions for Practice* (New York: National League for Nursing, 1967), p. 26.

[7] *Ibid.,* p. 33.

[8] Charlotte Towle: *The Learner in Education for the Professions* (Chicago: University of Chicago Press, 1954), p. 3.

give that is unique and that other members of the community do not have to offer to the same degree."

Nursing, as it is practiced today, is not always on a professional level. The writer believes, however, that nursing can and should qualify as a profession. This belief is supported by Towle,[9] who has included nursing in her list of professions.

To examine the possibility of nursing being a profession, certain characteristics of a profession and of professional practice have been selected for discussion. They include (1) ethical behavior, herein defined as a rigorous professional code and standard; (2) nursing care as a unique service to society; (3) professional competence; (4) understanding society; and (5) scholarly concern.

Although ethical behavior is demonstrated by individual members of a profession, each profession has a code that serves as a guide to the individual. In 1950 such a code was formulated by the American Nurses Association (ANA). It was revised in 1960 and again in 1968. A copy can be obtained from the ANA. One point emphasized in the code is that a profession has attitudes toward the recipients of its service that are essential to giving service in ways that are helpful.

What are some of the attitudes of the nursing profession toward the patient?

One attitude of those in professions having as their purpose helping people is respect for every person as an individual human being with dignity and rights. Every person has and retains his dignity and rights whatever his state in life, his religion, color, national origin, economic status, age, state of health, or personal habits. True respect for the dignity and rights of the individual is demonstrated in many ways. The person is treated with kindness, thoughtfulness, and courtesy. Service, whether it be for, to, or with the individual, is given in a way that meets the needs of the individual. Moreover, service is continued as long but only as long as it is required. The person who is sick is allowed to be sick, but as soon as he is able to resume the management of his own affairs he is encouraged to do so. Emphasis is on helping the individual to identify his strengths and resources and on assisting him in utilizing them rather than taking over and acting for him. When the latter is necessary, as it sometimes is, the reason should be to meet a need of the patient and not to meet a need of the nurse. An important objective is to identify and meet the needs of the patient in ways that are appropriate to the person and his situation. The behavior of the patient is recog-

nized to have a cause and to serve a purpose. Respect for him as an individual demands that an effort be made to consider the meaning of his behavior and to act accordingly.

Another attitude that the truly professional person has is acceptance that the recipient has needs, physiological, psychological, social, intellectual, and spiritual, that must be met if he is to survive and be productive. At times one need may take precedence over others; however, when the nurse is attending to a priority need, other needs should not be ignored. It is the responsibility of the profession to try to identify what needs it is prepared to meet and how it can go about meeting them.

A third attitude of a professional person is that he is not only responsible but also accountable for his actions. Despite the practice in the past for hospitals and physicians to be held responsible and accountable for the care of patients, recent legal decisions have also held nurses to be responsible and accountable for making decisions and for the outcome of these decisions. When the welfare of the patient is in jeopardy, a nurse may be held accountable for injury incurred by him, unless she can show that she acted appropriately.

To recapitulate, nursing as a profession is concerned with the welfare of the individual as an individual. It professes to respect the rights and dignity of each and every patient. It recognizes that each patient has needs, some of which can be met through the practice of nursing. It accepts the premise that each patient has the right to participate to the degree that he can in plans for his welfare. Although practice of nursing involves doing to, for, and with the patient, it further involves assisting him to become independent of the services of nursing as soon as he is able to do so. The profession has as a general objective the meeting of the needs of the patient, in distinction to meeting its own needs—that is, either those of the individual nurse or those of the profession. The above list of attitudes characteristic of a profession is not exhaustive, nor is it meant to be. Rather the intention has been to examine some of the attitudes fundamental to a profession. To the extent that these attitudes influence positively the practice of nursing, nursing can be said to be a profession. Morally and legally, professional persons are responsible and accountable for their actions.

The second characteristic of a profession is that it has some services or skills that are unique to that profession and that other members of the community do not have to the same degree. Despite some investigation and discussion, nurses are not in agreement about which skills are unique to nursing.

---

[9] *Ibid.,* p. 3.

What skills or services does the professional nurse have that other members of the community do not have to the same degree?

One view is that the area that is unique to nursing is the giving of physical care. Those who espouse this view do not mean, nor do they intend to mean, that nursing is limited to the physical care of the patient. When it is, it is a mechanical or technical procedure, just as any service to people may be. Physical care is made professional by the manner in which it is provided and by the degree to which the nurse identifies and meets other needs of the patient. Nurses too often fail to respect the importance of physical care to the patient, both to his immediate welfare and as a means of establishing a helping relationship with him.

Another view is that nurse-patient communication is the essential element in nursing care.[10] Those who believe that the critical element in nursing is the nature of nurse-patient communication would rightly say that the manner in which physical care is given is a form of communication.

Most nurses agree with Florence Nightingale that control of the external environment of the patient is a nursing responsibility.

Differing points of view about what is unique to nursing can be in part reconciled by remembering that nurses, like other members of the American culture, tend to look at the part away from the whole and to want a single answer to each question or problem. Perhaps this pitfall could be avoided if the needs of the patient were identified and priorities established for what is important in the care of a patient at a particular time. Care would then be planned in terms of the needs of the patient. Those needs for which the professional nurse possesses competence would be met by the practice of nursing. Those for which she lacked competence would be referred to or performed by others, such as the physician, social worker, occupational therapist, or clergyman.

PROFESSIONAL COMPETENCE

The third characteristic of a profession is that it demands a high degree of competence, both in knowledge and in skill, in its practice. No one denies that nursing requires a high degree of skill. There is less agreement as to how much or even what knowledge is required. Towle[11] quotes Tyler as emphasizing "that it is in the nature of a profession that it bases its technique

of operation upon principles rather than upon rule-of-thumb procedures or simple routine skills." Nursing faces the task of identifying the principles on which the practice of nursing is based. Because this has not been done very well, this is an area where the status of nursing as a profession is weak. There is little doubt that the welfare of the patient often depends on the exercise of considerable judgment on the part of the nurse. Basic to making valid judgments is a body of knowledge of the principles on which judgment is based. Studies presently underway as well as those of the future will in time lead to the identification of these principles.

Another decision to be resolved by the nursing profession is the degree to which the newly graduated nurse is able to function at the time he or she enters the profession. Should the graduate be able to function more or less independently in all or some settings with a minimum amount of supervision, or should he or she require a period of orientation by an employing agency before being able to function effectively? In the past the goal of education in nursing has been the first. Currently there is movement toward the second.

UNDERSTANDING SOCIETY

McGlothlin[12] says "Thus, the practitioner in every profession needs social understanding to do his work well. He needs it even in the introductory phases of his practice to provide a framework within which he can accumulate and interpret the experience he gains. He needs it to relate his practice to the larger social issues which face the profession and its society."

Among the reasons for a nurse to understand society and social issues is that she can better appreciate the significance of her contribution to society as well as what society's needs are.

Only a few of the many problems with which nursing has a concern are listed below. Not all are of equal significance. How and where should nurses be educated? How does nursing fit into the health care system in the United States? How does society cope with a rapid shift of rural populations to cities? How do health agencies meet the demands placed on them by Medicare and Medicaid? What effects have mass communication media had on man's expectations and sophistication? How has industrialization changed the hazards to which man is exposed? How has the fact that people are coming to view health care as a right rather than a privilege affected the demands made on the health care system? What effect will regional

[10] Jean E. Johnson, Rhetaugh G. Dumas, and Barbara A. Johnson: "Interpersonal Relations: The Essence of Nursing Care," *Nurs. Forum,* 6:325 (Summer) 1967.

[11] *Op. cit.,* p. 5.

[12] *Op. cit.,* p. 25.

medical planning have on nursing and what influence will nursing have on it? How will the fact that the average length of life has increased affect the kind and number of health facilities required? How will the rapid expansion in knowledge and technical developments influence the practice of nursing? What are the health needs of various cultural groups and how can they best be met? Why are recent biological discoveries of concern to all? The purpose of the above list has been to raise and not to answer questions. Some, but not all of them, will be discussed later.

SCHOLARLY CONCERN

As a service profession, nursing has stressed skill in providing care for patients. Only recently have an increasing number of nurses emphasized the need for having a considerable body of identifiable knowledge. It is possible to base actions on intuition and experience and for them to be appropriate. Knowledge, however, is essential for the identification of the possible reasons for a patient's behavior as well as its significance. Decisions based on knowledge of the possibilities are more likely to be correct than when they are made according to rule or intuitively. Further, the improvement of nursing practice depends on studying present and new practices. In today's world one either goes forward or goes backward. There is no standing still. To cite one example, in one study [13] no nurses, doctors, or technicians working in a hemodialysis unit developed infectious hepatitis. Several nurses who assisted with this procedure on general wards developed it. Undoubtedly nurses performing the procedure in the specialized unit were more knowledgeable about the danger of hepatitis than those in the general wards.

In the preceding paragraphs nursing as a profession has been examined in reference to some of the characteristics of a profession. Although the discussion has not exhausted the possibilities, perhaps the reader will be stimulated to think about what being professional means and what nursing must do to be, or to become, a profession. Sometimes insight can be gained into what one does or ought to do by examining the views of persons who are not of the profession.

What are some of the roles of the nurse in patient care?

Recently sociologists have developed an interest in the role of the nurse in patient care.

They suggest that the actions taken by nurses in the care of patients can be classified under two roles. One, the therapeutic or instrumental role, includes all those actions directed toward the prevention and treatment of disease. The other is the expressive role or mother-substitute role. It includes all those activities directed toward creating an environment in which the patient feels comforted, accepted, protected, cared for, and supported. The emphasis in the performance of the expressive role is not on cure, but on care. Johnson and Martin [14] and Schulman [15] emphasize that the physical care of the patient is an important vehicle for communicating to the patient the concern of the nurse for his welfare.

Because the therapeutic role of the nurse has as its goal the prevention and cure of disease, discussion of the details of this role will be included in later chapters. Inasmuch as all patients experience the manner in which they are nursed, the expressive role of the nurse will be considered in some detail here. Johnson and Martin [16] state that the objective of the expressive role is the relief of tension in the group. The group is composed of the doctor, nurse, and patient. Though they do not so state, the group actually consists of all those who have some relationship to the patient, including the members of his family and his friends. They further state that, in any social system, certain problems must be solved if the system is to maintain itself. That is, it must move forward toward the accomplishment of a common goal and it must maintain internal equilibrium. They explain by stating that "relationships between the social system members must be harmonious and integrated and each member must feel good both within himself and toward other group members." They emphasize the importance of the nurse in this role by suggesting that it is here she is the expert and as such should give leadership. She stands as an intermediary between the patient and the doctor and what he does for and to the patient. If this view is accepted, the nurse also stands between the patient and the other persons who participate in his care. To fulfill this role, she must know what the common goal or objective is and give leadership to those working toward its achievement. She leads by utilizing her skills in such a manner that each person feels "good within himself and toward other members of the group." Johnson and Mar-

[13] John B. Eastwood, *et al.*: "Hepatitis in a Maintenance Hemodialysis Unit," *Ann. Intern. Med.*, 69:59–66 (July) 1968.

[14] Miriam M. Johnson and Harry W. Martin: "A Sociological Analysis of the Nurse Role," *Amer. J. Nurs.*, 58:374 (March) 1958.

[15] Sam Schulman: "Basic Functional Roles in Nursing: Mother Surrogate and Healer," *Patients, Physicians and Illness*, E. Gartley Jaco, ed. (New York: The Free Press, 1958), pp. 528–37.

[16] *Loc. cit.*, p. 373.

tin[17] emphasize that the physical care of the patient is important because it gives the nurse an opportunity to reduce the tension of the patient and to promote good feeling.

Schulman [18] compares the feeling that the nurse should have for her patient as being similar to the feeling of a mother for her child. The early phase of the mother-child relationship is largely physical and marked by tenderness and compassion. The mother tends her child and stands between him and harm. She comforts him and soothes his hurts. As the child grows and develops in his ability to care for himself, she encourages him to become independent of her. The mother gives of herself and of her material resources to meet his needs, because he is her child.

Johnson and Martin [19] state that the expressive role of the nurse can be carried too far and that the needs and wants of a patient can be so gratified that he prefers sickness to health. As in other situations, multiple factors contribute to the preference of the patient for sickness to health. The nurse should not assume that she is necessarily the one who is responsible for the patient's behavior. She should examine her behavior to be sure that she is not contributing to the situation. The physician usually is responsible for indicating to the patient that he is not trying to get well and that his behavior is not acceptable. The nurse has the responsibility for recognizing the signs indicating that the patient is finding the secondary gains of illness preferable to returning to the healthy state and for supporting the physician and the patient when the physician decides the time has come to help the patient move toward recovery.

A second problem in the practice of the expressive role concerns the nurse. She must have and convey to the patient a very real concern for his welfare and at the same time develop in herself the ability to evaluate objectively both his behavior and the effect of her own behavior on him. She may find that in one instance she was too supporting and in another she withdrew her support too soon, or that she was too permissive or too limiting. She may also find that she felt so strongly with the patient that she was unable to give him the support he needed to consider his alternatives or to do what he knew he had to do. Psychologists emphasize that the more the person is concerned with himself, the less he is able to be concerned with others. The nurse contributes to the welfare of the patient when she not only is able to communicate to him her interest in and concern

for his welfare, but also maintains enough objectivity to evaluate his needs and act in the manner that is best suited to meet them.

What do patients want from nursing?

A study performed by Abdellah and Levine [20] to determine what patients want from nursing provides some answers to the above question. In summarizing their study, they say that a patient wants:

1. To be treated as an individual, that is, he wants his care to be personalized rather than depersonalized
2. An explanation of his care
3. To be considered as a partner in his care
4. To have his behavior as a sick person accepted as a part of his illness
5. To be treated with thoughtfulness, kindness, and firmness

The Patient as a Person

How can the care of the patient be personalized?

Basic to the treatment of each patient as an individual is respect for him as a person. This respect is demonstrated in many ways. The treatment of each patient with the same courtesy that one expects from one's associates goes a long way toward establishing the fact that the patient is an individual. This courtesy should be extended to the patient's family and friends. They have a right to be concerned about the patient and his welfare as well as a role to play in his recovery. An effort should be made to allow the family to express their feelings and to interpret their behavior in the light of its meanings. The effect of their behavior on the patient should also be evaluated. When some change is necessary, explanations should be in terms of the needs of the patient and recognition should be given to the interest of the family in the welfare of the patient.

If the nurse accepts the fact that she has a responsibility for the welfare of the patient, she will intervene when the quality or quantity of visiting is likely to be detrimental to his interests. An exaggerated, but true, example of the abdication by the nurse of her responsibility to protect the patient from harm is illustrated by the following anecdote. Mary Lively, age 17, was hospitalized on Friday night. She had been in an automobile accident and had two crushed lumbar vertebrae and some superficial scalp wounds. On the following Sunday she and her

[17] *Ibid.*, p. 374.
[18] *Loc. cit.*, p. 530.
[19] *Loc. cit.*, p. 376.

[20] Faye Abdellah and Eugene Levine: "What Patients Say About Their Nursing Care," *Hospitals*, 31:44 (Nov. 1) 1957.

roommate had 84 visitors. When Mary's mother visited her in the evening, she found Mary in a state of near collapse. When Mrs. Lively complained, she was told that it was the responsibility of the family to regulate visitors. Though she had visited Mary in the morning, she had not been in the hospital at the time when most of the visitors arrived. She had asked that a sign be placed on the door indicating that not more than two visitors be admitted at a time. The visitors cooperated. They lined up and entered the room two at a time until the room was full. The conclusion that the nurse in this situation had lost sight of her responsibility to protect the patient and that she failed to exercise reasonable judgment is an understatement. Moreover, patients other than those immediately involved must have suffered.

One unique characteristic of each person is his name. Therefore a way to show respect for an individual is to call him by his name and title. Despite a trend toward informality, an adult should be called by his surname preceded by the appropriate title, that is, Mr., Mrs., or Miss. Unless there is a specific and identified reason, an adult should not be addressed by his first name. Certainly first names should not be used to indicate that the social or economic status of the patient is less than that of those who care for him. Calling an elderly person "Grandma" or "Grandpa" may express affection, but it may also be interpreted by the patient to indicate a lack of respect for him and his potential. Some elderly persons bitterly resent being called "Grandpa" or "Grandma" by anyone except their grandchildren. A patient who is addressed by his first name or who is nameless does not always express his resentment openly, but this does not mean that he fails to feel resentment.

Respect for the individual is expressed by the nurse when she greets the patient when entering his presence and includes him in any conversation carried on in his presence. Other courtesies too often neglected include asking the permission of the patient when it is necessary to interrupt his activities or his care. His care should not be interrupted unless it is absolutely necessary. Respect for the patient as an individual also includes sensitivity to his feelings. This is expressed when the nurse tries to modify her behavior so that the patient knows that she appreciates how he feels. She tries to avoid being excessively cheerful in the presence of a downcast or depressed patient. On the other hand, she also avoids being depressed herself.

Respect for the patient is evidenced when his suggestions, opinions, and concerns are treated with courtesy and thoughtfulness. It is also evi-

denced when the nurse protects him from unnecessary embarrassment by protecting his modesty and by helping him prepare for the visit of his doctor or family.

Respect for the patient is demonstrated by creating an environment in which the patient is able to express his feelings and by interpreting his behavior as an expression of an unmet need or needs and then acting appropriately. Sometimes a patient is demanding and aggressive because he feels depersonalized. He fights to be recognized as a human being. The patient may relax when he is certain that he can depend on the nursing staff to meet his needs as an individual.

The nurse is likely to find individualization of each patient's care easier if she has some awareness of her own values as well as of her biases and prejudices. No one is completely free of prejudice. When an individual knows what he values and what his biases and prejudices are, he may be able to limit their effect on the care he provides the patient. For example, Mrs. Laura, a public health nurse, took pride in being unprejudiced. One day as she was thinking about how unsuccessful she had been with the Hill family, she thought. "How could anyone be successful with those hillbillies?" As she talked about her experience later, she said she was shocked to learn that she too had prejudices and thought of people not as individuals but as stereotypes. After she recognized what she had been feeling, she was better able to manage her feelings and as a result to enlist the cooperation of Mrs. Hill.

Although numerous situations in which care of a patient was or was not individualized could be cited, only three will be presented. In the first situation, failure to meet an obvious or overt need of the patient contributed to the patient's feeling of depersonalization and to failure of the nursing personnel to experience satisfaction. In the second situation, the nurse recognized and met a covert need of a patient. The last illustrates why it is impossible to individualize care by rule.

The first patient, Mrs. Devoted Family, had undergone major surgery several days previous to the incident cited below. Following her operation, both she and her family expressed their concern about her progress openly and volubly. One of her less serious complaints, from the point of view of the personnel, was that her feet were cold. Though she complained to everyone who participated in her care, nothing was done to relieve her discomfort. Her family took their mother's discomfort seriously and bought her a lovely, white, wool shawl, which they placed over her feet. A few days later the shawl was discarded with the bed linen. Naturally, Mrs. Family and her children were upset. The nursing staff responded by saying that they had no responsibility for the personal belongings of the patient; nothing could be done to recover the shawl. In this instance the simple procedure of placing a bath blanket over Mrs. Family's feet might have been sufficient to relieve her discomfort. Mrs. Family might well have had her feelings of importance enhanced had the nurse placed a blanket over her feet in such a manner that the patient knew that the nurse wanted her to be comfortable. Moreover, the manner of the nurse might also have suggested that if the blanket did not accomplish the objective there were other things that she could and would do. She could give Mrs. Family a hot-water bottle (if her condition permitted) or ask her daughter to bring her some bed or ankle socks. In any event the patient's feeling of depersonalization might have been reduced by any one of several simple acts. As it was, both the patient and her family felt that Mrs. Family was neglected. She had suffered a double injury—cold feet and a lack of appropriate action to correct her discomfort as well as the loss of a valued possession. These feelings were strengthened by the loss of the shawl and failure of the nursing staff to appear to make any effort to retrieve it. The nursing staff was also deprived because they failed to achieve any sense of satisfaction in the care of Mrs. Family.

The next patient is Mr. Johnson. In the care of Mr. Johnson the nurse recognized and responded to a need that the patient was unable to express directly. Mr. Johnson was a middle-aged, obese man with a diagnosis of far-advanced carcinoma of the lung. He was allowed bathroom privileges and permitted to sit in a chair as he desired. Patients who were up and about were expected to take their own sponge baths. Showers and bathtubs were not available. One busy morning just before noon his nurse stopped to check with Mr. Johnson to see whether or not he had taken his bath. In response to her inquiry he said, "I did the best I could." The nurse might have said, "I'll make your bed, or send the aide in to do it." She, however, interpreted Mr. Johnson's statement as saying, "I was not able to take a very good bath and I'd like to be given one." She thought a moment about his reply and realized that although he was up and about even a small amount of exertion caused Mr. Johnson to be short of breath. She got a basin of warm water and *gave* him a bath. As she was bathing him, he lay back against his pillows, sighed, and relaxed, saying, "This is the first bath that I've had since I came here."

The third patient is Mrs. Willow. Mrs. Willow was a young-middle-aged woman who some months earlier had had a radical mastectomy for cancer of the breast. The cancer had since metastasized to her spine and now impinged on her spinal cord. She was unable to control the movements of her lower extremities. Slight movement or jarring of her body resulted in muscular spasms accompanied by severe pain. Mrs. Willow was in the hospital for the purpose of determining the amount of a curarizing drug that would control the muscular spasms without paralyzing the muscles of respiration. After spending three days in a ten-bed ward, she was moved to a double room and was placed in the bed next to the door. She spent her days sitting in bed and guarding herself each time someone came into the room. Her general expression was that of a frightened fawn. In this instance the head nurse at the daily nursing care conference talked with the group about Mrs. Willow. Together they worked out ways to protect Mrs. Willow from avoidable suffering. A sign was placed on the door to warn those who were entering to avoid jarring her bed. The dietary aide was asked to call a nurse when Mrs. Willow's tray was ready rather than to deliver it to the room. As soon as the patient in the bed away from the door was discharged, Mrs. Willow's bed was moved. A special procedure was planned with Mrs. Willow so that her bed linen could be changed without causing her unnecessary discomfort. Other procedures were also modified. Suggestions were recorded on the "Nursing Care Record" so that the information about Mrs. Willow's special needs could be communicated to all members of the staff.

Though there was no possibility of cure in the instance either of Mr. Johnson or of Mrs. Willow, both these patients benefited from thoughtful and creative nursing. In both these instances the nurses also experienced satisfaction, inasmuch as they concentrated on and were able to improve the situation of the patient. In the care of these patients, nurses demonstrated their concern for the welfare of the patient largely through physical care, and they exercised judgment in the realm that is nursing. In neither instance was the amount of time involved great. In fact, time was probably saved in the care of Mrs. Willow.

How can nurses prepare patients for what to expect?

In addition to the wish of the patient to be treated as an individual, Abdellah and Levine [21] found that he wants an explanation of his care. Another way this may be said is that he wants to know what to expect and what is expected of

[21] *Loc. cit.,* p. 48.

him. Wertham,[22] a psychiatrist, in discussing his own experience as a patient, made the following comments: "Medical and surgical patients need psychological advice about how they should act, what their experiences mean; they need psychological preparation for what to expect; they need guidance, so that they can make the best of their possibilities."

Preparing the patient for what to expect includes acquainting him with such hospital routines as when meals are served and medicines administered, when his friends may visit or telephone him, and how to call the nurse. He should be informed about those aspects of his care requiring some change in his behavior. For example, he is to stay in bed until seen by his physician, or he is free to move about and go to the solarium, or he should stay in his room. Most persons who are ill are more or less anxious; they frequently need to have instructions repeated a number of times, as high levels of anxiety interfere with the ability to learn. Because the patient often has questions about his illness and the plan of therapy, the nurse will find it helpful to know what information the physician has given the patient. Even when the physician has given the patient a careful explanation of his disease and of what is required in its treatment, he may have failed to comprehend what was said. When the nurse knows what the patient has been told, she can answer his questions or refer them to his physician with the expectation that she is relieving rather than creating further tension.

Part of preparing the patient for what to expect is to determine what the patient expects and wants to know. Patients are frequently subjected to unnecessary anxiety, unless time has been taken to determine what their expectations are. To illustrate, Mrs. Fox, who had had heart surgery two weeks previously, was found lying on a cart in the hall outside the room where cardiac catheterizations were performed. The nurse who stopped to greet her learned that she had "been waiting for hours," and that she expected "to be stabbed in the back" without benefit of anesthesia. The fact that the catheter was to be introduced through an arm vein made her suffering quite unnecessary, had someone taken the time to determine her understanding of the procedure and to correct her misinformation. Moreover, she might have been less apprehensive if someone had stayed with her.

Determination of what the patient expects and wants to know helps to prevent giving him information that suggests problems or difficul-ties he has not anticipated. Wertham [23] makes this point in regard to his own situation. A surgeon made the comment to him that phlebitis seldom affects the arms. Previous to this time the possibility that his arms might be involved had not occurred to him, and it became a source of worry. He found himself trying to detect pain first in one arm and then in the other.

How can a patient participate as a partner in his care?

A patient is helped to be a partner in his own care when he is prepared for what to expect and for what is expected of him. When he is able to help himself by such activities as exercising, deep breathing, and coughing, he knows that he has a part in his recovery. Moreover, appraisal of how long a painful procedure will take and comments indicating progress help to keep the patient informed about how long he has to continue to brace himself. Further, both types of comments assure him that the person who is performing the procedure is aware of his needs. He is then better able to follow instructions relative to his part in the procedure.

A patient is often asked to assume responsibility for aspects of his own care. When this is done, he should be told that he is encouraged to take this responsibility because it furthers his recovery. Too often patients gain the impression that they are asked to bathe themselves or ambulate because the nurses are too busy or do not want to care for them rather than because activity is part of their therapeutic regime.

At other times patients wish to retain certain responsibilities or privileges. These are sometimes denied them without adequate thought being given to the reason for the refusal or to the value that the responsibility has to them. To illustrate, Mrs. Lottie Gamely had disseminated cancer of the breast which had metastasized to the cervical spine. She was in more or less constant pain and was very fearful lest any activity increase it. Her husband brought her some tablets of Empirin [24] compound, which she planned to take as needed. In the course of giving her care, the nurse discovered the Empirin in her bedside table. Before removing the medication, she talked with Mrs. Gamely's physician. The decision was made to leave the drug at the bedside because it gave Mrs. Gamely the feeling that she had some control over her pain.[25] The possibility of any harm resulting was negligible. Later, this patient expressed her

---

[22] Fredric Wertham: "A Psychosomatic Study of Myself," *When Doctors Are Patients,* Max Pinner and Benjamin Miller, eds. (New York: W. W. Norton & Company, Inc., 1952), p. 115.

[23] *Ibid.,* p. 117.

[24] Trade name for tablets containing phenacetin, 0.15 g (gr. 2½); acetylsalicylic acid, 0.23 g (gr. 3½); and caffeine 30 mg (gr. ½).

[25] In some hospitals selected patients assume responsibility for taking their own medications.

feeling that she was a partner in her care. This was revealed when the nurse told Mrs. Gamely that she was going on vacation and that she had enjoyed working with her. Mrs. Gamely responded by saying, "I've enjoyed working with you, too."

The satisfaction of the wish of the patient to be considered a partner in his care depends on the belief that each individual, sick or well, has a right to participate in plans concerning his welfare. The nurse has a responsibility to provide the individual with the information he needs in order to consider his alternatives, to carry out his decision after it is made, or to change his mind. Sometimes a patient is pressed to make decisions that he is unable or unprepared to make. If he feels that he is censured or blamed for failing to make the "right" decision, he may be unable to change his mind. Physicians and nurses sometimes forget that a patient may be asked to adjust to or make a decision about a procedure that may affect the entire course of his life and to do it quickly. Human beings tend to react to change with anxiety. Excessive anxiety makes the objective evaluation of his situation by the patient difficult, if not impossible.

In the practice of nursing, the nurse will see persons whose diseases require prompt action and yet who refuse to have treatment. Mrs. Youthful Thirty-Five was such an individual. She was found to have an ulcer on the left labia majora, which on examination proved to be cancer. Her physician explained why she should have a resection of the labia, and she entered the hospital to be prepared for surgery. On the morning of her operation she told Miss Noll, the nurse who was preparing her for surgery, that she had changed her mind. She would not have the operation. Miss Noll related the information to the surgeon. He came to see Mrs. Thirty-Five and calmly reassured her that she was free to decide whether or not she would have the operation. He tried to convey to her that he understood her feelings and that should she change her mind the operation could be performed at a later time. He encouraged her to remain in the hospital for a few days, so that the ulcer could be treated medically.

He left orders for sitz baths and dressings, as the lesion was draining. A plan was made to encourage Mrs. Thirty-Five to talk about her fears but not to force her to do so. Careful attention was given to her physical care. Her doctor saw her regularly. About a week later she decided to have the operation. It was not easy even then. She had had, however, an opportunity to consider her alternatives and to come to the decision that the operation was preferable to allowing the disease to progress.

In addition to the patient wanting to be treated as an individual, to have an explanation of his care, and to be considered as a partner in his care, Abdellah and Levine found that he wants to have his behavior as a sick person accepted as part of his illness and to be treated with thoughtfulness, kindness, and firmness. Mr. Tenny, a young man who had suffered a cervical cord injury when struck by a car, expressed this desire when he said, "I've been difficult, I know. But then doctors and nurses ought to understand how difficult this whole experience has been for me."

CREATING AN ENVIRONMENT OF TRUST

Though it is not stated explicitly in Abdellah and Levine's study, the patient wants to feel he can trust those responsible for his care. The confidence of the patient is built on his being accepted as an individual and on the confidence of the nurse in her ability to meet his needs. It is facilitated by the way his care is provided, by its timing, and by attention to details of his care, especially those that are important to him. It is strengthened by keeping promises and by keeping the patient informed about the status of those that take time to fulfill. For example, Mr. Samuel was promised a high-low bed. When the nurse called the storeroom, she learned that one would not be available for several hours. She relayed this information to Mr. Samuel. Later, when it had not arrived at the expected time, she called the storeroom and then told Mr. Samuel that the bed was on its way. The fact that the nurse kept Mr. Samuel informed helped to develop his confidence that she was concerned with his welfare.

The nurse may not always be able to fulfill all the expectations of the patient, nor is she always responsible for the fact that they are not met. She is responsible for trying to determine what they are and for considering them in his care. Most persons who are sick enough to require medical and nursing care suffer some degree of anxiety. When they are hospitalized, the environment is strange and frightening. A sick person should not be expected to be at his best. Despite his illness, he remains a human being and should be treated with courtesy and thoughtfulness. Interest in him as a person, concern for his welfare, kindness, and a desire to be helpful should all contribute to his confidence that his needs will be met.

CONCEPT OF PATIENTS' RIGHTS

Some of the rights of patients have been presented earlier. Chiles [26] states four rights. They

[26] Robert E. Chiles: "The Rights of Patients," *New Eng. J. Med.*, 277:409–11 (Aug. 24) 1967.

are (1) the right to privacy, (2) the right to pain, (3) the right to truth, and (4) the right to die. He includes under the right to privacy the right to keep his own counsel. He should not be expected to expose himself emotionally any more than he is expected to be exposed physically. The environment should be such that he feels accepted and respected.

In discussing the right to pain, Chiles does not mean that the patient should be subjected to unnecessary or cruel pain. Rather, pain should be accepted as a warning and a plea that the patient be taken seriously. Whatever its cause, pain indicates that something is wrong and that the patient is suffering.

The right to truth and the right to die will be considered elsewhere. Chiles is of the opinion that patients who want the truth should have it. If persons were certain that they could have the truth when they want it, at least some of them would be saved needless worry. Those with serious illness would then have someone to share their suffering.

CONCEPT OF PATIENTS' NEEDS

On what should the patient's nursing care be based?

The nursing care of each patient should be based on his individual needs. Briefly stated, patient needs determine patient care. This statement implies that the needs of the patient should be assessed and the assistance he requires identified. From the data collected, a nursing diagnosis can be established. The nursing diagnosis serves as a basis for the formulation of a nursing care plan directed toward the accomplishment of immediate and long-term goals. Because needs of the patient are seldom static, regular re-evaluation of the plan is essential if his needs are to continue to be met.

In the following chapters the basis for understanding each of the needs of the patient will be discussed in some detail. As the various needs are discussed, the fact that a human being functions as a whole should not be lost from sight. A disturbance in the capacity of an individual to meet one or more needs affects the whole person, not just a part of him. Moreover, a disturbance in the capacity of the individual to meet one need may interfere with his ability to meet other needs. Except in the terminal stages of an illness, however, the patient can be expected to be able to meet some of his needs without the aid of others.

For nursing care to be based on the needs of the patient, it is obvious that the nurse must be able to identify what they are. She must have an understanding of what is meant by the term

need, as well as which needs take priority. Moreover, to understand how needs are affected by illness and how to assist the patient in meeting his needs, some knowledge of the mechanisms used for defense and protection against changes in the environment is necessary. Knowledge of the mechanisms utilized to limit and to repair injury or disturbance is also essential. Finally, assessment of the success of the patient in meeting his own needs depends on knowledge of the behavior that indicates he is or is not successful.

What are some areas of understanding that are essential to fulfilling the concept "Patient needs determine patient care"?

Murray's [27] definition of need is paraphrased by King [28] as follows: "a concept that stands for a force of some nature in the brain region, an organizing force that affects thinking, knowing, perceiving in such a way as to change an existing, unsatisfying situation in certain directions. Each need is accompanied by a particular feeling or emotion, and even though sometimes weak or momentary, it usually persists and gives rise to overt behavior or fantasy, which may change the external circumstances sufficiently to appease or satisfy the organism and still the need."

Needs must be satisfied if the organism is to carry on one or more of the activities of life. These activities may be classified as (1) use of food and oxygen with the release of energy, (2) response to the environment, (3) growth, (4) reproduction, and (5) productivity. Needs may arise from, or be met at, any of the levels of organization of the human being—biochemical, cellular, systemic, psychological, interpersonal, and social.

According to Gordon, four basic phenomena of the nervous system make it possible for man to adapt, to survive, and to satisfy his needs in an ever-changing environment. They are pain, hunger, fear, and rage.[29]

CLASSIFICATION OF NEEDS

Though needs may be listed in endless detail, they will be considered in five broad categories. They are the (1) physiological, (2) safety, (3) psychological, (4) social, and (5) spiritual needs. All living beings have needs. On the cel-

[27] Henry A. Murray: *Explorations in Personality* (New York: Oxford University Press, 1938), pp. 123–24.
[28] Stanley H. King: *Perceptions of Illness and Medical Practice* (New York: Russell Sage Foundation, 1962), p. 43.
[29] Gerald Gordon: "To Live or Not to Live with Your Job," *Nurs. Forum,* **1:**38 (Winter) 1961–62.

lular level they are similar for all organisms. Man differs from other living beings in his psychological, social, and spiritual needs. The needs common to all species are sometimes referred to as basic or survival needs. These are the requirements that must be met to maintain life. Basic needs are prepotent, or take precedence, over others. Another way this concept can be stated is that needs are organized in a hierarchy with lower needs demanding satisfaction first. They must be satisfied before other needs are manifested and given attention. For example, physiological needs must be met to some degree before psychological needs can be expressed. Even among the basic needs some are more urgent than others. Some physiological needs, such as the need for oxygen, take precedence over the need for food or water. Knowledge of the fact that some needs are more important to survival than others has implications for the practice of nursing. For example, the patient who is acutely short of oxygen is unlikely to be interested in food, much less in conversation or other intellectual activities. Even more significant, his survival may well depend on correction of his oxygen deficit. Most students have at some time tried to study when they were cold, hungry, or angry and found that they were unsuccessful until they put on a sweater, had something to eat, or recovered from their anger.

Material relating to all needs will be integrated throughout. There are, however, a few general points in regard to safety that bear emphasis at this time.

One relates to the patient, another to the unsafe act, and a third to the responsibilities of those caring for the patient. Safety as related to the patient has two aspects: (1) a real danger or threat to his welfare and (2) his feeling that he is safe or in danger. Threats to the safety of the patient may have their origin in either his internal or external environment. As an example, the life of the patient is threatened by any condition that deprives him of some substance required by his cells or by failure to remove excesses of supply or products of metabolism. The life of the patient may also be endangered by conditions in the external environment such as extremes in temperature or radioactive substances or rays. What the person regards as being unsafe depends on his past experience and the unknown elements in his situation. A patient who interprets his symptoms as indicating the presence of a disease such as cancer is likely to be frightened during the period of diagnosis. Another patient feels unsafe when his light is not answered promptly. He wonders whether or not he can depend on help, should he really need it.

A general threat to safety is what Chapman [30] calls the unsafe act. According to Chapman, all accidents have their origin in an unsafe act. Knowledge of certain facts about unsafe acts contributes to their control. Few unsafe acts result in injury and still fewer result in death. The person who is responsible for an accident is not always the one who is injured. Sometimes the relationship between the unsafe act and the accident is not immediate or direct. Moreover, an accident may result from a series of unsafe acts. This point is illustrated by the instance of the man who was killed by an iron bar falling from an open window. The first unsafe act was the construction of a building with windows opening directly over the street. The second was the use of an iron bar to prop a window open. The third was failure to remove the bar from the window sill preparatory to opening the window. When the effect of an unsafe act is delayed the identification of who is responsible may be difficult, if not impossible.

A similar example, though less serious in outcome, occurred in General Hospital. The physician wrote the following order: "phenobarbital 30 mg t.i.d. to be administered by subcutaneous injection." The order was transferred to a medicine card and written on the Kardex by a ward clerk. The head nurse initialed the medicine card. The nurse caring for the patient administered phenobarbital tablets, U.S.P., instead of the more soluble form, sodium phenobarbital, U.S.P. Although no harm came to the patient, his safety was threatened by a series of unsafe acts. The one person in the series who was not negligent was the ward clerk.

The control of accidents depends on knowledge of the potential dangers and of the human factors entering into the performance of unsafe acts. Accident prevention takes planning, preparation, and instruction so that people may learn what the dangers are and develop the attitude that accidents can and should be prevented. Their prevention is the responsibility of everyone. In terms of the second example, each person had a responsibility to assure the patient's getting the correct drug in the correct form.

What factors alter the capacity of the individual to tolerate the frustration of a need?

The capacity of the individual to tolerate frustration of one or more needs depends on a number of factors. One factor is the adequacy of his structures and processes for meeting the need and for adapting to change. This is exemplified by the brain-damaged individual, such as one who has had a stroke, who may have very little tolerance for frustration. He becomes

[30] Albert L. Chapman: "The Anatomy of an Accident," *Public Health Rep.,* **75**:630 (July), 1960.

excited or upset when faced with minor difficulties. A general anesthetic reduces the ability of the person to adapt the caliber of his blood vessels to changes in position. The child who is born with a defect in the structure of his heart may be unable to meet the need of his tissues for oxygen during exercise. In general the individual can tolerate the frustration of a need better if the condition that is responsible develops slowly rather than rapidly. Time allows the organism an opportunity to adapt to the change both by altering its requirements and by initiating mechanisms that increase the effectiveness with which it utilizes its supplies. The capacity to tolerate frustration, particularly of psychological needs, depends also on the degree to which the need has been met in the past, especially in early life. Because illness involves the failure to meet one or more needs, the capacity of the sick person to tolerate frustration of his needs is often limited. For example, the patient who is in the period immediately following a major operation is unable to anticipate and adapt to changes in his environment. Changes such as moving him from the stretcher to the bed, or loud noises, may be followed by a fall in blood pressure. Until he fully recovers from the anesthetic, he must be protected from falling out of bed. Until he is up and about, procedures to maintain the patency of his airway are required. Until his alimentary canal can tolerate food and fluids, they must be administered parenterally.

The meeting of needs also depends on the availability of supplies or materials. For example, the requirement for oxygen cannot be met unless there is oxygen in the atmosphere. The need to be loved and to give love cannot be met unless love is available.

As has been previously implied, the capacity of an individual to meet his needs depends on processes and mechanisms that in health are regulated so that their action is appropriate, effective, and constructive. Structures and processes are required for the regulation of intake, distribution, use, storage, output, and elimination of excesses of supply or of waste products resulting from activity. Not only are individual processes regulated so that a need is met, but each process is regulated so that it is integrated into the activities of the total individual. In man many structures and functions may be involved in satisfying one need. To illustrate, the physiological need for water involves structures and processes whereby a deficit of water is recognized and is translated into the sensation of thirst. Further, coordinated activity is required to obtain, drink, and absorb water into the blood stream. Many more processes are involved in the distribution of water to the

cells, in its temporary storage, and in the elimination of an excess by the kidney.

To assist the nurse in collecting data, a guide is placed at the end of the chapter. The purpose of this guide is to provide a basis for the organized collection of data required to make a nursing diagnosis. Not all the information suggested is available for every patient, nor is it always necessary. Some of it may be obtained from the patient's hospital chart and medical history or from his family or physician. Moreover, continuous assessment is essential. As the patient recovers or fails, his needs change. As a consequence, his nursing care requirements also change.

To collect the information required to make a nursing diagnosis, knowledge and skill in the field of interpersonal relationships, as well as in the observation and interpretation of the signs and symptoms indicating deviations from normal functioning and behavior, are essential. After the data are collected, they should be analyzed and the problems that can be met through the practice of nursing identified. Problems outside the province of nursing or that are shared with other disciplines should be referred to the appropriate persons. The welfare of the patient often depends on the coordination of the activities of all who have a part in his care. In fact, the patient's care cannot be said to be truly comprehensive without it.

For example, to meet the food requirements of a patient, persons from a number of disciplines combine their efforts to make the proper food available to the patient. The physician prescribes the diet. The dietitian translates the prescription into food and is responsible for its preparation and serving. When the patient requires formal dietary instruction, this is frequently the responsibility of the dietitian. The nurse prepares the patient for his meal and feeds him, when necessary. She answers his questions about his nutritional needs, or his diet, or refers them to the physican or dietitian. The nutritional needs of many patients are met by each individual nurse, physician, and dietitian, performing his functions. When problems arise, however, their solution may depend on the combined efforts of the nurse, dietitian, physician, patient, and even the members of the family.

To illustrate, Mary Ellen Cliff was a young woman with a diagnosis of rheumatoid arthritis. She ate very little and consequently was weak, lacking in energy, thin, and frail looking. She was cared for at home by her mother and a visiting nurse who visited her twice a week. In the course of her visits the nurse learned that Mary Ellen ate poorly. She discussed this problem with Mary Ellen's physician, who said that her weakness and lack of energy were directly related to inadequate food intake. He prescribed a high-calorie diet and said that he would again talk to Mary Ellen about the importance of eating. To evaluate Mary Ellen's food pattern, the nurse asked her to keep a record of her food intake for three days. The nurse gave Mary Ellen and her mother instructions about how to make the study and told how the information was to be used. As a result of the study, the nurse's previous suspicion that Mrs. Cliff was an indifferent and unimaginative cook was borne out. Part of the problem stemmed from poorly prepared and unattractively served food. The nurse arranged for a consultation with the agency dietitian. The dietitian talked with the physician, and then she planned a diet that included foods Mary Ellen liked and that if eaten would be adequate to her needs. She also suggested that the nurse take some recipes with her that Mrs. Cliff might try to use. Mary Ellen was encouraged to try to eat even when she did not feel like it. After six months of continued effort Mary Ellen had gained 10 lb and her appetite had improved considerably. She was able to be out of bed and was beginning to think about seeking employment. Mrs. Cliff's cooking, though not in the gourmet class, was much improved. In this particular instance the nurse carried much of the responsibility for the instruction and the management of the patient and her mother. The solution of the problem, however, depended on the cooperative efforts of the members of several disciplines.

In the preceding sections of the chapter consideration has been given to the nature of professional nursing and the needs and wishes of patients. In the following section the concept of the nursing process will be presented.

The Nursing Process

What is it? How is it defined?

Although the outward and visible signs of nursing are what the nurse does for, with, or in behalf of a patient, her actions are based on a series of intellectual processes that are not directly visible. Together these intellectual activities and nursing actions are called the *nursing process*. Despite the recent introduction of the term, there is nothing new about the nursing process. What is new is the attempt to identify nursing problems and the steps taken to bring about their resolution. Essentially it is neither more nor less than a systematic method of problem solving, which includes actions intended to resolve or mitigate a problem. Thoughtful and

knowledgeable nurses have always used it. The nursing process is based on the scientific process. The foundation for the scientific process was laid by philosophers such as Sir Francis Bacon and Sir Isaac Newton. It was further developed and refined by the great scientists who followed them. The general rules followed by the scientist are (1) observe and choose facts, (2) form a hypothesis that links the facts together, and (3) carry out a sufficient number of experiments to prove or disprove this hypothesis.[31]

These three general rules have been further defined and clarified to include the activities involved in the nursing process. Before a model of the nursing process is developed, two other models will be presented.

Knowles [32] states that "the most significant characteristic of the professional nurse is her ability to make decisions about nursing care. What she does—her Doing—is her most public and identifiable activity, but if it is to serve her patients' needs it must be the end product of a conscious process which reflects her educational background and experience." Knowles [33] presents a model in which she uses five words as keys to the process: (1) discover, (2) delve, (3) decide and plan nursing approaches, (4) do, and (5) discriminate.

Although Knowles' five D's are easy to remember, they do not cover all aspects of the decision-making process. Neither do they provide for the establishment of criteria or standards by which the solution(s) to nursing problems can be judged. This is an important aspect of nursing and one that has not been done. Further, the word *discriminate* is intended to imply evaluation. Unfortunately, the two terms are not synonymous. To evaluate the results of the process should therefore be added, as well as to alter the plan in light of new information or as the condition of the patient changes.

A comparison between Knowles' model and Griffiths' [34] conventional model of the decision-making process is given in Table 1-1.

Nite and Willis [35] consider the nursing process to include four different, though interrelated, groups of activities. They are to (1) identify the patient's nursing problems, (2) state

[31] Disproving a hypothesis may be as great a contribution as proving it.

[32] Lois Knowles: "Decision Making in Nursing—A Necessity for Doing," in *ANA Clinical Sessions, 1966* (New York: Appleton-Century-Crofts, 1967), pp. 248–49.

[33] *Ibid.*, pp. 248–49.

[34] Daniel E. Griffiths: *Administrative Theory* (New York: Appleton-Century-Crofts, 1959), p. 94.

[35] Gladys Nite and Frank N. Willis, Jr.: *The Coronary Patient* (New York: The Macmillan Company, 1964), p. 35.

TABLE 1-1

Knowles' Model	Griffiths' Model
1. Discover	1. Recognize, define, and limit the problem
	2. Analyze and evaluate the problem
	3. Establish criteria or standards by which solution will be evaluated or judged as acceptable and adequate to the need
2. Delve	4. Collect data
3. Decide and plan nursing approaches	5. Formulate and select the preferred solution or solutions. Test them in advance
4. Do	6. Put into effect the preferred solution
	a. Program the solution
	b. Control the activities in the program
5. Discriminate	c. Evaluate the results and the process

nursing objectives directed toward solution of the nursing problems, (3) make a plan of care designed to achieve the objectives, and (4) evaluate the effectiveness of the plan.

The nursing process, as developed by the author and clinical nursing colleagues is as follows:

STEPS

1. Observe
2. Measure and quantify
3. Communicate
4. Classify data—organize facts into related groups
5. Predict
6. Infer
7. Formulate hypothesis
8. Develop a plan of care (involve the patient and his family as is appropriate)
   Decisions to be made
   8.1 State the patient's nursing needs and translate them into objectives of care
   8.2 Establish priorities
   8.3 Consider possible approaches and alternative solutions
   8.4 Select appropriate nursing methods
   8.5 Make an appropriate time plan
   8.6 Coordinate plan with the plans for other patients in group
   8.7 Coordinate and integrate all activities entering into the overall plan of therapy
   8.8 Anticipate future needs
9. Carry out plan—the doing or visible part of the nursing process

STEPS

   9.1 Inform the patient of the details of the plan so that he will know what to expect and what is expected of him
   9.2 Carry out the plan (intervene)
10. Evaluate the plan and change as indicated (includes acting on interpretation of data as well as new information)

For an example of the scientific process, see Gagne.[36]

STEPS IN THE NURSING PROCESS— A DISCUSSION

The first three steps in the nursing process are for the purpose of gathering information about the patient and his situation. Communication is discussed in Chapter 7 and will not be considered here.

OBSERVE

Throughout the history of modern nursing the value of observation has been recognized. Florence Nightingale wrote, "For it may safely be said, not that the habit of ready and correct observation will by itself make us useful nurses, but that without it we shall be useless with all our devotion." [37]

Observation is the act of noting and recording facts or occurrences in language or code. Observations involve the real. They are made by using the five senses: sight, hearing, touch, smell, and taste. Instruments can be utilized to increase the ability of the senses to obtain information as well as to measure and quantify the information obtained. Observation is a description, not an interpretation, or judgment, or evaluation. Certain difficulties enter into the making of observations. These include a tendency to interpret and evaluate rather than to describe. When the word of others has to be taken, the likelihood of error is increased. There are limits to the ability of any person to observe accurately, remember, and report. Past experiences influence what an observer "sees," for what he sees depends in part on what is in the environment and in part on what he is. There is always the possibility of overlooking or underestimating significant clues as well as misinterpreting or overestimating their importance. As an experiment, note the ways in which different people describe and interpret a similar incident or statement.

Skill in observation can be increased by systematic and regular practice. This practice can be done in any setting from an aquarium

[36] Robert M. Gagne: "Elementary Science: A New Scheme of Instruction," *Science*, **151**:49–53 (Jan. 7), 1966.

[37] *Op. cit.*, p. 160.

to a zoo. Group practice followed by a comparison of notes is useful in improving observational skills.

Facts about the individual patient, how he interprets his situation, and what his expectations are for himself and for others can be obtained by purposeful conversation with him and with the members of his family. Purposeful conversation as a tool in nursing care of the patient is discussed in Chapter 7. For students who wish to read further in this area, references have been included in the References for Chapter 7.

REPORT AND RECORD OBSERVATION

In reports or records of observations, what has been noted should be described as carefully and specifically as possible. The kinds of questions the description of the observation should answer are the following: What was seen? Heard? Touched? Smelled? Tasted? What quantity? Quality? Where? When describing what a patient says, use his exact words as far as is possible. Judge what is recorded by the following concept. The value of an observation depends on the integrity and detachment with which it is made and on its specificity.

CLASSIFY DATA

To increase the likelihood that the data collected may be of benefit to the patient, it should be classified according to some system. An example of a classification technique, a data-gathering guide, follows the discussion of the nursing process.

PREDICT OR FORETELL

After making observations and classifying them, the next step is to try to predict or foretell the possible outcome of the patient's nursing problems as well as the efforts made to solve or relieve them. Some predictions will be reasonably accurate, whereas others may be less so. For example, a patient who has had an appendectomy and is up and about and eating well can be expected to recover. The nurse can predict with some assurance that if the patient who has had a stroke or has been burned is kept in good alignment, he is less likely to develop contractures than one who is not. The patient who knows medication will be given promptly if he has pain generally requires less medication than the one who is uncertain.

CLINICAL INFERENCE—DEFINITIONS AND TYPES

The term *inference* can be defined quite simply as a conclusion arrived at by reasoning from a fact or facts that are known. Ham-

mond [38] defines an inductive inference as the process of reasoning from a specific fact or facts to the general case. Katherine Kelly [39] defines clinical inference as "making a judgment about the state of the patient and/or the nursing needs of the patient."

For a more complete discussion of clinical inference in nursing, see the series of papers published in *Nursing Research* beginning in the summer of 1966. Depending on a variety of factors, inferences may be perfect or imperfect, theoretical or empirical, and statistical or intuitive. Hammond [40] states that "Nearly all of our actions are based upon imperfect inductive inferences based on uncertain, probabilistic information. . . . our inferences are normally 'uncertainty-geared'." He [41] further states that many inferences made by nurses about the state of the patient are empirical and intuitive rather than theoretical or statistical.[42] The nurse is faced with the problem of correctly inferring the state of the patient from uncertain and incomplete data. Though she lacks theoretical knowledge, she is expected to make judgments on the medical state of the patient. This requires that she think not only like a nurse but like a doctor. The studies of Hammond and his associates indicate that the inferential tasks of the nurse are highly complex. Further, the nurse often needs far more knowledge than is generally appreciated.

To illustrate, Mrs. David has a pituitary tumor removed. Shortly after the operation she regains consciousness and appears to be recovering as expected. She complains of thirst and voids from 500 to 700 ml of urine every 1–2 hr. What do these observations mean? Certainly the fact that Mrs. David knows who and where she is are favorable signs. What does the fact that she says that she is thirsty and voids 500–700 ml of urine every 1–2 hr mean? Unless the nurse knows that these signs accompany a deficiency of the antidiuretic hormone, a real possibility is that this patient may die as a result of excessive loss of water from the blood.

HYPOTHESIS—WHAT IS IT?

The next step in the nursing process is to formulate a hypothesis or a number of them.

[38] Kenneth R. Hammond: "Clinical Inference in Nursing: II. A Psychologist's Viewpoint," *Nurs. Res.,* **15**:27 (Winter) 1966.
[39] Katherine Kelly: "Clinical Inference in Nursing: I. A Nurse's Viewpoint," *Nurs. Res.,* **15**:24 (Winter) 1966.
[40] *Op. cit.,* p. 28.
[41] *Ibid.,* p. 30.
[42] Empirical inference—one based on past experience. Theoretical inference—one based on knowledge. Intuitive inference—the knowing of something without conscious learning. Statistical inference—relationship established by mathematical treatment of data.

A simple definition of *hypothesis* is that it is an educated guess. Feibleman [43] states that "A hypothesis is a proposition which seems to explain observed facts and whose truth is assumed tentatively for purposes of investigation." For example, several hypotheses might be suggested to explain Mrs. David's large urine output. One is that she was overhydrated during the surgical procedure. Another is that she has diabetes insipidus. A better guess is that the trauma incurred during the operation resulted in swelling with pressure on the tissues surrounding the neurohypophysis. As pressure increased, release of the antidiuretic hormone decreased—a condition that is readily treated when recognized.

To clarify and summarize, two further examples are presented. Mrs. Smart is lying quietly in bed. Her hair is neat and she has polish on her fingernails. On her bedside table is a picture of a little boy. These are observations or facts. What inferences can be made from these facts? Are there enough facts to conclude that the little boy is her son? He may not be; he may be her nephew or grandson or the child of a friend. What are her feelings toward him? What other *facts* must be known before these questions can be answered? To emphasize, through observations, the *facts* in a situation are determined. These facts have value inasmuch as they are accurately and clearly described.

Sometimes the data available are inadequate to explain the event; then an educated guess, or hypothesis, may be made. For example, a man whose blood pressure is 90/60 arrived in a hospital emergency room following an automobile collision. There is a large wound in his right arm from which he has been bleeding. Though his normal blood pressure is not known, from the known facts the inference that he is in shock is reasonable. What is fact and what is assumed to be fact, however, should be kept clearly in mind. As new evidence is uncovered, new or different interpretations may be required.

MAKE DECISIONS

Based on the data collected and their meaning, the nurse makes one or more decisions. Stated simply, she makes up her mind about what the patient's nursing needs are. In the instance of Mrs. David, she notes the disparity between her intake and output. She also knows that if output continues to exceed intake the patient will soon be in serious trouble. The nurse has a number of alternatives. She can continue to observe the patient and see if the condition corrects itself. She can encourage Mrs. David to drink as much fluid as she can.

She can report her observation to the physician. Because the nurse knows that after surgery performed in the region of the neurohypophysis increased urine output and marked thirst indicate a decreased release of ADH, she decides to report her observations to the physician.

After the nurse has decided what the patient's nursing needs are, she translates them into nursing objectives and establishes priorities. As part of the decision-making process, the nurse considers the patient's wants and wishes as well as her own interpretation of what his needs are. For example, Mrs. Giat is unconscious. Among her nursing needs are such requirements as maintaining a clear airway, preventing skin breakdown, maintaining fluid intake, maintaining good body alignment, and others. She states the needs as objectives and decides which takes first priority, second, and so on. Actually all are important.

CONSIDER POSSIBLE APPROACHES AND
ALTERNATIVE SOLUTIONS

For each objective the nurse must consider what approaches she can use to achieve it. After she has identified the possibilities, she then selects the one or ones that appear to be most feasible.

At this point she is or should be ready to continue through the rest of the nursing process. The remaining steps should be clear as stated in the outline. From the above discussion it should be evident that sound nursing practice is based on a high level of intellectual activity.

COMPONENTS OF NURSING PRACTICE

To emphasize the complex nature of nursing practice, two nursing leaders will be quoted.

Abdellah [44] summarizes the *elements* in the practice of nursing as follows:

1. The continuous mastery of human relations, including the mastery of technical and of managerial skills needed to take care of patients
2. The ability to observe and report with clarity the signs and symptoms and deviation from normal behavior that a patient presents (this element would include the mastery of basic communication skills)
3. The ability to interpret the signs and symptoms that indicate deviations from health. A nursing problem exists in a situation involving patient care, a possible solution to which is found through the services that are the functions of nursing
4. The analysis of nursing problems, which will guide the nurse in carrying out nursing func-

[43] James K. Feibleman: "The Role of Hypotheses in the Scientific Method," *Perspect. Biol. Med.*, 2:335 (Spring) 1959.

[44] Modified from Faye G. Abdellah *et al.: Patient-Centered Approaches to Nursing* (New York: The Macmillan Company, 1960), p. 26.

tions, and the selection of the necessary course of action that will help the patient attain a goal that is realistic for him, as she plans for total patient care

5. The organization of her efforts to assure the desired outcome; effective patient care would thus result when the nurse is able to help the patient to return to health or what can be approximate normal health for him; this process may be referred to as nursing diagnosis and treatment

In an attempt to delineate the components of nursing practice, Kreuter [45] lists the following: (1) providing nursing care, (2) coordinating the care given not only by nurses but also by the members of other professions, (3) planning for the continuity of care not only within the hospital or agency but also with other community agencies, (4) evaluating the care of the patient, and (5) directing others in the care of the patient, including members of the family. Kreuter further emphasizes that nursing care includes the activities performed directly with the patient and those performed away from the patient but in his behalf.

In this chapter nursing as a profession and the broad role of the nurse have been reviewed. Because the writer believes that nursing has the responsibility for assisting the patient to meet needs that he is unable to meet by himself, a concept of need has been briefly explored. Because nursing is a complex activity, the nursing process has been outlined and discussed. A nursing guide for collecting data about patients has been outlined. By meeting the nursing needs of the patient, the nurse contributes to his welfare by what she does and by how she cares for him.

A GUIDE FOR DATA COLLECTION AND THE NURSING SKILLS REQUIRED TO MEET PATIENTS' NEEDS

ASSESSING THE NEEDS OF THE PATIENT
FOR NURSING

1. The general objectives toward which the nursing care of each patient is planned
   1.1 To personalize the care of each patient
   1.2 To ascertain, support, and maintain his capacity for meeting his physiological, psychological, social, and spiritual needs as well as recognizing his strengths and limitations
   1.3 To protect the patient from the threats to his safety, comfort, and well-being
   1.4 To support, comfort, and sustain the patient and to ease his suffering during all phases of illness
   1.5 To assist in the restoration of the patient to the fullest capacity of which he is capable
   1.6 To consider the members of the family of the patient and his friends as persons who have a legitimate interest and a role to play in his well-being
   1.7 To assist the patient and his family in planning for care required after discharge

GUIDE FOR ASSESSING THE NEEDS OF
THE PATIENT

1. Personal information
   1.1 General impression
   1.2 Patient's and family's perception of his illness and how he should be treated
   1.3 Apparent degree of illness
      1.31 Acutely ill, seriously ill, critically ill, improving, convalescent, failing to improve

   1.4 Cerebral activity [46]
      1.41 Mental status [47]
         1.411 Oriented
         1.412 Disoriented
      1.42 Level of consciousness [47]
         1.421 Fully conscious
         1.422 Inattentive
         1.423 Drowsy
         1.424 Confused
         1.425 Stuporous
         1.426 Comatose
   1.5 Previous experience with illness in hospital _____
      Previous experience with illness at home _____
   1.6 Age _____ Sex _____
   1.7 Drugs
      1.71 Drugs used
      1.72 Drug sensitivities
   1.8 Problems with communication
      1.81 Language
         1.811 Does not speak English _____
               Speaks _____
         1.812 Inability to speak _____

[46] Although the following characteristics of cerebral activity might appropriately be included under the "Physical and Physiological Status" heading of this guide, they are elaborated here because of their importance to the nurse in assessing the priority of needs of the patient.

[47] For definition of these terms, the reader is referred to glossaries of neurological and psychiatric terms.

[45] Frances R. Kreuter: "What Is Good Nursing Care?" *Nurs. Outlook,* **5**:302 (May) 1957.

1.813 Impediment
in speech _____
1.814 Hearing
impairment _____
1.815 Other _____
1.82 Manner in which
patient communicates
satisfaction or
dissatisfaction _____
1.83 How does he seem
to relate to others? _____
1.9 Cultural differences that
may affect his attitudes,
food preferences, expectations, modesty pattern,
time orientation, or
customary sleeping
garments _____
1.10 Religion _____
1.101 Does he wish to see
minister, priest,
rabbi? _____
1.102 Religious practices
with which he desires
assistance _____
1.11 Education and intellectual
level
1.111 Level of schooling _____
1.112 Interest in learning _____
1.113 Hobbies and recre-
ational interests _____
1.114 What does the
patient like to talk
about? _____
1.115 Prejudices _____
1.116 Aspirations _____
1.12 Role and place in family
1.121 Position in family _____
1.122 Position in
community _____
1.123 Apparent image of
himself. How does he
answer the questions
Where am I? What
am I? Who am I? _____
1.124 How does his family
appear to regard
him? _____
1.125 Is there anything in
the family relation-
ship that may have
an effect on the
patient? _____
1.1251 Favorable _____
1.1252 Unfavorable _____
1.126 Is there a relative or
friend who may be
helpful in meeting
the patient's needs? _____
1.127 If he has no family,

what resources are
available as a
substitute? _____
1.128 Who is the head of
the family? _____
1.13 Residence _____
1.131 Place of birth _____
1.132 Present residence _____
1.133 Travel (especially
overseas—recent or
in the past) _____
2. Social and economic status
2.1 Occupation and position _____
2.2 Insurance
2.21 Hospital _____
2.22 Medical _____
2.23 Income _____
2.3 Adequacy of income to meet
needs _____
2.4 Adequacy of housing _____
3. Emotional status [48]
3.1 Apprehensive _____
3.2 Anxious _____
3.3 Agitated _____
3.4 Restless _____
3.5 Irritable _____
3.6 Shy, timid _____
3.7 Withdrawn _____
3.8 Depressed _____
3.9 Discouraged _____
3.10 Happy _____
3.11 Demanding _____
4. Patient's expectations
4.1 How does he view his role
as a sick person? _____
4.2 What does he expect of those
who care for him? _____
4.21 Nurses _____
4.22 Doctors _____
4.23 Others _____
4.3 How does he expect his
family to behave? _____
4.4 How does he think his illness
should be treated? _____
4.5 What does he want to know
and do? _____
5. Previous experience and background that may be factors in his
reactions and his expectations _____
5.1 Previous hospitalizations _____
5.2 Previous care by nurses _____
5.3 Life experiences _____
6. Personal habits (which of these is

[48] See Footnote 47. These terms are intended to assist the nurse in identifying the nature of the emotional needs of the patient, to enable her to formulate the most effective plan or approach possible. Their purpose is not to label or categorize the patient but rather to help the nurse better understand and describe his behavior as a necessary first step to assisting him in coping with his illness.

the patient able to perform for himself, with which does he require assistance, which must be performed for him?)

6.1 Mouth care
    6.11 Dentures   ————
    6.12 Brushing teeth   ————
6.2 Bathing
    6.21 Modifications   ————
6.3 Hair (clean, dirty, tangled, matted)   ————
    6.31 Shampoo   ————
    6.32 Combing   ————
    6.33 Wig or hairpiece   ————
6.4 Nails (clean, dirty, long, short)   ————
6.5 Beard   ————
6.6 Bowel or defecation habits
    6.61 Usual time   ————
    6.62 Time of last defecation   ————
    6.63 Abnormalities   ————
        6.631 Constipation   ————
        6.632 Diarrhea   ————
        6.633 Incontinence   ————
    6.64 Dependent drainage   ————
        6.641 Colostomy   ————
        6.642 Ileostomy   ————
        6.643 Fistula   ————
        6.644 Draining wound   ————
6.7 Sleep and resting habits
    6.71 Rest periods   ————
    6.72 Sleep   ————
        6.721 Usual time for retiring   ————
        6.722 Usual hour for arising   ————
        6.723 Any assistance or modifications that he requires to get adequate sleep   ————
6.8 Food habits and pattern   ————
    6.81 Likes, dislikes, preferences   ————
    6.82 Timing of meals when at home   ————
    6.83 Any ideas about food that may have a bearing on patient's food intake   ————
7. Exercise
    7.1 Active or sedentary habits   ————
    7.2 Usual forms of exercise   ————
    7.3 Limits of exercise   ————
        7.31 Paralysis   ————
        7.32 Weakness   ————
        7.33 Prosthesis   ————
8. With what daily activities of living does the patient require help?

8.1 Eating   ————
8.2 Bathing   ————
8.3 Dressing   ————
8.4 Getting out of bed   ————
8.5 Walking   ————
8.6 Bathroom   ————
8.7 Uses crutches, braces, wheelchair, walker, etc.
9. Physical and physiological status
    9.1 Height ———— Weight ————
        (lean, normal, overweight)
    9.2 Vital signs:
        Temperature ————
        Pulse ————
        Respiration ————
    9.3 Blood pressure   ————
    9.4 Condition of skin
        9.41 Intact   ————
        9.42 Breaks or wounds   ————
        9.43 Dry   ————
        9.44 Moist   ————
        9.45 Wrinkled   ————
        9.46 Tense   ————
        9.47 Bruised   ————
        9.48 Rash   ————
        9.49 Flushed   ————
        9.50 Pale   ————
        9.51 Jaundiced   ————
        9.52 Ulcers or sores   ————
        9.53 Edematous areas   ————
    9.5 Teeth
        9.51 Own teeth   ————
        9.52 Edentulous   ————
        9.53 Dentures   ————
    9.6 Vision
        9.61 Good   ————
        9.62 Defective   ————
        9.63 Blind   ————
        9.64 Prosthesis   ————
    9.7 Eyes
        9.71 Conjunctiva   ————
        9.72 Lids   ————
    9.8 Hearing
        9.81 Good   ————
        9.82 Impaired   ————
    9.9 Body alignment   ————
    9.10 Position   ————
    9.11 General sensation   ————
        9.111 Sensory deficit   ————
        9.112 Inability to detect changes in temperature   ————
10. Needs with which the patient requires assistance
    10.1 Maintenance of oxygen supply   ————
        10.11 Clear airway   ————
        10.12 Assistance with breathing   ————

10.13 Additional supply of
oxygen _____
    10.131 Mask or
    catheter in
    proper
    position _____
    10.132 Mask
    comfortable _____
    10.133 Tent tucked
    in _____
10.14 Evidence of general
oxygen deficit _____
10.15 Difficulty in breathing _____
10.16 Signs or symptoms
indicating deficit of
of oxygen _____
10.2 Maintenance of water
balance _____
10.21 Intake _____
10.22 Output _____
10.23 Weight _____
10.24 Condition of skin
and mucous
membranes _____
10.25 Thirst _____
10.3 Nutritional needs _____
10.31 Interference with
capacity to eat _____
    10.311 Anorexia,
    nausea,
    vomiting _____
10.32 Condition preventing
absorption of food _____
    10.321 Diarrhea _____
10.4 Capacity to maintain
excretory function
10.41 Urine _____
    10.411 Voids _____
    10.412 Indwelling
    catheter _____
    10.413 Color, odor,
    appearance of
    urine _____
10.42 Bowel _____
10.5 Special observation of urine
10.51 Glucose _____
10.52 Acetone _____
10.53 Specific gravity _____
10.54 Color _____
10.55 Odor _____
10.56 Filter _____
11. Capacity to maintain motor
function
11.1 Difficulty in swallowing _____
11.2 Difficulty in walking _____
11.3 Difficulty with grasping _____
11.4 Motor incoordination _____
11.5 Motor instability _____
11.6 Motor weakness _____

12. Ability to maintain appropriate
position and body alignment _____
13. Therapeutic measures and devices
13.1 Blood transfusions _____
13.2 Indwelling catheter _____
13.3 Cast _____
13.4 Nasogastric or gastric
suction _____
13.5 Surgical procedure _____
13.6 Barron pump _____
13.7 Tracheostomy _____
13.8 Other _____
14. Signs and symptoms associated
with a disease state
14.1 Pain $\begin{cases} \text{Location} \\ \text{Quality} \\ \text{Severity} \end{cases}$ _____
14.2 Fever
14.3 Abdominal distention _____
15. Medical diagnosis _____
16. Condition of physical environment
16.1 Equipment used in the care
of the patient _____
16.2 Furnishings _____
16.3 Floors—clean and dry _____
16.4 Room temperature and
ventilation _____
16.5 Lights _____
17. Safety precautions
17.1 Side rails _____
17.2 Low bed _____
17.3 Other _____
18. What instruction does he require?
19. What problems does he have in
accepting the goals that are
possible for him?
20. What aspects of the medical care
plan have a bearing on the
patient's needs for nursing?
20.1 Diagnostic measures
20.2 Therapy
21. Which aspects of the patient's care
require assistance from members
of other disciplines?
22. What care and service is he likely
to require following his discharge
from the hospital? Need for
continuing care?
23. What nursing skills are necessary
to meeting the patient's needs? [49]
(intellectual as well as doing skills)
23.1 Observation of health status
of the patient
23.2 Skills of communication
Verbal
Nonverbal
Written
23.3 Knowledge

[49] Abdellah *et al.*, *op. cit.*, pp. 17–19.

Physical sciences
Biological sciences
Social and behavioral sciences
Nursing sciences
23.4 Teaching of patients and
families
Spontaneous teaching
Planned individual instruction
Spontaneous group teaching
Planned group teaching
23.5 Planning and organization of
work
Individual patient care
Group care of patient
Emergency or stress situation
As a nursing team member
As a health team member
23.6 Use of resource materials
Hospital records
Medical records
Reference materials
Library
23.7 Use of personnel resources
Patient, family, and friends
Medical staff
Dietary staff
Technical staff
Social service staff
Occupational therapy staff
Physical therapy staff

Hospital administrative staff
Community agency staff
Clergy
Other professional nurses
Nursing auxiliary
23.8 Problem solving
Implementing plan for care
Evaluating care given
23.9 Direction of work for others
Planning
Assigning
Teaching
Supervising
Evaluating
23.10 Therapeutic use of the self
Identification of own feelings
Identification of own needs
Establishing own goals
Personal
Nursing care
Professional
Assessment of own growth
toward goals
Use of moral and ethical
values consistent with
professional nursing
23.11 Nursing procedures
Ingestion
Instillation
Injection

REFERENCES

BOOKS

Bennis, Warren G., Benne, Kenneth D., and Chin, Robert: *The Planning of Change,* 2nd ed. (New York: Holt, Rinehart and Winston, Inc., 1968).

DeGowin, Elmer L.: *Bedside Diagnostic Examination,* 2nd ed. (New York: The Macmillan Company, 1969).

Feinstein, Alvan R.: *Clinical Judgment* (Baltimore: The Williams & Wilkins Company, 1967).

Field, Minna: *Patients Are People: A Medical-Social Approach to Prolonged Illness,* 3rd ed. (New York: Columbia University Press, 1967).

Maslow, Abraham H.: *Motivation and Personality* (New York: Harper and Brothers, 1954).

Wiedenbach, Ernestine: *Clinical Nursing: A Helping Art* (New York: Springer Verlag New York, Inc., 1964).

Yura, Helen, and Walsh, Mary B. (editors): *The Nursing Process: Assessing, Planning, Implementing, and Evaluating* (Washington, D.C.: Catholic University of America Press, 1967).

PERIODICALS

Nursing as a Profession

ANA Committee on Ethical, Legal and Professional Standards: "Code for Nurses," *Amer. J. Nurs.,* 68:2581–85 (Dec.) 1968.

Conference: "The Nature of Science in Nursing," *Nurs. Res.,* 18:388–410 (Sept.–Oct.) 1969.

Fleming, Donald: "On Living in a Biological Revolution," *The Atlantic,* 223:64–70 (Feb.) 1969.

Houle, Cyril O.: "The Lengthened Line," *Perspect. Biol. Med.,* 11:37–51 (Autumn) 1967.

Lancaster, A.: "The Reluctant Profession," *Int. Nurs. Rev.,* 14:25–32 (Nov.–Dec.) 1967.

Levine, Myra E.: "The Pursuit of Wholeness," *Amer. J. Nurs.,* 69:93–98 (Jan.) 1969.

Selden, William K.: "The Development of Professionalism in the Allied Health Field," *JAMA,* 206:1545–47 (Nov. 11) 1968.

The Nursing Process

Berggren, Helen J., and Zagornik, A. Dawn: "Teaching Nursing Process to Beginning Students," *Nurs. Outlook,* **16**:32–35 (July) 1968.

Komorita, Nori I.: "Nursing Diagnosis," *Amer. J. Nurs.,* **63**:83–86 (Dec.) 1963.

Leminen, Aili: "The Theory of Nursing," *Int. Nurs. Rev.,* **14**:63–70 (Nov.–Dec.) 1967.

Levine, Myra Estrin: "Adaptation and Assessment: A Rationale for Nursing Intervention," *Amer. J. Nurs.,* **66**:2450–53 (Nov.) 1966.

McPhetridge, L. Mae: "Nursing History: One Means to Personalize Care," *Amer. J. Nurs.,* **68**:68–75 (Jan.) 1968.

Nadler, Gerald, and Sahney, Vinod: "A Descriptive Model of Nursing Care," *Amer. J. Nurs.,* **69**:336–41 (Feb.) 1969.

The Patient

Ewell, Charles M., Jr.: "What Patients Really Think About Their Nursing Care," *Mod. Hosp.,* **109**:106–108 (Dec.) 1967.

Parry, Wilfrid H.: "Accidents and the Elderly," *Nurs. Times,* **63**:138–39 (Feb. 3) 1967.

Rous, Peyton: "The Fly in the Social Ointment," *Perspect. Biol. Med.,* **11**:1–8 (Autumn) 1967.

Smith, Dorothy M.: "A Clinical Nursing Tool," *Amer. J. Nurs.,* **68**:2384–88 (Nov.) 1968.

Smith, Dorothy W.: "Patienthood and Its Threat to Privacy," *Amer. J. Nurs.,* **69**:508–13 (Mar.) 1969.

Tarnower, William: "Psychological Needs of the Hospitalized Patient," *Nurs. Outlook,* **13**:28–30 (July) 1965.

The Role of the Nurse

Johnson, Dorothy E., Wilcox, Joan A., and Moidel, Harriet C.: "The Clinical Specialist as a Practitioner," *Amer. J. Nurs.,* **67**:2298–2303 (Nov.) 1967.

Mussallem, Helen K.: "The Changing Role of the Nurse," *Amer. J. Nurs.,* **69**:514–17 (Mar.) 1969.

2

Historical Perspectives

All theories have a life history. They start tentatively, grow piece-meal, and slowly become mature. Then they can successfully handle new facts and also have considerable predictive value. But sooner or later a discrepancy appears between fact and theory. Then the theory will become modified, perhaps will entirely disintegrate, to be succeeded by something new.[1]

The Nature and Scope of Disease

    What are the factors influencing the prevalence of given diseases?

    What are the theories of disease causation?

The Health Care System in the Twentieth Century

What agencies are involved in health care?

    What are the factors influencing delivery of health care?

    What changes have occurred in health problems in the twentieth century?

MOST people take health for granted. They accept minor ailments without complaint as long as they do not interfere with daily activities or are not interpreted as being of serious import. The hope that life and good health can be continued indefinitely appears in different forms throughout recorded history. There is accumulating evidence, however, that the maximum life span for each species is predetermined.[2] What has been accomplished is to increase the number of persons who approach the maximum by decreasing the mortality rate among infants, young children, and those in middle age.

Over the centuries in the parts of the world where the quantity and quality of food is adequate, water is clean, and modern medical care is available, the average length of life has been extended from about 18 years for ancient man to 70.4 years in 1967.[3] Another indication of increased longevity in Michigan is the percentage dying before and after 45 years of age. In 1900, 56 per cent died before 45 years of age, whereas in 1966 only 15 per cent died before age 45. In other words, in 1966, 85 per cent of

individuals dying were more than 45 years of age at the time of death.[4]

Support for the belief that disease will not soon be eliminated is provided by Perkins,[5] who states that despite sufficient knowledge and experience to eliminate "smallpox (almost certainly); tuberculosis, syphilis, typhoid fever, cholera (probably); malaria (perhaps)," man has never eradicated a single communicable disease. Some authorities use the term *eradicate* to mean to control or limit to an irreducible minimum rather than to eliminate.

Furthermore, as infectious diseases have been controlled, the incidence of diseases of middle and later life have increased. Although it is possible to delay the onset and slow the progress of these diseases, whether or not they can be entirely eliminated is open to question. Furthermore, these diseases are not new. What is new is their relative frequency.

Death rates in certain chronic and infectious diseases are given in Figure 2-1.

Despite increases in knowledge and skills, much remains to be done. A high quality of health care is not available to all people equally. Much is yet to be learned about the prevention,

---

[1] Lester S. King: *The Growth of Medical Thought* (Chicago: University of Chicago Press, 1963), p. 232.

[2] Leonard Hayflick: "Human Cells and Aging," *Sci. Amer.*, 218:32–37 (Mar.) 1968.

[3] Metropolitan Life Insurance Company: *Statistical Bulletin*, 49:3 (Feb.) 1968.

[4] *1966 Michigan Health Statistics* (Lansing: Michigan Center for Health Statistics, Michigan Department of Health), p. V.

[5] James E. Perkins: "Can Tuberculosis Be Eradicated?" *Public Health Rep.*, 78:422 (May) 1963.

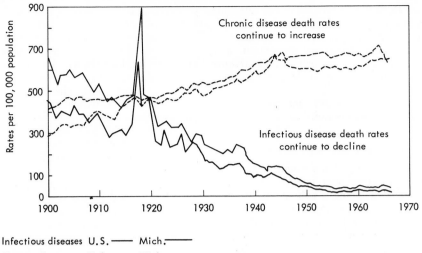

Infectious diseases U.S. ——— Mich. ———
Chronic diseases   U.S. ----- Mich. ----

FIGURE 2-1. Death rates in certain chronic and infectious diseases in Michigan and the United States, 1900–1966. The following diseases are included (International Classification Seventh Revision Detailed List Numbers in parentheses): chronic diseases—cancer (140–205), diabetes (260), vascular lesions affecting the central nervous system (330–334), diseases of the heart (400–443), chronic and unspecified nephritis (592–594), ulcer of the stomach or duodenum (540–541), and cirrhosis of the liver (581); infectious diseases—typhoid fever (40), scarlet fever (50), whooping cough (56), diphtheria (55), tuberculosis (1–19), dysentery (45–48), malaria (110–117), syphilis (20–29), measles (85), pneumonia and influenza (480–493), diarrhea, enteritis, and ulceration of intestines (543, 571, 572). [Source of United States data: *Building America's Health,* Vol. III, Table 36, and *Vital Statistics of United States,* Vols. I and II (U.S. data for 1966 not available). Source of Michigan data: Michigan Center for Health Statistics, Michigan Department of Public Health.]

causes, and treatment of a number of important diseases. Even when knowledge is available, people do not always use it. In many diseases the individual is as or more important than the causative agent(s). One problem is the development of habits and practices conducive to health as well as the control of the external environment.

Past and present experience demonstrates that some diseases can be fairly well controlled despite a lack of knowledge. Dubos [6] states that smallpox vaccination and the sanitary measures were introduced despite a lack of scientific knowledge. Yet they probably had more far-reaching effects on public health than modern scientific medicine.

A twentieth-century example of a group of people using empirical means to control bubonic plague is cited below. They have no understanding of why what they do limits the spread of plague. Their practices are based on observation and interpretation of apparent cause-effect relationships and not on scientific knowledge.

[6] René J. Dubos: "Scientists Alone Can't Do the Job," *Saturday Review,* **50**:68 (Dec. 2) 1967.

For example, bubonic plague is still endemic in Kurdistan. The plague season begins in September and lasts until May. When the villagers note an increase in the rat population in September, they move from the village to the center of a field. Although the villagers do not know that fleas transmit plague from the sick rats to man, the move from the village to the field is successful because it removes the people from the habitat of the sick rats and the vehicle of transmission of the plague, the flea. Plague is controlled, not because the people understand how plague is transmitted, but because the increase in the rat population is regarded as an omen of an impending epidemic of a deadly disease.[7]

The Nature and Scope of Disease

What are the factors influencing the prevalence of given diseases?

Among the factors interacting to determine

[7] Pierre Gascar: "Died of Plague: Ramsara's Daughter, 14 Years," *World Health,* **11**:12 (May–June) 1958.

the threats to health as well as to the selection of measures to prevent and treat them are (1) level of knowledge and technology; (2) theories of disease causation, prevention, and treatment; and (3) social beliefs and circumstances. All these have undergone marked change from ancient to modern times. They also differ not only in different parts of the world but in our own country.

LEVEL OF KNOWLEDGE AND TECHNOLOGY

Until the beginning of the twentieth century, progress in medicine was uneven and slow.[8] In fact modern medicine is only about 30 years old, as it dates its beginning from the development of sulfonamide by Domagk. In the past 30 to 40 years, the increase in knowledge and technology, although based on earlier discoveries, has been greater than the total of all past centuries.

What are the theories of disease causation?

Some theories date back to the beginning of mankind. Others are of recent origin; none has been entirely relegated to the past.[9] Some of the important theories are as follows:

1. Disease is caused by the evil influence of supernatural powers.
2. Disease is punishment for sin and the result of the wrath of an essentially righteous god.
3. Disease is part of the natural order and can be explained on a rational basis.
4. Disease is caused by the epidemic constitution of the atmosphere, miasmic influences, and filth.
5. Disease is caused by a germ.
6. Many diseases require not only a necessary condition (a microbe or other agent) but also a sufficient cause.
7. Disease results from the interaction of multiple factors.
8. Disease results from a disturbance in the adaptive capacity of the individual. This theory will be discussed in Chapter 3.

DISEASE IS CAUSED BY THE MALIGN INFLUENCE OF SUPERNATURAL POWERS

The first, or demonic, theory, though probably the oldest theory of the causation of disease, has not been entirely eliminated. Usually

this theory is expressed in one of three ways. Living persons (witches) have the power to cause disease in other living persons (witches were believed to have an evil influence because of supernatural powers). This power is exercised in different ways: The witch casts a spell on someone whom she dislikes, or a man has some power such as the evil eye. Even today one may hear an expression of the belief that one person is able to harm others by supernatural powers. Sam Thrill says, "You had better stay away from me; I always bring other people bad luck."

A second form of the demonic theory is that disease is caused by the spirits of disembodied dead. This idea is the basis for some of the burial rites practiced by primitive peoples. It is not unknown today, however.

A third expression of the demonic theory is that disease results from superhuman abilities of inanimate objects. Stones, trees, animals, and natural events are ascribed special qualities that enable them to act in a malevolent fashion.[10]

When a demon is held to be responsible for disease, prevention and treatment are directed toward the demon rather than the person who is sick. The principal methods employed are exorcism, evasion, and sacrificial propitiation. The individual who is possessed of a devil is beaten or given a vile-tasting medicine. Trephining (making a hole in the skull) was originally performed to provide an avenue of escape for the demon who had taken over the body of the sick person. Evasion, or avoiding the demon, is achieved by rituals that are prescribed to prevent contact between the potential victim and the evil spirit. The people of Kurdistan, by moving from the village to the field, were practicing a form of evasion. Sacrifices are made to appease the god who is believed to cause the epidemic. The sacrifice is really a bribe. The man makes the sacrifice not to atone for wrongdoing but to prevent an evil spirit from harming him.

DISEASE IS PUNISHMENT FOR SIN

A second theory of disease causation is that disease is incurred by the wrath of an essentially righteous god as a punishment for sin. Winslow states that this concept of disease causation reached its height among Semitic peoples and is best expressed in the Old Testament. This belief, however, was not limited to the Hebrews. The Hindus believed the epidemic of plague (1896–1897) was a punishment imposed on them by their god Siva. "Sin-caused" disease was treated

[8] Lowell T. Coggeshall: *Planning for Medical Progress Through Education.* A report submitted to the Executive Council of the Association of American Medical Colleges (Evanston, Ill.: Association of American Medical Colleges, 1965), pp. 3–4.

[9] Cordelia W. Kelly: *Dimensions of Professional Nursing,* 2nd ed. (New York: The Macmillan Company, 1968), pp. 422–47. Significant social, nursing, and medical developments in different historical periods are summarized in this work.

[10] Charles-Edward Amory Winslow: *The Conquest of Epidemic Disease* (Princeton, N.J.: Princeton University Press, 1943), p. 34.

by making atonement sacrifices to the offended god. Earlier modes of treatment, i.e., magical practices to appease demons, were condemned in this era. The theory of disease as a punishment for sin introduced a new concept, as it is based on a universal law.[11]

The Hebrews also gave cleanliness a spiritual value. Early man had practiced bathing for reasons of comfort. Other ancients such as the Egyptians required those entering temples to be clean, but the Hebrews had the most clearly formalized rules of hygiene institutionalized in their religion. Their hygienic laws are spelled out in the Book of Leviticus. They include practices relating to food, personal hygiene, clothing, diseases, and environmental sanitation. Without these laws there is doubt that the Jews would have been able to escape from Egypt.

DISEASE IS PART OF THE NATURAL ORDER

The first known reference to the idea that events in the universe can be explained on a rational basis appeared in the sixth century B.C. in the writings of the Ionic Greeks. Again in the words of Winslow,[12] "The Hebrews gave us a universe of moral law; but the Greeks clearly visualized for the first time in human history a universe of natural law." Thus the Greeks introduced a new way of thinking about disease. They stressed observation as a tool for learning about disease and advocated looking at the patient rather than assuming that his disease was something imposed on him from without by another being.

DISEASE IS CAUSED BY THE EPIDEMIC CONSTITUTION OF THE ATMOSPHERE, MIASMIC INFLUENCES, AND FILTH

In the period between Hippocrates and Pasteur, emphasis was on epidemic constitution of the atmosphere, miasmic influences, and filth. According to this theory, disease is propagated by the air, diseased persons, and goods transported from infected places. One or more of these agents was employed to explain epidemics occurring in various parts of the earth. For example, when plague was destroying a large part of the population of the world, the pandemic was explained on the basis that the immediate cause was a malign conjunction of planets over the Indian Ocean. They produced "corrupt vapors, raised up and disseminated through the air by the blasts of the heavy and turbid southerly winds." [13] References to atmospheric conditions as factors in the cause of dis-

ease are not unknown at the present time. Natural disasters, inasmuch as they disrupt measures taken to protect water and food supplies, can be sources of epidemic disease. What the individuals do at the time, however, depends on what they believe about the source of illness. If one believes that the cause of the illness is borne on a "turbid southerly wind," nothing much can be done to avoid disease. If, however, one believes that, when water and sewage pipes are broken, there is a possibility of drinking water being contaminated with pathogenic microorganisms contained in human feces, then measures such as boiling the water or treating it with chlorine are rational.

By *miasmic influences* one means that the air is poisoned or polluted by vapors rising from swamps, marshy grounds, and putrid or decaying matter. Because miasmic influences were held to be particularly dangerous at night, houses were often tightly sealed during the hours of darkness. Application of the theory of miasmic influences to the care of the sick resulted in sealing the sick person and his entire family in the house. As a result of sealing the house, disease-producing air was prevented from escaping into the atmosphere. This also prevented contact between the sick person, inanimate objects used in his care, and the members of his family and members of the community.[14] Because it usually increased the degree of contact among family members, sealing the house practically ensured that every family member would contract the disease. In the recent past persons who were ill with certain infectious diseases, as well as their human and animal contacts, were confined for the longest usual incubation period. Although current practices vary somewhat in different legal jurisdictions and with different diseases, restriction of the movement of persons is usually limited to those who are sick with the disease. The movement of contacts, that is, persons who are exposed and who are susceptible, may be limited during the longest usual incubation period. If, by the end of the incubation period, the contacts are well, restriction on their movements is lifted. Such practices as placarding the house have been discontinued.

The theory that epidemic diseases were caused by the constitution of the air, miasmic influences, and filth may appear to be strange. Considering, however, the state of knowledge and the conditions under which people lived during the Middle Ages, the theory was reasonable. It is difficult, if not impossible, for the modern-day middle or upper-class American to imagine the conditions of filth under which

---

[11] *Ibid.*, p. 36.
[12] *Ibid.*, p. 55.
[13] *Ibid.*, p. 182.

[14] *Ibid.*, p. 190.

people lived. People living in cities were crowded together. Provisions for safe water and food supplies, as well as for the disposal of human wastes, were limited and exceedingly primitive. There were exceptions, however. Before the time of Christ, the Romans had developed a public water supply and a sewage disposal system. The latter continues in use to the present time. Throughout the rest of the world, because of the lack of modern sanitary facilities for human excreta, filth was everywhere.[15] Though it is now known that pathogenic microorganisms are discharged in the body excreta and are spread by flies or by contact with the excreta, this was not known in the early nineteenth century. In keeping with the ideas of the time, diseases such as typhoid and cholera were believed to be transmitted by emanations from the filth. Facilities for bathing and for maintaining general cleanliness were lacking. Furthermore, similar conditions still exist in some parts of the world. While traveling, the writer observed people using the same ditch as a source of water for drinking and cooking, for washing clothes, and for disposal of excreta. Overcrowding and limited provisions for personal and community hygiene are not unknown in large cities of the United States.

Not only did social conditions in the past provide a reasonable basis for the theory that infectious diseases were caused by the state of the external environment, but a number of pandemics occurred. In Europe of the Middle Ages, epidemics of plague, syphilis, and cholera killed vast numbers of people. In the famous London plague of 1665, 68,596 Londoners died. Such a terrifying event called for drastic action. Consequently, it is not surprising that, besides sealing the family and person dying from plague into the house, dogs and cats were killed, as they were believed to be the source of the disease. Because of lack of knowledge of plague or its mode of transmission, flea-infested rats were allowed to run free.

By the end of the eighteenth century, plague, which had been a major threat to the populations of Europe for 400 years, was no longer a serious problem. It had been recognized as being contagious and measures appropriate to its eradication were undertaken. The incidence of human plague has been rising in the Republic of Vietnam and was high in 1968.[16]

Although there were a number of serious pandemics during the Middle Ages and Renais-

sance, they have not been confined to these periods in history. References are made in the Old Testament to ancient pestilences sent by God to punish people for having sinned against Him. The last great pandemic occurred during World War I when influenza spread to all corners of the earth. More people died as a result of influenza than from battle injuries. In the United States few people escaped, and because of the rapidity with which influenza spreads, entire families were ill at the same time.

Measures instituted to control the spread of disease during each pandemic depended on the state of knowledge and the prevailing theories of disease causation. Although some of the practices, based on the belief that the constitution of the air and filth caused disease, were irrational in the light of present-day knowledge, some were sound. The observation that disease and filth were associated led to the great sanitary movement, first in England and shortly thereafter in America. By the beginning of the nineteenth century the modern public health movement had been born. The fathers of this movement were lay people and social reformers. Among the names referred to with some frequency in the literature are John Howard (eighteenth century) and Edwin Chadwick (early nineteenth century). Neither was a physician. John Howard was a sheriff who discovered that the conditions in the jails for which he was responsible were appalling. When one reads about the sanitary procedures that he instituted, they appear to be elementary. At the time they were put into effect, however, they were most progressive. Walls were to be whitewashed each year. The walls were to be washed and cells ventilated regularly. Hot and cold water was to be made available to the prisoners for bathing. Clean clothes were also to be lent to prisoners, if necessary.

Chadwick, who was a social reformer, studied living conditions in the slums of London. His studies led to administrative reform and to laws relating to conditions affecting the health of the poor. His report, *Condition of the Labouring Population of Great Britain,* was published in 1842. It served as the basis for the sanitary reform that spread over the civilized world. In the early years of industrialization in England, living conditions were indescribably bad. One source of information is the novels of Charles Dickens. He not only wrote about the horrible social evils of the time but lent powerful support to the social reformers. In the United States, Shattuck [17] made a similar contribution.

[15] For an account of the sanitary conditions in England and other parts of the world, Winslow, *op. cit.,* pp. 236–66, "The Great Sanitary Awakening" is highly recommended.

[16] "Plague," *World Health* (June) 1969, p. 25.

[17] Lemuel Shattuck: *Report of the Sanitary Commission of Massachusetts, 1850* (Cambridge: Harvard University Press, 1948).

With the development of sanitary and housing codes to protect the life and welfare of the people, laws were passed to protect the quality of food, the supply of water, and the work and home environment. Later, as workers organized to promote and protect their rights, hours of work were shortened. Conditions under which women and children could work were defined. The right of the worker to a living wage was established. Machines not only enabled the worker to increase the production of goods, but by sharing in the rewards of increased production he was able to improve his standard of living and his health status. Members of groups such as fraternal organizations joined together to provide for insurance for their families in the event of death. Later, commercial insurance companies were formed for this purpose and the types of insurance were expanded to cover other kinds of human disaster.

Shortly after Chadwick's report was published, another event contributed to knowledge of the practical importance of cleanliness to health and recovery from disease. Florence Nightingale went to Turkey where the Crimean War was in progress (1853–1856). Aided by 37 assistants, she was able to reduce the death rate of soldiers hospitalized in Scutari from 42 to 2 per cent. Miss Nightingale had knowledge neither of germs nor of antibiotics. Previous to her appearance, cholera and dysentery ran rampant among the men who were hospitalized. She and her assistants used soap, water, clean linen, and humane care, with the result that she accomplished more than the entire British Medical Department in saving the lives of British soldiers. Though Miss Nightingale was the first to reduce the death rate among soldiers by reducing the incidence of infection, she was not the first to note the disastrous effects of infections among soldiers. An early Greek historian, Thucydides, wrote, "Appalling too was the rapidity with which men caught the infection; dying like sheep if they attended one another; and this was the principal cause of mortality."

Not too long after the close of the Crimean War, the American Civil War (1861–1865) was fought. As in the Crimean War, infectious diseases were responsible for a high mortality rate. Dysentery, typhoid fever, and tetanus killed more men than the wounds of battle. Approximately 300,000 men died and two thirds of them died, not from wounds, but from disease.

At the time Miss Nightingale was saving lives in Scutari by instituting hygienic and humane care, Pasteur was disproving the theory of spontaneous generation and developing the germ theory of disease. As is usually true when new ideas are proposed or discoveries are made, Pasteur was not solely responsible for either accomplishment, as the theory of spontaneous generation had been questioned earlier. What is important, however, is that, as a result of the work of Pasteur, the idea was accepted that living beings, no matter how small, had their origin, not from dead or decaying matter, but from other similar beings. Translated into the germ theory of disease, a specific microorganism is a necessary condition in the development of each infectious disease. Anthrax does not develop unless the anthrax bacillus is present. The natural culmination of the germ theory of disease was Koch's postulates. They are a set of criteria that can be utilized to prove that a specific microorganism does or does not cause a specific disease.

Without improvements in the power and precision of the microscope many of the discoveries supporting the germ theory could not have been made. It might be added that without the technological developments of the nineteenth and twentieth centuries much less would be known about the cause, prevention, effects, and treatment of a great number of diseases. In the period following the discoveries of Pasteur and Koch, the attention of scientists was on identifying the specific agents responsible for disease. The sanitary movement, which was introduced by the social reformers, now had a scientific basis.

The germ theory, along with related accomplishments, encouraged the hope that for each disease a specific causative agent could and would be identified. With knowledge of the cause, specific preventive and curative measures would follow; in some instances, this has happened. For example, although diphtheria has probably existed in epidemic form since the earliest times, it was not until 1826 that a French physician, Bretonneau de Tours, placed the clinical diagnosis of diphtheria on fairly firm ground. The diphtheria bacillus, or Klebs-Löffler bacillus, was seen and described by Klebs in 1883 and established as the cause by Löffler in 1884. From his observations of patients and animals with the disease, Löffler postulated that the bacillus secreted a diffusable toxin that was responsible for many of the effects of the disease. After this theory was proved by other investigators, the toxin was used to stimulate animals (the horse) to produce antitoxin. The antitoxin was found to provide passive immunity against diphtheria and, when administered early in the course of the disease, to hasten recovery and prevent serious complications.

Unfortunately, the relationship between cause, prevention, and cure does not fall so neatly into place with many infectious diseases. An effective preventive measure was available for smallpox before its cause was known, and although the disease can be prevented, there are no specific methods available for its treatment. In the twentieth century vaccines have been developed that are effective in the prevention of a number of other diseases, including poliomyelitis, tetanus, measles, and whooping cough. There is no method available to cure either poliomyelitis or whooping cough. Both must run their course. Tetanus can be treated with antitoxin, provided treatment is instituted early enough. For many infectious diseases there are no specific methods that are effective in either prevention or cure.

Only a few of the accomplishments of the nineteenth century have been reviewed. As one reads about them, one cannot help but be impressed with their significance to health. In the first half of the century foundation for a sanitary revolution was laid. In the second half the reason for sanitation was discovered and the germ theory of causation of infectious disease was shown to be valid.

In addition to the importance of the germ theory to the control of infectious diseases, it was equally important to the development of modern surgery. During the twentieth century surgical techniques have been developed to the point where almost all organs are subject to surgical intervention, including the successful transplantation of some organs from one person to another.

THE CONCEPT OF NOT ONLY A NECESSARY CONDITION BUT A SUFFICIENT CAUSE

Unlike the examples cited above, some agents do not cause disease on a single exposure and sometimes do not result in disease after repeated exposures. Not only do some etiological agents require repeated exposures over a period of time, but the development of a particular disease may depend on the presence of one or more other factors. These observations have led to the concept of the necessary and sufficient cause.[18] According to this concept, some diseases do not develop in the absence of a specific agent. The agent itself may or may not be pathogenic enough, that is, be powerful enough, to induce disease. For example, the disease tuberculosis does not develop in the absence of the *Mycobacterium tuberculosis*. Therefore, the *Mycobacterium* is a necessary etiological factor in tuberculosis. As a rule, tuberculosis does not develop on a single exposure to the disease but

[18] Edward S. Rogers: "Man, Ecology, and the Control of Disease," *Public Health Rep.,* **77**:756 (Sept.) 1962.

requires multiple exposures. Moreover, other conditions such as undernutrition are required to provide sufficient condition for the development of tuberculosis. In epidemiological terms, tuberculosis requires both a necessary and a sufficient cause for disease to occur.

MULTIPLE FACTORS IN DISEASE CAUSATION

. In many of the chronic degenerative diseases the "necessary" condition for their development is not known, if such a factor exists. They appear to be the result of multiple factors, some of which have their origin in the individual and others in the external environment. Before disease develops the sum total of all the factors must be sufficient to damage the cellular machinery and cause disease. Because chronic degenerative diseases require months or years to develop, assessment of the degree to which each factor is responsible is difficult. Further, some agents such as alcohol and tobacco are among the "multiple factors" contributing to the etiology of a number of diseases. For example, the continued inhalation of tobacco smoke is associated with a number of harmful effects and shortens the life span in human beings. Among the important diseases having a higher incidence among persons who smoke cigarettes than among nonsmokers are coronary artery disease; cancer of the lung, mouth, lip, larynx, pharynx, and esophagus; and pulmonary diseases including emphysema, pneumonia, and influenza. Agreement has not been reached about how tobacco smoke produces its harmful effects. Because not all persons who smoke develop the above disorders and some who do not smoke do, tobacco smoke is not a necessary condition in their development. It can be assumed, however, that in persons who do develop one of the above disorders, cigarette smoking combined with other factors is "sufficient" to cause disease.

Not all the factors contributing to the development of chronic disease are necessarily of a physical or chemical nature, nor are they of extrinsic origin. Apparently, the genetic constitution of an individual predisposes him to some diseases and protects him from others. Psychological and social stresses can also impose strain on the capacity of the individual to cope with physical and chemical agents. Therefore, when multiple factors appear to be involved in the causation of disease, the extent to which each factor—physical, chemical, genetic, microbiological, psychological, and social—is responsible in a given individual varies. When these and other factors combine so that the total effect is sufficient to interfere with cellular processes, disease results. In the person whose genetic constitution predisposes him to a given disease, less in the way of other factors is required than in individuals who are not so predisposed. Conversely, an individual who is not predisposed to a given disease can develop it, if one or more other etiological factors are sufficiently intense.

DISEASE RESULTS FROM A DISTURBANCE IN THE ADAPTIVE CAPACITY OF THE INDIVIDUAL

This theory will be discussed in detail in Chapter 3 and throughout the remainder of this text.

The Health Care System in the Twentieth Century

An adequate discussion of the basic health services in the United States is outside the scope of this book. An outline of the components of a basic system is provided. A brief review of methods of financing health care and some of the related legislation will follow. For those interested in further information, references are included at the end of the chapter.

Rogers summarizes, as shown in Figure 2-2, a health status scale, the focus of which is the major forms of health service. He does not include home care or nursing home care, both of which provide for a significant number of people. Community health centers located in areas where people live are being developed to serve people in periods A, B, and C. Depending on their functions, they are staffed by nurses, technicians, and other health professionals. All the activities included in Figure 2-2 are functions of the government—local, state, or federal. Some, such as the operation of health facilities, hospitals, clinics, and visiting nurse services are under voluntary auspices as well. In the mid and far west United States, some hospitals run by local governments are financed on a basis simi-

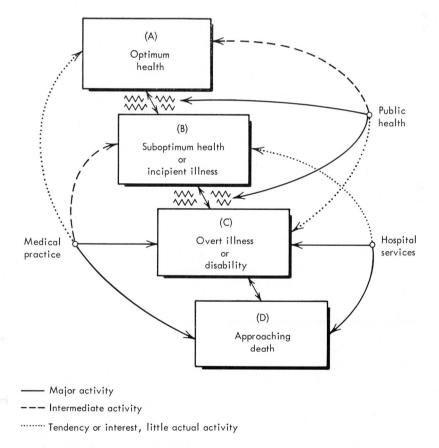

—— Major activity

‒ ‒ ‒ Intermediate activity

.... Tendency or interest, little actual activity

FIGURE 2-2. Health status scale showing focus of major forms of health service. Solid line, major activity; dashed line, intermediate activity; dotted line, tendency or interest, little actual activity. (Adapted with permission of The Macmillan Company, from *Human Ecology and Health*, Fig. 24, p. 176, by Edward S. Rogers. Copyright © Edward S. Rogers, 1960.)

lar to voluntary hospitals as they receive minimal support from local taxation.

What agencies are involved in health care?

Health agencies may be classified according to the nature of the controlling body—official or voluntary. Official agencies are controlled by some branch of the government—national, state or local. Voluntary agencies are of two general types—nonprofit and proprietary. As the term implies, *voluntary* agencies are sponsored by some organization such as a religious body or a group of public-spirited citizens. They are supported by their users plus by contributions of services by religious or other persons. When income is insufficient to cover costs, additional funds are donated by individuals or groups such as the United Community Fund, a religious group, or private citizens.

Proprietary agencies are operated for the profit of their owners. To make a profit, either cost to the patient is high or the standard of services suffer. To date many nursing homes are proprietary in nature. A hope for the future is that they will be integrated into the nonprofit health care system.

In addition to the classification of hospitals by ownership or type of controlling body, they may be classified by the type of patients treated. Thus they may be general or specialized. General hospitals provide care for people with a variety of medical problems. Specialized hospitals limit their clientele to some group or type of patient or problem.

Just as hospitals may be sponsored by the government or by voluntary agencies, so may public health agencies. Although voluntary agencies carry out other activities, their major function is to provide nursing care for patients who are sick at home.

What are the factors influencing delivery of health care?

Many other changes are taking place affecting health as well as the ability to deliver health benefits to people. In a limited discussion it is not possible to present all the advances or to predict those to come. Three areas—knowledge, technology, and changes in attitude—have been selected for brief consideration. References are suggested for those who wish to pursue these and other areas more comprehensively.

KNOWLEDGE

At one time a learned person could know all that was known. Presently no one person can know all about one field, such as nursing, law, or medicine. This fact has led to specialization and in some instances to subspecialization. Thus in nursing there are those who are "coronary care nurses" and "cardiac surgery nurses." These nurses learn a great deal about the needs of patients who have a particular type of illness. They are able to anticipate possible problems, to interpret changes in cardiac status, and to initiate measures that may be life saving. All the above are desirable. However, like other specialists, they can forget that a person is more than a heart (or any other organ). As an example, Mr. Sams, who suffered a severe myocardial infarction, was placed in an intensive coronary care unit. All the modern equipment was applied so that his status could be continuously evaluated. Despite receiving what was thought to be excellent care, he suffered because nurses and physicians talked about him. They seldom talked to or with him. He was frightened by what was said and by the concentration on machines and the intensity with which they were observed. Although specialization is not of itself responsible for depersonalization, each person must keep in focus the fact that it is a person, not an organ, that is receiving care.

One further problem will be mentioned: the lag between discovery of knowledge and its application. The reasons for this lag are varied. They range from sloth, greed, resistance to change, ignorance, and lack of money, to honest disagreement.

An example of a lag in the application of knowledge to the prevention of disease is typhoid fever. The history of the control of typhoid fever can be traced through changes in its importance as a cause of death. In 1905 typhoid fever caused more deaths than any other infectious disease. Moreover, the death rate was higher than it needed to be, as the rate was much higher in the United States than in Europe. Although typhoid fever decreased steadily as a cause of death after 1900, not until 1919 was there a sharp drop in its incidence.

TECHNOLOGY

One of the factors contributing to increased knowledge has been the technological developments of the past and present centuries. Once the source of power was animals and men. Now it is machines. Many unskilled, semiskilled, and even skilled activities are performed by the machines. These changes have brought about others, some of which either create health problems or contribute to them. Other examples include the shortening of the work week in a work-oriented society, movement from a rural to an urban society, and lengthening the period when children are dependent on their parents for support.[19]

CHANGES IN ATTITUDES

1. Prior to the twentieth century, with the exception of the indigent, most persons who were ill were cared for at home. In the past 50 years the number of hospital beds have been quadrupled. After World War II, the number of beds in federal hospitals increased sharply. After 1950, the most marked increase was in hospitals providing short-term care. Among the reasons for the increase is the fact that hospitals are no longer looked on as places to go to die. Rather they are expected to give sophisticated diagnostic and therapeutic care, thereby restoring the patient to the best possible state of health.

2. There is increasing emphasis on the development of facilities and services. Thus there is a trend toward building medical complexes that provide services for people in all stages of the health-sickness and disability continuum. There are facilities for diagnosis, treatment, care during critical stages of illness, convalescent care, and, as needed, rehabilitative and/or long-term care. An indispensable aspect is an arrangement whereby patients can move from one facility to another as their condition dictates. There is also a trend toward taking health centers to people rather than requiring people to go to distant centers.

Within the hospital itself, patients may be assigned to different areas depending on the type and degree of illness. For example, a patient may be admitted to a diagnostic unit. Later he is transferred to the operating room for a surgical procedure. From there he goes to a recovery room or to an intensive-care unit. With the concentration of patients having particular needs in a localized area, specialized equipment can be readily available and nursing personnel can develop a high degree of competence in the care of patients. This plan has some possible disadvantages. Unless provisions are made for continuing care, the patient may be transferred from one area of the hospital to another much as if he were going from one foreign country to another. What appears to the patient to be an abrupt change in expectations for him may increase his anxiety and his sense of depersonalization. With adequate planning

[19] In an advertisement in the *New York Times* (July 30, 1968, p. 80), William A. Emerson, Jr., editor of *The Saturday Evening Post,* said that the most critical domestic problems of our time are the rapid urbanization of our society, the pollution of air and water by human and industrial wastes, and radioactive materials.

and follow-through the patient does not have to experience these feelings. Certainly a real effort should be made to interpret a move from an intensive-care unit to a convalescent-care unit as a major step in progress from sickness to health. Provision should also be made for the personnel in the intensive-care unit to follow the progress of the patient.

Another possible danger in assigning patients to units on the basis of stage of diagnosis or degree of illness is that patients who appear to be less acutely ill or convalescent will be neglected. Care may be limited to meeting physical needs, the administration of medicines and treatments, and the performance of diagnostic tests. The period in which a patient is undergoing diagnosis is often characterized by anxiety. Perhaps the most important statement to be made at this point is that the priority of needs differs with different degrees of illness but that all sick people have needs. These needs should be identified and plans made to satisfy them.

HOME CARE

Another trend stimulated by the cost of medical and hospital care is movement toward caring for less acutely ill patients in their homes. *Home care,* as it is called, is a boon to the person who requires one or more professional services but does not require all the facilities of a hospital for the acutely ill. In many communities chronically ill persons can receive the care they require at home. To illustrate, Mrs. Albert, aged 35, has a chronic neurological disorder, multiple sclerosis. She has four young children ranging in age from 1 to 14 years. Though she required hospitalization at the onset of her illness, she is able to spend most of her time at home. In addition to medical supervision, she is visited daily by a visiting nurse who supervises her activity and exercise. A physical therapist visits her once a week to evaluate the effect of her activity program. The nurse has taught Mr. Albert to administer a preparation of the adrenocorticotrophic hormone by intramuscular injection. The nurse consulted the agency dietitian about how to help Mrs. Albert plan a low-fat diet. An occupational therapist is available but has not been consulted, because Mrs. Albert is kept busy supervising the children and the household. Because the Visiting Nurse Service also provides household aides, one is assigned to assist Mrs. Albert. Because the number of services and amount of care required by Mrs. Albert are great, even home care is expensive. One of the values of home care that cannot be measured in terms of money is that Mrs. Albert fulfills within the limits of her ability her role as wife and mother. For many persons home care may not play as vital a role, but it does make it possible for the person to live a more nearly normal life.

There is also a trend toward caring for patients in the terminal stages of illness at home and toward keeping the patient active as long as is practical. To do this, the family must be emotionally and physically able to care for the patient at home. The willingness of the family to have the patient at home is perhaps the most important factor in determining whether the patient can be cared for at home. Mrs. Lottie Gamely is a good example of how a seriously disabled person may be cared for at home. Despite being bedridden and unable to turn in bed without help, she remained at home until the week before her death. During her last months she maintained her role as mother to her children—one aged eight, the other ten. Before they left for school in the morning she checked them in the same manner as do healthy mothers. She saw to it that they performed their household chores and did their homework. She comforted them and she disciplined them. Household help was required. Medical and nursing care was available and provided.

Besides remaining useful, the patient's needs are often easier to meet at home than they are in the hospital. Food prepared at home is more palatable than hospital food. Visiting by friends and relatives is easier. The schedule and timing of the activities of the day are likely to be familiar. Medical and nursing supervision is necessary to the success of home care. They are required not only for the patient's safety but so that the strain on the family is not excessive. There is always the possibility that the patient will be neglected or become a sick-room tyrant. Neither is desired or desirable. It is also essential to be able to transfer the patient to the hospital when necessary.

Hospital personnel including physicians tend to minimize the problems faced by the chronically ill patient after he is discharged from the hospital. The result is that not all patients who require assistance at home are referred to the Visiting Nurse Service or other community agencies for guidance. The amount and type of assistance needed vary. Not all patients require as much help as Mrs. Albert or Mrs. Gamely; some require more. Further, no single type of service will meet the needs of all persons or even the same person at different periods in his life.

Among the factors leading to the development of voluntary health insurance plans and health-related legislation are (1) increased acceptance that health is the right of all segments of the population and (2) the rising cost of medical care. To cope with the problem of cost, a number of voluntary health insurance plans have been developed. In general, these plans are one of three types: insurance to protect against an acute disabling illness, insurance to pay the cost of a major or catastrophic illness, and insurance to prevent the loss of income during illness. Benefits are often limited to a stated period of hospitalization and exclude certain diseases. A few plans such as the Health Insurance Plan of Greater New York are complete. Insurance plans may be nonprofit or commercial. The best known nonprofit plan is Blue Cross (hospital insurance) and Blue Shield (doctor insurance). One form of income insurance is sick leave. An employed individual is allowed a set number of days each year when he may be absent from work without the loss of his wages or salary. In some situations sick leave is cumulative. With the increase in the incidence of long-term illness, insurance covering extended periods of illness and providing income is of great importance. Many persons between the ages of 18 and 65 do not have this type of insurance available to them at costs they can afford to pay.

HEALTH-RELATED LEGISLATION

Legislation has also been directed toward protecting the working conditions of people and providing financial support following injury or disease.

WORKMEN'S COMPENSATION

The first workmen's compensation law was enacted in 1910. It covered injuries caused by accidents. Later amendments included programs to protect the worker from diseases resulting from health hazards.

SOCIAL SECURITY ACT OF 1935 [20]

As a result of the depression that began in 1929, the fact that industrial workers were not always able to protect themselves against unemployment was recognized. In 1935 the Social Security Act was passed. It had three provisions based on the principle that society has an obligation to provide for the security of its people. The first provision was for unemployment compensation to be handled by the states. The second was establishment of an annuity that was to be paid at age 65 or on retirement of its members. The third provided for special cate-

[20] Information about who qualifies for health insurance for the aged may be obtained from the Superintendent of Documents, U.S. Government Printing Office, Washington, D.C., 20402. Price, 25 cents.

gories of needy persons including the aged, the blind, the crippled and disabled, and dependent children. In this law the government assumed responsibility for helping people provide for the future. In the intervening years the number of persons covered and the benefits have been increased.

MEDICARE–MEDICAID

In 1965 the Social Security Act was further amended to provide specified health services to those 65 years of age or older as a right through the application of social insurance principles.[21, 22] At the same time under Title XIX monies were made available on a matching basis to states for various categories of needy people. When the two social security amendments of 1965 took full effect, about 25 per cent of the population was covered.

In addition to discussing the conflicting principles of health care as a right and health care as a concession, Burns[23] considers other principles facing the health professions:

1. Availability of appropriate health services to all people. In the discussion of this point, Burns[24] makes a plea for giving children wherever they live priority in health care.
2. Attention should be given to high-quality medical services.
3. There should be an orderly organization of health services. What this principle means is that all services from the promotion of health and the prevention of disease to rehabilitation should be provided. Unnecessary duplication of services should be avoided.
4. Finally, attention should be given to economy in the use of health services.

Burns[25] emphasizes the last principle by quoting the New York Academy of Medicine: "the importance of using the nation's resources in the most effective and economical manner consistent with the enhancement of individual dignity and high standards of care." Although an adequate discussion of this point is outside the scope of this chapter, increasing attention is being given to it. How and who provides care, and where it is given, as well as the appropriate use of persons with different levels of preparation, is being studied. Increasingly, machines and unskilled workers are being used to deliver supplies and equipment to sites where they are

to be used. Use is being made of a variety of machines such as computers, monitors, and teaching machines. None of these replaces people, but they supplement and make it possible for people to utilize their time more effectively. As new hospitals and health centers are built or remodeled, attention is being given to the placement of general services so that the time and effort of personnel is utilized to the best advantage. In *Public Health Reports*[26] an experiment to reduce the cost of hospital construction and remodeling has been reported. In earlier experiments, silo-shaped buildings have been tried in an effort to keep each patient equally close to the nurse.

In some areas neighborhood centers are being developed to provide a variety of services to the community, such as the identification and referral of sick or probably sick for medical attention, instruction in normal nutrition or diabetic care, supervision of pregnant women, well baby care, day care for preschool children, and activity centers for all age groups from the young to the aged.[27] The effectiveness of these centers has been increased by involvement of people living in the area in the planning and conduct of the centers. One nurse with the assistance of persons recruited from the neighborhood provides a variety of health and social services to a group of people who might otherwise be neglected.[28] Appropriate medical and social services must be available for referral.[29]

THE HEART DISEASE, CANCER, AND STROKE AMENDMENTS OF 1965

In all, the 89th Congress passed 15 health-related laws.[30] Among these laws is the heart, cancer, and stroke amendment. What this law does is to set "forth a program for education, research, training and demonstrations in the fields of heart disease, cancer, stroke, and related diseases."[31] It also encourages cooperative arrangements among physicians and medical institutions to provide patients with the latest advances in the diagnosis and treatment of these diseases. Three features of this act are of the most significance. (1) It provides funding for regional programs without respect for polit-

[21] Eveline M. Burns: "Policy Decisions Facing the United States in Financing and Organizing Health Care," *Public Health Rep.*, 81:676 (Aug.) 1966.

[22] One of the probable outcomes of Medicare is the upgrading of nursing homes. For patients to be eligible for Medicare, a home must meet defined minimum standards.

[23] *Op. cit.*, pp. 679–83.

[24] *Ibid.*, p. 680.

[25] *Ibid.*, p. 682.

[26] "Experiment in Hospital Construction," *Public Health Rep.*, 83:558 (July) 1968.

[27] Marion K. Sanders: "The Doctors Meet the People," *Harpers Magazine*, 236:56–62 (Jan.) 1968.

[28] Nancy Milio: "Project in a Negro Ghetto," *Amer. J. Nurs.*, 67:1006–1009 (May) 1967.

[29] The June 1968 issue of the *American Journal of Public Health* is devoted to community health planning, comprehensive health planning, and an evaluation of regional medical programs.

[30] Edward H. Forgotson: "1965: The Turning Point in Health Law—1966 Reflections," *Amer. J. Public Health*, 57:934–46 (June) 1967.

[31] *Ibid.*, p. 936.

ical boundaries. (2) It requires that cooperative arrangements be made among major medical centers, that is, a medical school and its teaching hospitals with clinical research training, continuing education, and demonstrations of patient diagnosis and treatment. (3) It requires periodic evaluation of the initial operation before more funds can be allocated for its continuance or expansion. For a more comprehensive discussion of this law, see the reference cited (Footnote 30) or a copy of the law.

Although nursing is not directly referred to in the law, nurses in leadership positions as well as some physicians realize that the intent of the law could not be carried out without nurses' active participation. As a result they are participating in the regions in planning and carrying out activities implied by it.

OTHER LAWS HAVING AS THEIR PURPOSE THE
PROTECTION OF THE PUBLIC

Among other laws passed by the 89th Congress, some were amendments of previous laws and some were new, such as the Cigarette Labeling Law. These laws have as their general purposes (1) protection from health hazards in the environment, (2) making health facilities and services available to people, and (3) increasing the knowledge and skill of health service personnel.

Health legislation is far from new, for laws having implications for health have been passed since the beginning of this century. Many city, state, and even federal laws have been enacted for the purpose of protecting the general public from agents causing injury and disease. Examples include laws or regulations to control traffic, housing and building construction, water supplies, food handling, the preparation and serving of food in restaurants, and sewage disposal. Pure food and drug laws protect the quality of food and drugs.[32]

One of the best-known laws regulating drugs is the Harrison Narcotic Act of 1914, which regulates the importation, manufacture, sale, dispensing or prescribing, and use of cocaine and opium and all their derivatives. The new synthetic preparations known to cause addiction are also included. Although the Harrison Act was intended to be regulatory, it is administered as if it were criminal or prohibitory in nature. In a discussion of the need for the reassessment of the problem of drug addiction, Murtagh[33] makes a plea for changes that will make it possible to treat the drug addict as a medical rather than legal problem. Although the intent of the Harrison Act is to protect society, it has also created problems in relation to drug addiction.[34] To protect the public health from unscrupulous drug manufacturers, the Federal Food, Drug and Cosmetic Acts were passed first in 1906 and revised in 1938, 1962, and 1967.

What changes have occurred in health problems in the twentieth century?

Four methods have been utilized to indicate health status: infant and maternal mortality rates, life expectancy, mortality and morbidity rates, and the state of health of people. Each has its advantages and disadvantages. Although the increase in life expectancy has leveled off since 1950, on the average, man lives longer than any time in history. According to Dublin,[35] the average age to which each of the following lived was (1) prehistoric man, 18 years; (2) the Roman, about 22 years; (3) American, 1789, 35.5 years (Massachusetts or New Hampshire); (4) American, 1900–1902, 48.2 years; (5) American, 1957, 69.3 years; and (6) American, 1967, 70.4 years. Massachusetts and New Hampshire were the only states that kept records in 1789.

In addition to life expectancy rates, a common method of determining health status is to compare the leading causes of death. Mortality statistics have been relied on because they are the easiest to obtain and are the most complete. Presently their value is being challenged, as autopsies are performed on less than half of those who die. The diagnosis of the cause of death can be incorrect. At best, mortality statistics tell the cause of death. They do not provide information about the quality of the life of the person who died or what effect the disease had on his life. Despite their disadvantages, mortality statistics are used to make decisions about where money and effort should be concentrated in the study and treatment of disease.

Because they continue to be emphasized, nurses should be familiar with the leading causes of death and with the changes that have occurred in this century. See Figure 2-3, which demonstrates clearly the changing pattern.

Because Figure 2-3 is a composite of the leading causes of death, there are certain important facts that it does not show. Increasing attention is being given to the infant mortality rate, which is higher in the United States than in a number of other countries. Infant (see

---

[32] See Louis S. Goodman and Alfred Gilman: *The Pharmacological Basis of Therapeutics*, 3rd ed. (New York: The Macmillan Company, 1965), pp. 32–33.

[33] John M. Murtagh: "Dilemma for Drug Addicts," *America*, **108**:740–42 (May 25) 1963.

[34] For a fuller discussion of the Harrison Narcotic Act, see Goodman and Gilman, *op. cit.*, pp. 1723–25.

[35] Louis I. Dublin: *The Facts of Life from Birth to Death* (New York: Macmillan Company, 1951), p. 389.

FIGURE 2-3. Death rates for the ten leading causes of death, 1900 and 1965. [Source: U.S. Department of Health, Education, and Welfare, National Center for Health Statistics: *Facts of Life and Death* (Washington, D.C.: U.S. Government Printing Office, 1967), p. 14.]

Table 2-1) and maternal death rates have long been considered to be a significant index of the health of a community. Although accidents are the seventh most frequent cause of death for all age groups, they are the first cause for ages 1 through 44 years. Neither suicide nor homicide appears in the first ten causes, yet both are among the first ten between the ages of 5 and 44 years, and suicide is eighth in the 45–64 age group. Cirrhosis of the liver is increasing in

TABLE 2-1

Death Rates for the Ten Leading Causes of Death in 1900 and Death Rates for These Same Causes in 1965 *

Rank, 1900	Cause of Death and Category Numbers of the Seventh Revision of the International Lists, 1955		Rate per 100,000 Population	
			1900	1965
	All causes		1,719.1	943.2
1	Influenza and pneumonia, except pneumonia of newborn	(480-493)	202.2	31.9
2	Tuberculosis, all forms	(001-019)	194.4	4.1
3	Gastroenteritis	(543,571,572)	142.7	4.1
4	Diseases of heart	(400-402,410-443)	137.4	367.4
5	Cerebral hemorrhage and other vascular lesions affecting central nervous system ("stroke")	(330-334)	106.9	103.7
6	Chronic nephritis	(592-594)	81.0	†
7	All accidents	(E800-E962)	72.3	55.7
8	Cancer and other malignant neoplasms	(140-205)	64.0	153.5
9	Certain diseases of early infancy ‡	(760-776)	62.6	28.6
10	Diphtheria	(055)	40.3	0.0

* Adapted from U.S. Department of Health, Education, and Welfare, National Center for Health Statistics: *Facts of Life and Death* (Washington, D.C.: U.S. Government Printing Office, 1967), p. 13.
† Not comparable because of change in classification.
‡ Birth injuries, asphyxia, infections of newborn, ill-defined diseases, immaturity, etc.

incidence; between the ages 25 and 44 it is seventh and between 45 and 64 years it stands fifth as a cause of death. These differences are important for they represent threats to the lives of people who are either in the productive period of their lives or have not yet had a chance to be productive. Frequently those who are between the ages of 25 and 65 have a responsibility for others.

Conditions such as suicide, homicide, and cirrhosis of the liver further indicate that the quality of the lives of the people involved may have been unsatisfactory. The stigma attached to these conditions may adversely affect the lives of members of their families. None of these statistics includes any information about the effects of the use and misuse of widely publicized drugs.

With the exception of influenza and pneumonia, all the other leading causes of death are chronic diseases or accidents. They differ from the acute infectious diseases inasmuch as they are more likely to be accompanied by a lengthy period of temporary or complete disability.

SIGNIFICANCE OF DISABILITY

As indicated above, disease is important not only because it shortens the lives of people but perhaps even more so because it disables them. According to *Facts of Life and Death*,[36] heart

[36] *Op. cit.,* p. 29.

conditions are the most common cause of disability. Almost as many people are disabled by arthritis and rheumatism. Other frequent causes of disability are mental and nervous conditions, asthma and hay fever, hypertension without heart involvement, conditions of the genito-urinary and digestive systems, visual impairments, impairments of the musculoskeletal systems, diabetes, varicose veins, peptic ulcer, and partial or complete paralysis. Some of these disorders such as arthritis and rheumatism are responsible for years of human misery as well as loss of productivity.

Although disability occurs at all ages and in both sexes, its incidence rises with age. At all ages it is higher in women than in men. See Figure 2-4.

Rather than merely examining lists of diseases, a trend is developing to examine the agents and/or conditions contributing to disease.[37] Some, such as tobacco smoking, are factors in a variety of disorders, including cancer of the lung and larynx, emphysema, and coronary artery disease. Alcohol causes acute and chronic intoxication, cirrhosis of the liver, toxic psychosis, gastritis, peripheral neuritis, heart damage, and pancreatitis. There is evidence that it is a factor in cancer of the mouth, larynx, pharynx, and esophagus. It is also well known that alcohol is an important etiological

[37] Milton Terris: "A Social Policy for Health," *Amer. J. Public Health,* **58:**5–12 (Jan.) 1968.

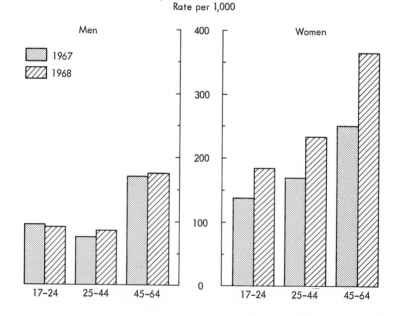

FIGURE 2-4. Incidence of disability for personnel of the Metropolitan Life Insurance Company, first quarter 1967 and 1968. [Reproduced by permission from *Metropolitan Life Insurance Company Statistical Bulletin,* 9:10 (June), 1968.]

agent in suicide, automobile accidents, and injuries and deaths caused by violence.

THE NATIONAL HEALTH SURVEY

There has been increasing interest in determining the health status of the people. In 1956, Congress established the National Health Survey and charged it with collecting the facts about national health problems and the level and extent of medical care. To gather data, two types of activities were initiated: the health interview survey and the health examination survey. The purpose of the health interview survey interviews is to measure the social dimensions of health. The health examination survey collects "precise physiological and diagnostic data by means of comprehensive clinical examinations with objective measurements and tests." [38] In the beginning representative samples of adults ages 18–79 were examined. In the second part of the study 7,000 children 6–11 were examined. In addition to the above, data were also collected from health facilities.[39]

Although no attempt will be made to summarize all the data gathered in this study, a few will be cited. In 1964, civilian nonhospitalized persons experienced more than 3 billion days of disability because of injury or illness. About 2 million people in the United States know that they have diabetes. A substantially larger number have symptoms generally attributed to diabetes but have not been so diagnosed. From this study information was obtained about the relationship of economic status to health and illness [40] (see Chapter 3).

Summary

In historical perspective, health hazards are determined by conditions in the environment and man's genetic constitution and practices. In much of the world, health hazards of the twentieth century are the same as they have been for centuries. In the United States and other industrialized countries they have changed as the environment and man's behavior have changed. At the beginning of the century the threats to health were mainly infections, some of which were brought under control by sanitary disposal of human wastes and clean food and water supplies. Programs of education resulted in the immunization of people against diphtheria, pertussis, tetanus, poliomyelitis, and measles. Although old threats to health continue, new ones, mostly of man's making, have increased to the point where they dominate. During the twentieth century legislation and social changes have promoted the idea that health is a right and that the community has a responsibility to provide facilities that promote health.

[38] Forrest E. Linder: "The Health of the American People," *Sci. Amer.*, **214**:24 (June) 1966.

[39] *Ibid.*, p. 24.

[40] *Ibid.*, p. 25.

REFERENCES

BOOKS AND PAMPHLETS

Abdellah, Faye G., and Levine, Eugene: *Better Patient Care Through Nursing Research* (New York: Macmillan Company, 1965).

Alcott, Louisa May: *Hospital Sketches,* edited by Bessie Z. Jones (Cambridge, Mass.: Harvard University Press, 1960).

American Hospital Association: *The Extended Care Unit in General Hospital* (Chicago: American Hospital Association, 1966).

Bullough, Vern L., and Bullough, Bonnie: *The Emergence of Modern Nursing,* 2nd ed. (New York: Macmillan Company, 1969).

DeFoe, Daniel: *The Plague in London* (London: George Bell & Sons, 1889).

Duffy, John: *Epidemics in Colonial America* (Baton Rouge: Louisiana State University Press, 1953).

Garrison, Fielding H.: *History of Medicine,* 4th ed. (Philadelphia: W. B. Saunders Company, 1929).

Griffin, John R., Weeks, Lewis E., and Sullivan, James H.: *The McPherson Experiment Expanded Community Hospital Service* (Ann Arbor: University of Michigan, Bureau of Hospital Administration, 1967).

Haggard, Howard W.: *Devils, Drugs, and Doctors* (New York: Harper and Brothers, 1929).

Rowntree, Leonard G.: *Amid Masters of the Twentieth Century Medicine* (Springfield, Ill.: Charles C Thomas, Publisher, 1958).

Rutstein, David D.: *The Coming Revolution in Medicine* (Cambridge: M.I.T. Press, 1967).

Somers, Herman M., and Anne R.: *Medicare and the Hospitals: Issues and Prospects* (Washington, D.C.: Brookings Institution, 1967).

PERIODICALS

Facilities

Abdellah, Faye G., and Strachan, E. Josephine: "Progressive Patient Care," *Amer. J. Nurs.,* **59**:649–55 (May) 1959.

Callahan, Enid Bailey: "Extending Hospital Services into the Home," *Amer. J. Nurs.,* **61**:59–62 (June) 1961.

Cherkasky, Martin: "Patient Services in Chronic Disease," *Public Health Rep.*, 73:978–81 (Nov.) 1958.

Georgopoulos, Basil S.: "The Hospital System and Nursing: Some Basic Problems and Issues," *Nurs. Forum*, 5:8–35 (No. 3) 1966.

Greenberg, Sidney M., and Rogers, Theresa F.: "Study Uncovers 'Unnecessary' Long-Term Stays in a Short-Term Hospital," *Hospitals*, 41:76–82 (Nov. 1) 1967.

Kaplan, Jerome: "The Day Center and Day Care Center," *Geriatrics*, 12:247–51 (Apr.) 1957.

Kinney, John M.: "The Intensive Care Unit," *Bull. Amer. Coll. Surg.*, 51:201–356 (Oct.) 1966.

Rogatz, Peter, and Crocetti, Guido M.: "Home Care Programs—Their Impact on the Hospital's Role in Medical Care," *Amer. J. Public Health*, 48:1125–33 (Sept.) 1958.

Rosenfeld, Leonard S., Feldman, Joseph G., and Stuckey, Ronald B.: "Pre-Medicare Utilization of Home Health Services in a Metropolitan Area," *Med. Care*, 5:85–99 (Mar.–Apr.) 1967.

Sargent, Emilie G.: "Evolution of a Home Care Plan," *Amer. J. Nurs.*, 61:88–91 (July) 1961.

Schwartz, Doris: "Nursing Needs of Chronically Ill Ambulatory Patients," *Nurs. Res.*, 9:185–88 (Fall) 1960.

Strauss, Anselm: "The Intensive Care Unit: Its Characteristics and Social Relationships," *Nurs. Clin. N. Amer.*, 3:7–15 (Mar.) 1968.

Veney, James E.: "Home Care: An Introduction," *Inquiry*, 4:3–4 (Oct.) 1967. Entire issue devoted to home care.

Wegmiller, Donald C.: "Long-Term Care," *Hospitals*, 42:93–94, 96 (Apr. 1) 1968.

Wilkiemeyer, Diana: "Unbinding the Homebound," *Amer. J. Nurs.*, 66:1803–1805 (Aug.) 1966.

Health Care Planning

Astley, Verna Jo: "Regional Health Planning," *Mich. Nurse*, 41:12–13 (Jan.–Feb.) 1968.

Boffey, Philip M.: "Health Crisis: LBJ Panel Calls for Reshaping American Medicine," *Science*, 158:1160–62 (Dec. 1) 1967.

Editorial: "Comprehensive Planning for Health Services: Past, Present, and Future Considerations," *Amer. J. Public Health*, 58:1–3 (Jan.) 1968.

Glasser, Melvin A.: "Planning for Hospital and Extended Care Facilities: Issues of Public Policy," *Amer. J. Public Health*, 57:1728–34 (Oct.) 1967.

Holder, Lee, and Deniston, O. Lynn: "A Decision Making Approach to Comprehensive Health Planning," *Public Health Rep.*, 83:559–68 (July) 1968.

Kent, James A., and Smith, C. Harvey: "Involving the Urban Poor in Health Services Through Accommodation—The Employment of Neighborhood Representatives," *Amer. J. Public Health*, 57:997–1003 (June) 1967.

Kurtagh, Cathryn: "Nursing in the Life Span of People," *Nurs. Forum*, 7:298–307 (No. 3) 1968.

Kissick, William L.: "Effective Utilization: The Critical Factor in Health Manpower," *Amer. J. Public Health*, 58:23–29 (Jan.) 1968.

"Medical Care: The Current Scene and Prospects for the Future," A Symposium in Honor of I. S. Falk, *Amer. J. Public Health, Suppl.*, 59: 1–76 (Jan.) 1969.

Morris, Robert: "The City of the Future and Planning for Health," *Amer. J. Public Health*, 58: 13–22 (Jan.) 1968.

Prindle, Richard A.: "Health Aspects of the Urban Environment," *Public Health Rep.*, 83:617–21 (July) 1968.

Rice, Dorothy P.: "Estimating the Cost of Illness," *Amer. J. Public Health*, 57:424–40 (Mar.) 1967.

Winston, Ellen: "Health-Welfare Partnership in Programs for Low Income Groups," *Amer. J. Public Health*, 57:1100–1106 (July) 1967.

Legislation

Coe, Rodney M., *et al.*: "The Response to Medicare," *Public Health Rep.*, 83:271–76 (Apr.) 1968.

Editorial: "The Personal Meaning," *Nurs. Outlook*, 16:21 (Jan.) 1968.

Marks, Anna E., and Malo-Juvera, Dolores: "Implementing a Medicare Program in a Private Hospital," *Nurs. Outlook*, 16:26–28 (Feb.) 1968.

Maureen, Sister: "The Impact of Federal Legislation on Home Health Services," *Amer. J. Public Health*, 57:1147–52 (July) 1967.

Peterson, Paul Q.: "The Impact of Recent Federal Legislation on Personal Health Services," *Amer. J. Public Health*, 57:1091–93 (July) 1967.

Pope, Irene: "Medicare—Impetus for Change," *Nurs. Outlook*, 16:34–35 (Jan.) 1968.

Popick, Bernard: "Social Security Disability Insurance Benefits," *Amer. J. Nurs.*, 69:553 (Mar.) 1969.

Siegel, Fanny F.: "Medicare and Its Opportunity for Nursing Leadership," *Nurs. Forum*, 5:95–108 (No. 3) 1966.

Tierney, Thomas M.: "The Continuing Partnership," *Nurs. Outlook*, 16:22–24 (Jan.) 1968.

Vanderwarker, Richard D.: "Meeting the Demands of New Health Care Legislation," *Hospitals*, 41:36–39 (Dec. 1) 1967.

Research

White, Kerr L.: "Research in Medical Care and Health Services Systems," *Med. Care*, 6:95–100 (Mar.–Apr.) 1968.

Wolfensberger, Wolf: "Ethical Issues in Research with Human Subjects," *Science*, 155:47–51 (Jan. 6) 1967.

Technology

Barnett, G. Octo: "Computers in Patient Care," *New Eng. J. Med.*, 279: 1321–27 (Dec. 12) 1968.

Mesthene, Emmanuel G.: "How Technology Will Shape the Future," *Science*, 161:135–43 (July 12) 1968.

3

The Health-Illness Spectrum

Health of mind and body is so fundamental to the good life that if we
believe men have any personal rights at all as human beings, then they
have an absolute moral right to such a measure of good health as society and society alone is able to give them.   ARISTOTLE

Determining Objectives for the Health Professions

The Maintenance and Promotion of Health: The First
Objective

How is health defined?

How can positive health, or high-level wellness, be
promoted?

What are the factors influencing health?

The Prevention of Disease: The Second Objective

What is the nature of disease?

How can diseases be prevented?

What is the nurse's role in prevention?

Care of the Sick: The Third Objective

What are the aims, objectives, and problems?

ALTHOUGH health and illness are often viewed
as separate entities, they are not. All aspects of
life, which begins with conception and ends in
death, are interrelated. The theoretical framework for this and later chapters is that in health
man is able to adapt successfully to his environment. In illness his adaptive capacity is limited
in some way. In the words of Dubos,[1] ". . . the
states of health or disease are the expressions of
the success or failure experienced by the organism in its efforts to respond adaptively to
environmental challenges." Later he says that

Human life is thus the outcome of the interplay
between three separate classes of determinants,
namely: the lasting and universal characteristics of
man's nature, which are inscribed in his flesh and
bone; the ephemeral conditions which man encounters at a given moment; and last but not least,
man's ability to choose between alternatives and to
decide upon a course of action.[2]

Determining Objectives for the
Health Professions

The objectives of the health professions are
(1) the maintenance and promotion of positive
health or of a high level of wellness, (2) the

[1] René Dubos: *Man Adapting* (New Haven: Yale
University Press, 1965), p. xvii.
[2] *Ibid.*, pp. xviii–xix.

prevention of disease and (3) the care and cure
of the sick. When cure is improbable, the goal
in the care of the person is to maintain and
support his strength and hope so that he remains a whole and, insofar as possible, a contributing member of society.

Each objective will be examined in terms of
some of the problems, past and present, that
contribute to and interfere with its achievement.
From an examination of the past and present-
day health problems, perhaps a foundation can
be laid for thinking of birth, growth, and maturation, health, disease, and death as phases of
life. Dunn[3] emphasizes the relationship of
health and disease by saying that "it is essential
to shift from considering sickness and wellness
as a dichotomy toward thinking of disease and
health as a graduated scale." What Dunn calls
high-level wellness is at one end of the scale,
whereas death is at the other. The problems
that are presently known as disease, as well as
those existing in the past, are related to conditions in the society of the time. Most of the
health problems of today have always existed.
As a matter of fact, writers such as Gordon[4]
indicate that the broad categories of disease

[3] Halbert L. Dunn: "High-Level Wellness for Man
and Society," *Amer. J. Public Health,* 49:787 (June)
1959.
[4] John E. Gordon: "Changing Accents in Community Disease," *Amer. J. Public Health,* 53:142 (Feb.)
1963.

have not changed to any extent over the years. What has changed is the degree to which a given disease is a significant cause of morbidity and mortality. These changes have come about largely because of alterations in the relationship of man to his environment. Some present-day health problems result not so much from failure but from accomplishment. For example, as infections and other conditions that were responsible for a high infant mortality rate have been brought under control, the ailments that are common in older adults have increased in incidence. Many, if not all, health problems have an ancient history. For example, though evidence of coronary artery disease has been found in the mummies of ancient Egypt, it was not recognized as a problem by the ancient Egyptians. What is identified as a problem depends on its incidence in relation to other problems.

The Maintenance and Promotion of Health: The First Objective

How is health defined?

Health is the norm and is the first objective toward which the efforts of the health professions are directed. Beyond general agreement that health is more than a lack of disease, definitions of health do not go very far toward establishing the specific nature of health. There are undoubtedly many reasons for this. One is that health is not easily measured. A disease may be well established or even far advanced before a person has signs or symptoms indicating that he is ill.[5]

Perkins[6] defines health as "a state of relative equilibrium of body form and function which results from its successful dynamic adjustment to forces tending to disturb it. It is not a passive interplay between the body substance and forces impinging on it, but an active response of body forces working toward readjustment." Francis[7] extends the concept of adequate structure and function by adding *adequate reserve*. Adding the term *adequate reserve* to the definition, an individual can be presumed to be in a state of health as long as he is able to adapt to changes in his environment in such a manner that structure, function, and reserve capacity are preserved. In fact, he is likely to appear to be

healthy as long as his reserve capacity is sufficient for him to carry on his usual activities.

Besson[8] includes the environment in his definition of health and changes the emphasis. He states,

Optimal health is not a condition of an individual, but a state of interaction between self and environment. It is a ceaseless struggle between a basically hostile environment and a series of defenses we are endowed with and which we add to when necessary. The homeostatic balance of forces is our goal and this may be accomplished by decreasing the threat of the environment or by raising the capability of the host to defend himself.

Thus Besson, Dubos, and others emphasize that one of the outstanding characteristics of the healthy individual is his capacity to adapt to a constantly changing environment. Through appropriate adjustments in behavior, the individual maintains the nutrition of his cells and responds to his environment in such ways that injury is prevented. Adaptation occurs at all levels of organization. In unicellular organisms, the cell carries on all life processes. In multicellular organisms, some cells specialize, and with specialization, some of the capacity of these cells to adapt is lost. For example, the growth potential of nerve and muscle cells is so small that it is of little practical significance. Cellular specialization, however, is to the overall advantage of the individual. It makes him better able to find food and water, escape his enemies, and modify the environment so that it meets his needs. All cells retain one common characteristic—they carry on the biochemical activities essential to metabolism. Although all cells are capable of adapting to changes in the supply of food, those with a high rate of metabolism are quickly injured by marked deprivation.

In addition to the capacity to adapt the rate of metabolism to the supply of nutrients, some cells can respond to a change in the environment by undergoing cell division. For example, following a small injury to the skin or mucous membrane, the epithelial cells multiply and repair the damage. More extensive breaks are repaired by fibrous connective tissue. Exposure to low oxygen tension, such as occurs at high altitudes, results in an increase in the number of erythrocytes in the blood. Erythrocyte and hemoglobin levels are also higher in children who have the type of congenital heart disease in which there is a mixing of venous and arterial blood. Some cells, such as muscle cells, adapt to a change in activity by increasing or decreasing their size.

---

[5] The World Health Organization's definition of health: the state of complete physical, mental, and social well-being and not merely the absence of disease or infirmity.

[6] W. H. Perkins: *Cause and Prevention of Disease* (Philadelphia: Lea & Febiger, 1938), p. 21.

[7] Thomas Francis, Jr.: "Research in Preventive Medicine," *JAMA,* **172:**994 (Mar. 5) 1960.

[8] Gerald Besson: "The Health-Illness Spectrum," *Amer. J. Public Health,* **57:**1904 (Nov.) 1967.

Survival of the cell and maintenance of its function are dependent on conditions in the cell's immediate fluid environment. It is from this environment that the cell obtains a continued supply of nutrients and into which it discharges its wastes. For all cells, this immediate environment is a pool of water in which a variety of substances such as sodium chloride and glucose are dissolved. For unicellular organisms, such as the amoeba, the fluid environment is a pond or puddle of water. For man and other large multicellular organisms, blood, lymph, and interstitial fluid form the immediate environment of the cells. These fluids are known as the internal environment, in distinction to the external environment, or the world outside the skin and mucous membranes, because cavities lined with mucous membranes are in reality outside the body proper. The fluids composing the internal environment not only serve individual cells as such but are the medium by which all body cells are united to and affected by the activities of all other cells within the entire organism.

HOMEOSTASIS: THE CONCEPT OF BALANCE OF THE INTERNAL ENVIRONMENT

Because of the importance of the internal environment to the activities of cells, many adaptations are involved in maintaining its constancy, within well-defined limits. These mechanisms were named *homeostasis* [9] by Cannon.[10]

Although the complexity of the internal environment of cells has only recently become known, the idea that it had an influence on human behavior is a very ancient one and is found in many civilizations. Regardless of the civilization into which a man is born, his level of intelligence or education, or the period of history in which he lives, man has always tried to explain his own nature, his environment, and his place in the latter. It is natural for man to think about his relationship to his fellow man and the nature of illness and evil. For example, the Navaho Indians believe that health will be granted them when they "live in accord with that which is called mountain soil, and the pollen of all the plants." [11]

Hippocrates, and later Galen, taught that man was composed of four humours. Man was healthy when these humours were in correct balance; disease was the result of unbalance.

This doctrine is based on the concept that the universe is composed of four elements: fire, water, earth, and air. Man, as part of the universe, was seen as composed of the four humours that corresponded to the four elements of the earth: blood (fire), phlegm (earth), yellow bile (air), and black bile (water). This theory was expanded by later physicians. They believed that when one humour dominated the others, it determined the physical and emotional characteristics of a man. Terms derived from this concept are still used to describe the behavioral characteristics of people. Thus a jolly, optimistic person, inclined to be fat, is said to be sanguine; one who is slow-moving and not easily aroused is described as phlegmatic; one who is easily angered or quick-tempered is choleric; and one who is depressed, peevish, or solitary is melancholic.

This theory of body fluids was not challenged until 1858, when *Cellular Pathology* was published by Virchow. As a result of this work the cell was recognized as the important entity in health and disease. In 1878 Claude Bernard introduced the concept that cells live in the fluid that bathes them. This fluid—blood, lymph, and tissue fluid—he called the *milieu intérieur*. He believed that all vital activities have but one objective, the maintenance of the stability of the *milieu intérieur*.

Cannon further elaborated and extended the scope of the work of Bernard. Like Bernard, he considered the stability of the internal environment its most important feature. He emphasized that although the blood and other fluids were constantly absorbing materials from the external environment and from the cells the composition of these fluids was maintained constant within limits. In describing his concept of how the constancy of the internal environment was maintained, he states, "The coördinated physiological processes which maintain most of the steady states in the organism are so complex and so peculiar to living beings—involving, as they may, the brain and nerves, the heart, lungs, kidneys and spleen, all working coöperatively—that I have suggested a special designation for these states, *homeostasis*." [12] He elaborated further that the term does not imply stagnation but rather variation within limits. Conditions are maintained within limits as long as the individual is capable of making appropriate adaptations to change.

MAINTENANCE OF HOMEOSTASIS

The maintenance of homeostasis depends on a variety of elements. Substances required by cells must be available in adequate quantity. Material supplies include water, oxygen, and a

[9] Some authorities object to the term *homeostasis,* as it implies a static rather than dynamic state. Some prefer the term *homeokinesis.*

[10] Walter B. Cannon: *The Wisdom of the Body,* revised and enlarged ed. (New York: W. W. Norton & Company, Inc., 1939), p. 24.

[11] René Dubos: *Mirage of Health* (New York: Harper and Brothers, 1959), p. 4.

[12] Cannon, *op. cit.,* p. 24.

variety of nutrients, including sources of calories, tissue-building materials, electrolytes, and regulators not synthesized or present in the body. The intake, storage, and elimination of excesses of supply are regulated so that the level of each substance is maintained within well-defined limits. Conditions that must be maintained within limits include osmolality, blood pressure, level of glucose in the blood, cation-anion balance and concentration, hydrogen ion concentration, and body temperature. Conditions in the external environment must be within the limits to which man can adapt. For example, man's capacity to adapt to extremes of temperature, high altitude, starvation, and physical trauma is limited. However, man is able to live in some hostile environments by adapting them to his needs.

Because of their size and complexity, multicellular organisms require specialized structures to supply cells with needed materials, to remove the waste products of metabolism, and to maintain the constancy of the internal environment. The healthy organism is capable of responding to disturbances in such a manner that damage is prevented or repaired. The kinds of structures that fulfill this function include the following:

1. Structures that absorb required substances from the external environment and, when necessary, modify them so that they can enter the internal environment. For example, oxygen is absorbed into the blood unchanged. The air from which oxygen is taken, however, requires conditioning. Nutrients usually require reduction to simpler forms before they can be absorbed and provision for elimination of indigestible substances is also necessary. Materials enter or leave the external environment through semipermeable membranes that separate the internal from the external environment. These semipermeable membranes act to protect the internal environment from too rapid change or from the entrance of potentially harmful or nonusable particles.
2. Structures that transport materials from points of entry to cells and from cells to points of elimination or exit such as the heart and blood vessels.
3. Structures that store or eliminate excesses of intake and by-products of metabolism. For example, glucose is stored as glycogen in the liver and muscles; much of the excess is stored as fat. Excess sodium is normally excreted in the urine.
4. Structures that make movement in the external environment possible. They enable the individual to seek food and water, to alter

the environment to suit his needs, to overcome or avoid danger, and to find a mate.
5. Structures that reproduce themselves—to replace worn-out cells, to repair injury, or to produce a new organism.
6. Structures that protect the organism from injury.
7. Finally, structures that regulate and integrate the activities of all individual cells and aggregates of cells so that the organism functions as a whole.

Mechanisms and Requirements for Regulation and Integration of Bodily Processes

The regulation and integration of bodily processes require that the organism has (1) receptors that function in such a way that the organism recognizes disturbances in its internal or external environment and (2) structures that communicate information about these disturbances to a center or centers that receive it, evaluate it, and initiate messages that are communicated to the appropriate effector cells. The effector cells are muscle or gland cells. Upon stimulation, they act to correct the disturbance. In following chapters the mechanisms for the maintenance of, and disturbances in, various homeostatic conditions will be discussed in some detail.

According to Cannon, the regulation of homeostatic mechanisms is primarily controlled by the sympathoadrenal system. Danger or its symbols, whether in the external or internal environment, result in activation of the sympathetic nervous system and the adrenal medulla. Changes occur that prepare the organism for flight or fight. Cannon also states that the sympathoadrenal system is responsible for regulating the processes whereby the resulting disturbances are repaired. According to his view, the parasympathetic nervous system is largely concerned with the regulation of activities relating to nutrition.[13]

In addition to nervous control of homeostatic mechanisms, hormones also play an important role. Their production is directly or indirectly subject to control by the hypothalamus. In some instances the action of a hormone enhances the action of the nervous system. For example, epinephrine and norepinephrine support the action of the sympathetic nervous system. Although the function of the adrenal steroids has not been completely elucidated, their presence is essential to the reaction of the body to changes in either the internal or external environment and to the response of the body to injury. They play a role in the regulation of a variety of homeostatic activities. In the absence of the

[13] *Ibid.,* pp. 263–85.

adrenal steroids, the individual reacts ineffectively to even moderate changes in activity, environmental temperature, illness, and physiological, psychological, or other stresses. The adrenal steroids have been demonstrated to play a role in the regulation of water, mineral, and glucose metabolism.

Other hormones such as insulin, thyroxin, parathormone, and antidiuretic hormone also function in homeostasis. Insulin is necessary for the utilization of glucose and directly or indirectly for the metabolism of fat and protein. Thyroxin regulates the rate of cellular metabolism and parathormone the level of calcium in the blood. The antidiuretic hormone participates in homeostatic regulation of water by increasing the rate at which water is reabsorbed by the renal tubules. No mention has been made of the role of the adenohypophysis in governing its so-called target glands or of its function in growth. The purpose has not been to review in detail all the structures that function in the control of homeostasis but rather to indicate the complex nature of its regulation.

For the organism to continue to maintain and restore homeostasis, it requires both defenses against injury and mechanisms whereby damage can be repaired. In health, physiological adjustments counteract either an increase or decrease in a bodily activity to prevent excessive change. Change in one direction is counteracted by the initiation of a mechanism acting in the opposite direction. Most physiological activities are regulated by negative feedbacks. In regulation by negative feedback, a change in one direction is counteracted or opposed by a change in the opposite direction. In other words, the reaction to change is negative to the stimulus.[14] By way of contrast, in a positive feedback system, a change causes more of the same. As an example, in a negative feedback, ingestion of glucose causes a rise in the level of glucose in the blood. The rise acts as a stimulus to the blood glucose lowering mechanism, and the blood glucose falls. In a positive feedback system, ingestion of glucose causes the blood glucose to rise even when it is already higher than normal. To summarize, a negative feedback system is self-correcting. A positive feedback system is self-perpetuating. Most homeostatic mechanisms are regulated by a closed-loop (continuous-circuit) negative feedback system.

See Chapter 6 for discussion of the body's defense mechanisms.

The organism's capacity to meet its physiological needs results from the fact that the cells, tissues, organs, and systems, as well as the entire organism, can respond to disturbances in the environment in such a manner that injury is prevented or damage is corrected.

To summarize and to clarify the concepts of homeostasis, the four features of homeostasis as outlined by Cannon will be stated and then applied to one condition of homeostasis, the maintenance of blood pressure. The characteristic features of homeostasis are as follows: [15] (1) To maintain constancy in an open system continually subjected to disturbance, some mechanism to prevent change is required; (2) the maintenance of a steady state requires that any tendency to change is automatically met by increased effectiveness of mechanisms to resist change; (3) regulation of any homeostatic condition may require one or more mechanisms acting at the same time or successively; and (4) homeostasis does not happen by chance but is the result of organized self-government. These postulates are illustrated by citing the instance of Mr. Brave. He was awakened at night by pain in his upper abdomen and a feeling of nausea. Shortly after awakening, he vomited what he and his wife described as a bowlful of bright red blood. Both were frightened. Mrs. Brave called the family doctor, who suggested that Mr. Brave be taken to the hospital. When he was admitted to the hospital his blood pressure was 120/76. This was his usual blood pressure and is well within the normal range. Let us suppose that he had lost 450 ml of blood and examine the maintenance of arterial blood pressure as a homeostatic function.

Arterial blood pressure is one factor in maintaining tissue perfusion. It is dependent on agencies acting to elevate it, balanced against those acting to lower it. Arterial blood pressure depends on the relationship of the blood volume to the capacity (capacitance) of the chamber (blood vessels) that holds it and the force with which the blood is driven into the arteries. The viscosity of the blood is also a factor in that a viscid fluid offers more resistance to being moved than does a thin or watery one. All these factors can be altered so that blood pressure is raised or lowered or maintained. In terms of Cannon's first postulate, the loss of blood tends to disturb the relationship between the volume of blood and the size of the chamber in which it is contained. Because Mr. Brave is able to maintain his blood pressure within normal limits, there must be some mechanism operating to counteract the effect of blood loss.

The second postulate suggests further that as blood continues to be lost and the tendency for the blood pressure to fall is increased the mechanisms elevating blood pressure must become increasingly active. For example, the heart beats

[14] Arthur C. Guyton: *Textbook of Medical Physiology,* 3rd ed. (Philadelphia: W. B. Saunders Company, 1966), p. 9.

[15] *Op. cit.,* pp. 299–300.

more rapidly and the arterioles increase the resistance to the flow of blood by constriction. The heart responds to the increase in resistance by contracting with greater force. For the time being, blood pressure is maintained. A point of considerable importance is that some persons maintain their blood pressure for a time despite large losses of blood, only to have it fall suddenly to a dangerously low level. This emphasizes the necessity for acting on the knowledge that, although individuals differ in their capacity to adapt, there are limits to this capacity. No single measure of the status of a patient should be considered to be infallible or apart from other evidence.

The third postulate states that there must be a number of agencies acting together or successively to regulate a homeostatic condition. Review of physiology reveals that both the heart and blood vessels are no exception. They are regulated by the autonomic nervous system and by hormones as well as by other chemicals, such as angiotensin, the activity of which depends on a substance secreted by the kidney. Blood volume is also regulated by a number of mechanisms. All these will be discussed in detail later in connection with shock and hypertension. A number of factors interact to prevent the fall of Mr. Brave's blood pressure.

The fourth postulate states that the changes following disturbances in homeostasis do not happen by accident but that disturbances in physiological processes call forth specific responses. This implies that there are receptors stimulated by change, and when these receptors are stimulated, a set of reactions is initiated to correct the disturbance. To illustrate by analogy, in any city in which the services are organized to meet the needs of the communiy, a call to the fire department brings forth firemen and fire-fighting equipment. Unless the fire is a big one or is in a critical area, the amount of equipment delivered is likely to be limited. It may or may not bring the police. In the instance of Mr. Brave, the stimulus initiating changes in his behavior was the loss of blood and what the loss of blood meant to him. Receptors sensitive to the level of the blood volume initiated impulses that resulted in the activation of mechanisms to maintain or to prevent the fall in his blood pressure. Thus Mr. Brave was protected against the harmful effects of blood loss.

At this point it should be clear that Mr. Brave was able to maintain his blood pressure because of multiple agencies acting to overcome the blood pressure-lowering effects of blood loss. In addition to those cited, other mechanisms served either to reduce blood loss or to protect him from its effects. Contraction of blood vessels at the site of bleeding, combined with the tendency of the blood to clot, served to protect Mr. Brave from further blood loss. Even the fact that he felt faint was protective. Because of this feeling he lay down, decreased his activity, and eliminated the need to move blood against gravity. His anxiety was protective because it spurred him to do something about his situation. In general, then, homeostasis was maintained because Mr. Brave was able to regulate supplies and processes in such a way that excesses were eliminated and deficits corrected.

With this review of homeostasis, it should be evident that its maintenance depends on the capacity of the individual to adapt or respond to changes in his environment in such a fashion that injury is prevented or damage is repaired. The environment is defined to include all internal and external factors affecting existence, growth, and welfare. For man it includes not only the fluid environment of his cells but his external environment as well—physical, emotional, intellectual, and social. Some of the aspects of environment may be temporary and some permanent; whatever they are they affect the entire organism.

NURSING FUNCTIONS

As indicated, in health the needs of the cells are met automatically by the integrated and coordinated activity of all the cells, including those in specialized facilities. In illness the capacity of the individual to cope with disturbances in his environment in such a manner that his needs are satisfied is reduced. In patients with medical-surgical diagnoses, the incapacity frequently lies in an inability to meet one or more physiological needs. Many of the activities of the nurse in the care of these patients are directed toward (1) gathering information about the nature of the internal environment of the patient, (2) modifying the external environment so the adaptations the patient is required to make are within his capacity to make, (3) supporting the efforts of the patient to adapt or to respond, and (4) providing him with the materials required to maintain the constancy of his internal environment.

ADAPTATION: THE CONCEPT OF BALANCE
WITH THE EXTERNAL ENVIRONMENT

The preceding discussion considered in some detail the manner in which each individual adapts to his environment. Not only are changes in function possible, but over a period of time alterations in structure may occur. The capacity to modify structures so that the organism is better suited to a particular environment is one of the truly remarkable features of living organisms. How this comes about is not completely understood. Observations have made it clear, however, that biological adaptation is one of the most necessary characteristics of life. Some traits confer on certain individuals an advantage over other individuals; that is, they favor their adaptation and survival in a particular environment and make them more likely to reproduce their kind than individuals who do not possess such traits.

There are numerous examples of successful structural and functional adaptations in nature. Birds, adapted to living in the desert, conserve water by excreting solid urine. Certain sea birds have developed salt-excreting glands that enable them to drink sea water. Despite kidneys that are less efficient in removing salt than man's, they are able to maintain the concentration of salt in their extracellular fluid at about the same level. Man, having no comparable structure, is unable to use sea water. When he drinks it, he dehydrates himself by using body water to eliminate the excess salt into his urine. The dehydration is further increased by the diarrhea that results from the high concentration of magnesium in the sea water.[16]

Another example of an environmental condition favoring the survival of organisms with certain traits is observed in England. In rural areas a certain species of moth is commonly found to be light-colored. In industrial areas the dark variety predominates. The light-colored moths are conspicuous on the soot-blackened trunks and branches of trees. Because they are easily identified by birds they are eaten as they appear and do not have much opportunity to multiply, whereas the dark species escape notice and survive.

Occasionally an abnormality serves as an asset in a particular environment. Sickle cell anemia is one such condition. For some reason it confers, or is associated with, some characteristic that increases resistance to malaria. In malarious areas of Africa sickle cell anemia is advantageous to the individual because it increases his chances of survival. In nonmalarious areas, such as the United States, it has no survival value.

At times the capacity of certain organisms to adapt has been a disadvantage to man. For example, the fact that mosquitos have developed resistance to DDT and other insecticides enables them to survive and makes the eradication of malaria difficult. A similar case is *Staphylococcus aureus*, of which strains resistant to penicillin have come to predominate. For a brief time, infections caused by this organism were brought under rapid control, but the capacity of the *Staphylococcus* to adapt has en-

abled it to survive. Not all species, however, have been successful in adapting to change. The mammoth dinosaurs are extinct because they were unable to adapt to changes from a tropical to a temperate climate or, what appears to be more likely, to a reduction in the amount of food available.

In general, man has the capacity to adapt to a wider range of conditions than do other species. There are a number of explanations for his ability to adapt to different conditions. He is able to modify his external environment to his needs, as well as to foresee future needs and to make plans that enable him to meet them. Though many species are restricted geographically to a limited area, man can roam the earth or live out his life span in the place where he was born. In either situation he alters his environment to suit his needs. His capacity to adapt the environment to his needs increased greatly when he began to build shelters, make clothing and fire, cultivate plants, and domesticate animals as sources of food and power. In modern times the adaptations of the environment have been further increased by the achievement of a high degree of refinement and efficiency in industrial and agricultural methods and tools.

In addition to adapting his environment to his needs, man adapts in all aspects of his life. These adaptations may be temporary or permanent. An example of a temporary protective biological adaptation is the capacity to tan the skin. Tanning on exposure to the sunlight offers some protection to the deeper layers of the skin. Persons whose skin does not tan run the risk of sunburn on each exposure to the sun. The fact that the races that developed in the tropics have dark skins whereas those in northern countries have fair skins is believed to represent a more permanent type of adaptation of the skin to environmental conditions.

Many other examples can be cited of ways in which man has adapted to climate, geographical location, physical activity, and disease. Body build appears to be influenced by climate and by the type of activities in which the individual customarily engages. The short, stocky frame of the Eskimo and the layer of fat under his skin serve to prevent heat loss. The heavy muscles of the manual laborer or the professional wrestler illustrate an adaptation to activities requiring muscular activity. Enlargement of the myocardium in essential hypertension is another illustration of biological adaptation to increased work. One of the factors enabling man to live at high altitudes is that he adapts by increasing the number of erythrocytes and the quantity of hemoglobin in his blood.

Man adapts to some pathogenic microorgan-

[16] Knut Schmidt-Nielsen: "Salt Glands," *Sci. Amer.*, 200:109–16 (Jan.) 1959.

isms by developing an immunity to them. For some microorganisms, such as the virus causing smallpox, he has been able to develop a vaccine that causes his body to produce antibodies that protect him from the disease. Others, either because they have diminished in virulence or because man has developed some resistance to them, do not cause as much damage as they once did.

A universal adaptation, that is, one that is common to all groups of people, is to the type of food available in an area. Whatever plant or animal is most abundant is utilized as the principal food. In some areas of the world one or possibly two plants are utilized as the basic food: potatoes, rice, and wheat. In others the principal food is corn, a fruit, or meat. The manner in which food is prepared reflects its abundance or scarcity and the means that are available to prepare it. For example, meat may be added to vegetables or sauces for flavor or to make a little go a long way. Because man takes his food habits with him wherever he goes, he may continue to select and to prepare foods in a certain way despite changes in his environment or in the availability of specific foods. In fact, changes in food habits are made only with difficulty. A common observation is that persons migrating from one area of the world to another adopt a new language but continue to cling to old food habits.

FACTORS INFLUENCING THE CAPACITY
TO ADAPT

Among the factors influencing the adaptive capacity of an individual are his genetic constitution, the extent to which his needs have been met in the past, his level of learning, his anatomical integrity, and his age. Genetic constitution, or heredity, determines the potential and the limits for the growth and development of both structure and functions in the individual. Through influencing the biochemical activities of cells, genes affect the capacity of the organism to adapt to changes imposed on it from within or from without. The effects of genes range from the activity of enzyme systems in cells to body build and the pigmentation of the skin. Some abnormalities are transmitted by genes and are incompatible with life. Some are evident at birth; some appear early in life; and others do not make their appearance until late in life. An abnormality may be seriously handicapping or produce little or no disability. An example of a disorder in which a defective gene has been identified is the sickle cell trait. In other diseases, such as diabetes mellitus and essential hypertension, heredity appears to be a factor, but the exact nature of transmission is less certain.

The adaptive potential is determined by heredity. Whether or not the individual achieves his potential depends on a variety of factors. Very important is the extent to which his physiological as well as psychological needs have been met in the past, most particularly in his early life. An inadequate intake of high-quality proteins in infancy and early childhood predisposes to liver disease and may impair intellectual capacity. A child who is seriously deprived of love is susceptible to failure to develop emotionally.

How well an individual achieves his adaptive potential also depends on how he has learned to satisfy his needs and to react to stress as well as to conditions to which he has been exposed. Experiences along the way may predispose the individual to health or to disease later in his life. For example, repeated streptococcal infections may predispose a person to rheumatic fever and the rheumatic fever to a reduction in the capacity of the heart to adapt. As a result of the effects of repeated illness, as well as of the attitudes of his parents and others during periods of illness or health, he may come to prefer illness to health. His schooling may be interrupted and his incentive to learn impaired.

A study reported by Rosenthal and Jacobson [17] indicates that expectations of teachers have an effect on the intellectual gains made by children as well as on their general behavior. The results of this study indicate that adaptation is influenced by the expectations of others.

The level of learning influences the flexibility of the individual. In general, educated persons are more adaptable than noneducated ones.

Anatomical integrity affects the capacity to adapt. As examples, the individual who has been brain-injured may be less able to cope with emotional and physical stress than a healthy person. A child with a defective intraventricular septum may not achieve full mental or physical growth. Neither will he be able to be as active as a healthy child. Depending on the nature of the environment, an individual achieves or fails to achieve his intellectual and physical potential.

Age—A Factor in Adaptability

Adaptability is generally greatest in youth and young middle life and least at the extremes of life. In infants and young children, the capacity to adapt is limited by the fact that not all organs and systems are fully mature. At birth the kidneys, nervous system, and immunological systems are not fully developed. For example, the kidney of the young infant is not able to concentrate urine as efficiently as during youth and adult life. As a consequence of the imma-

[17] Robert Rosenthal and Lenore F. Jacobson: "Teacher Expectations for the Disadvantaged," *Sci. Amer.*, **218**:19–23 (Apr.) 1968.

turity of his nervous system and lack of experience he is unable to evaluate his external environment and to modify it in terms of his needs.

One of the infant's more serious deficiencies is the immaturity of his immunological system. The very young child is more susceptible to and more seriously affected by infectious agents than older children and adults. His immunological system has to develop before it recognizes harmful agents and reacts to them by forming antibodies. As a result of immaturity, the infant, and to a lesser extent the child, depends on others for his safety and welfare.

In the later years of life adaptive capacity declines. Not all the factors in this process are fully understood. One seems to be a lessening of the reserve capacity of vital organs and with it the inability to cope with rapidly increasing loads. There is also a decrease in response to agents of disease such as bacteria. Infections, such as pneumonia, may be accompanied by few of the changes ordinarily associated with this disease. Fever may be absent or the temperature only slightly elevated.

CHARACTERISTIC FEATURES OF ADAPTATION

Whatever the power of the individual to adapt, adaptation is characterized by a number of features. As stated previously, one is that adaptation involves the entire organism. Mr. Brave illustrates this concept. He awakened with a feeling of nausea and vomited a large amount of bright red blood. After he vomited, he saw the blood and was frightened. He called his wife, who called his physician, who asked him to go to the hospital—which is a social response to medical knowledge and equipment. Mr. Brave's fear or anxiety was so great that he did not delay putting himself under the care of his physician. Neither was it so great that he was immobilized. His body was also reacting. His sympathoadrenal medullary system constricted his peripheral blood vessels. He looked pale and felt cold, dizzy, and faint. He lay on the bed until the ambulance arrived. His heart and respiratory rates increased. Although the picture is not complete, enough has been presented to emphasize the point that Mr. Brave reacted as a whole individual.

A second feature of adaptation is related to time. Given time, an organism is able to adapt to a greater degree of stress than it can when it is called on to adapt suddenly. In the instance of Mr. Brave, had he lost small amounts of blood over a period of time he would have been able to tolerate a lower hemoglobin level than when he lost blood rapidly. With a slow loss of blood he would probably have tolerated a hemoglobin of 4 g (25 per cent) or less without exhibiting manifestations of marked circulatory distress at rest. In contrast, with a rapid loss of blood, a hemoglobin of 50 per cent is accompanied by manifestations indicative of a serious impairment in the blood supply to vital tissues. There are a number of explanations for the differences in behavior of an individual following the slow and rapid loss of blood. In contrast to a rapid loss of blood with a slow loss, blood volume is not diminished and the tissues have time to adapt to a decrease in oxygen supply. With a sufficient decrease in the oxygen, signs and symptoms of circulatory distress appear. They include palpitation, rapid heart rate, shortness of breath, and possibly dizziness. Depending on the extent to which the hemoglobin level is diminished, these manifestations may appear with activity and disappear with rest or be present much of the time.

A third feature of adaptation is that the more flexible the organism is in its capacity to adapt, the greater is its capacity to survive. If, for example, the only mechanism available to adapt to the loss of blood was by constriction of blood vessels, man would be much more vulnerable and much less able to survive injuries involving blood loss than he is. Flexibility is as significant in psychological and social adaptation as it is in physiological responses. An illustration of the adaptation to available materials and climate is observed in the building of houses. Among the materials utilized in the building of houses are snow, wood, cement, cinders, sand, clay, aluminum, steel, glass, and skins of animals. Houses vary in size from one room to a hundred or more. Depending on climate and availability of fuel, they may be airy or almost airtight. Their shapes are varied. In fact, any adequate description of the varieties in manner in which man has adapted materials to his need for shelter would be impossible to list in this volume.

A fourth feature of adaptation is that the organism generally, though not always, uses the mechanism that is most economical of energy. The fact that adaptation also requires energy should not be overlooked. Adaptation is usually integrative in character and is usually the best that the organism can do at a given time. In illness there is always some decrease in the capacity of a person to adapt. The sick person is not at his best, and allowance should be made for his inability to cope with his environment and the resultant frustration of his needs.

A fifth feature is that the adaptive response may be adequate to the situation or it may be deficient, excessive, or inappropriate. To illustrate, following a meal, the blood sugar rises. In the healthy individual, as the blood sugar rises, insulin is secreted and glucose is removed from the blood by the liver and converted to glycogen.

Some glucose may be temporarily stored in the muscles and areolar connective tissues. Approximately two hours after a meal, the level of sugar in the blood drops to, or slightly below, the fasting level. As the level of glucose in the blood drops, mechanisms responsible for its fall are counteracted and the level of glucose in the blood rises to the normal range for the fasting blood glucose. (One of Cannon's characteristics of homeostatic mechanism.) An elevation in the level of glucose that is sustained above the upper limits of normal is usually caused by a relative or absolute lack of insulin.

To sum up, adaptation enables living organisms to respond to changes in their environment in such a manner that injury is prevented or damage is repaired. Although all living organisms possess the power of adaptation, not only species, but also individuals of the same species vary in their capacity to adapt.

How can positive health, or high-level wellness, be promoted?

As stated earlier, the promotion of health is accepted as a desirable objective. However, very little is known about how to measure health or even how to achieve or maintain it. In much of the literature little or no distinction is made between the promotion of health and the primary prevention of disease. Although knowledge and techniques are available to enable the physician to identify and categorize various diseases, there is little information and few techniques to aid him in distinguishing among and classifying different degrees of health. If the goal, to promote a "high level of wellness," is to be accomplished, at least some health workers will need to shift their emphasis from death and disease to health and its fulfillment.[18]

For want of more definitive knowledge, conditions contributing to healthful living will be considered as facilitating the accomplishment of the objective "to promote health" and the measures more directly related to the prevention of specific diseases as facilitating the accomplishment of the objective "to prevent disease or disability from disease." The discerning reader will note that there is some overlapping between the two.

The Commission on Chronic Illness [19] lists the following as among the most important components of healthful living:

Nutrition—adequate, safe, and well-distributed

[18] Iago Galdston: *The Meaning of Social Medicine* (Cambridge: Harvard University Press, 1954), p. 32.

[19] Commission on Chronic Illness: *Chronic Illness in the United States.* Vol. I. *Prevention of Chronic Illness* (Cambridge: Harvard University Press, 1957), pp. 9–10.

food supplies as well as appropriate levels of personal nutrition.

Mental hygiene—beginning at an early age, it is important that the individual develop an equanimity in the face of the natural and inevitable frustrations of living; appreciation of the values of family life; acceptance of oneself and one's limitations.

Adequate housing—including proper safeguards against accidents for persons of all ages, and particular safeguards for children and for the aged and handicapped.

Moderate and well-balanced personal habits—restraints in use of alcohol and tobacco, sufficient rest and an appropriate amount of exercise, careful attention to personal hygiene.

A useful and productive role in society.

General education and education specifically for health.

A safe and healthful working environment.

Recreation, including access to recreational opportunities and facilities on the one hand, and proper balancing of recreational activities against satisfying work on the other.

A sense of personal security, related to such things as access to health services; legalized provisions for minimum wages and some sort of job security; provision for income maintenance during illness or following retirement.

To this list may be added another concept— that is, a system of values that serves as a guide to action. Beginning at an early age, the individual should be helped to develop a sense of purpose in his life, that is, who and why he is and where he is going. His goals should be based on a wholesome appreciation of the rights and dignity of his fellow man.

The promotion of health is both an individual and a social responsibility. Whenever a large group of people live in a limited area, regulations are necessary to protect the general welfare. The individual has a responsibility to cooperate in protecting not only his own rights but those of others.

One of the best-known and -organized efforts in the field of health promotion is the well-baby clinic. The baby is examined regularly and the mother is given guidance in his care. Data are available by which the growth and development of the child can be measured. This information is useful in reassuring the mother that her baby is developing normally; in turn it may contribute to the mother's being more relaxed in the care of her baby. It may also be the basis for unnecessary anxiety, unless both the mother and the health worker know and accept the fact that there is much variation in the rate at which babies grow and develop. When the development of the baby is in some respect abnormal, the mother can be aided in modifying his care so that his health is promoted. For example, the baby may be gaining weight too rapidly. In addition to recognizing that obesity is undesirable, the mother may require support to modify his food intake. Attendance at the well-baby clinic also provides an opportunity to immunize the baby against diseases such as measles, smallpox, and diphtheria. Thus, through services provided to the baby and his mother, the healthy development of the baby is promoted.

Knowledge of the factors assisting in the promotion of health will undoubtedly increase in the future. Contributions from the fields of biochemistry, biophysics, psychology, sociology, and anthropology can be expected to provide a basis for a greater understanding of what health is and how it is measured and promoted than is now available. Among the questions being explored by social scientists are how to impart information about health so that it is effective, how to change attitudes, and how to improve communication between and among various groups.

As with other members of society, the nurse has a personal responsibility to promote her own health. As society expects the contributions of an individual to be commensurate with his education and opportunities, the nurse has more responsibility than the ordinary citizen to promote her own health. She also has a responsibility as a citizen to promote community projects such as improved housing and slum clearance that contribute to the general health and welfare of the entire community. As a professional nurse she also works with individuals and groups to help them raise their standards of health.

What are the factors influencing health?

Some of the hazards to health in an urban, industrialized society were presented in Chapter 2. They will be referred to as they predispose to specific diseases. A group of related conditions —economic status, education, and general standard of living—also affect the health of the population.

For example, nonwhite Americans have a shorter life-span than white Americans. Besson [20] states that the southern Negro's life is 17 years shorter than his white counterpart's. His wife is four times as likely to die in childbirth, and his mortality rate from tuberculosis is four times that of his white neighbor.

In 1965, the infant mortality rate per 1,000 live births for white babies was 21.5; for nonwhite babies it was 40.3. The difference in maternal mortality rates was even greater, as it was 21.0 for white mothers and 83.7 for nonwhite mothers.[21]

Walker [22] quotes a study conducted by the National Office of Vital Statistics in which the death rate ratio is correlated with income. Those with the lowest income have the shortest life expectancy; those with the highest income have the longest life expectancy. Professional men and businessmen listed in the 1950–1951 *Who's Who In America* have lived longer than men in the general population.[23] College graduates live longer than noncollege graduates. Clergymen, teachers, and lawyers live longer than the average. Linder [24] states that the National Health Survey statistics "confirm clearly and in quantitative terms the generally accepted idea that there is a positive relation between poor health and low income." People with incomes of $2,000 per year had more days of disability than those in the next higher bracket and so on.

Antonovsky [25] reviews a large number of life expectancy studies. These studies show that over the course of history, whatever index is used and the number of classes considered, the lowest class has the poorest life expectancy. Furthermore, the class differences are greatest in young and middle adulthood and tend to disappear after age 65.[26]

One further example will be cited. Each year in its annual report, the Department of Health of the City of Detroit summarizes the vital statistics for the city in a map. The divisions of the map correspond to the census areas. To orient the reader to the map, the "Central City," which includes the downtown area, Figure 3-1, is the section bounded on three sides by the Grand Boulevard and on the fourth by the Detroit River. According to a study made by the Southeast Michigan Council of Government,[27] approximately 230,000, or 14 per cent, of the population of the city of Detroit live in the area bounded by the Grand Boulevard. The extent to which overcrowding exists in this area is emphasized by a number of conditions. Another study showed that much of the land space, which is 11 per cent of the total area of Detroit, is used for commercial and industrial purposes. Even more telling is the fact that the Central

[20] *Op. cit.,* p. 1904.

[21] U.S. Department of Health, Education, and Welfare, National Center for Health Statistics: *Facts of Life and Death* (Washington, D.C.: U.S. Government Printing Office, 1967), p. 9.

[22] Gerald Walker: "Good News for Go-Getters!" *This Week Magazine, The Detroit News,* June 12, 1960, pp. 4–5.

[23] Metropolitan Life Insurance Company: *Statistical Bulletin,* **49**:3 (Jan.) 1968.

[24] Forrest E. Linder: "The Health of the American People," *Sci. Amer.,* **214**:28 (June) 1966.

[25] Aaron Antonovsky: "Social Class, Life Expectancy and Overall Mortality," *The Milbank Memorial Fund Quarterly,* Part 1, **45**:31–73 (Apr.) 1967.

[26] *Ibid.,* p. 67.

[27] Southeast Michigan Council of Government: *Population and Occupied Dwelling Units in the Detroit Region* (Detroit: Southeast Michigan Council of Government, July 1, 1967).

CITY LIMITS

ALTER ROAD · GRATIOT AVENUE · VAN DYKE AVENUE · EAST McNICHOLS · WEST McNICHOLS · WOODWARD AVENUE · HARPER AVENUE · EAST GRAND BOULEVARD · WOODWARD AVENUE · DETROIT RIVER · LIVERNOIS AVENUE · GREENFIELD ROAD · FULLERTON AVENUE · TIREMAN AVENUE · M. C. RR · W. GD. BOULEVARD · W. GD. BLVD · E. GD. BLVD.

HAYES · PHILLIP · HOUSTON

Population 83,200
Birth 13.6
Deaths: Total 8.4
Inf. mortality 18.6
Heart disease 339.0
All cancer 159.9
Lung cancer 26.4
Leukemia & blood ca. 6.0
Pneu. – influ. 13.2
Violence 56.5
Cirrhosis of liver 14.4
Tuberculosis 1.2

Population 73,300
Birth 11.6
Deaths: Total 10.8
Inf. mortality 24.6
Heart disease 447.5
All cancer 215.6
Lung cancer 32.7
Leukemia & blood ca. 6.8
Pneu. – influ. 19.1
Violence 65.5
Cirrhosis of liver 8.2
Tuberculosis 8.2

Population 99,500
Birth 18.2
Deaths: Total 10.3
Inf. mortality 14.3
Heart disease 418.1
All cancer 198.0
Lung cancer 13.2
Leukemia & blood ca. 10.1
Pneu. – influ. 27.1
Violence 64.3
Cirrhosis of liver 17.1
Tuberculosis 1.0

Population 99,700
Birth 13.6
Deaths: Total 11.2
Inf. mortality 24.3
Heart disease 498.5
All cancer 234.7
Lung cancer 41.1
Leuk. & blood ca. 10.0
Pneu. – influ. 21.1
Violence 50.2
Cirrhosis of liver 14.0
Tuberculosis 5.0

Population 92,400
Birth 16.5
Deaths: Total 9.4
Inf. mortality 19.0
Heart disease 363.6
All cancer 197.0
Lung cancer 45.5
Leukemia & blood ca. 6.5
Pneu. – influ. 16.2
Violence 54.1
Cirrhosis of liver 32.5
Tuberculosis 4.3

Population 201,300
Birth 21.9
Deaths: Total 21.1
Inf. mortality 28.3
Heart disease 422.3
All cancer 175.4
Lung cancer 42.7
Leuk. & blood ca. 6.0
Pneu. – influ. 69.5
Violence 24.8
Cirrhosis of liver 4.5
Tuberculosis

Population 109,400
Birth 18.2
Deaths: Total 18.6
Inf. mortality 50.3
Heart disease 667.8
All cancer 290.3
Lung cancer 53.7
Leuk. & blood ca. 104.7
Pneu. – influ. 137.1
Violence 46.6
Cirrhosis of liver 32.0
Tuberculosis

Population 80,300
Birth 18.9
Deaths: Total 14.3
Inf. mortality 34.2
Heart disease 504.4
All cancer 261.5
Lung cancer 36.1
Leuk. & blood ca. 5.0
Pneu. – influ. 87.2
Violence 36.1
Cirrhosis of liver 17.4
Tuberculosis

Population 120,000
Birth 15.2
Deaths: Total 36.7
Inf. mortality
Heart disease 516.0
All cancer 230.1
Lung cancer 49.2
Leuk. & blood ca. 4.2
Pneu. – influ. 83.3
Violence 120.7
Cirrhosis of liver 76.5
Tuberculosis 27.5

Population 194,900
Birth 23.2
Deaths: Total 10.3
Inf. mortality 38.3
Heart disease 348.4
All cancer 170.9
Lung cancer 38.0
Leuk. & blood ca. 7.7
Pneu. – influ. 41.0
Violence 78.5
Cirrhosis of liver 23.1
Tuberculosis 9.2

Population 89,800
Birth 19.4
Deaths: Total 10.8
Inf. mortality 17.8
Heart disease 418.7
All cancer 219.4
Lung cancer 40.1
Leukemia & blood ca. 2.2
Pneu. – influ. 33.4
Violence 50.1
Cirrhosis of liver 23.4
Tuberculosis 4.5

Population 63,600
Birth 18.0
Deaths: Total 18.5
Inf. mortality 21.0
Heart disease 432.4
All cancer 206.0
Lung cancer 37.7
Leuk. & blood ca. 4.7
Pneu. – influ. 33.0
Violence 51.9
Cirrhosis of liver 17.3
Tuberculosis 1.6

Population 72,300
Birth 18.0
Deaths: Total 12.1
Inf. mortality 28.4
Heart disease 426.0
All cancer 204.7
Lung cancer 36.0
Leuk. & blood ca. 9.7
Pneu. – influ. 48.4
Violence 92.7
Cirrhosis of liver 26.3
Tuberculosis 8.3

Population 87,500
Birth 19.6
Deaths: Total 11.8
Inf. mortality 26.8
Heart disease 482.3
All cancer 180.6
Lung cancer 27.4
Leuk. & blood ca. 2.3
Pneu. – influ. 32.0
Violence 107.4
Cirrhosis of liver 25.1
Tuberculosis 12.6

Population 85,400
Birth 17.1
Deaths: Total 10.1
Inf. mortality 21.2
Heart disease 394.6
All cancer 195.6
Lung cancer 36.3
Leuk. & blood ca. 14.1
Pneu. – influ. 19.9
Violence 58.5
Cirrhosis of liver 15.2
Tuberculosis 2.3

Population 87,400
Birth 16.2
Deaths: Total 8.9
Inf. mortality 14.1
Heart disease 337.5
All cancer 211.7
Lung cancer 48.0
Leuk. & blood ca. 14.9
Pneu. – influ. 21.7
Violence 57.2
Cirrhosis of liver 17.2
Tuberculosis 3.4

VITAL EVENTS WHICH OCCURRED TO DETROIT RESIDENTS IN 1966   Provisional

Rates for the City of Detroit

Estimated Population, July 1, 1966 – 1,640,000

Rates

Births	19.0
Deaths: Total	11.7
Infant mortality	28.0
Heart disease	442.8
All cancer	208.8
Lung cancer	39.9
Leukemia and blood cancer	7.9
Pneumonia and influenza	42.4
Violence	78.4
Cirrhosis of liver	27.9
Tuberculosis	9.6

Maternal mortality—6.8 per 10,000 live births

the mother may require support to modify his food intake. Attendance at the well-baby clinic also provides an opportunity to immunize the baby against diseases such as measles, smallpox, and diphtheria. Thus, through services provided to the baby and his mother, the healthy development of the baby is promoted.

Knowledge of the factors assisting in the promotion of health will undoubtedly increase in the future. Contributions from the fields of biochemistry, biophysics, psychology, sociology, and anthropology can be expected to provide a basis for a greater understanding of what health is and how it is measured and promoted than is now available. Among the questions being explored by social scientists are how to impart information about health so that it is effective, how to change attitudes, and how to improve communication between and among various groups.

As with other members of society, the nurse has a personal responsibility to promote her own health. As society expects the contributions of an individual to be commensurate with his education and opportunities, the nurse has more responsibility than the ordinary citizen to promote her own health. She also has a responsibility as a citizen to promote community projects such as improved housing and slum clearance that contribute to the general health and welfare of the entire community. As a professional nurse she also works with individuals and groups to help them raise their standards of health.

What are the factors influencing health?

Some of the hazards to health in an urban, industrialized society were presented in Chapter 2. They will be referred to as they predispose to specific diseases. A group of related conditions —economic status, education, and general standard of living—also affect the health of the population.

For example, nonwhite Americans have a shorter life-span than white Americans. Besson[20] states that the southern Negro's life is 17 years shorter than his white counterpart's. His wife is four times as likely to die in childbirth, and his mortality rate from tuberculosis is four times that of his white neighbor.

In 1965, the infant mortality rate per 1,000 live births for white babies was 21.5; for nonwhite babies it was 40.3. The difference in maternal mortality rates was even greater, as it was 21.0 for white mothers and 83.7 for nonwhite mothers.[21]

Walker[22] quotes a study conducted by the National Office of Vital Statistics in which the death rate ratio is correlated with income. Those with the lowest income have the shortest life expectancy; those with the highest income have the longest life expectancy. Professional men and businessmen listed in the 1950–1951 *Who's Who In America* have lived longer than men in the general population.[23] College graduates live longer than noncollege graduates. Clergymen, teachers, and lawyers live longer than the average. Linder[24] states that the National Health Survey statistics "confirm clearly and in quantitative terms the generally accepted idea that there is a positive relation between poor health and low income." People with incomes of $2,000 per year had more days of disability than those in the next higher bracket and so on.

Antonovsky[25] reviews a large number of life expectancy studies. These studies show that over the course of history, whatever index is used and the number of classes considered, the lowest class has the poorest life expectancy. Furthermore, the class differences are greatest in young and middle adulthood and tend to disappear after age 65.[26]

One further example will be cited. Each year in its annual report, the Department of Health of the City of Detroit summarizes the vital statistics for the city in a map. The divisions of the map correspond to the census areas. To orient the reader to the map, the "Central City," which includes the downtown area, Figure 3-1, is the section bounded on three sides by the Grand Boulevard and on the fourth by the Detroit River. According to a study made by the Southeast Michigan Council of Government,[27] approximately 230,000, or 14 per cent, of the population of the city of Detroit live in the area bounded by the Grand Boulevard. The extent to which overcrowding exists in this area is emphasized by a number of conditions. Another study showed that much of the land space, which is 11 per cent of the total area of Detroit, is used for commercial and industrial purposes. Even more telling is the fact that the Central

[20] *Op. cit.*, p. 1904.

[21] U.S. Department of Health, Education, and Welfare, National Center for Health Statistics: *Facts of Life and Death* (Washington, D.C.: U.S. Government Printing Office, 1967), p. 9.

[22] Gerald Walker: "Good News for Go-Getters!" *This Week Magazine, The Detroit News*, June 12, 1960, pp. 4–5.

[23] Metropolitan Life Insurance Company: *Statistical Bulletin*, 49:3 (Jan.) 1968.

[24] Forrest E. Linder: "The Health of the American People," *Sci. Amer.*, 214:28 (June) 1966.

[25] Aaron Antonovsky: "Social Class, Life Expectancy and Overall Mortality," *The Milbank Memorial Fund Quarterly*, Part 1, 45:31–73 (Apr.) 1967.

[26] *Ibid.*, p. 67.

[27] Southeast Michigan Council of Government: *Population and Occupied Dwelling Units in the Detroit Region* (Detroit: Southeast Michigan Council of Government, July 1, 1967).

VITAL EVENTS WHICH OCCURRED TO DETROIT RESIDENTS IN 1966

Rates for the City of Detroit   Provisional

Estimated Population, July 1, 1966 – 1,640,000

Rates	
Births	19.0
Deaths: Total	11.7
Infant mortality	28.0
Heart disease	442.8
All cancer	208.8
Lung cancer	39.9
Leukemia and blood cancer	7.9
Pneumonia and influenza	42.4
Violence	78.4
Cirrhosis of liver	27.9
Tuberculosis	9.6

Maternal mortality—6.8 per 10,000 live births

District data blocks (roads shown on map: CITY LIMITS, WOODWARD AVENUE, GRATIOT AVENUE, VAN DYKE AVENUE, EAST McNICHOLS, WEST McNICHOLS, LIVERNOIS AVENUE, GREENFIELD ROAD, FULLERTON AVENUE, TIREMAN AVENUE, M.C. RR, HOUSTON, HAYES, PHILLIP, HARPER AVENUE, ALTER ROAD, EAST GRAND BOULEVARD, E. GD. BLVD., W. GD. BOULEVARD, W. GD. BLVD., WOODWARD AVENUE, DETROIT RIVER):

	Pop. 99,700	Pop. 99,500	Pop. 92,400 (M)	Pop. 80,300 (L)	Pop. 201,300 (N)	Pop. 109,400 (K)
Birth	13.6	18.2	16.5	18.9	21.1	18.2
Deaths: Total	11.2	10.3	9.4	14.3	11.1	18.6
Inf. mortality	24.3	14.3	19.0	34.2	28.3	50.5
Heart disease	498.5	418.1	363.6	504.4	422.7	667.8
All cancer	234.7	198.0	197.0	261.5	175.4	276.3
Lung cancer	41.1	33.2	45.5	36.1	42.7	50.7
Leuk. & blood ca.	10.0	10.1	6.5	5.0	7.7	13.7
Pneu. – influ.	21.1	27.1	16.2	87.2	69.5	104.7
Violence	50.2	64.3	54.1	89.7	47.7	137.1
Cirrhosis of liver	14.0	17.1	32.5	36.1	24.6	46.9
Tuberculosis	5.0	1.0	4.3	17.4	4.5	32.0

	Pop. 83,200 (J)	Pop. 73,300	Pop. 85,400 (I)	Pop. 89,800	Pop. 87,400 (H)	Pop. 63,600 (E)
Birth	13.6	11.6	17.1	19.4	16.2	18.0
Deaths: Total	8.4	10.8	10.1	10.8	8.9	10.5
Inf. mortality	18.6	24.6	21.2	17.8	14.1	21.0
Heart disease	339.0	447.5	394.6	418.7	337.5	432.4
All cancer	159.9	215.6	195.6	219.4	211.7	206.0
Lung cancer	26.4	32.7	36.3	40.1	48.0	37.7
Leuk. & blood ca.	6.0	6.8	14.1	2.2	14.9	4.7
Pneu. – influ.	13.2	19.1	19.9	33.4	21.7	33.0
Violence	56.5	65.5	58.5	50.1	57.2	51.9
Cirrhosis of liver	14.4	8.2	15.2	23.4	17.2	17.3
Tuberculosis	1.2		2.3	4.5	3.4	1.6

	Pop. 194,900 (D)	Pop. 72,300 (C)	Pop. 87,500 (B)	Pop. 120,000 (A)
Birth	23.2	18.0	19.6	15.2
Deaths: Total	10.3	12.1	11.8	9.9
Inf. mortality	38.3	28.4	26.8	39.7
Heart disease	348.4	426.0	482.3	516.5
All cancer	170.9	204.7	180.6	239.2
Lung cancer	38.0	36.0	27.4	42.0
Leuk. & blood ca.	7.7	9.7	2.3	4.2
Pneu. – influ.	41.0	48.4	32.0	83.3
Violence	78.5	92.7	107.4	120.7
Cirrhosis of liver	23.1	26.3	25.1	27.5
Tuberculosis	9.2	8.3	12.6	

Map districts labeled: A, B, C, D, E, F, G, H, I, J, K, L, M, N, O, P

City contains only 4 per cent of the dwelling places of the community and 22 per cent of them are vacant. Much of the housing in the area is in various stages of deterioration and a not inconsiderable portion is unfit for human habitation.[28] Though the population in the area decreased in the period between 1960–1966, most of the decrease was in the adult population.[29]

As is to be expected, the population of the Central City not only lives under inadequate and overcrowded conditions, but many individuals have marginal or inadequate incomes. It is estimated that in 1960, 41 per cent of the families receiving aid to dependent children and 44 per cent of those persons receiving old age assistance lived in this area.[30] Like other large cities, Detroit is working on slum clearance and on improving the standard of housing for all its citizens. In general, though, both in housing and in income, those living in the Boulevard area are poor in comparison to those living in the remainder of the city. Many of the problems of the area are compounded because few of the underprivileged have had an opportunity to acquire educations adequate to secure employment in a modern industrialized society.

Granted that factors other than housing, education, and income have a bearing on the health status in the community, examination of the map reveals that on most counts the health of the people living inside the Boulevard suffers in comparison to the health of persons living in other areas of the city. The area with the highest infant mortality rate (census area K) has a rate almost four times that of the lowest. As stated earlier, maternal and infant mortality rates are generally accepted as an index of the standard of health in the community. The ma-

[28] Detroit Area Planning Committee of the United Community Services of Metropolitan Detroit: *Social Services in Detroit's Central City,* Sept. 1960.

[29] In the interval since this study was made some of the poorest houses have been replaced by middle- and upper-income housing. A number of hotels have been converted into residences for the aged. The 1970 census will undoubtedly indicate considerable change in the character of the population.

[30] Detroit Area Planning Committee of the United Community Services of Metropolitan Detroit, *op. cit.,* p. 8.

ternal mortality rates for the different areas is not shown. With the exception of cancer in one area, the mortality rate for all diseases listed on the map is also higher. The differences in the mortality rates from tuberculosis are particularly striking. In 1966 in census area N, 1 person per 100,000 died from tuberculosis, whereas in census area K, 32 died.

The high rate of crime occurring in the Central City is a reflection of the mental health of the community. Another difference in the various census areas is the extent to which violence, which includes traffic accidents and homicides, is responsible for death. In census area K, almost three times as many persons die as a result of homicide as in the adjoining census area P. The incidence of homicide in census area K is forty times greater than in J.

Although these statistics tell what the causes of death are in the city of Detroit, they do not tell the quality of the lives of the people who died or continue to live. What are the conditions in the environment that lead to alcoholism and thence to cirrhosis of the liver and to homicide, suicide, and other forms of violence? The promotion of health includes solving these as well as other problems.

Although most studies performed in the past do show an inverse relationship between socioeconomic status and mortality, authorities are not all agreed about why this relationship exists. Nor do authorities agree as to whether the inverse relationship is limited to infectious diseases or is also true in chronic diseases. To examine the nature and extent of the relationship of socioeconomic status and mortality, Stockwell[31] reviewed the 1949–1951 death records for the residents of Hartford, Connecticut, and Providence, Rhode Island, using two different approaches. By both methods, he confirmed that there was indeed a marked inverse relationship between socioeconomic status and mortality. He also found that the exact nature and extent of the relationship between the two factors vary between cities and with the methods

[31] Edward G. Stockwell: "A Critical Examination of the Relationship Between Socioeconomic Status and Mortality," *Amer. J. Public Health,* **53**:956–64 (June) 1963.

FIGURE 3-1. Detroit, Michigan, population, birth, and death rates by census areas, 1966. Estimated population, July 1, 1966, was 1,640,000; population by census area is estimated also. All figures refer to rates: birth and death rates per 1,000 population; infant mortality per 1,000 live births; over rates per 100,000 population. Total rates for entire city: births, 19.0; deaths (total), 11.7; infant mortality, 28.0; heart disease, 442.8; all cancer, 208.8; lung cancer, 39.9; leukemia and blood cancer, 7.9; pneumonia and influenza, 42.4; violence, 78.4; cirrhosis of liver, 27.9; tuberculosis, 9.6; maternal mortality per 10,000 live births, 6.8. (Source: Detroit Department of Health.)

used to study the relationship. In the light of the above, the conclusions about the relationship of the health of the population of the Central City of Detroit to the socioeconomic and educational status are probably valid. Neither the exact relationship nor all the factors involved have been established.

The Prevention of Disease:
The Second Objective

The second objective of the health professions is the prevention of disease. In the prevention of disease, actions are taken to forestall the development of disease or injury. In diseases already established, procedures are instituted to prevent disability or to delay its progress.

What is the nature of disease?

DEFINITION OF DISEASE

The first part of this chapter has considered the nature of health and some of the factors influencing it. This part will consider disease. Whenever considering disease, however, the nurse should keep uppermost in her mind and actions Besson's injunction [32] that professionals deal "more with people and less with patients . . . more with the human conditions, and less with formalin fixed pathology . . . more with the sociocultural hazards than with the biological ones . . . more with a continuum of care, less with the episode of sickness." As a personal

[32] *Op. cit.*, p. 1904.

opinion, no one approach to the care of people, sick or well, should be excluded. At one time one is more important than another. Man is at the same time a biological, sociocultural, and psychological being.

In contrast to health, disease is a state in which the individual is no longer in a state of equilibrium with the forces in his external and internal environment (see Figure 3-2). Francis [33] expresses this concept of disease in the following statement: "disease is a reaction to a stress which extends beyond the bounds of individual reserve and adaptability." Engel [34] defines disease as "failures or disturbances in the growth, development, functions, and adjustments of the organism as a whole or of any of its systems." Engel [35] also emphasizes the importance of defining disease as a natural phenomenon.

To clarify differences between a state of health and of disease, the essential features of each are summarized below.

ETIOLOGICAL AGENTS

In the preceding sections some of the factors influencing the capacity of the organism to respond to disturbances in its environment in ways that prevent disequilibrium have been considered. Disease has been defined and methods of prevention considered. However, success depends not only on the capacity of the individual to react appropriately but on the

[33] Francis, *loc. cit.*, p. 994.
[34] George L. Engel: "A Unified Concept of Health and Disease," *Perspect. Biol. Med.*, 3:459 (Summer) 1960.
[35] *Ibid.*, p. 469.

WHAT IS HEALTH?

1. In health, structure, function, and reserve are adequate.

2. Disturbances in the environment (internal and external) are within the capacity of the organism to respond or adapt to successfully. The organism is able to cope successfully with changes in its internal or external environment.

3. Responses to disturbances in environment are adequate and appropriate. They protect from injury.

4. As a result of a dynamic state of equilibrium, constancy of the internal environment is maintained within limits.

5. Adaptation is successful in preventing damage or in repairing it and in maintaining adequate functioning.

6. Survival, growth, reproduction, and productivity are facilitated.

WHAT IS DISEASE?

1. In disease, structure, function, or reserve are inadequate. (May be one or all.)

2. Disturbances in the environment (internal and external) are outside the capacity of the organism to respond or adapt to successfully. At the time of death, all adaptive powers are lost.

3. Responses to disturbances in the environment are inadequate, excessive, or inappropriate. They may be sources of injury.

4. It results in failure to maintain constancy within limits; that is, function is outside limits.

5. Disequilibrium in one area may lead to disturbances in function in other areas.

6. Adaptation is unsuccessful in some respects; that is, there is failure of adaptation at some level, including survival.

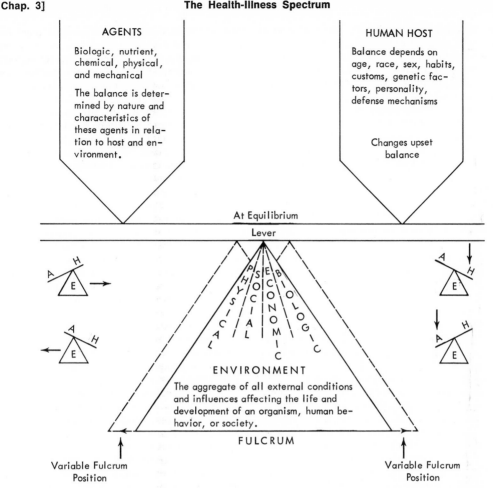

AGENTS

Biologic, nutrient, chemical, physical, and mechanical

The balance is determined by nature and characteristics of these agents in relation to host and environment.

HUMAN HOST

Balance depends on age, race, sex, habits, customs, genetic factors, personality, defense mechanisms

Changes upset balance

At Equilibrium

Lever

PSYCHOLOGICAL SOCIAL ECONOMIC BIOLOGIC

ENVIRONMENT

The aggregate of all external conditions and influences affecting the life and development of an organism, human behavior, or society.

FULCRUM

Variable Fulcrum Position

Variable Fulcrum Position

FIGURE 3-2. Simplified illustration of factors influencing health equilibrium. (Reproduced with permission of The Blakiston Division, McGraw-Hill Book Company, Inc., from *Preventive Medicine for the Doctor in His Community*, 3rd ed., 1965, p. 49, by Hugh R. Leavell and E. Gurney Clark.)

nature of the agent eliciting the response and on the interaction of both elements. Moreover, neither health nor disease results from a single factor. Rather both health and disease are the consequence of the interaction of many factors within the host and its environment—physical, biological, psychological, and social.

Engel [36] states that agents or conditions placing strain on the adaptive capacity of the individual are of four general types: (1) agents causing injury by their physical and chemical properties, (2) physical and chemical agents required for cellular processes that result in injury when they are supplied in insufficient quantities,[37] (3) living agents including microorganisms and parasites, and (4) psychological stress.

[36] *Op. cit.*, pp. 478–83.
[37] Some required substances can also cause injury when they are ingested in excessive quantities.

The disease-producing power of a pathogenic agent depends on the following: (1) its nature and characteristics, (2) its ability to maintain life and potency, (3) its ability to gain entrance and to establish itself in the host, (4) its source and reservoirs, and (5) vehicles and conditions for its dissemination. These factors are of importance in diseases caused by physical or chemical agents as well as those caused by living organisms. Knowledge of these factors contributes to the prevention, control, and treatment of disease, as well as to the identification of a disease-producing agent and its removal from the environment or the reduction of its effects. The application of the preceding to physical and chemical agents is made in Chapter 4 and to living agents in Chapter 5. In addition to the preceding, certain other factors influence whether or not pathogenic agents are able to cause injury. Highly virulent micro-organisms may overwhelm the host before he has an opportunity to mobilize his defenses. A chemical agent may be so concentrated that many cells are injured and death is inevitable. A physical injury may be so violent that all vital processes are immediately and completely depressed. For example, a head-on collision in an automobile may result in the sudden death of all its occupants. A single exposure of a susceptible individual to influenza is usually sufficient to cause disease.

NATURAL HISTORY OF DISEASE

Another way to view disease (or health) is to examine its natural history. The term *natural history* is defined as the course taken by disease from beginning to end—that is, (1) the factors in the initiation of the disease, (2) the possible course of the disease to cure or to death, and (3) how environmental and genetic factors modify the course.[38]

It can be seen in Figure 3-3 that the development of a disease takes place in two periods. During the first, the prepathogenic period, the host, agent, and environment interact to produce a stimulus. It is during the prepathogenic period that measures should be instituted to prevent a disease or delay its onset. During the second, the pathogenic period, disease develops. It is during this period that the clinical manifestations of the disease become evident. Depending on the balance among the host, agent, and environment, the individual may fully recover, may be partially or completely disabled, or may die.

METHODS OF STUDYING DISEASE

One way in which disease may be studied is to focus attention on the disease. When this is done it is described in terms of (1) the causative factors—such as direct, remote, necessary and sufficient, permissive, conditioning, inciting, predisposing, precipitating, and perpetuating; (2) the mechanisms whereby the disease-producing agent produces its effect—such as hereditary, biochemical, physiological, psychological, social; (3) the nature of its onset—sudden or gradual; (4) the characteristic signs and symptoms; (5) the predicted outcome or prognosis; (6) the preventive measures; and (7) the therapeutic measures. Although individuals who are sick are unique, diseases are not. They occur in classes or groups having common characteristics. Many persons may

have the same disease. The cause and manifestations of a disease as well as the methods by which it is effectively prevented and treated are similar in individuals who have the disease. For example, smallpox is caused by a specific virus. Although manifestations vary in degree of severity, they are similar in all individuals who contract smallpox. Smallpox is effectively prevented by one attack of the disease or by vaccination. Treatment of the person who has smallpox is nonspecific inasmuch as no curative measures are available to shorten or modify the severity of the illness.

Another approach to the study of disease is to use the methods of epidemiology. The term *epidemiology* may be defined very simply as medical detection. The same general methods are used in the identification of the person or persons responsible for a crime. A more comprehensive definition of *epidemiology* is stated by Frost:[39] "the science which considers the occurrence, distribution, and types of diseases of mankind, in distinct epochs of time, at varying points on the earth's surface, and secondly, will render an account of the relations of these diseases to inherent characteristics of the individual, and to the external conditions surrounding him and determining his manner of life."

The term *epidemiology* had its origin in and relates to its use in identifying the community factors in epidemic diseases. Paul[40] states that "epidemiology is concerned with measurements of the circumstances under which diseases occur, where diseases tend to flourish, and where they do not. . . . epidemiology deals with circumstances involving more than one person, a group of people upon whom something has been thrust. . . ." The group may be small or large.

As the science of epidemiology has developed, workers in the field have come to appreciate that the same techniques and questions are useful in the study of noninfectious diseases, such as mental illness and atherosclerosis. In the epidemiological approach to disease not only the sick but also the well are studied. Answers are sought to questions such as the following: Who is sick? Who is well? What are the characteristics of those who are sick? Of the well? What are the etiological agents? What are the characteristics of each causative agent? What are the factors in the environment bringing the susceptible host and the etiological agent or agents together? The answers to these questions serve as the basis for other questions.

[38] Huber J. Van Peenen: *Essentials of Pathology* (Chicago: Year Book Medical Publishers, Inc., 1966), p. 22.

[39] Kenneth F. Maxcy (ed.): *Papers of Wade Hampton Frost, M.D.* (New York: The Commonwealth Fund, 1941), p. 494.
[40] John R. Paul: *Clinical Epidemiology*, revised edition (Chicago: University of Chicago Press, 1966), p. 4.

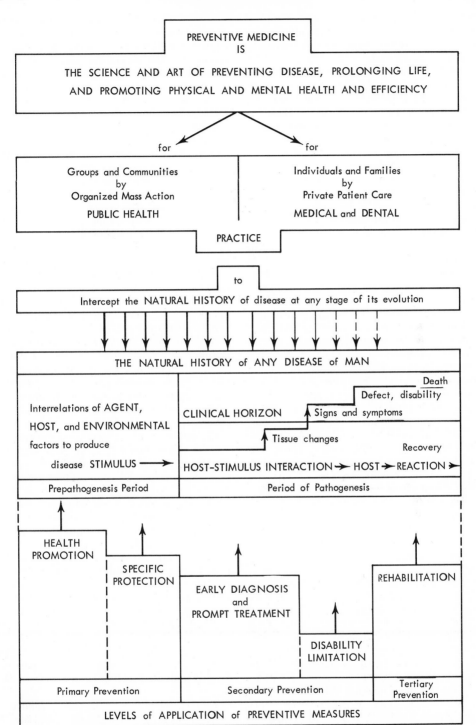

FIGURE 3-3. Diagram showing the application of preventive medicine. (Reproduced with permission of The Blakiston Division, McGraw-Hill Book Company, Inc., from *Preventive Medicine for the Doctor in His Community*, 3rd ed., 1965, p. 27, by Hugh R. Leavell and E. Gurney Clark.)

Which of the factors that have been identified as contributing to the development of the disease can be controlled? How can this control be most effectively applied?

A third approach to the study of disease is to focus attention not on the disease per se but on the person who is ill. In this approach some of the questions include the following: How has this disease come about? What effect does it have on the cells, tissues, and organs? Why did this particular person develop this particular illness at this time? What purpose, if any, does this illness serve the person? What purposes do the changes, physiological and psychological, serve in the adjustment of the individual to the causative factors in the illness?

To illustrate, a group of people become ill. Using the first approach, i.e., the study of the causative agent, the disease is described as having a sudden onset; the cause is *Staphylococcus aureus,* which releases an enterotoxin; the enterotoxin induces acute gastroenteritis; the signs and symptoms associated with the gastroenteritis include severe nausea, vomiting, diarrhea, and prostration. In most persons who are affected, the symptoms last only a few hours. Of the 100 persons who developed symptoms, 98 recovered promptly. The other 2 died. Using the second or epidemiological approach, the persons who became ill were of all age groups above the age of 2 years. About two hours previous to the onset of symptoms they had all eaten ham at a community supper. Those who ate roast beef did not become ill. No one else in the community suffered the same symptoms. Further investigation revealed that the day was very hot and that the ham was sliced and was not refrigerated after it was cooked. The woman who sliced the ham had an infected finger. Both of the persons who died were elderly men.

In the third approach to the study of disease, attention is centered on each sick individual. The responses of each person are subject to investigation and evaluation. For example, both Marie Skinny and her date John Robust ate ham. Marie was only mildly sick, while John was severely ill. Marie convalesced slowly, whereas John recovered promptly. Elderly Mr. Claro died, whereas equally elderly Mrs. Claro suffered only a few minor symptoms. Questions arising include the following: Why should John who was sicker than Marie recover more promptly than Marie? Why did Mr. Claro die and his wife recover? Some answers to these and other questions are easy to obtain. Others require extensive knowledge of the individual, his capacity for response, and what has happened to him throughout his lifetime. Because of insufficient knowledge, some questions cannot be answered at this time. The fact that John

was sicker than Marie may or may not be completely explained by the fact that she ate sparingly of the ham whereas John ate not only his serving but the remaining portion of Marie's. Certainly it does not explain why her recovery was prolonged. That Mr. Claro died may be explained in part by the fact that he had a diseased heart, but other factors may well have been of importance.

All these approaches to the study of disease and its effects are important. Knowledge of the causes and manifestations of a particular disease is necessary to the recognition of illness caused by it and to the introduction of measures to limit its effects. The epidemiological approach aims at the identification of those elements within or without the individual that are subject to control and the institution of measures to protect the population from harmful agents. As a result of study of incidents such as the community supper cited here, laws governing the handling of food have been enacted. Educational programs have been instituted to inform people of the procedures that are necessary for their protection. The fact that food poisoning continues to occur when conditions combine not only to introduce the *Staphylococcus aureus* but to favor its multiplication introduces the human factor. This brings the discussion to a summary of the third factor in the study of disease, that is, the individual. In the United States information is widely disseminated about the conditions favoring food poisoning. Why, then, should food be handled in such a manner that food poisoning occurs? The answers here are to be found in individual human beings. Each human being is an important factor in when, how, and why he becomes ill.

The incident of the community supper also serves to emphasize another concept that has been receiving increased emphasis in the literature. That is, any situation, including illness and recovery from illness, depends on the interaction of multiple factors. When the factors placing strain on the individual are within his adaptive capacity, he remains well. When they exceed his adaptive capacity, illness results. The nature of his illness, the degree of his illness, and the speed with which he recovers can also involve multiple factors.

To this point health has been defined and some of the ways it can be measured and promoted have been considered. Disease has also been defined, and general ways of studying it have been presented.

How can diseases be prevented?

To appreciate the tremendous contributions of preventive medicine, it is essential to be aware of some of the conditions in the world before the middle of the nineteenth century and some of the changes that have taken place in the Western world since that time. It is essential to understand that the conditions basic to health do not prevail throughout the world. In the larger part of the world the major health problems continue to be malnutrition, lack of sanitation, and inadequate medical care. In contrast, in the countries of the world where the supply of food is abundant, the sanitary facilities are adequate to the needs of the population, and a high standard of medical care is available, the problems are those with which Americans are familiar. These will be reviewed later in another context. Lest anyone conclude that the dangers to health in the external environment of man have been brought under final control, they should read *Time Magazine*, "Environment Versus Man" (September 26, 1960, pp. 66–68). In this article the questions "What is in the air? What is in the water? What is in the food?" are raised. Almost the entire January 1964 issue of the *American Journal of Public Health*, including a supplement, is devoted to "Man— His Environment and Health." Review of current periodicals reveals increasing concern for man's environment and health. James [41] reflects the views of many authorities in the following:

To an increasing degree, man is becoming the major cause of his own illness and death. Following our unbelievable progress against the epidemic diseases of the past, we see the emergence of a host of major chronic diseases as the key health problems of our day. At present, unable to attack these illnesses by the familiar methods of isolating an organism or producing a vaccine, we are faced with the need to understand their relationship to certain environmental factors that appear to increase greatly their danger to us as individuals.

STAGES IN THE PREVENTION OF DISEASE

Review of the history of the development of knowledge of the prevention of disease reveals that progress was made in three stages. In the first stage the environment was rendered safe and the individual was protected from harmful influences in the environment. In this period applications of knowledge of bacteriology and immunology were made. Sanitation of food and water supplies and immunization against smallpox, diphtheria, and other diseases were important contributions of the first stage to the health of the public.

In the second stage some diseases were

brought under control by the introduction of new drugs and vaccines. Drugs have made a significant contribution to the control of such diseases as tuberculosis, syphilis, and pneumonia. Hope that diseases such as tuberculosis and syphilis would be eradicated by the so-called wonder drugs has been replaced by the sobering knowledge that even today good control of any infectious disease depends on the constant application of all the available knowledge. Drugs have not proved to be the complete answer to the control of disease. Moreover, the value of an agent in the control or cure of an infectious disease is sometimes difficult to evaluate. To illustrate, the death rate from diphtheria, pneumonia, and tuberculosis had all dropped before modern methods of prevention and treatment were known. As infectious diseases have come under control, noninfectious diseases have increased in incidence. Whereas infectious diseases ranked first as the cause of death in 1900, heart disease has now taken that place.

The challenge of the third and present era of prevention is, therefore, the prevention of noninfectious diseases. These are the diseases that have their highest incidence in maturity and the later years of life. Whereas some diseases, such as cholera, typhoid, and malaria, have been controlled largely through changes in the environment, some infectious as well as noninfectious diseases require changes in the behavior of individuals as well. As examples, immunization against diphtheria, measles, poliomyelitis, and smallpox requires the cooperation of individuals. This cooperation results from sustained educational programs directed toward changing the behavior of individuals. The prevention of diseases such as lung cancer and coronary artery disease depends on changing both the environment and the attitudes and habits of individuals.[42]

PRIMARY PREVENTION

Francis [43] classifies the areas of true prevention as follows: (1) protection from exposure to harmful physical and chemical agents, (2) correction of dietary deficiencies and excesses, and (3) prevention of infectious diseases by specific measures and sanitary social procedures. To this list should be added (4) development in the individual of habits and attitudes that lessen his chances of developing certain diseases.

Francis [44] states that the first area applies primarily to occupational health. Certainly

[41] George James: "Emerging Trends in Public Health and Possible Reactions," *Public Health Rep.*, 80:580 (July) 1965.

[42] Milton Terris: "A Social Policy for Health," *Amer. J. Public Health*, 58:5 (Jan.) 1968.
[43] *Op. cit.*, p. 994.
[44] *Ibid.*

much has been done to create and enforce standards contributing to health and safety in factories and in other places of employment. Machinery is constructed with the safety of the worker in mind, and he is provided with clothing that is designed to protect him from the hazards of his particular job. In addition, educational programs are conducted to teach employees how to work safely and what to do in the event a fellow worker is injured. Campaigns are conducted to increase their interest and pride in their safety record. Workmen's compensation laws and various types of insurance protect the health of employees by establishing and enforcing safety standards. Insurance also provides a means of support for employees and their families in the event of injury incurred while they are at work. Equally important to those who are permanently disabled is provision for their continued support.

Medical and nursing departments have been developed to promote the health of workers and to prevent injury and disease. Much of the educational work is done by these departments.

Another form of exposure to a harmful agent is smoking, not only of cigarettes but of tobacco in any form. There is substantial evidence to support the thesis that smoking is an etiological agent in many diseases. The present state of knowledge of these health consequences can, in the judgment of the Public Health Service, be summarized as follows: [45]

1. Cigarette smokers have substantially higher rates of death and disability than their nonsmoking counterparts in the population. This means that cigarette smokers tend to die at earlier ages and experience more days of disability than comparable nonsmokers.
2. A substantial portion of earlier deaths and excess disability would not have occurred if those affected had never smoked.
3. If it were not for cigarette smoking, practically none of the earlier deaths from lung cancer would have occurred; nor a substantial portion of the earlier deaths from chronic bronchopulmonary diseases (commonly diagnosed as chronic bronchitis or pulmonary emphysema or both); nor a portion of the earlier deaths of cardiovascular origin. Excess disability from chronic pulmonary and cardiovascular diseases would also be less.
4. Cessation or appreciable reduction of cigarette smoking could delay or avert a substantial portion of deaths which occur from lung cancer, a substantial portion of the earlier deaths and excess disability from chronic bronchopulmonary diseases, and a portion of the earlier deaths and excess disability of cardiovascular origin.

The elimination of smoking involves not only the changing of the attitudes and behavior of smokers but also the economics of tobacco growers, manufacturers, advertisers, and others. Even when a health hazard has been identified, its solution does not necessarily follow immediately. One of the problems of present-day preventive medicine is to help man realize that he is more and more responsible for his own health problems. With this knowledge useful methods of attack can be developed.

Attention has been extended to evaluating dangers to the general public growing out of the pollution of the air by gaseous wastes. Impetus has been given to the study of this problem by the London and Donora air disasters. According to Breslow and Goldsmith,[46] public health authorities have been slow to recognize the potential dangers of air pollution. Because of public pressure they are, however, being forced to give their attention to it. According to Thomas,[47] urban air pollution stems from two different sources. One, the London type, is primarily coal smoke, which contains appreciable amounts of sulfur dioxide combined with a more or less dense fog. The other, the Los Angeles type, is primarily automobile exhaust gases. It contains none of the components of the London smog. The irritating and damaging compounds result from the action of sunshine on the substances contained in exhaust gas. Many cities have to cope to some degree with both types of air pollution. The prevention of air pollution is currently under study. According to Thomas,[48] prospects are good for understanding and eventually controlling it.

A different but no less dangerous source of air pollution originates with explosions of atom and hydrogen bombs and from the use of radioactive materials in hospitals and in industry. The effects of ionizing radiation and some of the factors in its control will be discussed in Chapter 4. One cannot, however, ignore the possible long-term effects of repeated exposure of large segments of the population to ionizing radiation. The pollution of the air, whether by coal smoke, automobile exhaust gases, or radioactive materials, illustrates how the external environment created by man threatens his health.

An example cited by James [49] is fluoridation of water. Public health officials know that there

[45] U.S. Department of Health, Education, and Welfare: *The Health Consequences of Smoking* (Washington, D.C.: U.S. Government Printing Office, 1968), pp. 3–4.

[46] Lester Breslow and John Goldsmith: "Health Effects of Air Pollution," *Amer. Public Health,* 48:913 (July) 1958.

[47] Moyer D. Thomas: "New Understandings from Current Atmospheric Pollution Research," *Amer. J. of Public Health,* 49:1664–65 (Dec.) 1959.

[48] *Ibid.,* p. 1668.

[49] *Op. cit.,* p. 583.

are more effective ways of preventing dental caries. The reason for supporting fluoridation is that none of the other methods works in the population as a whole. Fluoridation is the only practical method acceptable to the population that prevents dental caries to a major degree. Thus preventive measures must be both acceptable and effective.

The second aspect of primary or true prevention, the correction of dietary deficiency or excess, will be considered in Chapter 12.

The third aspect of true prevention is the prevention of infectious disease by specific measures and by sanitary social procedures. Prevention of these diseases will be discussed in Chapter 5.

Many city, state, and even federal laws have been enacted for the purpose of protecting the general public from agents causing injury and disease. Examples include laws or regulations to control traffic, housing and building construction, water supplies, food handling, the preparation and serving of food in restaurants, and sewage disposal. Pure food and drug laws protect the quality of food and drugs.[50] Other laws were discussed in Chapter 2.

Primary prevention depends on understanding and controlling the factors contributing to the development of disease. It also depends on the availability of procedures to remove noxious agents from the environment, to prevent their entry into the organism, or to neutralize their effects after they enter. Whether or not the appropriate techniques are available depends on both the status of knowledge and the resources available to procure the necessary supplies, equipment, and persons possessing the skills required to utilize current knowledge and techniques. For example, one of the deciding factors in whether a community can have sanitary water supply and a safe method of disposing of its wastes is whether or not it has or is willing to spend the money to build and to equip suitable facilities. Moreover, money is required to provide the necessary staff to operate the facilities after they are built, and persons with a variety of knowledges and skills are required to operate and maintain them so that they accomplish their purpose. Furthermore, the population must accept the need for these facilities and know how to use them. Use of a particular preventive measure depends in part on the knowledge of the group or individual that the measure is available and effective. The group must also accept a particular procedure as being necessary and desirable. Whether a facility or change in behavior will be adopted by a group

of people depends on the degree to which its performance takes into account local customs, habits, and beliefs. For example, Towle [51] reported a study of the administration of vaccines by injection to a group of people living in India. He states that in the early part of the study most of the candidates for immunization were men. After making this observation, the investigators placed a screen in such a position that the women could be hidden from the view of men. Following this adjustment the number of women seeking immunization did not differ materially from the number of men.

SECONDARY PREVENTION

In those persons who develop long-term or chronic illnesses, emphasis is on the prevention of disability and the delay of the progress of disease already established. Although disability may follow any illness, it is associated more frequently with long-term illness. There is objection to the term *chronic illness* because it suggests hopelessness rather than emphasizing the possibility of improving the situation of the individual. Chronic illness differs from acute illness in the intensity and length of course. Although the chronically ill person may have periods in which he is acutely ill (severe degree of illness and short, or limited, course), the degree of illness tends to be less marked and the course more prolonged than in an acute illness. Acute illness can terminate in full recovery or death or develop into a chronic illness. In our present state of knowledge, prevention of disability because of the progress of chronic disease is frequently the most that can be accomplished. However, in many patients, limiting the damaging effects of a chronic disease and instituting a program that enables the person to utilize his strengths may make the difference between an active and useful life and one of complete invalidism.

What is the nurse's role in prevention?

The nurse has a significant role in the promotion of health and the prevention of disease. Nurses in clinics and physicians' offices are often the first to see the patient. The patient may report symptoms or matters of concern to the nurse, because they hesitate to trouble a physician or because they feel safer telling the nurse. When the nurse's orientation is toward the person as a person she may be able to help him identify practices that predispose to chronic illness. Depending on a host of factors, the patient, nurse, and physician working together may be able to develop a workable plan for changing the patient's behavior.

---

[50] See Louis S. Goodman and Alfred Gilman: *The Pharmacological Basis of Therapeutics,* 3rd ed. (New York: The Macmillan Company, 1965), pp. 31–32.

[51] Richard L. Towle: "New Horizon in Mass Inoculation," *Public Health Rep.,* **75**:471–76 (June) 1960.

Nurses who work with children or adults, whatever the setting or their state of health, have an educational function. As examples, they can determine whether or not patients have been immunized and encourage them to follow appropriate immunization schedules. They should participate in instruction of the patient and his family about how to prevent disease. They should lend their support to as well as contribute to community health programs.

Although there is believed to be enough knowledge, were it applied, to delay or prevent the development of some of the common chronic diseases, many persons either do not have the necessary information or they do not use it. As a consequence, cancer of the lung and cervix as well as other preventable diseases develop. Further, though early cancer of the cervix is curable, it all too often is discovered after extensive disease is present. Like other members of the health professions, the nurse is a case finder, for with early diagnosis cure may be possible. Even when it is not, much can be done to prevent the progression of chronic disease and to limit the amount of disability.

The prevention of disability in the person who has a potentially disabling illness or injury involves knowledge of the factors in the development of the disability and what can be done to prevent or minimize it. Prevention of disability also depends on the ability to identify and help the person utilize his psychological, intellectual, physical, economic, and spiritual resources. It requires a knowledge of the facilities available in the community to assist him and knowledge of how to use them. With the imaginative and intelligent use of even limited resources, much can often be done to prevent unnecessary disability and to restore the disabled person to greater usefulness.

Care of the Sick: The Third Objective

The third objective of the health professions is to care for the sick. Sooner or later in the life of every individual sickness becomes a reality. Depending on the nature of the causative agent or agents and the capacity of the individual to respond, he may be mildly or seriously ill. He may recover promptly or experience a lingering illness. He may die suddenly or slowly. He may recover spontaneously without, or even in spite of, treatment or he may die despite excellent and intensive therapy.

In the American culture there is a tendency to equate recovery from illness with success and chronicity or death with failure. This attitude toward illness undoubtedly contributes to emphasis on the leading causes of death as major health problems and to less stress on the causes and effects of sickness. Little attention is paid by many individuals to health per se, as it is more or less taken for granted. As indicated earlier, the health professions are preoccupied with disease and death rather than with health and fulfillment.

What are the aims, objectives, and problems?

Therapy in illness is directed toward three objectives: (1) to cure the sick person, (2) to modify the course of the disease so that its progress is slowed and disability is limited, and (3) to modify the effects of disease so that the person is maintained in as active and comfortable a state as is possible for as long as he lives. This includes assisting him to a peaceful death.

CURE—AN OBJECTIVE OF CARE

The accomplishment of the first objective depends on two factors—the availability of a method of treatment and the capacity of the sick person to respond appropriately. The tendency toward recovery may be so great that the patient gets well with no treatment or despite meddlesome or harmful treatment. One aspect of an appropriate response to treatment is the desire of the patient to recover. A seriously ill or frail patient may be saved by specific and energetic therapy combined with the strong desire to recover.

APPROACHES TO THERAPY

One approach to the cure of disease is to attempt to eradicate the disease-producing agent. Elimination of the etiological agent may be accomplished by administering a chemical or physical agent capable of reaching and destroying it or the diseased tissue without affecting healthy tissue. Examples include the use of antibiotic and chemotherapeutic agents to eradicate microorganisms and the use of x-ray or the radioactive isotopes in the treatment of malignant neoplasms. Surgery is effective in eradicating disease by correcting structural defects or by removing diseased tissues.

Cure may also be effected by supplying a substance normally produced in the body in response to disease. An example of specific antiserum is diphtheria antitoxin, which is successful in the treatment of diphtheria. In patients who respond to substances that are not usually harmful, relief may be effected by limiting the contact of the patient with the harmful agent or by counteracting his abnormal response. The person with hay fever can prevent or lessen the severity of an attack by eliminating from his environment substances to which he has a sensitivity. He may also lessen the severity of his reaction by taking an antihistamine or epinephrine.

When a disease is the result of the lack of a substance required in the body economy, cure may be effected by increasing the supply of the substance that is deficient. For example, scurvy is cured by adding ascorbic acid to the diet. Sometimes the physiological disturbance occurring as a result of disease is so severe that the body is unable to restore balance or overcome the disease without aid. In these instances, needed materials are supplied to support body responses or defenses. For example, the temperature of the body may rise to a level that, if continued, will produce cellular damage. Cold sponges or antipyretic drugs may be administered to reduce the temperature until such time as effective body controls are re-established.

MODIFYING THE COURSE OF THE DISEASE TO LIMIT DISABILITY

That complete cure of disease is not always possible is well known. In some conditions, such as acute poliomyelitis, recovery from the acute infection may be complete, but there may be some degree of residual disability. In others, such as cerebrovascular accident, the patient may recover with or without disability, but the primary disease, atherosclerosis, remains. In these patients complete restoration to the pre-illness state may be impossible but the effects of the disease may be modified so that disability is minimized. The limitation of disability is one of the exciting challenges of today. Its achievement depends on the evaluation and use of the patient's strengths and assets, psychological as well as physical, and a program of education and work whereby the patient learns to use all his resources constructively. Accomplishment requires that both the nurse and the patient be aware of, accept, and work toward realistic or reasonable goals.

The prevention of unnecessary disability depends on the intelligent nursing of the patient during the acute phase of his illness. Months of therapy may be required to correct the effects not of disease or injury but of inadequate care. During the period of rehabilitation of the patient, nursing contributes to the progress of the patient in many ways. The patient is helped by an attitude of realistic optimism. He can be encouraged to try, even when his efforts are faltering. The nurse may find it difficult to decide when the patient should try to act for himself and when she should do things for, or help, the patient. In her sympathy for the patient she may forget that struggle is essential to growth or she may become impatient when the

patient is discouraged or depressed. The chicken that escapes from the egg shell does so because it struggles. The chicken that does not struggle dies. The patient is helped in his struggle when the nurse gives recognition to the fact that he is trying and that he is having difficulty. Recognizing his successes and helping him to accept his failures also contribute to his emotional support. For some patients a source of irritation may act as a stimulus. For example, elderly Mrs. Elm was irascible and depressed following a stroke, or cerebrovascular accident. Her nurse noted that she was a perfectionist who was greatly irritated by a crooked window shade or picture. Each day the nurse, unobtrusively but purposefully, pulled a window shade out of line. This seemingly minor event strengthened Mrs. Elm's feeling that nothing would be done correctly if she was not there, and she began to make an effort to recover. The nurse was successful in helping Mrs. Elm because she was able to motivate her toward recovery. She concentrated on identifying what Mrs. Elm needed and not on her failure to conform to her own expectations of how a patient should respond. Some judgment is required on the part of the nurse to assess the ability of the patient to perform so that he is not pushed beyond his capacity. Both thought and experience are required to learn when to wait and when and how to encourage the patient to continue his efforts. Physical and emotional readiness are both important factors in rehabilitation.

The family of the patient is also important to his rehabilitation. They can be a help or a hindrance depending on their relationship with the patient and on their understanding and acceptance of the program planned for the patient. The nurse can help them to accept what can be and is being done for the patient. They, too, need support to watch a patient struggle. They are more likely to be cooperative when they understand the plan of care and the what, how, and why of their contribution.

As a result of increased interest in rehabilitation, patients who have disorders associated with serious degrees of limitation of function are living more active lives than ever before in history. Some of them are self-supporting, drive cars, go to ball games and dances, take vacation trips, marry, rear families, and carry on lives that are as active as those of persons not physically handicapped.

DEATH A REALITY

For all persons the time comes when recovery and rehabilitation are no longer possible, for one of the realities of life is death. To some it comes quickly. To others it comes slowly in the form of a lingering illness. Some have a short life span, others a long one. In the American culture, extreme measures to prevent or to delay death for as long as possible are not at all unusual. Talk of death is avoided and elaborate efforts may be made to protect the sick from knowledge that death is a possibility. That these efforts sometimes, if not frequently, fail is indicated by the following letter written by Mrs. Carol Willis, who was dying from cancer.[52]

Boston, New York

Dear Editors: The epidemic of articles by cancer victims in the last few years leads even the most unscientifically minded observer to conclude there must be some correlation between people dying of cancer and the urge to appear in print.

Without exception the cancer patient is portrayed as a martyr, deeply suffering, but led at last through his troubles to realize the big things in life. All his trivialities are swept away, he appreciates the wonders of nature as never before, a change has come over his character so he is now a reformed person, he has turned again to God, and he keeps his temper.

I think it is time we let down our hair and told the truth. We have the urge to rush into print all right, but we who are dying of cancer are not martyrs or saints or holy folk. Frankly, if the truth were told, we embarrass our friends, and we often bore them.

Our first emotion is that of anger. We go through a "few nights of apprehension and hot weeping," but once over those we are surprised, shocked and angry. That this fate should be meted out to us— Us, of all people—seems hardly fair. We look around at our friends and neighbors and wonder why we have been singled out for this lingering, painful death. "Why me, O Lord, why me?" We forget that for every one of us who suffers others go free; we should be glad they are spared, not angry at our own destiny, deserved or undeserved. After all, why *not* us O Lord? We are no martyrs —heavens, no.

Cancer is not a pleasant way to die. It is too endlessly prolonged, too excruciatingly painful. Yet through that last, the pain, we learn we can take more than we even thought possible. We may rail, in spite of ourselves, when pain mounts; but if it subsides enough to be bearable we feel happy and relieved, like the woman whose girdle felt so comfortable when she took it off. I am not recommending extreme pain as a method of increasing pleasure or making us grateful for small comforts, but it does make us more able to bear the later heights of pain we will have to go through.

We embarrass our friends, for Emily Post has provided no rules for conversation with the dying. We know our friends guard their tongues, and they force us to watch our words even more. Mentioning that we won't be here next year, or even perhaps next month, is not in good taste. We have to

talk about "when the children are grown" or "when this house gets too big for just the two of us," because the sensibility of our friends to death will not allow them to face what we face each minute: the fact of our dying.

We are quite likely to bore our friends with our preoccupation with illness. We are so wrapped up in ourselves we talk too much. For that reason, I never bring up my illness; but if I am seriously asked about it I am only too glad to talk. It is a great relief to unburden oneself occasionally, to have the fact that one is bearing pain appreciated. One of the kindest acts a friend can do for a dying man is to listen to him.

What do we answer to the casual, "How are you?" For a person who is dying to reply automatically "Fine" is ridiculous. I solved it by saying cheerfully, with a rising inflection, "Pretty good." Now that there is no longer any truthful affirmative answer I reply, as lightheartedly as I know how, "Coming along," and that takes care of that. We have to be particularly careful not to be a specter at the feast, lest we spoil others' pleasure.

I don't suppose I should admit this, but we are not saints. The canker of our death which always eats at us makes us impatient, intolerant of other people's troubles. In great pain, it is hard for us to show sympathy with a bad cold, a hurt finger or a headache. Surprisingly enough, we usually come through well here, but don't be disgusted with us if we can't produce too much emotion over your problem. Yours will go, ours won't.

I'm afraid that I have to admit that I'm often testy, irritated over my children's complaints over trivialities, even sometimes upset by my husband's kindnesses when they are ill-timed. He is, naturally enough, concerned over my dying wife; it is far harder on him than on me. He has to go on living; all I have to do is to die, and die as well as I can.

Yet I, too, have cared for me for a long time, and I find it extremely hard to face the end of my personality, the complete extinguishing of everything I planned. Thus we are both inwardly upset, and sometimes show it outwardly. So is it any wonder that life, instead of being the beautiful idyl painted by cancerous writers, sometimes stoops to the petty details of existence?

I've gone through it all; the early times of Hope, the Facing the Truth, the Grin-and-Bear-It stage, then Just Bearing It, and now the End-Is-Just-Around-the-Corner or Final Stage. I'm still angry about it all, for I think no one has ever loved living more or had more fun doing it than I, and I want it to go on. But if it can't, then I must be truthful and say there are a few advantages in living only half a lifetime. Besides the end of good, death also means an end to tribulations—no more holding in the stomach, no more P.T.A., no more putting up the hair in pincurls, no more Cub Scouts, no more growing old.

Sincerely,
Carol Willis

---

[52] Carol Willis: "Let's Tell the Truth About Dying," *Ladies' Home Journal*, 77:4 (Jan.) 1960. Reprinted by special permission of the *Ladies' Home Journal*, copyright 1959. Curtis Publishing Company.

Mrs. Willis died two weeks after writing this letter. Her husband found it among her effects after her death.

Fielding,[53] in an essay on the uses of fear, expresses Mrs. Willis' feelings very beautifully.

When death comes slowly, fear may come fast: it can spread a conspiracy in a home: bright-eyed, stiff-smiling, and truly fearful. A silence is engendered which isolates the dying person far more surely than his malady. Two languages begin to be spoken: one in the sickroom and the other in the remainder of the house; the bedroom door may become an iron lattice filtering off the light and truth of the household from him who is in most need of them. But if the fear is described and accepted, the conspiracy shrinks to its proper dimensions; it is confined to the bed, to one man and the not-terrible whisperings of his demise. As Jacques de la Rivière said:
"Peace lies only in the irremediable."

Although Mrs. Willis' letter is a personal statement of her own needs and feelings, other dying persons can be assumed to experience similar feelings. Fielding's remarks about death also support this view. Because persons who visited Mrs. Willis were concerned with their own feelings, they were unable to perceive her need for someone to listen to her. Failure to accept death as a part of life or as a natural event cut off meaningful communication between Mrs. Willis and her visitors. By denying death, they placed on Mrs. Willis the burden of modifying her behavior, so that she did not make them uncomfortable.

NURSING IMPLICATIONS

Conception, birth, health, disease, and death are all aspects of life. Of all, death engenders the greatest fear in most people. Even for persons who have great faith in an afterlife, death as the great unknown is often feared. It is feared not only by the person who is dying but by the living. All cultures from the most primitive to the most complex have rituals that center around the dying and the dead. In the care of the dying, the needs, feelings, attitudes, and beliefs of the living as well as those of the dying should be considered. From both the moral and legal point of view nothing may be done for the purpose of hastening the death of a person. There is, however, no requirement that extraordinary measures be utilized in prolonging the life of a patient when only pain and suffering lie ahead. Rynearson [54] states that the indispensable care of the dying patient includes food, fluids, good nursing care, appropriate measures to relieve physical and mental suffering, and opportunity to prepare for death.

Rynearson also summarizes criteria that should be met in the care of the dying. They are:

1. He should die with dignity, respect and humanity.
2. He should die with minimal pain.
3. He should have the opportunity to recall the love and benefits of a lifetime of sharing; he and his family and friends should visit together, if the patient so wishes.
4. He should be able to clarify relationships—to express wishes—to share sentiments.
5. The patient and relatives should plan intelligently for the changes which death imposes upon the living.
6. The patient should die in familiar surroundings, if possible; if not, then quietus should take place in surroundings made as nearly homelike as possible.
7. Finally, but importantly, there should be concern for the feelings of the living.[55]

The care of the terminally ill patient is shared by the patient's family, physician, nurses, social workers, and clergyman—minister, priest, or rabbi. When available, specialists in psychology, sociology, and anthropology can be helpful to those caring for the dying. Healthy people often hesitate about having a clergyman visit a seriously ill person for the first time. They fear that the patient will be frightened and give up hope of living. Some hospitals solve this problem by employing or arranging to have a clergyman visit all newly admitted patients, unless the patient specifically asks not to be visited by a chaplain. Visits are then continued as a regular service to the patient. Catholic patients usually expect to be visited regularly. Though non-Catholics find it hard to believe, most Catholics are comforted by having the sacrament of the sick.

Much of the care that the patient receives is given by nurses. Some of the things that a nurse can do to ease the suffering of the patient who is dying are listed by Sister Mary Hubert in "Spiritual Care for Every Patient." [56] Although Sister Mary Hubert is writing about the spiritual care of every patient, her suggestions are most pertinent to the dying—whether death is imminent or a long time coming. Her first suggestion is kindness, thoughtfulness, gentleness, and a "personalized warm concern." Second, she suggests "frequent contacts"; staying away from the patient is easier when one is afraid or the patient is irritable and demanding, but only through contact with the patient can the nurse express her real concern for him or be kind or thoughtful. Third, the nurse should understand

[53] Gabriel Fielding: "The Uses of Fear," *Harper's Magazine,* 224:94 (Feb.) 1962.
[54] Edward H. Rynearson: "You Are Standing at the Bedside of a Patient Dying of Untreatable Cancer," *CA,* 9:87 (May–June) 1959.

[55] *Ibid.,* pp. 85–97.
[56] Sister Mary Hubert: "Spiritual Care for Every Patient," *J. Nurs. Educ.,* 2:9–11, 29–31 (May–June), 1963.

her own attitude toward "the truths of human existence; life, suffering, old-age, and death." According to Sister Mary Hubert, suffering is one of the most frequently encountered facts of life and is the least understood. Her fourth suggestion, the encouragement of wholesome reading, may or may not be applicable. Certainly, encouragement of the patient to continue his interests and activities as long as he is able is to be recommended. Finally, by prayer—the nurse may pray with the patient, help the patient to pray, offer to say a prayer for the patient—the nurse may be able to convey to the patient her concern for him and his welfare.

PHYSIOLOGICAL AND HYGIENIC NEEDS OF THE DYING PATIENT

The hygienic and physiological needs of the dying are also of great importance and they should not be neglected. In debilitated patients, improvement of nutrition may by itself bring about a marked change in the outlook of the patient and in his ability to be active. The same is true when anemia is corrected. Exercise is usually encouraged. It prevents the loss of strength that accompanies inactivity and improves the appetite as well as the morale of the patient. Florence Nightingale in *Notes on Nursing* [57] expresses the wish that as much attention were paid to the effect of the body on the mind as the reverse. Later she stated that one of the common causes of death in chronic illness is starvation. [58] This is no less true today than it was in Miss Nightingale's day.

Attention should be given to the maintenance of other functions such as fluid intake, respiration, and elimination. As the patient fails, more and more of the daily activities of living, such as bathing and mouth care and protection of his skin against breakdown, will have to be assumed by others. Attention to details that give the patient comfort benefits not only the patient but the members of his family.

An aspect of dying that has received little attention in nursing literature and is implied in Mrs. Willis' letter is that death does not always occur quickly. The final day or days of dying may follow weeks or months of gradually declining health. During this period the patient not infrequently requires more and more physical care and emotional support. Because little or nothing can be done to effect cure, what could be done to relieve the anxiety of the patient and his family and provide physical comfort for the patient is neglected. The problem is intensified when doctors and nurses feel helpless or are angry with the patient for dying or with his demanding behavior.

AMERICAN CULTURE AND THE DYING PATIENT

In the American culture, the care of patients with fatal diseases or who are dying is made more difficult by the emphasis on cure as the primary objective of the health professions. In defining their role, patient, nurse, and physician all emphasize cure as an important criterion of success. When a patient recovers, nurses as well as doctors take credit for the patient's success. Moreover, patients, nurses, and doctors frequently expect not only that patients should get well but that they should recover quickly and pleasantly. When they do not recover or they die, the nurse and/or doctor feels that he must have failed in some respect.

In addition to being an agent in the cure of the sick person, nurses also expect to comfort the sick and to relieve their suffering. When they are unable to do this, they may feel that as nurses they are inadequate and feelings of anxiety are aroused. With anxiety the defenses of the person against anxiety are invoked. The psychological defenses of people sick or well are alike. Nurse and patient may both be using similar or different defenses against feelings of fear. Because the burden for adapting behavior is on the nurse, she must have some insight into her own feelings about death and dying. When she has come to terms with her own feelings, she should be better able to concentrate on what the patient is feeling, even when he projects his negative feelings to her. She can allow the patient to talk about his feelings, be they of anger, remorse, guilt, or regrets. If, as Fielding says, the fear can be described and accepted, it can then be kept within bounds. Glaser and Strauss [59] state further that "Americans are characteristically unwilling to talk openly about the process of dying itself; and they are prone to avoid telling a dying person that he is dying. This is, in part, a moral attitude: life is preferable to whatever may follow it, and one should not look forward to death unless he is in great pain."

When the patient has reached that stage in his illness during which the goal in his care is to provide comfort, the nurse may wish to comfort him. At the same time she may be angry with him. She then feels guilty because nurses are taught to have kindly feelings toward the patient or because she is healthy and will continue to live. Her problems in caring for the patient are further compounded when the patient does not know or is not supposed to know

---

[57] Florence Nightingale: *Notes on Nursing: What It Is, and What It Is Not,* new edition, revised and enlarged (London: Harrison and Sons, 1860), p. 85.
[58] *Ibid.,* p. 92.

[59] Barney G. Glaser and Anselm Strauss: *Awareness of Dying* (Chicago: Aldine Publishing Company, 1965), p. 3.

that he is dying. She must be continuously on guard lest she reveal the true state of the patient to him.

The nurse is thus forced to use a variety of strategies against her unacceptable feelings. The nurse's own feelings of helplessness and despair may cause her to deny her feelings and to withdraw from the situation and refuse to care for the patient or she may try to relieve her own feelings by being excessively solicitous. She may treat him in an impersonal or cold manner (the cool, starched look). When the nurse is excessively disturbed by the predicament of the patient and feels too strongly, she may frighten the patient and be unable to be sufficiently objective [60] to support him emotionally.

As the condition of the patient deteriorates, he can be expected to become more and more dependent on those who are responsible for his care. How the nurse (or others) reacts depends on her ability to tolerate dependency in others. Chodoff [61] states that healthy persons often have ambivalent feelings with elements of hostility when they have contact with the helpless and disabled. In the patient who is in the terminal phase of a long-term illness such as cancer, there is no need for concern about the effects of long-term dependency on the nurse-patient relationship. The nurse must exercise judgment and sensitivity to the needs and feelings of the patient, so that he has done for him what comforts him and he is allowed and encouraged to do the things that he can and wishes to do.

Other problems to the nurse in the care of patients who die or are dying include the possibility that the nurse fears that the patient would not have died if she had acted quickly enough or in a different manner. When a patient dies unexpectedly or dies when the nurse is giving or assisting with his care, the nurse may feel that she was in some manner responsible. When a nurse is disturbed by any of these questions, she will do well to discuss the problem with someone who can help her explore the various facets of the problem.

Although there is a tendency on the part of the healthy to avoid even thinking about death, it is not always unwelcome to the person who is dying. Poets have put into words what experienced doctors and nurses know, that is, death is not always unwelcome or feared.

Walter Savage Landor's poem "On Death"

Death stands above me, whispering low

[60] The term *objectivity* is herein defined as the ability of the nurse to evaluate and meet the patient's needs in such a way that he is helped.

[61] Paul Chodoff: "A Psychiatric Approach to the Dying Patient," *CA*, **10**:30 (Jan.–Feb.) 1960.

I know not what into my ear;
Of His strange language all I know
Is, there is not a word of fear.

Alexander Pope in the first stanza of "The Dying Christian to His Soul" expresses a variety of feelings.

Vital Spark of heavenly flame!
Quit, O quit this mortal frame!
Trembling, hoping, lingering, flying,
O the pain, the bliss of dying.
Cease fond Nature, cease thy strife,
And let me languish into life!

John Donne, 1573–1631, in one of his sonnets says,

Death be not proud, though some have called thee
Mighty and dreadfull, for, thou art not so;
For, those whom thou think'st thou dost overthrow,
Die not, poor death, nor yet canst thou kill me.
From rest and sleep, which but thy pictures be,
Much pleasure, then from thee, much more must
    flow,
And soonest our best men with thee doe go,
Rest of their bones, and soules delivery.
Thou art slave to Fate, Chance, kings and desperate
    men,
And dost with poyson, warre, and sicknesse dwell,
And poppy or charms can make us sleep as well,
And better then thy stroke; why swell'st thou then?
    One short sleepe past, wee wake eternally
    And death shall be no more; death thou shalt die.

Another aspect of the care of the dying that engenders negative feelings relates to the extent to which life should be prolonged or death prevented. Though nurses are not responsible for making the decision that a given treatment should be instituted, withheld, or continued, they are affected by these decisions. For example, the nurse may be troubled when therapeutic measures are instituted that, though they have as their objective the prolongation of the life of the patient, appear to increase his suffering. The physician is responsible for informing the family of the condition of the patient and suggesting to them courses of action. Much of the care of the dying patient is given by nurses. They cannnot help but be affected by the decisions made relative to the patient.

NEEDS OF THE FAMILY OF A DYING PATIENT

As indicated, not only the patient and the nurse are affected but also the family and his friends. The family of the patient experiences feelings similar to those of the patient, and at the same time the patient requires their comfort, strength, and support. Even when family relationships have been good and family members have a basis for meeting the needs of the patient, they require comfort and emotional support. When the family relationships have not been good, the strain placed on the family by the illness may cause further difficulties. Particularly as the condition of the patient deteriorates, feelings of guilt and remorse may be awakened in family members. As a result they try frantically to compensate for past failures —real or imagined—in their relationship. Through their efforts to assist the patient, they try to reassure themselves of their devotion to the patient and of their own worth as human beings. The family needs support and a feeling that they are not alone. The nurse can help the members of the family fulfil their role by her acceptance of their behavior as having meaning, even when it seems to be unreasonable. The nurse cannot expect always to be able to change the behavior of the relatives of patients. She can show that she respects their feelings by listening to them and by treating them in a courteous, kind, and thoughtful manner.

When a patient dies unexpectedly, the family may need help in accepting his death. Conversely, when a patient has a prolonged illness and death is expected, the family may have difficulty in behaving as they are expected because they have already gone through the grieving process. Another factor that appears to influence the amount of grief is the social value of the person. In general, the young have greater social value than the aged. There is more grief for the young than for the old who have lived out a normal life-span.

NEW PROBLEMS

Although instances are recorded in the Bible of Christ bringing dead persons back to life, not until recent times has this been within the power of man (except in the patient who drowned). When an individual's heart stopped beating and his breathing ceased, he was pronounced dead. Some of us can remember the first instance in which a respirator was placed on a patient to keep him breathing. Now there are a considerable number of persons who are living and well whose hearts and breathing stopped and were restarted.

In an editorial, "When Do We Let The Patient Die?" [62] two questions are considered: (1) When is a patient dead? (2) For which patients do decisions have to be made?

Currently, there is discussion about when a patient is dead. According to the editorial the following signs are guides to the decision: (1) as in the past, when heart beat and respiration cease; (2) when there is no respiration for 5 minutes after the respirator is turned off (indicating medullary failure); (3) when the pupils

[62] J. R. E.: "When Do We Let the Patient Die?" *Ann. Intern. Med.*, 68:695–700 (Mar.) 1968.

of the eyes are fixed and dilated (indicating upper brain stem failure); (4) no spinal reflexes (cord failure); and (5) flat electroencephalogram (indicating damage to the cerebrum). Because cerebral function can return, it must be flat for at least 4 hours. In barbiturate poisoning and in hypothermia it should be flat for at least 24 hours. In young children it may be flat for several days and cerebral function may return.

The four patients for whom decisions have to be made are

1. The person in acute cardiac or respiratory arrest, requiring resuscitation immediately
2. The person whose prognosis is hopeless and who is maintained on supportive therapy
3. The person who is dying and is a potential donor of an organ—kidney, liver, pancreas, heart—to another dying patient
4. The person who is dying and whose life depends on the transplantation of a living organ or the use of an artificial organ

The decision that a patient is or is not dead and the decisions about what is to be done are the responsibilities of the physician. In the absence of a physician, nurses, firemen, policemen, and others are frequently expected to institute cardiac and respiratory resuscitation. When the nurse is responsible, she should know which patients are to be resuscitated and should have had practice in the proper techniques and in the use of equipment. Artificial respiration is described in Chapter 8.

Although nurses do not decide when supportive therapy is to be discontinued or which patients will serve as organ donors, they are touched by these decisions. As an example, a beautiful 4-month-old baby girl was brought into an emergency room. She appeared to have been suffocated. Heart beat and respirations had ceased. When the mother found the baby, she was not breathing but was warm. Despite the probability that her brain was seriously injured, resuscitation was undertaken. Her heart started beating and respiration was maintained with a respirator. On checking her EEG, it was and remained flat and her pupils were fixed and dilated. There were no spinal reflexes. Should supportive therapy be continued? The physician faced with this decision paced the floor of the intensive-care unit asking himself this question. Eventually he turned off the equipment. The baby continued to breathe for 3 or 4 hours. No nurse who was present was untouched. Each felt the anguish of the physician as he made the decision to disconnect the respirator. Each felt grief at the death of the baby. Each nurse also sensed the physician's feeling of helplessness and guilt for having the machines turned off and for not being able to save the baby.

The problem of the person who is dying and who has a suitable organ to transplant is, if anything, more difficult. To be transplanted, the organ must continue to be perfused with blood. Therefore, it must be removed while blood is circulating. Presently, rules or guidelines are being defined so that the rights of the donor will be protected.

As a basis for making decisions about life and death, physicians refer to Pope Pius XII who said that although ordinary means must be used in the treatment of the sick, extraordinary means are not required. This statement is of some help, but what is "ordinary" or "extraordinary"? That which is ordinary at one time and place may be extraordinary at another.

With the introduction of machines to take over body functions and organ transplants a host of other questions are arising. As an example, most of these procedures are extremely expensive. Among the questions to be answered is how will an organ transplant be paid for? Who will pay or how will biweekly hemodialysis be paid for? Who will be selected to live or to die?

In the recent past there has been and is a tendency either to neglect the care of those who are in the terminal phase of an illness or to use extraordinary measures to prolong life. There is the beginning trend toward emphasizing that much can be done to increase usefulness and comfort during the period in which the health of the individual declines. In some instances the patient is fully informed of the nature of his condition and what may be expected from the treatment. Attention continues to be on what can be done and on conveying to the patient that something can and will be done to help him. The emphasis here is not on cure, though this possibility is recognized, but on comfort and support of the sick person. The criterion for evaluating success is not, so much, how many are cured, but how long an individual is maintained in a reasonably comfortable and useful state.

To determine the needs of the dying and to assist those responsible for them, a number of studies have been done. Reports of studies as well as other materials are included in the References.

There are other ways of looking at the health problems that affect the practice of nursing. One is to examine some of the problems that arise out of illness and disability. These include some of the measurable costs of illness and disability to the community and to the individual. Hospitals, health departments, clinics, and all the services for the prevention and treatment of illness are costly and according to most predictions, are becoming more so. The individual wage earner who is ill often suffers complete or partial loss of income. He may have to go into debt to pay for his care or to care for the needs of his family. When the homemaker is ill and especially when there are children, a substitute mother may have to be employed. This may place a considerable financial burden on the family.

There are other losses that are more difficult to measure than the direct costs of the illness. These include the loss of productivity of a worker and sometimes of those who depend on his service or the product that he produces for their work. Who can place a monetary value on the loss of the homemaker from the home or the teacher from the classroom? Few substitute mothers or teachers can pick up where their predecessor left off and carry on fully. The adverse effects from the death or disability of a parent on growing children include the gamut from insufficient food and clothing to effects resulting from emotional deprivation and premature cessation of schooling. These things do not always happen, but they can and do occur. For example, Mrs. Alphonse, the 35-year-old mother of ten children, has severe, crippling rheumatoid arthritis. The children range in age from a few months to 12 years. During the last year and a half, Mrs. Alphonse has been in the hospital most of the time. The children have been cared for by grandparents filling in for a series of housekeepers, most of whom leave after a few weeks. Though the children have not been neglected physically, who can predict the effect of the absence of the mother from the home and exposure to a continuing state of anxiety about the mother and the costs of her care?

In addition to the problems created for children by death or disability of a parent, other members of the family are also affected. Women are now living an average of about eight years longer than their husbands. Among the problems that widows have to, or are likely to have to, face are adjusting to single living, coping with real or feared inadequacy of income to meet their needs and those of dependent children, and remaining in or changing their living arrangements. Older widows with little or no family, few friends, and no interests outside their families may have little incentive to continue living. Their purpose and meaning of life may be gone. The older, friendless widow is often lonely. Unless she has or can find a way to support herself emotionally and financially, she may have to depend on her children or the community for both types of support.

Nurses cannot solve all the economic and social problems arising out of illness, but they can be helpful to patients by being aware that they exist. They may also assist the patient by helping him to explore his resources and those in the community. With her special knowledge of the problems created by sickness, the nurse should be able to give constructive leadership to the community in its efforts to solve some of the problems arising as a result of illness.

Summary

In summary, the role of the nurse in the prevention of illness and conditions leading to illness and in its therapy includes

1. Knowledge required for the recognition of conditions or situations that are favorable or unfavorable to health.
2. Skill in instituting preventive measures and in supporting community efforts to institute these measures.
3. Recognition and use of the fact that disease prevention requires three general approaches: (a) maintenance of a healthy environment, (b) involvement of each individual in health maintenance, and (c) selection of methods of health protection that are acceptable and practical.
4. Knowledge required to identify the symptoms and signs indicating illness. This knowledge is essential in the nurse's role as a case finder.
5. Knowledge required to make judgments as to the urgency of the need of the patient for attention—Does he require the immediate attention of a physician? Should he be subject to careful observation? Can his needs be met at this particular time by the practice of nursing?
6. Knowledge required to make judgments as to the appropriate course of action; that is, to whom should the patient and his problem be referred?
7. Confidence to press for action when the condition of the patient appears to require it.
8. Knowledge of and competence in the practice of nursing. (See Chapter 1 for the steps in problem solving.)

REFERENCES

BOOKS

Agee, James: *A Death in the Family* (New York: Avon Books, 1957).

Brockington, Fraser: *World Health,* 2nd ed. (Boston: Little, Brown & Company, 1968).

Chekov, quoted in Trelling, L.: *The Experience of Literature* (New York: Doubleday & Company, Inc., 1967), p. 550.

Feifel, Herman (ed.): *The Meaning of Death* (New York: McGraw-Hill Book Company, Inc., 1959).

Fulton, Robert: *Death and Identity* (New York: John Wiley & Sons, Inc., 1965).

Goerke, Lenor S., and Stebbins, Ernest L.: *Mustard's Introduction to Public Health,* 5th ed. (New York: The Macmillan Company, 1968).

Gunther, John: *Death Be Not Proud* (New York: The Modern Library, 1953).

Harrington, Michael: *The Other America* (Baltimore: Penguin Books, Inc., 1962).

Irelan, Lola M. (ed.): "Low Income Life Styles" (Washington, D.C.: U.S. Dept. of Health, Education and Welfare, Superintendent of Documents, U.S. Government Printing Office).

Langley, L. L.: *Homeostasis* (New York: Reinhold Publishing Company, 1965).

Lenhoff, Edward S.: *Tools of Biology: Current Concepts in Biology Series* (New York: The Macmillan Company, 1966).

Katz, Alfred H., and Felton, Jean Spencer: *Health and the Community* (New York: The Free Press, 1965).

Kübler-Ross, Elisabeth: *On Death and Dying* (New York: The Macmillan Company, 1969).

Major, Ralph H.: *Disease and Destiny* (New York: D. Appleton-Century Company, 1936).

Morris, J. N.: *Uses of Epidemiology,* 3rd ed. (Baltimore: Williams & Wilkins Company, 1964).

Quint, Jeanne C.: *The Nurse and the Dying Patient* (New York: The Macmillan Company, 1967).

Rather, Lelland J.: *Disease, Life, and Man, Selected Essays by Rudolph Virchow* (Stanford, Calif.: Stanford University Press, 1958).

Reynolds, Frank W., and Barsam, Paul C.: *Adult Health Services for the Chronically Ill and Aged* (New York: The Macmillan Company, 1967).

Schwartz, Doris, Henley, Barbara, and Zeitz, Leonard: *The Elderly Ambulatory Patient* (New York: The Macmillan Company, 1964).

Sigerist, Henry E.: *Civilization and Disease* (Chicago: University of Chicago Press, 1943).

Simpson, R. R.: *Shakespeare and Medicine* (Edinburgh: E. & S. Livingstone Ltd., 1959).

Tolstoy, Leo: *The Cossacks—The Death of Ivan Illych, Happy Ever After,* Transl. by Rosemary Edmonds (Baltimore: Penguin Books, Inc., 1960).

Wilson, J. M. C., and Junger, C.: "Principles of Screening for Disease" *World Health Organ., Public Health Papers* No. 34, 1968. Available in the United States through the Columbia University Press, New York.

Wolstenholme, Gordon, and O'Connor, Maeve

(eds.): *Health of Mankind, Ciba Foundation 100th Symposium* (Boston: Little, Brown & Company, 1967).

Yamamoto, William S., and Brobeck, John R.: *Physiological Controls and Regulations* (Philadelphia: W. B. Saunders Company, 1965).

PERIODICALS

Adaptation

Baker, Paul T.: "Human Adaptation to High Altitude," *Science,* 163:1149–56 (Mar. 14) 1969.

Simpson, George G.: "The Biological Nature of Man," *Science,* 152:472–78 (Apr. 22) 1966.

Dying

Aring, Charles D.: "Intimations of Mortality," *Ann. Intern. Med.,* 69:137–52 (July) 1968.

Armiger, Sister Bernadette: "Reprise and Dialogue," *Nurs. Outlook,* 6:26–28 (Oct.) 1968.

Arnold, John D., Zimmerman, Thomas F., and Martin, Daniel C.: "Public Attitudes and the Diagnosis of Death," *JAMA,* 206:1949–54 (Nov. 25) 1968.

Biörck, Gunnar: "Thoughts on Life and Death," *Perspect. Biol. Med.,* 11:527–43 (Summer) 1968.

Bright, Florence, and France, Sister Luciana: "The Nurse and the Terminally Ill Child," *Nurs. Outlook,* 15:39–42 (Sept.) 1967.

Davidson, Ramona Powell: "To Give Care in Terminal Illness," *Amer. J. Nurs.,* 66:74–75 (Jan.) 1966.

Davis, Robert W.: "Psychologic Aspects of Geriatric Nursing," *Amer. J. Nurs.,* 68:802–804 (Apr.) 1968.

Easson, William M.: "Care of the Young Patient Who Is Dying," *JAMA,* 205:203–207 (July 22) 1968.

Editorial: "This He Said, Signifying What Death He Should Die," *Nurs. Outlook,* 16:19 (Oct.) 1968.

Garland, Daphne: "The Care of the Dying," *Nurs. Times,* 64:355–58 (Mar. 15) 1968.

Glaser, Barney C., and Strauss, Anselm L.: "Dying on Time," *Trans-Action,* 2:27–31 (May–June) 1965.

Kneisl, Carol Ren: "Thoughtful Care for the Dying," *Amer. J. Nurs.,* 68:550–53 (Mar.) 1968.

Maddison, David: "The Consequences of Conjugal Bereavement," *Nurs. Times,* 65:50–52 (Jan. 9) 1969.

Maddison, David: "The Nurse and the Dying Patient," *Nurs. Times,* 65:265–66 (Feb. 27) 1969.

Mead, Margaret: "The Right To Die," *Nurs. Outlook,* 16:20–21 (Oct.) 1968.

Quint, Jeanne C.: "The Dying Patient: A Difficult Nursing Problem," *Nurs. Clin. N. Amer.,* 2:763–73 (Dec.) 1967.

Shepard, Melba W.: "This I Believe About Questioning the Right to Die," *Nurs. Outlook,* 16:22–25 (Oct.) 1968.

Wygant, W. E., Jr.: "Dying, but Not Alone," *Amer. J. Nurs.,* 67:574–77 (Mar.) 1967.

Epidemiology

Feinstein, Alvan R.: "Clinical Epidemiology," *Ann. Intern. Med.,* 69:1037–61 (Nov.) 1968.

"*RN* Asks an Expert About Epidemiology," *RN,* 28:41–45, 88 (July) 1965.

Health and Disease

Aponte, Harry J.: "The Syndrome of Poverty: Children of Society's Ills," *Amer. J. Nurs.,* 66:1749–53 (Aug.) 1966.

Baumgartner, Leona: "How Will We Get Well and Keep Healthy?" *Nurs. Outlook,* 16:40–42 (Mar.) 1968.

Bendkowski, B.: "Incapacitating Diseases in the Elderly: A Survey in General Practice," *J. Amer. Geriat. Soc.,* 16:1340–45 (Dec.) 1968.

Bergner, Lawrence, and Yerby, Alonzo S.: "Low Income and Barriers to Use of Health Services," *New Eng. J. Med.,* 278:541–46 (Mar. 7) 1968.

Carter, Luther J.: "Development in the Poor Nations: How to Avoid Fouling the Nest," *Science,* 163:1046–48 (Mar. 7) 1969.

Christopherson, Victor A.: "Role Modifications of the Disabled Male," *Amer. J. Nurs.,* 68:290–93 (Feb.) 1968.

Cohen, Wilbur J.: "New Opportunities for Improving Health Care," *Postgrad. Med.,* 41:195–99 (Feb.) 1967.

Dubos, René J.: "Man and His Environment—Biomedical Knowledge and Social Action," *Perspect. Biol. Med.,* 9:523–36 (Summer) 1966.

Ennes, Howard: "A Crisis of Conscience in Health Care," *Amer. J. Public Health,* 58:1809–14 (Oct.) 1968.

Ford, Amasa B.: "Casualties of Our Time," *Science,* 167:256–63 (Jan. 16) 1970.

Gordis, Leon, Markowitz, Milton, and Lilienfeld, Abraham N.: "The Inaccuracy in Using Interviews to Estimate Patient Reliability in Taking Medications at Home," *Med. Care,* 7:49–54 (Jan.–Feb.) 1969.

Hudson, Robert P.: "The Concept of Disease," *Ann. Intern. Med.,* 65:595–601 (Sept.) 1966.

Kelman, Howard R., *et al.:* "Monitoring Patient Care," *Med. Care,* 7:1–13 (Jan.–Feb.) 1969.

King, Lester S.: "Signs and Symptoms," *JAMA,* 206:1063–65 (Oct. 28) 1968.

Kissen, David M.: "Physical Disease and Emotional Factors—An Approach to Prevention," *Nurs. Mirror,* 126:29–30 (Apr. 19) 1968.

Kupchik, George J.: "Environmental Health in the Ghetto," *Amer. J. Public Health,* 59:220–25 (Feb.) 1969.

Lasker, Gabriel W.: "Human Biological Adaptability," *Science,* 166:1480–86 (Dec. 19) 1969.

Lowenstein, Frank W.: "Iodized Salt in the Prevention of Endemic Goiter: A World-wide Survey of Present Programs," *Amer. J. Public Health,* 57:1815–23 (Oct.) 1967.

Magraw, Richard M.: "Interdisciplinary Teamwork for Medical Care and Health Services," *Ann. Intern. Med.,* 69:821–35 (Oct.) 1968.

Moses, Dorothy V.: "The Older Patient in the General Hospital," *Nurs. Clin. N. Amer.,* 2:705–14 (Dec.) 1967.

Murphy, Edmond A.: "A Scientific Viewpoint of Normalcy," *Perspect. Biol. Med.,* 9:333–48 (Spring) 1966.

Reid, Otto M., Arnaudo, Patricia, and White, Aurilla: "The American Health-Care System and the Poor," *Welfare in Review,* 6:1–12 (Nov.–Dec.) 1968.

"Science and the Citizen: Doctors' Dilemmas," *Sci. Amer.,* 218:49–50 (Mar.) 1968.

Shone, Dr.: "The Young Chronic Sick," *Nurs. Mirror,* 126:21–25 (June 28) 1968.

Thurlow, H. John: "General Susceptibility to Illness: A Selective Review," *Canad. Med. Ass. J.,* 97:1397–1404 (Dec. 2) 1967.

Twaddle, Andrew C.: "Aging, Population Growth and Chronic Illness. A Projection, United States, 1960–1985," *J. Chronic Dis.,* 21:417–22 (Oct.) 1968.

van Gindertael, Jean-Michel: "Pattern of Man's Life-Span Today and Tomorrow," *Nurs. Mirror,* 126:14–15 (Apr. 5) 1968.

Veith, Ilza: "Medicare in Utopia," *Perspect. Biol. Med.,* 11:91–110 (Autumn) 1967.

Weinstein, Morton R.: "The Illness Process," *JAMA,* 204:209–13 (Apr. 15) 1968.

Williams, Greer: "Needed: A New Strategy for Health Promotion," *New Eng. J. Med.,* 279:1031–35 (Nov. 7) 1968.

4

The Effects of Injurious Agents on Cells

The environment of the industrialized society is not only beclouded by products from the combustion of fuel, but it is also increasingly burdened by vast numbers of new chemicals of ambiguous potential used in medicine, agriculture, food processing, the cosmetic industry, and in vermin control. In addition, other products such as detergents, bleaches, and cleansing fluids—some highly toxic—are an essential part of the contemporary human environment.[1]

Basis for Control Measures	**Cellular Injury**
Objectives of Nursing	**What factors affect the degree of cell injury?**
	What are the causes of signs and symptoms?

IN Chapter 3 the various etiological agents were classified as those causing direct injury to cells and those inducing their effect indirectly through the mental apparatus. This chapter is concerned with the effects of certain physical and chemical agents on cellular function and the implication of this information to the practice of nursing. Physical and chemical agents have their origin in either the external or internal environment of the individual. Many of the harmful agents in the external and possibly in the internal environment are of man's own making. Moreover they are being created in increasing variety and potency. For a time we were occupied with the hazards of exposure to ionizing radiation. Too little attention has been paid to the possibility that other agents may be even more dangerous. Although some are, many of the noxious agents in the environment are not new. They are an augmentation of pre-existing natural hazards. For example, ever since lightning ignited a tinder-dry prairie or forest, man has been exposed to smoke. When man learned to use fire for his own purposes, he increased the intensity of his exposure by inhaling smoke from a campfire or a poorly constructed fireplace. Inventions such as the furnace and steam and diesel engines have increased the quantity of smoke spewed into the atmosphere. Though many cities have accomplished miracles

in controlling the contamination of the air with smoke, much remains to be done. Whatever the quantity of smoke in the air, many persons expose their respiratory tissues more or less continuously during their waking hours to tobacco smoke. The harmful effects of this practice are well documented.

Basis for Control Measures

General measures used in the control of potentially harmful physical and chemical agents do not differ in principle from those used in the control of microorganisms. Furthermore, living agents cause disease by their chemical and physical effects. Toxins formed by bacteria are poisonous chemicals. Control measures are based on information about sources of noxious agents, their vehicles for transmission, the forms in which they are harmful, and portals of entry as well as how they reach susceptible cells. Any information about the host making him or certain of his cells susceptible to a particular agent is also important. Some toxic agents do not cause any injury to the cell that is immediately apparent. Evidence that the individual was exposed to a particular agent may not appear for weeks or months or even years. To emphasize, injury by physical, chemical, or microbial agents depends on the agent, a susceptible host, and the environment.

---

[1] Wilson G. Smillie and Edwin D. Kilbourne: *Preventive Medicine and Public Health,* 3rd ed. (New York: The Macmillan Company, 1963), p. 275.

Objectives of Nursing

Some of the objectives of nursing derived from knowledge of the nature and effects of agents directly injuring cells are

1. To prevent exposure to harmful physical and chemical agents
2. To prevent injury to cells (or further injury)
3. To provide conditions essential to the recovery of the injured person
4. To gather the information required to evaluate the progress of the patient
5. To participate in community educational programs

Although this chapter is devoted to a discussion of the effects of injurious agents on the structure, function, and response of cells to injury, the fact that the total organism reacts or responds to the injury should not be forgotten. Whatever the nature or level of the response, it is directed toward overcoming the harmful agent, limiting and repairing the damage, and restoring the cell, tissue, and individual to health. When the total response of the individual is adequate and appropriate to the injury, it is beneficial. The nature and extent of the response depend on the nature and extent of the injury as well as the manner in which the individual perceives it and what his expectations are. Unless the injury is so great that death is sudden, the manifestations that are observed in the patient are often the result of complicated physiological and psychological changes set into motion by the effects of direct damage to cells. Thus injury to one part of the organism may induce a whole chain of reactions and involve parts far from the site of the original insult, including the entire individual. When these reactions are appropriate in quality and quantity to the injury, they promote recovery. They may, however, be sources of injury.

Cellular Injury

Survival of the patient who has suffered cellular injury often depends on the protection of damaged tissues until healing has taken place. Although the physician plans the therapeutic regime, the nurse is frequently responsible for its effectiveness. She makes many of the observations that are used to evaluate the response of the patient to disease and treatment. She helps to interpret both preventive and therapeutic measures to the patient and his family.

What factors affect the degree of cell injury?

Two general factors affect the degree of cell injury: the potency of the injuring agent and the susceptibility of the cell or individual to injury. Some chemicals, such as vitamin D, which is required, are harmful when too little or too much is ingested. Cyanide is highly toxic and wrecks the cell machinery in minute amounts. Other chemicals, such as silica, require excessive amounts and/or prolonged exposure to be harmful. Conditions within the host may act to protect him from or increase his vulnerability to certain chemicals. For example, the drug Thalidomide was supposed to be a mild and relatively safe sedative. It was safe when administered to adults, unless the adult happened to be a prospective mother who was in the early stages of pregnancy. Even then the drug appeared to be safe for the mother, but an unusual number of infants born of mothers who had taken Thalidomide during the first six weeks of pregnancy were born with a deformity called phocomelia (seal limb). Although the reason for the susceptibility of the embryo to Thalidomide is not known, the drug arrests and deranges the development of the embryo exposed to it. It is generally thought that drugs that produce fetal deformities exert their action at the time the affected part is undergoing differentiation. Some infants are only slightly deformed, whereas others were born with multiple anomalies, including serious deformities of all four extremities and of the viscera.[2] The nature and extent of deformity depend on the time of differentiation in the embryo in relation to the ingestion of the drug and its action. The differences between the effects of Thalidomide on the adult and embryo serve to emphasize that the susceptibility of the individual can be a factor in the effect of a chemical agent. In this instance, immaturity was the critical factor. In other instances, it may be something else.

The results of the action of Thalidomide also illustrate another principle in biology; that is, a cell can perform only as its biological properties allow. Despite the effect of Thalidomide on growth and development, insofar as is known, it has no power to alter structure after a given critical period in life. Chemical or physical agents can alter cell function, so that it is increased, inhibited, or fails. They can also alter cell structure, but they cannot make a cell perform a new function. For example, a muscle cell can be made to over- or undercontract or to fail to contract, but it cannot be made to secrete. Continued and unrelieved exposure of cells to agents increasing the activity of cells can be expected to result eventually in a failure of response. Simply stated, overstimulation leads to paralysis.

[2] Helen B. Taussig: "The Thalidomide Syndrome," *Sci. Amer.*, **207**:29–35 (Aug.), 1962.

Some physical and chemical agents may affect future generations by their chromosomal effect. Ionizing radiation may increase the rate at which undesirable mutations occur. Reports of studies of the chromosomal effects of LSD are conflicting and further study will be required to resolve this problem.[3] The fact that LSD causes undesirable effects in susceptible persons who ingest it is well documented.

Knowledge of the manner in which the various physical, chemical, and living agents injure cells is incomplete. However, injury may be brought about (1) by depriving the cell of something that it requires for its activities; (2) by crippling the cellular machinery, or, more specifically, by interfering with the action of the enzymes enabling the cell to utilize materials; and (3) by altering the nature of the proteins within the cells. The outcome depends on the degree of injury to the cell and its capacity to adapt. It will be influenced by the nature of the injuring agent, its concentration, and the length of time that cells are exposed to it. When the injury to the cell is not too great, the process may be reversible and recovery complete. With greater injury, the process may be irreversible and death of the cell may follow.

EFFECTS OF DEPRIVATION ON CELLS

One of the important causes of injury to cells is depriving them of something they require for optimum function. Cells may be deprived of an essential nutrient or of stimulation. The cell, like larger functioning units in the body, is capable of adapting to a decrease in the supply of nutrients or to a decrease in the functional demands made on it by decreasing its substance. As with other homeostatic mechanisms there are limits to which adaptation is possible. When the degree of deprivation is too great, the cell dies. The scientific term for the loss of substance, and with it a decrease in the size and functional capacity of a cell, tissue, or organ is *atrophy*. Some authorities include a decrease in the number of cells in a tissue in the definition of *atrophy*. For example, as a muscle atrophies it loses strength or becomes weak. In some instances atrophy can be prevented or reversed, if conditions leading to it are corrected soon enough. For instance, muscle atrophy that accompanies insufficient exercise can be reversed and the muscle can be restored to its former strength by exercise.

ATROPHY

Atrophy has many causes, some of which are physiological in origin. Others are the result of a pathological process. Atrophy is physiological or involutional when some tissue or organ diminishes in size as a result of the normal aging process. For the structure to maintain its youthful structure would be abnormal. For example, at the time of menopause, sexual organs, including the breasts of women, diminish in size. In old age all organs undergo some decrease in size. As a result elderly persons are not quite as tall as they were in their youth and they do not weigh as much. Shock[4] quotes a study made in Canada that illustrates the decline in weight from middle to old age. Men who weighed 167 lb at ages 35 to 40 years showed a decline in average weight to 155 lb at 65 years or older. They weighed 12 lb less at 65 than they did at 35 or 40 years of age. In a study made on a group of men in the United States, men who averaged 168 lb at ages 65 to 69 years weighed, on the average, 148 lb at the ages 90 to 94 years; that is, they lost approximately 20 lb during this period. Not only does the total body weight decrease, but individual organs decrease in weight after middle age. Shock[5] indicates that the average weight of the brain at autopsy drops from 1,375 g (3.03 lb) to 1,232 g (2.72 lb) between the ages of 30 and 90. Mrs. Sabin illustrates these changes very well. At 95 years of age she weighs only 145 lb. Her highest weight was 215 lb. She has lost about 2 in. in height. Her skin is loose and wrinkled, her hair thin and sparse. With her loss of tissue she has lost strength. She is no longer as energetic as she was in her youth. She spends her days in her rocking chair.

Classification of Pathological Atrophy

Pathological atrophy classified according to its etiology is (1) disuse, (2) deficient blood supply or ischemic, (3) pressure, (4) neurogenic, (5) endocrine, or (6) generalized atrophy.

Disuse atrophy is one of the forms commonly seen by the nurse. In some instances, disuse atrophy can be prevented or limited by the practice of nursing. In disuse atrophy there is a wasting of tissue, especially that of the muscle and bone. The development and maintenance of the size, strength, and composition of muscle and bone are influenced by the amount of strain placed on them. This is supported by the principle that, in nature, parts develop in proportion to the stresses and strains placed on them. In

[3] Robert S. Sparkes, John Melnyk, and Louis P. Bozzetti: "Chromosomal Effect in Vivo of Exposure to Lysergic Acid Diethylamide," *Science,* **160:**1343–44 (June 21) 1968.

[4] Nathan W. Shock: "The Physiology of Aging," *Sci. Amer.,* **206:**108 (Jan.) 1962.

[5] *Ibid.,* p. 108.

a tree the trunk is larger and stronger than the branches. The branches proximal to the trunk are larger in diameter than those distal to it. Patients may be allowed to lose weight and strength for the want of exercise. Inactivity and immobilization lead to muscle and bone atrophy. The results of the demineralization of the bone are known as osteoporosis and can be seen on x-ray. Sometimes the decalcification of the bone may proceed at such a rapid rate that calculi are formed in the urine. The weakness experienced by the patient who has been on bed rest is caused in part by generalized atrophy. A striking example of disuse atrophy can be observed by comparing the size of a limb that has been encased in a cast with that of its mate that was free. To minimize disuse atrophy, unless there is some contraindication, bed patients should be encouraged to exercise. All patients should have arms and legs put through the normal range of motion each day. This can be done as they are bathed. The nurse should exercise reasonable judgment. Motion should not be forced beyond the normal range nor should it cause pain. Patients who are able should be taught to do exercises such as wiggling their toes, moving the legs up and down in bed, and doing muscle-setting exercises. When the patient's condition permits, activities such as boosting or raising himself up in bed, reaching, and turning help to maintain muscle strength. For patients who are paralyzed or who are unable to get out of bed, strain on muscles and bones may be increased by the use of the standing board. The circoelectric bed makes this procedure easy to perform.

When the blood supply to tissue is deficient, the tissue adapts by undergoing atrophy. This will be further expanded in the discussion on pressure atrophy that follows.

Although pressure may have other effects, it predisposes to atrophy by causing ischemia. There are many examples of pressure causing atrophy by reducing the blood supply. For example, hydrocephalus is a condition in which cerebrospinal fluid accumulates within the ventricles in the brain, causing atrophy. As the fluid accumulates in the ventricles the brain tissue is stretched. This creates pressure on the blood vessels and with it a lessening of the supply of blood to the brain. Another example is the atrophy of glandular structures such as the kidney or liver following obstruction of a ureter or the common bile duct. As a result of the blocking of the duct, urine accumulates in the ureter or bile in the bile ducts. The accumulated fluid distends the ducts and causes back pressure. The distended ducts press on blood vessels and reduce the blood supply to the affected organ. If ischemia is marked, and if allowed to

continue, the functioning cells may die. With a decrease in the number of parenchymal cells, there is a decrease in the functional capacity of the organ.[6]

Loss of normal stimulation of tissues is accompanied by atrophy. When a muscle loses its motor nerve supply, it wastes or atrophies. For example, in anterior poliomyelitis, destruction of the motor horn cells in the spinal cord deprives muscles of normal stimulation and the muscles become flaccid or limp. Muscles permanently deprived of their motor nerve supply eventually degenerate. Injuries to the sensory nerves may have a similar effect.

Secretion by some endocrine glands is under the control of the anterior hypophysis. Atrophy of its target glands may result from failure of the anterior pituitary to produce its tropic hormones. Because of the negative feedback relationship of the anterior pituitary with its target glands, atrophy of a target gland can also be produced by the administration of large doses of its hormones.[7] To illustrate, atrophy of the adrenal cortex has been observed when large dosages of cortisone or hydrocortisone have been administered over a period of time. When thyroxin is administered in the absence of a thyroid deficiency, the thyroid gland adapts by decreasing its secretion of thyroxin.

Generalized atrophy is caused by a variety of conditions. It is most frequently associated with a lack of calories or from serious debilitating disease. An infrequent cause is destruction of the anterior pituitary gland following childbirth.

In a broad sense, atrophy occurs when the stimulation or nutrition falls below that required to maintain the optimum number, size, and strength of the cells. The factors initiating atrophy may be physiological or pathological. As an adaptive mechanism atrophy permits cells to survive unfavorable conditions. The nurse

[6] With stagnation of bile or urine, growth of bacteria is favored. Injury to the organ results from stagnation, ischemia, and infection.

[7] The relationship of the anterior pituitary to its target glands is essentially that of a system of negative feedbacks. The anterior pituitary produces a number of trophic (stimulating) hormones, each of which stimulates a specific endocrine gland. The gland so stimulated increases the secretion of its hormone. As the level of the hormone from the target gland rises, the secretion of the trophic hormone is depressed. The glands known to be under the control of the anterior pituitary are the adrenal cortex, the thyroid, and the gonads. The trophic hormones are ACTH (adrenocorticotrophic), TSH (thyrotrophic), and GSH (gonadotrophic). Some of the hormones secreted by the anterior pituitary, notably ACTH, have effects other than stimulation of target glands. The preceding is an oversimplified description of the relationship of the anterior pituitary gland to its target glands. The brain and liver both play a part in the system.

through the practice of nursing can help to prevent atrophy by encouraging and assisting the patient to exercise, by preventing and relieving pressure, and by assisting the patient in maintaining his food intake.

EFFECTS OF INCREASED NUTRITION AND ACTIVITY

Just as cells have the capacity to adapt to lessened nutrition or strain by decreasing in size or number, they have the capacity to respond to an increase in nutrition and activity by an increase in size and/or in number of cells. The term *hypertrophy* is used to indicate an enlargement in the volume of parenchymal tissue. *Hyperplasia* denotes an increase in the number of cells. Whether cells undergo hypertrophy or hyperplasia depends in part on whether or not they are able to regenerate or reproduce themselves. Highly specialized cells, such as nerve, skeletal, and cardiac muscle, and, to a lesser extent, smooth muscle, do not proliferate and they thereby respond to stimuli for increased function by hypertrophy.

Both hypertrophy and hyperplasia are adaptive and they are beneficial when they enable the cell (organ) to meet increased demands for function. Furthermore, both are organized processes. Possibly hypertrophy occurs because the capacity of the cell for anabolism is greater than it generally uses. With a higher rate of anabolism there is an increase in the storage of materials in the cell and the cell becomes larger. In terms of function, hypertrophy increases the capacity of the cell to do work.

HYPERPLASIA

Hyperplasia, which involves the multiplication of cells, is a somewhat more complex process than hypertrophy. In hyperplasia two cells are derived from one cell. Hyperplasia is physiological. It occurs only in response to a need, the process is organized, and it is terminated when the need is met. Daughter cells are similar to those from which they derive, which means that they are differentiated. Hyperplasia is possible because cells have a built-in capacity to grow and to multiply.

The capacity of cells to undergo hypertrophy or hyperplasia varies greatly among different organs. The skeletal muscles and the myocardium increase their size by undergoing hypertrophy. The kidney and liver increase their size by undergoing both hypertrophy and hyperplasia.

HYPERTROPHY

There are many examples of hypertrophy. The bulging muscles of the wrestler or the weight lifter are examples of hypertrophy of skeletal muscles in response to increased work. The same adaptation may be observed in the person who has lost the function of his lower extremities and uses his arm and shoulder muscles as legs. Hypertrophy also enables the myocardium to move the blood against an increase in resistance such as is produced by stenosis of a heart valve or of the aorta or by arteriolar constriction in essential hypertension. These disorders are examples of adaptations to a pathological process enabling the organism to survive. Unfortunately, the capacity of the individual to nourish the increase in muscle tissue may not keep pace with the increase in size. Eventually the muscle becomes ischemic and fails.

Smooth muscle also undergoes hypertrophy when its work is increased. For example, hyperplasia of the prostate gland obstructs the urethra, causing increased resistance to the flow of urine. The smooth muscle of the urinary bladder wall responds by increasing the size of the muscle fibers. For a time this results in a sufficient increase in force to move the urine through the narrowed urethra. In time, the bladder wall may reach several times its normal thickness. Although capacity to undergo hypertrophy is adaptive, in this instance the stimulus is pathological. Hypertrophy of the pyloric muscle, with a narrowing or stenosis of the outlet of the stomach, occurs in infants of two to three weeks of age. The infant manifests projectile vomiting, rapid loss of weight, and constipation or obstipation.

Hypertrophy can be expected to develop in any muscle in which the muscle is called on to increase its work over that which it normally does. Hypertrophy is adaptive when it enables the organ to perform a greater amount of work. It is maladaptive when it narrows the lumen of a tube.

Hyperplasia and hypertrophy may occur together. Following the removal of one kidney, the other one enlarges. The enlargement is caused by a combination of an increase in the size of the tubules and an increase in the number of cells lining them. The capacity of the bone marrow, the lymphoid tissue, and the reticuloendothelial tissue to undergo hyperplasia enables the organism to cope with infection, restore blood cells after blood loss or abnormal destruction of blood cells, and adapt to living at high altitudes.

The extent to which any organ or tissue can respond to a stimulus for an increase in function is limited. A factor in this limitation is the ability to increase the blood supply in proportion to the increase in the amount of tissue. To illustrate, hypertrophy of the myocardium is limited by the capacity of the coronary arteries to provide a supply of blood adequate to its needs. The increase in bulk demands an increased supply of nutrients. Moreover, as the heart muscle enlarges, it causes pressure on the small vessels and thereby decreases circulation. The consequence is an ischemic heart muscle and, eventually, failure. In summary, hypertrophy and hyperplasia are adaptive responses to an increase in stimulation, which may be either pathological or physiological. As a consequence of these responses an organ or part can increase the amount of work it performs. Without this adaptive capacity, life would be greatly shortened by many diseases and would not be possible in some environments.

METAPLASIA

Besides being able to adapt to environmental conditions by increasing the size and/or number of cells, some types of cells are able to adapt by a process known as metaplasia. In metaplasia one type of tissue is changed to another. Metaplasia involves two factors. The tissue must contain incompletely differentiated cells that have the potential for maturing into different types of cells and the environment of the cells must be unfavorable to the type of cell normally found in the tissue. For example, the different types of epithelial tissues have their origin in a common cell, the basal cell. When conditions are unfavorable to a given type of epithelial tissue, it is transformed to a type better suited to the particular environmental conditions. Squamous cell epithelium usually replaces other types. Conditions predisposing to epithelial cell metaplasia include chronic irritation by physical and chemical agents, certain vitamin deficiencies, and direct exposure of a mucous membrane to the external environment. For example, the mucous membrane in the trachea undergoes a transformation to squamous cell epithelium following a tracheostomy. The capacity to undergo metaplasia enables the cell or tissue to survive unfavorable conditions.

OTHER ALTERATIONS IN GROWTH

Agenesis

Although cells may adapt to unfavorable conditions, they may fail to develop or lose their capacity to proliferate. The failure of an organ or tissue to develop in the embryo is known as agenesis. Literally translated, *agenesis* means "without beginning." Occasionally an individual is born with only one of a pair of organs such as the kidney. This individual may very well live a normal life span. However, when neither kidney develops, life after birth is shortened to a few days or weeks. When the organ is one that is essential to life, death occurs at or before birth.

Aplasia

The functional or reserve capacity of a tissue or organ may be inadequate either because of failure to develop sufficient tissue or because the tissue is destroyed by an injurious agent. This condition is known as *aplasia* (the adjective is aplastic), which means "without formation." A lesser degree of aplasia, in that some tissue is present, is hypoplasia. In hypoplasia, the amount of tissue is insufficient to meet the functional requirements of the body. For example, as a consequence of failure to develop or as a result of exposure to toxic agents, the bone marrow may be aplastic or hypoplastic. A child may be born with aplastic or hypoplastic bone marrow. He may develop a disease or be exposed to an environmental condition causing partial or complete destruction of the bone marrow. There are many agents capable of injuring bone marrow. Among them are x-rays and radioactive materials and bone marrow poisons such as benzene. Evidence of an aplastic or hypoplastic bone marrow can be obtained from low blood cell counts and from biopsy of the bone marrow. As a consequence of hypoplasia, the individual not only is unable to adapt to conditions requiring an increase in the number of blood cells but may not be able to manufacture enough cells to meet his ordinary needs. The person whose bone marrow is aplastic can do neither.

The normal cell has the capacity to adapt to increased or decreased supply of materials or stimulation by increasing its size and strength (hypertrophy) or by decreasing its size and strength (atrophy). The integrity of the structure is further protected by the capacity of some cells to proliferate (multiply) and to undergo hyperplasia. Certain cells are able to protect themselves by differentiating into a type of cell better suited to the environmental conditions to which they are exposed. Failure of cells to proliferate whether because of a low growth potential or a deficiency or absence of tissue robs the individual of an important means of defending himself against injury.

EFFECTS OF THE FAILURE OF THE CELL MACHINERY

Despite an adequate supply of materials, the cell may be unable to utilize them in a normal manner. This failure may result from (1) the lack of an enzyme that catalyzes an essential step in the use of a nutrient (the lack of the enzyme may result from a defective gene), (2) the toxic effect of a chemical or bacterial poison on an enzyme or enzyme system, or (3) the effect of physical agents such as heat, cold, or radioactive materials on cellular machinery. When a cell is unable to utilize nutrients, the outcome depends on a number of factors, including (1) the nature and intensity of the injuring agent, (2) the period of time over which the cell is exposed to the injuring agent, and (3) the condition of the cell itself at the time of the injury. Depending on the interaction of these factors, the injured cell may recover fully, be crippled, or die. The sequence of events that follow cellular injury is as follows: First, (1) the chemical activity within the cell is altered; (2) cellular function is impaired; and (3) the structure of the cell is altered. In sudden and overwhelming injuries there may be less structural change than in those that are of long standing. Knowledge of this fact is utilized when tissue is prepared for microscopic examination. It is quickly frozen or treated in such a way that structural changes are minimized. When the structure of the tissue and cells is preserved, the comparison made between it and so-called normal cells is meaningful.

DEGENERATION

Disorders associated with a deterioration in the activities within the cell are called degenerations. In the various forms of degeneration, different substances accumulate within the cells. In some types the name is descriptive of the substance accumulating within the cell. In others it is descriptive of the appearance of the cell. Thus in fatty degeneration, fat accumulates within the cell. In cloudy swelling, changes take place that, as the name suggests, cause it to appear cloudy instead of clear. When a degenerative process is terminated during the phase in which chemical activity is alerted, it may be reversed and the cell restored to normal. This presupposes that the changes do not overwhelm the cellular enzymes, especially those in sensitive tissues, beyond the point of recovery. After structural changes occur, the cell goes on to necrosis or death. When there are blood vessels, blood cells, and connective tissues in the area of the necrotic cells, they respond with inflammation.

Infiltration Induced

Healthy cells may also be damaged by being overloaded with metabolites; the resulting condition is known as an infiltration. In infiltration the cell is damaged. Despite many possible disturbances in intermediary metabolism, the most common are those involving fat, glucose, amyloid, and calcium. Disturbances in the metabolism of glucose are discussed in Chapters 12 and 19, Part A. Disturbances in the metabolism of fat are usually of one of two types. One or both types may be present in a tissue at one time. Although the mechanisms by which they affect tissue are different, they are both known as fatty infiltration. In the first type, adipose tissue cells undergo hyperplasia. They are found in organs or in parts of organs where they are not normally present. They infiltrate the tissue rather than the cells. In the other, fat particles enter (infiltrate) cells and displace cellular elements. In severe obesity, adipose tissue cells undergo hyperplasia and infiltrate tissues in which they are not normally found. For example, some fat is ordinarily found around the base of the heart; however, in severe obesity adipose tissue cells infiltrate the muscle. They do not enter the muscle cells, but they lie between muscle fibers. They neither cause cellular degeneration nor provoke an inflammatory response. Because of their number, they occupy space and interfere with function by their mechanical effect.

Adipose tissue may also fill space left by the atrophy of the parenchyma of organs. Replacement of parenchymatous tissue by adipose tissue sometimes follows normal involution of organs, such as the thymus at puberty. It is also associated with pathology. Atrophy of muscle, especially when it results from a loss of the nerve supply to the muscle, may be accompanied by an increase in adipose tissue. When this happens the affected extremity may maintain its normal size, despite the loss of muscle tissue. With the loss of muscle, the function of the extremity is lost.

In the other type of fatty infiltration, lipids enter the cells of the organ and displace its normal elements. Cells may be so overdistended by fat that they rupture. One organ in which this type of fatty infiltration occurs is the liver. Though fatty infiltration of the liver may develop rapidly, it usually develops slowly. In the United States the most common cause of fatty infiltration of the liver is chronic alcoholism. In chronic alcoholism the principal source of calories may be ethyl alcohol. The etiology of fatty liver is disputed. The current most popular theory is that alcohol affects the DPN $\rightleftharpoons$ DPNH system so that DPNH [8] is greater than DPH; entrance of acetyl Co A into Krebs cycle is impaired, and the two carbon fragments are shunted toward fat synthesis. In parts of the world where the supply of high-quality proteins is deficient and malnutrition is made more severe by diarrhea, a disease called kwashiorkor is common among young children. One of its striking features is fatty degeneration of the liver. One of the problems in the care of the

[8] DPN is an abbreviation for diphosphopyridine nucleotide. The reduced form is abbreviated to DPNH.

patient who is alcoholic is to encourage him to eat foods such as meat, milk, eggs, and cheese. In regions where high-quality proteins are not available in sufficient quantity, the first problem is to supplement the available food with protein and to do this inexpensively as well as in an acceptable form. The other is to teach mothers how and why the new food should be used.

Ingestion of poisons, such as phosphorus, is followed by the rapid development of fatty degeneration. Though the liver is perhaps the most common site of fatty degeneration, other organs such as the heart muscle may be affected. Fatty degeneration of the heart is a serious complication of diphtheria and of marked and long-standing anemia, particularly pernicious anemia. Phosphorus poisoning has become infrequent, because phosphorus is no longer used in matches. Diphtheria is easily prevented by immunization. Patients with pernicious anemia can be protected by adequate treatment. In the latter two conditions, the nurse contributes through participating in public and individual education and by assisting with the required procedures.

Despite the importance of disorders characterized by fatty infiltration of vital organs, the disease with the highest incidence in which disordered metabolism of lipids is strongly implicated is atherosclerosis. The effects of this disorder will be considered in Chapter 10.

Infection Induced

In infections such as empyema, tertiary syphilis, and tuberculosis, a starchlike substance known as amyloid is deposited in the cells of the body. The organs most likely to be affected are the kidneys, spleen, liver, and adrenal glands. Similar to fatty degeneration, amyloid degeneration usually develops slowly and does not cause acute cellular degeneration or stimulate an acute inflammatory response. It does result in atrophy of the cell, probably as a result of interference with cellular nutrition. Symptoms resulting from the failure of function depend on the extent of damage to the affected organs. Though a number of organs may be involved, death is usually from renal failure.

What are the causes of signs and symptoms?

The signs and symptoms accompanying cellular injury depend on the degree of injury to cells as well as the extent of injury. They are modified by the nature of the injuring agent. The signs and symptoms are, however, those that result from (1) the inflammatory response (see Chapter 6), (2) the effect of the injury on the tissues or organ, (3) disturbances secondary to those induced either by the inflammatory response or by the disturbances in function of the injured organ, and (4) the total body response to the injury.

In those conditions in which cellular injury is sufficiently great or prolonged, death of the cell occurs. Throughout the course of life, body cells die and are replaced. For example, epithelial cells of the skin and mucous membranes, as well as blood cells, mature, live out their life span, and die. However, when a group of cells die not as a result of aging but from some injury, the condition is known as necrosis. It usually results from a lack of oxygen. Terms such as *gangrene* and *infarction* also imply death of cells but have more specific meanings. *Gangrene* is ordinarily used to indicate the death of a large section of an organ, an entire organ or part (such as a portion of the bowel, the appendix, or gallbladder), or an extremity such as a hand or leg.

Gangrene may be classified as wet or dry. Wet gangrene develops in those conditions in which there is fluid in the tissue. It occurs in disorders in which there is an obstruction of the venous return from a tissue or an organ. In dry gangrene, death of tissue results from obstruction of the arterial circulation. As a consequence the tissue becomes dehydrated and shriveled. It is blackened and mummified in appearance. The area of dead tissue is usually clearly demarcated from the living tissue by a red zone of granulation tissue.

The term *infarct* is used to indicate a localized area of necrosis resulting when the blood supply to an area falls below the ability of cells to survive. Infarction results from the obstruction of an artery at a point where both the main blood supply and the collateral circulation are blocked. It also occurs when the tissue requirements are raised above the capacity of the diseased vessels to deliver blood. Although an infarction may occur in any tissue, those that require a large supply of blood and/or have a poor collateral circulation are particularly vulnerable. Organs in which infarctions are commonly found are the brain, heart, kidney, and lung.

The consequences of an infarction depend on its location and extent. A large infarct in a vital organ such as the heart, lung, or brain may be responsible for sudden death. When the infarcted area is small enough for the function of the organ to be maintained, it is healed by fibrous tissue substitution, that is, by the formation of scar tissue. Residual effects will depend on its size and location. The reserve capacity of the organ will, however, be reduced in proportion to the amount of loss of parenchymal tissue.

ISCHEMIA

Ischemia is a condition in which the quantity or quality of blood delivered to the tissues is insufficient to supply their needs for oxygen and nutrients under varying degrees of activity. At one extreme, sufficient oxygen is delivered to meet ordinary but not unusual needs. At the other, barely enough blood is supplied to maintain life even at complete rest.

CAUSES

Ischemia may be generalized or limited to a small area of tissue. Generalized ischemia results from (1) the failure of the heart as a pump; (2) a lack in the quantity or quality of the blood; (3) generalized and excessive resistance of arterioles to the flow of blood; (4) excessive dilatation of veins which increases their capacity to hold blood and thereby reduces the amount of blood returned to the heart; and (5) failure of the lungs to oxygenate blood. In all these conditions cell nutrition suffers.

Localized ischemia can be of intrinsic or external origin. The most common intrinsic causes of ischemia are arterial occlusion and interference with the venous return which will be discussed in Chapters 10 and 11. A less usual cause of ischemia is Raynaud's disease. Arteries supplying the hands and/or feet respond to cold or to other stimuli by constricting so greatly that no blood can pass through them to the tissue. As a consequence, the involved areas are blanched and painful. Because the attack is brief, tissue necrosis seldom occurs. Small areas of ulceration of the skin sometimes do develop. The frequency of attacks can be reduced by preventing exposure to inciting agents, such as cold.

Among the common extrinsic causes of ischemia are prolonged sitting; the resting of a part of the body, particularly a bony prominence, against a firm surface; and casts and bandages that are too tight. Swelling of tissues, as the result of either edema or inflammation, reduces the capacity of vessels to carry blood. The effects of swelling develop more rapidly in solid tissue or those surrounded by a nonexpansible wall such as a cast or the skull. Any increase in tension in tissues lessens the capacity of veins to remove blood from the area. Unless corrected, the swelling that results leads to a decrease or even an interruption of arterial blood supply. Neoplasms also cause ischemia by pressing on either arteries or veins. Changes in the function or structure of arteries and/or veins are frequent causes of ischemia.

EFFECTS

Although marked and prolonged ischemia leads to the death of cells, cells differ greatly in their capacity to tolerate it. The suddenness with which ischemia develops also influences the outcome. Cells maintaining a high metabolic rate, such as those in the brain, tolerate ischemia poorly. Cells adapt to slowly developing ischemia by reducing their metabolic rate and cellular substance; that is, they atrophy. This adaptation is successful *only* as long as the tissue nutrition is maintained at a level high enough to sustain the life of the cells and the cells are not stimulated to function beyond this point. Tissues rendered ischemic by one cause have a smaller tolerance for other ischemia-inducing conditions than do normal tissues. For example, Mr. Brown, who has occlusive vascular disease in the arteries in his legs, is more susceptible to the effects of pressure on his heels than is his roommate, who has healthy arteries. When death of cells does occur, continuity of structure may be maintained by the formation of scar tissue. With the loss of parenchymatous cells, the reserve capacity of the organ is reduced and with it the capacity to adapt to changes in the environment.

Although ischemia is a factor in many illnesses, its effects on the skin and muscle will be discussed at this time. Ischemia of the skin results from a single cause or multiple causes. Whatever the etiology, it acts to cause a localized tissue anoxia. As stated earlier, external pressure on the skin, edema, occlusive arterial disease, and failure of venous return are common causes. Generalized undernutrition, particularly of protein and ascorbic acid, increases the susceptibility to ischemia. For reasons not completely understood, tissues deprived of their sensory nerve supply have increased susceptibility to ischemia. Because the sensory nerve supply to the tissue is part of the warning system, its loss diminishes the capacity of the individual to detect and evaluate threats of injury to the tissue. Cells supplied by end arteries are particularly susceptible to ischemia. Those with a double blood supply or a well-developed collateral circulation have some protection.

Bedsores

One of the most persistent problems resulting from localized areas of ischemia of the skin are bedsores or decubiti. Conditions predisposing to their development include (1) immobilization, (2) pressure over bony prominences, (3) undernutrition, (4) lack of sensory nerve supply, and (5) edema of the tissues. With the increase in persons living into the 65-and-over age group, the number of persons who are particularly susceptible to decubiti is increased. Furthermore, decubiti are not necessarily a terminal event, as some 31 per cent of patients studied by Bliss et al.[9] who developed decubiti were discharged from the hospital.

One of the factors contributing to pressure on vulnerable tissues is immobilization. The healthy person changes his position with great frequency. Even at night he may change it many times. As a result of debility, serious illness, or the application of restraints to keep a confused or disoriented patient in bed, the patient may not be able to move about. Deeply unconscious patients may not move at all. Further, interference with movement is not limited to the patient who is bedfast, for patients who are placed in chairs may not move all day.

Whether the patient sits or lies, the weight of his body is borne by tissues covering bony prominences. The skin and subcutaneous tissue are compressed between the bony prominences and the mattress or chair seat. When the patient lies on his back the points of greatest compression are the shoulders, sacrum, and heels. Weight may also be borne by the back of the head of babies and patients who do not use a pillow. In patients who sit, the weight of the trunk and head is borne by the ischial tuberosities.[10] The patient lying on his side bears his weight on his hip, knees, ankle, and shoulder. In the absence of a pillow, the weight of the head may be concentrated on his ear. Approximately 7 pounds of pressure per square inch of surface on the tissue is sufficient to shut off the blood supply. In some patients tissue necrosis may occur in as little as thirty minutes.

Patients in a sitting position, be it in a bed or chair, are susceptible to a second type of pressure, shearing pressure. As the patient slides down in the bed or chair the skin and subcutaneous tissues lag behind the bony prominences, which move in a forward direction until the sacrum bears the weight of the body. As the bone passes over the tissue, it damages or even destroys small blood vessels. When patients are pulled up in bed without being lifted, the shearing force is applied in the opposite direction. The injury to the tissues may be further increased by incorrect massage.[11]

The most successful treatment of bedsores is their prevention.[12] The first step in prevention is the identification of patients who are most likely to develop them. Next is the institution of measures to minimize pressure on susceptible areas. The importance of prevention is emphasized by the fact that curing a decubitus ulcer may cost from $2000 to $10,000.

To test the effectiveness of a variety of methods used in the prevention of decubitus, Bliss and McLaren [13, 14, 15] studied a number of them. They report that measures such as massage, soap and water, witch hazel, pHisoHex, and silicone are ineffective. Despite the belief to the contrary, sweat and urine do not cause sores if the patient continues to move about. They remind the reader that some of the worst pressure sores occur on the heels, one of the driest areas of the body. Sweat and urine can cause the skin to be irritated, wet, and soggy, however. Among the other devices that Bliss and McLaren found to be of limited value included sheepskin, nylon pads, and sponge rubber mattresses. These devices were helpful with patients with limited predisposition to decubiti but not with those who were seriously predisposed.

Regular turning every two hours was not successful or practical with geriatric patients as 50 per cent of these patients developed trunk sores. Some patients were confused and uncooperative and some, such as patients in congestive heart failure, could not or would not move. Regular turning was successful with patients with cord injuries where patients were positioned on pillows and there was a regular turning team.

Bliss and McLaren found two different types of mattresses to be successful. The first is a mattress that molds itself to the shape of the body, such as an air or water mattress. The second is a large cell alternating-pressure mattress.[16] This mattress consists of alternating plastic or rubber tubes or cells. The cells are arranged so that they lie either transverse or parallel to the length of the bed. The air cells are connected to a pump which causes alternate cells to inflate and deflate. See Figure 4-1 in which the cells are transverse to the bed. Bliss and McLaren [17] reported that during the test period no patient placed on a mattress with transverse cells developed decubiti on either

[9] Mary R. Bliss, Rhoda McLaren, and A. N. Exton-Smith: "Preventing Pressure Sores in Hospital: Controlled Trial of a Large-Celled Ripple Mattress," *Brit. Med. J.*, 1:394 (Feb. 18) 1967.

[10] Elizabeth C. Clay: " 'Operation Pressure Sore' 1," *Nurs. Times*, 64:394 (Mar. 22) 1968.

[11] *Ibid.*, p. 394.

[12] Elizabeth C. Clay: " 'Operation Pressure Sore' 2," *Nurs. Times*, 64:429 (Mar. 29) 1968.

[13] Mary R. Bliss and Rhoda McLaren: "Preventing Pressure Sores in Geriatric Patients," *Nurs. Mirror,* 123:379–82, 395 (Jan. 27) 1967.

[14] Mary R. Bliss and Rhoda McLaren: "Preventing Pressure Sores in Geriatric Patients," *Nurs. Mirror,* 123:405–408 (Feb. 3) 1967.

[15] Mary R. Bliss and Rhoda McLaren: "Preventing Pressure Sores in Geriatric Patients," *Nurs. Mirror,* 123:434–37, 444 (Feb. 10) 1967.

[16] There is also a small cell mattress.

[17] *Op. cit.*, p. 382.

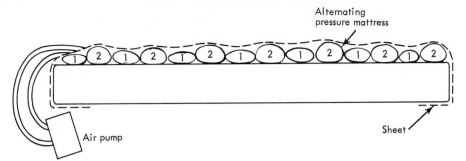

FIGURE 4-1. Diagram of large cell ripple mattress showing transverse cells. An alternating pressure mattress is a plastic (or sometimes rubber) air mattress, rather like a beach mattress, but connected to a motorized air pump that causes different parts of it to be alternately blown up and let down underneath the patient. All the cells labeled 1 are connected to the motor by one set of tubes and all those labeled 2 by another. Once every five minutes the 1 cells inflate while the 2 cells deflate; then the 2 cells inflate while the 1 cells deflate. The body thus rests first on the row of 1 cells and then on the row of 2 cells, so that the points of support, and therefore of pressure, are constantly being changed.

trunk or heels. They also found that the mattress with the cells parallel to the length of the bed was highly effective in preventing trunk sores. It was ineffective in preventing heel sores as the type of mattress used was not long enough to protect the heels. Mattresses are available that do protect the heels.

When an alternating pressure mattress is used, only one sheet is used to cover it, and it is tucked in loosely. The effectiveness of the mattress is progressively reduced by each additional layer of linen. The sheet should be free of wrinkles and crumbs. To encourage the patient to move, the top bed covering should be loose. Wrist and ankle restraints are to be avoided. When they are used, they should be removed at frequent and regular intervals and the patient moved. Whatever type of mattress is used, it must be properly placed on the bed. The mattress itself requires protection. The effectiveness of mattresses inflated by air or water depends on maintaining the integrity of the covering. A pin inserted to attach a light cord or tubing can ruin a mattress. The pump must also be kept working properly.

A recent innovation is the flotation bed. There are a number of types. One consists of a plastic tank which fits on a standard hospital bed frame. It is filled with water and covered with a heavy sheet of plastic. In another, a plastic bag of water is placed in the tank. In both types the linen is placed on the bed in the usual way. Because the patient "floats" on water, his weight is evenly distributed rather than being concentrated on bony prominences.[18]

[18] Joan Noonan, and Lawrence Noonan: "Two Burned Patients on Flotation Therapy," *Amer. J. Nurs.*, 68:319 (Feb.) 1968.

Another flotation device is a square pad filled with a gel the consistency of human fat; one example of this is the Stryker Floatation Pad. The pad is large enough to protect the sacrum of bed patients and the ischeal tuberosities of sitting patients. It can be moved from the bed to chair as the patient moves from one to the other. To prepare the bed for the flotation pad, a sponge-rubber mattress with a 16-inch square hole in the center and covered by a fitted sheet is placed on the mattress. The pad is placed in the hole. Like a water or air mattress the flotation pad accommodates itself to the contours of the part of the body resting on it. Just as with other pressure-relieving devices, the skin of the patient should be checked regularly to determine its condition. No matter how effective such aids are, their ultimate success depends on the competence of the professional staff utilizing them.

When a patient is in bed pressure can also be minimized by keeping the patient as flat as possible. A triangular-shaped pad is available to elevate the legs just enough to reduce pressure on the heels, or a thin pillow can be placed under the legs, just raising the heels from the bed. Care should be taken to prevent a ridge from pressing the tissue proximal to the heel. Provided the support extends far enough up the lower leg, preferably to the popliteal space, the broad surface on which the legs rest tends to distribute the weight.

A turning frame such as the Stryker or Foster frame is used particularly for a patient with neurological injuries to prevent and treat bed-sores as well as to immobilize him. The patient must be turned regularly and frequently enough to prevent prolonged pressure.

In addition to the preceding, attention should be given to the patient's intake of food, with particular attention to protein—meat, eggs, fish, cheese, milk—and ascorbic acid—orange juice, green leafy vegetables—and other fruits and vegetables.

When the skin breaks down, the first line of defense of the body is disrupted, and bacteria have a portal of entry. The situation may be further aggravated by the loss of tissue nutrients from the area.

Devices that reduce the incidence of bed-sores are those preventing the continued concentration of pressure on tissue and distributing the weight of the body over a wide area. A variety of pads and mattresses have been designed to accomplish these objectives. Success in the prevention of decubiti depends on the identification of susceptible patients and the proper use of appropriate measures to limit and relieve pressure.

As stated earlier, the best treatment is *prevention*. The first step is in identifying patients who are likely to develop them and in instituting preventive measures. Susceptible areas should be observed for reddening around a blackened area. The initial break in the skin may be no more than the size of a common pin head. Generally the area is painful and the pain is similar to that accompanying blistering of the heel. In patients with edema of the sacrum and buttocks, large areas can be denuded in a matter of a few hours.

The difficulty in curing bedsores is emphasized by the number of measures advocated. They range from the use of comb honey and raw or refined sugar to coating the area with some type of drug. The same measures as are used in prevention are basic: (1) mobilization of the patient, (2) measures to minimize pressure on susceptible and affected areas, (3) providing the patient with an adequate intake of protein and ascorbic acid, (4) treating the wound aseptically as well as keeping it clean and dry, (5) bladder training and the use of an external condom if the patient is incontinent, (6) prevention of tissue edema, (7) exposure of the wound to air and ultraviolet light, (8) débriding the wound surgically or by packing it with dry gauze, and (9) cleansing the wound by placing the patient in a tub of water. Large wounds may require skin grafting. As implied earlier, measures utilized in the treatment of decubiti are legion.

In addition to conditions such as bedsores in which tissues are undersupplied with blood, the entire blood supply to an area may be shut off by acute arterial obstruction. When the venous return is adequate, the tissue becomes pale and cold, and pain is experienced in the area. Tissue breakdown follows unless the condition is rapidly corrected.

Muscle Ischemia

Ischemia of muscle is frequently the result of a partial or complete occlusion of an artery. The most marked manifestation in acute ischemia is pain. Although a lack of oxygen to the tissues may be responsible for the pain, just why pain occurs is not completely clear. There is, however, no doubt about the reality of pain. When occlusion is complete, the pain continues for a day or two and then subsides. When the ischemia is relative rather than absolute, the pain is initiated by any condition increasing the need of the muscle for oxygen or food. This can be physical exercise, such as walking or running, or it can be an emotional state, such as anger or fear. The pain is relieved by rest. The ease with which the pain is precipitated depends on a number of factors, one being the degree to which the circulation to the tissue is compromised. When the pain occurs in an extremity, it is referred to as claudication. When the myocardium is involved, the condition is known as angina pectoris. The basis for the pain is the same in both instances. Arteries supplying the muscle of the heart or the extremities are unable to adapt the supply of blood to the requirement of the tissues for nutrition.

When the ischemia of the muscle is complete, death of tissue or infarction occurs. The pain that follows the sudden obstruction of an artery supplying a muscle is variously described by patients as being boring, crushing, clamplike, or cramping. Unlike the pain induced by activity in the patient with a relative ischemia of a muscle, it is not relieved by rest. Necrosis of muscle and associated tissues ensues. The extent of the necrosis and the outcome depend on the amount of tissue deprived of its blood supply and the adequacy of the collateral circulation. The symptoms and signs include those of inflammation—both general and local—and those arising from the effect the injury has on the affected organ. The general signs and symptoms, such as fever, leukocytosis, and increased sedimentation rate, usually start about the second day and continue for two or three days. Prolongation beyond this time usually indicates that complications are developing.

The responsibilities of the nurse in the care of patients with the occlusion of arteries supplying various organs will be considered in Chapter 10. However, these patients have a reduction in their capacity to adapt the supply of blood to the needs of the ischemic tissue. With impaired blood supply the tissue is susceptible to necrosis. Therefore, the tissue should be protected from conditions that increase its nutritional requirements, such as heat or exercise. When possible, measures to increase the flow of blood are instituted.

Effects of Venous Obstruction

Because venous pressure is relatively low in comparison to arterial pressure, veins are more easily obstructed than are arteries. When the venous return is obstructed, blood is delivered to the tissue but is not removed. As previously stated, in arterial obstruction the problem is one of supply. In venous obstruction, it is one of pickup and return. In venous obstruction or insufficiency, the blood remains in the tissue longer than is usual. The hemoglobin loses its oxygen, the quantity of reduced hemoglobin in the area is increased, and the tissue takes on a bluish tinge, or is cyanotic. The increase in filtration pressure that accompanies venous obstruction increases the amount of fluid in the interstitial space and causes swelling. This further obstructs the venous return and interferes with lymphatic drainage. A vicious circle is initiated. As the venous pressure rises, filtration pressure also rises, which further adds to imbalance between the quantity of fluid leaving the vascular system and returning to it and increases the swelling. Eventually, tissue fluid pressure may equal the filtration pressure, and the blood flow to the area ceases. Venous stasis plus the diminishing arterial circulation to the tissues favors bacterial growth. With the growth of bacteria, tissues are liquefied and putrefaction occurs. As the products of bacterial growth and the necrotic tissue are absorbed, the patient becomes toxic. Inflammation with its signs and symptoms develops in the area adjacent to the necrotic tissue. Tissues in a confined space are particularly susceptible to venous obstruction.

Signs and symptoms indicating obstruction to the venous return are swelling, coldness, cyanosis or pallor, numbness and tingling, and failure to be able to move exposed fingers or toes. The numbness and tingling and the inability to move are caused by pressure on sensory nerves. Unless the pressure is relieved promptly, irreversible nerve damage is likely.

Venous obstruction is commonly caused by a condition that interferes with venous return and at the same time allows arterial blood to enter. The tight-fitting cast or bandage is a good example. Another is the abdominal hernia. A loop of intestine is trapped in a hernial ring. This leads to obstruction of the venous return and, unless treated promptly, to gangrene of the trapped bowel. Surgery is usually required to reduce the hernia (removal of the bowel from the ring). When an extremity is in a cast or bandage, excessive swelling can often be prevented by elevating the limb.

TRAUMA

In addition to ischemia, physical agents are one of the most common causes of cellular necrosis. They include a variety of agents—trauma, extremes of temperature, electricity, and radioactive rays. Although trauma is used to denote any type of agent producing emotional or physical shock, it is used here to indicate a physical force. Trauma is capable of causing all degrees of tissue injury from relatively minor abrasions to disrupting the continuity of tissues. *Abrasions* are lesions resulting from the scraping of epithelial cells from the skin or mucous membrane by friction. They are produced by pulling or pushing the area over a rough surface. The skinned knee of the child who falls on a sidewalk is an example. Abrasions of the skin can be caused by pulling a sheet from underneath a patient without lifting or turning him. The same effect can be produced by pulling (dragging) a patient over sheets when moving him. Obese or heavy comatose patients who are difficult to move and turn are most likely to suffer from this treatment. Besides causing unnecessary discomfort, an abrasion robs the patient of one of his primary barriers to infection, that is, intact skin. In the care of the patient, attention should be given to the protection of the skin and mucous membranes from ill-advised friction, by rolling or lifting the patient as dictated by his condition and needs. As discussed earlier, injury to underlying tissues is also caused by the shearing force.

CONTUSION OR BRUISE

Injury to deeper layers of tissue is termed a *contusion* or *bruise*. Contusions are caused by the application of force to tissue, thereby causing injury to the underlying structures. Contusion frequently results from striking a part of the body against a hard object such as a table or chair. In a contusion there may be extensive damage to soft tissues, including blood vessels, with subsequent bleeding into the tissues. The surface layer of skin or mucous membrane may or may not be ruptured. Particularly in debilitated patients, a bruised area may serve as the site favorable to the growth of pathogenic bacteria. Free blood in the tissues provides food for their growth, and swelling interferes with the body's ability to increase the number of leukocytes in the area. In all individuals, blood escaping into the soft tissue acts as a foreign body and induces an inflammatory response. Pain on pressure or movement of the tissue is usual.

Contusion of the Brain

In traumatic injuries involving the skull, the brain may be contused or bruised. Contusions of the brain occur even in the absence of skull fractures. The bleeding may create further injury by increasing intracranial pressure. Sometimes the volume of blood escaping from the blood vessels is insufficient to cause a significant increase in intracranial pressure, but the clot that forms attracts and holds water. Venous bleeding is likely to increase intracranial pressure more slowly than does arterial bleeding. Bleeding into the space between the dura and the skull also takes time to increase intracranial pressure. (See Chapter 15, Part B.) The dura is tough and resists separation from the skull. Days or weeks may elapse after the injury before signs of increased intracranial pressure are seen. An injury unique to the brain is the so-called contrecoup, in which the bruise occurs at a site other than at the point at which the skull suffers trauma. A contrecoup injury is most likely to occur when the body has been in motion at the moment of injury and the head is brought to an abrupt stop by the injuring force. As an example, a contrecoup injury may occur when the head strikes the windshield in an automobile accident. The same type of injury may result from a fall. The course of events in the development of a contrecoup injury can be simulated by taking a full pail of water and walking rapidly—a sudden stop will cause the water to splash. Emergency-room nurses, as well as those caring for patients who have suffered head injuries, should be alert to the possibility that the brain has been bruised despite absence of obvious injury to the scalp or skull. Identification of the site of injury depends on careful observation of the signs and symptoms presented by the patient. Changes in level of consciousness and of vital signs should be reported without delay. Because the brain is susceptible to edema after it is shaken (concussion) or bruised, the patient should be encouraged to lie quietly, and care should be taken to protect the head from jarring or sudden movements.

LACERATIONS

Lacerations, injuries in which there is a disruption of the surface-layer tissue, also result from trauma. Lacerations not only disrupt natural defenses but may be accompanied by contusions and bleeding. Attention should be paid to minimizing the contamination of the wound and, if necessary, to controlling bleeding. The wound may be contaminated with one or more microorganisms, including *Clostridium perfringens* (*B. welchii*) and *Clostridium tetani.*

Both *Clostridium tetani* and *Clostridium perfringens,* and other types of clostridia, are widespread in nature. Because they form spores, they are protected against unfavorable environmental conditions such as drying and change in

temperature. They are anaerobic and grow on devitalized tissues. After *Clostridium tetani* or *perfringens* is able to establish itself in a tissue and elaborate its toxin, it is able to maintain the conditions necessary to its growth. *Clostridium perfringens* and other gas-forming organisms cause extensive damage at the site at which they enter the tissue. Gas in the tissues is not always caused by the clostridia, however, for certain other bacteria, notably gas-forming strains of *E. coli,* also may be responsible. To prevent conditions that favor the growth of these microorganisms, accidentally incurred wounds should be thoroughly cleansed and débrided of foreign bodies and necrotic tissue. Persons who have been previously immunized for tetanus are given a booster dose. Physicians disagree about whether or not patients should be given tetanus antitoxin, as some patients who receive it develop tetanus and others develop severe hypersensitivity reactions.[19]

Because tetanus antitoxin is contained in horse serum, individuals who are to receive it should be tested for sensitivity previous to its administration. Tetanus toxoid has been demonstrated to be effective in establishing an active immunity. Like other antigens, tetanus toxoid takes time to produce immunity. Because injuries in which tetanus is a possibility are common, immunization with tetanus toxoid is included in most immunization programs. Booster doses at regular intervals are necessary to maintain the level of immunity.

Unlike tetanus, there is at this time no effective way to protect individuals from gas gangrene by either active or passive immunization. Protection depends primarily on thorough cleansing and débridement of the wound. Sometimes despite thorough cleansing of the wound, gas gangrene develops. The usual incubation period is from one to four days, though the range is from six hours to six weeks. The onset of gas gangrene is often heralded by a severe pain in the affected part and a sweetish, foul odor. Bubbles of gas may be seen in the drainage from the wound. Because gas gangrene progresses rapidly, the area around the wound should be inspected regularly. Though this is usually done by the physician, the nurse should be alert to symptoms and signs such as pain in the injured part and the characteristic odor, both of which indicate the possible development of gas gangrene. The physician should be notified promptly, as the life or limb of a patient depends on the promptness with which treatment is instituted.

To summarize, trauma injures tissue by removing surface cells; by crushing tissues,

[19] "Tetanus Prophylaxis," *Brit. Med. J.,* 4:635 (Dec. 16) 1967.

including blood vessels; and by disrupting the continuity of tissue. The terms used to indicate the type of injury resulting from trauma are, respectively, *abrasion, contusion,* and *laceration.* Trauma predisposes to further ill effects by disrupting the body's first line of defense against microorganisms: the intact skin and mucous membranes. By devitalizing tissues it renders them liable to infection by one or more types of clostridia. Prevention of infections by these organisms can usually be accomplished by passive and active immunization against *Clostridium tetani* and by thorough cleansing and débridement of the wound.

HYPOTHERMIA

A second physical agent causing cellular (tissue) injury is a low temperature, or cold. Healthy cells can survive the gradual reduction of temperature to 20°C (68°F). Esophageal temperatures below 78°F are associated with an extremely poor prognosis. When tissue is actually frozen, further injury is caused by the formation of ice crystals. Hypothermia is accompanied by metabolic acidosis and physiological hypotension. Exposure to moist cold over a long period of time damages capillary endothelium and increases its permeability. As fluid leaks into the tissues, the erythrocytes are concentrated in the capillaries with the result that they tend to pack in clumps and obstruct the flow of blood. When these changes occur in the feet, the condition is known as immersion or trenchfoot. Trenchfoot was a serious problem during World War II, as the men were exposed to cold, damp weather for extended periods of time. Although the men had waterproof boots, their feet were kept in a dampened condition by perspiration. Because the external environment was cold, their feet were both damp and cold, and the capillaries of the feet were injured, with the consequences described above. During the Korean conflict a new type of boot developed in Iceland was used to protect the feet.

HYPERTHERMIA

Just as there are lower limits to temperatures that are tolerated by cells, there are also upper limits. The range varies from 30° to 45°C (88° to 114°F). Temperatures over 108.5°F are tolerated by tissues for only a short time. Though tissue damage may not be observed immediately, evidence of tissue injury may appear later. At autopsy persons who die from hyperpyrexia are found to have local hemorrhages and degeneration of tissue throughout the body. Just how heat damages the tissue is not fully understood. A principle of chemistry applying to the effect of temperature on the tissue is that the speed of chemical reaction is directly proportional to the temperature. Chemical reactions proceed more rapidly at higher temperatures than they do at lower temperatures. This principle applies to reactions catalyzed by enzymes as well as to those in test tubes. With each degree of temperature elevation, the metabolic rate goes up approximately 7 per cent. Hypermetabolism may be accompanied by the accumulation of acid metabolites in the cells and by a relative anoxia and lack of nutrients to support metabolism. Another explanation is that because enzymes are protein in nature, they, like other proteins, are inactivated by excessive heat. Tissue proteins may also be coagulated. The fact that arteriosclerotic tissue tolerates increases in temperature poorly may be the result of the inability to supply nutrients and oxygen in amounts needed by the tissue. Because tissues can be and are injured by heat, the nurse should protect the patient from injury by being certain that applications of heat are within the tolerance of the tissues. Individuals who are fully conscious and whose sensory nerve and blood supply are adequate are less likely to be injured than persons who have a deficit in either nerve or blood supply. All patients should, however, be protected from the danger of burning. Patients whose arterial circulation is impaired should be protected from temperatures that are harmless to persons with a normal circulation. (See Chapters 10 and 13.)

Thermal burns are one of the important and common causes of injury to tissue. Few persons escape minor burns from time to time. Serious burns are one of the most difficult types of injury to treat successfully. Burning is responsible for approximately 7,000 deaths per year in the United States.[20] Moyer[21] estimates that approximately 6,000 hospital beds are occupied the year around by persons who have been scalded or burned. Burns were responsible for approximately one third of the deaths at Hiroshima. Because of the high incidence of burning among children, burn centers are being established in the United States for the care of these children. According to some estimates at least one half of the burn injuries could be prevented by reasonable care. In the year 1963, 72 persons living in one large city died as a result of burns. Thirty-nine of the deaths were caused by careless smoking. Eighteen of the victims were chil-

[20] *Statistical Bulletin,* Metropolitan Life Insurance Company, 48:6 (Jan.) 1967.
[21] Carl A. Moyer: "Burns and Cold Injury," *Surgery, Principles and Practice,* 3rd ed., Carl A. Moyer et al., eds. (Philadelphia: J. B. Lippincott Company, 1965), p. 377.

dren under six years of age. Thirteen of them had been playing with matches. Twelve persons were burned in fires resulting from drying clothing too close to a heater. This report does not include other causes of burning or the number of persons who, though burned, recover. Some of these individuals spend months in the hospital before they recover. Among other incidents in which carelessness or a lack of reasonable foresight resulted in serious burns are the following: A small child is scalded by pulling on the handle of a pan containing boiling water. A woman wearing a loose-sleeved negligee reaches over a lighted stove. A child or an adult steps into a tub of scalding water. An entire family dies in a fire having its origin in defective wiring. A 14-year-old boy is seriously burned in a fire started by the throwing of gasoline on smoldering rubbish. A middle-aged man dies in a fire started by a lighted cigarette.

CLASSIFICATION OF THERMAL BURNS

Over the course of history a variety of classifications have been employed to express the extent of tissue damage resulting from burns. The most recent classification is simply (1) partial-thickness injury to the skin and (2) full-thickness injury to the skin. The older classification identifies burns by degrees of injury: first-degree burns—erythema; second-degree burns—death of the epidermis, with the appendages of the epidermis remaining viable in the dermis; third-degree burns—death not only of the epidermis, but of its appendages in the dermis; and fourth-degree burns—charring or carbonification of the skin. First- and second-degree burns are partial-thickness burns. Third- and fourth-degree burns are full-thickness burns. The seriousness of a thermal burn depends not only on the depth of the burn but on its extent.

ELECTRICITY AS A CAUSE OF BURNS

Electricity causes cellular injury in a variety of ways. It produces cellular necrosis by direct coagulation of proteins and by changes in the polarity of cells, which result in an increase in their permeability. Furthermore, resistance to the passage of the electric current through a tissue produces heat that has the same effect on the tissue as any other heat. The basis for diathermy is that tissues are heated as an electric current passes through them. Depending on how the electric current is distributed through the tissue, diathermy may either heat a tissue or destroy it. In either instance a high-frequency alternating current is passed through the tissue from one electrode to another. See Figure 4-2. Death from exposure to an electric current is usually caused by its effects on the heart and brain tissue. Exposure of the heart to 110-volt electric current alternating at 60 cycles per second induces ventricular fibrillation, because one of the stimuli is bound to come at the end of the refractory period when the heart is most susceptible to fibrillation. In contrast, an electric current may be used to stop ventricular fibrillation or to initiate contraction in a heart that has stopped beating.

EFFECTS OF RADIATION

Radiation is another form of physical energy capable of injuring cells. Radiation may be classified as rays that can be seen, that is, light rays; those that can be felt, or heat rays; and those that cannot be detected by any of the five senses. All may also be classified as to their length. In the discussion that follows, the effects of ultraviolet rays and of ionizing radiation, neither of which can be seen, will be considered. According to some authorities, ultraviolet rays also induce ionization in exposed tissues.

ULTRAVIOLET RAYS

Sunburn may be caused by the ultraviolet rays from the sun or from a lamp. These burns range from a mild erythema of the skin through second-degree burns. Fever and leukocytosis are not common unless the burns are severe. However, the cornea and conjunctiva of the eye are very sensitive to ultraviolet light and short exposures may produce keratitis (inflammation of the cornea) and conjunctivitis. The eyes can be protected from ultraviolet light by dark glasses. However, they do not protect the eyes from infrared rays. Persons who wear dark glasses should be instructed not to lie and look

A. To heal tissue   B. To destroy tissue

FIGURE 4-2. Diffuse and concentrated distribution of electric current passing through tissue in diathermy.

at the sun because of the danger of burning the retina. In the past, numbers of people have become partially blinded by staring at the sun during an eclipse. The pupil of the eye remains open because of the lack of light, and infrared rays concentrate on the retina, causing serious burns.

Persons who tan can protect themselves from sunburn by gradually increasing exposure to the sun. Tolerance is built up by starting with a limited exposure and extending the time by ten minutes or so each day. A number of factors modify the length of exposure to ultraviolet light that can be tolerated. Blondes and red-heads are much more sensitive to ultraviolet rays than are brunettes. Some never tan. Young infants and children are susceptible to burning and are unable to protect themselves. Concentration of ultraviolet rays is increased by reflection. Therefore, exposure is greater during activities such as boating or swimming. Because ultraviolet rays pass through clouds, sunburn is possible on cloudy days. Though the shade from trees provides some protection against sunburn, protection is only partial. Exposed areas are therefore liable to sunburn even when a person is shaded by a tree.

Prolonged or extended overexposure of the skin to the rays of the sun intensifies the rate at which it ages. It also predisposes to carcinoma of the skin. The incidence of carcinoma of the skin is higher among those living in tropical climates than those living in temperate or arctic regions. It is also higher among farmers and sailors than among those who work indoors. Great-grandma's sunbonnet and long sleeves served a useful purpose; they protected her skin from the sun. Other factors such as wind may increase the tendency to aging and carcinogenesis.

IONIZING RADIATION

Because of the extensive use of ionizing radiation, as well as its awesome potentialities, everyone should have some knowledge of its nature, uses, and dangers and of some of the methods man can use to protect himself from its effects. Since its discovery, the uses of ionizing radiation have greatly increased. It was first used primarily in medicine for diagnosis, treatment, and research. Now, industry is developing it as a source of power. Its capacity as an agent of destruction has been amply demonstrated and is well known. Depending on its use and the precautions taken in handling it, ionizing radiation can be either a boon to mankind or the source of man's destruction. The latter possibility raises philosophical and ethical questions that are of serious import. Some of the problems arising out of the peaceful uses of

atomic energy include the protection of those who work with it, as well as the protection of the general population from atomic wastes. Questions requiring answers include the following: What effects will raising the level of ionizing radiation in the atmosphere have on the length of life and health of the people now alive? What effects will it have on future generations? How can it be used and the population protected?

Some answers or clues to answers to the preceding questions, as well as to others, are being obtained from experimental work with a variety of animals. Knowledge of the effects of massive generalized doses of ionizing radiation as well as those of small, but repeated, doses on man are also being studied. The populations who were exposed at Hiroshima and Nagasaki and in the Marshall Islands have been and are being studied. Workers in laboratories, where accidental spillage of radioactive materials has occurred, have also been subjected to intensive and extensive study. Knowledge of the local effects of small, but repeated, exposure to ionizing radiation has been obtained from a variety of sources. One important source has been physicians who pioneered in the use of x-ray and radium. For example, *The AMA News* for August 10, 1959, carried an article about Dr. Emil Grubbe, aged 84, who had pioneered in the use of x-ray. The event that occasioned the article was that Dr. Grubbe had undergone his ninety-second operation for cancer. In this operation he had the first and fourth fingers of his right hand removed. Previously he had lost part of his left hand, nose, and jaw. Cancer had developed as a result of Dr. Grubbe's exposing himself to Crooke's tubes in 1895. Knowledge has also been obtained from the effects radiation has had on industrial workers. For example, girls were employed to paint the dials of watches with radium salts. In the process, they moistened the brushes that they used by placing them in their mouths. Radium and thorium contained in the paint were absorbed and stored in the bones of the girls. Eventually they developed cancer of the nasal sinuses and osteogenic sarcoma. Though from the point of view of the girls, their families, and society, the situation was a tragedy, it had one positive aspect. Useful information was gained about the long-term effects of low-level exposures to internal emitters of radiation.

Although this chapter is primarily devoted to agents that injure tissue cells and the manner in which cell function is altered, the use of ionizing radiation in therapy and diagnosis will also be included. Whatever the source or the reason for exposure to ionizing radiation, the effect on living tissue is the same. There is a transfer of energy, which, if the concentration is sufficient, has a destructive effect on the growth and reproduction of cells.

Before discussing the effects of ionizing radiation, some of the terms used in the discussion will be defined.

Ionizing radiation "is an electromagnetic radiation consisting of photons or particulate radiation (consisting of electrons, neutrons, protons, etc.) usually of high energy, but in any event capable of ionizing air, directly or indirectly." [22] Hardy [23] simplifies the definition. He says, "In the simplest terms, ionizing radiation separates the target molecule into ions, or removes an ion from the molecule." Warren [24] defines ionizing radiation as follows: Ionizing radiation may be defined as particles of electromagnetic waves moving so fast that they knock electrons from atoms or molecules of matter.

Alpha rays (alpha particles) are particulate ionizing radiation consisting of helium nuclei traveling at high speed.[25]

Beta rays (beta particles) are particulate ionizing radiation consisting of electrons or positrons traveling at high speed.[26]

Gamma rays are x-rays originating in the nuclei of atoms.[26]

Roentgen rays are x-rays usually produced by bombarding a (metallic) target with high-speed electrons in a suitable device.[26]

X-rays (sometimes x-radiation) are electromagnetic ionizing radiation.[27]

Neutrons (or neutron rays) are neutral particles of electricity found in the nuclei of atoms.

Protons are positively charged particles of electricity.[28]

Isotopes are atoms of an element having an identical number of protons and orbital electrons but differing in weight because the number of neutrons in their nuclei differs. All isotopes of the same substance have the same atomic number. They may be stable or unstable.[29]

Radioactive isotopes are those in which the nucleus undergoes spontaneous disintegration with the production of new elements and three types of rays—alpha, beta, and gamma rays.[30] Some radioactive elements such as radium occur in nature; others are produced artificially. In the process of degeneration, a radioactive isotope may form another radioactive isotope or it may decompose immediately to a stable atom.

Half-life is the period of time it takes one half of the atoms of a radioactive element to disintegrate or to become stable. The half-life of different elements varies from a few seconds to several billion years.[31]

Rad is the unit of radiation dose. It is 100 ergs absorbed per gram of the absorber. Therapeutic doses are measured in hundreds or thousands of rads. Diagnostic dosages are usually in millirads as it is desirable to minimize exposure.[32]

Despite the tendency to think of ionizing radiation as something new, it has existed since the beginning of time. Sources of natural radiation include cosmic rays and the crust of the earth. Exposure is greater at high than at low altitudes and in regions containing uranium and thorium deposits. Although the extent to which the general population is exposed differs, everyone is and always has been exposed to radioactivity. To illustrate sources, Table 4-1 lists the gonadal dose of irradiation in the United

TABLE 4-1

Source	Annual Dose Rate (Millirads Per Year)
Natural background	85–106
Medical radiology (1957)	19
Miscellaneous source (TV, shoe x-rays, etc.)	1
Occupational exposure (1959)	0.5
Fallout: Average value over five year period 1955–1959	2.4

Kingdom.[33] From this table the reader can see that by far the greatest exposure to ionizing radiation is from natural sources. This does not mean, however, that radioactive rays may not do harm, because they may. Protection from the

[22] U.S. Department of Commerce: *Permissible Dose from External Sources of Ionizing Radiation*, Addendum to National Bureau of Standards Handbook 59 (Washington, D.C.: U.S. Government Printing Office, 1954), p. 2.

[23] James D. Hardy: *Pathophysiology in Surgery* (Baltimore: Williams & Wilkins Company, 1958), p. 191.

[24] Shields Warren: *The Pathology of Ionizing Radiation* (Springfield, Ill.: Charles C Thomas, Publisher, 1961), p. 3.

[25] U.S. Department of Commerce, *op. cit.*, p. 4.

[26] *Ibid.*, p. 3.

[27] *Ibid.*, p. 2.

[28] Armand Joseph Courchaine: *Chemistry Visualized and Applied*, 2nd ed. (New York: G. P. Putnam's Sons, 1957), p. 14.

[29] *Ibid.*, p. 19.

[30] *Ibid.*, p. 99.

[31] *Ibid.*, p. 100.

[32] Edith H. Quimby: *Safe Handling of Radioactive Isotopes in Medical Practice* (New York: The Macmillan Company, 1960), p. 10.

[33] "Since the Beginning of Time: Radiation," *World Health*, **15**:5 (Jan.–Feb.) 1962.

effects of ionizing radiation depends largely on controlling sources that are made and/or used by man.

All radioactive material, whether in the form of electromagnetic rays (gamma rays) or particles such as the alpha or beta particles or neutrons, has the same effect on tissues. Delario [34] states that all radiations directly or indirectly produce their tissue effect through ionization. Regardless of its source, all ionizing radiation acts by a single mechanism that evokes an identical tissue change. The tissue change resulting from exposure to ionizing radiation is degeneration. If the effect on the tissue is marked, cells undergo necrosis. Although the effect on cells is the same, the power of various rays and particles to penetrate tissue or other materials differs. A curious fact is that the less they are able to penetrate, the more ion pairs they produce in the tissues through which they pass. Alpha particles, which have the least penetrating power, produce more ion pairs than do either beta particles or gamma rays. However, because gamma rays and neutrons have the greatest penetrating power, they are by far the most damaging type of radiation. Because alpha particles are filtered by air or a single sheet of paper, they are unlikely to have an opportunity to come in contact with much tissue. Likewise, the extent of damage caused by beta particles is limited by their poor power of penetration. They cause superficial injuries when tissues are exposed to them. Furthermore, beta particles may cause serious injury when they are ingested or inhaled in large quantities as after an atomic explosion. Likewise they can affect tissues in the interior of the body when they are introduced by a cut or injection. Unlike alpha and beta particles, gamma rays and neutrons can traverse the entire body.

The various types of radiation, their sources, their tissue-penetrating power, and what protects against each of them as well as potential hazards are summarized in Table 4-2.

Despite differing degrees of sensitivity, all living things are sensitive to the injuring effect of ionizing radiation. An early misconception was that it injured animals, particularly man, but has had little if any effect on plants. To test the validity of this belief, Woodwell [35] and others designed experiments in which they exposed plants to ionizing radiation. From these studies, they learned not only that plants are sensitive to ionizing radiation of an intensity sufficient to injure human beings but that dif-

ferent plants have different degrees of sensitivity. For example, pine trees are more sensitive than oak trees and weeds are highly resistant. Moreover, when a forest is destroyed by ionizing radiation, it upsets the ecological system in the forest. As an illustration, white oak trees were more sensitive to irradiation than some of the insects living on them. Therefore, though not all trees were killed by radioactivity, those remaining died because they were stripped of their leaves by the proportionately larger numbers of insects. There were, obviously, many other similar imbalances. One implication of these studies relates to the disposal of atomic wastes. Life in any area exposed to sufficient radioactivity to injure man is liable to destruction.

All cells are equally damaged by ionizing radiation, but those with large numbers of dividing cells are more susceptible than those with resting cells. Nondividing cells are frequently able to repair the radiation-induced damage, whereas cell division prevents such repair and often multiplies radiation injury. Many of the radiated cells will not die until they try to divide, and this may occur sometimes as long as several months or years after exposure to radiation. The effects of exposure to ionizing radiation may be classified as (1) more or less immediate somatic effects, (2) delayed somatic effects, and (3) genetic effects. The genetic effects are those in which damage is done to the chromosomes. They are not manifested in the exposed individual but appear in future generations. Despite its destructive effects, ionizing radiation in controlled amounts is useful as a therapeutic agent, in the diagnosis of disease, and as a source of energy.[36]

Not only do tissues vary in their sensitivity to ionizing radiation but the degree to which any tissue is sensitive can be altered to some extent. Any condition, such as hyperthyroidism or fever, elevating the metabolic rate increases tissue sensitivity. The reverse is also true. A decrease in metabolism is accompanied by a decrease in sensitivity. Sensitivity is also related to the degree of cellular differentiation and to the ability of the tissue to reproduce. The more highly differentiated a cell or tissue, the more resistant it is to the effects of radiation. The greater the capacity of the tissue to reproduce, the less its resistance is to the effects of radiation. This fact helps to explain the sensitivity of bone marrow and germ cells to irradiation. Cells undergoing reproduction are particularly sensitive when they are in the prophase of mitosis. Immature cells are more sensitive to irradiation than are mature cells.

[34] A. J. Delario: *Roentgen, Radium, and Radioisotope Therapy* (Philadelphia: Lea & Febiger, 1953), p. 61.

[35] George M. Woodwell: "The Ecological Effects of Radiation," *Sci. Amer.,* **208:**40–49 (June) 1963.

[36] Robert Plant: "The Dangerous Atom," *World Health* (Jan.) 1969, p. 15.

TABLE 4-2

Type of Radiation	Sources of Particles or Rays	Mode of Exposure	Penetrating Power	Protection Against	Potential Hazards
Alpha particles	Helium nuclei traveling at high speed	Ingestion; inhalation; through breaks in the skin; introduction into a body cavity or tissue in diagnosis or treatment	Minimal—completely absorbed or stopped by a few centimeters of air or a thin piece of paper	Very easily absorbed; distance; shielding; rubber gloves; filtration mask; protective clothing	Because of limited penetrating power, alpha particles are essentially harmless unless inhaled or ingested
Beta particles	Electron particles of small mass carry a negative charge; radioactive nuclei; emitted by ^{131}I, ^{198}Au, ^{226}Ra	As above	Only a few millimeters of tissue at most; 2 mm thickness of brass; 1 mm of lead	Easily absorbed; as above; copper and aluminum filters	Local tissue injury at site of application including tissues to which beta particles are applied in the interior of the body; when ingested or inhaled in sufficient quantities causes injury as listed below

Gamma rays	1. Roentgen rays or x-rays produced by bombarding a metallic target with high-speed electrons
	2. X-rays originating in the nuclei of atoms, e.g., ^{198}Au, ^{226}Ra
		As above, plus exposure to rays in the environment; scatter x-rays from diagnostic or therapeutic x-rays	Great; can traverse, that is, pass through, the entire body	Penetrates several inches of metal; lead is commonly used for shielding; concrete	1. Prompt effects
					  a. Hematopoietic system
					  b. Gastrointestinal system
					  c. Nervous system
					2. Delayed effects
					  a. Genetic aberrations
					  b. Induction of malignant neoplasms
					  c. Reduction in the life-span
					  d. Other effects such as (1) sterility (2) cataracts

Neutrons or neutron rays; uncharged particles	Cyclotron and from the so-called atomic pile; atom bomb (nuclear fission and transmutation)	1. Explosion of atom bomb 2. Persons working with neutrons 3. During therapy	Passes; in general very penetrating	Very penetrating—concrete slows down	See gamma rays

Factors that must be taken into consideration when evaluating the possible total effects of radiation include the likelihood of injury to the tissues exposed to irradiation, the function of these tissues, and the period of time over which the radiation is absorbed. The effects of a single large dose may be quite different from those resulting from small repeated exposures applied over a period of time. The effects of irradiation also are modified by the size of the area exposed.

Because this is the era of the atomic bomb, as well as the limited use of total body irradiation in medicine, the nurse should have some knowledge of the effects of exposure of the entire body to ionizing radiation. Radiation of the entire body produces a number of effects that differ from those that accompany local exposure to radiation.[37] Moreover, in addition to injury from radioactivity, those who are in the area of an atomic bomb explosion may suffer from flash or thermal burns or be injured by falling debris. Though given less publicity and attention, the effects of blast and burns may be more serious and cause more injuries than those of ionizing radiation. They are also more difficult to protect against. The seriousness of injury from ionizing radiation depends on distance from the site of the explosion and the extent to which the persons are shielded. If a group of people are at the same point, those who are out in the open will suffer the greatest exposure. Next will be those who are shielded by natural objects or who are in buildings made of brick, concrete or metal. Those who suffer the least exposure will be those in tunnels, caves, and air raid shelters. Scientists believed that at Nagasaki and Hiroshima the explosion was an important factor in the injuries that were suffered. Those who were injured by ionizing radiation were found in a relatively small area. As a consequence, they believed that ionizing radiation released by the atom bomb would be harmful only to those in a limited area. The Bikini test proved that they were wrong. Fishermen in a boat called the *Fortunate Dragon* 110 miles from the site of the explosion suffered from the effects of total body irradiation. Some died.

According to Warren,[38] irradiation of the entire body with massive doses, such as occurred in Hiroshima and Nagasaki, results in unconsciousness, and death occurs shortly after exposure. Unless the person who receives a dose of total body irradiation is so heavily irradiated that he dies from damage to the brain or he is

burned or is struck by flying debris, he may not be immediately aware of the fact that he has been injured. Depending on the seriousness of the injury, symptoms may appear in a few minutes or be delayed for eight to ten days. The early symptoms may last for a brief period and then return sometime between the fifth and twentieth days. The effect is similar to that of skin reactions following local applications of irradiation.

Early symptoms are those of nausea, vomiting, and diarrhea. Increased capillary and cell permeability throughout the body leads to a progressive loss of fluid and electrolytes with the development of shock. Death occurs in a few days. Bleeding into the skin and mucous membranes occurs. It is evidenced by petechiae and ecchymoses of the skin as well as frank bleeding from the mouth and gastrointestinal tract. One of the factors in the bleeding is a depression in the level of circulating thrombocytes. The leukocytes also disappear from the blood, and this decreases the resistance of the person to infection. Because of their longer life span, erythrocytes do not disappear as rapidly as do the other blood cells. Ulcerations in the gastrointestinal tract provide portals of entry for bacteria. With the decrease in resistance, infection follows. Weakness and fever are a consequence of the infection and the malnutrition that result from the nausea and vomiting. In patients who survive, fever and weakness may persist for months. During the period of recovery, patients should be protected from infection and all forms of stress, including physical exertion.

Because it is assumed that after any exposure there is some permanent injury, radiation injury may be cumulative over the life-span.[39]

Other effects of radiation result from less intense exposures to ionizing radiation. They may follow the use of ionizing radiation therapy as well as its use in destruction. Some of the effects such as the induction of malignant neoplasms, the reduction in the life span, and genetic aberrations may take months, years, or generations to make their appearance. They may result from a single or multiple exposures.

The effects of total body irradiation can be summarized as

1. Prompt effects (within a few days or weeks)
   a. None—exposure of entire body to less than 200 rads or superficial injury from exposure to alpha or beta particles
   b. Hematopoietic form (200 to 400 or 500 rads)

---

[37] Total body irradiation has been employed to destroy leukemic cells or to depress the immunologic mechanisms. One of the serious problems in the care of these patients is the prevention of a fatal infection.
[38] Warren, *op. cit.*, p. 16.

[39] Mark Barnett: "The Nature of Radiation and Its Effect on Man," *Nurs. Clin. N. Amer.*, 2:17 (Mar.) 1967.

(1) Lymphopenia
(2) Leukopenia
(3) Anemia
(4) Loss of immune response
   c. Gastrointestinal form (400 or 500 to 1,000 rads)
     (1) Nausea, vomiting
     (2) Diarrhea
     (3) Ulceration and infection
   d. Central nervous system form (greater than 1,000 rads)
2. Delayed effects (months or years)
   a. Genetic aberrations
   b. Induction of malignant neoplasms
   c. Reduction in life-span
   d. Other effects
     (1) Sterility
     (2) Cataracts

Skin damage may result from exposure to any form of ionizing radiation. At the site of exposure, the first evidence of injury is erythema or redness occurring 24 to 48 hours after exposure. Later, edema, vesiculation, and exfoliation (peeling) occur, leaving the skin denuded. Deep ulcers that heal poorly may form. Loss of hair, and brittleness of the nails also occur.

In those who have received a lethal dose of irradiation, no treatment is known that is effective in preventing death or in restoring the person to health. Those who have lesser exposures benefit from blood transfusions, antibiotics, protection from infection, maintenance of nutrition and of water and electrolyte balance, and emotional support. Because of widespread knowledge of the possible harmful effects of ionizing radiation, emotional support is essential. Lapp's [40] account of the 23 Japanese fishermen who were injured as the result of the Bikini explosion tells of the reactions of these men, their families, and the members of the community to the exposure of the fishermen to total body irradiation. It is well worth reading for it emphasizes the psychosocial effects of ignorance and misconceptions on the behavior of people as well as some of the very human effects of a catastrophe. The men were treated as if they were carriers of a contagious plague by their fellow townsmen.

Persons who are exposed to total body irradiation, as the result of either an explosion of an atom bomb or the accidental spillage of atomic materials, and those who are exposed to ionizing radiation over extended periods of time are liable to varying types of injury. Patients who are treated with ionizing radiation may also be injured, but they are usually protected by screening of untreated areas and by

the control of the size of the dose that is administered. Disorders requiring extensive exposure of the body or exposure of sensitive tissues are likely to be accompanied by evidence of tissue injury. The types of injury that may occur were summarized earlier but will be repeated for emphasis. They include (1) direct injury to the skin, (2) injury to the blood-forming organs, (3) the initiation of malignant neoplasms, (4) the production of cataracts, (5) decreased fertility, (6) harmful genetic mutations, and (7) decreased life-span.

In the following section the use of ionizing radiation in the diagnosis and treatment of disease will be considered. In the hands of the well-trained physician who understands both the uses and dangers of ionizing radiation, it may be used to benefit the patient. In the hands of the untrained or the unscrupulous, there are few forces available to mankind that can cause more harm and human misery. The public is partly protected by laws regulating the use and availability of radioactive isotopes. They are not as well protected from the misuses of x-radiation. The physician who has special training has credentials he can present, if necessary, to the patient. Should the patient have any doubt about the competence of a physician, he should ask to see the physician's credentials. The nurse as a citizen and as a health educator has a responsibility for educating the public about the uses and abuses of x-radiation. She should have at least enough knowledge to appreciate its dangers and benefits. She should have some basis for protecting herself and for aiding others to protect themselves.

The use of irradiation for the preservation of food is being explored but has not yet been accepted by the Food and Drug Administration as being safe. Arguments supporting its use are presented in three letters in *Science*.[41]

The most common form of ionizing radiation employed in medicine is x-ray. Though x-rays are utilized in therapy, they have their most frequent use in diagnosis. X-rays, like light rays, sensitize photographic plate on contact. Because they penetrate body tissues in inverse proportion to the density of the tissues, dense tissues filter out a higher proportion of the x-rays than do less dense ones. Therefore, when a body containing tissues of varying densities is placed between the source of x-rays and a photographic plate, dense tissues appear as light areas on the plate and less dense tissues appear as darkened areas. To outline hollow organs such as the esophagus or stomach, contrast can be obtained by filling the organ with a radiopaque substance such as barium sulfate or an

[40] Ralph E. Lapp: *The Voyage of the Lucky Dragon* (New York: Harper and Brothers, 1957 and 1958).

[41] "Letters," *Science,* **160**:483–85 (May 3) 1968.

iodine-containing compound. Contrast can also be obtained by removing fluid from a cavity and replacing it with oxygen or air. X-rays of the brain or spinal cord are made by removing the cerebrospinal fluid and then replacing it with air or oxygen.

X-rays may also be focused on a special screen after they pass through the body. This procedure is known as fluoroscopic examination. It is used to follow the progress of certain procedures such as cardiac catheterization and the reduction of fractures.

Gamma-emitting radioactive isotopes are also used in diagnosis. An isotope such as iodine 131 is administered orally or intravenously. Though it is largely a beta emitter, enough gamma rays are formed to penetrate the overlying tissues and be counted by a radiation-sensitive instrument located outside the body or be converted into a series of dots on film or paper. When the latter procedure is used it is called a scan as a brain scan or thyroid scan. These tests are based on the fact that stable and radioactive isotopes behave in the body in a similar manner. As an example, thyroid tissue removes iodine from the blood and concentrates it within itself. Iodine 131 is useful in determining the activity of the thyroid gland as well as in locating distant metastasis in thyroid cancer. In some of the scanning tests patients should be prepared to remain in a fixed position.

Following the administration of an isotope, body fluids or secretions may be examined in a similar manner. Urine may be checked to determine the rate of excretion of iodine 131. Sellars [42] lists 12 different radioisotopes administered internally for diagnosis and treatment. In addition to including the half-life of each isotope, the test for which it is used and its purpose, and its mode of elimination, she indicates the type of precautions required.

Because procedures for the preparation of patients for diagnostic tests vary from one institution to another, directions will not be detailed here. Each nurse is responsible for determining what is required for each patient and for being certain that the patient understands what is being done and what is expected of him. Printed directions are of help, especially for patients who are undergoing diagnosis on an outpatient basis.

Many of the same sources and methods of application can be used in therapy as well as in diagnosis. When selecting the source of radiation to be used in the treatment of a given patient, the physician considers many factors including the location of the tissue to be treated,

the tolerance of adjacent tissues, and the rays or particles available for use. Therapy may be administered externally through the skin and tissues over the organ, or be applied directly to the organ, or be administered internally. Whatever method of application is used, the effect on exposed tissues is the same. When the dosage is small, it leads to moderate degeneration of cells. When it is large, cells undergo necrosis.

In the use of ionizing radiation in therapy, the physician has to consider the fact that exposure to ionizing radiation delays wound healing. When ionizing radiation is administered previous to a surgical procedure, time must be allowed for the tissue to recover. Following surgery, treatment must be delayed to allow time for healing to take place. For example, when x-ray therapy is employed for a patient who has been treated surgically, treatment is delayed until wound healing is well under way.

Ionizing radiation, whether applied as rays or particles, has a local as well as a general or systemic effect. Evidence of the local effect is presented by changes in the skin through which the radiation passes. Although modern methods of treatment lessen the number of patients having marked skin reactions, the application of radiation through the skin to neoplasms is always accompanied by some changes in the skin. The physician is responsible for preparing the patient and his family to expect reddening and possibly some desquamation of the skin. The fact that the nurse knows that this is expected and takes it as a matter of course is supporting to the patient. Any expression of surprise may lead to doubts as to whether the treatment is being properly applied or is producing the expected effect. Furthermore, the changes in the skin should be spoken of as a reaction rather than as a burn. The term *burn* may suggest carelessness, which the term *reaction* does not. Because the reaction is temporary, the use of this word is also reassuring. The use of correct terminology helps to protect the patient from unnecessary stress.

After a large dose of radiation, the skin develops an active erythema that disappears in a few days. A week or so later the erythema reappears. This time it develops gradually but increases in intensity until it resembles a severe sunburn. Blistering and desquamation may take place. In severe reactions the area may be very painful and continue to be painful for about a month. Examination of the skin and underlying tissue reveals degeneration of cells in the epidermis. Small blood vessels, especially the arterioles, also undergo degeneration. Some of the vessels are thrombosed. Capillary permeability is increased, and the tissue is hyperemic. In six or eight weeks the skin begins to regenerate.

[42] Jacqueline H. Sellars: "Clinical Applications of Unsealed Radioisotopes," *Nurs. Clin. N. Amer.,* 2:66–67 (Mar.) 1967.

The appendages of the skin, such as the hair follicles and the sweat glands, do not regenerate. The resulting skin is thin and pigmented. The underlying tissue has a poor blood supply. When the injury is severe, skin atrophy, dryness, telangiectasis (dilated veins), and hyperkeratosis are common.

When the method used to administer radioactive rays or substances is such that damage to the skin is minimal, special care of the skin may not be required. If there is an obvious reaction, the skin requires special care. The tissue is susceptible to pressure, trauma, and infection. Gentleness is essential. Because the skin is fragile, washing should either be omitted or be limited to the use of clear water. Oily substances should not be placed on the skin unless specifically ordered by the physician. Oil prevents the evaporation of perspiration and predisposes to maceration of the skin by keeping it moist. The skin should be protected from the effects of pressure from bed coverings or clothing by the use of bed cradles and lightweight, loose clothing.

Outpatients should be directed to wear loose clothing. No corsets, girdles, or garter belts should be worn by patients being treated over the trunk. Tape should not be placed on the skin in treated areas. With the exception of cornstarch, powders should not be applied to the skin exposed to irradiation during the period of therapy. Many commercially prepared powders contain zinc. The radioactive rays or particles ionize zinc or other ionizable substances. These ions produce further injury of the skin.

If the skin breaks down, it must be treated aseptically. Patients treated on an outpatient basis should be warned against exposure of the treated areas to the rays of the sun, as they increase the damage to the skin. The patient should also be instructed not to remove marks placed on the skin by the physician because they serve as guides to treatment. Nurses should assume responsibility for making certain that patients understand the instructions given by the physician. Repetition is necessary to learning for those who are under severe stress.

The reactions of mucous membranes are similar to those of the skin. Erythema occurs first. When the reaction is severe, it may be followed by the formation of a tough adherent grayish white membrane. Some disturbance in function is to be expected. When the mouth is irradiated, secretion by the salivary glands may be depressed or the glands destroyed. Soreness makes it difficult for the patient to eat. A mouthwash of lidocaine (Xylocaine) applied before each meal increases his comfort while eating. When the patient is especially uncomfortable, 5 ml

lidocaine may be left at the patient's bedside to be used as needed.[43] Mucous membranes react more quickly than the skin, but the reaction does not last long and the mucous membranes of the mouth heal fairly rapidly.

Irradiation of the pharynx results in dysphagia, which may be relieved (if the physician agrees) by gargling with aspirin. Irradiation of the esophagus causes dysphagia and soreness in the chest. Patients who have heavy pelvic irradiation may develop an extremely painful proctitis.

Some isotopes can be temporarily or permanently implanted. At one time the only available isotope for implantation was radium or its emanation, radon 222, which is a gas. Among those now available are cobalt 60, cesium 137, iridium 192, tantalum 182, gold 198, and Iodine 125.[44] Whether the seeds or applicators are temporarily or permanently implanted depends on the half-life of the isotope and the organ being treated.

As stated earlier, patients who are treated with ionizing radiation may have systemic as well as local reactions during treatment. Depression of the bone marrow is accompanied by leukopenia, anemia, and thrombocytopenia. One type of systemic reaction is sometimes referred to as irradiation sickness. A number of factors contribute to its development. They include the location and intensity of the treatment and the emotional state of the patient. Treatments over the abdominal organs are more likely to be accompanied by systemic reactions than are those over other parts of the body. The symptoms presented by the patient include anorexia, nausea, vomiting, and diarrhea. These symptoms are seldom of serious import, but they add to the discomfort of the patient. There are a number of theories about the cause of the symptoms in radiation sickness. Some authorities believe the symptoms are caused by the effect of ionizing radiation on the bone marrow, lymph nodes, and gastrointestinal mucosa. Others believe that emotional factors are primarily responsible. Those who support the latter view point out that patients have many fears, some of which are aroused by the treatment itself and the meanings that it has. This theory is supported by the large number of agents used in the treatment of radiation sickness. The specific value of any of them is doubtful and their value may lie in the enthusiastic attitude of the physician.

[43] Marian S. Welsh: "Comfort Measures During Radiation Therapy," *Amer. J. Nurs.,* **67**:1881 (Sept.) 1967.
[44] Elizabeth B. Kendall: "Care of Patients Treated with Sealed Sources of Radioisotopes," *Nurs. Clin. N. Amer.,* 2:98 (Mar.) 1967.

Whatever the cause of the symptoms, patients are usually very miserable. They have difficulty in eating and are often worried by this fact. They lose food and fluids through vomiting and diarrhea. When these symptoms are severe, they can lead to dehydration and electrolyte imbalance. Intravenous fluids may be necessary to restore hydration and electrolytes. Compazine, an antinausea drug, may be prescribed. For some patients the food intake may be increased by adjusting the times at which meals are served. The patient who is treated early in the morning may be able to eat in the late afternoon or early evening. Food likes and dislikes should be given special consideration. This is no time to try to reform the food habits of the patient. A bottle of "Coke" or ginger ale may not meet all his nutritional requirements but either provides glucose and water. Adjustments made in the timing, or in the foods served, also help to convey to the patient the concern for his welfare. The objectives toward which the patient's care should be directed include the following: to minimize the undesirable effects of ionizing radiation and to provide the patient with support and comfort. For further suggestions about nursing actions in the care of patients with nausea and vomiting, see Chapter 12.

The nurse should also take into account the method by which radiation therapy is being applied. When therapy is given by x-ray or cobalt 60, the patient should be prepared to be placed in a room by himself. He should know that there is a small window in the room through which he can be seen at all times and that there is an intercommunication system that will enable him to talk to the person responsible for his treatment. In the care of patients in whom an applicator containing a radioactive element, such as radium or its salt radon, or cobalt 60, is placed directly in the organ, the nurse has additional responsibilities and objectives. They include the following: (1) to care for the patient in such a manner that the applicator stays in place; (2) to prevent the loss of the radioactive element, usually radium; (3) to notify the physician who is to remove the applicator at the proper time; and (4) to protect the personnel (and others) from the harmful effects of radiation.

To illustrate the accomplishment of the objectives stated, the care of Mrs. Erie, who was treated for cancer of the cervix by the implantation of radium, will be presented. Mrs. Erie was prepared psychologically and physiologically for the treatment. She knew what to expect and what was expected of her. Measures were instituted the day before the procedure was to be done to cleanse her intestinal tract and vagina. She was taken to the operating room for the actual insertion of radium. Radon, with a half-life of less than four days, might have been used. On her return she was to lie quietly and to avoid unnecessary movement in order to keep the applicator in the position in which it was placed. An indwelling catheter had also been inserted, so that she would not have to use the bedpan for urination.

Mrs. Erie's physician had explained to her why she needed to lie still. Because she was a very conscientious person, she scarcely moved. As anyone who has tried knows, lying in one position is very tiring. Mrs. Erie's back ached and she was generally uncomfortable. To reduce the backache, the nurse slipped her hand under the small of Mrs. Erie's back. She helped her move her legs and encouraged her to move her arms. She answered Mrs. Erie's light promptly and visited her frequently. The nurse performed those tasks for Mrs. Erie that Mrs. Erie could not do for herself. One of the objectives that the nurse considered very important was to make what was for Mrs. Erie a trying time less difficult. To protect herself, the nurse maintained a distance of at least a yard between herself and the patient when she was not actually giving care.

In addition to providing care for the patient, the nurse has a responsibility to prevent the loss of radium. The specific procedures in the prevention of the loss of radium vary from institution to institution and with the part of the body into which it is placed. However, there should be a regular system for informing all who care for the patient that the patient is under treatment. There should also be a system for saving and checking dressings after they are removed and before they are discarded. If the applicator containing the radium escapes the cavity in which it was placed, it should not be replaced, but the physician should be notified immediately. If the radium is applied in an area where it may be dislodged by movement, the patient must remain quiet until it has been removed.

Depending on the site of implantation, a patient may or may not need special treatment after the removal of the applicator. In this instance, Mrs. Erie had a profuse vaginal discharge for which her physician prescribed mild antiseptic douches.

Some of the instructions to the patient have been presented. Outpatients who are undergoing therapy should be impressed with the importance of keeping their appointments. It is understandable that the patient may be reluctant to return when he is beginning to recover from the effects of the previous treatment.

Just as the Japanese fishermen were feared, the patient or his family may fear that the patient is radioactive. The only time a patient is a possible source of danger is when he has received a therapeutic dose of ionizing radiation, either by implantation or other internal means. Furthermore, the danger lasts only as long as the applicator is in the body or until the half-life of the isotope has elapsed. Even during this period no one needs to be concerned if two principles are obeyed: (1) the time spent with the patient is limited and (2) a distance from him is maintained.

Two latent effects that are particular hazards to the person who handles and works with radioactive materials are radiation-induced cancer of the skin and leukemia. Dr. Grubbe and other physicians who pioneered in the use of x-ray and radium developed carcinoma of the skin of the hands. In some instances the neoplastic changes occurred fairly early. In others it was delayed for years. Leukemia is twice as frequent among physicians as it is in the general population. In Great Britain, where more stringent precautions are taken to prevent exposure of physicians, the incidence of leukemia among physicians does not differ greatly from its incidence in the general population. Employed by those who know and respect its dangers as well as its uses, it can be controlled and utilized to benefit mankind. In the hands of the ignorant or careless it may be a lethal weapon both for the user and for his victims. Protection from the hazards of radiation is important both for those who work with it and for patients. As stated previously, standards have been set for the protection of both workers and patients from the harmful effects of radioactivity. Some of these have been enacted into law.

The following principles, if acted upon, serve as guides to protection. Nurses are responsible for protecting patients and their relatives as well as themselves and their assistants. Ionizing radiation may injure tissue without producing immediate effects. When the degree of injury is small, the effects may not be evident for weeks, or even months or years. Its effects are cumulative. Some tissues are more sensitive than others. Because of the sensitivity of the gonads to radiation, special precautions should be taken to protect them in both patients and personnel. The effects on the gonads include the possibility of mutations of germ cells and of sterility.

Effective protective measures are based on shielding, distance, and time or length of exposure. The measures that are necessary depend on whether the source emits rays or particles. Because rays have the greatest power of penetration, lead-impregnated walls or materials are required for protection. Most radioactive isotopes are primarily beta emitters. To affect deeper tissues they must be taken into the body by ingestion or inhalation or be introduced by injection. Otherwise, their effect is primarily on the skin. Knowledge of what happens to the isotope in the body as well as its half-life is also important. For example, radium salts or strontium 90 are stored in bone. Because both have a long half-life, they may initiate changes that result in cancer of the bone or in leukemia. Last, the quantity of radiation to which the individual is exposed can be determined. This is of particular importance to personnel employed in radiotherapy or who care for patients who are receiving radioisotope therapy. Badges containing material sensitive to radioactivity are worn and examined at regular intervals. Should they indicate excessive exposure, procedures can be initiated to find the cause and to limit the exposure of the individual who has been exposed excessively.

Nurses who are responsible for the care of patients receiving ionizing radiation need to be concerned for their own protection only when patients are receiving treatment with radium or radioactive isotopes. As stated earlier, the principal source of harm from beta-emitting particles is from ingestion or inhalation of these materials. Protection is afforded by distance, shielding, the length of exposure, and checking. Provided the nurse is conscientious about carrying out appropriate protective measures, she does not have to worry about being harmed.

For nurses who do not work in x-ray departments or in radioisotope laboratories, the usual sources of contact with ionizing radiation are limited to (1) radioactive isotopes that are to be administered to or implanted into a patient and (2) the patient who is being treated, and his excretions. In the handling of radioactive materials protection is afforded by shielding and distance. They are transported in lead containers with long handles, which enables the person to keep the container at a distance. If the material is to be ingested, the patient removes the glass from the lead container and drinks the "cocktail" previously prepared in the isotope laboratory. After the glass is emptied, it is rinsed by the patient and replaced in the container. Radium is also transported in a lead-covered case and kept at a distance by a long handle.

In the care of patients receiving internal therapy with radioisotopes, the nurse protects herself by limiting the time she spends in close contact with the patient and by the way in which she handles equipment. Bed linens or other materials subject to contamination are handled without shaking so that a minimum of dust is raised. Thorough hand washing and keeping the nails short and clean are important. The Japanese fishermen referred to previously were found to have large amounts of radioactive materials under their fingernails. Measures such as wearing monitoring badges are for the protection of the individual against the cumulative effects of repeated exposure. They also serve to remind personnel of hidden danger. Because some of the isotopes such as ^{131}I are excreted in the urine and feces, the nurse should check to determine whether urine or feces should be collected and saved for the duration of the half-life of the isotope. Contamination of linen, the floor, or equipment should be checked by the radiation department. They should also supervise the cleaning of the floor should it be contaminated. The patient should either be confined to bed or be in a private room. In working with radioactive materials, the nurse should remember that an unsafe act may endanger not only herself but many other persons. Finally, relatives and visitors of patients should be instructed so that they can visit safely and comfortably.

Fields and Seed[45] list the essential rules for handling patients who are receiving radioactive isotopes. Quimby[46] also discusses the use of radioactive isotopes in medicine and the precautions that should be taken in hospitals. Many of the points relative to protection have previously been made but will be repeated for the sake of emphasis. Protection should take into account the length of the half-life of the isotope, the size of the dosage administered to the patient, and the route of excretion. To illustrate, the effective half-life of ^{131}I is six days. When it is administered as a tracer dose, the amount given is very small. It is excreted in the urine. No precautions need be observed in the care of the patients, but the urine should be saved in special bottles for checking. Because the drug is given by mouth, breakfast is limited to toast and coffee, and other food is withheld for three hours to allow time for the absorption of iodine. The study also requires that the patient should not have been receiving an iodine-containing drug within the past two weeks. Because the patient who is treated with ^{131}I receives a larger quantity of the isotope, precautions should be observed in his care. The precautions include the wearing of rubber gloves when giving direct care and the protection of the mattress and pillows with rubber covering. Linens used by the patient should be saved and checked. The urine of the patient should be saved and sent to the laboratory for checking. Should any be spilled, the radiological laboratory should be called to superintend the cleaning up.

The rules for the handling of patients receiving radioactive isotopes are usually made by the radiologist and/or the health physicist. They are applied by those who care for patients. The measures required are simple, but they will be ineffective unless they are strictly followed. Quimby[47] cites a well-known observation that persons are likely to be very careful when they first work in a new project and to become careless later. Certainly knowledge of how to protect oneself should make the nurse more comfortable in the care of patients and, in turn, improve the quality of the care of the patient. In caring for a patient who is undergoing radiation therapy, the nurse should work quickly without seeming hurried. An attempt should be made to reduce the patient's feeling of isolation by frequent short visits. Diversional therapy such as reading, radio, television, or handiwork may be helpful to those patients who feel well enough to enjoy them.

More specific directions for the management of patients under treatment with radioactive isotopes are contained in the References.

In addition to radioactive isotopes, a number of chemicals are used in medicine as cytotoxic agents. They include (1) alkylating agents, (2) antimetabolites, (3) plant alkaloids and antibiotics, (4) hormones, and (5) miscellaneous agents. Although the specific manner in which these agents act is different, they all cause death of cells. As with ionizing radiation, the most rapidly dividing cells appear to be the most sensitive. These include the cells found in the bone marrow, mucous membranes of the gastrointestinal tract, skin, and hair follicles. Because of their effects, these drugs are used in the study of cellular processes and in the treatment of certain types of malignant neoplasms. Possible toxic effects include (1) stomatitis; (2) nausea, vomiting, and diarrhea; (3) loss of hair; and (4) the suppression of the bone marrow. When a patient is treated with large doses of one of these drugs, he becomes highly susceptible to infection. To protect him, reverse isolation procedures may be instituted or the patient may be placed in a Life Island Isolator. Measures used in the care of patients undergoing radiation therapy are also applicable to patients undergoing chemotherapy.[48] For information about cytotoxic drugs, see Goodman and Gilman.[49] There is voluminous specialized literature on cancer chemotherapy.

[45] Theodore Fields and Lindon Seed (eds.): *Clinical Use of Radioisotopes*, 2nd ed. (Chicago: Year Book Medical Publishers, 1961), pp. 341–51 and 362–74.

[46] *Op. cit.*, pp. 11–35 and 56–97.

[47] *Ibid.*, p. 35.

[48] For a description of the care of the patient in a Life Island Isolator, see the References at the end of the chapter.

[49] Louis S. Goodman and Alfred Gilman: *The Pharmacological Basis of Therapeutics*, 3rd ed. (New York: The Macmillan Company, 1965), pp. 1345–79.

CHEMICAL POISONS OF EXTRINSIC ORIGIN

A variety of chemical agents may injure or destroy tissues and cells. Their effects may be direct or indirect. For example, cyanide is a highly effective poison, because it blocks the action of the respiratory enzymes in the cell. As the result of this action, cells are unable to release the energy from nutrients required for their activities. Death from cyanide poisoning is certain and occurs in a matter of minutes. The only method of prevention is to avoid the inhalation or ingestion of chemicals containing cyanide.

Certain chemicals coagulate cellular proteins. Examples include phenol and formaldehyde.

Carbon monoxide is also a powerful poison, but it causes its effect indirectly. Despite the presence of carbon monoxide in air contaminated by gases containing products of combustion, it seldom reaches dangerous levels except in confined spaces such as houses, where defective heating devices are used, or tunnels for automobile traffic. Little attention has been given to the inhalation of carbon monoxide during smoking.[50] The poisonous effect of carbon monoxide is caused by the ease with which it combines with hemoglobin. Hemoglobin has 300 times the affinity for carbon monoxide that it has for oxygen. Consequently, when carbon monoxide is present in the blood, it readily combines with hemoglobin. The hemoglobin is unavailable to carry oxygen, and cells are deprived of their oxygen supply. In the treatment of carbon monoxide poisoning, patients are placed in an environment containing a high concentration of oxygen. When the partial pressure of the oxygen in the alveoli is increased, the quantity of oxygen going into solution in the blood is also increased. More important, however, is the effect of the law of mass action; that is, the speed or rate of chemical reaction is proportional to the concentration of each of the reacting substances. According to the law of mass action, the quantity of oxyhemoglobin can be increased by increasing the amount of oxygen available to combine with the hemoglobin. When patients who have suffered carbon monoxide poisoning are treated with high concentrations of oxygen, a mask is the most satisfactory method of administration. When other methods are employed, particular attention should be paid to ensuring adequate concentrations of oxygen. When oxygen is administered by catheter, it should be replaced at least every six to eight hours or more frequently, if necessary, to maintain its patency. When it is administered in a tent, the canopy should be kept well tucked in in order to maintain the concentration of oxygen in the inspired air at a high level. In addition, every effort should be made to maintain the patency of the airway. (See Chapter 8.) To be of value the oxygen must be inhaled and have an opportunity to be absorbed.

FAT SOLVENTS

A group of toxic chemicals employed in industry and in the home are the fat solvents, which have their effect in fatty tissues. Benzene, because of its affinity for bone marrow, causes death relatively quickly. Other fat solvents such as chloroform or carbon tetrachloride are concentrated in the liver, kidney, and brain and produce tissue necrosis in the affected organs. Because fat solvents are volatile and are used in the drycleaning industry, special precautions are necessary to protect workers. Protection of patrons from the danger of fat solvents was one of the problems that had to be solved before "do-it-yourself" drycleaning establishments could be made relatively safe. Precautions should also be taken by those who use these agents at home. Directions on containers should be followed explicitly. One way to limit the quantity inhaled is to work out of doors. Drycleaning fluids should be stored out of reach of children, and bottles of "spot removers" should be stored away from medicines and food. Had Mr. Curly and his wife followed this rule, he might have been spared a long hospitalization and permanent renal injury. One night he awakened with indigestion. He went to the medicine cupboard and drank what he thought was a popular remedy for indigestion. Instead it was a drycleaning agent. As a result of the toxic effect of the solution and delay in treatment, Mr. Curly experienced gastroenteritis, injury to the liver, and permanent and serious injury to his kidneys.

A third source of chemical poisons is bacterial toxins and enzymes. (See Chapter 5.)

HEAVY METALS

A fourth group of toxic chemicals are the heavy metals such as mercury, arsenic, and lead. Although mercury harms cells in other parts of the body, death is usually from its effect on the kidney. Small quantities of mercury in the form of organic compounds are used as diuretics, because they inhibit enzyme systems concerned with the reabsorption of sodium ions and fixed anions. Toxic dosages of mercury salts cause necrosis of the renal tubules and result in failure of kidney function.

The effects of arsenic are widespread: it damages the brain, heart, bone marrow, and kidneys. One of the interesting points about arsenic is

   [50] John R. Goldsmith: "Environmental Epidemiology and the Metamorphosis of the Human Habitat," *Amer. J. Public Health,* **57:**1536 (Sept.) 1967.

that in times past, it was the favorite agent in fact and fiction to eliminate one's enemies.[51] Arsenic is an ingredient in insecticides, rat poisons, and crabgrass killers. Children should be protected from the danger of accidental poisoning by proper handling and storage of supplies of arsenic-containing compounds and by the substitution of less toxic agents.

Lead, a chemical commonly used in industry, causes widespread effects when inhaled or ingested. Young children are particularly likely to be exposed to lead poisoning. The source of the lead is materials in the environment of the child—nails, flakes of old paint, painted plaster, or any surface covered with a paint containing lead. The child chews the lead-containing material.[52] A little lead appears to do no harm, but it is stored in the bones, where it accumulates. In the hot summer months when more vitamin D is available, the turnover of calcium and lead from the bones to the blood is more rapid than in colder months of the year, thus raising the level of lead in the blood. Other factors may also be involved. The effects on the nervous system, especially the brain, are marked. To prevent lead poisoning the use of paints containing lead should be avoided. Treatment with disodium calcium versenate, if instituted early, is effective in removing the lead and in preventing brain damage. Poisoning from arsenic, gold, mercury, and, with the exception of lead, other heavy metals can be effectively treated with Bal.[53] Nurses should be familiar with the location of the nearest poison center. If the container from which the poisonous material was taken is available, the name of the product and/or its constituents can be given to the center by telephone so that proper treatment can be initiated promptly.[54]

ALCOHOLS

A fifth type of poisonous chemical is methyl alcohol, commonly called wood alcohol. It is a highly toxic substance that produces its effect indirectly. It is converted first to formaldehyde and then to formic acid. Methyl alcohol is thought to be toxic by virtue of conversion to formaldehyde. Formic acid itself is nearly innocuous. Acidosis results from the inhibition of aerobic metabolism (in particular the enzyme lactic dehydrogenase) with accumulation of

organic acids, especially lactic acid. In nonlethal doses, methyl alcohol causes blindness by injuring the retina. During prohibition, poisoning from methyl or wood alcohol was not uncommon. An article in a recent newspaper indicated that the number of illegal stills in operation has been increasing and with them there has been an increase in the number of persons poisoned by wood or methyl alcohol. Ethyl alcohol differs from methyl alcohol in one respect: It takes smaller amounts to induce inebriation. Although the effects of the long-term excessive use of ethyl alcohol are not within the scope of this chapter, alcoholism is an increasing problem in the United States. Despite its absence from mortality tables, many authorities consider alcoholism to be one of the major health problems. Alcoholism is not a new problem, nor is it one that is unique to industrialized societies.

INSECTICIDES, RODENT AND WEED KILLERS

A sixth type of noxious chemical is the insecticide and rodent and weed killers, all of which are man-made. Each year more of these chemicals are added to the list of substances available to kill insects, ants, and rodents. Because some of these chemicals are highly toxic and chemically stable, they are threats to both man and nature. They are prepared in the form of dusts, sprays, and aerosols. About 350 million pounds of pesticides are used each year in the United States. Because of the large quantity used, there has been an increase in the level of certain toxic compounds in the environment. Pesticides have on occasion caused the widespread destruction of wildlife. Acute insecticide poisoning is responsible for about 150 deaths a year. About half the deaths are among children. In the state of California alone as many as 1,100 instances of acute insecticide poisoning have occurred among agricultural workers in a single year.[55] Aerosol preparations carry with them an additional danger, as the containers can explode if damaged or heated. Because these chemicals are relatively new, there has been little or no time to evaluate their long-term effects on human health. Depending on the form in which they are employed, these chemical agents may be inhaled, be ingested, or contaminate the skin. For example, in Limbow, U.S.A., for three consecutive nights just preceding a Fourth of July celebration the entire town was dusted with DDT powder to kill the mosquitoes. Great billowing clouds of dust blanketed the area, thus exposing all the inhabitants to a potentially toxic chemical. Similar programs are carried out in large cities for the con-

[51] Joseph Kesselring: "Arsenic and Old Lace," *Best Plays of the Modern American Theatre*, 2nd series, by John Gassner, ed. (New York: Crown Publishers, 1947), pp. 459–510.

[52] "Lead Paint in Chicago," *Time*, **82**:36 (Aug. 9) 1963.

[53] Trade name for dimercaprol, U.S.P.

[54] For a more complete discussion of the action of heavy metals, see Goodman and Gilman, *op. cit.*, pp. 943–75.

[55] "Science and the Citizen," *Sci. Amer.*, **209**:64 (July) 1963.

trol of Dutch elm disease. There is growing concern about the extent to which residues in food constitute a health hazard. Laws have been passed in some states prohibiting the use of DDT.

In the area around Limbow, U.S.A., many of the wells have been rendered unfit for use by either human beings or animals by chemicals containing nitrogen. Over a period of years commercial fertilizers containing large quantities of nitrogen have been employed in enriching the soil. Because nitrogenous compounds are highly soluble, each rain carries them further into the subsoil. Eventually the nitrogenous chemicals reach the water supplying the wells. Although the high nitrogen content of drinking water does not appear to harm mature animals, it causes a serious illness in immature animals, including human infants.

To evaluate the possible hazards of chemical weed killers, pesticides, and insecticides and to formulate principles governing their use, a number of experts have been studying the problem. Among them have been members of FOA and WHO meeting jointly to consider problems in relation to their use. In the United States, the President's Science Advisory Committee prepared a report calling for reforms in the use and control of chemical pesticides. Among the recommendations made by the committee are that (1) the government transfer responsibility for all the health aspects of the pesticides to the Department of Health, Education, and Welfare (some are now controlled by the Department of Agriculture); (2) a data-gathering system be developed to monitor pesticide levels in the environment; and (3) the federal agencies cease area spraying with long-lived insecticides, except when required to control vectors of disease. The third recommendation has been put into effect. Moreover, this committee commended Rachel Carson for alerting the public to the hazards associated with the indiscriminate use of pesticides.[56]

FOOD ADDITIVES

Another possible chemical hazard about which there is little real information is the chemicals that are added to food to preserve it or to improve its palatability or appearance. These chemicals may be added at the time a food is processed or during the growing stage. As a simple example, coloring is used to create pink ice cream or green lime sherbet. Stilbestrol is administered to chickens or beef cattle to improve the quality of the meat and to lessen the cost of weight gain. Although none of these practices is believed to be hazardous to man, over the years they may be.

[56] *Ibid.*, p. 64.

DRUGS

Drugs are chemicals that, when administered in appropriate amounts, are expected to be beneficial. For some, the margin between the effective therapeutic dose and the toxic dose may be wide. For others, the margin may be very small. At one time, it was believed that there was a threshold of exposure to certain physical and chemical agents below which no harmful effects occurred. Scientists, therefore, tried to establish safe levels of exposure. It is now known that some agents have delayed effects that may be manifested months or years after the initial exposure to the substance. As a consequence, the concept of safe level of exposure has been replaced by the "permissible dose." Basically, permissible dose means that the possibility that exposure to a particular agent will cause harm is slight. At times the condition of a person alters the quantity of the drug that he can tolerate. For example, acetylsalicylic acid (aspirin) is a drug found in every medicine chest—and possibly in almost every purse. Few people are aware of the toxic potentialities of aspirin. Yet when a child finds a bottle of a hundred or so aspirin tablets and eats them, the acetylsalicylic acid can cause fatal acidosis. Occasionally an individual is so sensitive to aspirin that one 5-grain tablet can cause serious effects or even death. A laxative taken to treat a digestive upset may cause the perforation of an inflamed appendix. The concept that certain drugs are safe and that within limits all drugs are safe is being replaced by the concept that safety is a relative matter. Furthermore, safety cannot always be judged by the immediate effects of a drug.

INDUSTRIAL POISONS

Some of the hazards associated with the exposure of the population of cities and industrial areas to pollution of the air was presented in Chapter 3. Water in some areas is also rendered unfit for human use and dangerous to fish by detergents and industrial wastes. In industry, a variety of chemicals are potential sources of danger against which workers require protection. They include arsenic, thallium, beryllium, aliphatic hydrocarbons, nickel, chromium, asbestos, and benzol. Although a number of sources of injury to cells have been cited, there are others and the number will undoubtedly be increased in the future. According to Lee,[57] a conservative estimate of the number of new potentially toxic chemicals added each year is at least 500. Because many chemicals are stable (they do not deteriorate into harmless com-

[57] Douglas H. K. Lee: "Environmental Health and Human Ecology," *Amer. J. Public Health*, Part 2, **54**:8 (Jan., Suppl.) 1964.

pounds) and are highly toxic, increasing attention is being devoted to regulating their use and to devising ways of protecting the population from unnecessary exposure to them.

As emphasized in succeeding chapters, failure to maintain the concentration and distribution of components of body fluids within limits has an adverse effect on cellular function. Marked alterations are incompatible with life. Cellular function and structure depend on the regulation of physical and chemical conditions within the organism so that neither too much nor too little is present.

TOBACCO

No discussion of noxious chemicals is complete without some mention of the effects of cigarette smoking. Over the last decade or so increasing attention has been devoted to the question of the relationship of cigarette smoking to the genesis of disease. Hammond [58] discusses a number of studies, including one of his own, that were made to discover answers to the above question. One of the reasons for interest in the problem was that the incidence of bronchogenic carcinoma, a disease that had once been relatively rare, was known to be rising rapidly. Hammond [59] discovered in his study that not only was the incidence of cancer of the lung higher among cigarette smokers but the total death rate from all causes among this group was far higher than among nonsmokers. He states that this finding is the most significant of all. Though the death rate is lowest among nonsmokers, those who stop smoking have a longer life expectancy than those who continue to smoke. There is also an adverse relationship between the number of cigarettes smoked and life expectancy. The more cigarettes smoked, the shorter the life-span.

In January 1964, the Surgeon General of the United States released a report based on a long series of major research projects establishing smoking as a significant health hazard. More recent reports support earlier findings.

PHYSICAL AND CHEMICAL AGENTS OF INTRINSIC ORIGIN

In the preceding discussion, some of the physical and chemical agents found in the external environment having a deleterious effects on the structure and functions of cells have been presented. Cellular injury may also be caused by physical or chemical agents of intrinsic origin. It may result from the abnormal distribution or concentration of one or more body constituents

[58] E. Cuyler Hammond: "The Effects of Smoking," *Sci. Amer.*, 207:39–51 (July) 1962.
[59] *Ibid.*, p. 42.

or from the failure of one or more steps in the utilization of substances within the cell. The latter is usually caused by the lack of one or more enzymes or by some condition interfering with their action. As a consequence, substances that are necessary to the body economy or that are the product of a step in metabolism accumulate within or around the cells. Chemically inert substances may act as foreign bodies and provoke an inflammatory response. In addition, chemically active substances may also alter chemical and physical conditions within the cell and have an adverse effect on the activity of cellular enzymes. The effects of the accumulation of normal or abnormal products within or around cells can be summarized as follows: (1) As they accumulate they occupy space, thereby encroaching on normal cellular constituents. (2) They alter the physical and chemical conditions in and around the cell, thereby interfering with the activity of enzymes. Some of these conditions are reversible when detected early. If they are allowed to progress, they lead to death of parenchymal cells and all that their loss implies.

DISTURBANCES IN CALCIUM AND PHOSPHORUS METABOLISM

Like other body constituents, calcium and phosphorus are subject to disturbances in their metabolism. Normally they exist in the blood plasma in a concentration very close to saturation. About one half of the plasma calcium is in an ionized form and the other half is bound to protein and is therefore in a colloidal form. The latter serves as a reserve supply that can be added to or subtracted from as needed. Phosphorus also exists in the plasma in differing states. These include the phospholipids and ester lipids and inorganic phosphorus in the form of mono- and dibasic phosphate ions. There is a reciprocal relationship between the levels of calcium and phosphate ions in the blood. When the level of one is raised, that of the other is depressed. The product of their levels must be kept below a certain point or precipitation of calcium occurs.

Knowledge of the factors entering into the regulation of calcium and phosphorus is incomplete. Because of their reciprocal relationship, anything that affects the level of one also affects the level of the other. Their levels in the plasma, however, represent a balance between intake and output. Absorption of calcium from the gastrointestinal tract is increased by vitamin D_2, or calciferol. Calciferol also increases the excretion of phosphates in the urine. Although authorities are not in complete agreement as to the action of parathormone, it is believed to regulate the excretion of phosphates by the kidney and absorption of calcium from the gut and bone. When the level of phosphates in the plasma falls, the calcium level rises. The source of the calcium is either from absorption from the gastrointestinal tract or from the bone. Although discussion of the metabolism of calcium and phosphorus in the bone is not planned here, the bone serves as an important reserve supply of both.

ABNORMAL CALCIFICATION

Abnormal calcification may take place when tissue is diseased or in certain types of disturbances of calcium and phosphorus metabolism. There are many conditions in which calcification of diseased tissues occurs. The ultimate effect depends on the tissues affected and the effect that the calcification has on the functioning capacity of the involved or related organs. For example, calcification of fibrous tissue in an old tubercle or thrombus is an expected reaction of the body to a particular type of injury. It is also regarded as beneficial rather than harmful. Calcification of the medial layer of middle-sized arteries results in the so-called pipestem arteries. This type of calcification is relatively harmless. In contrast, calcification of the pericardium, which sometimes fo'lows tuberculosis or pneumococcal pericarditis, causes great harm. The firm wall formed around the heart limits its ability to dilate and therefore to fill during diastole. This condition is known as constrictive pericarditis. Calcification of the heart valves following the healing of rheumatic fever contributes to their rigidity and deformity and their failure to open or close properly.

Disturbances in the metabolism of calcium and phosphorus may result in the calcification of normal tissues. As was stated earlier, calcium and phosphorus are in the blood in a nearly saturated solution. Any condition that increases the level of one or the other or that decreases their solubility favors precipitation. For example, calcium is more soluble in an acid than in an alkaline solution. Consequently, calcification is more likely to occur in those tissues where alkaline conditions exist. According to Hopps,[60] these are most likely to be in the stomach, lungs, and kidneys. In the stomach, following secretion the cells secreting hydrochloric acid are left with an excess of hydroxyl ions and are therefore relatively alkaline. In the kidney tubule, cells are in an alkaline state after the excretion of acid phosphate. The effect on the patient depends on which organ is calcified. Other conditions favoring calcification of normal tissues are hyperparathyroidism, the excessive intake of calciferol, and primary disease of bone associated with excessive decalcification of the bones. In nursing, knowledge that excessive intake of vitamin D may result in pathology should serve as a basis for instructing parents and patients to limit the dosage of vitamin D to that prescribed by the physician. This is the instance where some is good, but more is definitely not better.

LITHIASIS

Another pathological condition resulting from the precipitation of calcium and phosphorus and sometimes other blood constituents is the formation of concretions or stones. The terms used to indicate their formation or presence are *lithiasis* and *calculi*. Stones are formed in hollow organs and their ducts, primarily in the biliary and urinary tracts. Though their composition varies, they are generally composed of calcium, phosphorus, and organic matter. The formation of stones depends on two factors: (1) a focus, usually of organic materials, and (2) a soluble substance in solution that precipitates on the organic particles such as bacteria, epithelial cells, or tissue debris. The substance that precipitates depends on the constituents of the fluid in the hollow organ or duct. For example, calculi formed in the gallbladder may be composed of cholesterol, calcium, or bilirubin or a mixture of two or more of these substances. Those formed in the urinary tract are most likely to be of calcium oxalate.

The effects of lithiasis depend on such factors as the size of the stones and the structure in which they are located. Small stones generally cause more trouble than large stones, because the small stone is more likely to move into a duct and cause obstruction and muscle spasm. Muscle spasm is accompanied by severe cramping pain, which is referred to as colic. The patient with a stone in the common bile duct accompanied by pain is said to have biliary colic. The patient with a stone in the ureter has renal colic. In both instances, the pain is thought to be caused by the muscle spasm induced by obstruction and stretching of the tube. The pain, which is often accompanied by some degree of shock, is severe, often exquisitely so.

If the stone remains in the duct, it also causes obstruction. The consequences of the obstruction depend, in part, on its location. An obstruction in the cystic duct from the gallbladder may cause pressure on the blood supply of the duct and be followed by gangrene of the gallbladder and spillage of bile into the peritoneal cavity. Obstruction of the common bile duct or a ureter interferes with the drainage of the liver or the kidney, respectively. This leads to pressure and stasis and, if unrelieved, to infection and eventu-

[60] Howard C. Hopps: *Principles of Pathology*, 2nd ed. (New York: Appleton-Century-Crofts, 1964), p. 125.

ally to the atrophy or necrosis of the affected organ. Other effects will depend on the function of the organ.

Methods of Therapy

At this time there is no known method of dissolving calculi that are already formed. Because fat in the stomach initiates a reflex initiating contraction of the gallbladder, patients who are subject to biliary colic are advised to restrict their intake of fat. The nurse can assist the patient by helping him to learn what foods to include or reject from his diet. For patients who have, or who are predisposed to, renal calculi, teaching them to maintain an adequate, or even a high fluid intake, may help to keep the urine diluted and thus prevent the formation of stones. When a patient is admitted in acute colic, measures should be taken to relieve his pain as rapidly as possible. This usually involves the injection of an analgesic such as morphine or Demerol Hydrochloride [61] and an antispasmodic such as atropine, scopolamine,[62] and/or papaverine. Prescription of the drug or drugs to be used is the responsibility of the physician. The nurse is responsible for making the needs of the patient known to him and for instituting prescribed therapy as soon as possible.

BODY FLUIDS

One further source of injury to cells is the patient's own secretions and body fluids. As stated earlier, blood escaping from blood vessels causes damage by occupying space, by irritation and by increasing the number of osmotically active particles in the area. There is usually an inflammatory response in tissues into which there has been bleeding. Interstitial fluid or lymph, when it accumulates in excessive quantities, interferes with tissue nutrition because it occupies space.

Digestive juices are also capable of causing cell injury when they escape from the gastrointestinal tract or when the balance between the resistance of the mucous membrane lining the tract and the digesting action of the secretion is upset. Gastric, pancreatic, and intestinal juices contain protein-splitting enzymes. When they come in direct contact with cells, these enzymes break down the protein constituents of cells into polypeptides or amino acids and thereby disrupt the structure of cells. The digesting action of the various secretions is modified by their pH. In health, gastric juice is acid, and secretions in the intestine are alkaline. A prolonged or marked lowering of the pH of the gastric juice is a frequent finding in peptic ulcers. Although ulceration may occur any-

where along the alimentary canal, the stomach, the proximal portion of the duodenum, and the large intestine are the most common sites. Ulcerative disease of the large bowel is often disabling. Not all the factors responsible for ulceration along the alimentary canal are understood. In many instances multiple factors probably interact to disturb the balance between the digesting action of the juices in the stomach or intestines and the efficiency with which the mechanisms for the protection of the mucous lining act. The results of this failure are disruption of cell structure and the formation of sores opening to the surface of the mucous lining of the alimentary canal. The size and depth of the ulcers vary with the location, acuteness of the condition, and other factors.

Specific therapy of ulceration along the gastrointestinal tract is directed toward providing conditions favorable to healing. To the extent to which the ulceration is related to the patient's way of life, healing and continued good health may also depend on the identification and control of predisposing factors. Thus Mrs. Johns, who has an active duodenal ulcer, is admitted to the hospital for treatment. She is thereby removed from her usual environment. In addition a therapeutic regime is instituted to accomplish two general objectives. One is to decrease the motor and secretory activity of the alimentary canal and the other is to decrease the digesting power of the gastric juice. As soon as Mrs. Johns is well enough, a program of instruction is begun that will help her learn to manage her life and disease so that the possibility of future ulcerations is decreased. The problems associated with the therapy of the patient with peptic ulcer are described more fully in Chapter 12.

Digestive juices also have a destructive action on cell proteins of structures outside the alimentary canal. Pancreatic enzymes, when activated by a reflux of bile into the duct of Wirsung, digest the pancreas. This serious condition may be induced by obstruction of the ampulla of Vater by biliary calculi or by scar tissue. Fistulae, especially those from the small intestine, usually heal with great difficulty. Sometimes they are of great size. Healing is facilitated by preventing digestive enzymes from coming in contact with body tissues. This is not easy.

An abnormal opening such as an ileostomy or colostomy allows the intestinal contents to escape onto the abdominal wall. Unless appropriate measures are instituted, breakdown of the skin is inevitable. The situation is more acute when the feces are fluid than when they are solid, as the watery state brings the enzymes in contact with the skin. The proper application of an ileostomy or colostomy bag reduces this

---

[61] Trade name for meperidine hydrochloride.
[62] Also known as hyoscine hydrobromide, B.P.

possibility to a great extent. Other measures are discussed elsewhere.

Continued exposure of the skin to urine predisposes to its breakdown. The skin does not tolerate being wet over long periods of time as this predisposes the skin to maceration and lessens its resistance to destructive agents. In addition, with standing, urea contained in urine is decomposed by bacteria to ammonia, a highly irritating substance. When urine escapes onto the skin, prevention of irritation depends on the conscientious use of measures designed to prevent urine from coming in contact with the skin or to remove it by washing the exposed areas of the skin with soap and water and changing the bed linen promptly.

ADAPTATION AS A SOURCE OF INJURY

Earlier the capacity to adapt structure and function was discussed as a means of the survival of the individual or species. It can also be the cause of disease or injury. Among the first to make the relationship between adaptive responses and the etiology of disease was Claude Bernard. He proposed that disease could result when a response was faulty in degree or magnitude or when in correcting one defect other responses were initiated that resulted in injury. As an illustration, direct injury to cells causes an inflammation. When the inflammatory response is excessive, swelling may impede the flow of blood and tissue nutrition may be so greatly impaired that cells die from a lack of nutrients and oxygen. When a sufficient number of parenchymal cells are killed, scar tissue proliferates and as it matures it shortens. Tissues may be deprived of their blood supply and tubular organs are obstructed. As a consequence of the inflammatory process and scar tissue formation, more harm may be done to the involved organ than the initial injury caused.

As another example, hypoxia acts as a stimulus to the formation of erythrocytes. Possibly, in some instances, the disease polycythemia vera is initiated by hypoxia. The capacity to increase the number of circulating erythrocytes at high altitudes and in certain congenital defects of the heart is homeostatic. In the absence of an appropriate stimulus and when the number of cells formed is excessive and continued, the condition is maladaptive.

Another concept of the relationship of adaption to disease causation was introduced by Selye, who proposed that the organism undergoes certain stereotyped general and local adaptive reactions to injury irrespective of its cause. To the extent to which these responses are appropriate in kind and degree, they assist the sick person in coping with the injury and its effects. Although Selye classified the phases of the adaptive response to illness under different names, they have come to be called the stage of injury or the alarm reaction, the "catabolic" phase and the "anabolic" phase. (See Chapter 6 for a discussion of the response of the body to injury.) Selye further suggested that certain diseases are "diseases of adaptation." According to Selye, these diseases are not the result of some external agent such as a microbe, but they result from the inability of the body to cope with injury by appropriate adaptive responses.[63] These diseases may involve the body tissues or the structures regulating the metabolic responses to injury. Thus, in addition to the body tissues, the nervous system, the anterior hypophysis, or the adrenal cortex may be involved. Disturbances in adaptation may be manifested during any stage of its metabolic response to injury. Thus disturbances in adaptation occur during the stage of the "alarm reaction." Evidence of shock is not at all uncommon among individuals who have experienced severe injury of various types. In certain acute fulminating infections, such as an infection caused by the meningococci, the alarm reaction may be profound. On examination the adrenal cortex is found to be destroyed by hemorrhage into the cortices of both glands.

Disorders of adaptation may also occur during the other stages of the "adaptive" syndrome. Thus there are disorders of adaptation during the catabolic phase of the general adaptation syndrome. Lesions similar to, but not identical with, those induced by the injection of large doses of aldosterone into animals are observed in a great variety of human diseases. These include disseminated lupus erythematosus, diffuse collagen diseases, dermatomyositis, psoriasis, acute and chronic nephritis, ulcerative colitis, as well as in a number of allergic states such as asthma and allergic rhinitis and certain psychiatric states.

Similarly, disorders may result from failure of adaptation during the anabolic response to injury. Many patients, particularly those with wasting diseases, go through the early stages of illness satisfactorily only to falter in the anabolic (restoration-of-body-tissue) stage. The malnourished and seriously burned or injured patient may have a prolonged anabolic phase. Ill health in chronic illnesses, such as rheumatic fever or arthritis, may also be prolonged by failure to adapt during the anabolic phase of illness.

[63] Hans Selye: *The Stress of Life* (New York: McGraw-Hill Book Company, Inc., 1956), p. 128.

From the work of Selye and other investigators, there are now known to be changes occurring in the body that represent the body's reaction to injury. Inasmuch as they are appropriate in kind and degree, they facilitate survival and recovery. When they are excessive, inappropriate, or inadequate, they can be sources of disease.

IATROGENIC DISEASE

The term *iatrogenic* has its origin from *iatros,* "physician"; *iasthai,* "to cure or heal"; and *genesis,* "the beginning or origin." Therefore, iatrogenic disease is defined as disease having its origin in treatment of disease. Accordingly, bedsores are iatrogenic when they are associated with immobilization prescribed in treatment of disease. Phocomelia induced by Thalidomide is iatrogenic, as is aplasia of the bone marrow following therapy with cytoplastic drug. A single catheterization can, through injuring the mucosa of the urethra or bladder or by introducing microorganisms, result in cystitis. Illness induced by a misinterpretation or a careless remark is also a source of iatrogenic illness that can be as incapacitating as some of the structural injuries induced by physical and chemical agents. From the preceding examples, iatrogenic disease is a common event. It can occur in any situation in which disease is being treated. Nurses have a responsibility to be alert to evidence indicating adverse effects of a treatment. They also have a responsibility to observe safety precautions as indicated.

Summary

In this chapter some of the causes and effects of injury to cells have been presented. Emphasis has been on the nature of the pathological changes rather than on the agents causing the injury. Agents leading to cellular injury may have their origin in the external or the internal environment of cells or from within the cell itself. Injury to the cell may result from a deficiency of, or an excess of, or imbalance among substances required by the cell or substances useful to the organism in its activities. Cellular injury may be induced by agents interfering with machinery of the cell for utilizing nutrients or by alteration of the nature of the proteins within the cell. Within limits, cells are capable of adapting to unfavorable conditions. They do this by undergoing atrophy or hypertrophy or hyperplasia or by altering the character of cells. Furthermore, cells reverse the changes induced by injury provided the structure of the cell itself is not altered.

In relation to tissue injury, the nurse has a responsibility to prevent injury by forestalling conditions leading to further injury. The responsibilities of the nurse encompass a variety of activities ranging from public education to the direct care of the sick. Public education includes activities such as teaching how to protect children from accidental poisoning and what to do should poisoning occur or be suspected. Some of the activities in the care of the sick to prevent injury or to protect already injured tissues have been indicated. More will be included in later chapters.

REFERENCES

BOOKS (that should be useful in most chapters; they will not be repeated in other chapters)

Anderson, W. A. D. (ed.): *Pathology,* Vol. 1, 5th ed. (St. Louis: The C. V. Mosby Company, 1966).

Anderson, W. A. D., and Scottie, Thomas N.: *Synopsis of Pathology,* 7th ed. (St. Louis: The C. V. Mosby Company, 1968).

Beeson, Paul B., and McDermott, Walsh (eds.): *Cecil-Loeb Textbook of Medicine,* 12th ed. (Philadelphia: W. B. Saunders Company, 1967).

Best, C. H., and Taylor, H. B.: *The Physiological Basis of Medical Practice,* 8th ed. (Baltimore: The Williams & Wilkins Company, 1966).

Brunner, Lillian Sholtis, *et al.: Textbook of Medical-Surgical Nursing* (Philadelphia: J. B. Lippincott Company, 1964).

Crawford, T.: *Modern Trends in Pathology,* 2nd series (New York: Appleton-Century-Crofts, Inc., 1967).

Davis, Loyal (ed.): *Christopher's Textbook of Surgery,* 9th ed. (Philadelphia: W. B. Saunders Company, 1968).

Fuerst, Elinor, and Wolff, LuVerne: *Fundamentals of Nursing,* 4th ed. (Philadelphia: J. B. Lippincott Company, 1969).

Gius, John Armes: *Fundamentals of General Surgery,* 3rd ed. (Chicago: Year Book Medical Publishers, 1966).

Gordon, Malcolm S., *et al.: Animal Function: Principles and Adaptations* (New York: The Macmillan Company, 1968).

Guyton, Arthur C.: *Textbook of Medical Physiology,* 3rd ed. (Philadelphia: W. B. Saunders Company, 1966).

Harrison, T. R., *et al.* (eds.): *Principles of Internal Medicine,* 5th ed. (New York: Blakiston Division, McGraw-Hill Book Company, Inc., 1966).

Harvey, A. McGehee, *et al.* (eds.): *The Principles and Practice of Medicine,* 17th ed. (New York: Appleton-Century-Crofts, 1968).

The Health Consequences of Smoking, 1968 Supplement to 1967 Health Service Review (Washington, D.C.: U.S. Department of Health, Education, and Welfare, Public Health Service).

MacBryde, Cyril Mitchell (ed.): *Signs and Symptoms: Applied Pathologic Physiology and Clinical Interpretation,* 4th ed. (Philadelphia: J. B. Lippincott Company, 1964).

Moyer, Carl A., *et al.* (eds.): *Surgery: Principles and Practice,* 3rd ed. (Philadelphia: J. B. Lippincott Company, 1965).

The Pesticide Review, 1967 (Washington, D.C.: U.S. Department of Agriculture, Agricultural Stabilization and Conservation Service).

President's Commission on Heart Disease, Cancer and Stroke: *Report to the President,* Volumes 1 and 2 (Washington, D.C.: Superintendent of Documents, U.S. Government Printing Office, 1964 and 1965).

Report of the Advisory Committee to the Surgeon General of the Public Health Service: "Smoking and Health," *U.S. Department of Health, Education, and Welfare, Public Health Service, Public Health Service Publication* No. 1103, (Washington, D.C.: Superintendent of Documents, U.S. Government Printing Office).

Robbins, Stanley L.: *Pathology,* 3rd ed. (Philadelphia: W. B. Saunders Company, 1967).

Shafer, Kathleen Newton, *et al.: Medical-Surgical Nursing,* 4th ed. (St. Louis: The C. V. Mosby Company, 1967).

Shires, G. Tom: *Care of the Trauma Patient* (New York: The Blakiston Division, McGraw-Hill Book Company, Inc., 1966).

Smith, Dorothy W., and Gips, Claudia D.: *Care of the Adult Patient,* 2nd ed. (Philadelphia: W. B. Saunders Company, 1967).

Sodeman, William A., and Sodeman, William A., Jr. *Pathologic Physiology,* 4th ed. (Philadelphia: W. B. Saunders Company, 1967).

Talso, Peter J., and Remenchick, Alexander P.: *Internal Medicine* (St. Louis: The C. V. Mosby Company, 1968).

BOOKS (more or less specific to this chapter)

Buschke, Franz (ed.): *Progress in Radiation Therapy,* Vol. 3 (New York: Grune & Stratton, Inc., 1965).

Lifton, Robert: *Death in Life: Survivors of Hiroshima* (New York: Random House, 1968).

Moss, William T.: *Therapeutic Radiology* (St. Louis: The C. V. Mosby Company, 1965).

PERIODICALS

Decubiti

Merlino, Anthony F.: "Decubitus Ulcers: Cause, Prevention and Treatment," *Geriatrics,* 24:119–24 (Mar.) 1969.

Silver, Christine: "Prevention of Pressure Sores," *Nurs. Mirror,* 126:22, 25 (Mar. 1) 1968.

Electrical Injuries

Battig, Charles G.: "Electrosurgical Burn Injuries and Their Prevention," *JAMA,* 204:1025–29 (June 17) 1968.

Environmental Hazards

Abelson, Philip H.: "Progress Toward Abatement of Air Pollution," *Science,* 160:257 (Apr. 19) 1968.

Abelson, Philip H.: "How Man Shapes His Environment," *Amer. J. Public Health,* 58:2043–49 (Nov.) 1968.

Ashenburg, Norman J.: "The Effects of Air Pollution on Health," *Nurs. Outlook,* 16:22–25 (Feb.) 1968.

Baron, Robert Alex: "Noise and Urban Man," *Amer. J. Public Health,* 58:2060–66 (Nov.) 1968.

Goldman, Stanford: "Aging, Noise and Choice," *Perspect. Biol. Med.,* 12:12–30 (Autumn) 1968.

Sanderson, James T.: "Occupational Noise," *Occup. Health,* 18:61–71 (Mar.–Apr.) 1966.

Stead, Frank M.: "II. What Man Can Do Technologically To Restore His Environment," *Amer. J. Public Health,* 58:2050–59 (Nov.) 1968.

Toxic Chemicals

"Alcoholism in Industry and Family," *Lancet* 2:1179 (Nov. 30) 1968.

Abrams, Arnold, Gagnon, John H., and Levin, Joseph J.: "Psychosocial Aspects of Drug Addiction," *Amer. J. Public Health,* 58:2142–55 (Nov.) 1968.

Editorial: "Disease Drugs Cause," *New Eng. J. Med.,* 279:1286–87 (Dec. 5) 1968.

Edwards, Clive A.: "Soil Pollutants and Soil Animals," *Sci. Amer.,* 220:88–99 (Apr.) 1969.

Fishbein, Morris: "The Problem Drinker," *Postgrad. Med.,* 41:232 (Feb.) 1967.

Horn, Daniel: "Current Smoking Among Teenagers," *Public Health Rep.,* 83:458–60 (June) 1968.

Hyman, Samuel, and Greengard, Joseph: "Self-Poisoning and Accidental Poisoning," *Postgrad. Med.,* 41:578–84 (June) 1967.

Johnson, Paul E.: "Health Aspects of Food Additives," *Amer. J. Public Health,* 56:948–51 (June) 1966.

Knott, David H., Beard, James D., and Wallace, James A.: "Acute Withdrawal from Alcohol," *Postgrad. Med.,* 42:A109–A114 (Dec.) 1967.

Owens, John, *et al.:* "Nursing the Drug Addict," *Nurs. Times,* 64:584–85 (May 3) 1968.

Pattison, E. Mansell: "Differential Diagnosis of Alcoholism," *Postgrad. Med.,* 41:A127–A132 (June) 1967.

Poplar, Jimmie F.: "Characteristics of Nurse Addicts," *Amer. J. Nurs.,* **69**:117–19 (Jan.) 1969.

Rubin, E., *et al.:* "Alcohol, Other Drugs, and the Liver," *Ann. Intern. Med.,* **69**:1063–67 (Nov.) 1968.

Samter, Max, and Beers, Ray F.: "Intolerance to Aspirin," *Ann. Intern. Med.,* **68**:975–83 (May) 1968.

Sapira, Joseph D.: "The Narcotic Addict as a Medical Patient," *Amer. J. Med.,* **45**:555–88 (Oct.) 1968.

Schafer, M. L.: "Pesticides in Blood," *Residue Rev.,* **24**:19–39, 1968.

Soto, A. R. and Deichmann, W. B.: "Major Metabolism and Acute Toxicity of Aldrin, Dieldrin and Endrin," *Environ. Res.,* **1**:307–22 (Dec.) 1967.

Waller, J. A.: "Holiday Drinking and Highway Fatalities," *JAMA,* **206**:2693–97 (Dec. 16) 1968.

Irradiation

Croft, D. N.: "Radioisotopes in Clinical Medicine," *Nurs. Times,* **64**:1416–18 (Oct. 18) 1968.

Jamison, Andrew: "Irradiated Foods: FDA Blocks AEC, Army Requests for Approval," *Science,* **161**:146–48 (July 12) 1968.

Kautz, Harold D., *et al.:* "Radioactive Drugs," *Amer. J. Nurs.,* **64**:124–28 (Jan.) 1964.

Levin, Sheldon G., and Stoms, Richard K.: "Natural Background Gamma Radiation Dose Rate Measurements in Michigan, Colorado, and Minnesota," *Amer. J. Public Health,* **59**:102–109 (Jan.) 1969.

Little, John B.: "Environmental Hazards: Ionizing Radiation," *New Eng. J. Med.,* **275**:929–38 (Oct. 27) 1966.

Little, John B.: "Cellular Effects of Ionizing Radiation," *New Eng. J. Med.,* **278**:308–15 and 369–76 (Feb. 8 and 15) 1968.

Mangan, Helen M.: "Care, Coordination and Communication in the Life Island Setting," *Nurs. Outlook,* **17**:40–44 (Jan.) 1969.

"Radiation," *World Health,* pp. 3–29 (Jan.) 1969.

"Radioactive Pollution: Minnesota Funds A.E.C. Standards Too Lax," *Science,* **163**:1043–44 (Mar. 7) 1969.

Raventos, Antolin: "X-Rays in Pregnancy," *Amer. J. Nurs.,* **66**:1308–11 (June) 1966.

Wares, Elizabeth: "Cathetron," *Nurs. Times,* **64**:1585–87 (Nov. 22) 1968.

Welsh, Marian S.: "Comfort Measures During Radiation Therapy," *Amer. J. Nurs.,* **67**:1880–82 (Sept.) 1967.

Trauma

Curry, George J., McLaughlin, Harrison L., and Murphy, James Peter: "The Severely Injured Patient," *Postgrad. Med.,* **42**:291–97 (Oct.) 1967.

Jarvinen, Klaus A., and Jarvinen, Päivi H.: "Falling from Bed as a Complication of Hospital Treatment," *J. Chronic Dis.,* **21**:375–78 (Aug.) 1968.

Jolles, Keith E.: "First Aid for Road Casualties," *Nurs. Times,* **64**:886–89 (July 5) 1968.

Kossuth, Louis C.: "Immediate Care to Vehicle Accident Victims," *Postgrad. Med.,* **41**:407–13 (Apr.) 1967.

Markush, Robert E., *et al.:* "Motor Vehicle Accidents in the United States (1906–1964)," *JAMA,* **203**:88–94 (Jan. 8) 1968.

"Road Accidents," *World Health,* pp. 3–35 (Feb.) 1969.

Thomas, Sally: "Fat Embolism—A Hazard of Trauma," *Nurs. Times,* **65**:105–108 (Jan.) 1969.

Worman, Leonard W., Yount, Carol J., and Jacobs, Lois E.: "The Care of Patients with Gunshot Wounds," *Amer. J. Nurs.,* **63**:93–96 (Feb.) 1963.

OTHER

"Symposium on Stones," *Amer. J. Med.,* **45**:649–783 (Nov.) 1968.

5

The Control of Infections

From the most ancient times peoples have taken measures to protect themselves against the introduction of diseases from without. Among the most elaborate codes of this kind in the written history of man are the regulations enunciated in the Hebrew scriptures, chiefly in the Book of Leviticus.*

Overview

What are some of the general characteristics of infectious diseases?

What are the nurse's responsibilities in the control of infectious disease?

History of Infectious Diseases and Control Efforts

Man and Microorganism: The Concept of Ecological Equilibrium

What are some of the causes and effects of disturbing the ecological equilibrium between man and microorganisms?

What are some of the factors influencing host susceptibility?

The Pathogenic Microorganism

What information about a pathogenic microorganism is required to control its spread?

After microorganisms are established, how do they cause disease?

What are some of the factors in the environment that bring the agent and the host together?

Transmission of Infectious Disease

The Course and Control of Infectious Disease

What are the stages in the course of an infectious disease?

What are some of the characteristic manifestations in acute infectious disease?

What kinds of activities or procedures are required for the control of acute infectious diseases?

The Planning of Nursing Care for Patients with Infectious Diseases

How are viruses classified? What are some of the characteristic responses to viral invasion?

What are some of the implications of the physical and chemical characteristics of viruses to nursing?

Overview

MAN lives in a world populated with many forms of life, some of which threaten his existence. Not all living forms are directly visible, though their effects can be observed. Neither are all forms of invisible life, or microbes, harmful. As a matter of fact, relatively few microorganisms are harmful or disease-producing. Many are highly beneficial to man. Although disease-producing agents are regarded as enemies, they are as much a part of nature as man.

Disease-producing organisms are called pathogens, and the diseases they cause are called infectious diseases. Authorities once defined infection as a condition resulting from the

entrance of microorganisms into the tissues of the body causing injury and subsequently tissue reactions. The term *infection* indicates that microbes are present in the body and multiplying. There does not have to be evidence of pathology.

What are some of the general characteristics of infectious diseases?

Although infectious diseases have a number of similar characteristics, they are also very different from one another. One characteristic common to all is that a pathogenic microorganism is a necessary condition to the development of disease. It may or may not be sufficient to cause disease, however. The microorganism may be a virus, rickettsia, bacterium, yeast, mold, protozoan, or other parasite. The microbe is capable of being transmitted from a reservoir,

---

* *World Health,* 11:7 "Photo Essay: First Report on the World Health Situation," (Nov.–Dec.). 1958.

usually another human being, but it may be an animal, to a susceptible host. The infectious disease may occur with great frequency and be readily transmissible, such as the common cold, or it may occur infrequently and only under special conditions. It may be self-limiting, that is, run a relatively predictable course and be self-terminating; or it may have no point at which it terminates naturally but continues indefinitely. It may induce a more or less permanent immunity or be characterized by repeated attacks. The infectious process may be relatively mild or wreak great destruction. For some reason not understood, different microorganisms have a predilection for specific organs or tissues of the body. The period of time required by different microorganisms to establish themselves in the body and induce disease varies from hours to many months and possibly years.

Despite emphasis in the past on the necessary condition, the germ, it is now known that an equally significant factor is the susceptibility of the host. Susceptibility to some infectious diseases can be lessened by vaccines and other immunizing agents.

Communicable disease is an illness caused by a specific infectious agent or its toxic products that is transmitted directly or indirectly from an infected person or animal to a susceptible host.

Carrier is an apparently well person in whom pathogenic microorganisms live and multiply without apparent ill effect.

Contamination indicates the presence of pathogenic or disease-producing microorganisms on inanimate objects. The term *contamination* is often used to indicate the possibility rather than the known presence of microorganisms.

Endemic means that a disease is continuously present in a community.

Epidemic is a temporary and significant increase in the incidence of a disease at a given time.

Nosocomial infection is an infectious disease arising within the hospital or other institution.

Pandemic is a world-wide epidemic.

Sporadic means that disease occurs occasionally and its incidence is low.[1]

What are the nurse's responsibilities in the control of infectious disease?

In this chapter, information has been selected to further the understanding of the nurse of some of the important problems involved in the control of diseases caused by microorganisms.

No attempt will be made to describe in detail all the infectious diseases to which man is heir. Four diseases that are problems in the United States will be used to illustrate points being made, but not all information about each disease will be included. Emphasis is on the prevention and control of an infectious disease rather than on the care of the patient who is sick. The nursing of the person who is ill with an infectious disease has two general aspects, the care of the person who is sick and the prevention of the spread of disease to the nurse and others. As in the control of infectious disease in the community, measures employed can be classified as:[2]

1. Preventing spread
2. Increasing the resistance of the new host
3. Minimizing the ill effects of cases that have not been prevented

To fulfill her responsibilities in the control of infectious disease the nurse requires a body of knowledge that will enable her to

1. Keep abreast with changes in knowledge of the factors in the control of infectious disease
2. Develop procedures and practices based on the knowledge required for the protection of patients, personnel (including self), and the community
3. Evaluate, or participate in the evaluation of, practices employed in the control of infectious disease
4. Accept changes in established procedures when change or changes are indicated
5. Carry out procedures that are for the protection of all concerned
6. Develop and/or participate in the hospital or agency educational program
7. Participate in the hospital or agency program to control infection:
   7.1 By identifying problems in the control of infection
   7.2 As a participating member of the committee on infections
      7.21 Report to the committee problems in the control of infections
      7.22 Report to the nursing staff the deliberations of the committee
      7.23 Make suggestions in the committee on the problems and possible solutions
   7.3 By making suggestions to the nurse member of the committee on the prob-

---

[1] For a more complete list of definitions of terms relating to infectious disease, see John E. Gordon (ed.): *Control of Communicable Diseases in Man,* 10th ed. (New York: The American Public Health Association, 1965), pp. 13–22.

[2] Gaylord W. Anderson, Margaret G. Arnstein, and Mary R. Lester: *Communicable Disease Control,* 4th ed. (New York: The Macmillan Company, 1962), p. 47.

lems and proposing suggestions as to
how the problems might be solved
8. Recognize that in the present state of
knowledge the control of some of the
troublesome infections is complex
   8.1 Be prepared and willing to cooperate in
   investigating the source of infections
   and in correcting conditions that appear
   to be responsible
9. Act as a case finder
10. Participate in community programs of
prevention
11. Participate in the education of the public
in supporting the rational use of antimicrobial agents

Anderson and Himmelsbach [3] emphasize that
effective infection control depends on continuing and unwavering practice of medical asepsis.
Furthermore, Anderson and Himmelsbach,[4]
Streeter, Dunn, and Lepper,[5] and other authorities recommend that a nurse be assigned the
responsibility of infection surveillance. Responsibilities of the surveillance or infection-control
nurse include such activities as case finding; the
collection and analysis of data about the incidence, location, and other factors relating to
infection; inspection of the environment; education of personnel; and institution of preventive measures. In other words, this nurse spends
her entire time in case finding and in developing
and instituting measures designed to keep the
hospital infection rate at a minimum. In addition, this nurse might well be held responsible
for determining whether or not patients have
been immunized for smallpox and other diseases that can be prevented by vaccines and
other immunizing agents.

An important part of the work of nurses
employed by schools, health departments, and
visiting nurse associations is case finding and
the prevention of infectious disease.

The preceding is indeed an imposing list of
responsibilities. To fulfill them, the nurse requires knowledge, experience, interest in learning, and a willingness to alter her practice when
new discoveries indicate the need for change.
In addition, the effective control of an infectious
disease frequently depends not on the nurse
alone or on a single measure but on the cooperation of a large proportion of the community
and a variety of procedures.

One of the essential elements in the effective
control of infectious disease is application of the

concept: A change in practice is difficult if not
impossible to effect, unless the person who desires to bring it about understands what the
beliefs and values are that support existing
practices. Understanding of this concept is important in the United States because of the
diverse character of the population. Furthermore, more and more nurses are traveling to
distant lands to assist people to improve their
health practices. Because not all persons have
the same beliefs or system of values, one of the
elements in the success of nurses working with
peoples from different cultures is the ability to
put into practice this concept.

History of Infectious Diseases and Control Efforts

Throughout the course of history, five infectious diseases—plague, smallpox, cholera,
typhus, and yellow fever—have been the great
killers. None has been entirely eradicated, as
there are pockets of infection for each of them
in various parts of the world. As long as reservoirs of infection remain, there is always the
possibility that one of the preceding diseases
can become epidemic.[6] Egypt has experienced
four sizable epidemics of typhus. The latest one
began in 1956.

In 1959 when a world-wide smallpox eradication program was initiated, there were 81,444
cases reported. The number has fluctuated since
then, with 99,599 cases in 1964. According to
WHO figures, the number of cases in 1968 was
68,023. Smallpox is endemic in six countries of
Asia, almost all of Africa, and Brazil, Colombia,
and Peru.[7] Although not included as one of the
great killers in history, diphtheria has also been
responsible for the deaths of large numbers of
persons. As with other infectious diseases,
control of diphtheria depends on the continued
application of appropriate measures including
the immunization of susceptible persons with
toxoid.[8]

Infectious Diseases of the Present

Among the infectious diseases having a high
morbidity rate in the United States are some of
the acute infectious diseases of childhood (such
as mumps and chickenpox), acute infections of

[3] Louise C. Anderson and Clifton K. Himmelsbach:
"The Nurse: First Line of Defense Against Infections,"
Hospitals, 41:84–98 (Oct. 1) 1967.
   [4] *Ibid.*, pp. 88–98.
   [5] Shirley Streeter, Helen Dunn, and Mark Lepper:
"Hospital Infection—A Necessary Risk?" *Amer. J.
Nurs.*, 67:527 (Mar.) 1967.

   [6] "WHO, What It Is, What It Does, How It Works,"
World Health, 15:4 (July–Aug.) 1962.
   [7] World Health Organization: "Nineteenth World
Health Assembly—2," *WHO Chron.*, 20:276–77 (Aug.)
1966.
   [8] Toxoid is a toxin altered by removing its toxo-
phore but retaining its immunogenic group. In other
words, a toxoid is antigenic. It immunizes against a
toxin but is nontoxic to the recipient.

the respiratory system (the common cold, influenza, pneumonia), acute infections involving the gastrointestinal system, and infectious hepatitis. Other more serious infectious diseases include syphilis, gonorrhea, tuberculosis, staphylococcal infections, and infections caused by the normal inhabitants of the alimentary canal. Rheumatic fever, though not directly caused by the group A beta-hemolytic streptococci, is the most important sequela of this infection.

Diseases that have not been problems in the United States may be introduced by men returning from Vietnam. They include malaria, diarrheal diseases, melioidosis, tropical sprue, plague, arbovirus infections, dengue, leptospirosis, intestinal parasites, and other tropical diseases.[9]

In other regions of the world, factors such as climate predispose to, or eliminate, the possibility of diseases such as malaria. Although there is a large number of infectious diseases, a few are of great significance because they affect a large number of people and have serious effects. In terms not only of the number of people involved but also of its debilitating effects, malaria continues to be a health problem in some parts of the world. According to the "Little Dictionary of Infectious Diseases," [10] 250 million people had malaria in 1955 and 140 million had it in 1962. In 1958, Ethiopia experienced an epidemic of malaria. Three million of the population of 18 million had the disease and 100,000 persons died. Most of those who were sick were between the ages of 5 and 20 years, but some were younger. In some families, every member was ill.[11] By 1965, 77 per cent of persons who had lived in malarious areas were living where malaria had been eradicated or where eradication [12] was in progress.[13]

In Tanzania, 23,000 people are preventing malaria by replacing ordinary table salt with salt containing 1.38 per cent chloroquine.[14]

Not only is the mosquito a vector for the malarial parasite, but it requires the mosquito for part of its life cycle. In eradication projects, attempts have been made to eliminate the mosquito by spraying malarious areas with insecticides such as DDT (dichlorodiphenyltrichloroethane). Unfortunately, some mosquitoes have become resistant to DDT, thus greatly complicating the problem of eradication. Further, some of the *P. falciparum* strains have become resistant to the 4-aminoquinolines.

Even when malaria has been brought under control, keeping it under control is a continuous process. The mosquitoes that are a necessary intermediary in its transmission remain. Travelers, either citizens or foreigners, who are infected can serve as reservoirs. It is not always possible to identify malaria carriers, as some may carry the parasites as long as 30 years. With or without manifestations of overt disease, there may be infectious parasites in the blood.

Among other diseases causing ill health and disability are leprosy, trachoma, yaws, and onchocerciasis, or river blindness. There are approximately 10 million persons throughout the world who have leprosy. About 500 million persons have trachoma, which causes total blindness in about 1 per cent of its victims and economic blindness in about 4 per cent. Yaws is a widespread disfiguring disease affecting large numbers of people in Asia. Onchocerciasis is caused by a minute worm transmitted to man by a black fly. When these worms invade the eye, they cause blindness. Some 200 to 300 million people are believed to be infected.[15]

Africa has all the diseases known elsewhere and one or two all her own. Malaria exists almost everywhere, yaws and smallpox are not yet eradicated, tuberculosis is widespread, leprosy yields slowly to modern methods of treatment, pockets of sleeping sickness still remain, while parasitic diseases such as schistosomiasis and onchocerciasis tend to increase. Children from one to five years of age die in great numbers from infections and diseases due to malnutrition. Only in parts of the cities is there a piped supply of safe water or adequate facilities for the disposal of human wastes.[16]

The purpose of presenting this brief survey of some of the more important infectious diseases in the world of today is not to provide the nurse with the information required to work in a program of control but to emphasize that infectious diseases continue to be a real threat. They are important as causes not only of mortality but of serious degrees of morbidity. In areas where diseases such as malaria and bilharziasis are endemic, progress in raising standards of living is impeded because of the large number of people who are affected with these serious and debilitating diseases.

[9] David N. Gilbert *et al.;* "Potential Medical Problems in Personnel Returning from Vietnam," *Ann. Intern. Med.,* **68:**662 (Mar.) 1968.

[10] "Little Dictionary of Infectious Diseases," *World Health,* **15:**5 (July–Aug.) 1962.

[11] "Malaria Epidemic Strikes in Ethiopia," *World Health,* **13:**39 (May–June) 1960.

[12] The objective of eradication is to wipe out, or abolish, an infectious disease. In contrast, the objective of control is to prevent a disease from becoming a problem, that is, epidemic.

[13] World Health Organization: "Malaria Eradication in 1965," *WHO Chron.,* **20:**286 (Aug.) 1966.

[14] "Around the World: Salt Against Malaria," *World Health,* (Mar.) 1969, p. 34.

[15] "Little Dictionary of Infectious Diseases," *op. cit.,* p. 5.

[16] "The Crucial Problem," *World Health,* **21:**6 (July) 1968.

For a variety of reasons, the incidence of specific infectious diseases varies from one part of the world to another. Because of similarities in sanitary procedures, standards of living and medical care, and climate, similar diseases are problems in the United States and western Europe. Diseases caused by inadequate sanitation, such as typhoid fever, cholera, and dysentery, have been brought under control. Experience indicates, however, that any real lapse in the application of methods of control can result in an outbreak of typhoid fever or of any infectious disease that has been controlled.

Discoveries Contributing to Reduced Incidence of Certain Infectious Diseases and Increases in Others

In the nineteenth and twentieth centuries, a variety of discoveries has contributed to the reduction in the incidence of infectious disease. In some instances the problem of control of some diseases has increased. Included among the more important discoveries are the following:

1. Sanitary measures could effectively control the spread of enteric diseases.
2. A necessary condition in the etiology of some diseases is a germ.
3. Techniques have been developed to identify many but not all microbes.
4. Immunity to some diseases can be induced:
   a. By injecting antibodies specific for the disease (temporary or passive immunity).
   b. By introducing antigenic substances (active acquired immunity).
   c. By having the disease (active acquired immunity).
5. Some diseases can be cured by antimicrobial agents. For example, penicillin cures syphilis.
6. Some diseases are transmitted by an insect vector, and in some instances the microbe also spends part of its life cycle in the insect.
7. Discovery and use of measures to eliminate insect and animal reservoirs.
8. Improvement in living conditions, including nutrition and improved housing, has enhanced resistance or decreased exposure to some infectious diseases.
9. Some germs have developed resistance not only to one but to a number of antimicrobial agents.
10. Some pathogenic microorganisms inhabit carriers and can be disseminated to susceptible persons and cause disease.
11. Some airborne diseases are spread by droplets and others by droplet nuclei.

All of the above are of significance in any program of control of infectious disease. Each will be considered later in relation to the control of specific microorganisms.

Man and Microorganism: The Concept of Ecological Equilibrium

Despite a large body of knowledge about microbial agents and how they reach their potential hosts, many questions remain to be answered. Among the most intriguing questions to be answered are the following: Why was the incidence of some infectious diseases decreasing before the advent of specific immunizing and microbial agents? Why can organisms which are usually nonpathogenic cause disease? Why can virulent pathogenic agents be present in the tissues of man and not at the same time be accompanied by evidence of clinical disease? Though the answers to these questions are still incomplete, enough is known to be able to say with confidence that infectious diseases are similar to many other diseases; their development depends on the host, the etiological agent or agents, and the factors in the environment that bring the agent and host together.

Before a healthy baby enters the birth canal, he is free of microorganisms. Beginning with birth and continuing throughout his lifetime he acquires, and develops a relationship with, a variety of microorganisms. Depending on the host and microbe, their relationship varies all the way from one of mutual benefit to the production of serious disease in the host. The state in which a host and microbe live in a mutually beneficial relationship is known as symbiosis. For example, microorganisms living in the alimentary canal obtain their nutrients from its contents. They also synthesize vitamin K, a nutrient their human host cannot synthesize. The relationship is symbiotic because man and microbe both profit from the arrangement.

A second type of relationship between the host and his microorganisms is called commensalism. The microorganisms are dependent on the host, but they neither injure nor benefit it. The microorganisms of the normal flora in the gastrointestinal tract have been generally classified as commensals. Though these organisms are generally harmless, there is increasing evidence that under certain conditions they can cause infectious disease. According to McDermott,[17] the microorganisms forming the normal flora of the gastrointestinal tract are more important in the cause of infectious disease than

[17] Walsh McDermott: "Inapparent Infection: Relation of Latent and Dormant Infections to Microbial Persistence," *Public Health Rep.*, 74:498 (June) 1959.

is the *Staphylococcus*. Apparently the condition of the host is an essential factor in determining the type of relationship between it and the commensals.

A third type of relationship is known as **parasitism**. In this relationship, one organism derives significant benefit from the other. In the instances in which the commensals cause disease, they become parasitic. Of the organisms living in a parasitic relationship with the host, some are able to live independent of the host as well as with it. These are known as facultative parasites. Staphylococci and streptococci are examples of facultative parasites. Other microorganisms are dependent on the host for survival and for propagation. They are known as obligatory parasites. An example is the *Treponema pallidum*. It dies very quickly after leaving the body; it has never been cultivated, with certainty, outside the human body.

What are some of the causes and effects of disturbing the ecological equilibrium between man and microorganisms?

The relationship existing between man and his microbes is an excellent example of the concept that adaptation is basic to survival. As a result of adaptations, both man and microorganisms exist in a state of ecological equilibrium. Anything tending to disturb the equilibrium in favor of man (the host) leads to a reduction in the incidence of disease. Any disturbance in the state of equilibrium favoring the microorganism increases the incidence of disease. Survival of the microbe depends on its maintaining and reproducing itself without destroying its host. Microorganisms have been successful in doing this. For example, when a group of people are exposed to a microorganism for the first time, both the attack and mortality rates are high. In a group who has lived with the same microorganism for a long time, both the attack and the mortality rates tend to be low. The late Theobold Smith summarized this point in a much quoted statement, "Whenever you find a parasite that has affected a given host over a long period of time, you will find that the infection does not interfere with the survival of the host and is of low virulence." Dubos [18] cites a number of examples of populations that suffered great losses on their first exposure to smallpox. After smallpox was introduced into North America, whole villages of Indians were decimated. Historians believe that had it not been for smallpox and other acute communicable diseases the Indians would have been able to resist colonization more effectively than they did.

[18] René Dubos: *Mirage of Health* (New York: Harper and Brothers, 1959), p. 78.

The results of the adaptation of man to his microbes, and vice versa, are also illustrated by the effects of tuberculosis among successive generations of Indians living on the Qu Appelle Valley Reservation.[19] In the first and second generations, many individuals experienced acute forms of the disease. By the third generation, though the disease was still epidemic, it showed a tendency to localize in the lung. Glandular involvement, a manifestation of high susceptibility, had fallen to 7 per cent. In the fourth generation, evidence of tuberculosis occurred in less than 1 per cent of the schoolchildren. When an ecological equilibrium develops between two living organisms, it is not permanent. Thus the incidence may be altered at any time by a change in the susceptibility of the host or in the virulence of the microorganism.

Interest in the factors influencing the ecological equilibrium between the host and his microorganisms has been stimulated by a number of observations. The incidence of diseases caused by microorganisms that were once believed to be relatively harmless has risen greatly. Microbes that were once susceptible to antimicrobial agents are now resistant to them. More attention is being paid to the observation that, in some individuals, the host is an important factor in whether or not an infection develops and in its outcome. Therefore a question that is being asked with increasing frequency is, "Why does the host develop or resist disease?" Perhaps one of the reasons that this question has been neglected is that it is a difficult one to answer—another is that man prefers to look outside himself for answers to troublesome questions.

Man has for centuries been able to alter his external environment and adapt it to his needs. Now he is able to alter his internal environment as well. Through the use of antimicrobial agents, he is able to change the nature of the normal flora of his body.

All living organisms live in ecological equilibrium with other living organisms. This concept is as true of microorganisms as of multicellular plants and animals. The members of an ecological system live in competition with each other. Competition is particularly keen for food. The growth and multiplication of one species may suppress the growth and multiplication of another species. For example, despite the bad reputation of the fox as a chicken thief, he functions in nature to control the population of rodents. When, because of disease or overhunting, the fox population is decreased excessively, the population of rodents rises. When, in contrast, the population of foxes exceeds the supply

[19] *Ibid.*, p. 71.

of food, they become susceptible to disease and raid neighborhood chicken yards. Death from starvation also helps to reduce their number.

In the gastrointestinal tract many microorganisms live in a state of equilibrium not only with their host but with each other. Apparently, when this equilibrium is not disturbed, the growth of some species tends to suppress that of others. Exactly how this is accomplished is only beginning to be understood. When the balance among the microorganisms is disturbed, some species may grow and multiply in excess and may therefore cause disease. For example, the tetracycline antibiotics inhibit the growth and multiplication of the gram-negative bacteria forming part of the normal flora of the intestinal feces. Tetracycline-resistant organisms include yeasts, fecal streptococci, *Proteus,* and *Pseudomonas.* There are instances reported in the literature in which death was caused by *Candida albicans,* a yeast. As the bacterial count diminishes, the microorganisms resistant to the tetracyclines flourish and the total count of microbes may actually increase. Sprunt and Redman [20] obtained evidence to support the hypothesis that the interrelationships among the microbes in the nasopharynx act to maintain the status quo. Previous to antibiotic therapy, the nasopharynxes of patients studied were found to be colonized with alpha streptococci. After therapy was started, the streptococci disappeared and were replaced by other potential pathogens such as *Pseudomonas aeruginosa,* staphylococci, and slow-growing gram-positive coccibacilli. When the antimicrobial therapy was stopped, the streptococci returned, indicating that alpha streptococci inhibit the growth of other bacteria. In the nasopharynx, alpha streptococci are commensals. Located in other parts of the body, such as the heart valves, they are pathogens.

In a paper titled "Inapparent Infection," McDermott suggests two other possibilities for the increase in the incidence of certain infections.[21] During his lifetime, man acquires and carries certain microorganisms. Some of these organisms may be in a dormant or in a latent state. McDermott distinguishes between dormant and latent infections as follows: In a dormant infection the microorganisms can be demonstrated to be present, but they are not causing disease. Carriers of *Salmonella typhosa* and *paratyphi* and *Corynebacterium diphtheriae* are classic examples. McDermott also suggests that the organisms comprising the respiratory and intestinal flora, the so-called commensals,

may also be viewed as dormant infections. McDermott uses the term *latent infection* for situations in which organisms cannot be demonstrated by methods now available but in which overt disease later develops. A familiar example is that of herpes simplex (cold sores). The virus remains within the cells of the body. Cold sores appear only when conditions are right, that is, when the person has a fever, is overexposed to sunlight, or is menstruating.[22]

Tuberculosis sometimes recurs in persons who have been "cured" of the disease. Although the recurrence may be a new infection, it is thought that it is usually a reactivation of the previous infection. McDermott believes that microorganisms are able to assume a state in which they are protected from the effects of microbial drugs.[23] In this state the presence of microorganisms in the tissue cannot be demonstrated. However, the protective state allows them to survive. When conditions again favor their resuming the vegetative state, they do so. Perhaps one of the reasons for the increasing incidence of tuberculosis among people over 50 years of age is that the microorganism was acquired earlier in their lives. At the time the tubercle bacillus entered the body it assumed a latent state. Later when the condition of the host was favorable, the *Mycobacterium tuberculosis* multiplied and caused active disease. Though tuberculosis has been used as an example, this capacity to assume a protective state is not limited to the *Mycobacterium tuberculosis.* All the reasons for microorganisms going into the dormant or latent state are not known. In some instances drug therapy may be a factor. The capacity to become latent is an adaptation enabling microorganisms to survive.

What are some of the factors influencing host susceptibility?

As stated previously, three factors are involved in the development of an infectious disease. They are the host, the microbe, and the environment that brings the host and microbe together.

DEFINITIONS

Susceptibility can be defined as conditions making an individual more or less liable to a condition or disease. Conversely, *resistance* decreases his liability. From observation some people appear to be more and others less susceptible to certain diseases than others. What actually constitutes susceptibility is not well understood.

Although host factors were known to play

---

[20] Katherine Sprunt and Winifred Redman: "Evidence Suggesting Importance of Role of Interbacterial Inhibition in Maintaining Balance of Normal Flora," *Ann. Intern. Med.,* 68:579–90 (Mar.) 1968.

[21] McDermott, *op. cit.,* pp. 485–89.

[22] *Ibid.,* p. 489.

[23] *Ibid.,* p. 490.

a part, in the past emphasis has been placed on the number and virulence of germs as the significant factor. With the use of immunosuppressive and cytotoxic drugs in organ transplants and in the treatment of cancer, it has been learned that almost any microbe can cause disease if the defensive physiological responses are sufficiently depressed. Thus coliforms, diphtheroids, yeasts, and other organisms that are usually nonpathogenic cause endogenous infections. To reemphasize, a microbe is a necessary condition in the development of an infectious disease. Whether it is "sufficient" to cause disease depends on the relationship of host, germ, and environment. To express the relationship of host and germ, Stewart[24] rewrites Theobald Smith's equation:

$$\frac{\text{Severity of}}{\text{disease}} = \frac{\text{Number} \times \text{virulence of organisms}}{\text{Susceptibility of host}}$$

The three elements—host, germ, and environment—might be expressed as three circles, as in Figure 5-1.

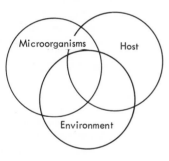

FIGURE 5-1. Overlapping elements in disease causation.

Among the factors in host susceptibility are heredity, state of nutrition, hormonal balance, age, sex, the integrity of the host's defense mechanisms, other diseases, as well as competitive microflora colonizing the skin and alimentary canal. *Commensals* may "starve out" or suppress virulent germs. Susceptibility to disease also depends on the past experience of the individual with a given microorganism or its antigens.

Host resistance to a number of important infectious diseases can be increased by vaccines and other immunizing agents. The nurse should keep herself informed about which diseases can be prevented and the schedule required to maintain immunity to each. The nurse as well as the

physician has a responsibility to determine the immune status of individuals under their care. This responsibility is not limited to nurses employed in well-baby clinics and schools but applies to all nurses. The nurse should act on the dictum that the best form of treatment of any disease is its prevention.

HEREDITY

Most of the information about genetic factors in immunity comes from animal experiments. Susceptibility to and the type of lesion developed in tuberculosis differ from one animal species to another. Susceptible or resistant strains of animals have been developed by inbreeding. Among human beings, the sickle cell trait offers some protection against malaria. Studies of twins indicate the possibility of a genetic factor in tuberculosis. When one of a pair of heterozygous twins develops tuberculosis, the chances of the other twin having it is 1 in 3. In homozygous twins the chances are 3 out of 4.[25]

NUTRITIONAL STATUS

An association between nutritional status and the incidence of certain infections is well known. The lack of resistance particularly to skin infections of the poorly controlled diabetic patient is common knowledge. Ischemia predisposes to infection of tissues. The observation that the incidence of certain infections rises when the nutritional level of a group falls is well documented. During both World Wars I and II the incidence of tuberculosis in Europe rose. Following each war, the incidence fell.[26] Although undernutrition was only one of the factors, the diseases that were common in the concentration camps in Europe during World War II were skin ailments, bronchopneumonia, staphylococcal infections, and pulmonary tuberculosis.[27] These conditions were caused by the microorganisms that were common in the European community. The conditions under which the people lived combined to reduce their resistance and render them susceptible to the microbes with which they lived. Following the war many of these people improved with little or no treatment. In other words, balance between man and his microorganisms was restored so that they could live together in a state of peaceful coexistence.

[24] G. T. Stewart: "Limitations of the Germ Theory," *Lancet*, 1:1079 (May 18) 1968.

[25] *Ibid.*, p. 1080.
[26] Bernard D. Davis *et al.: Microbiology* (New York: Harper & Row Publishers, 1968), p. 853.
[27] René J. Dubos and James Hirsch: *Bacterial and Mycotic Infections in Man,* 4th ed. (Philadelphia: J. B. Lippincott Company, 1965), p. 22.

HORMONAL BALANCE

Cortisone and its related analogues diminish resistance to tuberculosis probably by suppressing the inflammatory response. The use of cortisone in the treatment of a variety of diseases is believed by some authorities to contribute to the increase in infections caused by microbes of the normal flora. Persons whose adrenal cortices hypersecrete the glucocorticoids also have an increased susceptibility to infection.

AGE

With a few exceptions, resistance to disease develops with age. Prophylactic immunization of infants is ineffective for about two months. Babies are temporarily protected by antibodies from their mothers. By the time children have reached puberty, they have developed an immunity to many diseases. Although youngsters become immunized to a number of diseases by the age of puberty, this immunity is a coincidence and is not attributable to a cause-and-effect relationship. For some reason not understood, susceptibility to tuberculosis begins to be evident in the teens and wanes in the late twenties. A second peak begins about the age of 50 and continues through the last three decades of life. According to a recent newspaper report most of the patients hospitalized in a city hospital for tuberculosis were over 50 years of age. Age is also an element in susceptibility to staphylococcic infections as they are more common in the very young and in the old.

SEX

There are many other factors appearing to influence susceptibility to infection. For some of these, that they do is based more on observation than on a clear understanding of why they do. For example, sex influences susceptibility to infection. Males appear to be more susceptible to pneumonia and epidemic meningitis than are females, whereas females are more susceptible to scarlet fever and typhoid fever. Females between the ages of 15 and 25 are more susceptible to tuberculosis than males. After the age of 30 the incidence among men becomes progressively higher so that the incidence among older men exceeds that of women. About one third of the men are alcoholics; a poor state of nutrition may be a factor.

In the following outline the characteristics of the host entering into the development of an infectious disease are summarized. The routes by which microbes (or other agents) penetrate the first lines of defense are also included.

1. Characteristics of *mechanisms of defense* of the host
   a. Anatomic and physiologic barriers to the entrance of microorganisms (discussed in Chapter 6)
      (1) Intact skin and mucous membranes
      (2) Structures and functions that protect the entrances to the respiratory and gastrointestinal tract
      (3) Character of secretions and body fluids
         (a) pH (acid pH inhibits bacterial growth)
         (b) Lysozyme produced by leukocytes is found in tears, saliva, and other body fluids; it lyses bacteria and is bactericidal
         (c) Properidin system
         (d) Bactericidins
         (e) Agglutinins
         (f) Opsonins
      (4) Anatomic barriers within the tissues
         (a) Continuous matrix
         (b) Fibrin barrier
   b. Cells (discussed in Chapter 6)
      (1) Microphages (neutrophils—highly mobile, quickly responding, somewhat vulnerable)
      (2) Macrophages
   c. Antibodies—past experiences (discussed in Chapter 6)
      (1) Antitoxin—directly neutralize toxins
      (2) Antibacterial or antiviral antibodies combine with a specific substance at the surface of a virus or bacterium and produce a new surface about which leukocytes can spread and more easily ingest the microorganism
   d. Inflammatory response (discussed in Chapter 6)
   e. Other host factors
      (1) Heredity (genetic)
      (2) Age
      (3) Sex
      (4) Nutritional state
      (5) Hormonal balance
      (6) Inhibition of virulent strains by normal flora
2. Routes of spread after a microbe has penetrated the first line of defense
      (1) Intercellular spaces—direct extension to contiguous tissues
      (2) Lymphatics
         (a) Arrest at lymph node
         (b) Spreads from the lymph node through lymphatics to blood stream
      (3) Blood stream

(4) Ingested by macrophages but not destroyed—carried to other parts of the body

(5) Spillage or escape from a hollow organ
   (a) Direct extension
   (b) Perforation of the hollow organ

The Pathogenic Microorganism

What information about a pathogenic microorganism is required to control its spread?

To answer the questions "Who protects whom from whom?" and "How?" certain information about the pathogenic microorganism is required. Among the characteristics that should be considered are the microorganism's capacity to survive outside a host, its infectivity and invasiveness, as well as its pathogenicity and virulence. It is possible for a single organism to establish itself and cause disease, but an increase in the number is generally believed to increase the chances of disease. Some of the characteristics of microorganisms influencing their ability to survive and to establish themselves are (1) morphology; (2) physiology, including nutritional and temperature requirements; (3) resistance to physical and chemical agents; (4) pathogenicity, virulence, invasiveness, and (5) toxin production. These points will be further clarified in the discussion of specific microorganisms.

MORPHOLOGY

The morphology of microorganisms influences their ability to survive and to establish themselves. Some germs such as those causing botulism, tetanus, and gas gangrene are spore formers. They are unusually resistant to heat, drying, and chemicals. Many bacteria form capsules that offer some protection against the body defenses. In some instances the capsules determine the virulence of the microbe. As an example, the pneumococcus is dependent on its capsule for its pathogenicity. The protein coat of the virus not only protects the nucleic acid core but is necessary for it to enter the cell.

PHYSIOLOGY, INCLUDING NUTRITIONAL AND TEMPERATURE REQUIREMENTS

In general the principles of biochemistry are the same for all living organisms. All microorganisms require oxygen and nutrients for metabolism. Enzymes are required to catalyze chemical reactions which are required for the release of energy and for other activities including reproduction and protection from hostile agents. Similar to other living organisms, some microbes have special requirements. Many of those that are pathogenic to man grow best under circumstances that are similar to man's internal environment. For the particular requirements of a specific microorganism, see a textbook of microbiology.

RESISTANCE TO PHYSICAL AND CHEMICAL AGENTS

Some of the factors influencing the resistance of microorganisms to physical and chemical agents have been previously mentioned. A variety of physical and chemical agents have been used to remove or destroy pathogens before they have an opportunity to enter the body. With the introduction of the antimicrobial agents that can be administered internally, some infectious diseases can be combated after they are established. Despite a high degree of effectiveness when first introduced, some antimicrobial agents lose their effectiveness in certain infections after a period of time.

Why should a once-effective agent become ineffective? For example, why should penicillin, which was once highly effective against the *Staphylococcus aureus,* become ineffective? There are a number of possibilities: (1) As susceptible strains are killed, resistant strains multiply without competition and come to predominate. (2) New strains develop as a result of mutation. (3) Infectious drug resistance develops. Because an example of the first type has been previously cited, it will not be discussed further. In mutation a change occurs in the genetic material that results in a resistant strain. As stated, resistant strains have a competitive advantage over the nonresistant ones.

The third possibility, infectious drug resistance, was first reported in Japan in 1959. Watanabe [28] defines infectious drug resistance as "a process whereby the genetic determinants of resistance to a number of drugs are transferred together and at one stroke from a resistant bacterial strain to a bacterial strain, of the same species or a different species, that was previously drug-sensitive, or susceptible to the drug's effect." Experimental evidence suggests that the resistance factor (R) responsible for infectious drug resistance is episomal in character as the R factor is usually located in the cytoplasm and rarely in the chromosomes.

From the clinical point of view infectious drug resistance is important because

[28] Tsutomu Watanabe: "Infectious Drug Resistance," *Sci. Amer.,* **217:**20 (Dec.) 1967.

1. Resistance is developed to multiple drugs. The first patient to be studied had dysentery caused by shigella and was resistant to four drugs: sulfanilamide and the antibiotics tetracycline, streptomycin, and chloramphenicol.

2. Susceptible bacteria can be made resistant to a number of antimicrobials in contact with bacteria carrying the R factor. A wide variety of gram-negative bacteria can be infected. The R factor can be transferred from commensals to highly virulent organisms and vice versa. Many of the organisms developing infectious drug resistance cause serious diseases. Bacteria developing resistance to multiple drugs and passing R factors to other bacteria include, in addition, shigella (dysentery), salmonella (one species causes typhoid fever), *Vibrio cholerae* (cholera), *Pasturella pestis* (plague), and *Pseudomonas aeruginosa* (purulent infections). According to Watanabe,[29] 90 per cent of the organisms causing urinary tract infections now carry R factors. They include *E. coli, Klebsiella,* citrobacter, and *Proteus.* The last group is part of the normal flora of the large intestine. Though the R factors do not appear to be transferable to gram-positive bacteria such as the streptococcus and staphylococcus, a similar type of infectious resistance to drugs has been reported for staphylococci.[30]

The diseases caused by resistant organisms become more difficult to treat. Further, the infecting organism does not need to be resistant at the time it enters the body as it can be rapidly infected by R factors from bacteria normally found in the large intestine. Prevention of multiple drug resistance is therefore of great importance.

Within the last thirty years a variety of antimicrobials have been discovered that have been effective in the treatment of some infectious diseases. After a period of use, these agents lose their effectiveness against some bacteria. With repeated use some individuals have become sensitive to them. According to Weinstein,[31] it takes from five to ten years before enough is known about an antimicrobial drug to use it effectively. Following the introduction of a new antimicrobial, it is used extensively. Then the results are critically evaluated. During the time that elapses between discovery and the stage of

rational use a number of mechanisms favor the survival of the bacteria:

1. Most antimicrobials are bacteriostatic rather than bactericidal.
2. Resistant organisms develop as a result of mutation.
3. Resistant strains multiply and come to predominate as a consequence of destruction of susceptible strains.
4. Infectious drug resistance develops.

PATHOGENICITY, VIRULENCE, INVASIVENESS

The character of a microorganism also influences its disease-producing capacity. Terms used to describe attributes of microorganisms, which enable them to cause disease include *pathogenicity, virulence,* and *invasiveness.* The term *pathogenicity* refers to the capacity of a microorganism to cause disease. The meningococcus is pathogenic for man but under natural conditions is not pathogenic for animals. As implied earlier, virulence is relative, because the host is a significant factor in disease. Depending on host factors, an organism may be highly virulent in one person, mildly virulent in another, and latent in still another.

Despite the tendency to use the term *virulence* as a synonym for *pathogenicity,* it adds the concept of degree of disease-producing capacity. For example, some strains of staphylococci have a greater power to produce disease, that is, greater virulence, than others. Certain viruses, such as those causing influenza, increase in disease-producing power or virulence when they pass rapidly from one susceptible person to another.

Invasiveness refers to the capacity of microorganisms to enter the tissues of the host, multiply, and spread to adjacent tissues or to distant parts of the body. Microorganisms vary greatly in their power to invade and disseminate themselves throughout the body. At one end of the scale are the noninvasive toxin producers, such as the organisms of tetanus and botulism, and at the other end are the highly invasive organisms of plague and anthrax. Most microorganisms that have any degree of invasiveness have some sort of capsule or protective covering. The capsule appears to protect the microorganism against the defense mechanisms of the host. Without its capsule, the germ is quickly destroyed by the phagocytes. Even viruses have a protein "capsule" surrounding the central core of DNA (deoxyribonucleic acid). The protein capsule attaches itself to the cell, but only the DNA enters. After the DNA multiplies within the cell, the cell must build protein to surround the DNA before the cell ruptures and releases the

---

[29] *Ibid.,* p. 26.
[30] *Ibid.,* p. 26.
[31] Louis Weinstein: "The Present Status of Antimicrobial Therapy with Special Emphasis on Host Determinants of Response to Treatment," *Med. Times,* 96:106 (Feb.) 1968.

virus. Without the protein capsule, viruses cannot cause disease.[32]

After microorganisms are established, how do they cause disease?

As indicated earlier, pathogenic microorganisms may be present in the tissues without causing manifestations of disease. For clinical evidence of the disease to appear, the organism must not only establish itself in the host but multiply in sufficient numbers to overcome host resistance and to induce tissue response. Whether or not the microbe is successful in causing disease depends on the relationship of its virulence, invasiveness, and numbers to the nonspecific and specific resistance of the host. After the microorganism is successful in establishing itself, that is, after it becomes adapted to a susceptible host, it may then induce local and systemic effects, by one or more mechanisms. Some bacteria, such as the diphtheria bacillus, secrete water-soluble toxins that are distributed by the blood to all regions of the body. These exotoxins are responsible for the systemic manifestations of disease in botulism, tetanus, diphtheria, and gas gangrene. They are highly specific, as each exotoxin acts as an antigen stimulating the body to produce a specific antitoxin (an antibody) that neutralizes a specific toxin.

The exotoxin not only stimulates the antibody-producing mechanism of a victim of a disease, but it can be used to stimulate an animal, such as a sheep or a horse, to produce antitoxin. Serum obtained from an animal treated with toxin, therefore, contains the specific antibody or antitoxin, and it can be used to confer a passive immunity, that is, to neutralize toxin in the blood of an infected host. To protect a person who has a disease caused by an exotoxin-forming microbe, the antitoxin must be given early, for after a toxin has combined with cellular constituents, antitoxin is of little or no benefit. Persons with a disease, such as diphtheria or tetanus, must receive antitoxin at once if they are to benefit. Nurses acting as case finders may be responsible for getting patients under medical care. In an epidemic of diphtheria in one large city, a school nurse was credited with recognizing the possibility that the children who were sick had diphtheria. When her suspicions were verified, sick children were treated with antitoxin, and measures were undertaken to prevent the spread of diphtheria to others by immunizing schoolchildren and other contacts. A modified toxin can also be used to stimulate the production of antitoxin

by the individual. The toxin may be converted to toxoid by a chemical such as formalin. Because the immunity produced as a result of disease or vaccination is relative rather than complete, Anderson *et al.* suggest that the term *resistance* might be preferable.[33]

Although the general manifestations occurring in tetanus, diphtheria, and botulism differ, the specific exotoxins produced in each of these diseases cause injury to the nervous system. The exotoxin of diphtheria also injures the myocardium. Each of the exotoxins varies in degree of toxicity; however, exotoxins are among the most highly poisonous substances known.

The local effects of microorganisms producing exotoxins vary. *Clostridium botulinum* does not cause injury by the growth of microorganisms in the alimentary canal or in the tissues but by an exotoxin produced by the microorganism growing in bland vegetables or fish canned at temperatures insufficient to kill *Clostridium botulinum* spores. There is no local growth of microorganisms to cause injury. Fortunately, the exotoxin is easily destroyed by boiling vegetables such as home-canned corn, beans, or peas for five minutes before they are eaten. Commercially canned vegetables are rarely sources of botulism because they are subjected to high temperatures during the process of canning.

Clostridium tetani also causes little local effect. It does not grow on living tissue and is a strict anaerobe. Tetanus has been known to occur after small or insignificant wounds have healed. For the *Clostridium tetani* to grow, however, there must be some necrotic tissue.

In diphtheria the local manifestation consists of superficial ulceration of mucous membrane, usually located in the nasopharynx, pharynx, or larynx. The ulcerated tissue is covered by a membrane, which may extend through the glottis into the larynx and tracheobronchial tree, where it can cause death by suffocation.

In addition to exotoxins, bacteria also form substances known as endotoxins. Endotoxins differ from exotoxins in that they are not liberated in appreciable amounts during the life of the bacterial cell, but they are released as the cell degenerates. Endotoxins also differ from exotoxins in that they are not specific to a given microorganism. They appear to be a fairly homogeneous group of substances that probably cause injury by a similar chemical grouping. In experimental animals these endotoxins cause similar physiological effects. Among these changes are severe shock and fever. The implications to nursing of both these conditions are discussed elsewhere.

---

[32] Gunther S. Stent: "The Multiplication of Bacterial Viruses," *Sci. Amer.,* **188**:39 (May) 1953.

[33] Anderson *et al., op. cit.,* p. 38.

Many microorganisms have the power to invade healthy tissues. Not all the factors that enable microorganisms to invade tissues and to disseminate themselves throughout the body are known. Some of the substances that are formed by bacteria and that facilitate their spread are not directly toxic. They play a role in the infectious process by protecting microorganisms from the defense mechanisms of the body or by enabling them to spread throughout the tissue. For example, many pathogenic staphylococci produce a substance called coagulase. Coagulase plus certain factors in the blood serum interact to form fibrin clots in small blood vessels supplying the infected area. It is a factor in the formation of fibrin walls around areas of tissue infected by the staphylococcus. The fibrin wall serves to protect the staphylococcus from the defenses of the body and from antistaphylococcic drugs and thereby favors their persistence in the tissues.

Clostridium welchii produces collagenase and lecithinase. These substances dissolve collagen and lecithin and thereby facilitate the spread of microorganisms throughout the tissue.

Hemolysins and leukocidins dissolve erythrocytes and leukocytes, respectively. Streptokinase has the opposite effect of coagulase. It digests coagulated plasma and is thought to be an important factor in the spread of organisms such as hemolytic streptococci throughout the body. It has been used experimentally to digest blood clots formed in blood vessels in disease.

A group of enzymes, formed by certain bacteria and known as hyaluronidases, act as spreading factors because they have the power of increasing the permeability of tissues. Hyaluronidase is sometimes added to fluids administered subcutaneously to increase tissue permeability and, as a consequence, to increase the rate at which the fluid is absorbed.

To summarize, the following characteristics of microorganisms or their products may enhance pathogenicity

1. Polysaccharide capsule inhibits phagocytosis
2. Toxin production
   2.1 Exotoxin
   2.2 Endotoxin
3. Other substances
   3.1 Coagulase
   3.2 Streptokinase
4. Other factors
   Number, virulence, and invasiveness are sufficient to overcome local body defenses. Reaches a tissue where it is able to establish itself, grow, and multiply.

The outcome of the struggle for survival between an individual host and an invading microbe depends on many factors. These include the state of the defense mechanisms of the host and his capacity to respond promptly and appropriately to microorganisms. The microorganism must be able to find a vehicle or mode of transmission, a portal of entry, and tissue that provides an environment suited to its needs and be able to establish itself, grow, and multiply. Whether or not it induces general or local evidence of disease also depends on a number of factors. It may be able to produce an exotoxin that is not neutralized before it combines with susceptible tissues or produce other substances that enable it to destroy tissue cells. These cells may be either parenchymal or blood cells, particularly leukocytes.

Although microorganisms forming exotoxins tend to remain at the site at which they enter the tissue, other microorganisms behave differently. Some multiply at the point at which they enter the host. They break down the local tissue defenses and spread to contiguous tissues before being disseminated by the blood and lymph. Others have little or no effect at the site of entry but are carried to distant points by blood and lymph. The microorganism may be free in the blood or it may be a passenger in a macrophage, because the macrophage was successful in ingesting the microbe but unable to destroy it. Macrophages may disseminate the tubercle bacillus throughout the body because they are able to ingest but not destroy them. Whatever the specific mechanisms, microorganisms can be distributed to, and set up secondary infections far from, the point of origin. The routes by which microorganisms and their products may be disseminated throughout the body were summarized on page 118.

What are some of the factors in the environment that bring the agent and the host together?

Besides a pathogenic microorganism and a susceptible host, conditions in the environment must be such as to bring the two together if an infectious disease is to develop. Many of these factors have been discussed earlier. Bilharziasis has increased in incidence as a result of vast systems of irrigation constructed to improve living standards. Some authorities say that it is the most common and important parasitic disease in man as it affects the young and causes a high degree of disability. Conditions required for the propagation of the snail in which the *Schistosoma* (a flatworm) spends part of its life cycle are provided. The eggs of the organism are voided or defecated into the water by infected persons. They hatch, and the larvae enter a suitable fresh-water snail. After a period of time, free-swimming larvae leave the snail. They pierce the skin of a person wading, working, or swimming in the water. From the site of entry, they are carried by the blood to the liver, where they mature. The essential point here is that customs and habits, i.e., discharging human excreta wherever convenient and the provision of suitable conditions for the propagation of a pathogenic microorganism, provide the conditions in the environment required to transmit the disease. The practices of working, wading, and swimming provide the final conditions necessary to spread the disease. Control of bilharziasis could be effected by the sanitary disposal of urine and feces.

A variety of conditions in the environment facilitate or prevent the transmission of a pathogenic microorganism to man. They include such factors as customs, climate, geography, sanitary procedures, housing, neighborhoods, and the adequacy of health facilities. For those diseases to which immunity can be developed, the proportion of susceptibles to nonsusceptibles is a significant factor in the control of spread.

In the preceding sections, three factors in infection, the susceptible host, the germ, and the environment, were explored. In the following part, the elements involved in getting the organism from its source to a susceptible host will be considered.

The Transmission of Infectious Disease

THE RESERVOIR

Granted a susceptible host, a pathogenic microbe and an environment conducive to bringing the infectious agent and host together, there must be a reservoir or source of a microbe. In a strict sense, a reservoir is a storage receptacle. In microbiology the term is used to indicate not only a storage site but a place where microbes grow and propagate. Reservoirs of pathogenic microorganisms include the tissues of people, animals, and insects, as well as human wastes and food and water contaminated by them.

Human reservoirs include apparently well persons who harbor pathogenic microorganisms, persons in the prodromal stage of illness, and those who are mildly, as well as those who are seriously, ill. The apparently well person whose mucous membranes or secretions are found to contain virulent microorganisms is called a carrier. The reasons that some individuals become carriers are not well understood. Diseases in which carriers serve as reservoirs include typhoid fever, diphtheria, and infections

caused by the staphylococcus and streptococcus. After recovery of the individual from typhoid fever, the biliary tract can continue to act as a source of typhoid bacilli. Virulent diphtheria bacilli, staphylococci, or streptococci can be found on the mucosa of persons who have not experienced an apparent infection.

Persons who are ill with an infectious disease are reservoirs or sources of virulent microorganisms. The number of germs available for dissemination does not necessarily correspond with the stage or degree of illness. For example, the most infectious stage of measles is the prodromal stage, that is, before the rash appears and when the eyes and nose are weepy. The degree of illness apparently does not prevent the individual from being a source of microbes. Therefore a person who shows little evidence of illness or one who has symptoms only a short period of time can still be a source of infection. For example, not all persons who have poliomyelitis during an epidemic are diagnosed as having the disease. Fewer still become paralyzed. Yet persons who are not aware of having had poliomyelitis can be demonstrated to have antibodies in their blood. Terms such as *inapparent infection, missed cases,* and *abortive cases* are used to describe the situation in which an individual apparently reacted to a virulent germ without experiencing the expected manifestations of the disease. The extent to which communicability is related to degree of illness is not known.

In addition to people, animals may serve as reservoirs of infection. Although animal reservoirs are not as important in the United States as they once were, some diseases such as Rocky Mountain spotted fever, tularemia, and psittacosis are transmitted to human beings by animals. In some parts of the world they are of considerable significance. Diseases such as plague and malaria are examples previously cited. Diseases of animals to which human beings are susceptible are known as zoonoses. The zoonoses are important not only because they are animal diseases that are transmissible to man but because they add to the problem of disease control. As an example, a tick is the reservoir for the rickettsiae causing Rocky Mountain spotted fever. Besides man, a number of animals, some of which are wild, are susceptible to this disease. Obviously the eradication of all infected animals is difficult. Another disease difficult to eradicate is yellow fever because wild monkeys serve as reservoirs.

Besides living reservoirs, inanimate substances may be sources of pathogenic microbes. As examples, food and water can be reservoirs for some microorganisms such as the staphylococcus, streptococcus, and typhoid bacillus. In hospitals hand lotions and ice cubes have been found to be contaminated with pathogenic microorganisms.

MODE OF ESCAPE FROM RESERVOIR

For the infectious process to succeed, a microorganism must not only have a reservoir but also a mode of escape from it. The avenues of escape from the reservoir include the respiratory, gastrointestinal, and urinary tracts and open lesions of the skin. In some instances escape of the microorganism from the reservoir depends on some other living organism such as an insect.

The most common natural avenue of escape for microorganisms is the respiratory tract. Droplets of secretions containing microorganisms located on the respiratory membranes are driven out with the expired air and by coughing, talking, and sneezing. Although large droplets quickly settle to the floor, the moisture surrounding small droplets may evaporate, leaving the nucleus containing bacteria or viruses suspended in the air. These droplet nuclei may be held aloft or wafted in air currents for considerable periods of time and for appreciable distances.[34]

Most of the pathogenic microorganisms discharged from the gastrointestinal tract are expelled with the feces. In addition to the normal flora of the intestinal tract, which can under certain circumstances cause disease, the feces may contain organisms causing typhoid and paratyphoid fever, cholera, and amebic dysentery. Worms or their eggs may also be contained in the feces and, when ingested, cause disease. The control of infectious diseases of the gastrointestinal tract has been accomplished largely by providing sanitary facilities for the discharge of feces and by controlling water and food supplies. The same facilities also serve to prevent the dissemination of microorganisms contained in the urine. Open lesions serve as a route of escape either by direct contact with a sore or by contact with its discharge.

VEHICLE OF TRANSMISSION

After a microorganism has escaped from the reservoir, it must have a vehicle for its transmission to a susceptible host. The simplest mode of transmission is direct contact. The microorganism is passed directly from one person to

[34] For a complete discussion of transmission of respiratory infections among human beings, see Richard L. Riley and Francis O'Grady: *Airborne Infection* (New York: The Macmillan Company, 1961).

another either by droplets, by droplet nuclei, or by a body surface of the susceptible host coming in direct contact with infected tissue. For example, Mary Sue arises in the morning with the "sniffles," which she interprets as a cold. After she goes to school she sneezes, spraying droplets of nasal and pharyngeal secretions in all directions. Children in the room inhale the droplets as well as droplet nuclei, and within a few days many of the children have colds. The usual mode of transmission of syphilis is by the tissues of the susceptible host coming in contact with a lesion containing the *Treponema pallidum.*

Microorganisms may also be passed indirectly from one person to another by means of air currents, contaminated dust, hands, water, food, or objects. The indirect transmission of microorganisms will be illustrated in the discussion of staphylococcal infections later in the chapter. Some microorganisms such as the typhoid bacillus may be transmitted on the feet or bodies of insects such as the fly. To be transmitted indirectly, microorganisms must be able to survive for at least a time outside the body of the host. Organisms such as the *Treponema pallidum* and the gonococcus are fragile and survive for only brief periods outside the body. They are therefore unlikely to be transmitted by indirect contact. In contrast, the typhoid and tubercle bacilli are capable of living for extended periods of time outside the host. They may therefore be transmitted indirectly.

PORTAL OF ENTRY

Besides requiring a portal of exit from the reservoir and a vehicle for transmission, microorganisms must be able to find a portal of entry into the new host. The same structures, that is, the respiratory tract, mouth, skin, and mucous membranes, that are sites for the escape of microorganisms are also portals for their entry into the host. However, before a microorganism can cause disease, it must get past the defenses that guard each of these structures. The reader is referred to Chapter 6. Even when the microorganism makes its way past these defenses, the specific resistance of the individual may be sufficient to overcome the microorganism so that disease does not occur.

SUMMARY OF SIX FACTORS ESSENTIAL TO THE INFECTIOUS DISEASE PROCESS

As a summary, the six factors listed by Anderson, Arnstein, and Lester[35] as being

[35] Anderson, *et al., op. cit.,* p. 19.

essential to the infectious disease process are again given here:

ESSENTIAL FACTORS IN SUSCEPTIBILITY	SUMMARY OF COMPONENTS OF ESSENTIAL FACTORS
1. A causative or etiological agent (a necessary condition)	Viruses Rickettsia Bacteria Spirochetes Protozoa Fungi
2. A reservoir or source of the causative agent	Human beings Animals, including insects

3. A mode of escape from the reservoir	Respiratory tract—
	  sputum
	  droplets
	  droplet nuclei
	Alimentary canal—
	  feces
	Genital tract—
	  secretions
	Urinary tract—urine
	Skin lesions—drainage
	Blood

4. A mode of transmission from the reservoir to the potential new host	Vehicles—air
	     dust
	     food
	     water
	     blood
	     fingers
	     insects

5. A mode of entry into the new host	Respiratory tract, mouth, skin or mucous membrane
6. A susceptible host	

Factors affecting the susceptibility of the host to any type of illness have been considered earlier. One critical characteristic is the degree to which the individual is or is not immune to the pathogenic microorganism. Immunity is seldom absolute. Whether or not disease results from exposure to a pathogenic microorganism depends on the interaction of the host and the microorganism.

These steps or links in the chain in the infectious disease process have been listed because if any one is absent or missing infection or infectious disease will not occur. One aspect in the practice of nursing is the prevention of the spread of infectious disease to others including nurses. In the prevention of the spread of infection, one of the first questions that the nurse should ask and answer is, "Who should be protected from whom?" How?

The Course and Control of Infectious Disease

What are the stages in the course of an infectious disease?

The course of infectious disease is usually divided into three stages. The first, or incubation, period is the time that elapses between the entrance of the microorganism into the body and the appearance of clinical signs and symptoms. In terms of the microorganism, the incubation period is the time it takes it to adapt to the host and achieve a rate of multiplication sufficient to cause evidence of disease. The length of the incubation period is different for each acute communicable disease but is constant for a particular disease. As examples, the incubation period for measles is 10 to 14 days and not longer than 21 days. In meningococcus meningitis, it varies from 2 to 21 days. In those diseases in which not only a specific microorganism (a necessary condition) but other factors (sufficient cause) enter into their development, the length of the incubation period may be difficult to determine. For example, the virus of herpes simplex may be present in the tissues for an extended period of time without any indication of its presence. When the individual develops a cold or has a fever, a cold sore appears. The length of the incubation period for tuberculosis is also variable. It depends on such factors as age, state of nutrition, and other factors.

The next stage is the period of illness. As with the incubation period, the length of the period of illness is predictable for a given disease but varies from one type to another. A self-limiting disease may run its course in a few hours or extend for a few weeks at most. The old saying "If a cold is treated it lasts two weeks and if it is not treated it lasts 14 days" applies here. Most of the acute communicable diseases are of relatively short duration. Some diseases such as tuberculosis may continue to be active for months or years. As in noninfectious diseases, the degree and severity of illness vary from one individual to another. Some individuals have antibodies in their blood indicating that they must have reacted to a given microorganism, but they have no knowledge of ever having had the disease. Other individuals experience mild attacks, whereas in still others the course of the disease is so rapid and so severe that the patient becomes ill and dies within a few hours. When the course of a disease is unusually rapid and the manifestations are unusually severe and uncontrollable, it is said to be fulminating.[36] For

[36] The term *fulminating* can be applied to any disease in which the manifestations are unusually severe and which progresses in a short time to death.

example, John Harvey felt fine yesterday. This morning he awakened with a shaking chill, feeling very ill. He had a fever that continued to rise. Despite intensive therapy, he died less than 24 hours after the onset of his illness. He was diagnosed as having fulminating pneumococcal pneumonia, type III. At the onset of his illness he was not a weakened old man but a healthy and robust young one. Despite the possibility of an infectious disease being fulminating, the tendency toward recovery is strong in most acute communicable diseases.

The onset of the period of illness of acute communicable diseases is usually marked by a prodromal period. During the prodromal period the individual has early manifestations of the impending illness but does not have the specific signs and symptoms. One of the problems in the control of diseases such as measles is that the manifestations indicating the onset of illness are similar to those of the common cold. Moreover, the individual is more infectious during the prodromal phase than he is later. This morning when Mary Sue went to school with "just a cold," she might well have been in the prodromal phase of measles or another acute communicable disease.

Following the onset of illness, the individual experiences a period in which the specific manifestations of the particular illness are evident and he is sick. Depending on the nature of the disease and the person who is ill, he may go into the third stage of the infectious illness which is the period of convalescence and may recover completely; or he may develop complications; or he may die.

What are some of the characteristic manifestations in acute infectious disease?

During the period of illness most patients have fever. The fever may be constant, intermittent, or remittent. A fever is said to be constant when the amount of variation is less than 2°. It is remittent when it varies more than 2° but does not drop to normal. It is intermittent when the temperature varies above and below normal levels. The type of fever, the degree of elevation, and the length of time it persists are reasonably characteristic for each disease. For example, in untreated pneumococcal pneumonia following a shaking chill, the temperature rises rapidly. It can be expected to remain elevated to from 38.8°C (102°F) to 40°C (104°F) for five to nine days. The fever then falls rapidly, that is, by crisis, to below normal. Unless the patient develops a complication, the temperature does not again rise above normal, and from that point on the patient recovers rapidly. When the temperature does not fall within the expected period of time, or if it rises above normal after the crisis, a complication such as lung abcess or empyema is suspected. Accurate determination and recording of the temperature are important in assessing the progress of the patient toward recovery. Although some deviation from the expected pattern does not always indicate that the patient is developing complications, it may.

Along with fever, the patient can be expected to have an elevation in pulse and respiratory rates. Other signs and symptoms are more or less characteristic for each disease. The illness is terminated when the body's defense mechanisms are sufficient to overcome the causative agent. For example, in diphtheria recovery occurs when sufficient antibodies are formed to neutralize the exotoxin. With the neutralization of the exotoxin, the phagocytes are then able to overcome the diphtheria bacilli.

In some infectious diseases, notably typhoid fever, the patient may appear to be recovering only to have a recurrence of symptoms. Usually the course of the second illness is not as severe, nor does it last as long as the original attack. Recurrence of infection in patients treated by antimicrobial agents also happens. Apparently the antimicrobial drug suppresses but does not kill the microbe. The recurrence is caused by the multiplication of the microorganism following the termination of drug therapy.

Not all infectious diseases are self-limiting. The period of illness in some diseases, such as tuberculosis, may depend as much or more on conditions within the person who is ill as it does on the virulence and invasiveness of the microorganism.

During convalescence, which follows the period of illness, the patient returns to health. Its length will depend on how long the patient has been ill as well as on how well his general condition was maintained during the illness. Some illnesses are more debilitating than others. For example, though the period of illness from influenza may not be unduly long, patients often complain of being weak and easily fatigued for weeks. In the past when patients with typhoid fever were starved, convalescence was delayed until their nutritional status was improved. Attention to nutrition during the period of illness as well as in the period of convalescence is important.

The requirements of the patient who has an infectious disease should be evaluated in the same manner as for persons with other illnesses. Particular attention should be paid to the person who is isolated. Many, but not all, patients who are isolated feel rejected by nursing and medical personnel. Because drainage from an

ulcer on her leg contained virulent staphylococci, Mrs. Lilac was placed on isolation precautions. Because no single rooms were available, the curtains were drawn about her bed.
At 11 o'clock in the morning a nurse opened
the curtains to speak to Mrs. Lilac. Her breakfast tray was still sitting on her bedside table
and her bed was in complete disarray. When
the nurse spoke to Mrs. Lilac, she burst into
tears. As she sobbed, she spoke of her feelings
of desolation at being deserted. "You would
think that I had leprosy or something. What do
I have that makes everyone afraid and avoid
me? It must be awfully bad."

Not all patients who are isolated, however,
feel neglected. Mrs. Solo, who was also screened
from other patients in a large ward, thanked
the nurse for making it possible for her to have
privacy. The differences in the responses of the
two patients related to differences in their perception of a similar situation.

The nurse, too, should examine how she feels
about the particular illness. It is not uncommon
for nurses to express fear of diseases such as
tuberculosis or syphilis. Nurses should also
know how they feel about people who have
these diseases. Although one cannot always
completely change one's feelings, they are easier
to control when one knows what they are. Some
fears arise from ignorance of the manner by
which specific infectious diseases are spread and
from not knowing what can be done to prevent
their spread.

The role of the nurse in meeting the psychological needs of patients has been discussed in
Chapter 7. During the period when the patient
is acutely ill, attention should be directed toward
conserving his energy, providing comfort, relieving symptoms associated with fever, and
maintaining his fluid intake and, if possible, his
intake of food. Rest should be provided and unnecessary stimulation avoided. Because fever
activates the herpes virus, cold sores on the lips
and face of the patient may cause him discomfort. Camphor ice or some type of bland or
mildly stimulating ointment, prescribed by the
physician, should be applied as necessary. Unless the patient breathes through his mouth, his
mouth will remain clean and moist if his fluid
intake is adequate, and he should be given
whatever assistance he requires to maintain his
fluid intake. Mouth care is important to the
comfort of the patient even when the mouth appears to be clean. During illness and convalescence, the patient should be protected from
unnecessary exposure to other infectious agents.

During convalescence, the needs of the patient will not be particularly different from those
of the patient undergoing a surgical procedure

or some other illness. Some patients, especially
those having had typhoid fever or diphtheria,
may continue to discharge virulent bacteria.
Precautions designed to protect others may
therefore have to be continued during or after
the period of convalescence.

The Control of Infectious Disease

*What kinds of activities or procedures are
required for the control of acute infectious
diseases?*

Activities that are useful in the control of
infectious disease are directed toward the accomplishment of three objectives. These objectives, as stated by Burrows, are (1) to reduce
or to eliminate the reservoir of infection, (2)
to break the chain between the reservoir and
the susceptible host, and (3) to reduce the number of susceptible people in the community.[37]
Anderson and his associates [38] add to the list
of objectives: to minimize "the ill effects of
cases that have not been prevented."

REDUCING THE RESERVOIR OF INFECTION

As stated earlier, the reservoirs of infection
include human beings who are carriers or who
are ill with the infectious disease, animals
including insect carriers, and human wastes.
Human beings may be isolated or quaran-
tined during the period of illness and for as
long as they carry virulent microbes. In some
infectious diseases, the number of human reservoirs may be reduced by treating the disease. One reason, though not the only one, for
treating patients who have tuberculosis in hospitals is to remove them from the community,
where they may be a source of infection to
others. Since the introduction of antimicrobial
agents, the length of hospitalization has been
shortened. Patients must continue treatment for
varying periods of time on an outpatient basis.
Therapy of the patient who has tuberculosis
has two aims. One is to eradicate the reservoir.
The other is to help the patient learn a way of
life that will enable him to live in healthful coexistence with the *Mycobacterium tuberculosis*.
Even before the days of the antituberculosis
drugs, the tuberculosis process was arrested in
many patients by a program of rest—both mental and physical—a nutritious diet, and attention
to individual factors in each patient. The atmosphere in the sanitarium is calm and un-

[37] William Burrows: *Textbook of Microbiology,*
19th ed. (Philadelphia: W. B. Saunders Company,
1968), p. 307.
[38] *Op. cit.,* p. 47.

hurried. Because the individual patient is a key factor in his recovery, he is taught early the nature of his disease and what his part is in recovery and in maintaining health. He also learns how to protect others. The program of therapy serves to assist the patient not only to arrest the tuberculous process but to learn a way of life that will enable him to keep his disease under control.

Surgical therapy has made a contribution to the eradication of the reservoir in tuberculosis. Some surgical procedures result in temporary or permanent collapse of the affected area in the lung. In either event the purpose is to assist the body in healing diseased tissue. When the disease process is localized in one organ or part of an organ, the diseased tissue may be removed surgically. For example, when tuberculosis involves one kidney and not the other, the diseased kidney is usually removed. In pulmonary tuberculosis, a part of or an entire lung may be removed. In some instances, portions of both lungs may be excised. Eradication of the reservoir by surgical removal of the infected tissue is not limited to tuberculosis, as persons who are typhoid carriers can sometimes be cured by cholecystectomy.

The most important measures available to control tuberculosis are the antimicrobial drugs. Although Goodman and Gilman [39] list a number of drugs, they state that the primary ones used singly or in combination are isoniazid, streptomycin, and aminosalicylic acid. When antituberculosis drugs were first introduced, the hope was entertained that man now would have a means of effectively and easily eradicating tuberculosis. Despite the fact that the original expectations have not been realized, the mortality rate and to a lesser extent the morbidity rate continue to fall in the United States. Parry [40] states that tuberculosis is the most important disease in the world. He estimates that there were 50 million active cases in 1966 and that 3 million die each year. Further, in Great Britain, drug-resistant tuberculosis is increasing despite a decrease in morbidity and mortality rates. Although it is possible to cure tuberculosis, cure is not certain. Therefore regular follow-up is essential to discover reactivated disease process.

Case finding is important but is not an end in itself. It is done so that patients who have tuberculosis can be identified and brought under treatment. The initiation of prompt and effective treatment, not only with antimicrobial drugs

but with measures designed to improve the resistance of the host to tuberculosis, is imperative. The earlier the disease is discovered, the easier it is to prevent damage.

Antibacterials are also useful in the eradication of reservoirs in other infectious diseases. Among diseases treated with success are syphilis, gonorrhea, and bacillary infections, as well as infections caused by the pneumococcus, meningococcus, and hemolytic streptococcus.

Animals also act as reservoirs of disease. Animal reservoirs may be reduced or eradicated by killing diseased animals. For example, in the past, bovine tuberculosis was a problem in dairy cattle. After methods for the identification of tuberculous cattle were developed, programs were instituted to identify and to destroy diseased animals. Farmers, however, were resistant to the program of testing because diseased animals were destroyed. To farmers, the problem was a matter not of public health but of economics. They did not find it easy to accept as a fact that healthy-looking cows were diseased and must be sold for a price far below their value as producers of milk. The program has, however, been effective in eradicating bovine tuberculosis among cattle and therefore among human beings. When the reservoir of disease is in one or more species of wild animals, the problem of eradication is difficult. Eradication of the *Anopheles* mosquito eliminates not only a reservoir of malaria infection but its mode of transmission as well.

Sewage serves as a reservoir for some types of microorganisms. One of the problems in urban living is the disposal and disinfection of human wastes. As populations concentrate in an area in larger and larger numbers, the problem of protecting people from their own excreta increases. Articles in journals devoted to public health emphasize the need for dealing with this problem. In one midwestern state, many of the wells are presumed to be contaminated because the water has a high nitrogen content from barnyard wastes. The high level of nitrogen in the water is of itself dangerous to babies and to immature animals. There is also the possibility that the water in these wells contains pathogenic microorganisms.

BREAKING THE CHAIN BETWEEN HOST AND RESERVOIR

Although a considerable discussion has been, and will be, devoted to the value and methods of breaking the chain of events leading from the reservoir to the susceptible host, community efforts are highly important. They include such activities as the filtration and chlorination of water supplies, the pasteurization of milk, the

[39] Louis S. Goodman and Alfred Gilman (ed.): *The Pharmacological Basis of Therapeutics,* 3rd ed. (New York: The Macmillan Company, 1965), p. 1335.

[40] Wilfrid H. Parry: "Tuberculosis: A World Problem," *Nurs. Times,* **62**:1454 (Nov. 4) 1966.

supervision and inspection of food and food handlers, and the destruction of insect vectors.

REDUCING THE NUMBER OF SUSCEPTIBLE PEOPLE

The third method in control of disease is to reduce the number of persons in the community who are susceptible to the disease. This may be done by administering antibodies (*passive immunity*) or by stimulating the person to form his own antibodies by administering a vaccine or other immunizing agent. Sometimes antibodies are administered to persons sick with a disease in order to modify the course of the disease. Whether or not the person develops an active immunity depends on the time the antiserum is administered in relation to the onset of the disease, as well as other factors. The immunization procedures that are most effective are those most nearly like the natural process. Immunizations for smallpox, poliomyelitis, mumps, and measles, in which living, but attenuated, viruses are administered and for tetanus and diphtheria, in which attenuated toxin is injected, are at the present time most successful. Killed organisms are not usually as effective as live ones. A problem that has to be solved before a vaccine can be administered to human beings is making it both effective and safe. The most important test that a vaccine must pass is that of safety. Although there is no such thing as absolute safety, the element of risk should be far below the risk involved in having the disease.

Influenza vaccine, which induces a temporary immunity, is useful in preventing the rapid spread of influenza throughout a community. A problem with influenza virus is that there are many strains. One strain does not necessarily protect against another. Vaccines, such as those for typhoid fever, typhus fever, and yellow fever, are often advised for persons traveling into communities where these diseases are endemic.

Authorities in public health point out that the control of an infectious disease does not depend on the eradication of all the reservoirs of infection or the immunization of all who are susceptible. They do not underestimate the desirability of this goal, but they are aware of how difficult total eradication is to attain. The spread of an infectious disease can be quite effectively controlled provided a sufficient proportion of the population is immune to it. In a community of persons who are susceptible to a given infectious disease, the disease spreads by geometrical progression; that is, one person infects two persons, and two people infect four, and so on until all susceptible persons in the community develop the disease. This formulation is theoret-

ical, not actual, as one person may be the source of infection for many persons. If, in contrast, only half of the people in a community are susceptible, then of each two persons exposed only one develops it. Instead of spreading rapidly through the community, the infectious disease spreads slowly.

Anderson et al.[41] state that diphtheria can be controlled in a community, provided 50 per cent of the children are immune. For this percentage to be effective, the children must be distributed among all age groups. An occasional case of diphtheria will develop, but the disease will not become epidemic. The community runs a risk of an epidemic when the number of susceptibles is allowed to rise.

THE IDENTIFICATION OF SUSCEPTIBLE PERSONS

Although tests are not available in all instances, the identification of persons who have reacted to specific microorganisms or their antigens is useful in the selection of persons for immunization procedures. For many diseases, such as measles and smallpox, no special test is necessary, because all persons are presumed to be susceptible unless they have had a known attack of the disease. The immune reaction, a slight swelling and reddening at the site of inoculation, in smallpox, indicates that the person who was vaccinated is immune.

The tests that are available for the identification of persons who have or have not reacted to specific antigens are of two types. In one, a specific toxin is injected into the skin to identify the presence or absence of neutralizing antibodies. In the other, antigenic material is injected intradermally to identify skin-sensitizing antibodies. For example, the Schick test is used to identify persons who have antibodies against diphtheria toxin. A minute quantity of toxin is injected into the skin. Persons lacking the neutralizing antitoxin develop, within 24 to 48 hours, a swollen, reddened lesion at the site of injection. These persons are said to have a positive Schick test and are susceptible to diphtheria. Those who do not react to the toxin have sufficient antibodies to neutralize the toxin. This does not necessarily indicate, however, that they have a high level of immunity to diphtheria, though they may.

In contrast, in tuberculosis, antigenic material is injected to demonstrate the presence or absence of a tuberculous infection by determining whether or not there are skin-sensitizing antibodies in the skin. The test is based on the fact that the tissues of an individual who acquires a tuberculous infection react to the proteins of

[41] *Op. cit.*, p. 81.

the tubercle bacillus in a characteristic way. The primary use of tuberculin testing is to determine the size of the reservoir of tuberculosis in the community. Two sources of material are available for tuberculin testing. One is an extract of the tubercle bacillus, which is called old tuberculin, or simply OT. The other is purified protein derivative, or PPD. It is prepared by growing tubercle bacilli on special synthetic media. Whether the material is injected into the skin (Mantoux), scratched into the skin (Von Pirquet), or applied as a patch test (Vollmer), an area of induration is interpreted as a positive reaction and a nonindurated area as a negative reaction. A positive reaction indicates that the person has at some time reacted to the tubercle bacilli; that is, he has experienced a tuberculous infection. As a consequence, his skin contains sensitizing antibodies that react with the injected antigenic material to produce a delayed hypersensitivity reaction. Because a positive test does not indicate whether or not the person presently has active tuberculosis, those who have positive tuberculin tests then have a chest x-ray.

DIAGNOSIS

The diagnosis of infectious disease is based on three types of findings, not all of which are present in every instance. The first and most definitive diagnostic finding is the identification of the causative organism. Somewhat less certain, but highly useful in diagnosis, are the manifestations of illness presented by the patient. Third is the identification of specific types of responses to microorganisms.

IDENTIFICATION OF THE CAUSATIVE ORGANISM

In a number of infectious diseases the identification of the causative organism is essential not only to proper treatment of the patient but to the protection of noninfected individuals. For example, a diagnosis of tuberculosis carries with it the possibility that long-term treatment will be required and the possibility that others will be infected. The tubercle bacillus may be found in the sputum, gastric washings, or urine. Verification may require that one or more of the above be injected into a guinea pig.

Among other infectious diseases in which a positive diagnosis can be made by the identification of microorganisms are typhoid fever, bacterial and amebic dysenteries, bacterial pneumonias, and staphylococcal and streptococcal infections. The nurse frequently is responsible for collecting body discharges to be examined for pathogenic microorganisms. The inside of the container to be used for the specimen should be sterile at the time the collection is made. The discharges and containers should be handled in such a way that the outside of the container is kept clean. The nurse should protect her hands from contact with potentially contaminated material. Finally, she should thoroughly wash her hands after the collection procedure has been completed.

MANIFESTATIONS OF THE ILLNESS AS AN AID TO DIAGNOSIS

Although many of the manifestations in infectious disease are similar from one disease to another, the pattern of signs and symptoms is fairly characteristic for each disease. Frequently there are one or two effects that are pathognomonic of a particular disease. For example, swelling at the angle of the jaw and pain on swallowing sour food, such as pickles, are characteristic findings in mumps. When the patient is at least moderately ill and there are other patients in the community with the same infectious disease, the problem of diagnosis may be relatively easy. When the manifestations presented by the patient are not very marked and there are but few other sick persons, then the problem of diagnosis may be difficult.

IDENTIFICATION OF SPECIFIC TYPES OF RESPONSES TO MICROORGANISMS

A third method used in the diagnosis of the presence of specific infections is the serological test. In persons who are infected by the *Treponema pallidum,* certain immunochemical changes take place in the blood that can be determined by appropriate procedures. Because similar changes can be temporarily induced by a number of other disorders, such as infectious mononucleosis, malaria, and virus pneumonia, a patient can have a positive serological test and not have syphilis. A long-term disease, lupus erythematosus is frequently accompanied by a positive serological test despite the absence of syphilis.

Skin-sensitizing antibodies are also formed in response to certain other microorganisms. For example, the pathological changes that occur in blastomycosis are often similar to those of tuberculosis. A patient may be found on x-ray to have pathology similar to that of tuberculosis and yet to have a negative tuberculin test and no tubercle bacilli in his sputum or gastric washings. Injection of antigenic material into his skin from the organism causing blastomycosis may reveal sensitization to it.

To this point, the factors influencing the nature of man's relationship to the microorganisms in his environment have been presented. Although man has been able to control a few microbes, he has not been able to eradicate them. In the past, applications of the germ theory have led to remarkable progress in controlling some diseases. In recent years, the germ theory is being extended to include the fact that man is as important as the germ. Infection remains a health problem. Though infectious diseases that are problems differ from one another, the questions to be asked are similar.

The Planning of Nursing Care for Patients with Infectious Diseases

The Patient with a Virus Disease

There are a larger variety of viruses than any other microorganism causing disease. They are responsible for many human, animal, and plant diseases as well as for a high percentage of acute illness among human beings. To illustrate their frequency, at least 150 viruses are associated with the common cold.[42] Not only do viruses cause minor illnesses, but they cause serious diseases such as smallpox, yellow fever, and hepatitis. Because they are known to cause some forms of cancer in animals, the possibility that they are involved in some human cancers is being investigated.

Among the developments that have contributed greatly to knowledge of viruses are electron microscopy, x-ray diffraction techniques, and the discovery by Enders, Weller, and Robbins [43] that the poliomyelitis virus could be grown in animal as well as human tissue culture. Previous to the work of Enders *et al.* techniques had been developed so that many viruses were grown in fertilized eggs and in cultures of embryonic cells. Much of the information about the relationship of the virus to the host has been obtained from the study of bacteriophages (viruses that attack bacteria).

Unlike bacteria that contain both RNA and DNA, viruses contain one or the other. The nucleic acid forms a central core and is protected by a protein coat that enables it to survive outside the cell and that contains the antigenic material. After a virus enters the cell, the protein dissolves. The DNA or RNA takes over the metabolic machinery of the cell to reproduce itself and to direct formation of protein to coat the new nucleic acid molecules. If the cell dies, it undergoes necrosis and the viruses

are released. If the cell lives, viruses may be released one at a time. In either event, the new viruses are free to enter other cells, where they multiply. In virus diseases signs and symptoms may be caused by the response of cells to the virus as well as to cell necrosis.

Although specific viruses prefer particular hosts and tissues, in experimental situations they can be induced to grow on the tissues of other animals. To grow, the virus adapts to the new tissue by selection. In the process, its virulence may be altered for the new or for the original host. As an example, when the smallpox virus is passed through a calf, it is attenuated, but it retains sufficient antigenicity to induce immunity to smallpox for a period of three or four years.

Differences in the incidence and severity of influenza during epidemics may be caused by changes in the virulence or a mutation of the influenza virus; or it may be caused by the number of susceptible individuals, as well as the degree of their susceptibility. To illustrate, a new variant of influenza A virus has been identified in Hong Kong. Although it is an influenza A virus, it is different enough from the previous strain that one does not confer immunity to the other. Because individuals had not previously been exposed to this virus, an epidemic occurred. The size of the epidemic and the degree of illness depended on the virulence of the virus and the degree of susceptibility of the people who are infected.

To summarize, the factors contributing to difficulty in studying viruses include the following: (1) they are small in size, (2) they propagate only in living cells, and (3) human viruses rarely grow in animals.

Although viruses tend to be of small size, some are as large as small bacteria. Others are so small that they cannot be seen without the electron microscope. Electron microscopy and other techniques have enabled scientists to increase knowledge of the anatomy, physiology, and chemical characteristics of viruses. For detailed information, see the References.

Human viruses rarely grow readily in animals. To grow and multiply, they have to adapt to the animal host. Although scientists working in different laboratories start with the same virus, they may not be working with exactly the same one at a later time. As a result, their findings may be at variance. The capacity of viruses to alter their character in nature has great practical significance. For example, a vaccine capable of inducing immunity to one strain may be useless in another closely related strain. A new vaccine must therefore be developed.

An interesting discovery that may have some

[42] John H. Dingle: "The Common Cold and Common Cold-like Illnesses," *Med. Times*, **94**:191 (Feb.) 1966.

[43] J. F. Enders, T. H. Weller, and F. C. Robbin's: "Alteration in Pathogenicity for Monkeys of Brunhilde Strain of Poliomyelitis Virus Following Cultivation in Human Tissues," *Fed. Proc.*, **11**:467, 1952.

implications in the prevention and treatment of virus diseases was made by Issacs about ten years ago. He discovered that some virus-infected cells produced a protein, which he called **interferon**. This protected cells from the viruses.[44] Although infected cells produce interferons, some viruses stimulate interferon production better than others. Interferons have two limiting properties: (1) Cells have to be treated with interferons before or very soon after infection if they are to be effective and (2) they are specific to an animal species. Interferons protect other members of the same species but are ineffective in other species. Interferons, if administered early enough, may prove to be of value in the prevention and therapy of some virus diseases. They do not kill the viruses already present, but they do prevent the formation of new viruses, thus limiting the extent and spread of the disease.

How are viruses classified? What are some of the characteristic responses to viral invasion?

Viruses may be classified in a number of ways: according to the type of nucleic acid in the core (RNA or DNA); according to their biological, chemical, and physical properties; or according to the type of symptoms they produce.[45]

When viruses are classified according to the symptoms that they induce, they can be placed in two large groups: those that induce generalized effects and those in which the primary effects of the virus are localized. Generalized diseases include smallpox, measles, chickenpox, and yellow fever. Many types of tissue serve as the primary site for infection in virus disease. The nervous system, the respiratory tract, the skin and mucous membranes, the eye, the liver, the salivary glands, and the lymph glands are all known sites of infection.

Cellular responses induced by viruses are of two types and can occur alone or in combination. Tissue invaded by a virus may undergo hyperplasia. A familiar example is the common wart. This ability to induce hyperplasia in tissues suggests the possibility that viruses may play a role in initiating some types of neoplasms as they do in some plants and animals. Hyperplasia may be followed by necrosis of cells. The lesions formed in smallpox are characterized by hyperplasia followed by necrosis. Necrosis can occur alone. The lesions in the anterior horn cells in poliomyelitis are charac-

terized by necrosis. In infections caused by viruses, damage to and rearrangement of chromosomes have been noted.

Viruses are capable of causing all degrees of infection. In an epidemic of diseases such as poliomyelitis, antibodies can be demonstrated in the blood of those who have not been ill as well as of those who have been. Depending on the epidemic, only some who are ill are paralyzed. The fact that the person is ill may be obvious, but the character of his illness may not be. Some virus infections are accompanied by different manifestations in different persons. For example, during an epidemic of common colds, some persons may have symptoms that are more or less typical of a cold, whereas others have symptoms of gastroenteritis.

Many viruses are capable of inducing immunity. For some virus diseases, vaccines have been prepared that are successful in establishing immunity. The oldest is the vaccine for smallpox. The diseases in which the virus travels through the blood stream to cause disease are the ones in which antibodies are most successful in preventing a second attack. For those in which the virus directly infects cells, as in influenza, it is more difficult to establish a lasting immunity. Diseases in which a variety of viruses appear to be involved, such as the common cold, may not be entirely preventable by immunization. Possibly this is not undesirable. Scientists have discovered that for a time after one virus infection an animal is not susceptible to infection by another. Why this happens is not known.

What are some of the implications of the physical and chemical characteristics of viruses to nursing?

Some of the physical and chemical characteristics of viruses have practical implications in the practice of nursing. Most viruses are destroyed by heating to 60°C (140°F) for 30 minutes. An important exception is the virus causing serum hepatitis. It is able to withstand heating to 60°C for 4 hours. Because it is highly infectious, as little as 0.01 ml of plasma can carry enough virus to cause disease or to contaminate a batch of pooled plasma. Persons without a history of hepatitis may be carriers of the virus. The virus of infectious hepatitis, although less resistant to heat, may also be transmitted in blood plasma. For this reason authorities generally recommend that needles, syringes, pipettes, and other articles contaminated by blood be sterilized by autoclave for 15 minutes. Because of the possibility of transmitting infectious and serum hepatitis, as well as for economic reasons, many agencies use disposable syringes, needles, and other equipment.

[44] Robert M. Freidman: "Interferons and Virus Infections," *Amer. J. Nurs.*, 68:542–43 (Mar.) 1968.

[45] For a detailed classification see Ernest Jawetz, *et al.: Review of Medical Microbiology*, 8th ed. (Los Altos: Lange Medical Publications, 1968), pp. 296–98.

To prevent infection of herself, the nurse should try to avoid needle pricks after drawing blood or giving injections. In the event that she does prick herself, she should report the fact to her supervisor, so that arrangements can be made for her to receive immune globulin.

The virus is known to be present in the feces and blood in infectious hepatitis. From the available evidence, the urine and nasopharyngeal secretions probably do not contain the virus. Because the likelihood of spreading is increased by overcrowding and contaminated food and water, preventive measures should be directed toward relieving overcrowding and the sanitary disposal of feces.

The virus of infectious hepatitis also withstands residual chlorine of 1 part to 1 million. The resistance of the virus of infectious hepatitis is of significance, as the virus leaves the body in the feces and is ingested from food and water. In large cities, however, the water supply is usually safe. The swimming pool in the back yard can be a source of infection unless care is taken to keep it clean and to disinfect the water. Poorly constructed and overcrowded camp sites are also hazardous. Some epidemics of hepatitis have had their origin in oysters and clams obtained from contaminated water and eaten raw or insufficiently cooked.

To prevent the spread of infectious hepatitis,[46] the American Hospital Association recommends that the patient be isolated until the jaundice subsides and that a gown be worn over the uniform. As for any infectious disease, provision should be made for the sanitary disposal of contaminated articles. Everyone who enters the room should wash his hands on leaving. If possible, the patient should have his own toilet.

In the care of the patient with a virus infection, the nurse has two general responsibilities. One of these is to meet the needs of the patient for nursing. The other is to prevent the spread of the disease to herself and others. The same principles apply to the spread of virus infections as to others caused by microorganisms. The fact that viruses are relatively resistant to conditions in the external environment should be taken into account when planning an effective method for preventing their spread. The only viruses that consistently leave the body in feces are enteroviruses, but the adenoviruses may. Others are spread in respiratory secretions. Andrewes [47] states that his experiments demonstrate that the common cold is spread by droplets rather than droplet nuclei. If this is true, a properly worn

mask on the person who has a cold should be reasonably effective in preventing its transmission to others.

The Patient with Syphilis: An Example for Patient Care Planning

The first infectious disease to be discussed is syphilis. The necessary condition, or the direct cause of syphilis, is a spirochete known as the *Treponema pallidum.* Syphilis illustrates the point that the host is an important element in who develops an infectious disease. Despite a marked decrease in its incidence in the 1950's, there has been a significant increase in the 1960's. In 1956, 6,399 cases of early syphilis were reported; in 1964, 22,969. Most of the increase was in teen-agers. Because many of the new cases were not reported, there may have been as many as 120,000.[48] In fact, the incidence of syphilis is still rising as there were more cases in 1968 than in 1964. Most of the ten possible explanations for the increased incidence cited by Jekel [49] do not indicate a change in the virulence of *T. pallidum.* Rather they indicate changes in society. Among reasons given are less money for the support of syphilis control programs, increased urbanization, treatment is given in doctors' offices rather than public health clinics,[50] greater mobility of people, an increased rate among teenagers, and greater consumption of alcohol. All the preceding stem from the community and the circumstances affecting individual behavior.

Despite the importance of the environment in the development of syphilis, it is an infectious disease. A necessary condition is *T. pallidum.* It is a fragile organism, rapidly killed by drying and by a temperature of 42°C (107.6°F). The *T. pallidum* is susceptible to cold, soap and water, and weak disinfectants. It is killed by penicillin. It requires conditions similar to those existing within the living human being. When a nurse cares for a patient who has syphilis, and she asks the question "Who is to be protected from whom?" the answer is that the nurse *may* require protection. More information is required, however, before the nurse can answer the question positively. If protection is required, then the next question is "From whom or what is protection required?" Because the organism is delicate and survives for only a brief period

---

[46] *Infection Control in the Hospital* (Chicago: American Hospital Association, 1968), p. 131.

[47] Christopher H. Andrewes: "The Viruses of the Common Cold," *Sci. Amer.,* 203:88–102 (Dec.) 1960.

[48] Sidney Olansky: "Syphilis—Rediscovered," *DM,* p. 3 (May) 1967.

[49] James F. Jekel: "Role of Acquired Immunity to *T. pallidum* in the Control of Syphilis," *Public Health Rep.,* 83:627 (Aug.) 1968.

[50] There is disagreement on this point, as some physicians believe that all patients should be treated in physicians' offices.

of time outside the host, objects coming in contact with the patient do not remain contaminated for long. This is especially true if the objects are dry. Since *T. pallidum* is sensitive to moderate degrees of heat and to weak chemical disinfectants, elaborate measures are not required for disinfection.

In syphilis, the reservoir or source of *T. pallidum* is the person who has syphilis in an infectious stage. The location of the reservoir depends on the stage of the disease. The reservoir, the mode by which the spirochete escapes from the reservoir, the mode of transmission, and the portal of entry will be discussed at the same time. The portal of entry is usually the skin or mucous membrane or the placenta from the mother to the fetus. Transmission is by direct contact, usually by sexual intercourse or kissing.

PRIMARY STAGE

The incubation period varies from two to ten weeks; different authorities cite varying figures. In any event, some time after the individual is exposed, a sore or ulcer, called a chancre, develops at the site where the organism entered the body. The chancre is accompanied by a "satellite bubo," an enlarged lymph node in the drainage area of the chancre. Because of the nature of its transmission, the chancre is likely to be located on the genitalia or the lip. Though the lesion is often described as a painless ulceration surrounded by a hard, raised edge, it may be painful and varied in appearance. The chancre is highly infectious, as it teems with spirochetes. The spirochetes can be identified under the microscope by dark-field examination. After the second week, two other tests may be used. One is the TPI, which is shorthand for *Treponema pallidum* immobilization. It measures specific antibodies to *T. pallidum* and closely related infections such as yaws. The second is simpler than TPI, as it does not require live organisms. It is known as the FTA-ABS or fluorescent treponemal antibody test. The patient's serum is added to killed *T. pallidum* and fluorescein-labeled antihuman gamma globulin is then added. This test also includes a step to absorb the serum with nonpathogenic treponemes. This absorption increases the sensitivity of the test and probably also the specificity.

Other serological tests are based on the presence of an antibody-like substance, sometimes called reagin, in the serum of a patient who has been infected by *T. pallidum*. Among the serological tests used in the past and the present are the Wassermann, Kline, Hinton, Kohlmer, Kahn, Mazzini, and VDRL (Venereal Disease Research Laboratory). Some, such as the Hinton, Kahn, Kline, Mazzini, and VDRL, are flocculation tests. These tests are based on the knowledge that when normal blood serum is treated with lipid antigen the particles remain dispersed. In serum containing reagin, aggregates or clumps of material are formed, particularly when it is shaken or centrifuged. Tests such as the Wassermann and the Kohlmer are complement-fixation tests. As in the flocculation tests, a positive reaction depends on the presence of reagin in the blood serum. These tests can be positive in unrelated disorders. Currently the VDRL test is used almost exclusively in routine diagnosis.

Fortunately, the length of the period of communicability can now be shortened by treatment of the patient with penicillin. According to Goodman and Gilman,[51] the rash begins to fade within 48 hours and is usually gone by 14 days. The serologic test usually becomes negative in less than 3 months after therapy has been completed.

SECONDARY STAGE

Whether or not treatment is given, the chancre heals. Some weeks later, in untreated patients, the secondary stage follows. In some patients this stage is so mild that it passes unnoticed, whereas in others the symptoms may be severe. Symptoms characteristic of the second stage include a generalized rash on the skin and mucous membranes, fever, sore throat, and malaise. The rash may be widespread, even involving the palms of the hands and the soles of the feet. The rashes on the mucous membranes of the mouth, anus, and genitalia are more significant than in other areas because these rashes tend to break down and form small superficial erosions called mucous patches. They, like the chancre, are teeming with spirochetes. The lesions on the anus and genitalia may hypertrophy and form moist condylomata.

Because of the large number of lesions, the secondary stage is the most infectious stage of syphilis. The fragility of the microbe, however, limits the mode of transmission to direct contact. Although authorities such as Anderson *et al.*[52] concede that transmission by fomites—food or toilet seats—is theoretically possible, it is highly unlikely. Babies born of syphilitic mothers may develop congenital syphilis, though they may not if the mother has had syphilis for several years or is adequately treated prior to, or during, the early stages of pregnancy. Babies born of syphilitic mothers do not have the first stage of syphilis. They may be stillborn or, if

51 *Op. cit.*, pp. 1221–23.
52 Anderson *et al.*, *op. cit.*, p. 463.

born alive, be in the secondary stage, or they may present no evidence of having syphilis. The lesions of the baby with secondary syphilis are also full of spirochetes.

Whatever the age of the patient, the nurse and other persons are the ones who require protection. This protection requires that contact with the lesion or lesions containing spirochetes be prevented as long as the patient is infectious. Rubber gloves should be worn to prevent the nurse from having direct contact with infectious lesions until the patient is rendered noninfectious by treatment. In the general care of adult patients, there may be few occasions when gloves are required. They should, however, be worn when handling a newborn baby who has secondary lesions. In the absence of effective treatment, congenital infections are not usually communicable for more than one or two years.[53] Patients who acquire syphilis after birth remain communicable for a period of from two to five years. The disease is most communicable during the first four years after infection. Mothers may transmit the infection to the fetus for as long as ten years after they are infected. The ability to transmit *T. pallidum* to others depends on continuing infection. Patients remain infectious only if they are not adequately treated.

LATENT SYPHILIS

Following the secondary stage of syphilis, the disease becomes latent. During this period there are no overt clinical signs or symptoms. The only way the majority of cases can be recognized is by serological testing.

Some of the syphilitic individuals will never have more sign of it than the positive serological test. However, in others the treponema invades some body structure, usually the cardiovascular system or nervous system. The period in which clinical symptoms are absent is called the latent stage. The outcome of latent syphilis varies. Some never develop tertiary disease. In others as much as 20 to 30 years elapse after infection before signs and symptoms appear. Occasionally the latent period may be very short. Recently a patient was admitted to a local hospital with an acute tertiary, or third, stage of syphilis. The course of the disease had been telescoped from the first to the third stage in just a few weeks. The physician who cared for this patient had not seen a similar patient in 20 years. Usually when syphilis is introduced into a new population, it runs a rapid course. Winslow[54] indicates that toward the end of the fifteenth

century an epidemic of syphilis swept over Europe with great deadliness.

The late lesion of syphilis is the gumma, which in the opinion of some authorities is a hypersensitivity reaction to *T. pallidum.*[55] It consists of vascular and perivascular changes followed by tissue necrosis and eventually scar tissue formation. It contains few or no spirochetes. The most common sites for late lesions are the nervous system, the thoracic aorta, and the eye, though practically any organ may be involved. Cardiovascular syphilis is the most incapacitating and fatal form.

In the past the late lesions of syphilis were not thought to contain the spirochete. Because patients with late syphilis improve following treatment with penicillin, this is regarded as evidence that spirochetes are in the tissues in a form that cannot be recognized by measures now available.[56] Gummas do not resolve with treatment, nor do other destructive lesions disappear. During the late stage of syphilis, the reservoir for the spirochete is the organ or tissue that is infected. The danger of infecting others by ordinary means is considered to be nonexistent. Because of the possibility of the blood containing *T. pallidum,* patients in any stage of syphilis are not permitted to be blood donors.

SUMMARY

When a nurse cares for a patient who has a diagnosis of syphilis, she should first learn whether or not the patient is in an infectious stage of the disease. If he is not, no special precautions are necessary. If he is, she should then ask herself "Who is to be protected from whom?" and "From what and for how long is protection necessary?" The answers to these questions should then serve as a basis for her actions. Nurses are frequently unnecessarily worried about the possibility of a patient's being infectious. When the nurse is in doubt, she should discuss her fears with the head nurse or with the patient's physician.

She should not delay seeking appropriate advice. If there is a real possibility that she has been infected, the sooner she is treated the better. Moreover, the problem should be resolved so the nurse can be spared needless worry.

Miss Slender illustrates the preceding situation. When handling wooden side rails from the bed of a patient in the tertiary stage of syphilis, she scratched a finger on a jagged edge of the side rail. From her knowledge of syphilis, her intellect told her she was not in any danger. Yet she was frightened. After worrying for a day or

[53] *Ibid.,* p. 462.

[54] Charles-Edward Amory Winslow: *The Conquest of Epidemic Disease* (Princeton, N.J.: Princeton University Press, 1943), p. 124.

[55] Olansky, *op. cit.,* p. 19.

[56] McDermott, *op. cit.,* pp. 493–97.

so, Miss Slender told her head nurse what had happened. Because Miss Slender was anxious, the head nurse told Miss Slender what she already knew, that she was not in danger. However, because she was concerned, the head nurse suggested that Miss Slender consult her physician. When Miss Slender saw her physician, he, too, told her that she was in no danger, but he administered penicillin as a prophylactic measure.

One point requiring emphasis when discussing nursing of the patient who has acquired syphilis is the nurse's own feelings about the disease and its mode of transmission. The nurse should be particularly careful to avoid making moral judgment or to allow her own values to interfere with care of the patient. The aim in treatment should be to enlist the cooperation of the patient so that he will continue treatment in order to prevent the late effects of the disease and to prevent its spread to others.

In answering the question "Who protects whom?" the answer includes more than the protection of the nurse from the infection. It includes the protection of the patient from the destructive effects of the disease and the prevention of the infection of others.

One problem that should be of concern is that the incidence of gonorrhea and infectious syphilis, especially among teenagers, is rising in the United States. In some states, consideration needs to be given to changing the law that physicians must have the consent of a parent or guardian to treat a teenager. Because of their reluctance to discuss the possibility of being infected with a venereal disease with their parents, some teenagers go untreated. They continue to be a danger to themselves and to others.

In the November 1960 *Public Health Reports* a brief report is made about seminars conducted on venereal disease during 1960 by the United States Public Health Service.[57] Among the conclusions that have pertinence to nursing practice were the following:

1. The knowledge and skills are available to reduce the incidence of syphilis to the point where this disease can be kept under control by nominal expenditures of money, time, and effort.
2. Action must be taken promptly.
3. The basic action is to find the newly infected person before he has a chance to infect others and to bring him under treatment.
4. Case finding requires the use of all community resources, including the patient. Another paper in the same issue of *Public Health Reports* describes a program for

training nurses to interview patients, so that they can participate effectively in case finding and in case holding.[58]
5. The suggestion was also made that informational and educational efforts should also be strengthened.

Briefly, the causative agent in syphilis is *T. pallidum*. It is a delicate organism that is well adapted to the internal environment of the human being. It is easily destroyed by conditions that vary in any degree from these conditions. The reservoir is the person who is infected. The period of greatest communicability is the first four or five years after the infection is acquired, though occasionally it may be as long as ten years. Transmission is by direct contact with tissues, including blood containing the spirochete. Prevention depends on sterilizing the reservoir or protecting others from contact with it. To eradicate the reservoir of infection, persons who are in the communicable phases of the disease must be identified and brought under treatment before they have had an opportunity to infect others. This is in their own interest as well as for the welfare of others. They must also be treated until they are cured. This requires follow-up and education. Nurses participate in all these activities.

Hospital-Acquired Infections

INCIDENCE

The problem of infection in hospitals is not new; it has been a problem for centuries. Not until the introduction of antisepsis and asepsis in the late nineteenth century were infections brought under some degree of control. The present concern about infections is caused by the observation that the incidence of infection in hospitals is higher than it was previous to the introduction of antimicrobial drugs. According to Reimann,[59] between the years of 1935 and 1947 the death rate from infections at the Boston City Hospital fell steadily. Since 1947 it has increased steadily. In 1957 there were four times as many patients with staphylococci in their blood stream as there were in 1935 and twice as many as in 1947. Reimann continues by saying that, prior to 1937, infections from gram-negative bacilli were rare and that they have increased at even a more rapid rate than have those caused by staphylococci. Following the introduction of new antibiotics, the incidence of *Staphylococcus aureus* again dropped.

[57] "A Current Look at Venereal Disease," *Public Health Rep.*, **75**:989–92 (Nov.) 1960.

[58] "The Venereal Disease Contact Interview," *Public Health Rep.*, **75**:1000–1006 (Nov.) 1960.

[59] Hobart A. Reimann: "Infectious Diseases," *Arch. Intern. Med.*, **106**:681 (Nov.) 1960.

In a 57-day study in which 491 infections were investigated, McNamara et al.[60] found that 16.3 per cent were hospital-acquired and that more than twice as many occurred on the surgical unit than on any other unit. The common sites of infection in percentages were respiratory tract, 39.2; wound and skin, 27.8; and urinary tract, 24. With one exception, in which the patient was being treated with immunosuppressive therapy, the urinary tract infections followed catheterization.[61] Gram-negative organisms caused 68.5 per cent and gram-positive organisms caused 16.4 per cent of the infections. Despite the increase in the number of infections caused by gram-negative bacilli, McNamara et al.[62] stated that the S. aureus still plays an important role in hospital infections. Altemeier [63] emphasizes the importance of infection among surgical patients. In a general hospital, from 40 to 65 per cent of the patients are treated surgically. Approximately 40 per cent of these patients have an established infection at the time of their admission or develop one during their hospital stay.

Barrett et al.[64] found that of 782 patients studied in early 1967, 122 had hospital-acquired infections and 206 had community-acquired infections. The nosocomial infections were more common among surgical patients and the community-acquired infections were more common among medical patients. Of 40 wound infections, only one was community-acquired.[65]

INFECTING ORGANISMS AND SITES

The organism(s) causing an infection is related to such factors as whether the infection is hospital- or community-acquired, the site and mode of infection, the state of health of the host, types of treatment, and mode of transmission. Respiratory tract infections are most commonly caused by pneumococci, streptococci, staphylococci, and aspirated gram-negative bacilli.

Skin infections are frequently caused by S. aureus, most of which secrete penicillinase, and some of which are resistant to methicillin. This staphylococcus also infects burned areas, although Pseudomonas infections are common. In fact, Pseudomonas infections may be more

common than appreciated as they thrive on moist surfaces.[66]

Urinary tract infections usually follow catheterization or some type of instrumentation of the urinary bladder. Within 96 hours almost all patients having an indwelling catheter have bacteriuria and from 10 to 20 per cent have bacteremia. The common organisms are streptococci, particularly enterococci, gram-negative bacilli, Proteus, and mixed infections.[67]

Gastroenteritis may be caused by salmonellae, staphylococcal food poisoning from enterotoxin, and, in newborns, some types of E. coli.

The findings of Streeter, Dunn, and Lepper [68] are similar to those previously cited. A variety of organisms are responsible for hospital infections. As in the other studies, the site of infection influenced the type of microbe(s) causing the infection. Staphylococcus aureus was most common in wound infections (36 per cent). In respiratory infections the most commonly cultured organisms were Pseudomonas aeruginosa and Klebsiella. In tracheostomy infections, the organism was Pseudomonas aeruginosa, and in urinary infections, E. coli. All of these, plus other organisms, were cultured from each of the four sites, sometimes singly but usually in combination with other microbes.

FACTORS PREDISPOSING TO NOSOCOMIAL INFECTIONS

In the preceding discussion some of the factors predisposing to nosocomial infections were indicated. Duma [69] summarizes them as (1) manipulative procedures including instrumentation, (2) treatment with chemical or physical agents that lower the resistance of the host, (3) presence of a debilitating disease, and (4) exposure to pathogenic microorganisms.

MANIPULATIVE PROCEDURES

Any procedure that causes a break in a barrier between the external and internal environment (skin or mucous membrane) deprives the patient of one of his defenses against infections. Thus surgical procedures of any type— cardiac catheterization, bladder catheterization and cystoscopy, spinal tap, paracentesis, tracheostomy, drainage tubes from any body cavity, intravenous infusions, parenteral injections, as well as others—provide a portal of entry for microorganisms.

[60] M. J. McNamara et al.: "A Study of the Bacteriologic Patterns of Hospital Infections," Ann. Intern. Med., **66**:481 (Mar.) 1967.

[61] Ibid., p. 482.

[62] Ibid., p. 480.

[63] William A. Altemeier: "Bodily Response to Infectious Agents," JAMA, 202:1085 (Dec. 18) 1967.

[64] Fred F. Barrett, Joan I. Casey, and Maxwell Finland: "Infections and Antibiotic Use Among Patients at Boston City Hospital, February 1967," New Eng. J. Med., **278**:6 (Jan. 4) 1968.

[65] Ibid., p. 7.

[66] "Pseudomonas Contamination Hard to Control," Hospitals, **42**:66 (Jan. 1) 1968.

[67] Richard J. Duma: "Management of Hospital Infections," GP, **39**:110 (Jan.) 1969.

[68] Streeter et al., op. cit., p. 531.

[69] Op. cit., p. 107.

CHEMICAL AND PHYSICAL AGENTS

Chemical and physical agents used in the treatment of disease predispose to infection by reducing the ability of the individual to respond to microorganisms. Some of the agents predispose to endogenous as well as exogenous infections. They include the introduction of prosthetic devices, x-ray therapy, immunosuppressive and cytotoxic chemicals, corticosteroids, and antimicrobial drugs. As discussed earlier, one of the ways in which antimicrobial drugs predispose to infection is by upsetting the ecologic balance among microbes. Thus fungus infections, usually *Candida,* ordinarily clear up when antibiotic therapy is discontinued.

PRESENCE OF DEBILITATING DISEASE OR
SERIOUS INJURY

Although any person may become infected, certain individuals are especially susceptible. They include the aged, the very young, the undernourished, and those who have been burned or whose tissues have been traumatized. Compound fractures (bone breaking the skin) are particularly liable to infection. Among the diseases in which infection is a constant threat are cirrhosis of the liver, chronic pulmonary disease, uremia, agammaglobulinemia or dysgammaglobulinemia, cancer, diabetes mellitus, hemolytic diseases, and dermatitis.

EXPOSURE TO PATHOGENIC ORGANISMS

Most of the organisms causing nosocomial infections, including the *S. aureus,* have a low degree of pathogenicity in healthy individuals. As a result of disease, trauma, or any condition causing a depression of body defenses, they can cause diseases that may or may not be serious. In the hospital the patient's chances of being exposed to infection are increased by the density of the hospital population. He may share a room with from 1 to 20 or more people. The number of hospital personnel and visitors spending time in his immediate environment further increases the possibility of his being exposed to infection. The areas in the hospital where infection rates are highest are those in which contact between patient and personnel is the greatest—newborn nurseries, recovery rooms, operating rooms, intensive-care units, and burn units.[70] Host susceptibility is undoubtedly a factor. Studies made on drugs, food, water, and equipment indicate that they may be contaminated with potential pathogens.

In this discussion some of the circumstances predisposing patients to hospital-acquired infec-

[70] *Ibid.,* p. 108.

tions have been presented. As stated earlier, all people including nurses are susceptible to infection. By identifying the circumstances that increase the likelihood of patients developing an infection, measures can be instituted to protect patients and personnel.

RESERVOIRS

Three general groups of people in the hospital act as reservoirs for microorganisms. The first group includes patients who are admitted for treatment of a septic condition or who are carriers of pathogens. The second group includes those patients who are negative at the time they are admitted but who acquire an infection after their admission to the hospital. The person may become a carrier or develop an infectious disease. The third group is comprised of the various members of the hospital personnel. They, too, may act as carriers or develop overt disease. According to Duma,[71] hospital personnel are the most important source of infection. Furthermore, these persons are likely to be carriers.

The results of a number of studies on carriers indicate that some persons do not easily become carriers. In some persons who do, the carrier state is persistent, whereas in others it is intermittent. The reasons for these differences are not well understood. In general, the highest rate of carriers is found among those persons in the hospital who are in closest contact with patients. The lowest rate is found among those who are farthest from the patient. As a consequence, the rate is highest among nurses and physicians and lowest among office personnel.

Not only may the carrier state be a problem to the nurse, but she, too, sometimes develops staphylococcic infections. In a study by Davies [72] on the incidence of staphylococcic infections among nurses at the London Hospital, he found that 16.4 per cent of the admissions of nurses to the infirmary were for staphylococcic infections. In the six years prior to the year in which the study was made, the percentage was 18.2 per cent. The study showed that the average length of time lost by each nurse was 8.5 days. Davies states that all the infections were of the soft tissues and were of the type that probably involved transmission by direct contact. The lesions were found on the face, neck, axilla, and upper limb. Almost 98 per cent of the organisms were resistant to penicillin. Davies questions the use of the scrubbing brush, because many of the

[71] *Ibid.,* p. 108.
[72] D. M. Davies: "Staphylococcal Infection in Nurses," *Lancet,* 1:644–45 (Mar. 19) 1960.

lesions were on the hands. Vigorous scrubbing may disrupt the skin and thereby provide a portal of entry for microbes.

MODES AND VEHICLES OF TRANSMISSION

FOOD

Food may serve as a vehicle for the transmission of microbes and their products and thus be a source of disease. An example of the first is the Salmonella group of bacteria and of the second is the enterotoxin of the *Staphylococcus aureus*.

Salmonellosis is a continuing problem. Salmonella can be transported by milk, poultry, and eggs. Some infections have been traced to nonfat dry milk. Skimmed milk must be pasteurized before it is dried. Cooking poultry and eggs kills the salmonella. Liquid feedings containing eggs should be pasteurized before ingestion. Some health departments suggest that poultry be washed and prepared in an area reserved for that purpose and that the area not be used for other food.

Although food poisoning can be a serious illness, it is not a staphylococcal infection. It is caused by an enterotoxin elaborated by certain strains of the *S. aureus*. Culture characteristics help to explain why these organisms are frequently implicated in food poisoning. They grow well at room temperature, as well as at body temperature. They are aerobic but grow under anaerobic conditions. Foods containing mixtures of egg and milk, such as cream pies, provide a good culture medium for *S. aureus*. If food is contaminated and allowed to stand at room temperature, the staphylococci multiply and in five to seven hours produce enough enterotoxin to cause gastroenteritis. To prevent poisoning from food contaminated by *S. aureus*, bakeries and restaurants are required to refrigerate all cream pies and other cream-filled desserts. Housewives should do likewise in the home. Because time is required for the staphylococcus to elaborate the enterotoxin, there is no danger from foods that are eaten as soon as they are prepared. Leftovers should be refrigerated promptly.

After the ingestion of the enterotoxin, the incubation period is short. It varies from 45 minutes to 6 hours. The more enterotoxin, the sooner symptoms appear. Acute prostration and even death may occur in debilitated patients. The main feature in therapy is to restore the fluid and electrolyte balance of the patient. As indicated above, prevention is based on prompt and adequate refrigeration of susceptible foods. Because the enterotoxin is heat-stable, heating the food after enterotoxin is formed is of no avail. The only procedures of value are to prevent the contamination of food and to refrigerate it if it is not eaten as soon as it is prepared. The sanitary handling of food lessens the chances of introducing microorganisms and refrigeration minimizes bacterial growth.

In addition to their ability to grow and multiply in simple culture media, staphylococci are able to survive for extended periods of time outside the host. Their great resistance to drying is emphasized by Colbeck.[73] His assistants were able to make cultures of staphylococci from sealed test tubes containing dried cultures that had not been subcultured in five years. The staphylococci were pathogenic. Eighteen hours after opening the tubes, Colbeck developed boils on two fingers; organisms recovered from the boils were the same phage type as those in the test tubes. Because the phage type was rare in Vancouver, the assumption was made that the source of the staphylococci was the old dried culture.

An application to nursing is illustrated by Fason[74] who studied the feasibility of reusing disposable tube-feeding bags. Failure to keep the formula under constant refrigeration was found to be responsible for unsafe bacterial counts, rather than the reused bags. Safe food depends on cleanliness in its preparation, pasteurization or adequate cooking, and refrigeration, particularly of meat, milk, fish, and eggs. Despite the apparent safety of properly cleaned bags, their reuse is not recommended.

WATER

Just as food may act as a vehicle for the transmission of pathogens, water may be also. Walter[75] found bedside pitchers to be highly contaminated. Ice cubes have also been found to carry pathogens. Bedside pitchers should have a wide neck so that they can be thoroughly cleaned and be of a type that can be sterilized and covered. Ice cubes should be handled with tongs.

EQUIPMENT

The patient in the hospital is exposed to a great variety of potential pathogens. One of the

[73] John C. Colbeck: "Environmental Aspects of Staphylococcal Infections Acquired in Hospitals: 1. The Hospital Environment—Its Place in the Hospital Staphylococcus Infections Problem," *Amer. J. Public Health*, **50**:472 (Apr.) 1960.

[74] M. Fitzpatrick Fason: "Controlling Bacterial Growth in Tube Feedings," *Amer. J. Nurs.*, **67**:1246–47 (June) 1967.

[75] Carl W. Walter *et al.*: "Bacteriology of the Bedside Carafe," *New Eng. J. Med.*, **259**:1198–1202 (Dec. 18) 1958.

ways in which exogenous organisms are transmitted to him is by way of equipment used in his care. Duma [76] and Christie and Ginsberg [77] list a great variety of materials in common use that may transmit microorganisms, including hand lotion, eye drops, multiple-use vials, and disinfectants. Among the devices used in the care of patients are respirators and other ventilatory assistive devices, especially those introducing an aerosol mist of less than five microns (μ). When respirators are used, each patient should have his own equipment and not just his own mouthpiece, nebulizer, and tubing.

The prevention of transmission of infection by equipment involves individualizing all parts that come in contact with the patient or his secretions. Equipment that is not discarded after use should be thoroughly cleaned by healthy, trained personnel who understand the importance of each detail and take pride in doing a competent job. As an example, postoperative pneumonia caused by *Pseudomonas* has been traced to anesthetic equipment and the people who clean it. All types of equipment from thermometers to cardiac bypass machines should be checked at regular intervals for the efficiency of disinfecting techniques.

When air conditioners are used in rooms where there is more than one patient, room air should not be recirculated. Inside air should be exchanged for outside air.

CATHETERIZATION

As stated earlier, catheterization and cystoscopy are all too often followed by bacteriuria and at times bacteremia. Santora [78] reviewed the literature on urinary tract infections. On the basis of this review she concluded that during catheterization and when an indwelling catheter is in place meticulous aseptic technique must be maintained. When the patient has an indwelling catheter, a sterile closed drainage system with an antiseptic added to the collecting container should be used. A rigid collecting container should be used for ambulatory patients. The tubing leading from the bladder should be below the level of the bladder but above the level of the urine. The meatus should be washed with a bacteriostatic agent. The area around the meatus should be cleansed at least twice daily with 1:1,000 aqueous benzalkonium chloride solution. To reduce trauma to the urethra, the smallest catheter possible should be used and the catheter should be generously

lubricated before it is inserted. Measures to increase the relaxation of the patient by asking her (him) to take a deep breath at the time the catheter is inserted generally decreases constriction of the urethra. To prevent pushing bacteria normally present in the terminal meatus into the urinary bladder, the urethra may be irrigated by inserting a sterile asepto syringe about three fourths of an inch into the urethra and irrigating it with one ounce of 1:1,000 aqueous benzalkonium chloride solution or an antibacterial lubricant may be used. To prevent the upward ascent of bacteria in the tubing, fluids should be forced when the patient can take fluids by mouth. When he can tolerate cranberry juice, he may be encouraged to drink it as it helps to keep the urine acid. Bacterial growth is inhibited in acid urine.

The protection of the patient who must be catheterized or who has an indwelling catheter is facilitated by measures (1) to prevent or limit the number of organisms introduced into the bladder, (2) to prevent trauma to the meatus and bladder, (3) to prevent the reflux of urine into the bladder, and (4) to maintain drainage from the bladder to the collecting container.

For a further discussion of catheterization, see Chapter 17.

AIRBORNE INFECTIONS

The air may become directly or indirectly contaminated and serve as a vehicle of transmission in any disease or carrier state in which pathogens are in the respiratory tract. Coughing, sneezing, and talking have been demonstrated to be accompanied by the discharge into the air of droplets of moisture of varying sizes. Because large droplets settle rapidly, doubt is cast on the importance of droplet infection as a vehicle of transmission. Droplet nuclei are, however, believed to be important because tiny dried particles or nuclei are suspended in the air. Because they are buoyant, they remain in the air currents and are carried by the air wherever the air goes. Riley [79] cites three studies in support of the theory that droplet nuclei and dust serve to transmit infection. The principal vehicle for the transmission of tuberculosis is said to be droplet nuclei. Air may also be contaminated by dust particles, which can carry staphylococci. Colbeck [80] states that the number of colonies of staphylococci cultured from the air can be doubled by moving a blanket rapidly from the top to the foot of the bed once a minute for five minutes. Blankets and sheets may be contaminated by drainage from a wound. The air is then contaminated by dust

[76] *Op. cit.*, p. 106–107.
[77] Jean E. Christie and Frances Ginsberg: "Seven Places Where Cross Infection Can Start," *Mod. Hosp.*, 110:142 (May) 1968.
[78] Delores Santora: "Preventing Hospital-Acquired Urinary Infection," *Amer. J. Nurs.*, 66:793–94 (Apr.) 1966.
[79] Richard L. Riley: "Air-borne Infections," *Amer. J. Nurs.*, 60:1247 (Sept.) 1960.
[80] *Op. cit.*, p. 470.

shaken from the bedding during procedures such as changing or straightening the patient's bed.

Not all investigators agree about the extent to which clothing and bed linens of patients with staphylococcic disease act as vehicles of transmission. There is, however, general agreement that they are heavily contaminated. Burnett et al.[81] state that among hospital personnel student nurses seem to be most vulnerable. Because their infections were found to be on exposed areas, this suggests transmission by contact. From this brief review of the mechanisms of transmission of the staphylococci, the fact that they are multiple and complex should be evident.

One of the most commonly used measures in the control of airborne infection is the wearing of masks. Masks are worn to accomplish two different purposes. One is to prevent the contamination of the external environment by microorganisms from the respiratory tract of the person wearing the mask. In terms of the links in the chain of the infectious process, the mask stands between the point at which a microorganism leaves the reservoir and the point at which it finds a vehicle for its transmission. This is the basis for wearing a mask in the operating room or in the newborn infants' nursery or for a patient with a cold, tuberculosis, or other respiratory infection wearing a mask. A mask may also be used to guard a portal of entry. In this instance, a nurse or doctor wears a mask to protect himself from microorganisms discharged by the patient.

According to Riley,[82] masks are more effective in preventing the escape of microorganisms from the reservoir into the external environment than they are in preventing the inhalation of droplet nuclei. The reason is that they catch the droplets of moisture in the expired air. Droplet nuclei, which form as the moisture evaporates, are smaller in size and are therefore more difficult to trap. Although the construction of a mask and the way it is worn determine its effectiveness, instances are all too frequent in which masks are improperly worn. Riley[83] states: "Furthermore, proper use of the mask depends on individual initiative and a high level of understanding, cooperation, and discipline."

Blair[84] describes in detail the construction of a face mask and outlines the procedure for wearing it. In general the mask should be constructed of a number of layers of material of dense porosity. It should be made of absorbent material so that it takes up moisture as it passes through. It should be clean when applied and discarded when removed. It should be replaced before it becomes wet. Most authorities suggest that a mask should not be worn longer than an hour or an hour and a half. It should cover both the nose and the mouth. It should be tied firmly in place. Some surgeons, such as Adams,[85] advocate the wearing of double-thickness masks. Howe[86] recommends that two masks be worn and that they be changed at one-and-one-half-hour intervals in long operations.

Although masks have been the most widely used device to control airborne infection, other measures are available. The concentration of microorganisms in the air can be reduced by ventilation. Florence Nightingale advocated ventilation as a measure in the care of the sick. It is still frequently neglected. Outdoor air may be laden with soot and dust, but it usually carries few microorganisms. Particularly in the operating room, air-conditioning systems may be used to remove the respired air and add clean air. Hart[87] recommends that ultraviolet light be used to sterilize the air in the operating room. One point that is too often neglected in the control of airborne infection is keeping doors closed. Air currents carry droplet nuclei wherever they go.

HANDS

The hands may act as vehicles in the transmission of virulent germs. The source of their contamination may be discharges from the nasal mucosa of carriers or discharges from open lesions, as well as urine and feces. Contamination of the hands may therefore result from direct contact with a lesion or its discharges or from contact with dressings covering septic wounds, bed coverings, or the clothing of the patient. Measures should be carried out to prevent the hands from being contaminated or to remove any microorganisms present on them.

To protect the person who is changing the dressings over draining wounds, rubber gloves should be worn. Koenig[88] recommends that all persons having contact with a patient with a staphylococcal infection wear gloves. The dress-

[81] W. Emory Burnett, et al.: "Program for Prevention and Eradication of Staphylococcic Infections," JAMA, **166**:1183–84 (Mar. 8) 1958.

[82] Riley, op. cit., p. 1248.

[83] Richard L. Riley: "Protective Measures—Reasonable or Ritualistic?" Nurs. Outlook, **7**:39 (Jan.) 1959.

[84] Esta H. McNett Blair: "Oh, for a Mask," Nurs. Outlook, **7**:40–42 (Jan.) 1959.

[85] Ralph Adams: "Prevention of Infections in Hospitals," Amer. J. Nurs., **58**:345 (Mar.) 1958.

[86] Chester W. Howe: "Prevention and Control of Postoperative Wound Infections Owing to Staphylococcus aureus," New Eng. J. Med., **255**:787–94 (Oct. 25) 1956.

[87] Deryl Hart: "Bactericidal Ultraviolet Radiation in the Operating Room," JAMA, **172**:1019–28 (Mar. 5) 1960.

[88] M. Glenn Koenig: "Staphylococcal Infections—Treatment and Control," DM, p. 29 (April) 1968.

ings should also be discarded in such a manner that no one handles them after they are removed. For example, they may be placed on several thicknesses of newspaper and wrapped so that the outside of the package is kept clean. Whatever technique is utilized, it should be based on the certainty that discharges from infected lesions are teeming with virulent microorganisms.

Because it is impossible to prevent contamination of the hands in all instances, hand washing is essential to the removal of microorganisms. To be effective, it must be performed properly and after each patient contact. Benson [89] describes in detail the hand-washing technique used at the Clinical Center, National Institutes of Health, Bethesda, Maryland. It will not be repeated here. The procedure described by Benson is for use on medical and surgical wards and not as part of the preparation for surgical operations. Hand washing, properly performed, is an essential step in the infectious process.

As in other areas some question the value of hand washing per se and believe [90] that a cleansing agent such as hexachlorophene is more important. As previously stated, too vigorous hand washing may traumatize the skin. In some individuals it may lead to dermatitis. There is agreement that the hands should be washed between administering care to each patient.

The control of staphylococcic disease is complicated by the fact that healthy carriers as well as patients with the disease are sources of infection. The objective of any program of control should be to limit contact of persons with active disease as well as healthy carriers with susceptible patients.[91] Streeter et al.[92] and others emphasize that a surveillance program is basic to any adequate system of infectious disease control.

THE CONTROL OF HOSPITAL-ACQUIRED INFECTIONS

SPECIFIC CONTROL MEASURES

Among the specific measures to control hospital staphylococcal infections suggested by Koenig [93] are

1. All hospital personnel who have active staphylococcal lesions, even if they are relatively minor

pustules or furuncles, should be excused from work and excluded from the hospital environment.
2. The indiscriminate use of antimicrobial agents must be abolished. Such agents not only increase the reservoir of hospital staphylococci, but render the particular patient to whom they are given susceptible to colonization with strains resistant to multiple drugs.
3. Patients with underlying diseases which predispose them to staphylococcal infections should not be admitted to hospitals on an elective basis. These would include patients with exfoliating skin diseases of mild to moderate degree who might be treated at home.
4. Local procedures which greatly increase the host's susceptibility to infection such as tracheostomies and venous cutdowns for the administration of blood, fluids or drugs should be used only when absolutely necessary and measures should be directed to prevent the contamination of these sites. Nasopharyngeal or tracheal suctioning should be done only when absolutely necessary and with care not to cause unnecessary trauma.
5. Agents which generally decrease host resistance such as corticosteroids, immunosuppressive agents and antineoplastic drugs should be administered judiciously and only for well defined reasons.
6. Patients with active staphylococcal infections should be isolated from other patients. Hospital personnel and visitors coming into contact with such individuals should wear gowns, gloves and masks to prevent them from acquiring and transmitting disease-producing strains.
7. The opportunity for infecting patients with exfoliating skin diseases, widespread burns or agranulocytosis should be minimized by the institution of protective isolation procedures.

As more is learned about specific microorganisms and how they are spread, practices in their control change. Authorities do not always agree about practices. As illustrations, whether a mask is worn and who wears it depends on how a disease is spread and who is to be protected. Whereas Koenig recommends the wearing of a mask for the prevention of the spread of staphylococcal infection, Infection Control in the Hospital 1968 [94] does not. The patient should be isolated and a clean gown worn. Gloves should be worn by the person having direct contact with the patient.

When the nurse has close contact with the patient and the organism is resistant to destruction, the clothing of the nurse may become contaminated. For this reason, the nurse wears a gown during the time she cares for the patient. In some hospitals anyone who changes or assists in the changing of dressings on septic wounds also wears a mask, gown, and gloves. To limit the danger of the spread of virulent

[89] Margaret E. Benson: "Handwashing—An Important Part of Medical Asepsis," Amer. J. Nurs., 57:1136–39 (Sept.) 1957.
[90] "Does Hand-Washing Really Prevent Cross-Infection," RN, 29:71–73 (June) 1966.
[91] Koenig, loc. cit., p. 28.
[92] Streeter et al., op. cit., p. 527.
[93] Koenig, op. cit., pp. 29–30.
[94] Op. cit., p. 131.

organisms from one patient to another, individual dressing trays or sets are recommended for each patient.

SPECIAL TECHNIQUES

Patients receiving cytotoxic and immuno-suppressive drugs are robbed to a greater or lesser extent of their ability to defend themselves against microbes. Burned patients are also especially vulnerable to infection. Laduke [95] describes devices and techniques for isolating an entire patient or part of him in a germ-free environment. The air entering the enclosure is sterile as is all the equipment. This device protects the patient from exogenous infections.

HOUSEKEEPING

Although nurses are no longer directly responsible for cleaning, they should utilize their knowledge to make certain that the environment is clean. One large area in the control of disease comes under the heading of housekeeping. Studies performed by a large number of investigators indicate that blankets, mattresses, bed linens, and other articles in a patient's environment become laden with resistant staphylococci. Sheets and pillowcases are usually sterile after they are laundered; soiled linen may, however, release virulent organisms in linen chutes and may be sources of infection for laundry workers. Each hospital should have a method for handling contaminated linen so that the worker is protected. Bed linens on the beds of patients with heavy discharges should be changed frequently enough to prevent heavy contamination with microorganisms. The time-worn custom of storing blankets in a common cupboard should, if it has not already been, be eliminated. Blankets should be washed and sterilized after the discharge of a patient. Because wool blankets withstand washing poorly, some hospitals are replacing them with blankets made of washable fabrics. In some hospitals, blankets are oiled to encourage particles to adhere to the fibers.

In some hospitals, mattresses and pillows are encased in plastic coverings. Because staphylococci are resistant to drying, plastic coverings should be sterilized between patients. Ordinary washing is not likely to be effective. In some hospitals, mattresses and pillows are sterilized between patients. Adams [96] emphasizes that a light cleansing with a brush dipped in lysol solution has little or no effect on organisms buried in the mattress (or in a plastic cover either). Dr. Howard E. Lind [97] is reported in *Time*

Magazine to have found old pillows carrying not only enormous numbers of bacteria but a wide variety of gross contaminants such as food and false teeth.

General cleaning techniques should include wet mopping or mopping with a mop treated with a substance that causes dust to adhere to it. The same general procedure should be observed in dusting. In the past the use of vacuum cleaners has been frowned upon because they stir up dust. Recently, there have been some references to types in which this factor is controlled.

The control of the spread of nosocomial infections is neither quick nor easy. The procedures that are available are not glamorous; no newspaper is likely to headline them as producing a miracle. They are based on the application of principles of hygiene and antiseptic and aseptic techniques. Everything that comes in contact with a patient, be it an oxygen tent or a mask or a bed sheet, should be treated as being contaminated. Measures employed in the control of nosocomial infections, should be based on the knowledge that the offending microorganism is ubiquitous and that it is resistant to drying.

SUMMARY

Hospital-acquired infections as well as other infections are a very old problem. The discovery of the sulfonamides and then of penicillin and other antibiotics encouraged the hope that man could be victorious in his struggle with microorganisms. Furthermore, some forms of therapy as well as serious injuries and debilitating diseases decrease the host's resistance to his own germs. As a result, the importance of considering all the steps in the infectious process when planning the control of a microorganism is emphasized. Nurses are not responsible for nosocomial infections becoming a problem. They are not solely responsible for their control. They do have a responsibility to participate on the infections committee, to cooperate in control measures, and to study ways to improve methods of control. They also have a responsibility to participate in educational programs in the institution so that more effective control measures can be instituted and effected. Specific methods useful in the destruction of microorganisms have not been discussed. References have been included in the References for those who are interested. The infections that are most prevalent at this time in the United States are different from those of the past. Antibiotic-resistant strains have flourished as a result of disturbance in ecological equilibrium among microbes. The indifferent application of medical and surgical asepsis contributes to spread. Host

[95] Marjorie Morrill Laduke *et al.*: "Germfree Isolators," *Amer. J. Nurs.*, 67:72–79 (Jan.) 1967.
[96] Adams, *loc. cit.*
[97] "Pillow Talk," *Time*, 76:56 (Nov. 14) 1960.

susceptibility is increased by extensive surgical procedures, the use of immunosuppressive agents, and advanced age.

The literature supports the point made earlier. An infection cannot develop in the absence of a germ, but in many instances the germ is not sufficient to cause an infection unless the resistance of the host is lowered. Moreover, environmental conditions must make it possible for the host to be exposed to the microbe. The extent to which each factor is important varies. Besides being responsible for both morbidity and mortality, each hospital-acquired infection costs someone at least $4,000.[98] To the extent an infection prolongs a patient's hospitalization, it prevents another patient from being hospitalized.

There are many questions and few definitive answers. For this reason the nurse must expect, and be prepared to take, responsibility for continued learning. In protecting herself and others she should ask the question "Who is protected from whom? Why? From what? How?" Even when answers to these questions appear to be adequate, they should be continuously explored in an effort to obtain more adequate ones.

[98] James T. Hicks: "Hospital-Acquired Infections: Part 1—Problems of Environment," *Hosp. Manage.,* **105**:27 (Jan.) 1968.

In addition to her role in the care of patients in hospitals, the nurse has a responsibility to educate persons in the hospital and out in the community in the use of hygienic measures to prevent the spread of infectious diseases. The following definition of *health education* is taken from "An Official Report of the American Public Health Association." [99]

Health Education—Health education is the process by which individuals and groups of people learn to promote, maintain or restore health. To be effective, the methods and procedures used to achieve this aim must take account of the ways in which people develop various forms of behavior, of the factors that lead them to maintain or to alter their acquired behavior, and of the ways in which people acquire and use knowledge. Therefore, education for health begins with people as they are, with whatever interests they may have in improving their living conditions, and aims at developing in them a sense of responsibility for health conditions, as individuals and as members of families and communities. In communicable disease control, it commonly includes an appraisal of what is known of a disease by a population; an assessment of habits and attitudes of the people as they relate to spread and frequency of the disease; and the presentation of specific means to remedy observed deficiencies.

[99] Gordon (ed.), *op. cit.,* p. 15.

TABLE 5-1

Summary of the Interrelationship of Factors that Produce Four Infectious Diseases in Man

	Staphylococcal Disease	Syphilis	Tuberculosis	Infectious Hepatitis
Causative agent	*Staphylococcus* (numerous strains)	*Treponema pallidum*	*Mycobacterium tuberculosis*	*Hepatitis virus*
Distribution	World-wide (ubiquitous)	Widespread, throughout the world	World-wide; incidence varies in countries and economic status of population	Endemic throughout the world; common particularly among children; many mild nonicteric cases; highest in fall and winter
Nature—characteristics				
1. Ability to survive outside living organism	More resistant to drying than most nonspore formers; virulent strains resistant to antibiotics	Fragile—exists outside host only moments; susceptible to penicillin; adequate treatment usually terminates communicability within 24 hr	Capable of long-term survival outside host; resistant to disinfection; acid-fast; susceptible to sunlight, ultraviolet light, and drying	Resistant to moderate degrees of heat as 56°C; not destroyed by pasteurization of milk; resistant to chemicals including chlorine, ether, Merthiolate, nitrogen mustard; storage at room temperature for 6 months and −10° to −20°C for

Factors that Produce Four Infectious Diseases in Man (*cont.*)

	Staphylococcal Disease	Syphilis	Tuberculosis	Infectious Hepatitis
				years; destroyed by heating to 100°C for 30 min and exposure to ethylene oxide (liquid or gas)
2. General description	Host susceptibility is an important factor in disease production; multiplies rapidly in tissues; causes necrosis and multiple focal abscesses; coagulase positive; staphylococci may survive within phagocytes	Highly infectious; systemic from the onset; overt manifestations in primary and secondary stages; characterized by years of asymptomatic latency; may or may not be followed by serious crippling		Varies; often in mild form in children; varies from necrosis of liver cells with preservation of reticulum framework and regeneration of liver in 8 to 12 weeks to destruction of liver with extensive fibrosis
3. Reservoirs—human and animal	Human beings, carriers as well as the obviously infected; possibly animals, contaminated objects, and articles	Man—organism contained in exudate from obvious or hidden lesions of primary or secondary syphilis	Primarily man, but in some areas diseased cattle	Human beings—feces and blood; shellfish—polluted water
4. Characteristic lesions	(1) Impetigo and pyoderma of infants, and umbilicus of newborn infant; (2) mastitis in postpartum patients; (3) wound infection in surgical patients; and (4) infections in debilitated patients superimposed on other conditions; skin manifestations of the disease in adults or older children may be furuncles, carbuncles, infected decubiti, and paronychia; other infections include pyelonephritis, endocarditis, parotitis, and pneumonia	Lesions of primary syphilis, chancre; secondary syphilis —moist condylomata, blood, semen, vaginal secretions during the infectious stages; late syphilis—gumma (few organisms)	(1) First infection—Ghon complex; exudative-type lesion spreading to the lymphatic node(s); the lymph node undergoes caseation necrosis and eventually calcification; (2) reinfection—chronic lesion with caseation necrosis and fibrosis; little or no involvement of lymph nodes	See general description
5. Vehicles and conditions of transmissions	Airborne droplets, or droplet nuclei; contact with heavily contaminated articles; at least one study discredits the importance	Direct contact by kissing, sexual intercourse, fondling of children, during primary and secondary stages of syphilis; prena-	Contact with persons with active disease; via droplets and droplet nuclei or via exudate or secretions from infected organs;	Fecal—oral route most common; food; shellfish; water; contaminated needles and instruments

Clinical Nursing

Factors that Produce Four Infectious Diseases in Man (*cont.*)

	Staphylococcal Disease	Syphilis	Tuberculosis	Infectious Hepatitis
	of contaminated articles as vehicles of transmission	tally through the placenta	milk from diseased cattle; usually requires extended and intimate exposure; persons living in overcrowded conditions have more opportunities for exposure	
Human host				
1. Age, sex, race 2. Heredity, personality 3. Habits, customs 4. Defenses—general and specific	Fair degree of immunity or resistance; susceptibility general, especially in newborn, elderly, debilitated, wounds, traumatized tissue, and burns	Susceptibility is universal as there is no natural immunity; one half of cases have onset between the ages of 15 and 24; incidence believed to be the same in both sexes; sexual promiscuity	Some family contacts avoid infection for a long period of time; susceptibility highest in children under 3 years; higher among the undernourished	Especially common among children of the lower socioeconomic group living under overcrowded conditions; unsanitary living conditions; polluted water
5. Portal of entry	Skin, wounds, respiratory tract	Mucous membrane, breaks in skin	Respiratory and gastrointestinal tracts; lung lesions probably most important	Mouth
6. Portal of exit	Open lesions	Chancre, mucous patches, moist condylomata, blood	Respiratory tract	Feces, blood
7. Immunity	Authorities disagree; normal healthy adult has some immunity; may be that hypersensitivity results from infection	None, except cannot be reinfected when infected	Degree varies with the individual	No natural immunity Passive immunity may be induced with human γ-globulin Attack of the disease when due to virus A
8. Duration of carrier	Varies with the individual; indefinitely in some; intermittently in others			Blood—unknown (at least 8 months); feces—weeks to months
9. Prevention	Meticulous practice of aseptic technique; no one with even minor lesions should be allowed to care for patients; some physicians prescribe strict isolation	Adequate treatment of those with disease, education	Treatment of those with disease as well as those recently converted; BCG is also effectively used in immunizing people who run a high risk of being exposed to tuberculosis	Gamma globulin—prevents jaundice; patients should wear pajamas to reduce contamination of bed linens; gowns when in close contact with bed or patient; handwashing—thorough; private

Factors that Produce Four Infectious Diseases in Man (*cont.*)

Staphylococcal Diseases	Syphilis	Tuberculosis	Infectious Hepatitis
			bathroom for patient; care in handling feces and equipment used in blood sampling and parenteral therapy; when possible disposable equipment should be used; a syringe when used should *never* be reused without sterilization; eliminate overcrowding; common among children in lower socioeconomic group; correct unsanitary conditions; avoid eating raw or insufficiently cooked shellfish

REFERENCES

BOOKS

Burdon, Kenneth L., and Williams, Robert P.: *Microbiology,* 6th ed. (New York: The Macmillan Company, 1968).

Burrows, William: *Textbook of Microbiology,* 19th ed. (Philadelphia: W. B. Saunders Company, 1968).

De Kruif, Paul: *Microbe Hunters* (New York: Harcourt, Brace & Company, 1932).

Diagnostic Standards and Classification of Tuberculosis (New York: National Tuberculosis and Respiratory Disease Association, 1969).

Horsfall, Frank L., and Tamm, Igor: *Viral and Rickettsial Infections of Man,* 4th ed. (Philadelphia: J. B. Lippincott Company, 1965).

Stead, William W.: *Understanding Tuberculosis Today* (Milwaukee, Wis.: Marquette University Press, 1969).

Thompson, Morton: *The Cry and the Covenant* (New York: Doubleday & Company, 1949).

Top, Franklin H.: *Communicable and Infectious Diseases: Diagnosis, Prevention, Treatment,* 6th ed. (St. Louis: The C. V. Mosby Company, 1968).

U.S. Department of Health, Education, and Welfare, Public Health Service Publication No. 1660: "Syphilis, A Synopsis" (Washington, D.C.: U.S. Government Printing Office, 1967).

PERIODICALS

Theories on and the Incidence of Infections

Calafiore, Dorothy C.: "Eradication of Measles in the United States," *Amer. J. Nurs.,* **67:**1871–74 (Sept.) 1967.

Finegold, Sydney M.: "Infections Due to Anaerobes," *Med. Times,* **96:**174–87 (Feb.) 1968.

Gilbert, David N., *et al.:* "Potential Medical Problems in Personnel Returning From Vietnam," *Ann. Intern. Med.,* **68:**662–78 (Mar.) 1968.

Gregg, Michael B.: "Communicable Disease Trends in the United States," *Amer. J. Nurs.,* **68:**88–93 (Jan.) 1968.

Macdonald, Norman: "Pneumonia Today," *Nurs. Times,* **64:**4–6 (Jan. 5) 1968.

Stewart, G. T.: "Limitations of the Germ Theory," *Lancet,* **1:**1077–81 (May 18) 1968.

Williams, R. Fraser: "Clinical Infection. 1," *Nurs. Times,* **63:**1572–74 (Nov. 24) 1967.

Youmans, John B. (ed.): "Symposium on Syphilis and Other Venereal Diseases," *Med. Clin. N. Amer.,* **48:**571–809 (May) 1964.

Hospital-Acquired Infections

"AHA-HIA. Conference Examines Clean Room Methods of Hospitals and Industry," *Mod. Hosp.,* **108:**63–64 (Jan.) 1967.

Altemeier, W. A.: "Bodily Responses to Infectious Agents," *JAMA*, 202:1085–89 (Dec. 18) 1967.

Altmeier, W. A.: "Control of Wound Infection," *J. Roy. Coll. Surg. Edinb.*, 11:271–82 (July) 1966.

Anderson, Louise C., and Himmelsbach, Clifton K.: "The Nurse: First Line of Defense Against Infections," *Hospitals*, 41:84–98 (Oct. 1) 1967.

Bentley, David W., and Lepper, Mark H.: "Septicemia Related to Indwelling Venous Catheter," *JAMA*, 206:1749–52 (Nov. 18) 1968.

Blenkiron, C. H.: "Baths and Bacteria," *Nurs. Times*, 64:927–28 (July 12) 1968.

Eickhoff, Theodore C.: "Hospital Infection Control Begins with Good Surveillance," *Hospitals*, 41:118–20 (Mar. 16) 1967.

Hicks, James T.: "Hospital-Acquired Infections: Part II—Problems with Personnel, Patients and Visitors," *Hosp. Manage.*, 105:47–50 (Feb.) 1968.

Huszar, Robert J.: "Air Curtains for Patient Isolation," *JAMA*, 207:549–51 (Jan. 20) 1969.

Kress, Bertha K., and Elliott, Marlene: "Isolated in a 'Life Island'," *Canad. Nurse*, 64:48–49 (May) 1968.

Louria, Donald B.: "Hospital-Acquired Fungus Infections Are on the Increase," *Hosp. Manage.*, 101:75–78 (Feb.) 1966.

Newsom, S. W. B.: "Hospital Infection from Contaminated Ice," *Lancet*, 2:620–22 (Sept. 14) 1968.

O'C., V.: "Cross-infection Control in Hospitals," *Nurs. Times*, 62:1700–1701 (Dec. 23) 1966.

Rubenstein, A. Daniel, and Morse, Leonard J.: "Study Reveals Hand Lotions May Be Source of Gram-negative Bacteria," *Mod. Hosp.*, 110:119 (Apr.) 1968.

Schaeffer, Robert L.: "Environmental Sanitation," *Hospitals*, 41:59–62 (Apr. 1) 1967.

Hepatitis

Gunn, Alexander D. G.: "Hepatitis," *Nurs. Times*, 62:1132–33 (Aug. 26) 1966.

Hillis, William D.: "Viral Hepatitis: An Unconquered Foe," *Milit. Med.*, 133:343–54 (May) 1968.

James, D. Geraint: "Viral Hepatitis—the Nurse's Occupational Hazard," *Nurs. Mirror*, 125:viii–ix (Dec. 29) 1967.

Koff, Raymond S., and Isselbacher, Kurt J.: "Changing Concepts in the Epidemiology of Viral Hepatitis," *New Eng. J. Med.*, 278:1371–80 (June 20) 1968.

Redeker, Allan G., and Yamahiro, Harry S.: "Viral Hepatitis," *Postgrad. Med.*, 41:21–29 (Jan.) 1967.

Malaria

Blaunt, Robert E.: "Malaria—A Persistent Threat," *Ann. Intern. Med.*, 70:127–29 (Jan.) 1969.

Neva, Franklin A.: "Malaria—Recent Progress and Problems," *New Eng. J. Med.*, 277:1241–52 (Dec. 7) 1967.

World Health Organization: "Preventing the Reintroduction of Malaria," *WHO Chron.*, 22:150–54 (Apr.) 1968.

Staphylococcal Infections

Bulger, R. J., and Sherris, J. C.: "Decreased Incidence of Antibiotic Resistance Among *Staphylococcus aureus*," *Ann. Intern. Med.*, 69:1099–1108 (Dec.) 1968.

Cluff, Leighton E., *et al.*: "Staphylococcal Bacteremia and Altered Host Resistance," *Ann. Intern. Med.*, 69:859–73 (Nov.) 1968.

Drutz, David J., *et al.*: "Bacterial Interference in the Therapy of Recurrent Staphylococcal Infections. Multiple Abscesses Due to the Implantation of the 502A Strain of Staphylococcus," *New Eng. J. Med.*, 275:1161 (Nov. 24) 1966.

Ellis, M.: "The Infected Hand," *Nurs. Mirror*, 123:i–iii (Oct. 28) 1966.

Gallivan, Gregory J., and Tovey, James D.: "Isolation for Possible and Proved Staph," *Amer. J. Nurs.*, 67:1048–49 (May) 1967.

Gonzaga, Antonia J., *et al.*: "Transmission of Staphylococci by Fomites," *JAMA*, 189:711 (Sept. 7) 1964.

Oldstine, Michael B. A.: "Hospital-Acquired Staphylococcal Infection," *Amer. Surg.*, 32:391–94 (June) 1966.

Shinefield, H. R., and Rebble, J. C.: "Current Aspects of Infections and Diseases Related to *Staphylococcus aureus*," *Ann. Rev. Med.*, 16:263–84, 1965.

Shooter, R. A., Stoodley, B. J., and Gordon, Barbara: "Control of an Outbreak of Sepsis Due to *Staphylococcus aureus* Phage-Type 52/52A/80/81, in Nurses," *Lancet*, 1:293–95 (Feb. 10) 1968.

WHO Expert Committee on Streptococcal and Staphylococcal Infections: "Streptococcal and Staphylococcal Infections," *WHO Chron.*, 22:483–88 (Nov.) 1968.

Tetanus

Gunn, Alexander D. G.: "Tetanus," *Nurs. Times*, 63:752–54 (June 9) 1967.

van Heyningen, W. E.: "Tetanus," *Sci. Amer.*, 218:69–73, 76–77 (Apr.) 1968.

Tuberculosis and the Atypical Mycobacteria

Amroliwalla, F. K.: "Tuberculosis Today: A Review," *Nurs. Times*, 64:1196–98 (Sept. 6) 1968.

Chapman, John S.: "The Atypical Mycobacteria: Their Significance in Human Disease," *Amer. J. Nurs.*, 67:1031–33 (May) 1967.

Guerrin, Robert F.: "Tuberculosis Hospital Staff Attitudes: Nurses and Nursing Assistants," *Amer. J. Public Health*, 56:37–49 (Jan.) 1966.

Johnston, Robert F., and Hopewell, Philip C.: "Chemotherapy of Pulmonary Tuberculosis," *Ann. Intern. Med.*, 70:359–67 (Feb.) 1969.

Kincade, G. F.: "Domiciliary Treatment of Tuberculosis," *Canad. Med. Ass. J.*, 95:818–20 (Oct. 15) 1966.

Myers, J. Arthur: "Tuberculosis in the Aged," *Postgrad. Med.*, 41:214–22 (Feb.) 1967.

NTA Ad Hoc Committee on Treatment of TB Patients in General Hospitals: "Infection Control: Infectiousness of Tuberculosis," *Nurs. Clin. N. Amer.*, 3:183–85 (Mar.) 1968.

Parry, Wilfrid H.: "Tuberculosis: A World Problem," *Nurs. Times,* **62**:1454–56 (Nov. 4) 1966.

South, Jean: "Impediments to TB Eradication," *Nurs. Outlook,* **15**:50–52 (Sept.) 1967.

"Tuberculin Tests Today," *Brit. Med. J.,* **2**:134 (Apr. 20) 1968.

Waaler, H. T.: "A Dynamic Model for the Epidemiology of Tuberculosis," *Amer. Rev. Resp. Dis.,* **98**:591–600 (Oct.) 1968.

Antimicrobial Agents and Vaccines

Ager, Ernest A.: "Current Concepts in Immunization," *Amer. J. Nurs.,* **66**:2004–11 (Sept.) 1966.

Datta, Naomi: "Infectious Drug Resistance," *Brit. Med. Bull.,* **21**:254–59 (Sept.) 1965.

Gamer, Mary: "Is Smallpox Vaccination Still Necessary?" *RN,* **31**:46–47 (Apr.) 1968.

Hutchison, D. A.: "Measles Vaccines," *Canad. Nurse,* **64**:26–27 (Jan.) 1968.

Kilpatrick, Robert: "The Sulphonamides," *Practitioner,* **200**:10–14 (Jan.) 1968.

Kundsin, Ruth B., and Walter, Carl W.: "Antiseptics and Disinfectants," *Practitioner,* **200**:15–22 (Jan.) 1968.

Sabath, Leon D.: "Drug Resistance of Bacteria," *New Eng. J. Med.,* **280**:91–94 (Jan.) 1969.

Smith, Stephen E.: "Biological Drugs and Vaccines," *Nurs. Times,* **63**:311–12 (Mar. 10) 1967.

Stewart, H. C., and Hughes, W. Howard: "Antibiotics," *Practitioner,* **200**:5–9 (Jan.) 1968.

Weinstein, Louis: "The Present Status of Antimicrobial Therapy with Special Emphasis on Host Determinants of Response to Treatment," *Med. Times,* **96**:105–17 (Feb.) 1968.

Virology and Virus Diseases

Horne, R. W.: "The Structure of Viruses," *Sci. Amer.,* **208**:48–56 (Jan.) 1963.

Parry, Wilfrid H.: "Influenza," *Nurs. Mirror,* **126**:29–30 (Jan. 26) 1968.

Parry, Wilfrid H.: "What Do We Know About Viruses?" *Nurs. Times,* **64**:1047–48, 1087–88, 1111, 1137–38, 1173 (Aug.) 1968.

"*RN* Asks an Expert About Virology," *RN,* **28**:67–70, 86, 90–91 (Nov.) 1965.

Weinstein, Louis, and Chang, Te-Wen: "Interferon: Nonviral Infections and Nonviral Inducers," *Ann. Intern. Med.,* **69**:1315–22 (Dec.) 1968.

Wood, William B., and Edgar, R. S.: "Building a Bacterial Virus," *Sci. Amer.,* **217**:60–66, 71–74 (July) 1967.

6

Defenses Against and Responses of the Body to Injury

> As the essence of things must always remain unknown, we can learn
> only relations, and phenomena are merely the result of relations.
>
> CLAUDE BERNARD

Overview

THROUGHOUT Chapter 5, emphasis was placed on the importance of the host in determining the infections that he develops. Reference was made to the fact that many of the manifestations associated with infection are caused by the responses of the individual to injury. This is not only true of infection but of injury attributable to any cause.

Some understanding of the physiological mechanisms by which the organism responds to injury is essential to planning and meeting the needs of sick patients. During the early stages of an acute illness or following a serious injury, the energy and the resources of the patient are concentrated on survival.

What are the nursing objectives in the care of the acutely ill?

1. To prevent further injury
2. To ascertain the degree and extent of injury as a basis for modifying nursing care
3. To support the patient and modify his environment and nursing care so that he can use his energy to recover (survive)
4. To observe the reactions of the patient so that his care can be altered as his needs change and that, inasmuch as is possible, complications can be prevented

5. To provide the patient with materials and services required during the various phases of illness
6. As the patient recovers, to shift responsibility to the patient for meeting his own needs

How does the body protect itself against injury?

Although emphasis is on the response of the organism after it is injured, a brief discussion of protective structures and functions follows. Body structure is protective. Boney cages shelter vital organs such as the brain, heart, and lungs. The eye is recessed in the skull and is further guarded by the nose and the outward jutting of the brow. Injury great enough to disrupt the continuity of bones is almost always accompanied by injury to underlying or surrounding structures.

Barriers against the entrance of foreign matter into the body include sensory receptors that are stimulated by conditions in the external environment, the intact skin and mucous membranes, mechanisms for conditioning air as it passes through the respiratory tract and for the removal of particles that do reach the alveoli, and mechanisms for the rejection of irritating substances from the gastrointestinal tract. The hydrogen ion concentration of secretions in the stomach, mouth, and vagina offers some protection against microorganisms. The presence of enzymes such as lysozyme injures the cell wall and causes the bacteria to lyse, mainly because of environmental conditions. Because secretions by glands in these organs are stimulated by irritation, there is an increased volume of fluid to dilute and wash away noxious agents.

Reflexes such as coughing, sneezing, vomiting, dodging, and blinking initiate activities enabling the individual to remove or avoid harmful agents. Often protection involves a number of mechanisms. For example, a particle of dust gains access to the cornea of the eye where it stimulates sensitive nerve endings in the cornea. Exquisitely severe pain demands relief, and the person suffering it is prompted to initiate measures for the removal of the foreign body. Simultaneously the lacrimal glands secrete tears that dilute the foreign material (when this is possible) and wash it away by flooding. Blinking of the eyelids distributes the tears over the eyeballs and tends to prevent the entrance of new particles. A person in whom the cornea and sclera are insensitive to pain or who cannot secrete tears lacks a primary defense mechanism. To prevent irreparable injury to the affected eye, this person must institute a regular schedule of procedures that substitute for the ones that have been lost. Because he does not suffer pain when a foreign body enters his eye, he must develop the habit of inspecting the sclera for redness several times a day. He should also consciously blink his eyes at regular intervals. He may have to bathe his eyes with saline solution. He should try to identify sources of injury and then utilize appropriate measures to protect himself against them. For example, on windy days or when there is the possibility of exposure to dust, he should wear goggle-type glasses.

As discussed in Chapter 4, cells can alter their size and strength in response to increased or decreased stimulation (hypertrophy-atrophy). Some can adapt to a change in the environment by undergoing metaplasia. The organs of most persons are capable of doing more work than they are ordinarily called on to do.

Even when the first lines of defense are penetrated, in some instances the body is able to destroy or localize an injuring agent. As an example, a cut in the skin allows pathogenic microbes to enter. The germs may be destroyed by local defense mechanisms before they are able to multiply. If they do multiply, they may never leave the site of entry because the body's localizing mechanisms are effective. One of the barriers to spread is hyaluronic acid, an intracellular cement of gel-like consistency. It is permeable to small particles such as water and electrolytes but less permeable to large particles such as bacteria, protein molecules, and cells. Other localizing factors will be discussed later.

Assuming that injurious agents get beyond the second line of defense, they may be destroyed or inactivated by reticuloendothelial cells in the lymph nodes, the spleen, or liver or destroyed by phagocytic cells in the blood. The body is further protected by the ability of the liver and kidneys to excrete bacteria and certain chemicals into the bile or urine. Depending on the effectiveness of the body's defense mechanisms, injuring agents may be eliminated without appearing to cause harm, may be localized to the site of injury, or may escape to be destroyed or eliminated at more distant sites or to cause overt injury.

Responses to Injury

Despite protective structures and the capacity to respond to the environment so that injury is prevented, injury to cells does occur. When cells are injured, survival depends on the capacity of the organism to react in such a manner that the injury to cells is limited and damage is repaired. As with other homeostatic mechanisms, there are limits to the capacity of any individual to withstand injury. The damage to the total organism or to a vital structure may be so great that death occurs immediately. At the other end of the scale, because human beings are thinking, learning, remembering, and feeling organisms, they sometimes respond to symbols of danger when no real threat exists. Responses to imaginary danger may be as incapacitating as responses to tissue injury.

In injury or illness of a serious nature, not only the cells in and around the site of injury but those throughout the entire organism participate in the response. Many of the manifestations observed in illness arise from the local and general responses of the organism to cell damage. They are initiated by a noxious agent sufficiently potent to cause direct injury to cells or to alert the mental apparatus to the possibility of serious danger. Similar to other homeostatic mechanisms, responses to injury may be excessive or deficient in degree or they may be inappropriate to the stimulus. As will be emphasized later, a response may be the cause of injury.

The stimulus initiating one or more of the responses to injury may be damaging to cell structure or a symbol implying danger to the individual. To illustrate, fire, by raising the environmental temperature above that tolerated by the tissue, injures the tissue. Cells in the burned area are affected by the products released by injured or killed cells and respond in ways that are protective. The pain associated with even a small burn acts as a stimulus for responses involving the entire organism. When more than a limited area of tissue is burned, the individual can be expected to respond on all levels of organization, from the biochemical level to the highest integrative centers in the brain. Some of these same reactions can be elicited by a situation in which fire is perceived as being a source of danger. Seeing a flame where none should be elicits behavior similar to that in which actual burning has occurred. Even a fire siren may alarm an individual who has recently experienced a severe burn.

Many of the responses occurring during illness are to injury or danger rather than to the specific agent. They are therefore nonspecific or stereotyped rather than specific. Though there are modifying factors, the magnitude of reaction is usually in proportion to the extent of the danger or injury. There are also patterns of response that can be attributed to particular etiological agents. For example, during the prodromal stage of the acute infectious diseases of childhood, the child is ill but the nature of the illness may be unclear for several days. Unless he develops a rash or some other feature of a specific disease, his illness will be attributed to a cold or a virus. Antibodies specific to the causative agent may be isolated from his blood. The final outcome in any illness depends on two general factors: the nature and extent of the injury and the appropriateness of the response of the individual.

Man has a remarkable capacity to respond to changes in his internal and external environment in such a manner that function is maintained within physiological and psychological limits. As long as disturbances do not exceed the adaptive capacity of the individual, energy is available for growth and reproduction and to alter conditions in his external environment. When conditions in the environment are such that the survival of the organism is threatened, energy is utilized to escape from, or to overcome, the injuring agent and to make necessary repairs.

Finally, through the use of his intellect, man evaluates and modifies his environment so that he protects himself against many potential dangers. Through the enactment and enforcement of laws, he regulates his own behavior and that of his fellows so that all are protected from disease and injury.

In general, the magnitude of a response to injury varies with the extent of the injury. Some agents inflict more damage and provoke a greater reaction than others, and injuries to certain body structures are accompanied by a greater response than are others. The charac-

teristics of the person who is ill also influence his response. Persons who are at the extremes of age usually respond less vigorously than do children and young adults. The response of persons in middle life is not as vigorous as that of young adults, but it is greater than that of the elderly. There are exceptions. Mrs. Malone, aged 96, is one. She experienced and recovered from pneumonia. At the height of her illness, she had a fever of 102°F. It is not uncommon for persons of advanced age to have little or no elevation in temperature in disorders commonly causing fever in younger persons. Males usually respond more vigorously than females, but the fact that vigorous young men respond actively does not mean that they have a higher recovery rate from serious illness than women do. In fact, there is some evidence that the reverse is true. As might be expected, the well-nourished react more actively than the poorly nourished and vigorous, healthy persons more than debilitated or sickly ones. In general, the vigor of homeostatic responses to illness or injury is greater in those with a good adaptive capacity and less in those whose adaptive capacity is deficient.

As stated earlier, the ultimate goal of the homeostatic responses to injury or to dangers perceived as sources of injury is survival. The attainment of this goal involves escaping from, or overcoming, noxious agents and repairing disturbances or damage that results. At the time the individual is threatened with, or suffers, severe injury or illness, a whole series of integrated reactions are initiated involving the neuromuscular, neuroendocrine, circulatory, respiratory, and reticuloendothelial systems. Structures and functions not immediately useful to survival are suppressed. The significance of the preceding to nursing will be indicated as the various responses are discussed.

Systemic Responses

NEUROMUSCULAR RESPONSES

One of the primary and earliest responses to threat of or actual injury is the alteration of position in space. There are, obviously, many other types of stimuli that result in movement. At the very minimum, this response depends on a receptor connected by nerve cells and fibers to an effector. Receptors contain cells sensitive to changes in the internal or external environment. The retina of the eye contains receptor cells sensitive to light. Effector cells are capable of some overt activity. These cells are of two general types, muscle and gland cells. Between the receptor and effector cells are efferent (sensory) nerve fibers that convey messages from the receptor cells to centers, groups of cells, in the spinal cord and brain where "decisions" are made. (See Chapter 15, Part B.) From the centers, messages are sent by way of efferent pathways to a few or to many effector cells. Alteration of position in space requires not only intact neuromuscular units but an adequate skeletal system. Joints must be functional so that areas of the body can be moved, and the bones must be sufficiently rigid to be moved by the muscles.

Response to danger or to injury by alteration of position in space may be manifested in one or more of three ways. One is to flee or run away. A second is to remain and fight the enemy. A third is to become immobile or freeze, by contracting opposing sets of muscles. Each type of reaction is appropriate in different situations. On awakening, Mr. All notes that his apartment is on fire and that the blaze is sufficiently large that fighting it is out of the question; to try is to court disaster. Immobility is even more inappropriate. To flee as quickly as possible is the only reasonable course of action. Under other circumstances, such as in the presence of a lion or a poisonous reptile, immobility is the only response likely to be successful.

Frequently the manner in which the individual reacts is entirely automatic. Sometimes a person is able to control the impulse to act and to make a conscious decision as to the most appropriate course of action. An illustration of more or less automatic behavior occurred when Mr. All, who had taken his son John with him as he left his burning apartment, found that John had returned to get his clothing. Although Mr. All had to go through flames, he returned to the apartment. Despite suffering painful burns, he was able to rescue his son and to protect him from the fire. He had no recollection of his actions or of what had happened to him. Had his reaction not been more or less automatic, he probably would not have been able to save his son.

An illustration of a situation in which a young woman was able to increase her chances of survival by making a conscious decision was recently reported. This young woman was trapped in a walk-in freezer. Despite feelings of panic, she remembered that freezing could be delayed by continued movement. To maintain her self-control and to keep herself moving, she concentrated on counting the cans of food stored in the refrigerator. Fortunately, her mother missed her before she suffered serious injury. She survived because she was able to act intelligently and to modify her behavior appropriately. One factor that was very helpful to her was the certainty that her mother would miss her soon enough so that she would be rescued in time.

Despite the value of "flight, fight, and freeze" to the past survival of the human species, the number of situations in which they now serve a useful purpose is quite limited. In fact, fight and flight are both modes of behavior that are disapproved of in the American culture. Persons who fight in public are censured or jailed for disturbing the peace. Those who openly flee are called cowards. This leaves only one mode of behavior, that is, immobility in circumstances eliciting a fight-or-flight response. Some persons are in a state of constant muscular contraction. They behave as if they are in a continuous state of danger. Persons who have a large number of muscles contracted are likely to appear tense or strained. In some persons, contraction may be limited to a group of muscles such as those of the back or neck. Sustained muscular contraction, even in the absence of motion, requires the expenditure of energy, and it results in fatigue and muscular pain. In some instances, it may predispose to disease.

MUSCULAR RESPONSE

In illness, sustained muscular contraction is not uncommon source of suffering. Headache is one of the most common complaints of people who are ill. One of the factors in its development may be spasm of the head and neck muscles. Backache, another frequent discomfort, results from sustained contraction of back muscles. Many other aches and pains of illness result from the effects of muscle tension. In a number of diseases, and following injury, a characteristic feature is increased muscular tension or even muscular spasm. For example, the person whose thyroid hypersecretes is in a continuous state of increased muscular tension. A small sudden noise initiates a startle reflex out of proportion to the stimulus. Disorders in which muscle spasm is a factor in pain include acute poliomyelitis, fractures, rheumatoid arthritis, peritonitis, biliary or renal colic, and menstrual cramps.

Measures used in prevention and treatment of muscular tension vary. They are usually directed toward one or more of the following objectives: (1) to lessen the degree of muscular spasm, (2) to relieve the pain, and (3) to remove the cause. Measures that relieve muscle spasm are likely to relieve the pain associated with it. For example, the application of moist or dry heat over an area of a painful muscle is a well-known practice in folk medicine. In acute poliomyelitis, muscle spasm and pain may be relieved by the application of moist heat. In rheumatoid arthritis, use of salicylates with or without the application of heat will often afford relief. A number of muscle-relaxing drugs are also available. Diathermy may be employed to relieve pain by the application of heat. (See Chapter 4 for explanation.)

Under some circumstances, muscle spasm can be relieved by the application of traction, that is, by the application of a force opposing muscle contraction. After a period of time the muscle becomes fatigued and relaxes. As an example, traction is frequently employed in the treatment of fractures (broken bones) in which the ends of the bones are displaced. Traction is applied to lessen muscle spasm by fatiguing muscles. As the muscles relax, the two ends of the bone return to their normal position with the two parts of the bone in normal alignment and the ends of the bone just touching each other. Should the traction be removed, the muscles again contract and displace the fracture. When traction is utilized in the treatment of a fracture, everyone, including the patient and members of his family, should understand why it must be continuously applied. They should also know what conditions must be met for it to be effective. Under no circumstances should it be removed or lessened without a prescription of the physician. Traction may also be prescribed in the treatment of muscle spasm associated with pressure on nerve roots. For example, it is used to relax the muscles of the back in low-back pain or to relax the muscles of the neck when pain is caused by pressure on nerves supplying spastic muscles. When a patient is placed in traction, the nurse should know why the traction is applied and whether it may or may not be released.[1]

When pain results from the spasm of muscles in ducts or tubular structures such as a ureter or the common bile ducts, an analgesic or muscle-relaxing drug may be required to relieve pain. Thus morphine or one of its substitutes with or without a smooth-muscle relaxant such as papaverine is administered to relieve the pain.

Because muscle tension frequently accompanies illness and its treatment, the nurse should develop the habit of looking for evidence indicating its presence as well as for conditions that predispose to its development. She should also develop skill in the performance of nursing measures that prevent and/or relieve muscle tension. Most of these are not difficult and require little complicated equipment. They do require a conviction on the part of the nurse that they are important to the welfare of the patient. One of the most important aspects is attention to the position and body alignment of the patient, not only when he is in bed but when he is up and about and sitting in a chair. Weak and flaccid muscles should be supported and protected from overstretching. When sup-

[1] See the References for descriptions of the types and methods of applying traction.

ports are required, they should support, rather than be held in place by, the patient. They should extend along the length of the part and they should be adjusted so that strain is not placed on another structure. For example, when a sling is applied to support an arm, it should extend the entire length of the forearm. It is not enough to support the arm at the wrist.

One of the most frequent causes of discomfort in the patient confined to bed is back pain. It can often be prevented by use of a firm mattress or by the simple procedure of placing a board under the mattress. Frequent changes in position also aid in the prevention of prolonged strain on back and other muscles. When a patient is required to lie on his back continuously, a support under the lumbar curve of the back may prevent stretching of back muscles. A properly placed footboard and a cradle to prevent bed covering from weighing on weakened extremities are other measures that protect muscles from spasm or overstretching.

No matter how comfortable a position is at the start, it becomes less so as time elapses. There should therefore be a regular schedule for changing the position of weak and helpless patients. At the time their position is changed, the arms and legs should be put through the normal range of motion. Exercise not only promotes muscular relaxation by relieving strain on muscles used by the patient to maintain his position, but it acts as a stimulus to relaxation. A well-given back rub will further contribute to muscular relaxation. Any attention to the comfort of the patient should facilitate relaxation. It is difficult to relax when one has to look at a bright light, listen to a noise, or be too cold or too warm and not be able to correct the situation. The nurse should be alert to possible sources of irritation and take appropriate steps to prevent or eliminate them from the environment of the patient.

Because the psychological and social climate of the patient has an effect on his physiological status, these too may be the source of muscular tension. There are many sources of muscular tension in the course of an illness, and no effort will be made to enumerate them all. The nurse should develop the habit of looking for evidence of it. When a patient looks relaxed and comfortable, he probably is. When he appears to be tense or in poor position, he is likely to be uncomfortable. The nurse should also be alert to conditions in the environment of the patient—physical, psychological, or social—that are likely to induce tension. She should then act to correct them.

The following illustrations represent two relatively common nursing problems whose solutions are not very complicated. The first is Mr.

All, who was introduced earlier. For the first two or three days after he was burned he paid little attention to his surroundings and showed no concern for anyone but himself. About the third day, he began to ask about his son John, who was hospitalized after the fire. Despite everyone's effort to reassure him that John was not badly injured and would soon be discharged from the hospital, he was obviously worried. Arrangements were made for John to visit him. When he saw that John's burns were really of a minor nature, he was much relieved. This one visit did what verbal reassurance could not do; it convinced Mr. All that John was alive and would completely recover from his injury.

About a week or ten days after Mr. All was burned, skin grafts were applied to his upper arms and neck, and he was instructed to lie still for three days as any movement might disrupt the contact between the skin graft and the underlying tissue. Because Mr. All understood and accepted the importance of remaining immobile to the success of skin grafting, he concentrated on lying quietly. Although he maintained the desired position, he experienced considerable muscular tension. Because the nurse knew that Mr. All was to lie in the same position for three days, she checked his mattress to be sure that it was firm and provided adequate support for him. To encourage Mr. All to relax, his back was rubbed at two-hour intervals by inserting a hand between the mattress and the lumbar region of his back, and he was assisted in performing leg exercises. He was encouraged to wiggle his toes and to flex and extend his foot at the ankle. The nurse made a real effort to anticipate his needs and to visit him frequently. Because he was in a large ward, she encouraged ambulatory patients to stop briefly to see if he needed anything. As is frequently true when the arms are immobilized, one of his greatest sources of discomfort was an itching nose. When the nurse observed him wiggling his nose, she offered to scratch it for him. During the period immediately following skin grafting, the objective given precedence in Mr. All's nursing care was to minimize the sources of physiological and psychological stress so that he could use his energy for recovery. His environment and nursing care were planned to meet this objective. Even so, he experienced discomfort. Despite the inability of the nurse to eliminate all of Mr. All's discomforts, she was able to minimize them and to make the experience more tolerable.

The second patient is Mrs. Carney, who had a radical amputation of the left breast. Her left arm was to be elevated in order to prevent swelling of the hand and arm. The positioning of the arm under circumstances such as Mrs. Carney's is based on the fact that water runs downhill. Therefore, distal parts should be higher than proximal parts. In terms of the particular structures the hand should be higher than the elbow and the elbow higher than the shoulder. Unnecessary muscle tension can and should be prevented by arranging and balancing supporting apparatus, including pillows, so that it will support Mrs. Carney's arm. Briefly stated, supports should support.

The capacity to alter his position in space has been one of the significant factors in the survival of man. It has enabled him to overcome danger, to find or produce food, to find a mate, and to alter his environment so that it is better suited to his needs. In illness, the neuromuscular system reacts to the implied as well as to the real injury. Inasmuch as this response is appropriate, it contributes to survival. Even when muscle tension is appropriate, it adds to the fatigue and pain of illness. When the response is inappropriate or excessive, it increases the suffering of the patient, and it may be a factor in the development of undesired complications or sequelae.

What is the nurse's role in helping the patient with a neuromuscular response?

The nurse can help to lessen the severity of the neuromuscular response and its attendant discomforts by

1. Removing noxious stimuli from the external environment that the patient, if able, would eliminate or remove himself. Some examples include bright lights, loud or sudden noises, overheated or underheated surroundings, inadequate ventilation, dripping faucets, blaring radio or television sets, overtalkative people, untidy surroundings.
2. Giving attention to the position of the patient and changing his position regularly.
3. Providing for a comfortable bed.
4. Relieving muscle tension by putting extremities through the normal range of motion and rubbing the back.
5. Performing therapeutic procedures to relieve muscular spasm such as warm, moist packs; administering prescribed pain-relieving medications and supervising traction.
6. Identifying the implications that the illness has to the patient and the use of appropriate resources to relieve him. Preparing the patient for what to expect and what is expected of him.
7. Modifying care of the patient in relation to the severity, extent, and phase of his illness. This implies accepting him and his behavior.

The seriously ill patient who is fighting for his life should not be required to make decisions or to be responsible for meeting his own needs. The patient is allowed and encouraged to be sick. He should be bathed, moved, turned, and assisted out of bed as his condition demands. He should be held responsible neither for deciding when he requires care nor for carrying it out. When the nurse gives care she should exercise judgment about its timing. When caring for a very ill patient, his welfare may demand that certain aspects of care be omitted or be given at a particular time. With some sick patients the nurse may have to say firmly and kindly, "I have come to give you a bath. You look miserable and the bath will help you to feel better," or "It is time for you to be turned to your other side or to get up." As the patient recovers, responsibility is shifted to him as he is able to assume it.

THE AUTONOMIC NERVOUS SYSTEM

The autonomic nervous system is that portion of the nervous system regulating and coordinating visceral activities as well as aspects of emotional and expressive behavior. Its primary function is to help maintain the stability of the internal environment. It is customary to discuss the autonomic and somatic portions of the nervous system as if they were functionally and structurally separate entities, but they are not. To quote Gellhorn,[2] "Work during the past two decades has made it abundantly clear that so-

[2] Ernst Gellhorn: *Principles of Autonomic-Somatic Integrations* (Minneapolis: University of Minnesota Press, 1967), p. ix.

matic sensory and motor functions, as well as visceral, are subject to fundamental regulation by hypothalamic and reticular mechanisms." Furthermore, though the postganglionic fibers of the visceral system have cell bodies located outside the brain and cord, the cell bodies and dendrites of the preganglionic fibers are in the hypothalamus, brain stem, and spinal cord. One functional difference between the somatic and visceral systems is that the somatic system acts more rapidly than the visceral.

In addition to centers regulating the autonomic nervous system, the hypothalamus has centers for the control of other activities not under the control of the autonomic nervous system. They include regulation of endocrine glands, regulation of body weight, and fluid and electrolyte regulation. Recent studies suggest that the autonomic nervous system may influence the reabsorption of sodium.

With the exception of the smooth muscle of the blood vessels, the muscle of the hair follicles, and the sweat glands, all visceral organs are innervated by both systems. Although the sweat glands are supplied by the sympathetic nervous system, they are cholinergic; that is, acetylcholine is released at the effector cell rather than norepinephrine. See Figure 6-1. The sympathetic and parasympathetic systems function so that visceral activity is regulated and the needs of the organism are met under differing conditions. Because the sympatho-adrenal system stimulates an organ under some circumstances and depresses it under others, some authorities postulate two different types of receptor substance in the effector cells—the

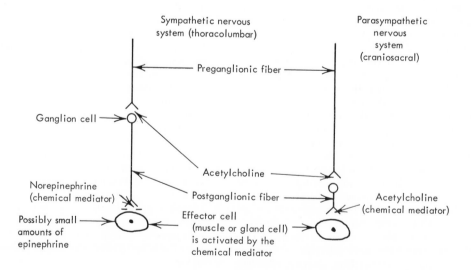

FIGURE 6-1. Peripheral structure of the sympathetic and parasympathetic divisions of the autonomic nervous system.

alpha and the beta receptor substance. Although the sympathoadrenal system is continuously active, it acts most intensely during stress and emergency situations. Many of the signs and symptoms observed in patients who are under acute stress are caused by sympathoadrenal activity. As examples, many of the signs and symptoms observed in early shock or hypoglycemia are caused by sympathoadrenal activity. Among the few generalizations that can be made about the autonomic nervous system is that under emergency conditions the sympathoadrenal system regulates those activities in which energy stores are utilized with the result that the individual is prepared for flight, fight, or freeze. Conversely, the parasympathetic nervous system regulates activities associated with conservation and restoration of energy stores. As stated earlier, the functions of the two systems are integrated and are not antagonistic to each other. It was once believed that the sympathoadrenal system always acted as a unit when the individual was in danger. It is now known, however, that a part can be activated independently of other parts. Thus it can regulate nonemergency functions such as body temperature.[3]

The parasympathetic nervous system consists of the third, seventh, ninth, and tenth cranial nerves and branches of the second, third, and fourth sacral nerves. There are no interconnections among the fibers forming these nerves. In the parasympathetic system, the ganglia lie in, or very close to, the organ that they stimulate with the result that preganglionic fibers are long and postganglionic fibers very short. There are very few connections among ganglia. The chemical mediator between the preganglionic fiber and the ganglion and the postganglionic fiber and the effector cell is acetylcholine. (See Figure 6-1.)

The preganglionic fibers of the sympathoadrenal system originate from cells in the thoracolumbar portions of the spinal cord. The preganglionic fibers branch in the vertebral ganglia. cells) lying peripheral to the spinal cord. Some are parallel to the cord, and others are located in the abdominal cavity or near an organ. Depending on their location, these ganglia are known as vertebral, collateral, or terminal. The preganglionic fibers of the sympathoadrenal system branch widely and often synapse with cells located in more than one ganglion. Preganglionic fibers branch in the vertebral ganglia. Some of the branches synapse with ganglionic cells, whereas others pass through the ganglia

to higher or lower vertebral ganglia or to collateral ganglia. Preganglionic fibers are generally relatively short and postganglionic fibers are long. One exception is the fibers supplying the adrenal medulla, as it is supplied with preganglionic fibers. Stimulation of the sympathetic nervous system results in stimulation of the adrenal medulla.

Another relationship exists between the sympathetic nervous system and the adrenal medulla. The chemical mediator between the sympathetic postganglionic fiber and the effector cell—muscle or gland—is norepinephrine. Epinephrine and possibly small amounts of norepinephrine are secreted by the adrenal medulla. Both these chemicals augment and prolong the action of the sympathetic nervous system. As in the parasympathetic nervous system the chemical mediator between the preganglionic fiber and the ganglion cells is acetylcholine.

The innervation of sweat glands is somewhat peculiar. Though anatomically they are part of the sympathetic nervous system, they are cholinergic; that is, the chemical mediator for the postganglionic fibers supplying sweat glands is acetylcholine. Depending on their orientation, some authorities classify the nerve supply to the sweat glands as parasympathetic, whereas others consider them to be controlled by the sympathetic nervous system.

One effect of increased sympathoadrenal activity deserving emphasis is that the seriously ill or injured patient is often unusually alert. Whereas a high degree of alertness is protective in a hostile environment, it may be an unnecessary source of stress to the patient who is under professional care. In fact, the climate surrounding the patient ought to be such that the patient can trust others to be responsible for his care. Conversations in the vicinity of the patient should take into account the possibility that the patient is overly alert. Nothing should be said that is likely to increase his anxiety. A useful rule is not to talk in the presence of the patient without including him in the conversation. (See Chapter 7.) Furthermore, noise, jarring, and other forms of unnecessary stimulation should be avoided, as the patient is likely to be unusually sensitive to them.

Some of the effects of activation of the two divisions of the autonomic nervous system are summarized in Table 6-1.[4]

As stated earlier, differences in behavior resulting from stimulation of the sympathoadrenal system are explained by proposing two different types of receptor substances. Some authorities

[3] Allan Hemingway and William M. Price: "The Autonomic Nervous System and Regulation of Body Temperature," *Anesthesiology*, **29**:694 (July–Aug.) 1968.

[4] For a more detailed summary, see Arthur C. Guyton: *Textbook of Medical Physiology*, 3rd ed. (Philadelphia: W. B. Saunders Company, 1966).

TABLE 6-1

Selected Actions Resulting from Activation of the Sympathetic and Parasympathetic Divisions of the Autonomic Nervous System

Site of Effector Cells	Activation of Sympathetic Division (Thoracolumbar) Tends to	Activation of Parasympathetic Division (Craniosacral) Tends to
Heart	Increase rate and output	Decrease rate and output
Coronary arteries	Dilate	
Blood vessels in nose, salivary glands, and pharynx	Constrict	Dilate
Cutaneous vessels	Constrict	
Bronchi	Dilate	Constrict
Gastrointestinal motility and secretion	Decrease (decreased peristalsis and muscle tone); constrict sphincters	Increase; relax sphincters
Glycogenolysis by liver	Increase	
Glands	Decrease secretion	Increase secretion
Sweat glands	Increase (some authorities classify this as a parasympathetic function)	
Pupil of eye	Dilate	Constrict
Ciliary muscles	Lessen tone; eyes accommodated to see at a distance	Contract ciliary muscles; eyes accommodated to see near objects
Mental activity	Increase	

suggest that norepinephrine affects only effector cells containing alpha receptors. Epinephrine affects both. See Table 6-2.

TABLE 6-2

Comparison of Effects of Stimulating Alpha and Beta Receptors

Alpha Receptor	Beta Receptor
Vasoconstriction	Vasodilatation in muscles
Dilatation of pupil	
Increased heart rate	
	Increased strength of heart contraction
Relaxation of intestine	Relaxation of uterine muscle
Conversion of glycogen to glucose	Bronchial relaxation

What is the nurse's role in helping the patient with a sympathoadrenal response?

The activity of the sympathoadrenal system can be expected to be increased in any patient who suffers an injury or illness threatening his survival. Major surgery, severe burns, overwhelming infection, frightening sounds or sights, myocardial infarction, pain, and many other conditions stimulate the activity of the sympathetic nervous system. Most, if not all, persons have experienced symptoms resulting from stimulation of the sympathetic nervous system. Mr. Brave (bleeding peptic ulcer), Mr. All (burned), and Mrs. Carney (amputation of breast) all had symptoms and signs indicating stimulation of the sympathetic nervous system. Both Mr. Brave and Mrs. Carney perspired profusely. All these patients had an increase in pulse rate. Mr. Brave complained that his heart pounded (palpitation). All breathed at a rapid rate. Though both Mr. Brave and Mrs. Carney lost blood, neither had an appreciable drop in blood pressure. Despite a loss of considerable volume of fluid into the burned area, and possibly in other tissue, Mr. All's blood pressure was maintained within normal limits. All three patients had some depression in gastrointestinal activity. In Mrs. Carney, diminished gastrointestinal activity was of short duration. In common with other patients who are seriously burned, Mr. All was predisposed to acute gastric dilatation. Consequently oral fluids were withheld for two days. When oral fluids were first prescribed, he was given 30 ml per hour for four hours. Because he did not complain of feelings of fullness, or of nausea, he was rapidly promoted to a full fluid and food intake.

Some degree of hyperglycemia may result from increased sympathoadrenal activity. On the third day after Mr. All was burned, his fasting blood sugar was 180 mg per 100 ml of blood. Because he was not known to have diabetes mellitus and his blood glucose returned to physiological limits after a few days, the elevation probably indicated an increase in the release of glucose from glycogen by the liver. Other factors, including increased secretion of glucocorticoids by the adrenal cortex, may have contributed to the increase in the level of the blood glucose.

Mr. Brave had some evidence of so-called paralytic ileus. His abdomen was distended and silent (absence of peristalsis). To prevent overdistention of his stomach, his physician prescribed nasogastric suction until peristaltic activity was re-established. On admission to the hospital, Mr. Brave was cold to the touch and pale; he appeared to be alert and anxious. These manifestations can all be ascribed to increased sympathoadrenal activity. Probably most patients have some increase in activity of the sympathoadrenal system at some stage of their illness. Even when illness is relatively minor, uncertainty about its cause or outcome may be a sufficiently potent stimulus to bring this about. When diagnostic or therapeutic procedures are perceived as indicating the possibility of a serious disease, or inducing pain, the likelihood of sympathoadrenal stimulation is further increased.

When a patient exhibits signs and symptoms indicative of increased sympathoadrenal activity, the nurse should seek answers to the following questions. Do the manifestations presented by the patient indicate that his illness is becoming more severe or that he is developing a complication? Are they the result of some physical or emotional stress associated with his illness or his personal life? Is there something in the environment of the patient that probably explains their presence? Has the patient undergone, what is for him, an unusual degree of activity? Are the symptoms and signs transitory or do they persist? As an illustration, suppose that Mr. Brave has an increase in his pulse and respiratory rate. Because he has a history of hemorrhage, he may be bleeding. Depending on other circumstances the nurse will look for additional evidence that he is bleeding or will modify his care in some way. Perhaps a visitor has stayed too long or Mr. Brave is anxious because his wife, whom he expected at 2, has not arrived by 5 o'clock. If Mr. Brave is out of bed for the first time after several days of bed rest, the nurse will assist him to bed. She may then allow him to rest for a short period of time and then recheck his pulse and respiration. If indicated, she will take his blood pressure. Whatever the stimulus is, Mr. Brave is responding to it by increasing his circulatory and respiratory rates. Appropriate action on the part of the nurse depends on taking into consideration the possible causes and acting in light of the one or ones that appear most reasonable.

Care planned to reduce the activity of the sympathoadrenal system should be based on two factors. One is that, within limits, physical activity tends to lessen the degree of activity of the sympathoadrenal system, and the other is that implied or imagined threats can act as stimuli initiating or augmenting its action.

Much of the nursing care given to relieve muscle tension will also tend to minimize sympathoadrenal activity. Care that increases the comfort of the patient promotes muscle relaxation. Within limits, physical activity has a similar effect. One of the values of early ambulation is that it decreases the intensity of the sympathoadrenal response. Patients whose condition allows them to get out of bed and to walk soon after injury or major surgical procedures usually have less pain and an earlier return of gastrointestinal activity than do those who are confined to bed for longer periods of time.

Not only does the sympathoadrenal system participate in the response of the individual to present and actual dangers to his survival, but it is activated by fear or anxiety initiated by implied or imagined threats to his well-being. When the nurse is successful in developing a trusting relationship with the patient, she can lessen the opportunities for him to imagine or magnify dangers in the situation. (See Chapter 7.)

Sympathectomy by surgical or chemical means is employed in the therapy of diseases of blood vessels in which vascular spasm is believed to be a factor. It is most commonly used in the treatment of essential hypertension, severe Raynaud's disease, and occlusive arterial disease involving the extremities. In surgical sympathectomy, a few to many pre- or postganglionic fibers of vertebral sympathetic ganglia are interrupted and a section of the fiber is removed. The number and location of the fibers to be excised depend on the disorder under treatment. Preganglionic fibers to collateral or terminal sympathetic ganglia may also be interrupted. In splanchnicectomy the preganglionic fibers to the celiac ganglia, the superior and inferior mesenteric plexuses, may be severed and removed. Instead of surgical interruption and excision of sympathetic fibers, a similar effect may be obtained by chemical means. There are a number of drugs that inactivate the autonomic nervous system by blocking the transmission of impulses through autonomic ganglia (ganglionic blocking agents). These drugs act by reducing the number of impulses reaching blood vessels and thereby reducing vascular tone and blood pressure. To evaluate the effectiveness of blocking agents the blood pressure should be taken in the lying, sitting, and standing positions. One undesirable effect of extensive surgical and chemical sympathectomy is that they limit the capacity to adapt the diameter of the blood vessels to changes in position. Blood pressure falls when the affected person assumes the upright position after having been in the recumbent position. The patient should therefore be instructed to assume the upright position slowly. When postural hypotension is severe, excessive pooling of blood in the legs may be prevented by wrapping them from instep to groin with elastic bandages.

SUMMARY

One of the factors in the survival of man has been his capacity to respond to threats of, or actual, injury by attacking or removing himself from danger. Many of the processes involved in these responses are under the control of the sympathoadrenal system. Because the sympathoadrenal system can be activated by any change in the external or internal environment that is perceived to be a threat to survival, most serious illnesses are accompanied by increased sympathoadrenal activity. Trauma, including surgical therapy, is a stimulus to increased sympathoadrenal activity. The effect on the patient is a decrease in those activities not immediately essential to survival and an increase in those that are. Thus the individual is more alert, his pupils are dilated, and he has increased muscle tension as well as an increase in heart and respiratory rate, increased sweating, and a rise in blood sugar. Activities not immediately es-

sential to his survival are depressed. Thus the alimentary canal is less active or may be temporarily paralyzed. Many of the discomforts and problems accompanying illness are caused by alterations in the activity of the autonomic nervous system. They should therefore be anticipated and dealt with by appropriate measures.

METABOLIC RESPONSES TO INJURY

In addition to muscular and visceral responses in illness that are largely regulated by the nervous system, there are also metabolic reactions to tissue injury. Even in these responses, the nervous system may participate in their initiation and regulation. Whereas muscular and visceral responses enable the organism to fight or flee its enemy, the metabolic responses have three objectives. They are: (1) to maintain the stability of the organism during stress, (2) to repair damaged tissues, and (3) to restore the body to normal composition and activity. The care of the patient should therefore be planned to assist him in achieving these objectives.

Both Moore [5] and Selye [6] have studied the metabolic responses to injury. Despite differences in terminology and emphasis, there are similarities between their findings.

Though there is overlapping between the various phases, Moore [7] describes convalescence as taking place in four phases. The first phase serves three purposes: (1) the release of amino acids and electrolytes into the extracellular fluid, (2) maintenance of the extracellular fluid volume, and (3) conversion of body fat as sources of energy. During the first phase there is rapid catabolism of lean tissue and fat. For about 6 to 24 hours after major surgery or a severe injury, water and sodium chloride are retained in the body. Until the patient is eliminating water and salt at a normal rate, overloading is possible. The danger of overloading is greatest among patients with heart disease or who are elderly. In the period immediately following major surgery or injury, careful attention should be paid to the rate at which solutions are introduced intravenously, to the type of solution, and to the relation of intake to output. Nitrogen, potassium, and phosphates are lost in the urine. Clinically the patient is characterized by all the reactions to an acute injury. Hemorrhage, pain, and fear augment the reaction. The patient has tachycardia and

[5] Francis D. Moore: *Metabolic Care of the Surgical Patient* (Philadelphia: W. B. Saunders Company, 1959), p. 27.

[6] Hans Selye: "The General Adaptation Syndrome and the Diseases of Adaptation," *J. Clin. Endoc.*, 6:117–230 (Feb.), 1946.

[7] *Op. cit.*, p. 27.

a slight fever which persist for two or three days. Unless he is storing water, he loses weight as the result of tissue catabolism.

The changes in nitrogen metabolism that are a part of the stress response have been extensively studied. As a result of this response, lean tissues undergo catabolism and large amounts of nitrogen and potassium are lost in the urine. The catabolic response cannot be reversed and may be intensified by forced feeding. It can also be induced by the administration of corticotropin,[8] or the adrenocorticoids. It occurs in any adrenalectomized animal who is maintained on the adrenocortical hormones.[9]

In nondiabetic persons who have a healthy liver, marked changes in glucose metabolism are not usually evident during stress, whereas the person who is diabetic usually has an elevation in blood glucose unless measures are taken to prevent it. The adrenocortical hormones and insulin are physiological antagonists. During stress the tolerance of the diabetic person for glucose is lessened. For a period following surgery, the diabetic patient requires more insulin than he does at other times. Following injury, considerable amounts of fats may be utilized as fuel. In patients who have diabetes mellitus, regular checking of the urine for glucose and acetone is therefore important.

Phase II, which Moore[10] calls the turning point, begins about the fourth day and continues for two or three days. Catabolism of tissue substance decreases, and preparations are made for anabolism. Clinically the patient appears improved. His appetite and spontaneous activity increase. He begins to be a bit less self-centered and more interested in the affairs of others. He shows some concern for his wife or for his roommate or for the man down the hall.

In phase III, or anabolic phase, which begins seven to ten days after an extensive injury, the person who has been injured restores his lean tissue. This phase involves the reconstruction of the lean tissues lost during the catabolic phase of illness. During this period, the person requires a generous dietary intake, and if he does not receive it, convalescence will be retarded as he will fail to gain the necessary weight, strength, and vigor. Wound healing continues normally, despite postoperative starvation.[11] Progress through phase III, depends,

however, on an adequate intake of calories and protein. Unless adequate calories and protein are available during this period, the recovery of the patient may be seriously delayed. A patient may require between 2,000 and 3,000 calories per day. Progress means not only that wound healing occurs normally, but that the patient gains weight and strength. Attention must be paid to the food intake of patients following surgical treatment, severe trauma, burns, and severe infections. The glass of milk in the refrigerator for a between-meal or evening snack is important and contributes to recovery provided it is consumed by the patient. Further, since many surgical patients are discharged some time between the seventh and tenth days, attention should be given to preparing them so that they understand the importance of eating sufficient amounts and variety of food. Eating may not be a serious problem for those whose appetite is good, but in the elderly or chronically ill, a real effort may be required to assure adequate food intake. In the patient who has been seriously burned, losses of protein during phase I may have been very great. Infection of the burned areas may have aggravated that loss. For example, despite the fact that Mr. All ate quite well, his food intake was augmented by tube feeding to the point where his gastrointestinal tract was unable to tolerate food. Despite heroic efforts to maintain his caloric and protein intake, he lost 20 lb during the first few weeks of his illness.

During phase IV, which may last for weeks or months, there is a return to full body weight and function. Fat deposits are restored, and the patient returns to work. During this phase the appetite of the patient may be very good. When he reaches his desired weight he may have to consciously limit his food intake in order to prevent an excessive gain in weight.

Many of the extensive studies of metabolic responses of human beings to injury have been made on young men undergoing a surgical procedure, but some studies have been made on individuals who have suffered fractures or burns. There is no reason to suppose that patients who are seriously ill with nonsurgical diseases do not also have a metabolic reaction. Response to injury is believed to be universal, and many, though not all, authorities believe it to be homeostatic.

Knowledge of the systemic response to injury, disease, or surgical therapy is essential to determining the requirements of patients who have suffered injury or acute disease. Unless the reactions of the patient are understood, treatment may interfere with rather than support the responses that promote recovery.

---

[8] Also known as adrenocorticotropin.

[9] James D. Hardy: *Pathophysiology in Surgery* (Baltimore: The Williams & Wilkins Company, 1958), pp. 15–16.

[10] *Op. cit.,* p. 42.

[11] G. M. Wilson, F. D. Moore, and R. P. Jepson: "The Metabolic Disturbances Following Injury," *Metabolic Disturbances in Clinical Medicine* (G. A. Smart, ed.) (Boston: Little, Brown & Company, 1958), p. 80.

The intensity of a metabolic reaction varies with a number of conditions. For example, the catabolic response is greatest in well-nourished young males. A less intense response occurs in females, the elderly, and the poorly nourished of either sex. The degree and type of trauma also influence the reaction. Minor trauma induces a less intense response than major trauma. Following minor trauma phase I is shorter. Phase II is scarcely noticeable, and the other two phases are passed through quickly. Burns and bone injury elicit a more vigorous response than can be predicted on the basis of the degree of injury. Extensive injury to soft tissues also adds to the severity of the reaction. Infection is a potent activator of the metabolic response. Fever may also be a factor. There is evidence that a marked and prolonged metabolic response to injury predisposes to the development of decubiti. Among the seriously injured, tissue breakdown may occur in a matter of hours. Care that can ordinarily be counted on to prevent the development of decubiti may be ineffective. Under these circumstances they result not so much from neglect as from the vigor of the metabolic response of the patient. Because seriously injured patients are predisposed to decubiti, protective measures should be instituted immediately. Because tissue breakdown can be far advanced before external evidence such as reddening of the skin occurs, preventive care should not be delayed until signs appear. (See Chapter 4.)

What is the nurse's role in helping the patient with a metabolic response?

The metabolic response to injury can be intensified by apprehension and pain and by other factors such as chilling, fever, and infection. The nurse has a responsibility to provide an emotional and physical environment that reduces undesirable stimuli to a minimum. Preoperative preparation of the patient for what to expect after operation, prompt attention to the relief of pain, gentleness in handling the patient, a quiet, nonstimulating environment, realistic expectations for and acceptance of the behavior of the patient—all should reduce the strain on the patient. The patient should be protected from too many stimuli from well-meaning friends and relatives, who stay too long or talk too much, who are too boisterous or come in too large numbers. The writer has seen newly operated and seriously ill patients exhausted by too many visitors or by those who remained too long. Conversely, a relative or friend whose presence comforts or quiets the patient should have an opportunity to visit the patient or be encouraged to remain. When the necessity arises to lessen the number

of visitors or the length of time that they stay, the interpretation should be in terms of the needs of the patient. The feelings of the visitor should be respected. The nurse may need to take initiative and use her ingenuity in accomplishing the reduction in the number of visitors. When necessary, something can be arranged to do to or for the patient that requires the visitors to leave. The nurse may suggest to the visitors that cards and letters are greatly enjoyed. However, the regulation of visiting should be based on the needs and condition of the patient.

Occasionally the problem of no visitors to a patient arises. The patient may be far from home or have no surviving relatives or friends. Visits from the doctors and nurses are then especially welcome. If a volunteer service worker is available, she or he may be utilized to meet needs of the patient that are ordinarily met by the family. In addition to visiting the patient she may write letters for him, read to him, shop for minor necessities, and the like. Of course, what the volunteer does should be adapted to the requirements of the patient. A friendly and sympathetic person who sits quietly by his bed may make a significant contribution to a seriously ill patient.

As a result of severe injury, major surgery, or serious illness, the person undergoes a variety of responses that are integrated by the neuroendocrine system. Among the changes are a series of metabolic responses by which the organism provides the materials for repair and restores itself to normal. These changes have been studied more extensively in animals and in patients who have been treated surgically than in patients with acute or chronic disease. The metabolic changes are characterized by a series of catabolic and anabolic changes that proceed through overlapping phases. In the earlier phases of the reaction elements associated with an intense reaction are youth, male sex, and good nutrition. Elements associated with a less intense reaction are advanced age, female sex, and undernutrition. Extensive surgery, burns, and fractures are accompanied by more intense and prolonged reactions than is minor injury or surgery. Apprehension, pain, and other circumstances associated with operative procedures intensify the response to injury. Through the intelligent practice of nursing, emotional and physical climate of the patient can be controlled so that harmful stimuli are minimized. The nurse should give attention to those observations indicating the state of the water and electrolyte balance. As soon as the patient is able to eat, his food intake should be noted and attention given to those patients who eat poorly. Patients who suffered wasting diseases before surgical treatment require special attention to improve their nutritional status. Intelligent application of the knowledge of the changes taking place after injury can shorten the convalescence of the patient.

Just what initiates or ends the metabolic responses is not known at the present time. The metabolic changes following surgery or injury are assumed to be the result of homeostatic mechanisms that function to maintain the circulating fluid volume so that tissues may be supplied with nutrients and oxygen. The catabolic changes liberate both water and materials from which energy may be obtained to maintain body processes. The changes occurring in the later phases of the response to injury restore the body to preinjury condition.

SELYE'S THEORY OF HOW THE BODY RESPONDS TO INJURY

Selye proposes that the responses of the tissues during injury are the result of the reaction of sensitive tissues to an increase in secretions of the adrenopituitary axis. Much of the data on which this theory is based has been obtained by subjecting rats to varying types of physical, chemical, and psychological injury. From these studies, Selye postulated that no matter what agent was used to cause injury, certain nonspecific stereotyped reactions occur in the stressed organism. Like Cannon,[12] Selye believes that homeostatic responses may cause disturbances in the internal environment. He also postulates that certain diseases may result from prolonged overactivity of homeostatic mechanisms. These he calls the diseases of adaptation. He includes among the diseases of adaptation the collagen fiber diseases and degenerative vascular diseases.[13]

According to Selye, increased endocrine secretion, particularly from the adrenopituitary axis, is responsible for the response of the organism to injury.[14] This response may be general or local or both. In either instance, it is nonspecific, because it may be elicited by any agent causing injury. The general response that Selye calls the "adaptation syndrome" takes place in three stages: (1) the alarm reaction, (2) the stage of resistance, and (3) the stage of exhaustion. The alarm reaction consists of two phases: (a) shock and (b) countershock. During the stage of shock and countershock the organism undergoes catabolic and other changes that result from the effects of the injury and response of the body to it. The "alarm reac-

tion" as described by Selye is similar to phases I and II of the metabolic responses to injury as described by Moore. During countershock, the organism is restored to its preinjury condition. In the stage of resistance the organism is adapted to the injuring agent. It can tolerate greater exposure to the injuring agent than can the nonadapted organism. Eventually, if the stress is continued, the animal loses its adaptation and goes into the stage of exhaustion. The stage of exhaustion is comparable to the shock of the earlier period.

Whether or not the animal goes through all phases of the adaptation syndrome depends on its capacity to react as well as on the intensity and continuance of the injuring agent. Any injury may be so severe that the vital processes of an individual are depressed to such an extent that death occurs immediately. Or he may die because his adaptive capacity is inadequate to cope with the injury. In contrast the individual may add to the damage by overreacting. Finally, when an injury is limited to a single insult and is within the adaptive capacity of the individual, recovery may be complete.

Selye believes that adrenocortical hormones not only affect the general responses of the organism but also modify the local response of tissue to injury. Further, the type of change in the tissues depends on whether the mineralocorticoids (aldosterone) or the glucocorticoids (cortisone) predominate. According to Selye, the mineralocorticoids are prophlogistic; that is, they stimulate the connective tissue to proliferate and enhance its inflammatory potential. In contrast, the glucocorticoids are anti-inflammatory or antiphlogistic. They inhibit proliferation of connective tissue and suppress the inflammatory process with the result that there is a reduction in the quantity of scar tissue formed in repair. Thus they may be prescribed in the treatment of rheumatic fever, rheumatoid arthritis, and other disorders in which an excessive or prolonged inflammatory response may lead to crippling scarring. Selye is of the opinion that the growth hormone from the anterior pituitary sensitizes the tissue to the mineralocorticoids. Other investigators do not agree that the changes in metabolism following tissue injury are caused solely by the action of the adrenocortical hormones.

Although the mechanisms of action of the adrenocortical hormones in response to injury are not known, these hormones are essential to the general response. Furthermore, cortisol and its analogues are used therapeutically to modify the local reaction of certain tissues to injury. See Figure 6-2 for a diagram summarizing body responses to stress.

Disorders of adaptation may occur at any

---

[12] Walter B. Cannon: *The Wisdom of the Body* (New York: W. W. Norton and Company, Inc., 1939), p. 22.

Selye, *loc. cit.*

[13] *Ibid.*, p. 127.

[14] *Ibid.*, pp. 119–20.

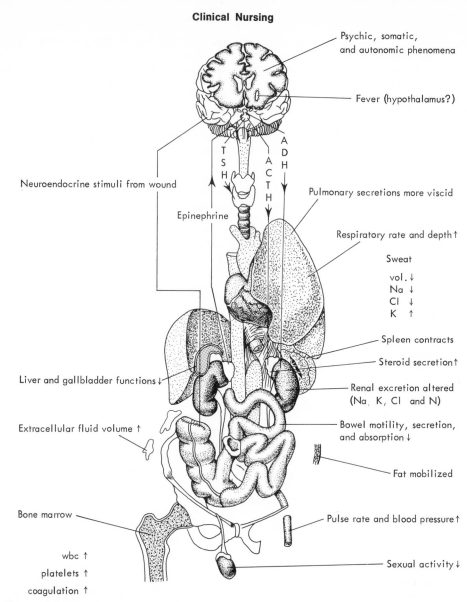

Psychic, somatic, and autonomic phenomena

Fever (hypothalamus?)

Neuroendocrine stimuli from wound

Epinephrine

T S H

A C T H

A D H

Pulmonary secretions more viscid

Respiratory rate and depth↑

Sweat

vol. ↓
Na ↓
Cl ↓
K ↑

Spleen contracts

Steroid secretion↑

Liver and gallbladder functions↓

Renal excretion altered
(Na, K, Cl and N)

Bowel motility, secretion, and absorption↓

Extracellular fluid volume ↑

Fat mobilized

Bone marrow

Pulse rate and blood pressure↑

wbc ↑

platelets ↑

coagulation ↑

Sexual activity↓

Figure 6-2. Reaction to stress. The first phase of surgical convalescence. Each system in the body participates in the total response to the stress of surgery, injury, or disease. Variations in response depend on the extent of surgery or injury and the severity of disease as well as the status of the patient prior to surgery or illness. In terms of metabolic responses, the chronically ill patient reacts to a lesser degree than does the previously well individual. Coordination of reactions to stress depends on the integrating roles of the nervous, circulatory, and endocrine systems. [After Hardy, courtesy of *Therapeutic Notes*, 67:203 (July–Aug.), 1960.]

phase of the "adaptation syndrome." As examples, rheumatic fever and rheumatoid arthritis occur during the catabolic phase. In other disorders the patient fails to progress into the anabolic phase. Patients in whom failure is most likely to occur are those with chronic debilitating conditions such as starvation, severe burns, large draining wounds, hyperthyroidism, Cushing's syndrome, and many others.

IMMUNOLOGIC RESPONSES

Whereas many of the responses to injury are nonspecific, most individuals also have, or are able to develop, resistance to specific microorganisms. The term *immunity* signifies a characteristic of the host that confers resistance to a specific agent. This characteristic is based on the ability of cells to distinguish "self" from "nonself" and to elaborate a specific agent that acts against foreign substances. The ability to recognize and to respond to foreign agents is certainly adaptive. It has contributed to survival of the species. Understandably enough, the first observations involving immune responses were made in relation to infectious diseases. Very early man noted that after a person experienced and recovered from certain diseases he never had them again. Instances are reported in which material was taken from a smallpox lesion and inoculated into a susceptible host with the hope that he would have a mild case of the disease. In 1798 Jenner reported that persons inoculated with material from a cowpox lesion could be effectively protected from smallpox. Later workers in the field such as Pasteur, Koch, Metchnikoff, and Ehrlich added to the knowledge of immunity. From the time of Pasteur to the present, considerable effort has been devoted to developing vaccines against specific diseases. As emphasized in Chapter 5, a number of deadly and/or crippling diseases can now be prevented by vaccines and other immunizing agents.

Schwartz [15] summarizes the developments in the field of immunology in the following:

The control of disease by immunologic means began in 1796, when Edward Jenner inoculated James Phipps with cowpox. Immunologic prophylaxis still flourishes, and the discovery that passive immunization prevents erythroblastosis is its latest triumph. Early in this century Clemens von Pirquet initiated another branch of immunology by establishing the principle that antibodies can be injurious. The central issues of clinical immunology, formulated in terms of these momentous discoveries, are the production of desired immunity and the elimination of undesired immune reactions. . . .

Recent developments stimulating the study of immunity include (1) the recognition of immunologic deficiency and its effects, (2) the overproduction of certain gamma globulins and of abnormal immunoglobulins (as an example, an abnormal protein is produced in myeloma, a malignant disorder of plasma cells), (3) the concept of autoimmune disease, and (4) the immunologic interference with organ transplants. The introduction of electron microscopy and fluorescent antibody techniques has made a considerable contribution to the understanding of the biochemical and physiological aspects of immunity and immunopathology.

As knowledge of the immune response has increased, the field has been greatly expanded. It is now known that some of the responses involve many structures: the phagocytic system, the thymus, the lymphocytes, and the plasma cells and their secretory products, the immunoglobulins. Further, the immune response is not limited to microbes and homografts but can be elicited by a vast number and variety of agents. Similar to other body responses, immunologic responses may be appropriate in kind and degree. They may also be inadequate (hypo), excessive (hyper), or inappropriate to the stimulus.

Adjuvant is any substance that enhances the response to an immunogen.

Allergen is a substance giving rise to hypersensitivity or allergy.

Allergy is an altered reaction of tissues to repeated contacts with antigenic agents. The tissues behave differently on exposure to a material than they did on earlier exposures.

Antibody is a protein formed in the body as a result of contact with an antigen. This humoral protein is an immunoglobulin. It can be detected by its ability to combine with an antigen.

Antigen is a substance that stimulates the formation of antibodies. It may be one of a variety of large molecules, many of them protein in nature, such as a part of a virus, bacterium, a foreign tissue cell, a fragment of a foreign tissue cell, or a polysaccharide. Lipids and nucleic acids are capable of becoming antigens after they combine with protein. With the exception of the erythrocytes and tissues sequestered from the blood stream, such as parts of the brain, the thyroid gland, and the lens of the eye, antigens stimulating the formation of antibodies are usually derived from another species or individual.

Atopy is an allergic disease of the wheal and erythema type in which there is usually a family history of allergic disease.

Autograft (selfgraft) is tissue transplanted from one part of the body to another.

Autoimmune disease is "any pathologic condition resulting from the interaction within the body of antibody or immunologically competent cells—immunocytes—on one hand and antigenic determinants carried by normal body components on the other." [16]

Bradykinin is a potent vasodilator that is re-

[15] Robert S. Schwartz: "Therapeutic Strategy in Clinical Immunology," *New Eng. J. Med.*, 280:367 (Feb. 13) 1969.

[16] Sir Macfarlane Burnet: "Concepts of Autoimmune Disease and Their Implications for Therapy," *Perspect. Biol. Med.*, 10:141 (Winter) 1967.

leased from the alpha-2-globulin fraction of the blood by the proteolytic enzymes.

Complement is a group of serum proteins, but not antibodies, that react with antigen-antibody complexes. Among the biological activities of complement as listed by Stroud [17] are the following: (1) increases capillary permeability, (2) causes neutrophil chemotaxis, (3) causes immune adherence of antigen-antibody complexes, (4) promotes phagocytosis, and (5) causes damage to membranes of mammalian cells, bacteria, and viruses and possibly to basement membranes.

Hapten is an incomplete antigen. It requires another substance to become antigenic. It reacts with an antibody but does not by itself stimulate antibody formation.

Heterograft (xenograft) is tissue transplanted from one species to another (goat to sheep). It is always rejected.

Histamine is a powerful vasodilator. Experimentally it has been demonstrated to produce asthma-like symptoms. It is a powerful stimulator of secretion of hydrochloric acid. It is found in mammalian tissues, especially mast cells. The breakdown of mast cells leads to liberation of histamine and serotonin.

Histocompatibility is the degree to which cellular antigens are alike in two animals of the same species. Histocompatibility is genetically determined.

Homograft (allograft) is tissue transplanted from one member of the same species to another (noninbred), as from one man to another. In the absence of immunosuppressive therapy, the tissue is rejected.

Hyperergy is an exaggerated tissue response. In allergy the tissues hyperreact.

Hypersensitivity is used interchangeably with allergy. Delayed-type hypersensitivity is one in which the reaction is delayed for several hours and may last for days. The delayed type is mediated by immunologically competent cells. Immediate-type hypersensitivity is a wheal and flare reaction that begins immediately on contact with the allergen and disappears promptly. The immediate type is mediated by humoral antibodies.

Hypoergy is a deficient tissue response to a given substance.

Immunity implies a protected state.

Immunogen is a substance stimulating the formation of antibodies.

Immunology is the study of the immune response.

Isoantibodies are antibodies acting against isoantigens.

Isoantigens are substances found in an individ-

ual that are antigenic in other members of the same species (as antigens in the red blood cells).

Isograft is tissue transplanted from one animal of a highly inbred strain to another of the same strain (genetically identical) or from one identical twin to another. The tissue is usually accepted.

Normergy is a normal tissue response to a given substance.

Reagin (homocytotropic antibody) is a skin-sensitizing antibody occurring in the skin of some persons who are allergic. These individuals have the immediate type of hypersensitivity. Reaction is characterized by a wheal and flare response about 20 minutes after the intradermal injection of antigen.

Serotonin is a powerful smooth-muscle stimulator and vasoconstrictor. Serotonin is formed in the argentaffin cells of the gastrointestinal tract and is transported by the blood platelets. It is found in the brain and many other tissues.

Tolerance is a state in which the immunological system does not react to a substance. Normally, an individual is tolerant of his own tissues.

IMMUNOGLOBULINS

The immunoglobulins are a heterogeneous group of blood proteins varying in molecular weight from 140,000 to 1 million. Antibodies are their most important members. Immunoglobulins (antibodies) are designated as IgG, IgA, IgM, and IgD. IgG was formerly called $7S_\gamma$. From the available evidence, antibodies appear to consist of two heavy (H) or long and two light (L) or short peptide chains joined by disulfide ($-SS-$) bonds. Immunoglobulins have two types of activity, antigenic and antibody. Their antigenic activity is used to distinguish one from the other. Both H and L chains probably contribute to the combining sites on the antibody molecule, but the H chain appears to have the most antibody activity. The L chain may contain the recognition site. The L chains are closely similar in all immunoglobulins, but the H chains serve to distinguish one class from the others. Antibody activity is specific to the antigen, stimulating its production. (For further description of antibodies, see the References.) Some authorities suggest that the first step in the formation of antibodies is the phagocytosis of antigen by the macrophages. They then transfer the information in a form of RNA or the antigen itself to the lymphocytes that synthesize antibodies.[18] The fact that a mixture

---

[17] Robert M. Stroud: "Complement and Disease," *Postgrad. Med.,* **41**:387 (Apr.) 1967.

[18] There are several forms of RNA, only one of which is postulated to act in the transfer of information for synthesis of antibody. See Chapter 15, Part A.

of leukocytes is more effective in antibody formation than lymphocytes alone supports this view.

STRUCTURE AND FUNCTION OF THE IMMUNOLOGIC SYSTEM

Clinical and experimental evidence supports the hypothesis that there are two interrelated immunologic systems. One is thymus-dependent; the other is thymus-independent. The thymus gland forms small lymphocytes that migrate to and are buried deep in the lymph nodes scattered throughout the body. They release cells known as immunoblasts into the circulation. These cells must pass out of the blood into the tissues before they can produce antibodies. This system mediates cellular responses such as hypersensitivity reactions and the rejection of skin grafts. Children born without a thymus gland have normal amounts of immunoglobulins, but they do not show hypersensitivity responses to various antigens. They either accept skin grafts from unrelated donors or reject them after a long delay.

In contrast, the thymus-independent or humoral system involves the immunoglobulins or circulating antibodies in the blood. Some authorities refer to this system as the gut-associated lymphoid-tissue system. The structures that may function in this way are the appendix and Peyer's patches. Others are not certain about the location of the tissue that plays a role similar to that of the thymus. These immunoglobulins are synthesized by fixed plasma cells in the lymph nodes and spleen and are secreted into the blood. Children with congenital agammaglobulinemia lack plasma cells and humoral antibodies, but they have normal cellular immunity.[19]

Both these systems are essential to combating a host of foreign substances, including not only microorganisms and homografts but a wide variety of other foreign agents.

In the words of Hall,[20] "in the absence of cell-mediated immune mechanisms the extravascular compartment, which means most of the body, has little in the way of an immunologically specific defence against bacteria and viruses in the early invasive stage of the disease process. For this reason, it seems proper to regard the evolution of cell-mediated immunity as an adaptive response to the major environmental threat, i.e., infectious disease." The rejection of homografts is, therefore, to be expected.[21]

[19] "Science and the Citizen. Dual Immunology," *Sci. Amer.,* **220**:43 (Feb.) 1969.
[20] J. G. Hall: "Effector Mechanisms in Immunity," *Lancet,* **1**:27 (Jan. 4) 1969.
[21] *Ibid.*

The thymus-dependent system reacts relatively quickly to microbes entering a tissue. Within four to five days after exposure, the lymphoid tissue produces large numbers of immunoblasts that pass into the affected tissue where they synthesize cellular antibodies. These antibodies help to limit the spread of infection from one cell to another. Immunoblasts may be of particular importance in the prevention of the dissemination of virus and certain types of bacterial infection in tissues.

Hall[22] discusses the relationship of cellular immunity to recovery from measles. Children with agammaglobulinemia recover from measles and develop immunity to them. In children treated with cortisone, the thymus-dependent system (cellular immunity) is eliminated. These children die from giant cell pneumonia and do not have a rash.

The thymus-independent system is slower acting and less accurate than the thymus-dependent system. It takes about ten days after exposure to invasive organisms for humoral antibodies to reach peak levels in the blood.

Occasionally an individual is born who has congenital agammaglobulinemia, a disorder in which there is a failure in the synthesis of gamma globulin. It is probably caused by a defect in the formation of plasma cells. Agammaglobulinemia falls into three categories:

1. Primary congenital—sex-linked, recessive—male children
2. Primary acquired—no clear-cut hereditary basis and may appear in either sex at any time in life
3. Secondary—to neoplastic disease, e.g., Hodgkin's, other malignant lymphomas, multiple myeloma, and chronic lymphatic leukemia

Syndrome of primary agammaglobulinemia includes

1. Recurrent pyogenic infections
2. Gastrointestinal symptoms (diarrhea; large, bulky, foul-smelling stools; and flat oral glucose tolerance curves)
3. Reticuloendothelial disorders
4. Arthritis and arthralgia

The ability of tissues to react to antigenic agents by synthesizing antibodies and to distinguish between self and nonself has many applications in the field of medicine. On the positive side, the capacity of tissues to react to foreign substances by forming antibodies enables the individual to become immune to (protected against) a variety of infectious agents. On the negative side, it increases the hazards of blood

[22] *Ibid.*

transfusion, limits the extent to which tissues of one individual can be successfully transplanted to another, and is responsible for a number of diseases. As examples, because the body is able to form antibodies against the virus causing smallpox, immunity to smallpox can be developed. Before blood can be safely transfused into an individual, the blood from the donor and the recipient must be matched to eliminate the possibility of the recipient's serum containing antibodies against the antigen in the donor's erythrocytes. Unless the donor is an identical twin or the recipient has agammaglobulinemia, or is treated with an immunosuppressive agent, the chances of tissue transplanted from one individual to another "taking" are negligible. The tissues of one individual are antigenic in another; that is, the tissues of the recipient recognize the tissue as "foreign" and form antibodies against it. This response is as normal as any response to a foreign antigen.

STAGES IN THE DEVELOPMENT OF IMMUNITY

As previously emphasized, body structures and functions prevent many foreign agents from penetrating the body's surface. After a germ or other foreign substance gains access to the internal environment, the body is faced with three tasks: capture, recognition, and response.[23] Capture, which is the first stage of the specific response to bacteria, involves at least three processes: ingestion (phagocytosis), intracellular killing, and digestion of antigens. Although capture is the first stage of the specific response, it will be discussed later in this chapter.

The second stage, recognition, is poorly understood. After lymphocytes have contact with a foreign antigen, they are able to recognize it as being different from its host. This means that the lymphocyte has some means of distinguishing between host and foreign chemical configurations. On subsequent exposures to the antigen the lymphoid cells "remember" that they have had previous contact with a specific foreign agent. The latter is called *immunologic memory*. According to Janeway,[24] immunologic memory is clearly associated with the small lymphocyte. The second time the lymphocyte has contact with an antigen, it responds more quickly and to a greater degree than it did the first time.[25] The third stage of response will be considered later.

ALLERGY

Like other homeostatic mechanisms, the immunological defense system can be a source of

disease. Two abnormalities, agammaglobulinemia in which the individual is unable to form humoral antibodies against foreign materials and absence of the thymus, have been previously mentioned. A far more frequent malady is allergy. The word *allergy* was introduced in 1907 by von Pirquet to describe altered reaction of tissues after repeated contact with microorganisms and antigenic agents such as foreign serums, tuberculin, and vaccine virus. Subsequently, the term *allergy* has come to include a large group of conditions in which the tissues or organs of a person respond on repeated contacts with a foreign material in a way that is different from the manner in which other members of the same species react. Allergy differs from beneficial immunological reactions in that it does harm to body tissues. Crowle[26] refers to allergy as an immunological mistake. It is immunity gone wrong.

Although the preceding has been the classic view of allergy, allergic responses are now thought to be beneficial in supporting the host's responses to microbial antigens. As an example, granulocytes, macrophages, and serum proteins including antibodies and complement accumulate at the site of a localized allergic response to microbes. Some types of microbes such as *Mycobacterium tuberculosis* can multiply in "nonactivated" macrophages, whereas they are destroyed in "activated" ones. It is also possible that delayed-type reactions enhance antibody formation.

Antigens

Antigens vary in their capacity to induce antibody formation from those that are seldom antigenic to those that almost always are. Horse serum induces hypersensitivity in a high percentage of instances on the first exposure to it. Poison ivy will eventually induce hypersensitivity, if exposure continues to be repeated. As indicated earlier, large molecules are more likely to be antigenic than small molecules. Chemically, antigens are usually proteins or polysaccharides, though they may be lipids or nucleic acids. According to one hypothesis, polysaccharides do not become antigenic until they attach themselves to a protein molecule. Lipids and nucleic acids must be attached to a protein molecule to be allergenic. A vast variety of substances are therefore potentially antigenic. Some of the more common ones are the plant pollens, animal danders, seafoods, berries, eggs, chocolate, and wheat. Foreign serums, tuberculin, and vaccine viruses as well as drugs such as penicillin, streptomycin sulfate, heavy metals, sulfonamides, iodides, and barbiturates

[23] Charles A. Janeway: "Progress in Immunology," *J. Pediat.,* 72:886 (June) 1968.

[24] *Ibid.,* p. 887.

[25] *Ibid.,* p. 886.

[26] Alfred J. Crowle: "Delayed Hypersensitivity," *Sci. Amer.,* 202:129 (Apr.) 1960.

are also common offenders. Antigens may be introduced in the body by injection, inhalation, ingestion, or contact with the skin.

Just as antigenic agents vary in potency, individuals vary in their capacity to become allergic or hypersensitive. Many of the common forms of allergy depend on a hereditary factor. What is inherited is not the allergic manifestation but the tendency to become allergic. For example, a parent has asthma; his child develops urticaria. Physical, chemical, and emotional factors also play a role in the development of allergy. They may be significant not only in inducing hypersensitivity but in prolonging a particular allergic response. Some persons appear to be hypersensitive to certain substances on their first contact with them. Others evidence great resistance to even common allergens. For example, some babies are unable to tolerate wheat or eggs from their first exposure to them. One theory advanced to explain this observation is that antigenic material is transferred from the mother to the fetus in utero.

In the more usual conception of allergy, the tissues most likely to become hypersensitive are those in contact with the external environment, that is, the skin and the respiratory and gastrointestinal tracts. Hall [27] states that immunoblasts are commonly observed in the parenchyma of the alveoli and the interstitial tissue of the gut. When there is a high concentration of antibodies in the circulating blood, circulatory collapse may follow re-exposure to the antigen. The tissues in which allergic responses are manifested are sometimes referred to as shock tissues. It is not known whether they have a greater tendency to become sensitized or whether they become sensitized because they have greater exposure to allergens.

IMMUNOLOGIC DISORDERS

Immunologic disorders can be classified in different ways, such as the length of time elapsing between exposure to an antigen to which the individual has been sensitized and the development of an allergic response. They may also be classified according to the mechanism underlying the response. Although Burdon and Williams [28] use the traditional classification, the immediate and delayed response, they emphasize that the mechanisms for the two types are different. The immediate type is mediated by humoral antibodies, whereas the delayed type is mediated by immunologically competent cells. Further, the immediate type of hypersensitivity

reactions may be either local or general. They may also be cytotropic (cell-stimulating) or cytolytic (cell-damaging) anaphylaxis.

Schwartz [29] classifies harmful immunologic mechanisms as (1) anaphylaxis, (2) cytolysis, (3) injury by soluble antigen-antibody complexes, and (4) delayed hypersensitivity.

IMMEDIATE-TYPE HYPERSENSITIVITY:
CYTOTROPIC TYPE

It can be noted that the immediate type of hypersensitivity can be induced by several types of antigens. Either genetic plus environmental factors or previous sensitization with a foreign protein or drug predisposes to it. In those disorders in which genetic factors play a role, sensitivity is said to be natural and the resulting diseases are called atopic diseases. They include infantile eczema, which is often followed in later life by respiratory allergies; hay fever; allergic rhinitis; and asthma. Other atopic allergies include urticaria, gastrointestinal allergies, and in some instances migraine headaches. Although the tendency to atopic allergy is a characteristic of an individual throughout his lifetime, the antigens to which he is sensitive and the manifestations of his atopic state may change.[30]

In atopic individuals an antibody, which is variously called the homocytotropic skin-sensitizing or reaginic antibody, or simply reagin, mediates the wheal and flare reaction. According to Schwartz,[31] reagin is IgE. In normal persons, it is present in millimicrogram amounts; in allergic individuals it is present in microgram amounts. IgE adheres to leukocytes and mast cells. An allergic reaction occurs when IgG bound to these cells comes in contact with the appropriate antigen. Subsequently, when these cells come in contact with the antigen, pharmacologic agents are released from the target cells. Histamine, serotonin, and bradykinin, among others, may be released. A lipoprotein called slow-reacting substance (SRS) is released by polymorphonuclear leukocytes.[32] These chemicals are responsible for the acute manifestations of allergy as they cause vasodilatation, increased vascular permeability, and smooth-muscle spasm. When vasodilatation is generalized, life-threatening hypotension, that is, anaphylactic shock, may occur. Anaphylactic shock may follow the parenteral injection of foreign serum and certain drugs such as penicillin. The specific manifestations of anaphylactic shock differ with each species.

[27] Hall, loc. cit.
[28] Kenneth L. Burdon and Robert P. Williams: Microbiology, 6th ed. (New York: The Macmillan Company, 1968), p. 479.

[29] Op. cit., p. 368.
[30] William B. Sherman: "Atopic Hypersensitivity," Med. Clin. N. Amer., 49:1599 (Nov.) 1965.
[31] Op. cit., p. 368.
[32] Schwartz, op. cit., p. 368.

Physiological Reactions

Although a cytotropic reaction including atopy involves the entire body, it is usually manifested by a specific or shock organ. Target organs are most frequently those that are in contact with the external environment. Interestingly enough, the lymphocytes and plasma cells are commonly observed in the alveolar parenchyma and the interstitium of the mucosa of the small intestine. Many of the manifestations of atopic disease occur in organs supplied by the autonomic nervous system.

Vascular Reactions

The characteristic vascular change is an increase in capillary permeability with loss of fluid into the interstitial spaces. The resulting edema may be noted as swelling of the face, eyelids, and lips. When edema of the larynx occurs, it may be an immediate threat to life as it impairs ventilation by obstructing the airway. When the blood vessels themselves are the shock or target organ, loss of fluid from the capillaries may be so great that blood volume is diminished sufficiently to cause a serious decrease in cardiac output and arterial blood pressure. When the capillaries are dilated, the skin is flushed or red. From the preceding it should be obvious that increased capillary permeability threatens the life of the individual by predisposing to laryngeal edema and loss of blood volume. Because the manifestations develop rapidly, the patient should be observed for flushing of the skin and any puffiness of the face, mouth, or eyelids. Any patient in whom these signs appear should be treated immediately. Epinephrine should be immediately available to be administered in situations where systemic reactions are a possibility.

Skin Reactions

When a small amount of antigen is injected into previously sensitized skin, a swelling with erythema or reddening occurs at the site. It is believed that the skin-sensitizing antibody sensitizes certain cells, particularly the mast cells and blood platelets. The capillaries dilate, causing local erythema. Then the arterioles dilate, causing the flare. The skin response is utilized in identifying hypersensitive individuals. As little as 0.1 ml of antigen diluted 1:10 is injected into the skin. Within a matter of minutes the reaction occurs. Knowledge that the individual is sensitized to the antigen may save him a life-threatening experience.

The typical skin lesion is known as a wheal or hive. Hives, which may be single or multiple, are localized areas of swelling caused by increased capillary permeability. They are red, hot, and accompanied by intense itching.

Although they can be seen on the skin, they may also occur in the gastrointestinal and tracheobronchial mucosa.

Itching, especially when generalized, is important not because it threatens the life of the individual but because it serves as a warning that a general systemic reaction is developing. When a patient has received a potentially antigenic drug such as penicillin, itching should be regarded as indicating the patient is developing a systemic response. The fact of itching should be immediately reported to the patient's physician. In any situation in which a generalized hypersensitivity reaction is a possibility, epinephrine should be prepared and be immediately available. Life-threatening allergic responses occur relatively infrequently. Therein lies a danger, for preparation may not have been made for this possibility.

Smooth Muscle Reactions

In target organs containing smooth muscle, the musculature contracts. In man, contraction of the musculature of the bronchi causes labored breathing characteristic of asthma. Increased contractions of the gastrointestinal musculature causes vomiting and diarrhea.

Mucous Membrane Reactions

Increased capillary permeability in the mucosa results in redness, swelling, weeping, and itching. Mucous glands hypersecrete mucus, thereby predisposing to obstruction of the tracheobronchial tree.

SOME ATOPIC ALLERGIES

There is a group of common human allergies, including nonseasonal vasomotor rhinitis, hay fever, infantile eczema, urticaria, and angioedema, as well as some migraine headaches and gastrointestinal disorders, having a number of features in common. They all appear to be based on a common predisposing hereditary factor. The characteristic lesion in the allergic tissues is the wheal or hive. In many instances, symptoms and signs appear promptly on exposure to the allergen. Injection of the offending allergen into the skin is followed by the immediate type of response.

There are some instances, however, in which individuals who are predisposed by heredity to become allergic do not develop signs and symptoms following exposure to an allergen for 12 to 24 hours. For example, Silas Cornflower has a positive family history for allergy, as his mother had urticaria when she ate strawberries or seafood. Injection of minute quantities of antigenic material from either strawberries or seafood results in a raised swollen area at the site of injection (wheal). Mr. Cornflower has asthma when he is exposed to dog dander, but his symptoms do not develop immediately on exposure. They are delayed for 12 to 24 hours after he is in close proximity to a dog. Skin tests do not show the immediate type of reaction. The mechanism in the delayed type of immunological responses must be different from that in the immediate type. How it differs is not known.

Hay Fever

In hay fever (seasonal vasomotor rhinitis) and nonseasonal rhinitis the mucous membranes lining the nose, related structures, and conjunctiva are affected. The manifestations include tearing and redness of the eyes, burning of both the eyes and nasal mucosa, sneezing, watery discharge from the nose, and obstruction to the passage of air by congestion of the nasal mucosa. The severity of symptoms varies from mild to so severe that the patient cannot get sufficient rest. Seasonal and nonseasonal vasomotor rhinitis differ principally in the antigens to which the person is sensitive. They include pollens—ragweed is a common offender and is responsible for seasonal vasomotor rhinitis —house dust, animal danders, drugs, foods, and the products of infection. With the exception of ragweed, all the other materials cause nonseasonal vasomotor rhinitis. Besides causing varying amounts of discomfort, vasomotor rhinitis predisposes to allergic asthma.

Allergic Asthma

In allergic asthma, the basic lesion is the same as in other allergic responses of the immediate type, but the lesions occur in the bronchial tubes. Three factors are commonly considered to be responsible for allergic asthma: (1) the inhalation of allergens, causing seasonal or nonseasonal asthma; (2) infection of the respiratory tract, causing intermittent or chronic symptoms; and (3) a combination of the first two. The same antigens causing allergic rhinitis may also be responsible for allergic asthma. Because of the variety of factors involved in allergic asthma, it may be seasonal, nonseasonal, or chronic.

Because the bronchi are involved in allergic asthma, there are three responses contributing to the development of symptoms: (1) increased capillary permeability in the mucosa lining the bronchi, (2) spasm or contraction of bronchial musculature, and (3) increased secretion of mucus. All these changes contribute to the interference with breathing—the major manifestation in asthma. At the onset of an attack, the patient is likely to feel that he is about to suffocate and his behavior may suggest that he is in a state of panic or acute anxiety. For example, Mrs. Pine, who had been hospitalized

for the treatment of asthma, developed an acute attack. She turned on her light. Before the nurse had time to reach her room, she called out for the nurse to hurry. Mrs. Pine appeared to be frightened and she did not want to be left alone. The feelings of suffocation accompanying an attack of asthma probably always engender feelings of fear and anxiety and may prolong the attack, after it is under way. Whatever the cause, cell injury results in the release of histamine and serotonin. Any serious threat to oxygen supply and to the removal of carbon dioxide can be expected to have a similar effect.

Emotional factors may also trigger attacks of asthma. As an illustration, one morning Mrs. Pine thought that she had been given a drug to which she was allergic and she developed a full-blown attack of asthma. What had actually occurred was that a laboratory assistant had drawn blood. The attack had been triggered by a thought rather than a material substance. It was no less severe, however. She required the same treatment as any patient experiencing an acute attack of asthma. During the attack Mrs. Pine sat with her feet hanging over the edge of the bed. She was supporting herself with her hands and arms in a winglike position. This position enabled her to make maximum use of her accessory muscles of respiration. Because bronchi dilate with inspiration and are smaller with expiration, air is trapped in the lungs, causing them to be distended and the chest to be in a continuous state of expansion. Therefore, the efforts of the patient are directed toward forcing air out of the lung during expiration. Expiration appears more labored than inspiration. Her (Mrs. Pine's) respirations were accompanied by a wheeze that was audible to her and to those who were nearby. Coughing was stimulated by an increase in the secretion of mucus. Therapy for an acute asthmatic attack is directed toward (1) depressing the allergic response, (2) dilating the bronchi, (3) decreasing the anxiety of the patient, and (4) correcting the conditions predisposing to asthma. When at all possible someone should stay with the patient who is in an acute attack of asthma. When only one person is available, the most reasonable course of action is to prepare and administer the prescribed drug or drugs. Some of the same drugs that are effective in treatment of anaphylactic shock are also useful in relieving an acute attack of asthma. These drugs include epinephrine, ephedrine sulfate, or hydrochloride, aminophyllin, U.S.P., B.P., isoproterenerol hydrochloride, and Tedral.[33] In a very acute attack, epinephrine is usually administered.

[33] Trade name for compound containing theophylline, 0.13 g; ephedrine hydrochloride, 24 mg; and phenobarbital, 8 mg.

Skin Reactions

Skin reactions characteristic of the immediate type of allergy include infantile eczema, erythematous rashes, exfoliative dermatitis, and hives.[34]

Urticaria or hives of the skin is most frequently associated with allergy to foods. Drugs may also be responsible.

Wheal and erythema reactions occurring along the gastrointestinal tract, combined with the contraction of smooth muscle, cause symptoms such as nausea, vomiting, and diarrhea. Gastrointestinal allergies are likely to be caused by ingestants such as seafood, wheat, or eggs.

IMMEDIATE-TYPE HYPERSENSITIVITY: CYTOLYTIC TYPE

A second harmful immune mechanism of the immediate type is cytolysis. Whereas in the cytotropic reaction cells are stimulated by the antigen-antibody in cytolytic or cytotoxic reaction, sensitized cells are directly injured. According to Schwartz,[35] the offending immunoglobulin is almost always IgG. The antigen may be of either intrinsic or extrinsic origin. An example of an intrinsic antigen is the Rh factor in the erythrocyte. An extrinsic antigen is penicillin. Whatever the offending antigen, coating of the cell with IgG makes it susceptible to damage by macrophages and other mononuclear cells. A series of changes occur that lead to the damage of red blood cells. Examples of disorders caused by cytolytic reactions are the hemolysis of red cells following the transfusion of mismatched blood, erythroblastosis in the newborn, some types of hemolytic anemia, thrombocytopenia, leukopenia, and a type of anemia induced by penicillin.

The Arthus Reaction

Another example of a cytolytic reaction is the Arthus phenomenon. An individual sensitized by repeated injections of a specific antigen may eventually respond to the same antigen by a localized inflammatory response at the site of the injection. Within 12 to 24 hours a centralized area of necrosis appears. The reaction requires large amounts of antigen in the tissues and circulating antibodies (IgG). In the presence of complement soluble antigen-antibody complexes are deposited in the blood vessels. As a result of their irritating effect large numbers of polymorphonuclear leukocytes enter the area and phagocytosize the antibody-antigen complexes. Protein-digesting enzymes are released. Platelets accumulate and blood clots.

The result is an area of hemorrhagic necrosis. Healing is by repair.[36]

A response that appears to be similar in many respects to the Arthus reaction is also mediated by soluble antigen-antibody aggregates. Instead of occurring at the site of injected antigen, the reaction occurs at a distant site such as in the kidney. Schwartz [37] states that insoluble aggregates of antigens and antibodies are formed when antibodies are mixed with appropriate antigens. When increasing amounts of antigens are added, however, some of the molecules of the aggregate are rearranged and form soluble complexes. Because of their size insoluble immune aggregates are rapidly removed by the reticuloendothelial system. Conversely, the soluble complexes are not easily removed from the blood and they penetrate the walls of blood vessels. Because they are highly vascular organs, the kidneys are frequent sites of injury. Soluble immune aggregates are deposited in the basement membranes of the glomeruli and activate the complement system. In response polymorphonuclear leukocytes enter the area and ingest the deposits. Lysosomal granules in the cell burst and release lytic enzymes, which then injure the basement membrane of the glomerulus.

From the preceding discussion, it should be obvious that there are a number of systemic and local allergic responses of the immediate type. The nature of the manifestations depends on whether or not the response is systemic or localized to an organ or part. The organs in which the manifestations are most prominent are those in direct contact with the external environment: the skin, the airway, and the gastrointestinal tract. The bone marrow may, however, be a primary site of reaction as well. In anaphylactic shock, the blood vessels throughout the body are affected. Two factors that seem to influence the nature of the response are the rate and site of exposure to an antigen. Most of the manifestations are caused by increased capillary permeability and by contraction of smooth muscle. Vascular collapse and obstruction of the airway as a result of edema of the larynx are the two most serious threats to the life of an individual. No person should be treated with a foreign serum or other type of antigenic agent without first determining whether or not he has been treated with it at some earlier time. Patients receiving horse serum should be tested previous to its administration by the injection of horse serum intradermally (into the skin). A reddening or flare indicates that the patient has been sensitized to horse serum.

---

[34] A number of terms are used to describe blisters. Blebs, vesicles, and bullae all imply blisters. Bullae are large blisters.

[35] *Op. cit.*, p. 368.

[36] Burdon and Williams, *op. cit.*, p. 495.

[37] *Op. cit.*, p. 368.

DELAYED-TYPE HYPERSENSITIVITY

Another harmful immunologic response is delayed hypersensitivity. The classic example is the response of the tissues to the tubercle bacillus. A similar type of reaction occurs in other chronic infections as well as in contact dermatitis. Although signs and symptoms usually occur within minutes after exposure to an antigen in the immediate type of hypersensitivity, there are a few exceptions such as serum sickness. In general, however, signs and symptoms are slower to develop in the delayed type than in the immediate type. In the immediate type the antibody circulates in the blood; in the delayed type it is bound to cells. The first is known as a humoral antibody and the latter as a high affinity or avidity antibody. Antibodies in the serum can be identified in and transferred in the serum.[38] Cellular antibodies cannot be transferred in the serum but require lymphocytes to which antibodies are bound.

Differences in the Lesions

Whereas the lesion in the immediate type of hypersensitivity usually develops within a few minutes and may disappear within a short time, the lesion of the delayed type of hypersensitivity reaction takes several hours to appear. It is similar inasmuch as the area is red, hot, and swollen. The swelling is firmer and lasts longer than it does in the immediate type of reaction. When the reaction is severe, tissue cells may be killed and cellular necrosis may be evident. The initial damage may result from the combination of the antigen and the antibody. Further injury may be caused by substances released by the necrotic cells. With cellular injury, tissues also respond by inflammation. This response will be discussed later in the chapter. The classical example of the delayed type of hypersensitivity is the response of the tissues to tuberculin. Anyone whose tissues have been sensitized to *Mycobacterium tuberculosis* and has had a Mantoux or similar test has experienced the delayed type of allergic skin reaction. When this reaction is marked, there is some degree of tissue necrosis.

Allergies of the Delayed Type

Allergies of the delayed type include contact dermatitis, poison ivy, drug allergies, and allergies of infections such as tuberculosis. According to Crowle,[39] the cavities forming in the lungs in tuberculosis appear to be the result of a delayed hypersensitivity reaction. Changes occurring in the tissues in a variety of other

[38] Transfer of humoral antibodies from an immunized to a susceptible individual provides passive immunity.
[39] Crowle, *op. cit.,* p. 133.

infections such as syphilis are believed to be attributable to hypersensitivity reactions. Symptoms in conditions such as athlete's foot may be the result of delayed hypersensitivity to the fungus causing the disorder. Following the administration of heterologous serum and certain drugs, including penicillin, changes take place in blood vessels that are characteristic of a delayed type of allergic response. The pathological changes in the blood vessels resemble those of periarteritis nodosa.

One of the most common examples of delayed hypersensitivity is contact dermatitis. Because of the frequency with which it occurs and its increasing incidence, contact dermatitis will be discussed in some detail. As a result of repeated contacts with a wide variety of simple as well as complex antigenic agents, including detergents, the skin becomes sensitized to an antigen. The agents that initiate or prolong dermatitis are numerous. The signs of dermatitis appear in sensitized skin from 12 to 48 hours after exposure to the antigen. They include (1) erythema and swelling, (2) oozing and/or vesiculation, (3) crusting and scaling, (4) thickening and evidence of repeated excoriation (the results of scratching), and (5) hyperpigmentation, scratch papule formation, and lichenification. The first three groups of signs occur during the acute phase and the latter two during the chronic phase of the disorder. The eventual outcome depends on the early identification and elimination of the cause. When contact dermatitis is allowed to persist, secondary changes follow and tend to prolong it.

Autoimmune Disease

Until recently most antigens were believed to be foreign substances that were introduced into, or entered, the individual from his outside environment. Some individuals, for reasons that are poorly understood, appear to lose their ability to identify their own tissues as being of themselves, for they react to certain of their own tissues as they would to foreign antigens. Diseases in which the body may possibly form antibodies against its own tissues are called autoimmune diseases. Though this theory offers an attractive explanation for the changes occurring in certain diseases such as rheumatic fever, multiple sclerosis, lupus erythematosus, periarteritis nodosa, and rheumatoid arthritis, it is largely unproved. One disorder usually cited as being caused by a hyperimmune response is Hashimoto's disease of the thyroid. A number of observations have been made that lend support to the theory that tissues can become antigenic and thus stimulate the formation of antibodies against themselves. In diseases such as rheumatic fever, the onset is frequently preceded by a streptococcal infection occurring approximately two to three weeks earlier. How the infection or the products of bacterial growth induce changes in tissue cells is now known. It has been shown that streptococcus and the myocardium possess a common antigen—a body response to the streptococcal infection is also a response against myocardial tissue. Antibodies are formed in response to this antigen; they combine with the ˙antigen and injure tissue cells. The damaged cells release histamine and possibly serotonin, both of which cause secondary changes that are possibly more damaging than the initial injury. Further destruction of healthy tissues may result from the contraction of scar tissue formed to replace dead tissue. One of the puzzling things about these diseases is that after they are initiated there is no sure way known to stop their progress.

Diagnostic Skin Tests

As previously stated, various body tissues may be sensitized to specific antigens. Because antibodies are frequently found in the skin, and it is conveniently located, the skin may be used (1) to identify individuals who are sensitized to horse serum or other antigens; (2) to check the effectiveness of certain immunization procedures, as the Schick test for diphtheria; (3) to trace the distribution of a disease such as tuberculosis in the community; and (4) to establish the nature of the diagnosis as an example to distinguish between tuberculosis and histoplasmoses.

Skin tests may be performed by injecting a dilute solution of the desired antigen into the skin or by placing a small quantity of the solution on the skin and abrading or scratching it with a hypodermic needle. The scratch test is believed to be safer than intradermal injection because the rate of absorption of the antigen is slower. In the intradermal test, 0.1 to 0.2 ml of a given dilution of the antigen is injected into the skin. In patients known to be or suspected of being hypersensitive, the dilution should be appropriately large. The patient or a member of the family should be asked if he has had the particular type of injection previously and, if he has, how he reacted to it. Skin reactions, similar to other allergic responses, may be immediate or delayed. The immediate reaction occurs within a few minutes after the antigenic material is injected and lasts only a short time; the area should therefore be subject to continuous observation. With a positive reaction, the skin becomes red or flushed. Careful observation of the site where antigenic material is injected is important if an immediate response is to be detected. When the patient is to receive an antigenic agent such as tetanus antitoxin (horse serum), detection of a positive response may prevent the patient from developing a serious response or even be life saving. A person who is found to be sensitized to horse serum and who requires tetanus antitoxin can be temporarily immunized by small but increasing doses of antigenic material. The first dose may be no larger than the initial test dose. The safety of the patient depends on identifying the fact that he is sensitive and on rigid adherence to the schedule for increasing the dosage and for its timing.

The skin reaction in the delayed type of hypersensitivity takes several hours to appear. It may or may not have been preceded by the immediate type of reaction. The skin at the site of the injection is red, hot, and swollen. The swelling is firm. The lesion lasts longer than it does in the immediate reaction.

In some skin tests, such as the Schick test, reddening of the skin indicates that the individual has not developed antibodies against the antigen. Antibodies protect the skin from the antigen rather than sensitizing it.

What is the nurse's role in helping the patient with an immunologic response?

Because allergic responses, however they are manifested, are the result of an immunological mechanism, preventive and therapeutic measures are based on similar principles and are directed toward the achievement of three objectives. The site of the response and the requirements of the individual patient influence the selection of specific preventive and therapeutic measures. These factors also influence the decision as to which objective takes priority at a given moment in time. The primary objectives are (1) to prevent or limit the exposure of the patient to antigens to which he may be, or is known to be, hypersensitive; (2) to relieve or mitigate the effects produced by a hypersensitivity reaction; (3) to increase the resistance of the patient to a specific antigen.

The accomplishment of the **first objective,** that is, to prevent or limit the exposure of the patient to antigens to which he is known to be, or may be, hypersensitive, depends on knowledge of what the common allergens are, what their sources are, how they are transported in the environment, and how they gain entrance into the organism. Actually, this is the very knowledge that forms the background for the prevention of the spread of infectious agents causing disease. Because not all persons are allergic to the common allergens, knowledge of the particular antigens to which the patient is hypersensitive is also useful. Some of the substances to which people are frequently hypersensitive have been previously mentioned.

Hypersensitivity to horse serum is so common, and so easily developed, that all persons are presumed to be sensitive to it unless they are shown not to be by skin testing. The use of skin testing in the identification of substances to which individuals are hypersensitive has also been discussed. Although skin testing is of value, it also has limitations. A reddened area indicates that the patient has antibodies for that antigen in his skin but it does not necessarily mean that he will have an allergic response when he is exposed to it. Why this is true is not known. Neither does the absence of a reddened area necessarily mean that the person is not hypersensitive to a particular antigen. Some persons have a high degree of hypersensitivity to an antigen, despite the absence of a positive skin reaction.

Because skin tests do not necessarily give complete information about the antigens to which an individual is hypersensitive, other methods have to be used in their identification. Perhaps the most important of these is the observation of a cause-effect relationship between contact with an antigen and the development of an allergic reaction on the part of the patient. Patients are often aware of these relationships. For example, Mrs. Cornflower knows that each time she eats strawberries she develops hives. In some instances an individual such as Mrs. Cornflower knows that if she eats one strawberry she becomes deathly sick. Her cousin Frank is able to eat a small serving of strawberries three or four times during the summer, but he has hives if he eats them more frequently. Nurses can help in identifying antigens when they observe and report events that are coincident. For example, Mrs. Batelman was hospitalized for treatment of an acute attack of allergic asthma. Following her recovery, her physician decided to remove some nasal polyps obstructing her breathing. Nasal polyps are a common sequela in allergic rhinitis. As part of her preparation for polypectomy, Mrs. Batelman was given ephedrine. Shortly thereafter, she began to wheeze and to show signs of a developing asthmatic attack. Despite the impending attack of asthma, the surgeon removed the polyps and the ephedrine was continued. Each time Mrs. Batelman received ephedrine, wheezing and difficulty in breathing were intensified. The nurse observed the apparent cause-effect relationship between the ephedrine and the difficulty in breathing exhibited by Mrs. Batelman. She brought her observation to the attention of the physician, who discontinued the drug. Mrs. Batelman's breathing improved and other evidence of asthma also cleared rapidly. Despite the usefulness of ephedrine in relieving asthmatic attacks in most individuals, in the instance of Mrs. Batelman it acted to trigger its onset.

Cause-effect relationships are frequently more difficult to establish than in the illustration cited here. To collect data, the patient may be instructed to keep a diary or a record of his activities, including what he eats, and to describe any abnormal responses. For example, Mrs. Bobbin learned from keeping a diary that she was allergic to an insecticide used to kill mosquitoes. She developed asthmatic symptoms each evening after an insecticide containing pyrethrum was sprayed just outside the porch where she sat in the evening.

When a food is suspected to be allergenic, a diary may be employed or the patient may be placed on an elimination diet. The elimination diet may be approached in different ways. The patient may be instructed to eliminate one food at a time and observe his response or to eliminate all commonly allergenic foods and then add them to his diet one at a time. Before adding a new food, he should note any response to the one just previously included in his diet. Occasionally all foods except those that are rarely antigenic may be removed from the diet and then the above procedure followed. The success of any type of elimination diet in discovering antigenic foods depends on the patient and/or the person who prepares his food understanding why the diet is prescribed and what is entailed in its preparation. It must be understood that it is the specific food and not its method of preparation that is important. The food must be eliminated in all forms. The following example has its origin in the days before electricity was supplied to every farmhouse. Mrs. Farwell brought her three-year-old son, Bobby, to University Clinic for the treatment of atopic eczema. In an attempt to identify the offending allergen, the physician prescribed a diet from which all forms of wheat were to be eliminated. Mrs. Farwell was duly instructed and appeared to be interested and cooperative. A week later she returned with Bobby. He was no better. The physician checked with Mrs. Farwell to determine whether she had carried out the instructions. He asked her if Bobby had had any bread. She replied, "No, none at all. I toasted every bit of it." Mrs. Farwell did not have a toaster and she did not usually toast bread unless a member of the family was ill. She believed that toast was more easily digested than untoasted bread and was therefore more suitable than bread for a sick person. The making of toast was a cultural response to illness.

Patients sometimes eliminate foods from their diet because they are, or believe that they are, allergic to them. Although the avoidance of one or two specific foods is not likely to cause malnutrition, the exclusion of many foods may, and this possibility increases in proportion to the number of foods eliminated. Occasionally an individual appears for medical attention who has eliminated almost all types of food from his diet. It is quite important that persons for whom elimination diets are prescribed understand that the diet is temporary.

Prevention of Acute Drug Reactions

Because of the possibility of an acute hypersensitivity developing after the use of drugs, certain precautions should be taken. Before any drug is administered to a patient, he should be asked whether he has any history of allergy in himself or his family and whether he has ever, to his knowledge, been treated with the drug to be used. Because of the common practice of treating infections in cows with penicillin, milk may contain penicillin. Persons who drink milk may be sensitized to penicillin without ever having been treated with it. For reasons not well understood, drugs applied to the skin are more likely to induce sensitivity reactions than those ingested or injected. When there is reason to suspect that an individual may be allergic, he should be tested for skin-sensitizing antibodies. When a patient inquires about the nature of a drug that he is receiving, the nurse should at least ascertain the reason for his question. In some hospitals, only the physician tells the patient what drugs have been prescribed. The practice of withholding information from a patient about the drugs he is receiving is being questioned. Some physicians now request the pharmacist to indicate on the label of the container the generic or trade name of drugs prescribed for and taken by the patient. Should the patient state that he is allergic to a given drug, it should be withheld until the physician has been notified. Even drugs such as aspirin can, in the occasional individual, be highly antigenic. When agents such as heterologous serum are administered, the patient should be skin-tested before the serum is administered, and a syringe containing epinephrine should be prepared so that it will be immediately available should symptoms develop. In all patient areas, emergency equipment including epinephrine, a tourniquet, an airway, oxygen, and intravenous equipment should be immediately available.[40] Despite the infrequency of anaphylactic reactions, they can cause death unless they are treated immediately. Patients who are treated as outpatients should remain at least one-half hour after the injection of any potentially antigenic agent.

[40] Richard A. Kern: "Anaphylactic Drug Reactions," *JAMA*, **179**:22 (Jan. 6) 1962.

The danger to the individual who receives an antigen to which he has been sensitized can be illustrated by Mrs. Johns, who had a serious reaction to penicillin. Fortunately for Mrs. Johns, she had not left her physician's office when she experienced systemic or anaphylactic shock. The reaction might have been prevented had either the physician who prescribed the penicillin or the nurse who administered it questioned her about her previous experience with penicillin. Failure to do so very nearly cost Mrs. Johns her life. Almost immediately following an injection of penicillin, she developed hives and had great difficulty in breathing; in a matter of a few minutes her blood pressure dropped sharply and she became unconscious. The physician injected epinephrine and applied artificial respiration. As soon as an ambulance could be obtained, she was taken to a hospital. When her condition improved, the doctor learned that she had had penicillin on two previous occasions. After the second injection she had had swelling, reddening, and itching at the site where it was injected. She had not remembered to tell her doctor of this. Unlike horse serum, skin tests to determine sensitivity to penicillin are unreliable. The only protection of the patient lies in regular questioning of each patient before therapy with penicillin is initiated.

Adaptation of the Environment

In addition to assisting in various ways with the identification of antigenic agents, the nurse is often responsible for the preparation of an environment that is as nearly free of antigenic agents as is possible. She may also be helpful to the patient in planning his home environment. Extremes should be avoided in adapting the home to the needs of the allergic person. The same general points apply whether the patient is in the hospital or at home. Frequently, stripping the bedroom of unnecessary dust-catching furniture and draperies is all that is required. Overstuffed furniture, draperies, pillows, mattresses with ordinary covering, and rugs serve as reservoirs for the accumulation of dust, and they should be removed or covered with an impervious material. Mattresses can now be purchased with plasticized coverings that prevent them from accumulating dust. They do not require further covering. The rest of the house may be furnished as desired. For older children and adults, airborne allergens are of considerable importance. House dust and pollens are common antigens. When furniture is purchased for the home, ease of cleaning should be kept in mind.

The patient can use a Dacron[41] pillow. Sponge rubber may be used, but in time it tends

[41] Synthetic fiber.

to take on dust, and some persons are allergic to rubber. Allergic patients often take their own pillows with them to the hospital. Despite the possibility of the patient's losing his pillow, he should be permitted to keep it and a concerted effort should be made to prevent its loss.

The air may be a source of dust and pollens. Hot-air systems without adequate filters circulate considerable dust. For persons who are allergic to dust, filters should be installed in systems circulating air. They require regular cleansing or replacement. Many persons who are sensitive to pollens can reduce exposure enough to keep themselves fairly comfortable by sleeping in an air-conditioned room. When this is not possible, a window fan combined with a paper or glass-wool filter will give some relief by reducing the pollen count and cooling the room. Keeping the windows closed also reduces the pollen count in the house. For patients who have severe hay fever or asthma, and who are able to afford it, a trip to an area in which the pollen count is low may be indicated. Before the advent of air conditioning, certain areas of the United States were havens for hay fever sufferers. Persons who are sensitive to fungi are advised to avoid damp climates. Damp basements can be dried by the use of dehumidifiers. Anyone who has worked in the emergency room of a large city hospital cannot escape being impressed by the number of patients who come in for treatment of asthma on a warm, moist summer evening. In fact, physicians and nurses can sometimes be heard to say, "This is an asthma night." Many persons who are allergic learn to identify substances and circumstances that activate their symptoms and can plan to avoid them.

Animal danders are another common cause of hypersensitivity. Hypersensitive persons should be advised against acquiring a dog or cat if they do not already have one. When there is a pet in the home its effect can be tested by removing it for a month or so. If the condition of the patient is improved, the patient and his family should be advised to dispose of the pet. Should there be no difference in the patient's condition, there is no reason to do so.

In the control of contact dermatitis, the same general principles hold. The first step is to identify the offending antigen or antigens and then to make a plan to avoid them. Because of the variety of contactants, this is not always as easy to do as to narrate. The importance of prompt action cannot be overestimated. Secondary changes including infection may cause more problems than the original dermatitis. Sometimes, as in the instance of a housewife who is allergic to detergents, protection merely involves wearing rubber gloves when using detergents or substituting soap for them. To avoid dermatitis, she may have to wear gloves every time she uses a detergent.

At other times the problem is more complicated. For example, streptomycin sulfate has been found to induce hypersensitivity in a high proportion of those who work with it either in its preparation in factories or in hospitals. This problem has been minimized because streptomycin is now supplied in disposable syringes. Rubber gloves should be worn by nurses and pharmacists when they handle it. Contact dermatitis can occur in persons who handle penicillin, but this does not occur as commonly as it does with streptomycin. The amount of either of these drugs required to cause a reaction in sensitive persons may be infinitesimal. In one hospital where nurses had become sensitized to streptomycin, it was necessary to assign them to units where patients did not receive streptomycin.

On occasion, a nurse may develop a sensitivity to other drugs. In the experience of the writer one nurse was so highly sensitive to morphine that she developed a dermatitis each time she prepared even a single dose of it. To continue in the practice of nursing she had to arrange to be relieved of any responsibility for administering morphine, or being near where the drug was prepared. In nurses who develop contact dermatitis, the problem of control is often difficult. Any measures that can be taken to prevent its development are well worth taking. When the possibility of exposure to a sensitizing agent exists, thorough washing with soap and water will serve to remove the agent and thereby reduce the intensity of the contact. For example, after exposure to poison ivy a shower should be taken as soon as possible. Although both soap and water should be generously applied, this should be accompanied by minimum rubbing of the skin as the antigen of poison ivy does not induce sensitivity unless it is rubbed into the skin.

The first step in the accomplishment of the objective to limit or prevent the exposure of the patient to substances to which he is hypersensitive is to identify the offending agent or agents. In some instances this can be accomplished by skin tests. In others, the antigenic agents cannot be identified by skin tests but may be by establishing a cause and effect relationship. This requires a form of medical detective work. The patient and others, including the nurse, try to identify the conditions associated with the onset of symptoms. The relationship of various elements to the patient's allergic manifestations can be tested by eliminating possible antigens one at a time from his environment and observing the results. In instances in which there is doubt, a suspected antigen may be further tested by its reintroduction into the environment of the patient. After the causative agent is identified, the next step is to plan how contact with the agent can be reduced or eliminated. Points to be considered include the nature of the antigen, its source or reservoir, vehicles by which it is transmitted, and portals of entry. The degree of sensitivity of the person is also a factor. In the person who is highly sensitive to an antigen, all exposure may have to be prevented. In the person who is less sensitive, restrictions on exposure may be less stringent.

When an allergic patient experiences an acute response to an allergen, his symptoms may be such that he is incapacitated or his survival threatened. At this time the **second objective**, to relieve or mitigate the allergic response, takes priority. The urgency of the situation depends on the type and acuteness of the reactions of the patient. Prompt and energetic treatment may be necessary to save the life of a patient in anaphylactic shock or in status asthmaticus. Protection from further exposure to foreign serum or to an antigenic drug and palliation of his symptoms may meet the major requirements of a patient with serum or drug sickness. The patient with hay fever (allergic rhinitis) may be miserable, but his life is not usually in danger.

Drugs have an important role in the prevention and relief of allergic responses of various types. One of the most generally useful drugs is epinephrine. It is believed to act directly on effector cells, stimulating some and inhibiting others. Because the action of epinephrine is similar to that of the sympathetic nervous system, it is said to be sympathomimetic. It antagonizes the effects of the parasympathetic nervous system (cholinergic), other cholinergic chemicals, and histamine. In disorders such as anaphylaxis and acute asthma it may be life saving. Epinephrine should always be in readiness in situations where an anaphylactic response is a possibility. Because of its powerful bronchial dilatory action, it is often effective in the relief of asthmatic attacks that are resistant to other drugs. It affords symptomatic relief in urticaria, serum sickness, hay fever, angioneurotic edema, and other similar allergic disorders. It may be administered by subcutaneous, intramuscular, or intravenous injection or by inhalation. The usual range of dosage for subcutaneous injection for adults is from 0.2 to 0.5 ml of a 1:1,000 aqueous solution. Despite the fact that epinephrine is dispensed in ampules containing 1 ml, a nurse should not give more than 0.5 ml without special instructions from the physician. Smaller dosages are indicated when the patient is receiving the drug for the first time. Patients with hyperthyroidism and hypertension are especially susceptible to the effects of epinephrine, and it is contraindicated in these conditions. In any patient, an overdosage of epinephrine predisposes the patient to ventricular fibrillation.

When epinephrine is administered by inhalation, the exact dosage is difficult to control. The delivery of epinephrine to the bronchi requires that the solution be converted to a fine mist. It also requires that the solution be at least 1 part epinephrine to 100 parts of water. A positive pressure machine and nebulizer may be used. An atomizer or nebulizer should be made entirely of glass or plastic. When the patient uses a hand-operated atomizer he may need considerable practice to coordinate squeezing of the bulb with inspiration. Proper coordination is necessary to deliver and distribute the drug through the tracheobronchial tree. Oxygen may be used in a nebulizer to convert the solution to a fine mist and distribute it to the desired area. Whether an atomizer, a mask, or a nebulizer is used, the drug is inhaled through the mouth. The patient should be cautioned against overusage, as it causes dryness of the throat and irritation of the tracheobronchial tree. Should irritation of the airway occur, the patient may have to discontinue inhalations for several days. The nurse should note the frequency with which patients inhale epinephrine, and if it seems excessive, she could caution the patient or bring her observation to the attention of the physician. Because swallowing epinephrine causes epigastric pain, the patient should be taught to wash his mouth after each administration. Sometimes the mucus that is expectorated is pink, due to changes in the color of the drug. Bleeding is not necessarily indicated.

Ephedrine may be used to relax the smooth muscle of the bronchi in asthma. It has an advantage over epinephrine because it can be administered orally. Theophylline, U.S.P. is also prescribed because it relaxes the smooth muscle in the tracheobronchial tree.

The antihistaminics are a group of drugs providing relief in a number of allergic disorders. Among those in which antihistaminics are most beneficial are hay fever, serum sickness, urticaria, drug reactions, and angioneurotic edema. These are all forms of allergy in which exudation is a significant factor. The antihistaminic drugs have two general effects believed to be important in the treatment of allergy. They are supposed to counteract the effect of histamine by displacing histamine from receptor sites in the cell. This effect is called the blocking action of the antihistaminic drugs. Some authorities question the validity of this concept of their action. The chemical structure of some antihistamines bears little superficial resemblance to histamine. Therapeutic dosages of these drugs cause some depression of the central nervous system; they have a sedative effect in some persons and in others they cause restlessness, insomnia, and nervousness.

Cortisone and ACTH have proved to be useful not only in the relief of symptoms in acute attacks of asthma, hay fever, allergic dermatitis, and drug reactions but also in the treatment of chronic states. In some patients the relief lasts only as long as the drug is administered, in others relief may continue for months or longer.

Itching is frequently referred to as a troublesome symptom of allergic dermatoses. Although itching does not threaten the life of the patient and does not always incapacitate him, it can cause him a good bit of discomfort and reduce his efficiency. Since the introduction of antihistaminic drugs, itching is often easier to control than it was in the past. In the care of the patient, the nurse may add to his comfort by the prevention of overheating of the room, as sweating increases itching. A cool environmental temperature reduces itching, whereas a warm one increases it. When wet dressings are ordered, at least 20 layers of gauze or an equal thickness of turkish toweling should be used. Dressings should be applied loosely and kept well soaked. One of the frequently used solutions is aluminum subacetate, or Burrows' solution, a mild astringent. To prevent increasing the concentration of the solution, water should be used to remoisten dried dressings.[42] When the patient is able to moisten his own dressings, he may be given some of the solution or water and a syringe so that he can keep his dressings moist. Though a nonporous material should be placed under the dressing to protect the bed, it should not be wrapped around the dressing. Interference with evaporation decreases heat loss and predisposes to elevating the temperature of the involved area. Before selecting material to protect the bed, the nurse should ascertain whether or not the patient is allergic to the material to be used.

Because most of the injury to the skin in allergic conditions is caused by scratching, every effort should be made to prevent and relieve the itching. The fingernails should be cut short. Sometimes the patient gets some relief

[42] When a solution is used repeatedly to moisten the same dressings, the concentration of the solution increases. Water evaporates but the solute does not and its concentration therefore rises.

by scratching the bed. Few symptoms are more unpleasant than itching. A patient with a severe dermatitis is likely to be irritable, because he is uncomfortable and has difficulty in obtaining rest and sleep. Whenever lotions or salves are applied to the skin in dermatitis, the nurse should observe the skin for signs of increasing irritation, that is, redness, swelling, or vesiculation, as some patients develop a sensitivity to the chemicals used in therapy.

Because contact dermatitis is likely to be a recurring problem, the patient should be taught to identify and to avoid agents in his environment to which he is sensitive. He should also be encouraged to institute palliative measures as soon as he notes the characteristic lesions on his skin. Scratching is to be avoided, as it excoriates the skin and predisposes to more itching as well as to infection. For many persons, contact dermatitis is a long-term problem. As in many other chronic disorders, control depends on the willingness and ability of the patient to carry out the preventive and therapeutic program.

To accomplish the **third objective**, that is, to increase the resistance of the patient to a specific antigen, the patient may be given small but increasing doses of an antigen over a period of time. The procedure for raising the resistance of the patient to a specific antigen is known as hyposensitization. In addition to the hyposensitization of a patient to foreign proteins, as previously discussed, some patients with hay fever benefit from being treated with offending pollens. Therapy is usually started two or three months before the expected onset of symptoms. They may be continued at four-week intervals throughout the year. The injected antigen stimulates the formation of what is known as the blocking antibody. The blocking antibody is distinct from the pre-existing sensitizing antibody. Increased tolerance for the antigen appears to be caused by the blocking antibody.

Knowledge of how hyposensitization to an allergen benefits the allergic patient is incomplete. Decreased sensitivity may in part be attributable to blocking antibodies, which are IgG immunoglobulins. Blocking antibodies are incomplete antibodies with the power to combine with antigen. They lack the ability to form insoluble antigen-antibody complexes.

Because emotional factors may predispose to, precipitate, perpetuate, or contribute to the development of complications, their significance in each patient requires evaluation. When emotional factors are of importance, the patient may require assistance in learning to identify situations aggravating his disorder and either avoid them or modify his reaction to them. For example, Mrs. Cornwall usually develops an asthmatic attack when she smells, or imagines she smells, cigar smoke. Because the physician believes that emotional factors are probably involved in precipitating and prolonging Mrs. Cornwall's asthmatic attacks, he explores this possibility with her.

Homotransplantation

One of the most publicized accomplishments of the last decade or so has been the ability to transplant whole organs from one person to another. Successful transplantation presents a variety of problems. One problem that has been solved for organs such as the kidney and the heart has been the development of techniques for removing an organ from one individual and placing it in another in such a manner that it is supplied with blood and is able to carry out its function. A second and less easily solved problem is obtaining a sufficient number of healthy and viable organs. In the case of the heart, a living heart must be obtained from a person who has died. References to the ethical problems raised by this procedure are included in Chapter 3.

The third problem, which will be discussed briefly, is created because tissues of one individual recognize those of another as being foreign. As a consequence, homografts are almost always rejected by the immunologic response of the recipient to the donor's antigens.[43]

To achieve success in homograft transplantation, histocompatible tissues must be used or some method found to induce a state in which the immune system fails to respond to foreign antigen or antigens. Because identical twins are genetically similar, a kidney or skin transplanted from one can be expected to be accepted by the other.

Another natural type of tolerance was reported by Owen in 1945. In cattle twins, vascular anastomoses frequently develop in utero. As a result, each twin of the nonidentical pair may have two different types of red blood cells, his own and that of his twin. He retains the two types of red blood cells throughout his life-span. Experimentally, animals can be made tolerant to foreign antigens during embryonic life.[44]

Hall[45] states that homografts present the immune mechanism with the same challenge as any foreign protein be it a virus or bacterium in a cell. The difference is in degree and not in kind, as homotransplanted cells are less antigenic than other foreign proteins. Another difference is that bacteria and viruses release

toxins that provoke acute inflammatory responses. Most authorities believe that the initial rejection of the homograft is caused by a delayed type of hypersensitivity. There is evidence, however, that humoral factors are eventually involved.

Following the transplantation of tissue, there is a more or less typical and predictable sequence of events. For a few days the transplanted tissue remains viable and its blood supply appears to be developing. In ten days to two weeks or more the graft becomes intensely inflamed, undergoes necrosis, and dies. A second graft from the same donor is more rapidly rejected than the first. The accelerated reaction is known as a "second-set" reaction. The second-set reaction is specific to the original donor and can be induced by prior inoculation of cells from the donor. Clark[46] states that rapid rejection is caused by humoral factors and that complement participates in the rejection of vascularized grafts. Chase[47] summarizes evidence that both delayed hypersensitivity and immunoglobulin may be involved in the rejection reaction. Chase[48] as well as others state that large organs such as the kidney are not rejected as fast as skin.

Medawar[49] says that the success of renal homografts is greater than expected. However, he doubts that any homograft will survive the lifetime of the host unless it develops a state of immune tolerance.

To achieve success in homograft transplantation, two methods are combined to increase the likelihood of the recipient accepting the donor's tissues. First, a donor is selected whose tissues have a minimum number of antigenic differences from the recipient. The fewer the foreign antigens that the recipient has to respond to, the greater the chance of success. Second, the recipient is altered in such a manner that tolerance to the foreign antigen is induced. Acting on the hypothesis that the lymphocyte is responsible for antibody formation, total body radiation may be used to destroy the lymphocytes. Irradiation must be administered before transplantation. If administered at the same time or after exposure to the antigen, radiation has little effect. Some of the drugs used in the treatment of leukemia such as 6-mercaptopurine and certain antibiotics are useful in suppressing immune responses. They may be used not only

---

[43] Sidney Leskowitz: "Immunologic Tolerance," *BioScience*, **18**:1030 (Nov.) 1968.
[44] *Ibid.*
[45] *Loc. cit.*, p. 27.

[46] D. Scott Clark *et al.*: "Effector Mechanisms in Renal Graft Rejection," *Surgery*, **62**:770–78 (Oct.) 1967.
[47] Merrill W. Chase: "Delayed Sensitivity," *Med. Clin. N. Amer.*, **49**:1633–35 (Nov.) 1965.
[48] *Ibid.*, p. 1633.
[49] P. B. Medawar: "Transplantation of Tissues and Organs: Introduction," *Brit. Med. Bull.*, **21**:98–99 (May) 1965.

to eliminate the initial response but to maintain tolerance to foreign tissues. A third method has been used to deplete the body's store of lymphocytes by draining the thoracic duct. Under certain circumstances antibody synthesis may be inhibited by overloading with antigen. This technique is called immunologic paralysis.

Prevention of or minimizing the immune response depends on limiting the number of antigens to which the recipient is exposed combined with altering the capacity to respond. The latter depends on understanding the role that various body components play. This includes not only lymphocytes but macrophages and other elements. Moreover, despite the importance of preventing the initial rejection of transplanted tissue, methods must be used to maintain continuing tolerance to foreign tissue.

Finally, with methods such as total body irradiation and with immunosuppressive agents the individual's capacity to respond to microorganisms is lost. Methods must be used to protect him from exposure to exogenous microbes. Protecting him from his own organisms is a more difficult problem. (See Chapter 5.)

For those who wish to pursue this subject in more detail, references are included at the end of this chapter. Because much research is in progress, future reports will undoubtedly be enlightening.

Summary

The discussion thus far has dealt with the immunologic tissue responses of the body, factors that incite them, and methods of predicting and controlling them. The capacity of the organism to produce antibodies is one of its mechanisms of defense against foreign invaders. It arises out of the capacity of the cells of the body to distinguish self from nonself. As with other mechanisms of defense, immunologic responses are useful when they are initiated in response to truly harmful agents and in the amounts required by the situation. They are harmful when they are initiated in response to harmless substances or when the response is deficient or excessive. There is some evidence to support the theory that many chronic diseases may result from immunologic responses. Recent studies of immune responses are adding greatly to understanding this very important defense mechanism. This is a completely new and exciting field in medicine.

In the care of patients with the diseases of allergy, nurses have an opportunity to assist in the identification of agents that act as antigens, they care for patients during acute phases of illness, and they help to prepare the patient to live with his disorder.

PHAGOCYTOSIS

Phagocytosis is a process whereby certain cells capture and ingest bacteria and other large particles such as tissue fragments and sometimes destroy them. Some microbes escape from the phagocytes and may destroy them. Some survive and even mutiply within the phagocyte. Sometimes the phagocyte acts as a vehicle to transport certain bacteria from one part of the body to another. For phagocytosis to occur, the particles must come in contact with the cell membranes. Globulin molecules called opsonins combine with particles and increase their likelihood of adhering to the phagocyte. After particles are ingested by the cells, lysosome granules within the cell break down and release digestive enzymes. This process of digestion requires the expenditure of energy. The utilization of glucose and oxygen goes up and the production of lactic acid rises. Attention to maintaining the nutritional state of the individual should help to support this extremely important defense mechanism.

MACROPHAGES

Phagocytic cells are classified according to size as macrophages and microphages. Macrophages are monocytic cells. They may be either fixed (stationary) or wandering. The largest source of wandering cells are lymphocytes, which change first into monocytes and then into macrophages. The fixed cells, tissue histocytes, are permanently located in the interstitial tissues of the reticuloendothelial system. They are concentrated in the sinusoids of the liver (Kupffer's cells) and the spleen, the lung, the lymph nodes, and the blood vessels, particularly the veins. Apperly [50] compares the fixed macrophages to the rural police, as they are scattered through the body at strategic points. They are highly phagocytic. They digest bacteria, foreign substances, worn-out red blood cells, and other cells, as well as remove certain dyes. They are also believed to form antibodies.

Macrophages are less numerous than the microphages but each cell has greater phagocytic power. They are characteristic of chronic infection and the stage of resolution in acute infection. In chronic infection, macrophages fuse to form giant cells.

An interesting observation is that some species of bacteria, especially those causing chronic infections, may not only be transported by macrophages and multiply in them but may remain dormant for months or years. This may help to explain the development of immunity in diseases such as tularemia. The macrophage may also serve as a vehicle for the transport of some bacteria such as *M. tuberculosis*.

MICROPHAGES

Microphages are granulocytes having their origin in the bone marrow. There are three types of granulocytes: neutrophils, eosinophils, and basophils. Of these the neutrophils are the most abundant. They are much more numerous than the macrophages, but their phagocytic power is much less. During phagocytosis granulocytes can be seen to lose their granules. These granules contain phagocytin, a substance released into the phagocytic vacuoles, which contain bacteria. Following infection with certain types of bacteria or the death of tissue, a leukocytosis-promoting factor is released. This substance stimulates the bone marrow to release large numbers of microphages, particularly neutrophils. From a normal of 5,000 to 9,000 the number may rise as high as 20,000 to 30,000 cells. The response to dead tissue is usually less than that to an acute infection by a pyogenic organism.

Although neutrophils are short-lived cells, living only three or four days, the healthy bone marrow is capable of replacing them in large numbers. Some drugs, such as aminopyrine, sulfanilamide, and nitrogen mustards, depress the bone marrow, so that following their administration the production of granulocytes may be diminished or even absent. As discussed in Chapter 4, radioactive materials, including x-rays, have a similar effect. The capacity of the bone marrow to tolerate chemical and physical agents depressing its activity places a limitation on their use in treatment. Injury to the bone marrow by aminopyrine and sulfanilamide occurs when it is hypersensitive to a particular agent. Not all persons, therefore, experience depression of the bone marrow after ingestion of these agents. In contrast, nitrogen mustard and ionizing radiation have a cytotoxic effect on cells. The nitrogen mustards contain two or more alkyl groups that react with some of the constituents of cells. Radioactive materials injure the cells by ionizing substances within them. Though cells vary in sensitivity, all cells are injured when they receive a large enough dose of either type of agent.

When the number of neutrophils is markedly deficient, the condition is known as agranulocytosis. A better term would be *granulocytopenia*. Granulocytopenia is a serious disorder because the capacity of the person to protect himself against microorganisms is impaired. Evidence of a loss of the capacity of tissues to protect themselves is seen as ulcerations in the mouth, pharynx, gastrointestinal tract, and vagina. When infection develops in the patient with agranulocytosis, his prognosis is very poor. Special precautions should be taken to protect these persons from infection.

Phagocytosis is not only an important mechanism of combating established disease, but it is important in preventing disease. In a healthy individual, the blood is highly efficient in destroying bacteria.

The effectiveness of phagocytosis is influenced by the structure of the tissues. Because dense tissues offer more opportunity for phagocytes to come in contact with bacteria or other foreign material than tissue spaces, phagocytosis is more efficient in them. Thus bacteria implanted in a solid tissue such as the gluteal muscle are more likely to be phagocytized than those placed in the peritoneal or pleural cavity.

Local Responses

INFLAMMATION

To this point, the body defenses involving the body as a whole have been discussed. In addition to these responses, cells at the site of injury also react to injury in a characteristic and more or less stereotyped fashion. Similar to the more widespread responses, the local reactions to injury serve to limit the area of injury, to prepare the area for repair, and finally to replace the damaged tissue. Because inflammation is one of the most common responses of the body to injury, knowledge of the mechanisms involved in inflammation provides a basis for understanding the changes that occur in a wide variety of infectious and noninfectious diseases. Essentially the response of the tissue injured by an antigen-antibody reaction is one of inflammation. Even in those conditions in which inflammation is not considered to be an aspect of the disease, it may play a role. For example, in some patients who have cancer the body responds to the neoplastic cells (new growth cells) much as it does to a foreign body, with the result that surrounding tissues are inflamed.

Inflammation may be defined as an active and aggressive response of tissue to injury. It involves the blood vessels, the fluid and cellular components of the blood, and the surrounding connective tissue. It is a useful response because it serves to destroy or neutralize the injurious agent and to prepare the tissue for repair. Inflammation may cause harmful effects by virtue of its location or by an ineffective, excessive, or inappropriate response.

Basic knowledge of the acute inflammatory process can be presented by tracing the history of the understanding of inflammation. Almost

20 centuries elapsed between the time the cardinal signs of inflammation were first described and the fundamental nature of the response was understood. Similar to knowledge in other areas, progress has been uneven and sometimes delayed by false steps and interpretations. In the first century, Celsus described the four cardinal signs of inflammation as rubor (redness), calor (heat), dolor (pain), and tumor (swelling). It was not until almost the end of the eighteenth century that John Hunter first established inflammation as a mechanism of defense. Cohnheim, a student of Virchow's, recognized the part that blood vessels play in inflammation. He also described the margination and emigration of leukocytes. The part played by the leukocytes in phagocytosis was established by the Russian zoologist Metchnikoff when his study of inflammation was published in 1901. Though knowledge of the biochemical changes in the inflammatory process was, and still is, incomplete, the discoveries of Metchnikoff established an understanding of the fundamental nature of the process. With the development of electron microscopy and the rabbit's ear chamber, knowledge of the process has been further expanded.

CAUSES OF INFLAMMATION

Despite a tendency to think of inflammation as a response initiated primarily by microbes, it can be induced by any agent causing injury to tissue cells. Only a few of the possible causative agents will be discussed. Essentially they all act to injure tissue cells. The surrounding tissue then responds with inflammation. How the various types of agents injure cells was presented in the preceding chapters. Physical agents that are common initiators of the inflammatory process are heat, cold, radiant rays including ultraviolet and infrared rays, radioactive rays, and trauma.

Chemical agents also act as irritants. They may be either extrinsic or intrinsic in origin or result from a combination of the two. Examples of extrinsic chemical irritants include strong acids and bases, insect bites, allergens, and the toxins manufactured by microorganisms. Chemical irritants of intrinsic origin are substances that are produced in the body. They may be normal substances, such as pancreatic juice that escapes from the gastrointestinal tract and comes in contact with tissues not protected from the digesting actions of its enzymes. Large areas of necrosis of the abdominal wall may occur in those who have the misfortune to have a fistulous tract from the small intestine to the surface of the body.

Perhaps the most common example of a body fluid that is "out of place" is blood. The body responds to blood that escapes into tissue from a break in a blood vessel as it does to a foreign body. Frequently soreness is the first sign of bleeding into a tissue. Soreness at the site of an intramuscular injection may result from the rupture of a small blood vessel during the insertion of a needle. Bruises caused by bumping furniture or other hard objects often pass unnoticed for a day or so and then come to attention because the area is painful.

Inflammation also develops in the tissue surrounding dead or necrotic tissue. In the degeneration of the dead tissue, products are formed that act as irritants. When the death of tissue is caused by the loss of its blood supply, the necrotic area may also serve as a site for the development of infection. The tissue, robbed of its blood supply, is no longer able to supply phagocytes to control microorganisms in the area. They are therefore able to establish themselves and grow and multiply in the tissue. For example, following infarction caused by the obstruction of a branch of the pulmonary artery by an embolus, Mr. Ash developed pneumonia. The original focus for the infection was in the infarcted tissue.

Products of metabolism may also act as irritants. They may be abnormal either in quantity or in kind or in the manner in which the body handles them. In gout, because of a defect in the metabolism of purines, uric acid crystals accumulate in the tissues about joints. The resulting inflammatory process is exceedingly painful. Because, according to folklore, gout is the result of high living, which it is not, persons who develop gout are often subjected to cruel jokes and ridicule.

Among other causes of inflammation are antigen-antibody reactions and neoplasms. From the preceding it is evident that a wide variety of agents can indeed initiate the inflammatory response.

ROLE OF BLOOD VESSELS IN INFLAMMATION

In the study of inflammation in the laboratory, immediately following the application of an irritant, blood vessels may be seen to constrict momentarily. Constriction is extremely transitory and is of no consequence. Following constriction, arterioles, then venules, and finally capillaries dilate, and more blood vessels come into view. Blood flows rapidly through the vessels and the tissue becomes bright red. This active increase in the flow of blood is known as hyperemia.

Associated with the greater blood flow is an increase in the filtration pressure of the blood and in the permeability of the capillaries with the result that a large volume of fluid, known as the inflammatory exudate, is moved into the interstitial space. In minor injuries, the increase in capillary permeability may be small so that little extra fluid escapes into the injured area. Neither is there an increase in the rate at which larger molecules in the blood plasma diffuse from the blood into the injured area. In more severe injuries, large molecules, most particularly proteins, escape into the inflammatory exudate in increased quantities. The effects of this loss of protein are not serious when the inflamed area is small. However, when the area is large, or when the loss continues over an extended period of time, the consequences may be serious. As an illustration, the patient who is burned may lose enormous quantities of proteins as well as of water and electrolytes into the burned area. Moreover, the absorption of chemicals released at the site of the burned or injured tissue may increase the permeability of capillaries throughout the body causing a generalized edema. Loss of fluid leads to a decrease in blood volume and concentration of the blood of the patient.

The extent to which fluid escapes into the tissue of the patient who has been burned can be illustrated by Mr. All. Examination of the intake and output record reveals that during the first 48 hours after he was burned the ratio of his fluid intake to output was 13,000 ml to 2,000 ml. Even when another 2,000 ml is added to his output to account for fluid lost by other avenues, he still lost at least 10 liters of fluid into the burned area. In addition to water, he lost protein and electrolytes. Human blister fluid contains about 4 g of protein per 100 ml of fluid. Because serum albumin is smaller in molecular size than the other blood proteins, a higher proportion of albumin is lost into the inflammatory exudate than of either globulin or fibrinogen.

The increase in filtration pressure plus the greater permeability of the capillaries upsets the balance between the quantity of fluid leaving the capillary and the quantity returning, in favor of the fluid escaping from the capillaries. The disequilibrium is further aggravated by the loss of protein from the blood plasma to the interstitial fluid. As protein is added to interstitial fluid, it increases its colloid osmotic pressure. When the quantity lost from the blood is large, the level of protein in the blood falls and with it the colloid osmotic pressure of the blood. The three factors contributing in varying degrees to the production of the inflammatory exudate may therefore be summarized as (1) the elevation of the filtration pressure of the blood, (2) the increased permeability of the capillaries, and (3) the increase in the colloid osmotic pressure of the tissue fluid in the area. The result is inflammatory edema.

Dilatation

As is often true, it is easier to describe what happens than to explain why it happens. However, the current explanation is that on injury cells release a chemical or chemicals acting either directly or reflexly to dilate the blood vessels and to increase their permeability. Sir Thomas Lewis first described such a substance, which, because of its similarity to histamine, he called the H-substance. Menkin [51] isolated a substance from the inflammatory exudate that he calls leukotaxine. It increases capillary permeability and in addition attracts leukocytes. Despite the ability of many chemicals to increase capillary permeability, convincing evidence that they are primarily responsible in inflammation is lacking.

Slowing of Blood Flow

During the early phase of the inflammatory reaction, the blood moves rapidly through the tissues. Later, depending on the severity of the injury, blood flow slows. The factors contributing to slowing include (1) the increased concentration of the blood in the capillaries that results from the loss of fluid into the inflamed area, (2) the increase in tissue fluid pressure which counteracts the increase in filtration pressure of the blood, and (3) possibly increased resistance to the flow of blood by the blood cells that adhere to the vascular endothelium.

With the slowing of the flow of blood, cells, especially the leukocytes, settle out of the main stream and line the vascular endothelium. This is known as the pavementing of leukocytes. Normally, the blood cells are carried in the axial stream with the leukocytes in the center and the smaller cells or erythrocytes surrounding them. The erythrocytes are separated from the vascular epithelium by a layer of plasma. In the inflammatory process, red cells tend to adhere together in clumps (blood sludge) that are larger than the leukocytes. They replace the leukocytes in the center of the stream. The leukocytes migrate peripherally, adhere to and enter the capillary wall, and pass between the endothelial cells by a process known as emigration. Because leukocytes accumulate in the injured area, they were believed to be attracted to the site by a process known as chemotaxis. Why they accumulate is questioned, as continuous observation shows that they move about at random.

Retardation of the blood flow may be so great that the blood moves forward only when the heart is contracting. This is one cause of a throbbing sensation. As long as some blood

[51] Valy Menkin: *Biochemical Mechanisms in Inflammation,* 2nd ed. (Springfield, Ill.: Charles C Thomas, Publisher, 1956), p. 11.

flow to the tissues is maintained, the process may be reversed and the tissues restored with little or no permanent harm. Blood flow, however, may be stopped by the formation of blood clots (thrombosis) in small vessels and by the pressure of inflammatory edema. Swelling caused by inflammatory edema is a particular hazard in tissues that have little space for distention, such as the brain or an extremity encased in a bandage or plaster cast. As the inflammatory edema increases, pressure on the small blood vessels increases, thereby decreasing their capacity to carry blood. The problem is aggravated by the fact that the venous return is restricted first, so that although blood continues to enter the tissue it adds to the swelling. Unless the condition is corrected, tissue pressure eventually exceeds the arterial pressure and the blood flow to the tissue ceases. When an extremity is involved, swelling, pain, numbness and tingling, bluish discoloration of the skin, coldness, and inability to move the part are warning signs. When the brain is affected, signs of increasing intracranial pressure develop. (These are discussed in Chapter 15, Part B.) Proper elevation of the extremity encased in a cast will often support the venous return enough to prevent excessive swelling.

To illustrate, Mrs. Willow suffered a fractured tibia in a traffic accident. The fracture was reduced and the leg was encased in a cast. She was placed in a bed in which the mattress was slightly depressed at the foot of the bed. A nurse found her crying with pain and begging for a "shot." Instead of administering medication, the nurse examined Mrs. Willow's toes and found them to be cold and swollen. She could move her toes only with difficulty. The nurse then elevated Mrs. Willow's leg so that gravity aided the venous return.[52] She also told Mrs. Willow that she expected that her pain would be relieved shortly by the elevation of her foot and leg, but if it was not, she would call her physician and obtain a prescription for a pain-relieving medication. Should elevation fail to relieve the pain, the physician would also be apprised of this fact, as the cast might have to be cut to relieve the pressure. In about half an hour the nurse returned to see Mrs. Willow. She was comfortable and about to begin eating her breakfast. Her toes were warm and she could wiggle them.

ROLE OF CELLULAR ELEMENTS

Neutrophils

The cells playing an active role in the acute inflammatory process have phagocytic action.

Of these the neutrophils are most important in acute inflammation, the eosinophils are increased in allergy, and the function of the basophils is not known. The neutrophil plays an important role in inflammation, both when it is alive and after it dies. It is actively phagocytic when alive; that is, it ingests, kills, and digests microbes and their foreign material. After it dies it releases proteolytic enzymes that digest not only other dead cells and bacteria but itself. Thus neutrophils aid not only in overcoming the injurious agent but also in ridding the area of debris. The latter process is an essential step in the preparation of the tissue for healing. Wood [53] postulates that dead neutrophils release a substance that is pyrogenic (fever-producing) when absorbed into the blood stream in sufficient amounts. If this hypothesis is correct, the neutrophil contributes not only to the local reaction but to the total response of the individual.

Macrophages

Both fixed and wandering macrophages have a number of important functions in inflammation. They act as scavengers. They phagocytize foreign bodies, cellular debris, and the more resistant organisms, such as *Mycobacterium tuberculosis* and fungi. They are called on to remove such substances as silica, talc, mineral oil, and sutures. They are essential to the reaction in tuberculosis as they form the epithelioid cells. They fuse to form giant cells, which are also found in the tubercle (the specific lesion of tuberculosis). They are necessary to the formation of fibrous connective tissue as they mature into fibroblasts.

Lymphocytes

The lymphocyte is the second most abundant leukocyte. It is smaller than the granulocyte and has a large nucleus with relatively little cytoplasm. It does not appear to be phagocytic to particulate matter.

As indicated in the discussion of immunity, lymphocytes play a role in immunologic responses. Small lymphocytes conditioned by the thymus recognize and are responsible for immunologic memory. Some authorities suggest that plasma cells originate from lymphocytes. It will be remembered that the plasma cells are the most active cells in the production of immunoglobulins.

Monocytes

Monocytes are less phagocytic than either granulocytes or macrophages.

---

[52] The nurse applied the second law of thermodynamics in which it is stated that energy runs downhill.

[53] W. Barry Wood: "Fever," *Sci. Amer.*, **96**:68 (June) 1957.

Summarizing the role of leukocytes in inflammation, leukocytes are essential to the inflammatory response. They function by phagocytosis (ingestion, killing, and digestion) of foreign bodies, bacteria, and the products of inflammation. Some of them form antibodies. Macrophages not only have a high phagocytic power, and form antibodies, but they contribute to the repair of the damage by maturing into fibroblasts and forming collagen. Without the power of phagocytosis the organism is at the mercy of any foreign invader. Not only do leukocytes increase in number in the injured area, but the number in the circulating blood is usually increased in all but minor injuries. The leukocyte count may reach 30,000 cells per cubic millimeter of blood or rise even higher in severe systemic reactions to infection or tissue injury. In acute inflammation, the rise is usually in the neutrophils, particularly in the less mature forms. As neutrophils mature the nucleus undergoes segmentation; therefore, the percentage of segmented cells drops when the number of neutrophils rises rapidly. In a few infections such as acute infectious mononucleosis and whooping cough, the lymphocyte count rises.

The number of leukocytes may also fall (leukopenia) in a number of infections. Infections in which this is true include typhoid fever, brucellosis, and malaria. As stated earlier, the count may be depressed in overwhelming infections or in any condition having a toxic effect on the bone marrow.

The reasons for leukocytosis are not known. It occurs not only in acute bacterial infections, such as pneumonia, but in conditions in which there is death of tissue, such as myocardial infarction and advanced malignant neoplasia. With leukocytosis there is often an associated increase in the sedimentation rate. The degree of increase in leukocyte count or sedimentation rate provides clues to the severity but not to the specific nature of the illness. Whether or not the level of the leukocytosis is in keeping with the apparent severity of illness is also significant. The obviously sick patient with a falling leukocyte count has a poor prognosis, for it indicates that the response of the patient is inadequate to the degree of illness.

In the preceding pages, the nature of the changes taking place in the blood vessels and in the blood cells occurring in inflammation have been considered. These changes have two purposes: (1) to destroy or localize the injuring agent and (2) to prepare the tissue for repair.

The dilatation and increased permeability of the blood vessels bring fluid to the area that contains antibodies and other substances to neutralize the toxins or to destroy the irritant. This fluid also dilutes the toxins and helps to restore homeostatic conditions by reducing the hydrogen ion concentration. It contains nutrients required for the release of energy and for the repair of cells. The leukocytes in the exudate phagocytose and destroy the irritant and the cellular debris.

SEQUENCE OF EVENTS FOLLOWING
TISSUE INJURY

The early changes that have been discussed proceed somewhat as follows: The tissue is injured by an inflammant—heat, cold, radiant rays, chemicals, trauma, microorganisms, antigen-antibody reaction, or some combination thereof. Almost immediately the blood vessels in the area dilate and capillary permeability increases. The extent to which these changes take place depends on the severity of the injury. Blood flow increases and there is an outpouring of fluid containing protein and leukocytes. The polymorphonuclear leukocytes are concentrated around the irritant. When the inflammatory response is initiated by bacteria able to reproduce themselves, the bacteria may at first overcome the leukocytes. Leukocytes, however, are poured into the area and eventually they turn the tide in favor of the body. In the process, however, tissue cells, bacteria, and leukocytes are killed. Fibrinogen that escapes from the blood is converted to fibrin. It forms a meshwork in the area. Antibodies are formed in increasing quantities and support the action of the phagocytes by neutralizing bacterial toxins. The wall of leukocytes surrounding the irritant deepens. The leukocytes are supported by a net formed of fibrin. The inner zone of leukocytes is composed of polymorphonuclear cells with lymphocytes, monocytes, and macrophages at the periphery. The area is bathed by a fluid rich in antibodies and nutrients. Obstruction of small blood and lymph vessels helps to block the spread of microorganisms. If the response is successful, the bacterial cells escaping from the area are phagocytosed in the blood and lymph. The central mass in the inflamed tissue is composed of dead cells and living and dead leukocytes and bacteria. These are digested. The entire zone of inflammation is called an abscess.

The abscess may rupture spontaneously or be opened. Drainage of the abscess to the outside facilitates healing by aiding in the removal of materials that would otherwise have to be digested and absorbed before healing can begin. Rupture of the abscess into a serous cavity, such as occurs in perforation of the appendix, leads to the dissemination of the contents of the abscess as well as those of the intestine into the peritoneal cavity, thus predisposing to localized or generalized peritonitis. Perforation with the development of peritonitis is one of the most serious complications in acute appendicitis. When leakage from the appendix is minimal, the body may be able to wall off the area with the formation of an appendiceal abscess.

Rupture of an abscess into the pleural space results in a condition called empyema, a disorder that is often resistant to treatment. Although the term *empyema,* when used by itself, usually refers to an accumulation of pus in the pleural cavity, it actually means a collection of pus in any natural body cavity. Therefore an accumulation of pus in the gallbladder is also empyema.

Understanding the nature of the walling-off process of inflammation is of importance in the practice of nursing. Premature or improper opening of an abscess may interfere with the mechanisms of the body for limiting spread of microorganisms and lead to their widespread dissemination. Manipulation of boils and pimples should be avoided until they have a well-defined area of pus in the center. Then they should be opened under surgical conditions. Care should be taken not to squeeze a pimple or a boil forcefully and the extruded pus should be prevented from coming in contact with the surrounding skin. Pus contains living bacteria and proteolytic enzymes that are able to digest both dead and living tissue. The combination of protein-digesting enzymes and viable bacteria predisposes to infection of the tissues with which they come in contact. Anyone changing dressings that cover draining wounds should protect himself by using instruments to handle the dressings or by wearing gloves.

In addition to draining at the surface, an abscess may terminate in other ways. When an abscess is small or the injury to the tissue structure is minimal, the products of inflammation may be digested and absorbed into the circulation. This process is known as resolution. Following pneumonia, healing takes place by resolution. Enzymes released by the degenerating leukocytes digest and liquefy the material in the alveoli. Much of the exudate is removed by coughing. Following recovery from uncomplicated pneumococcal pneumonia there is no evidence of past disease. The lung is restored to its original condition and there is no evidence of scar tissue having been formed.

Still another way an abscess may terminate is for it to drain to the surface of the body through a sinus or tract. A sinus differs from a fistula in that a sinus is a tract draining an abscess, whereas a fistula is a tract between two hollow organs or between a hollow organ and the outside. An example of a sinus is a tract from a mediastinal abscess to a bronchus. An example of a fistula is a tract or passageway between the rectum and the vagina or from the colon through the abdominal wall to the outside.

Ulcers and erosions may also result from an inflammatory process. They are alike inasmuch as the surface layer of tissue, skin, or mucous membrane is lost. They differ in that an ulcer extends through the covering membrane, whereas an erosion involves only the covering membrane. Examples of ulcers include peptic ulcers and varicose ulcers. A common site of an erosion is the cervix uteri. In the formation of ulcers and erosions, the body mechanism for maintaining the integrity of tissue breaks down and the tissue destruction follows. In most people the tissue lining the stomach and duodenum is protected from the digesting action of gastric secretions. Any condition that upsets the balance between tissue resistance and protection from the digesting action of the gastric secretions so that digestion is favored predisposes to peptic ulcer formation. Varicose ulcers are essentially the result of inadequate tissue nutrition.

FACTORS AFFECTING THE OUTCOME
OF THE INFLAMMATORY RESPONSE

The outcome of an inflammatory response depends on many factors including the agent responsible for injury to the tissues, the effectiveness of the individual's mechanisms of defense, and the specific tissues that are involved, as well as the nature and extent of the injury to the tissues. Factors influencing the capacity of an individual to respond to injury include his age and general state of health and nutrition. When microorganisms are responsible, the body may or may not be able to localize them. Some bacteria are difficult to localize because they manufacture an enzyme, hyaluronidase, that destroys hyaluronic acid. Hyaluronic acid, a mucopolysaccharide, is a gel-like ground substance that acts as a cement substance between cells and to hold water in interstitial spaces. It is a component of synovial fluid, vitreous humor in the eye, and Wharton's jelly in the umbilical cord. It is also a constituent of the capsules of certain types of streptococci, pneumococci, and other microbes. Because hyaluronidase destroys the tissue hyaluronic acid and therefore allows greater spreading of materials in the tissue spaces, hyaluronidase is called the spreading factor. Production of hyaluronidase by such organisms as the staphylococcus and streptococcus enables them to break down the continuity of the tissue as well as the fibrin clots formed in the area of infection. When microorganisms are successful in disrupting barriers to their spread, they are then able to penetrate the surrounding tissue and cause cellulitis. With a breakdown of the local barriers to their spread, organisms may also enter the lymph and blood channels. Fibrin clots in the small venous and lymph channels may delay the entrance of bacteria into the general circulation. Lymph nodes in lymph channels also act as traps to remove and phagocytize microbes and other particles as well as to respond with acute inflammation (lymphadenitis). When bacteria enter and are circulated in the blood, the condition is known as bacteremia. When bacteria enter and multiply in the blood the condition is called septicemia. In some diseases, such as typhoid fever, bacteremia characteristically occurs in a particular phase of the illness. In others, such as pneumonia, the appearance of bacteremia is an unfavorable prognostic sign. Septicemia is always a serious and often fatal disorder. In either bacteremia or septicemia, microorganisms may be distributed through the body and set up sites of infection distant from the original infection.

CLASSIFICATION OF INFLAMMATION

Any condition that modifies the nature of the inflammatory response or is useful in identifying something about it can be used as a basis for classification. Inflammation may be classified according to (1) the causative or etiological agent, (2) the characteristic type of exudate, (3) the location or site in which it occurs, and (4) the length of time the process has been in existence. Any classification of inflammation according to cause includes an endless variety of physical, chemical, and living agents. Some have their origin in the external environment and some in the internal environment of the individual.

Characteristic Types of Exudates

The character of the fluid exudate depends on the severity of the injury. In less severe injuries there may be very little exudate and what there is may differ very little in composition from normal interstitial fluid. As the severity of the injury increases, the damage to blood vessels increases and more components of the blood are found in the inflammatory exudate.

The inflammatory process may be classified according to the nature of the exudate. The exudate may be purulent, serous, serosanguineous, fibrinous, hemorrhagic, or catarrhal.

A **purulent exudate** is commonly known as pus. Although a number of other agents stimulate the production of a purulent exudate, it is most commonly associated with the so-called pyogenic bacteria. In these infections the exudate is rich in leukocytes. The purulent exudate or pus contains a large number of leukocytes,

together with tissue debris and the products of digestion by proteolytic enzymes released by dead and dying leukocytes. The thick creamy pus found in the spinal fluid of the patient with meningococcic meningitis is an example of a purulent exudate associated with a pyogenic infection. Another more common example is the pus associated with staphylococcal infections of the hair follicle or a wound or the material occurring in the center of a pimple or boil (furuncle).

A **serous exudate**, which occurs in mild injuries, is a watery fluid containing high protein derived from the blood or from the cells lining serous cavities and joint spaces. Perhaps the most common example of a serous exudate is the fluid found in the blisters or vesicles associated with second-degree burns. Mr. All had some blistering of his skin as a consequence of burns. These blisters contained a serous exudate. Another example of a serous exudate is the fluid that accumulates in the pleural cavity as a result of some types of pleurisy. This type of pleurisy is known as pleurisy with effusion. It is frequently caused by tuberculosis or by a malignant neoplasm in the lung.

Infections involving the peritoneum or the pericardium may likewise result in the production of a serous exudate. Pericarditis with effusion is likely to cause serious impairment in cardiac function. Relatively small amounts of fluid prevent the heart from dilating fully during diastole and interfere with the filling of the heart. This results in congestion of blood in the systemic venous circulation and reduces the quantity of blood available to circulate to the tissues.

In the more severe acute inflammatory processes, damage to capillaries may increase permeability to the extent that large molecules such as fibrinogen escape in the exudate. The fibrinogen is converted to fibrin and forms a sort of meshwork structure in the inflamed area. It also obstructs small lymph vessels and capillaries. Authorities disagree about the function of the fibrin. Some, such as Menkin,[54] believe that it prevents dissemination of organisms by providing a mechanical barrier to their spread. The fibrin probably acts to delay the spread of microorganisms by providing a sort of maze through which bacteria must pass before they can escape into the surrounding tissue. This maze also increases the likelihood of the bacteria coming in contact with phagocytic cells. The fibrin network may contribute to the difficulty of removing all microorganisms from tissues even when the microorganisms are sensitive to antibiotics. The network acts to protect

[54] *Op. cit.,* p. 111.

microorganisms by limiting their exposure to the therapeutic agents. Until the inflamed area is well walled off, it should be protected from trauma. **A fibrinous exudate** is characteristic of certain types of infections, such as pneumococcal pneumonia. The alveoli are filled with a fibrinous exudate containing large numbers of leukocytes. When the inflammatory process extends to the pleura, it causes the so-called fibrinous pleurisy. The fibrin on the surface of the pleura is sticky. Pain during breathing results from the pleural surfaces rubbing together. Though fibrinous pleurisy is an early finding in pneumonia, it also occurs in the absence of pneumonia.

Hemorrhagic Inflammations

In very severe inflammatory reactions, damage to the blood vessels may be so great that erythrocytes escape into the exudate. This may be observed as minute hemorrhages into the skin that are known as petechiae, which appear as small reddened areas in the skin. They are commonly found in subacute bacterial endocarditis. In fulminating infections the damage to blood vessels may be so great that bleeding into the subcutaneous tissues takes place. This gives the skin a dusky hue. The color of the skin is responsible for the black smallpox or meningitis of fact and legend.

Catarrhal Inflammation

Catarrhal inflammation occurs only in those tissues in which there are mucous glands—that is, in mucous membranes. The term is really a misnomer, but it continues to be used because of force of habit. The exudate from mucous membranes contains large amounts of mucinous material. It is one of the most frequent types of exudate because it is associated with inflammations of the respiratory tract. The clear mucinous exudate accompanying a common cold is an example. Mucous secretion may be increased by the exposure of the respiratory tract to chemical irritants such as those contained in smoke or smog.

Other Classifications

Inflammatory processes may also be classified according to the tissue or organ in which they are located. Students can recognize that the inflammatory process is involved when the suffix *itis* is added to the combining form indicating a tissue or organ. Inflammation of the trachea and bronchi, whatever the causative agent, is known as tracheobronchitis. The term *myositis* indicates that a muscle is inflamed. Myocarditis is used to indicate that the heart muscle is inflamed. Nephritis indicates that the site of inflammation is the kidney. None of these terms indicates the cause of the inflammatory process. The only information provided is that a particular organ is the site of an inflammatory process.

The inflammatory process may also be classified as to the length of time it has been in existence. This classification gives some clue as to the degree of activity of the process. Thus the terms *acute, subacute,* and *chronic* are used. Acute inflammations are those of recent origin and in which the process is active. The common cold is an example of a condition in which there is an acute inflammatory process. A recently incurred burn is another. An example of a condition that may go from the acute to the chronic stage is acute hemorrhagic nephritis. The kidney may recover fully following the acute phase of the disease or it may fail to do so and go into the subacute phase and finally into chronic nephritis.

Not all inflammatory processes are highly active at the beginning. Some inflammants are only mildly irritating and cause damage only by prolonged exposure. Such an irritant is silica. When it is inhaled into the lung, it sets up a simple inflammatory process in which the macrophage plays an important role. Because silica is indigestible, it cannot be destroyed by the macrophage. Macrophages, however, can wall it off by forming fibroblasts that mature into fibrous connective tissue. One particle of silica will not require a very large scar, but many particles do. Therefore, to prevent serious scarring of the lung, workers who are exposed to silica dust require measures that reduce the chances of inhaling dust.

CAUSES OF SIGNS AND SYMPTOMS

The signs and symptoms in inflammation depend in part on the degree of response of the host, the nature of the inflammant, and the site of the injury. Mild irritants, including psychogenic stimuli triggered by a symbol of injury, may produce only a transient inflammation lasting only a few minutes or hours, whereas severe injury may last for days, weeks, or even months. The response may be limited to a small area or may involve the entire organism.

The cardinal signs of inflammation are increased heat, redness, swelling, pain, and loss of function. The rise in the temperature is caused mainly by an increase in blood supply, though there may also be some increase in the metabolic rate. With the increase in blood flow in the area, the temperature approaches that of the interior of the body. The increase in blood in the area is also responsible for the redness. Although the increased quantity of blood contributes to the swelling, swelling or inflammatory edema is mainly caused by the accumulation of the exudate in the tissue. Swelling causes pain because of pressure on sensory nerve endings. Some authorities believe that toxic metabolites are also a factor in pain.

Loss of function is partly caused by pain, as motion increases pain. Muscle spasm in the injured area also serves to splint or limit motion of the part. For example, following spillage of the contents of the gastrointestinal tract into the peritoneal cavity, the muscles of the abdominal wall contract and act as a physiological splint. Even cuts involving skin over or near a joint induce some muscle spasm and a disinclination to move the joint because of the pain.

As a space-occupying mass, an area of inflammation may impinge on the circulation to an organ or obstruct a hollow organ or duct. For example, a localized area of inflammation of a structure within the cranial cavity may raise the intracranial pressure enough to deprive the entire brain of an adequate supply of blood. It may also cause pressure on the area of the brain where it is situated. An abscess in the mediastinum may interfere with swallowing by obstructing the esophagus from without. An abscess in the neck may obstruct the trachea by local pressure on it. In none of these examples does the inflammatory process directly involve the affected structures, but it causes its effects as a space-occupying mass.

In the description of inflammation thus far, emphasis has been on the local responses of tissues to injury. When only a relatively small number of cells are damaged, most, if not all, of the physiological response is in the region of injury. When, however, the products of inflammation are absorbed into the blood stream in sufficient quantities, the whole organism becomes involved. Although the nature of the etiological agent influences the severity and timing of the general physiological manifestations, they are not unique to a single class. Therefore the manifestations of illness resulting from the escape of the products of inflammation into the general circulation can be observed in Mr. All (burns), Mr. Hoffer (myocardial infarct), and Mrs. Carney (radical mastectomy —major surgery), as well as Miss Mallow, who has pneumococcal pneumonia.

Generalized Signs and Symptoms

One important group of symptoms includes fever and the symptoms and signs that commonly accompany fever. The degree and character of fever vary with the causative agent. Following a major surgical procedure or an acute myocardial infarction, the temperature rises a degree or two and remains elevated for no more than two or three days. It should then return to normal and remain within the normal range. If it does not, or if the temperature rises higher than expected, this usually indicates that a complication is developing. Because the pattern of fever varies with each acute infectious disease, no attempt will be made to describe them here. The pulse and respiratory rate are usually, though not invariably, accelerated in proportion to the increase in temperature. Weakness and general malaise—a general feeling of unfitness—are common. Anorexia, or loss of appetite, is frequent; headache, backache, and generalized aching are not uncommon. Nausea may occur, with or without vomiting or diarrhea. Leukocytosis and an increase in the erythrocyte sedimentation rate occur in a wide variety of acute conditions—with and without infection. Some infections, such as pneumococcal pneumonia, may be preceded by a chill in adults or by a convulsion in infants and young children. In other conditions, such as advanced tuberculosis, subacute bacterial endocarditis, and malaria, chills and fever may alternate with sweating (diaphoresis).

If the inflammatory process (1) continues for more than a few days, (2) is severe, (3) is associated with fever, or (4) is associated with the loss of considerable quantities of tissue substance or nutrients, weight loss may be marked. During fever, the metabolic rate is increased about 7 per cent for each degree of fever. With continued fever, the patient needs a substantial intake of calories to prevent weight loss. In long-continued inflammatory processes, particularly when associated with infection, the production of erythrocytes by the bone marrow may be depressed; normocytic anemia is a common finding in chronic infections.

Inflammation is one of a living organism's most important mechanisms of defense against injury. Inflammation is a defensive response to an injurious agent. It involves blood vessels; blood cells, particularly the leukocytes; tissue cells; the immunologic system; and cells of the reticuloendothelial system. It serves to neutralize, destroy, and limit the spread of inflammants and to prepare the tissues for repair.

The signs and symptoms accompanying the inflammatory process result from the response of the injured tissue and the person to injury as well as from the nature and severity of the injury. Inasmuch as the inflammatory process is a space-occupying mass, it may interfere with the function of organs. The signs and symptoms will depend on the extent to which function is disrupted. When sufficient products of the inflammatory process are absorbed, signs and symptoms indicating that the whole person is sick follow.

What is the nurse's role in helping the patient with an inflammatory response?

The specific therapy of any patient who has suffered cell injury and an accompanying inflammatory response will depend on such factors as the nature of the etiological agent and the extent of the injury and its location, as well as on the adaptive capacity of the individual. In general, therapy will be directed toward (1) assisting the patient to overcome or eliminate the causative agent, (2) supporting the inflammatory response, and (3) providing substances required for the repair of the injured tissues. Attention is also given to the prevention of further injury so that the individual may be restored to health.

In planning the therapy of the patient a number of principles serve as guides in the selection of specific measures. The **first principle**, when appropriately used, is that rest favors healing. How rest of an organ or part is achieved depends on its location and function. Both these factors—location and function of the affected part—are important in determining the degree of rest that it is possible to achieve. To illustrate, Mr. Carlos fractured his leg. Maintaining his leg at rest was relatively easy. It was placed in a cast or in traction with the two ends of the bone held in apposition. Mr. Carlos remained in bed until sufficient healing occurred. Even after he was out of bed he did not bear weight on his leg until healing was well under way or the leg was immobilized by a cast or brace. By way of contrast, despite the desirability of rest to the liver in the treatment of hepatitis, only relative rest can be secured. Mr. Devon,[55] who had a diagnosis of infectious hepatitis, was placed on a high-carbohydrate, high-protein, and low-fat diet. He was maintained at bed rest for several weeks in order to provide rest for the liver. Mr. Hoffer, who suffered a myocardial infarction, was also treated by bed rest for four weeks in order to reduce strain on the heart; then his physical activity was gradually increased.[56] Immediately following myocardial infarction, Mr. Hoffer was fed, bathed, and, inasfar as possible, protected from psychological and social stresses. Though bed rest is used less extensively than in the past, it is still believed to be an important form of treatment in infectious disease, in acute glomerulonephritis, and in acute rheumatic fever.

Bed rest is not without its hazards. As emphasized earlier, rest or lack of use of the body is accompanied by a loss of body substance and strength. Visceral and circulatory functions are depressed with the result that gastrointestinal function is disturbed and clotting of blood in vessels is favored. Respiratory excursions are lessened and this predisposes to atelectasis and pneumonia. Despite these and other disadvantages, the indications for rest may be sufficiently great for the physician to prescribe it. When bed rest is prescribed, the nurse has the responsibility to select appropriate nursing measures so that physical and psychological rest are achieved.

A **second principle** is as follows: Survival depends on an adequate circulation of blood to and from the tissue. The effectiveness of the inflammatory response as well as the life of the cells depends on (1) a continued supply of nutrients, leukocytes, antibodies, and other substances required by the tissue and (2) the removal of products of tissue metabolism as well as those of the inflammatory process. Heat in the form of dry or moist heat may be used to dilate the blood vessels. Because each tissue has a thermal death point, care should be taken to prevent burns. Moist heat is more dangerous than dry heat because it prevents evaporation. A temperature of from $40.5°$ to $46°C$ ($105°$ to $115°F$) is very hot.[57] Exposure of the tissue to $85°C$ for as little as ten seconds is sufficient to cause burning. With each degree that the temperature of tissue is raised, the metabolic rate goes up about 7 per cent. Patients with arterial diseases such as arteriosclerosis are sensitive to heat because they have a limited capacity to increase the delivery of nutrients to their tissues by dilating their arteries. Their ability to judge the temperature may also be defective. Should moist heat be applied to a patient with a diagnosis of arteriosclerosis, the temperature of the solution should be prescribed by the physician and should be checked with a thermometer. The dressings should be removed if the patient complains of pain and the physician should be notified. These patients should also be taught to check the temperature of bath water with a thermometer before stepping into the bathtub.

Heat is sometimes applied to extremities of patients in the form of a light cradle. Tissues can be protected by using a cradle in which the heat is controlled thermostatically. The

---

[55] Authorities disagree about the necessity for bed rest in the treatment of hepatitis.
[56] The time selected is to illustrate a point and is not intended to reflect any particular practice in treating patients following myocardial infarction.

[57] American Medical Association: *Handbook of Physical Medicine and Rehabilitation* (Philadelphia: The Blakiston Co., 1950), p. 174.

temperature should be maintained between 30° and 34°C (between 86° and 95°F) as this is the temperature at which maximum vasodilatation can be expected.[58] When a cradle with a thermostatic control is not available, the patient can be afforded some measure of protection by using light bulbs of 25 watts or less. Despite great care some patients have pain caused by muscle ischemia at environmental temperatures that are very little above ordinary room temperature. When this is true, the heat should be discontinued and the physician notified.

Maintenance of the venous return is also important to the nutrition of tissues. In inflammation, distention of tissues by the inflammatory exudate causes pressure on veins, thereby interfering with the venous return. Elevation of an extremity is an important measure in promoting venous return. An elastic stocking or bandage is also useful in supporting the venous circulation. Should signs and symptoms that accompany impaired circulation occur in an extremity encased in a cast or bandage, measures to relieve the situation must be instituted promptly if tissue injury is to be prevented.

Care directed toward the maintenance of the circulation of inflamed tissue is important. Observation of the signs and symptoms indicating the status of the circulation in the tissue is imperative if indications that the circulation is failing are to be detected early and appropriate measures instituted in time.

A **third principle** in therapy is to provide the patient with specific assistance to overcome the causative agent. This principle applies primarily to those conditions in which the causative agent propagates itself, or is a foreign body. At this time the main group of causative agents falling into the first category are microorganisms. There are two general, but specific, ways of attacking microorganisms or their products. One is to give the patient specific antibodies formed by an animal or another human being. The other is to administer a chemical that acts to weaken or to kill the microorganism. The use of specific therapy in the treatment of infectious disease is included in Chapter 5.

The **fourth principle** is to modify the tissue response in inflammation so that tissue injury is prevented. As in other body responses, the inflammatory reaction may be deficient or it may be excessive. In the first case, recovery may be threatened because the body is unable to overcome the irritant and prepare the tissue for repair. In the latter, the tissue is damaged by the excessive reaction. Agranulocytosis has been previously cited as an example of a condition in which the body response to injury may be inadequate. In individual patients in whom the inflammatory response is excessive, tissue damage may result. The control and effects of excessive swelling have been discussed. Necrotic areas are often repaired by fibrosis. Scar tissue may cause deformity of the affected tissue or organ. In disorders such as iritis, arthritis, and rheumatic fever, residual injury can sometimes be lessened by modifying the severity of the inflammatory response of the tissues. By limiting the exudative phase of the inflammatory response, tissue swelling is lessened. This contributes to the maintenance of the circulation to the tissues and therefore helps to prevent tissue necrosis. In the absence of tissue necrosis, fibrosis does not occur. To illustrate, in the treatment of iritis (inflammation of the iris of the eye) cortisone, hydrocortisone, or one of their synthetic analogues may be placed in the eye to reduce the severity of the inflammatory reaction and, as a consequence, the amount of scarring. Although authorities do not agree as to how the corticoids act, they reduce in some way the exudative response in inflammation. As a result, there is less tissue damage and a reduction in the amount of scar tissue formed in healing. Corticoids and salicylates are used in the treatment of arthritis and rheumatic fever for essentially the same reason.

The **fifth principle** is that healing cannot proceed until the inflammatory debris, foreign bodies, blood clots, necrotic tissue, and the like are removed. In simple inflammations, the products of inflammation may be digested and absorbed into the blood stream. The blood vessels and tissue may be repaired leaving little or no evidence of the past inflammation. In pneumonia, the exudate in the lung may be coughed up and the tissue repaired without leaving any sign of the past infection. In boils, wound infections, empyema, and other similar infections, as well as those in which foreign bodies are present in the tissue, recovery may be hastened by the evacuation of pus, tissue debris, or foreign bodies. The removal of necrotic tissue and foreign bodies is called débridement; sometimes, as with a boil, this may need to be done only once. In other disorders, such as a serious wound infection, repeated opening of the wound may be required to facilitate drainage. Such wounds may be irrigated with isotonic saline or some other solution to remove debris and pus. When irrigation is done, enough force should be used to remove the purulent material. Care should be taken to prevent contamination of other areas of the skin of the patient and of the nurse.

[58] R. W. Wilkins: "Peripheral Vascular Diseases Due to Organic Arterial Obstruction," *Cecil-Loeb: A Textbook of Medicine*, 12th ed., Paul B. Beeson and Walsh McDermott, eds. (Philadelphia: W. B. Saunders Company, 1967), p. 729.

The **final principle** in the treatment of the patient with an inflammatory response is that procedures should be instituted that help to support the patient in his reaction to his condition. The support should be both emotional and physiological, as one augments the other. No one is at his best when he is ill and he should not be expected to be. Moore and his associates [59] found that apprehension and fear before a surgical procedure were associated with a mild catabolic response. Attention to the needs of the patient and prompt relief of unnecessary pain should help to minimize suffering. Attention should be given to supplying the nutritional needs of each patient. There is evidence to indicate that in undernourished patients phagocytic ability is less than in those who are well nourished. Nutrients are necessary to the formation of antibodies and to the replacement of nutrients lost in the inflammatory exudate. Tissue substance lost as a result of the catabolic response to tissue injury must also be replaced by the food intake of the patient.

Water intake should be sufficient to replace that which is lost. Insensible perspiration may be increased by one liter or more in fever. Drenching diaphoresis may be responsible for the loss of one liter or more of water. A urine output of less than one liter usually indicates that the fluid intake of the patient is inadequate. This presupposes a normally functioning kidney.

Rest and reassurance may also be important ingredients in the care of the patient. The doctor usually orders the degree of activity that is allowed, but the nurse is the one who tries to modify his environment so that he is able to rest. Reassurance is discussed in Chapter 7.

Provided that the body is successful in removing, destroying, or neutralizing the injurious agent, the tissue goes on to repair the damage that has been done. Essentially the nature of repair is the same whether the continuity of the tissue is disrupted by a spontaneous process or by a carefully planned incision.

Repair

The question of whether repair is the final stage of inflammation or is a separate response to injury is really of little importance. What is significant is that repair is a response to injury in which the body attempts to restore the injured tissue to normal. How this is accomplished depends on the severity and type of the injury as well as on the tissues that have been injured. There are three general ways in which repair

may take place: healing by recovery, by regeneration, and by replacement with scar tissue.

In the discussion of possible outcomes of inflammation, the point was made that when injury to the tissue is minimal the products of inflammation are absorbed and the tissues are returned to their former condition. The restoration of tissue to its former state is known as recovery.

Regeneration

When the injury is more severe and cells are destroyed, repair may be accomplished by regeneration, a process in which cells are replaced by similar cells. Actually, regeneration of tissues such as the skin is a constant process. As the surface cells of the skin are shed, they are replaced by underlying cells, which are in turn replaced by cells at the base of the skin, each of which undergoes mitosis and divides into two. The process is carefully controlled, so that only as many cells are produced as are needed to replace those that are lost.

Regeneration of cells and tissues depends on two fundamental properties. One is the capacity of cells to proliferate or multiply. The other is the capacity of the organism to organize new cells into a functional pattern. Scientists have long been intrigued by the fact that animals, such as the salamander, are able to regenerate limbs following amputation. One of the factors in the regeneration of an organ is the ability of cells forming different types of tissue to regenerate at the same rate. In man different types of tissue cells reproduce at different rates. The problem is complicated by the fact that fibrous connective tissue regenerates more rapidly and under less favorable circumstances than other types of tissues. Therefore, even in tissues having the capacity to regenerate, healing may take place by scarring rather than by regeneration.

Not only is man incapable of regenerating limbs, but the capacity of his tissues to regenerate varies. As stated previously, highly specialized cells such as those in nerve and muscle tissues are incapable of regeneration. Injuries are repaired by replacement with microglia (a connective tissue in the nervous system) and fibrous connective tissue. By way of contrast, tissues having their origin in the mesenchymal tissues (those that form the supporting structures for the parenchymal or functioning cells) have a great capacity for regeneration. Surface and glandular epithelium, bone, and lymphoid tissue are also able to regenerate adequately.

The capacity to produce an adequate number of differentiated cells is only one aspect of regeneration. Another is the capacity to organize these cells into functioning units with the necessary blood, lymph, and nerve supply. A

[59] G. M. Wilson, F. D. Moore, and R. P. Jepson: "The Metabolic Disturbances Following Injury," *Metabolic Disturbances in Clinical Medicine*, G. A. Smart, ed. (Boston: Little, Brown & Company, 1958), p. 76.

good example of an organ in which the capacity to regenerate fails, not because cells do not proliferate but because the body is unable to properly organize them into functioning units, is the liver. The liver is susceptible to injury by a wide variety of agents: microorganisms; chemical poisons, such as chloroform or carbon tetrachloride; and undernutrition, as the liver is particularly susceptible to a lack of protein and of vitamin B in the diet. The liver fails to recover following injury not because liver cells do not have an adequate capacity to regenerate but because the body is unable to organize the cells around ducts. Despite the capacity to replace damaged liver cells, the resulting tissue is likely to be of little use. In a way, the liver is repaired much as a jerry-built house is constructed—a cell here and one there without thought as to where it should be placed to accomplish its function.

The third way in which repair is achieved is by the substitution of fibrous connective tissue for the injured tissue. When fibrous connective tissue is used in repair, it serves as a patch to preserve or restore the continuity of the tissue. It does nothing more. Therefore, when an injury to a vital organ is repaired by the substitution of fibrous connective tissue, the result is a decrease in the functional reserve in that organ. For example, a myocardial infarct heals by the formation of scar tissue. The extent to which the cardiac reserve is diminished will depend on the size of the scar. Following an attack of glomerulonephritis, scar tissue is formed to heal the kidney. The scarring may do more damage than the original disease process because as the scar tissue matures, it contracts and obstructs the flow of blood to the kidney. Functioning tissue dies as a consequence of loss of blood supply. In patients who die from the effects of glomerulonephritis, the kidney is frequently found to be a contracted mass consisting mostly of scar tissue.

The circumstances under which repair by the substitution of fibrous connective tissue occurs are (1) when conditions in the internal environment are unfavorable to mitosis, (2) when the quantity of tissue destroyed is too large for it to be replaced by regeneration of the cells in the area, (3) when highly specialized tissues have been destroyed, (4) when the rate at which parenchymal cells multiply is slow, and (5) when tissues are subjected to repeated injury.

As has been implied, healing by the formation of fibrous tissue serves a number of purposes. It restores the continuity of tissue after too great destruction of tissue. It walls off foreign bodies and disease processes such as tuberculosis. It reinforces weakened structures such

as aneurysms of the aorta and other large arteries.[60] Fibrous connective tissue also plays an important role in the healing of thrombosis, infarctions, osteomyelitis, and nephritis as well as of many other conditions. When thrombi form in veins, fibrous tissue serves to hold the clot at the site of formation and to repair the damage. Following an infarction, scar tissue maintains tissue continuity.

Similar to other homeostatic mechanisms, tissue repair by the formation of scar tissue is beneficial when the process is initiated by an appropriate stimulus and is sufficient to correct the damage caused by injury. Likewise it may also be the source of harm. The principal harmful effects of scar tissue are (1) the unnecessary replacement of parenchymatous tissue; (2) interference with the function or drainage of an organ; or (3) the cutting off of the blood or nerve supply to an organ; and (4) the formation of an excessive quantity of scar tissue.

Certain of the characteristics of scar tissue account for some of its potentially harmful effects. It is composed largely of collagen. When a scar is subjected to slight or moderate stress, it tends to shorten or contract. When it is subjected to much stress, it tends to lengthen. Contraction of the scar does no harm when it is in the abdominal wall and the quantity of scar tissue is not excessive. However, when scar tissue is formed in or around an organ, it can be expected to interfere with the function of the organ as it matures, as sometimes happens in the healing of third-degree burns or in arthritis. In these patients, attention to maintaining the extremities in the appropriate position so that deformities caused by contractures can be prevented may be a lasting service to the patient.

Scar tissue located in areas where it is subjected to repeated strain may lengthen or extend. Sites that are subjected to considerable pressure include the wall of the heart and the arteries. Especially when an infarct in the wall of the heart is large or when the heart is subjected to repeated infarction and the quantity of scar tissue is large, the collagen fibers in the scar may be stretched by the pressure created as the heart contracts. Because they are not elastic, after they are lengthened they do not return to their former state. This results in a bulge or aneurysm. This bulge reduces the mechanical efficiency of the affected ventricle. Instead of only one area of relatively low pressure, that is, the artery, there are two, the artery and the

---

[60] An aneurysm is a bulge or outpouching in the wall of an artery. It usually results when the wall is weakened by a disease such as arteriosclerosis or syphilis. As it distends, the wall of the artery thins and is further weakened. Fibrous connective tissue strengthens the wall.

distensible area in the wall of the heart. As the heart contracts, blood enters both the artery and the aneurysm. This increases the work of an already weakened heart.

Many of the general factors favoring tissue repair have already been indicated. They may be summarized as (1) a limited amount of injury and a high regenerative capacity of tissues, (2) an abundant supply of blood to the tissue as well as an adequate supply of protein and ascorbic acid, and finally (3) good health and youth. Regarding the last point, the most important practical difference between healing in the young and in the old is that the young tend to heal more rapidly than the old. The need for a good blood supply is obvious. Protein is necessary to supply the amino acids required for the formation of new tissue. Some authorities are inclined to interpret the metabolic response following injury as an adaptation by which the organism provides the tissues with the materials needed for healing. Because the metabolic response is greater in the young and healthy than in the old and feeble, perhaps this is one reason that they recover more quickly than do the old and feeble. Ascorbic acid, or vitamin C, is necessary for the formation of collagen—an essential element in fibrous tissue.

The presence of diseases such as uncontrolled diabetes mellitus or atherosclerosis delays repair. Though there is some disagreement among authorities about the effect of anemia on wound healing, it probably is not an important factor.

Local conditions in the injured tissue also have an effect on the healing. The exact nature of the stimulus to cellular proliferation is not known, but it is believed to be caused by a local factor or factors. As was emphasized in the discussion of inflammation, healing is delayed or prevented until the wound has been cleared of infection and any dead space has been obliterated. In the past, healing has been delayed by the introduction of foreign substances at the time the wound was made or treated. At various times throughout history, antiseptics and germicides have been placed in wounds to destroy microorganisms. It is now known that any agent potent enough to kill bacteria also kills body cells. Furthermore, before healing can proceed normally, all foreign material must be removed. Because it acts as a foreign body when introduced into a wound, talc is no longer used to powder gloves. A form of treated cornstarch or Biosorb cream and powder have been substituted for it. Though it is much less likely than talc to produce a foreign-body reaction, cornstarch can and does. Therefore, it should be used as sparingly as possible in powdering the gloves. The outer surface of the gloves

should be washed before the operation is started.[61]

The mechanism of injury also has a bearing on healing. A clean, incised wound free from infection is the most favorable to healing. Crushing wounds, fractures, especially those with much soft-tissue damage, and infection of wounds delay healing. They also are attended by the possibility of excessive scar tissue formation.

So that the reader may have some understanding of what is happening in a patient who is healing an area of injured tissue, the healing of a clean, incised wound will be briefly described. The process of healing all injuries is essentially the same. The principal difference between the healing of a clean, incised wound and an infected one, or one in which the tissue is subjected to longstanding injury, is in the quantity of scar tissue required to heal the defect. In a clean, incised wound only a small scar is required, which may form quickly; in other wounds, scarring may be extensive and delayed.

Preparatory to, and during, healing a number of things must be accomplished. The damaged cells and tissue debris must be removed. Bleeding must be stopped. The gap between the two severed edges of tissue must be bridged. As the surgeon makes the incision he works carefully. Though a small clot of blood or fluid exudate is necessary to fill the defect between the two sides of the wound, a large clot delays healing. Therefore, the surgeon carefully ligates (ties) the ends of each blood vessel as it is cut. Small vessels seal themselves by the formation of blood clots, which on retraction of the vessel form an effective plug in its end. The surgeon also facilitates healing by the careful approximation of like tissues to like tissues. As he completes his part in the healing of the wound, nature takes over.

Authorities usually describe healing as occurring in three phases. There is considerable overlapping among the various phases. They may all be going on at the same time in different parts of the wound. The first phase, which lasts from three to five days, is variously called the initial, the lag, the catabolic, and the inflammatory phase. These terms all have some virtue in that each describes some change or condition that is present in the tissues. The term *lag* has been used because the strength of the wound diminishes during this time. The term is, however, misleading because it implies that no changes are occurring in the tissue. This is not

[61] James D. Hardy: "Operative Surgical Care," *Surgery: Principles and Practice,* 3rd ed., Carl A. Moyer et al., eds. (Philadelphia: J. B. Lippincott Company, 1965), p. 263.

true, for exudation is increased and leukocytes accumulate in the area. Blood vessels dilate and the area becomes hyperemic. The fluid exudate and/or blood fills the space between the two edges of the wound and not only causes the edges of the wound to stick together but provides a meshlike framework for fibroblasts and budding capillaries. Materials essential to tissue repair accumulate. Fibroblasts appear and there is an increase in collagen. Without collagen, wound healing does not take place. Collagen does not form unless the proper materials and conditions are present. Capillary buds also begin to appear. Their formation coincides with the general catabolic response of the body as a whole. During this phase the patient looks and acts ill. Moore [62] calls this the stage of injury or the adrenergic corticoid phase.

After four or five days the leukocytes begin to disappear from the wound. About this time the fibroblasts can be observed to be actively proliferating. During this phase collagen is formed and the newly formed tissue is highly vascular. Because of its appearance, the new tissue is called granulation tissue. As the collagen fibers mature, they tend to shorten or contract. Early in the process of wound healing, epithelial cells migrate and later proliferate to cover the wound surface. With large wounds the epithelial covering may be very thin and delicate. Care should be taken when the wound

[62] *Op. cit.*, p. 28.

is dressed to protect these newly forming cells lest they be destroyed. In time, the scar, which was a bright pink, fades, because the blood vessels are squeezed out. The result is a mature scar, or a cicatrix.

When a wound is infected, suppuration occurs and healing is delayed. At one time infection was so common that surgeons thought it was necessary to healing. The type of pus that was believed to favor healing was called laudable pus. When pus is present, the wound is said to heal by second intention. Healing is delayed and more granulation tissue is required to fill the defect than in the absence of infection. Occasionally, either because of the nature of the wound or because of its disruption, secondary closure is necessary. This is known as healing by third intention.

Currently, knowledge of the factors involved in wound healing is incomplete. Questions as to what initiates the process and what terminates it have not been answered. In experiments with rats, Selye has been able to prevent scar tissue formation by the administration of cortisone and to augment its formation by administration of desoxycortisone. Exactly how cortisone, hydrocortisone, and related analogues act is not known. In rats, the different adrenal cortical hormones depress or enhance the inflammatory response that follows tissue injury.

Earlier in this chapter the changes occurring in the tissue in response to injury were described. In Table 6-3, changes that take place in the body as a whole and in the wound are

TABLE 6-3

Phase I	Neuro-endocrine	Psychological	Circulatory	Metabolism	Water and Electrolytes	Blood
A. Onset		Anxiety, fear				
		Guilt, shame				
		Frustration				
		Denial				
		Aggression: ill-tempered, irascible				
		Passivity: pitiable, complains, obsequious				
		Elation: neurotic level of function				
		Indecisiveness, vacillation				
		↓				

summarized and correlated with the signs and symptoms that can be expected in the patient and his needs during each phase. The length of each phase varies with the extent of injury to the tissue as well as with the capacity of the individual to respond. The summary is based on the changes occurring in a patient who has a clean, incised wound such as is made in the performance of abdominal surgery. Changes are less marked in conditions in which the extent of injury to tissue is less and is more marked in those in which there is greater injury to the tissue.

During the twentieth century, techniques have been perfected and the knowledge of the changes that take place in the body as a whole, as well as in the wounded tissue, has increased. With expansion in the fields of physiology and biochemistry, clues are being uncovered that can be expected to lead to a knowledge of the factors that initiate the healing process, regulate its course, and terminate it. Interest is also centered on the biochemical changes that take place in the body as a whole following injury and during illness. The preceding discussion re-emphasizes that the body acts as a unit. Biologically it gives priority to the injured tissue. As the understanding of these changes becomes more complete, care of the patient following injury can perhaps be planned to support body responses rather than to interfere with them. In other patients, such as those with glomerulonephritis or rheumatic fever, this knowledge may make it possible to limit the inflammatory

response, including subsequent scarring, so that tissue structure and function may be preserved.

In this chapter, mechanisms by which the organism responds to injury have been presented. Inasmuch as these responses are appropriate and adequate, the survival of the organism is facilitated.

Though the role of the nurse has been indicated throughout the chapter, objectives of her care may be summarized as follows: (1) To control, or to teach the patient to control, agents causing injury of the tissue. This includes many activities: the prevention of fires and automobile accidents, the protection of an allergic person from the antigen or antigens to which he is susceptible, the maintenance of asepsis in the operating room and cleanliness in the areas where patients reside, and the prevention of sunburn. (2) To provide the necessary conditions for the tissue response to be adequate to the needs of the situation. This too involves a variety of activities ranging from those that have to do with supporting the arterial or venous circulation to providing the necessary nutritional elements. Although points were illustrated in many instances by relating the content to events occurring in patients treated by surgical therapy, all persons who are ill undergo similar responses. They may be less obvious and are sometimes of a lesser degree. All illness, however, of whatever degree is compounded of injury and the response of the individual to the injury.

Summary of Some of the Responses to Injury [*]

Respiration	Alimentary Canal	Other	Wound	Needs of the Patient

Phase I	Neuro-endocrine	Psychological	Circulatory	Metabolism	Water and Electrolytes	Blood
B. Injury 2-4 days patient looks and feels sick	Sympatho-adreno-medullary response (1–12 hr) ↑ Norepi-nephrine ↑ Epi-nephrine	Surrender, abdication of respon-sibility Listless, sleeps, "regressive integration" Egocentricity Constriction of interests or lack of interest Emotional dependency, with am-bivalence toward those on whom dependent	Tachycardia ↑ Cardiac output ↑ Systolic blood pressure Vasocon-striction ↑ Diastolic blood pressure Splenic contrac-tion to maintain blood volume ↑ Blood volume	↑ Hepatic glyco-genolysis, hyper-glycemia	Water loss from lungs, skin sweat-ing	↑ Platelets and fibrinogen ↓ Prothrombin time Results in accel-eration of blood clotting ↑ Sedimentation rate (varies with blood content of fibrinogen
Catabolism exceeds anabolism	Adenohy-pophysis (anterior pituitary) ↓ ACTH Adreno-cortical response ↑ Glucocor-ticoids ↑ Cortisol (peak 6 hr)	Hypochon-driasis		↓ Adrenal choles-terol and ascorbic acid ↑ Gluconeo-genesis ↓ Cellular glucose utiliza-tion ↑ Protein catab-olism ↓ Protein synthesis Negative nitrogen balance Nitrogen excretion in urine increased; may lose 7–15 g per day in ordinary soft-tissue injury ↑ Fat mobi-lization (from fat depots) ↑ 17-hydroxy-cortico-		Leukocytosis Lymphocytes and eosino-phils diminish in number Hyperglycemia

Summary of Some of the Responses to Injury (*cont.*) °

Respiration	Alimentary Canal	Other	Wound	Needs of the Patient
↑ Rate and depth Bronchial dilation ↑ Oxygen consumption As a result of anesthesia, drugs, unconsciousness, immobility, and other effects of illness, increased secretion into and interference with mechanisms for clearing the tracheobronchial tree predispose to obstruction of the airway	Peristalsis decreased or absent for 12–48 hr No appetite	Skin: ↑ sweating (cholinergic) Immobilization and splinting of wound with pain Resistance to movement, tries to find a comfortable position Hypothermia first 12 hr or so, then fever should not be over 100°F for 24–48 hr, and then return to normal	Lag or inflammatory phase Strength of wound is low Exudation of fluid into the wound— contains leukocytes and antibodies; exudate also contains protein, mucopolysaccharides, and ascorbic acid from which collagen fibers are formed During this time tissue debris and foreign materials are removed; this phase may be prolonged by the accumulation of blood, pus, or any other material in the wound that must be removed before wound healing can take place	The specific regime for each patient is prescribed by his physician Oral food and fluids are withheld until peristalsis is restored; encourage deep breathing, coughing, and turning, exercises of the extremities, and ambulation; patient requires assistance and support; protect from unnecessary stimulation, provide for periods of rest and quiet, use analgesics and other measures to prevent unnecessary pain; the nurse should assume responsibility for the care of the dependent patient; observe vital signs, urinary output in relation to intake, and if intake is exceeding output to an unexplained degree, report observation to the physician Note time, onset, degree of elevation of fever; should it be over 37.7°C (100°F) or continue at or above this level longer than usual 24–48 hr, this indicates that an infection may be developing; for example, incipient infection is often characterized by a marked rise in body temperature to 38.3°C (101°F) or higher All abdominal and chest wounds should be supported when the patient coughs; excessive and ineffective coughing should be avoided as it may lead to the disruption of an abdominal wound

TABLE 6-3

Phase II	Neuro-endocrine	Psychological	Circulatory	Metabolism	Water and Electrolytes	Blood
	↑ Adrenal androgens (slight)			steroid excretion ↑ 17-keto-steroid excretion in urine		
	↑ Aldosterone			↑ 11-oxy-steroid excretion		
	Neurohypophysis ↓ ↑ ADH			Rapid weight loss	Sodium retention Potassium excretion	
					Water retention resulting in oliguria for approximately 12 hrs after injury	
					Diuresis may begin in 1–2 days Diuresis of water and salt	
Turning point 3-7 days Patient begins to look and feel better	Adreno-medullary signs past Adreno-cortical secretion returns to normal	Ambition with weakness "I feel better today" Interested in surroundings, grooming and visitors	Normo-tension Normal cardiac output	↓ 17-hydroxy-cortico-steroid excretion ↓ Nitrogen excretion Wound begins to acquire tensile strength (stitches out)	Potassium excretion Body water still slightly high	Eosinophils and other leukocytes normal

Summary of Some of the Responses to Injury (*cont.*) *

Respiration	Alimentary Canal	Other	Wound	Needs of the Patient
		↓ Gonad, secretion, amenorrhea, ↓ libido		
Normal	Bowel sounds return Appetite improves	Temperature returns to normal	Chemical and morphological changes occur in the wound leading to the formation of scar tissue and the healing of wound	During this period the patient may feel better than he actually is; he should be protected from overactivity and overstimulation; food intake should be encouraged; high-quality proteins and food containing ascorbic acid are of particular importance The patient should be encouraged to be up and walking

TABLE 6-3

Phase III	Neuro-endocrine	Psychological	Circulatory	Metabolism	Water and Electrolytes	Blood
Muscular strength returns 2-5 weeks	Normal	↓ Reintegration of personality Relinquishes: dependence egocentricity provincial reactions rebellion against dependency wants to go home ambulation no longer painful ambition with increasing strength ↑	Normal	Positive nitrogen balance Weight gain Anabolism exceeds catabolism Resynthesis of muscle tissue	Normal	Normal

Phase IV	Neuro-endocrine	Psychological	Circulatory	Metabolism	Water and Electrolytes	Blood
Fat gain several months	Normal	↓ Returns to work	Normal	Positive nitrogen balance, carbon and energy balance Normal strength	Normal	Normal

Summary of Some of the Responses to Injury (*cont.*) *

Respiration	Alimentary Canal	Other	Wound	Needs of the Patient
Normal	Absorption capacity returns	Needs adequate diet and exercise May attempt premature overwork	Wound broader, raised red scar, tensile integrity established and function of soft tissues resumed	Patient should not return to work involving heavy muscular exercise until this phase has been completed Normal strength returns Adequate intake of protein and calories; may need 2,000–3,000 calories per day; severely burned patients may need more; patients leaving the hospital during the seventh to tenth day may need to be instructed to eat well; without an adequate intake of food convalescence may be delayed

Respiration	Alimentary Canal	Other	Wound	Needs of the Patient
Normal	Normal	Looks underweight, at beginning Clothes fit loosely May tend to overeat Normal sexual function returns	During this time the wound loses its convex and reddened appearance; it becomes a concave, thin white line	The patient is able to return to his ordinary occupation The patient's food intake should exceed his energy output until desired weight is regained; when this has been acomplished, food intake should be balanced with energy output so that obesity is avoided

Henry D. Lederer: "How the Sick View Their World," *Patients, Physicians and Illness*, E. G. Jaco, ed. (New York: The Free Press, 1958), pp. 247–56.
Francis D. Moore: *Metabolic Care of the Surgical Patient* (Philadelphia: W. B. Saunders Company, 1959), pp. 25–48.
Ruy Perez-Tamayo: *Mechanisms of Disease* (Philadelphia: W. B. Saunders Company, 1961), pp. 452–57.

REFERENCES

BOOKS

American Physiological Society: *Handbook of Physiology*, Section 4. *Adaptation to the Environment* (Baltimore: Waverly Press, Inc., 1964).

Bajusz, E.: *Physiology and Pathology of Adaptation Mechanisms: Neural-Neuro-Endocrine-Hormonal* (New York: Pergamon Press, Inc., 1968).

Chapman, C. B. (ed.): *Physiology of Muscular Exercise* (New York: American Heart Association, 1967).

Dixon, Frank J., and Kunkel, Henry G. (eds.): *Advances in Immunology*, Vol. 9 (New York: Academic Press, Inc., 1968).

Ganong, William F.: *Review of Medical Physiology*, 4th ed. (Los Altos: Lange Medical Publications, 1969).

Gell, P. G. H., and Coombs, R. R. A.: *Clinical Aspects of Immunology*, 2nd ed. (Philadelphia: F. A. Davis Company, 1968).

Janeway, Charles A., *et al.: The Gamma Globulins* (Boston: Little, Brown & Company, 1967).

Larson, Carroll B., and Gould, Marjorie: *Calderwood's Orthopedic Nursing*, 6th ed. (St. Louis: The C. V. Mosby Company, 1965).

Lissák, K., and Endröczi, E.: *The Neuroendocrine Control of Adaptation* (New York: Pergamon Press, Inc., 1965).

Noback, Charles R.: *The Human Nervous System* (New York: McGraw-Hill Book Company, Inc., 1967).

Pirovsky, B.: *Autoimmunity and the Autoimmune Hemolytic Anemias* (Baltimore: The Williams & Wilkins Company, 1969).

Thomas, Lewis, Uhr, Jonathan W., and Grant, Lester: *International Symposium on Injury, Inflammation and Immunity* (Baltimore: The Williams & Wilkins Company, 1964).

Transplant. Partial Proceedings of the 1968 John F. Kennedy Symposium on Recent, Significant Developments in Medicine and Surgery. (Sommerville, N.J.: Medical Communications Inc., 1969.)

PERIODICALS

Immunology

Batchelor, J. R.: "Histocompatibility Systems," *Brit. Med. Bull.*, 21:100–105 (No. 2) 1965.

Cohen, E. P.: "On the Mechanism of Immunity—in Defense of Evolution," *Ann. Rev. Microbiol.*, 22:283–304, 1968.

Coombs, R. R. A.: "Immunopathology," *Brit. Med. J.*, 1:597–602 (Mar. 9) 1968.

Craddock, Charles G., *et al.:* "The Immune System, Immunoglobulins, and Some Disorders of the Lymphatic System," *Ann. Intern. Med.*, 64:687–708 (Mar.) 1966.

Gewurz, Henry: "The Immunologic Role of Complement," *Hosp. Practice*, 2:44–50, 54–56 (Sept.) 1967.

Good, Robert A.: "Disorders of the Immune System," *Hosp. Practice*, 2:38–53 (Jan.) 1967.

Holborow, E. J.: "The Genesis of Immunological Competence," *Lancet*, 1:1148–50 (May 27) 1967.

"Immunoglobulins and Disease," *Ther. Notes*, 74: 120–24 (Sept.–Oct.) 1967.

"The Immunological Orchestra," *Lancet*, 1:185–86 (Jan. 27) 1968.

"Immunology," *Nurs. Times*, 64:1244–45 (Sept. 13) 1968.

Jones, Barbara: "Inside the Coronary Care Unit: The Patient and His Responses," *Amer. J. Nurs.*, 67:2313–20 (Nov.) 1967.

Kretschmer, Roberto, *et al.:* "Congenital Aplasia of the Thymus Gland (DiGeorge's Syndrome)," *New Eng. J. Med.*, 279:1295–1301 (Dec. 12) 1968.

Lischner, Harold W., and DiGeorge, Angelo M.: "Role of Thymus in Humoral Immunity," *Lancet*, 2:1044–48 (Nov. 15) 1969.

"A Proposed Classification of Primary Immunologic Deficiencies," *Amer. J. Med.*, 45:817–25 (Dec.) 1968.

Nye, Alice Wade, *et al.:* "Sixteen Patients: Postoperative Nursing Experience with Heart Transplantation," *Amer. J. Nurs.*, 69:2630–34 (Dec.) 1969.

Schlossman, Stuart F.: "The Immune Response: Some Unifying Concepts," *New Eng. J. Med.*, 277:1355–61 (Dec. 21) 1967.

Singer, S. J., and Doolittle, Russell F.: "Antibody Active Sites and Immunoglobulin Molecules," *Science*, 153:13–25 (July 1) 1966.

Terry, William D.: "Structural Characteristics of Human Immunoglobulins," *Postgrad. Med.*, 41: 133–43 (Feb.) 1967.

"Thymus," *Ther. Notes*, 72:8–12 (Jan.) 1965.

Tomasi, Thomas B.: "Human Immunoglobulin A," *New Eng. J. Med.*, 279:1327–30 (Dec. 12) 1968.

Wilkinson, R.: "Gamma Globulins in Health and Disease," *Nurs. Times*, 64:725–28 (May 31) 1968.

Witebsky, Ernest: "Autosensitization: A New Concept in Pathology," *Ther. Notes*, 72:15–18 (Jan.) 1965.

Witebsky, Ernest: "Immunology: Views of the Past and Visions for the Future," *Canad. Med. Ass. J.*, 97:1371–77 (Dec. 2) 1967.

Neuroendocrine Responses

Beisel, William R., and Rapoport, Morton I.: "Inter-relations Between Adrenocortical Functions and Infectious Illness," *New Eng. J. Med.*, 280: 541–46 (Mar. 6) 1969, 280:596–604 (Mar. 13) 1969.

"Symposium on the Autonomic Nervous System," *Anesthesiology*, 29:621–827 (July–Aug.) 1968.

Wynn, Victor: "The Anabolic Steroids," *Practitioner,* **200**:509–18 (Apr.) 1968.

Immunosuppressive Agents

Berenbaum, M. C.: "Immunosuppressive Agents," *Proc. Roy. Soc. Med.,* **60**:125–28 (Feb.) 1967.

DiPalma, Joseph R.: "Drugs Used in Organ Transplants," *RN,* **32**:53–63 (Mar.) 1969.

Kiser, William S., and Kolff, Willem J.: "When Is Transplantation of Organs Feasible or Practical?" *DM,* 3–32 (Sept.) 1967.

Woodruff, M. F. A.: "Immunosuppression in Relation to Organ Transplantation," *Proc. Roy. Soc. Med.,* **60**:128–30 (Feb.) 1967.

Ethical Aspects of Transplantation

Hall, Jacquelyn H., and Swenson, David D.: Psychological and Social Aspects of Human Tissue Transplantation (Chevy Chase, Md.: National Clearinghouse for Mental Health Information, 1968).

Lister, John: "Medicine, Morals and Money," *New Eng. J. Med.,* **276**:971–72 (Apr. 27) 1967.

Murray, Joseph E., and Lynch, John J.: "Ethical Implications of Renal Transplants," *JAMA,* **200**:187 (Apr. 10) 1967.

Wound Healing

Ross, Russell: "Wound Healing," *Sci. Amer.,* **220**: 40–50 (June) 1969.

Allergic Responses

Cannon, Paul J.: "Antihistamines," *Practitioner,* **200**:53–64 (Jan.) 1968.

deGara, Paul F.: "Allergy's Widening Horizon," *Ann. Allerg.,* **26**:614–15 (Nov.) 1968.

Feinberg, Samuel M.: "Allergies and Air Conditioning," *Amer. J. Nurs.,* **66**:1333–36 (June) 1966.

7

The Psychosocial Aspects of Illness *

Canst thou not . . . raze out the written troubles of the brain,
And with some sweet oblivious antidote
Cleanse the stuff'd bosom of that perilous stuff
Which weighs upon the heart?

SHAKESPEARE, *Macbeth,* Act V, Scene 3

Overview

What factors must a nurse consider when dealing with a hospitalized patient?

Cultural Elements Having the Greatest Significance for the Practice of Nursing

How does the patient feel he ought to behave during his illness?

How does the nurse feel the patient ought to behave during his illness?

Psychological Elements Having the Greatest Significance for the Practice of Nursing

Nursing Care

How can the nurse identify the patient's emotional reaction to his illness?

How can the nurse minimize psychological stress through nursing intervention?

Overview

In the preceding chapters, the concept was developed that human beings have physiological and psychosocial needs that must be met if the individual is to survive, grow, reproduce, and be productive. Each person has a physical structure that not only enables him to react to change in his physical and social environment but also helps to determine the limits of his capacity for adaptation. Adaptation to change, within oneself or within the environment, is also dependent on the individual's intellectual and emotional capacity—his ability to identify, examine, and master problems. The over-all capacity for adaptation varies from individual to individual and within the same individual from time to time. In this chapter the content has been selected to provide the nurse with knowledge of some of the factors to be considered if the psychosocial needs of patients with medical-surgical problems are to be met. It is not within the scope of this book to discuss the causes and effects of serious disturbances in the interpersonal and social spheres of the individual. With most individuals, however, illness that requires medical attention causes

some disturbance in the person's interpersonal and social functioning. These disturbances arise out of the meaning that illness has for the person physically, emotionally, and intellectually. How he responds to his illness will also depend on the value that his family and culture place on the "sick role." His behavior is also influenced by the responses he receives in the hospital culture. In other words, how others treat him when he is ill depends on the interplay of meanings that he and significant others attach to his illness and behavior.

To provide a common understanding, the terms *psychology, society,* and *culture* will be defined.

Psychology is defined as a science that is primarily interested in the study of the individual as a thinking, remembering, imagining, feeling, and reacting person. Psychology looks at the behavior of individuals as a means of understanding the intrapersonal and interpersonal processes that stimulated the behavior. According to Lewin,[1] behavior and development depend on the state of the person and his environment. This means that in order to understand

[1] Kurt Lewin: *Field Theory in Social Science* (New York: Harper Torchbooks, 1964), pp. 239–40.

---

* This chapter revised by Jean A. Werner, M.N., R.N., Associate Professor of Nursing, Wayne State University, College of Nursing, Detroit, Michigan.

or predict behavior the person and his environment have to be considered as a unit composed of interdependent factors.

Society refers to the association of individuals in organized relationships of mutual dependence.[2] The system of a society, according to Biesanz,[3] includes the division of labor persisting within a certain time and place and the sharing of common goals. *Social* is an adjective used to describe the relationships of one person to another.

Culture, as defined by Biesanz,[4] is *"the learned portion of human behavior,* the ways of thinking, feeling and doing that man himself has developed as part of his environment."* This refers to understandings concerning the value of things, ideas, emotions, and actions. Thus culture even defines how one should feel in different situations—love of country, grief at the loss of something loved, and so on. Culture also defines how these emotions are to be expressed, within certain social contexts, and this mode of expression may vary from one culture to another.[5] Culture is peculiar to man in that it arises out of language communication.[6] Animals such as the wolf organize themselves into societies, but they cannot be said to possess a "culture."

Sciences such as sociology and cultural anthropology are those that deal with social action and the behavior of human beings. Together with psychology they are classified as behavioral sciences. Some appreciation of all three is important in nursing in order to understand man and his reactions to illness—not as an isolated individual but as an individual who is a member of a society and, in part, a product of his culture.

In recent years interest has increased in extending knowledge of the psychological and cultural factors that influence the acceptance, use, or rejection of health services. Many of the questions that have been and are being investigated are familiar to nurses. For example, why do some people seek medical attention at appropriate intervals whereas others do not? Even among those who appear to accept advice and follow instructions, cooperation may appear to be more complete than it actually is. The behavior among those who do not seek medical attention, or who ignore or reject advice, also varies. Some seek attention so late in the course of illness that little can be done to restore health or to reverse the disease process. Others seek attention and then openly or quietly refuse to follow recommendations or to permit themselves to be treated. On the other side of the coin, needed treatment may be difficult to obtain. By the time the individual is admitted to a treatment facility it is possible that the point of greatest possible recovery is past. Remotivation toward participation in treatment becomes an extremely difficult task for both the patient and the health team.

Answers to questions such as the following may provide clues for extending the use of available community services. For example, why did Mr. and Mrs. Earl respond to an extensive educational program by having their children immunized for poliomyelitis and diphtheria, whereas Mr. and Mrs. Gray did not? Why does Mrs. Far consider herself to be ill when she has a cold, whereas Mrs. Hays continues with her ordinary activities and resents any comments about her cold? What determines the individual's pattern of behavior when he is ill?

What factors must a nurse consider when dealing with a hospitalized patient?

Because illness involving hospitalization is usually regarded as an extremely disruptive situation by the patient and his family, the patient can be expected to experience fear and anxiety. Frequently these feelings are related to the individual's being placed in a dependent role, and the feelings may gain expression through regressive or seemingly infantile behavior. The hospitalization may be viewed by the patient as either a stressful situation or a crisis. Rapoport[7] distinguishes *stress* from *crisis* by stating that the concept of stress most often carries a negative connotation. In stress the person views his situation as a burden or load under which he will survive or break. Crisis, on the other hand, has a growth-promoting potential; it calls the person to new action, brings forth new coping mechanisms to meet the challenge, strengthens the person's adaptive capacity, and is thought to raise the individual's level of mental health. Stress, however, is thought to have great potential for reducing the individual's level of mental health.[8] How a patient views his illness depends not only on his inner resources but on how he is assisted to deal with the situation in which he finds himself. Nurses frequently can assist patients to view hospitalization either positively or negatively depending on how they relate to the patient.

[2] John Biesanz and Mavis Biesanz: *Modern Society,* 3rd ed. (Englewood Cliffs, N.J.: Prentice-Hall, Inc., 1964), p. 87.

[3] *Ibid.,* p. 87.

[4] *Ibid.,* p. 25.

[5] *Ibid.,* p. 44.

[6] *Ibid.,* p. 25.

[7] Lydia Rapoport: "The State of Crisis: Some Theoretical Considerations," *Crisis Intervention: Selected Readings,* Howard J. Parad, ed. (New York: Family Service Association of America, 1965), p. 23.

[8] *Ibid.,* p. 23.

If the preceding concepts are accepted, why do those who care for Mrs. Marks consider her behavior as cooperative, courageous, and sensible and describe her as a fine woman because she takes adversity without a murmur? Why, on the other hand, is Mrs. Crane's seemingly irrational behavior equated with stubbornness, ignorance, or stupidity? Why is she looked on as childish, demanding, and lacking in self-control and self-discipline? Why does Mr. Robbin resist every suggestion or effort to help him? Why does Mr. Nelson accept the care offered without question and make no extra demands on the nursing staff? Why is Mr. Nelson described as a good patient? Why do nurses like to care for Mrs. Marks and Mr. Nelson and avoid, when possible, the care of Mrs. Crane and Mr. Robbin? Why is one person satisfied with hospital care whereas another feels that the care received was unfeeling and inadequate?

Other questions arise out of the observation that there seems to be a direct relationship between the way a person perceives his illness and his chances for recovery. Why do some patients deal with their illness realistically and engage in treatment? Why do others react with feelings of fear, loathing, or dread that seems out of proportion to the nature of their illness and that may inhibit recovery? For example, why does Mr. Hall strive to recover from a severe stroke, whereas Mr. Donald, who appears to have had a slight stroke, makes little effort to recover?

A complete answer to any one of these questions is, of course, impossible without much more information about each individual and his life situation. However, these illustrations suggest three general questions. Why do people behave the way they do? What purpose does their behavior serve? How can this knowledge be used in the practice of nursing?

A general answer to these questions is that people behave as they do in order to meet obvious (overt) or hidden (covert) needs. Failure to satisfy a need results in behavior that is directed toward its satisfaction. This behavior may not always seem reasonable or rational to the observer in that it does not communicate clearly and concisely really what is *the need*. Yet, the goal of behavior is need satisfaction even though the behavior may fall short of obtaining the satisfaction desired. Much of the behavior that results in the satisfaction of needs is learned. What a person eats and enjoys depends, to some extent, on his family and cultural background. How he behaves when he is in a situation where food is not available in the form and amount he prefers is also partially dependent on past learnings. However, to add to the complexity of the individual, one cannot discount newly incorporated learnings.

Knowledge of family and cultural patterns is helpful in the identification of needs that can be met by nursing and in the selection of the manner in which care is provided. Obviously, the nurse cannot be expected to know or anticipate all the variations in a patient's expectations that may arise out of family and cultural patterns. The nurse should have enough understanding of the influence of her own family and culture on herself—regarding values, goals, expectations, and modes of expression—to be able to understand that similar influences also affect people in general. The nurse should also have knowledge of the characteristic features of several cultural groups and be prepared to consider the possibility that a patient's behavior may have cultural origins. Instead of categorizing the patient's behavior as abnormal or peculiar, the nurse may find that the patient is acting according to the dictates of his culture. Considered from this standpoint, his behavior is reasonable even though not in keeping with the nurse's personal standards for behavior given a similar situation.

According to Biesanz,[9] all cultures include an *economic system* that includes beliefs and practices governing the production, distribution, and consumption of goods and services. The economic system also encompasses the technology necessary to produce these goods and services. Every culture has a social structure that includes the family system, which, in turn, regulates sex behavior and defines rights and responsibilities regarding the procreation and education of children. Religion, systems of government, and general beliefs concerning "good" and "bad" are also included under social structure. Language, as mentioned previously, is necessary for the existence of culture and is, therefore, a universal element of cultures. Variations occur in cultures and seem to result from man's adaptability, creativity, intelligence, and accidents of original choices.[10]

Cultural Elements Having the Greatest Significance for the Practice of Nursing

Although all elements of culture may be significant in patient care at one time or another, there are some elements that are generally thought to be more significant than others. These are (1) language; (2) religion; (3) orientation to time; (4) food habits; (5) values as they relate to age and sex; (6) patterns of family organization and child care; (7) patterns of care during birth, sickness, and death; (8) patterns of sleep and personal hygiene; (9)

[9] Biesanz, *op. cit.,* p. 36–37.
[10] *Ibid.,* p. 39.

patterns of modesty; (10 methods of communicating satisfaction and dissatisfaction; and (11) values placed on individuality and personal achievement. Circumstances that influence cultural and subcultural differences in the United States include (1) place of residence—such as city or country, North or South, and segregated or integrated; (2) socioeconomic status; (3) place of birth—United States or foreign country; and (4) level of education, including professional education. As the level of education of people rises, differences among people tend to become less marked.

These elements serve as the basis for the way in which a given culture plans for and meets the problems that arise out of illness. They also affect the way in which an individual within a culture regards illness and what he does to prevent illness or to treat it. In other words, each person brings to every situation (1) a set of values, (2) a set of expectations, (3) a code of behavior—an internalized set of rules or standards that guide his conduct, (4) customs and ceremonies he observes, and (5) manner and vocabulary by which he communicates nonverbally as well as verbally with other people. An important aspect of communication in nursing is understanding the manner in which satisfaction and dissatisfaction are expressed. Without this information the nurse may have difficulty determining whether or not the patient's needs are being met.

To illustrate and clarify the preceding statements, a folkway that is characteristic of middle- and upper-income groups in Western society will be described. The situation is one in which Mr. and Mrs. Holt invite Mr. and Mrs. Questa for supper. The language and the manner in which the invitation is extended provide information about things such as the degree of formality, purpose, and others likely to be invited. Depending on these and other factors, each person will bring with him a unique set of expectations about how the guests and host and hostess should behave and be treated and what constitutes hospitality. They also have a set of standards to guide their conduct, a set of customs and ceremonies they observe, and even a terminology for communicating with each other.

When the expectations of both the host and the guest are the same, few problems arise. When expectations differ, the guest may arrive and find his host in his shirt sleeves and the hostess in the bathtub or find that the roast is dried out. The host and guests also have ways of expressing their satisfaction or dissatisfaction with each other. They may be sincere or they may try to cover up their true feelings. When they say good night, they may express

pleasure despite the fact that the evening was dull.

Although this illustration could be expanded further, enough detail has been presented to make the point that each individual has a set of expectations, a code that guides his behavior, customs he observes, and a terminology for expressing his meanings. Social functions are usually more mutually satisfying when the host and guests have similar expectations or when each is aware that the other has expectations different from his own and takes these into consideration. Moreover, when a host invites a comparative stranger into his home he attempts to learn something about this stranger. He attempts to apprise his guest of what to expect so that he can plan in terms of his needs. If the host values this relationship he does not show disrespect for his guest by ignoring or condemning practices that have value and meaning to the guest. For example, he does not serve pork chops to an Orthodox Jew. At the same time the host should be able to expect mutual respect from his guest. The guest, therefore, does not expect his host to serve cocktails if the host disapproves of alcoholic beverages.

In the care of the sick, the relationship between nurse and patient has some of the same overtones as the host-guest relationship, and yet there are important differences. The nurse is a member of a service profession, and the person who comes seeking that service is called a "patient." The nurse, by virtue of her education, is in a position to make a decision about whether or not she can render the service being sought. The sick person is seeking help for some personal problem and therefore does not have the expectation of mutual give-and-take that is part of the social encounter. It suffices to say that knowledge of the elements of culture should be helpful to the nurse in anticipating the patient's needs and in personalizing his care. In Chapter 12, attention will be given to the cultural aspects of food. Because of the limitations of the scope of this book, American patterns of child care and of childbirth will not be included.

Religion

Religion is an essential consideration in the care of each patient. A simple definition of religion is that it is man's idea of God and of his relationship to Him. It also includes the way in which man shows his respect and love for God. Respect for the person includes respect for his right to practice his religion. The nurse, physician, social worker, and teacher must accept the person's right to his own religious beliefs. Many people who are ill turn to their religion for solace. The nurse can be helpful by making it easy for the patient to see his pastor or a clergyman of his faith. The nurse also needs to have some understanding of what is important to the patient so that she can anticipate his religious needs. Thus the nurse contributes to the patient's welfare by supporting his right to his religious faith—this may include his faith and hope that his suffering is not in vain. The nurse also does what she can to ease the patient's suffering and to keep his hope alive. References are given at the end of this chapter that give more specific information about the major faiths.

Patterns of Family Organization

Patterns of family organization are important if one is to understand certain responses that patients have to patterns of care. Although all possible patterns of family organization cannot be described, knowledge about who is the head of the family, who is responsible in time of crisis such as illness, how the members of the family regard each other, and similar information may be helpful. In the United States we have three kinds of family life generally: patriarchal, matriarchal, and equalitarian. The last is a product of the twentieth century and is not generally seen in cultures other than our own. In the patriarchal family the husband makes the decisions. In the matriarchal family the wife is the head of the family and, therefore, makes the decisions. In the equalitarian family decisions are made jointly. To illustrate, the wife is behaving appropriately in the patriarchal family when she submissively accepts her husband's decisions. When she is ill or requires medical attention she should be expected to behave in a similar manner. It would be in error to expect a woman from a patriarchal system to behave in the same way as a woman who has been head of the family or who has supported herself for some length of time. She should not be expected to engage in decisions about plans for therapy or change without having an opportunity to ask her husband.

A certain amount of disruption in the family is to be expected when a member is ill. The degree of disturbance will depend in part on the role in the family of the person who is ill. According to Parsons and Fox,[11] illness of the mother is more disturbing to the rest of the family than is sickness of either the father or one of the children. They believe this is true because the mother provides the primary emotional support for the other members. Christopherson [12] states that the culture prescribes unique sex roles for men and women. When, for example, illness forces one to retreat from their usual sex role the results are potentially serious. Individuals frequently need help to cope with alterations in culturally prescribed roles that result from illness or disability.[13]

Until recently, the trend toward hospitalization of the sick has increased. This has been particularly true for those who are seriously ill or for whom the illness is prolonged. Reasons given for caring for patients in hospitals include the fact that specialized services and equipment are available and that the patients can be given care that would be impossible for them to have at home. Sometimes this is true. Sociologists also suggest other reasons for caring for the sick in specialized institutions. One of these is that it serves to protect the family from the disrupting effects of having a sick person in their midst. In a small two- or three-bedroom house the continued presence of a seriously ill person may place great physical and emotional strain on the family. A trend is developing, however, toward returning the sick to their homes earlier than has been the general practice in the immediate past. The success of this plan depends, among other things, on the patient, the nature of his illness, the family strengths, the attitudes of the members of the family toward each other and toward the illness, and their acceptance of the patient and the plan to care for him at home. It also depends on the provision of the kinds of services to the patient and his family that make it possible for him to be cared for, or to care for himself, at home. These services include medical and nursing care, physical therapy, housekeeping, and occupational therapy. Ambulance service may be provided to return the patient to the hospital for a needed service such as an x-ray or for hospitalization. In some instances, home care is easier for the patient and family to accept when they are assured that the patient will be readmitted to the hospital promptly should this be necessary.

Not all cultures care for their sick in the hospital. In fact they may look on the hospital as a cold and formal place that can in no way substitute for the presence of a loving family. For example, Saunders cites the instance of the young girl whose family would not permit her to be hospitalized for the treatment of tuberculosis because they believed that the sick should have the care and support of the family. The fact that the girl was capable of infecting the

---

[11] Talcott Parsons and Renée Fox: "Illness, Therapy and the Modern Urban American Family," *Patients, Physicians and Illness,* E. Gartly Jaco, ed. (New York: The Free Press, 1958), p. 239.

[12] Victor A. Christopherson: "Role Modification of the Disabled Male," *Amer. J. Nurs.,* **68**:291 (Feb.) 1968.

[13] *Ibid.,* p. 291.

family was of no importance to them. Neither did they believe that she might be given better care in the hospital than at home.[14] In other cultures, support is provided by one or more of the members of the family going to the hospital with the patient and staying until he is well. They may cook his meals and provide for his personal care. Probably one of the greatest values of this practice derives from the fact that the patient shifts his concern for his welfare to his family. They are there. They will be responsible. They will take care of him.

Practices in the care of the dying and the dead vary in different cultures all the way from placing the dying outside the village limits or deserting them to taking extraordinary measures to preserve life. Though the desertion of the sick and infirm seems cruel, in primitive societies this may be necessary to the survival of others. There are also those who question the kindness of taking extreme measures to continue life in the seriously disabled or diseased person.[15] In the American culture there is a tendency to protect the young from knowledge of death and from the dying. Many who die, die in hospitals, where they are separated from family members by equipment, procedures, and personnel. Most students of nursing have had little if any experience with death. Many adults are fearful in the presence of the dying person. Mrs. Carol Willis (see Chapter 3) was well aware of this when she said, "We embarrass our friends." She also said that one of the needs of the dying person is for someone to listen. As long as the nurse is primarily concerned with her own fears about death and dying, she cannot be an empathetic listener.

The attitude of those caring for the sick aged may be adversely influenced by the fact that, in the American culture, youth is the idealized state. In some cultures youth is considered to be a handicap and age is respected because it brings with it experience and wisdom. In these cultures the aged are given status rather than being relegated to the background.

Another factor influencing the status and role of an individual in his group is his sex. In some cultures the male has a higher status than the female, though the reverse is true in some cultures. In most cultures the relationships between the sexes are defined, as are the occupations and activities that are fitting for, or expected of, one and not the other. Appropriate behavior is also defined in terms of sex. For example, in the Anglo-American culture women may cry with-

out losing status. Men may not. In a society such as ours, what is acceptable behavior is subject to change. Not too many years ago "nice" women did not smoke cigarettes or wear trousers in public. Now they do both. To satisfy the patient's needs requires some knowledge of how he regards his role and what he considers is and is not proper for him to do.

Language

Language is, of course, necessary for communication. Even when two people speak the same language, difficulties in communication may arise out of the fact that although two people use the same words they may interpret them differently. Inflection, tone, and nonverbal behavior also contribute to giving a variety of meanings to words. Listening to what is said will help diminish distortions in communication. People in the hospital culture, including nurses, frequently are guilty of jumping to the conclusion that they understand exactly what the patient is trying to say even before the patient gets it said. This so-called "mind-reading ploy" is both infuriating and frightening because the patient tends to think what he wants is discounted, and he begins to wonder if he will be heard if something *really* important does arise. When people speak different languages, some means other than verbal communication must be used. If there is someone available who speaks the patient's language, he should be used as an interpreter. Suitable provisions must also be made to communicate with the patient who is unable to speak because of a defect in his nervous system or organs of speech. Sign language or writing may be used. Although nonverbal communication is always important, it becomes increasingly significant when caring for patients who are unable to send or receive messages through the use of speech. In such instances increased awareness of cultural factors —family and preillness patterns of the individual—is often helpful in achieving a better understanding of the person while he is in the hospital. Nursing care that is carried out in an attitude of kindness and true concern for the patient will do much to overcome barriers created by the lack of a common language.

Orientation to Time

Some problems in the care of patients arise out of differences in orientation to time and value placed on it. Orientation to time may be to the past, present, or future. This is illustrated in the literature of various peoples. For example, in our literature the ant spends the summer busily storing supplies for the coming

[14] Lyle Saunders: *Cultural Difference and Medical Care* (New York: Russell Sage Foundation, 1954), pp. 16–17.
[15] "A Way of Dying," *Atlantic Monthly,* **199**:53–55 (Jan.) 1957.

winter months, whereas the improvident grass-hopper dashes around enjoying himself. It is quite shocking to Americans to learn that there are cultures in which the ant is viewed as the foolish one and the grasshopper is wise. From the latter point of view, the present is what one has. Why expend effort for a time that may never be. A third orientation to time was held by some Chinese in bygone days. They believed that the future is behind one and therefore cannot be seen. They are said to have built pleasure gardens along the side of the streams where they sat facing downstream contemplating the past.

That not all Americans have the same view of time is borne out in a study by Koos.[16] In this study he found that respondents from class I (upper) looked toward the future; those from class II (middle) were primarily occupied with the present; and those in class III (lower) had little hope in either the present or the future. In general, middle-class Americans look at the present as better than the past, and the future is expected to be better than either. In another study, Saunders found that Spanish-speaking Americans who live in the southwestern part of the United States lived in the present or immediate past rather than in the past or the future. He states that this creates a problem in their medical care. How can they know whether they want a clinic appointment next week when they do not know how they will be feeling at that time? According to their perception of time, this is a logical conclusion. When they are talked into making clinic appointments, they may or may not keep them. If on the day of the appointment they feel well, they see no reason to keep it.[17]

Because of the trend in the American culture to consider the future important, Americans provide for old age and for illness and death by buying some type of insurance. People who fail, or are unable, to do this are generally considered to be improvident. As a result of the depression that began in 1929, the fact that industrial workers were not always able to protect themselves against unemployment was recognized. In 1935 the Social Security Act was passed. It had three provisions based on the principle that society has an obligation to provide for the security of its people. The first provision was for unemployment compensation to be handled by the states. The second was establishment of an annuity that was to be paid at age 65 or on retirement of its members. The third provided for special categories of needy persons including the aged, the blind, the

crippled and disabled, and dependent children. The Social Security Amendments of 1965 added Medicare and Medicaid, recognizing that there are increasing numbers of elderly people in this country where there are diminishing extended family systems that will assume responsibility for the aging. In this way the government has assumed responsibility for helping people provide for the future.

The other dimension of time is the value placed on it. Time is sometimes equated with success by Americans. It is generally believed to have value in achieving success, as it can be used with profit or it can be wasted. Sayings in the American language such as "Time waits for no man" or "Time is money" indicate this. When one is employed by another he most often sells his time rather than his productivity. He may punch a time clock when he arrives at and when he leaves his place of employment. An employee is usually paid for the number of hours rather than for the units of work. There is a tendency to judge efficiency in terms of the individual's ability to appear to be busy at any given moment. Nurses are judged by this standard. Most nurses are employed for 40 hours per week. The nurse who is busy is commended. The one who is not occupied in some task and is seen talking with patients is often viewed as using her time in a frivolous manner. There is probably more than one instance when a nurse has been interrupted in the course of talking with a patient about some meaningful feeling or problem. The interruption is prefaced too often by, "As long as you're not doing anything. . . ." The transmission of such values certainly encourages nurses to be utilitarian rather than humanitarian in their practice.

Because of the emphasis placed on the value of time in the American culture, it is not surprising that the sick person places great importance on having his medications and treatments at the time they are scheduled. The patient frequently judges the quality of his care by how closely nurses adhere to the schedule. As was seen in the previous paragraph, nurses themselves communicate that this is where the value lies. The patient not only brings some orientation to the value of time with him to the hospital, but he quickly has this orientation reinforced by the hospital value system. In our culture time carries elements of security, caring, and control, and violations of schedules may give rise to anxious feelings that gain expression through a wide range of behaviors. The hospitalized patient has the feeling that there is so little he can control—about the course of his illness or the nature of the treatment he will receive—that he tends to focus on those things, such as the nurse's punctuality, where he may

[16] Earl L. Koos: *The Health of Regionville* (New York: Columbia University Press, 1954), pp. 21–24.
[17] Saunders, *op. cit.*, pp. 117–22.

be able to exercise some controlling influence. For example, Mrs. Pope, who was hospitalized for an extended period, was allowed to spend weekends at home provided she arrange to have a nurse administer Acthar [18] by intramuscular injection both at 8 o'clock in the morning and in the evening. When the nurse was even a few minutes late, Mrs. Pope became very agitated, thus placing a strain on the nurse. In this instance the nurse recognized the importance of time to Mrs. Pope and made an effort to arrive a few minutes early. Our example does not help us understand exactly what time meant to Mrs. Pope; that would require further exploration based on the nurse's observation that Mrs. Pope became agitated when the nurse was late.

Sleep and Personal Hygiene Patterns

Some knowledge of the sleep patterns of the person may be useful when providing care. For example, the person may be accustomed to having a room of his own or to sharing his room with another. If the first person is in a large ward, he may have difficulty in sleeping, whereas the second may be lonely when he is by himself. This does not mean that the nurse may be able to alter the situation, but she can be understanding of the patient's difficulties. Perhaps more attention should be given to the patient's habits of personal hygiene than is often done. Not all people come from areas where a daily bath or shower is possible. Some even live where taking a bath entails a good bit of effort and planning. Old people, especially old men, may suffer itching of the skin when they bathe more than once or twice a week. Conversely, there are those who bathe daily and are upset when they cannot. This point can be illustrated by two brothers, Allen and Bert, who were seriously ill. Allen was much upset because his nurse insisted on giving him a bath every morning. Bert was upset for an entire day because he did not have a bath. In neither instance did the patient's physical welfare depend on whether or not he had a bath. Other aspects of personal hygiene that are sometimes neglected and at other times forced on reluctant or protesting patients include the opportunity to brush their teeth, to have their hair combed, to wash their hands after using the bedpan, and to have back care. The point here is to try to learn

something about the personal habits and expectations of the patient. When something in the nature of the illness of the person necessitates a change, then the cooperation of the patient should be enlisted. The nurse should assess those aspects of hygienic care that are essential to the welfare and peace of mind of the patient and modify the care accordingly.

Expression of Satisfaction and Dissatisfaction

There are innumerable ways in which people can express their satisfactions and dissatisfactions. Though either may be expressed directly, they may also be expressed indirectly. For example, a patient may smile and say that everything is fine and be sincere, or he may feel quite differently. Sometimes the nurse may detect something in the patient's tone of voice, expression, or position that tells her that everything is not fine. He may not wish to hurt her feelings, or he may want her approval, or he may feel that she is not really interested, or he may even feel that it is not safe for him to express his dissatisfaction directly. He may also express his dissatisfaction indirectly by being demanding or hypercritical. Sometimes only after the nurse has made considerable effort to develop a trusting relationship will the patient express his true feelings.

Place of Residence

Place of residence is another factor that influences the cultural and subcultural differences in people. In the United States there is less difference between city and country people than there once was. However, differences do continue to exist, particularly in those instances where a group is segregated or isolated, either by choice or by custom, from the remainder of the population. For example, some religious groups, such as the Mennonites and Amish, settle in communities in order to protect and maintain a way of life that is essential to the practice of their religion. Though the situation is changing slowly, Negroes living in rural areas in the South are isolated from the white population. One preliminary study of the behavior of hospitalized Negro patients being cared for by white nurses has been reported by McCabe.[19] Although she is careful to state that her conclusions are tentative, effective care of these patients appears to depend on the nurse's being aware of the patient's expectations of the nurse's behavior, as well as her own expectations. McCabe also indicates that to evaluate

---

[18] Acthar (adrenocorticotropic hormone) is a trade name for an extract of anterior pituitary glands, prepared for parenteral use in doses of 25, 40, and 80 U.S.P. units. It acts by stimulating the adrenal cortex to secrete all of its glucocorticoids and its mineralocorticoids at an increased rate. The average adult dose is 40 to 50 U.S.P. units daily. See a pharmacology textbook for further information about the action and toxicity of adrenocorticosteroids.

[19] Gracia S. McCabe: "Cultural Influences on Patient Behavior," *Amer. J. Nurs.,* **60:**1101–1104 (Aug.) 1960.

success in meeting the needs of Negro patients from southern rural areas, the nurse must know how they express satisfaction or dissatisfaction with their care. She emphasizes the importance of not stereotyping patients.

Implications of Socioeconomic Status

Despite the general conviction of Americans to the contrary, socioeconomic status does influence the expectations, aspirations, and way of life of Americans. Recent statistics indicate that it even influences life expectancy in that the lower the income, the shorter the life expectancy. It seems safe to conclude that anything in the life of the individual that is different from that of other individuals contributes to differences in expectations, codes regulating behavior, modes of expressing and satisfying needs, and the language used. If the point that individuals differ appears to be overstressed, it is because not only patient satisfaction but also that of the nurse depends, in part, on the identification and satisfaction of individual expectations of patients.

Values

One of the important aspects of culture is its system of values. Ruesch states that many values held in America have their origin in the fact that until very recently America was a pioneer country. Moreover, the early settlers were Puritans who placed a high value on plain living, industry, self-control, willpower, cleanliness, consistency, honesty, and the assumption of responsibility. In settling the country, survival often depended on such characteristics as strength, initiative, and hard work. There was little time for pleasure. Entertainment was organized around important events in life such as a wedding, a death, or a house building.[20]

According to Ruesch, the American value system is based on four premises: equality, sociality, success, and change. The ideal that all men are equal has its origin in the Judeo-Christian belief that all men are equal in the sight of God. This represents a change in culture. In the ancient world the attitude toward man was very different. In the words of Hamilton,[21] "In Egypt, in Crete, in Mesopotamia, wherever we can read bits of the story, we find the same conditions: a despot enthroned, whose whims and passions are the determining factor in the state; a wretched, subjugated populace;

a great priestly organization to which is handed over the domain of the intellect." The founders of our nation made their views clear in The Declaration of Independence when they said, "We hold these truths to be self-evident: that all men are created equal, that they are endowed by their Creator with certain unalienable Rights, that among these are Life, Liberty and the pursuit of Happiness." Lincoln re-emphasized the belief in equality of men in the opening sentence of The Gettysburg Address. One of the important issues in the world today stems from whose rights come first, the individual's or the state's, and from whom these rights are derived.

In application of the premise of equality to the practice of nursing, nurses are taught to give the same quality of care to all patients whatever their background, social condition, or disease. Because all patients are individuals, as are nurses, and each one is different from all others, perhaps the nurse can come closer to reaching the ideal of equality of care if she can accept the patient as a human being, recognize his dignity, identify behavior that provides clues to his needs, consider the meaning of his behavior, and plan his care to meet his needs. To do this, the nurse requires some knowledge of her own system of values.

The second premise on which Ruesch[22] says the American value system is based is that of sociality. By this is meant that the American tends to be guided in his actions by the opinions of his peers. He forms social groups in which he works to accomplish the goals of the group. He is responsive to the pressure of the group and is very much aware of his status in it. When called on to make a decision, he tends to think in terms of "What will the neighbors think?" As might be expected, health care and the way the individual behaves when he is sick is influenced by dependence on what he thinks is his neighbors' approval or disapproval of his actions. Koos' study cites the example of a woman who called a physician to see her child with the chickenpox, not because she felt it was necessary but because she did not want her friends to think that she was neglecting the child.[23] Children and adults are dosed with vitamins and patent medicines, not because there is objective evidence that they are required but because everyone is taking the preparation.

The tendency of Americans to form social groups is also evident in the health and welfare field. Organizations in the health field extend from those dedicated to research and investigation of the causes of, and education of the public about, the nature of a single disease to those in which a group of people come together

[20] Jurgen Ruesch and Gregory Bateson: *Communication* (New York: W. W. Norton & Company, Inc., 1951), pp. 94–134.

[21] Edith Hamilton: *The Greek Way* (New York: W. W. Norton & Company, Inc., 1930), p. 19.

[22] Ruesch, *op. cit.,* pp. 108–13.

[23] Koos, *op. cit.,* p. 71.

in order to provide emotional support for each other as they work toward the accomplishment of a single goal such as the loss of weight.

Moreover, the value of group action is so great that Americans voluntarily tax themselves for the financial support of numerous organizations. They do this by contributing to the individual organization or to the Community Chest. Individuals who devote time and effort to these organizations are accorded special status in the community. They may be both approved of and envied by their peers. Certain values influence defining the goals of these groups. For instance, the strong help the weak as long as the weakness is the result of age or some circumstance not within what society considers to be the control of the individual. Americans also place a high value on independence. Children are trained early to be independent. Dependence is accepted as concomitant to illness, but the patient is expected to work toward independence. If the individual is to receive continued assistance he can do so only by meeting the expectation of doing whatever is necessary to alter his situation for the better.

The need to be part of a group and for status is observable in the behavior of hospitalized patients. Persons who are hospitalized for long periods of time tend to form social groups on both formal and informal bases. Many extended-care hospitals make use of this fact when planning treatment programs. The formation of groups is encouraged as a way of providing channels through which patients can make their needs known and also get some of their needs met. For example, the need for status may be partially met by forming a group whose task is to give administration suggestions regarding patient care and general ward problems. Other groups may be used to help patients work through some feelings about illness and to prepare them for life outside the hospital. Frequently the latter groups are formed by and for individuals who share a common disability or problem. There are many examples in society of these kinds of groups—colostomy clubs, Alcoholics Anonymous, and the National Paraplegics Foundation are but a few.

Sometimes an individual achieves status by having an unusual condition or by having an unusual variation of an illness. On the other hand, the fact that he is different or does not conform to the usual pattern may cause the patient to become anxious. After he recovers he may boast to the neighbors that he had an illness that his doctors had not seen before, but during the illness he may have had a great deal of concern because he did not conform to the norm for any diagnostic category.

The American places high value on a healthy body, on youth, and on physical attractiveness. In general, we tend to devalue those who are weak (physically or emotionally), deformed, or unsightly. At times a person may be unable to accept necessary treatment because of the effect the treatment will have, or that he believes it will have, on his appearance, his capacity to function, or his acceptance by the group to which he belongs. The need to conform to the expectations of the group is illustrated also by the concern parents have that their children meet standards that are considered to indicate that the children are developing normally. This need to adhere to "the norm" results in unnecessary anxiety on the part of parents and, in turn, places pressure on the children. Children are also sensitive to pressure from their peer group to conform, as is illustrated in the instance of six-year-old Joey, a dark brunet, who played with light, blond children. Joey made his awareness of this difference clear when he said to his mother, "Mommy, when you were getting a boy, why didn't you get a light one?"

Recognition of the value that people place on approval from their peers, as well as their tendency to work in groups and to conform to group pressure, has significance in the practice of nursing. These are important factors to consider when the condition of the patient demands a change in his pattern of living. These factors also relate to that aspect of the role of the nurse whereby she attempts to relieve tension among the members of the treatment team. In this role, the nurse contributes to the care of the patient by helping members of the treatment team function more effectively as a team. It is also well to remember that in the American culture, for many people, it is more important to be liked than to like others. This is an unrealistic expectation, but the effect of this particular value system is observable. As a consequence, failure on the part of the physician or nurse to express approval may be interpreted by the patient as a lack of caring, concern, or liking or as disapproval. A hypothetical example is as follows: The nurse tells ten patients in the ward that they look very well this morning, but she overlooks giving the same message to the eleventh patient. The eleventh patient may interpret this in many ways, and one of the interpretations may be that the nurse is more fond of everyone else in the immediate group. Obviously, this does not mean that nurses have to treat everyone exactly the same, but they should not be too surprised if they are called on periodically to sort out patients' distortions about their intentions.

The third premise on which the American value system is based is success. Success is a yardstick by which the value of an individual is measured. This means there is generally a high value placed on achievement. There is little respect for those who rest on their oars or who are not considered to be productive. There is a tendency to believe that failure results from a lack of effort and that mastery of any problem is possible if sufficient effort and/or money is expended. Thus the chronically ill person, or one who has lost his job, loses status because he has not expended sufficient effort to stay well or be restored to health or keep or get a new job. This point may help to explain the fact that many health workers, including nurses, prefer to care for the acutely ill who get well quickly and avoid the care of the chronically ill, that is, those who fail to recover fully or quickly.

There is also a tendency to measure success in the various aspects of life. A baby is not just a baby who is thriving, but he is the biggest, the smallest, the fattest, the cutest, the cryingest, or the most voracious eater on the block. Mr. Lang was not just sick with pneumonia; he had the highest temperature, made the quickest recovery, and so on. Another measure used to indicate success is the tendency to emphasize the length of life and the status position achieved rather than the fullness or richness of it.

The fourth premise is that, for the American, life is not static but is in the process of change. The result is that the American is geared for action and is ready for change. He values adaptability and moves from one job to another to get experience, better pay, or higher status. Our "typical American" hopes that change will improve his chances of ascending the ladder of success. Popular magazines frequently carry articles about the mobility of American society and its causes and effects. Because change constitutes moving from the known to the unknown, it is accompanied by anxiety. The degree of anxiety one experiences depends on such things as the nature and magnitude of the change, the flexibility and adaptability of the individual or the society, and the meaning associated with the change.

The attitude toward change of the person from middle-class society is reflected in expectations about what constitutes adequate and appropriate medical care. When he is well, the middle-class individual is often willing to spend money to finance research into the causes and prevention of illness, and when he is sick he finds it difficult to understand why answers are so slow in coming. After all, he is spending money on such problems and wants results. He also looks for signs that his condition is improving, and when he does not find them or

learns that he cannot expect to change quickly for the better, he tends to become anxious and feels hopeless and helpless. The middle-class American also has great faith in the value of machines and drugs and somehow feels cheated if these are not used as part of his treatment. We see on television that this drug or that machine will fix things and return them to normal in less time than it takes to run the commercial. It is no wonder, then, that the person who comes for treatment expects rapid change back to his usual state of health and functioning and has difficulty accepting changes that permanently alter the "usual."

As a basis for discussion of the role of the sick person in the American culture, some of the values that relate to Ruesch's four premises —equality, sociality, success, and change— having to do with motivation have been discussed and illustrated. There are other values that are important to many Americans. Because the values held to be important by the individual influence his behavior, personalizing of patient care depends on some knowledge of what these values are. The nurse should remember that not all Americans value the same things. Understanding the place of cultural factors in reactions to illness is a principle that has application in all aspects of nursing. However, the previous examples are generalizations about middle-class culture and cannot be applied to specific individuals except as a guide for understanding one dimension of the person. Studies indicate that even in fairly homogeneous communities the values held differ from one socioeconomic group to another. For example, Hollingshead and Redlich [24] report that the type of psychotherapy that patients expect differs with each socioeconomic group. Patients from the upper socioeconomic groups expect and profit from insight therapy. They expect to learn about why they act as they do and to learn to modify their behavior. Those in the lower classes expect an authoritarian attitude on the part of the psychiatrist. They want the psychiatrist to tell them what to do. Hollingshead and Redlich qualify this by stating that there are individuals in the upper classes who cannot profit from insight therapy, whereas there are those from the lower classes who can. The authors of this study further state that psychiatrists, both because they come from the middle and upper classes and because they are trained to use insight therapy, seemed to find it difficult to work with patients from the lower classes.

Studies of the attitudes of nurses toward

24 August B. Hollingshead and Fredrick C. Redlich: *Social Class and Mental Illness* (New York: John Wiley & Sons, Inc., 1958), p. 345.

patients such as the one reported by Mac-Gregor [25] also indicate that nurses view patients in light of their own values. MacGregor concluded that the students' image of the upper-class patient tended to be that of a "spoiled, demanding, condescending person who may regard the nurse as a servant." The students' view of the lower-class patient was that of a "person who is more appreciative, respectful, and less demanding." These examples are cited not in criticism of either psychiatrists or nurses but to emphasize the point that each individual tends to evaluate the behavior of others in light of his own values and standards. This happens even when both individuals are from a similar, though not identical, culture. Of necessity this discussion has been brief, but perhaps enough detail has been presented so that the nurse can appreciate that each person tends to perceive his situation in light of his past learnings and experiences. It is easier to accept others who have similar values and standards of behavior than it is to accept those who differ. Individualization of the patient's care demands that the nurse try to see the situation through the eyes of the patient. She should realize that she can never see things exactly as the patient sees them, but she can be aware of the necessity for trying to understand as much about the patient as is possible.

How does the patient feel he ought to behave during his illness?

In addition to having values that are important in other aspects of the life of the individual, each culture or subculture establishes rules about what it regards as sickness and the behavior and responsibilities of those who are ill as well as of those who care for them. This is illustrated in the studies of the responses of Jewish, Italian, and Old Americans to pain that led Zborowski [26] to conclude that knowledge of culture is essential to the effective care of these patients. He found that the Jewish and Italian patients were more overtly emotional in expressing pain than were the Old Americans. Jewish and Italian patients differed in their response to treatment, however. When appropriate measures were instituted, the Italians were relieved of their pain and happy with the result. Jewish patients, on the other hand, were concerned about the possible implications of their pain to their future health and were reluctant to take pain-relieving medications. They were fearful that drugs might produce ill effects that would be manifested at some future time. To relieve Jewish patients' pain it was necessary to relieve their concern about what was causing the pain and to reassure them about possible delayed effects of the pain-relieving medication or about their illness. Though the observed behavior appeared to be similar for Italian and Jewish patients, the meaning was different. To be effective, the treatment had to take the meaning of the pain into account.

Zborowski [27] also found that the patient of Old American stock was similar to the Jewish patient inasmuch as he tended to be concerned about the implications of the pain to his future recovery. He differed from the Jewish and Italian patient in that he was undemonstrative in his reaction to pain. He also gave the impression of trying to report on pain; that is, he appeared to be trying to be an objective observer. When he was in severe pain, the Old American tended to withdraw from society. He might cry, but when he did he preferred to cry alone. He was observed to have a different pattern of behavior when he was with his family and friends than when he was with members of the professional staff. In the presence of his family and friends he tended to minimize his pain and to avoid complaining. On the ward he tried to cooperate with the staff and to behave as he thought he was expected to. He considered himself a part of the team—doctor, nurse, and patient—in which every member had a part to play and each member was expected to do his share.

Not only do each man's beliefs, customs, and value systems affect the way he behaves when he is ill, they also affect how he thinks he should be treated and how those who are responsible for his care feel about him and what they do for him. As in other areas involving human beings, multiple factors are often involved, and seemingly simple behavior may have complex meanings that are interrelated with other factors. Furthermore, the interpreter interprets in his own frame of reference. The patient who moans and groans when he has pain may be suffering from pain that is well-nigh unbearable, or he may feel that this is the way to bring his pain to the attention of those who care for him or that his family expects him to behave this way. He may be concerned about the pain itself or its implications for his future. The nurse who cares for the patient may have been brought up to believe that pain should be borne silently, or that it is appropriate to express it, or that after it is treated one should be satisfied. The manner in which the nurse

[25] Frances Cooke MacGregor: *Social Science in Nursing* (New York: Russell Sage Foundation, 1960), p. 101.

[26] Mark Zborowski: "Cultural Components in Response to Pain," *J. Social Issues*, 8:16–30 (No. 4) 1952.

[27] *Ibid.*, pp. 16–30.

treats the patient, and the extent to which she is able to be helpful to him, will depend in some measure on her understanding of the meaning that the situation has to the patient. Respect for the rights and dignity of man and the right of each person to participate in plans that concern his welfare are values that are sometimes lost in the conflict over other values.

An attempt has been made to establish the importance of knowledge of the beliefs, customs, and values of the providers of care as well as of those who receive it. It is not possible to discuss all aspects of the American culture, let alone the characteristics of its subcultures. One point that has not been introduced is that professional education creates certain barriers between those who serve and those who are served. As a result of professional education and experiences, the individual acquires a modified set of values, attitudes, vocabulary, and behaviors in regard to illness. Rather than reinforcing the distance between those who serve and are served, professional education should aim at assisting the learner to manipulate elements in the treatment environment so that these barriers are minimized.

How does the nurse feel the patient ought to behave during his illness?

Nurses, as well as patients, are people who have needs that require satisfaction. They, like other people, learn to satisfy their needs in ways that are socially acceptable to the family, group, and culture into which they were born. When they enter a school of nursing they bring with them the values, ideals, goals, and ways of behaving they have learned. Depending on their past experiences, they bring to nursing a set of expectations for what patients ought to be like and how they ought to behave. When the student is from the Anglo-American culture, she is likely to expect that patients will respond to treatment by getting well quickly and that patients will express satisfaction with and be grateful for their care. The nursing student also brings to nursing a set of expectations based on values she has learned. This includes what she believes a good nurse is, does, and ought to be able to accomplish. Through the course of her program the goals of the student and expectations for herself and for patients are modified or changed to conform more closely to those of her mentors. Brown [28] indicates that part of the difficulty in health care stems from the fact that health professionals do not effectively communicate with each other or with patients. Each professional group is more attuned to developing its own "uniqueness" than to understanding the needs of patients. This same author [29] goes on to state that "Most important, perhaps, among the causes of paucity of communication, is the fact that doctors and nurses are still trained almost exclusively to treat disease and to make patients physically comfortable. The concept of 'total patient care' is extensively promoted, but it is only in the initial stage of becoming an operational concept." As in other areas of nursing, all nurses need to improve their ability to identify and meet the psychosocial needs of patients through study, evaluation, and practice.

By this point the fact that illness and health have social and cultural definitions as well as biological and physiological ones should be clear. As a result of family, group, and cultural patterns the individual learns what to regard as health or sickness. He learns what he should do about sickness—what kinds of measures can be expected to be effective in warding it off or in curing it. He learns what his responsibilities are when he is ill and what he should expect from others including his family and the members of his culture who have special knowledge and skill in matters of health and disease. Those who are given status by a society by virtue of having special knowledge and skill in treating illness also have expectations, values, and ways of behaving that they accept as being appropriate. The more nearly those of the patient and the nurse or other professional persons agree, the more satisfactory services are likely to be and the more likely both individuals are to achieve satisfaction. Conversely, the greater the disparity between the client and the giver of service, the greater the possibility that the service will not be provided in a way that is satisfactory to the recipient. Moreover, this disparity can be a source of psychological stress to the patient.

As emphasized, the meaning that an illness has for an individual and what he does to prevent or to treat it are conditioned by the beliefs, customs, and values that he acquires from his family and the society in which he lives. These factors determine what man as a thinking, remembering, imagining being regards as illness and what he should do about it. Illness is, however, a personal as well as a cultural experience. When a person is ill, he responds in a variety of ways: intellectually, emotionally, physically, and physiologically. The degree of his response depends on a variety of factors, some of which include the causative agent, the way in which the person perceives the threat to his well-being,

[28] Esther Lucile Brown: "Meeting Patients' Psychosocial Needs in the General Hospital," *Social Interaction and Patient Care*, James K. Skipper, Jr., and Robert C. Leonard, eds. (Philadelphia: J. B. Lippincott Company, 1965), p. 15.

[29] *Ibid.*, p. 15.

and his biological, intellectual, and emotional resources. Some of his responses will be voluntary and others involuntary. Some of them will be highly individual. Whatever they are, they will be of value to the degree to which they are constructive and integrative and result in action that enables him to protect himself against, or to eliminate, danger. They are pathological to the degree that they are disorganized, inappropriate, exaggerated, and ineffectual.

Psychological Elements Having the Greatest Significance for the Practice of Nursing

In the discussion of the psychological aspects of illness, the following points will be considered: (1) the concept of homeostasis, (2) a definition of psychological stress, (3) some purposes served by intellectual responses to illness, (4) the differences in definition of the sick role as a source of psychological stress, (5) the emotional reactions of a person who recognizes he is ill, and (6) the emotional reactions of significant others to illness.

The Concept of Emotional Homeostasis

Although the concept of homeostasis was introduced by Cannon [30] to explain the constancy of internal physiological environment of cells in the body, psychologists have adapted the concept to encompass the emotional state. Thus used, *homeostasis* refers to a general condition of psychological integration.[31] As with physiological homeostasis, emotional homeostasis depends on having certain needs fulfilled. Whereas the supplies required to satisfy physiological needs are materials such as oxygen or water, those required to meet psychological needs are nonmaterial, though they may be represented, symbolically, by material objects. Psychological needs are the conditions, situations, actions, or effects of action that the individual perceives, experiences, and represents in his mind as having meaning. Depending on the situation and its meaning, the person may feel safe and protected, esteemed by others and himself, and loved. Conversely, in other situations he may feel threatened, unsafe, unesteemed, endangered, and unloved. The satisfaction of psychological needs depends on the person having structures that function in such a manner that he is able to perceive and evalu-

[30] Walter B. Cannon: *The Wisdom of the Body* (New York: W. W. Norton & Company, Inc., 1939), p. 22.
[31] Franz J. Kallmann: "The Genetics of Mental Illness," *American Handbook of Psychiatry* (New York: Basic Books, Inc., 1959), p. 178.

ate anything that impinges on his being. Psychological homeostasis implies, as does physiological homeostasis, the presence of processes or mechanisms that regulate, maintain, or restore emotional or psychological stability in a changing environment.

Agents that endanger psychological homeostasis may have their origin in either the internal or external environment of the individual. They are similar to agents that threaten physiological homeostasis in that they may result from an excess or deficit of supply. They differ from agents that threaten physiological homeostasis in that the individual responds not only to the agent itself but to what it symbolizes. Consequently, fear and anxiety can be engendered by harmless things. The individual feels and behaves in the presence of the symbol as he would if he were in the presence of the thing it represents to him. As a consequence of this phenomenon, much of what man fears is learned.

To illustrate, Mrs. Simon is afraid of dying. Despite her knowledge that her illness is minor and not considered to threaten her life, she has all the signs and symptoms commonly associated with terror. She has no understanding of why she is reacting in this way. Her fear does not diminish when she is given logical and reasonable explanations. Illness of any sort symbolizes total destruction to Mrs. Simon, and she responds to the symbolic meaning of illness rather than to the reality of the situation.

As in physiological homeostasis, individuals differ in their capacity to adapt. Many factors contribute to this difference. Some of these may be inborn, others may be learned, and still others may result from disease. For example, the capacity of the brain-injured child or adult to adapt to frustration is less than that of a healthy person. This must be recognized and the environment adapted so that expectations are kept within the person's ability to function. Though the capacity to tolerate psychological stress differs from one individual to another, all people have a limit. As stated earlier, there are many factors in illness that contribute to the disruption of psychological homeostasis, with the end result an increase in psychological stress.

PSYCHOLOGICAL STRESS

As a basis for the discussion of the causes of psychological stress, Engel's definition of stress is quoted: "Psychological stress refers to all processes, whether originating in the external environment or within the person, which impose a demand or requirement upon the organism, the resolution or handling of which necessitates work or activity of the mental apparatus before any other system is involved or activated."[32]

It is difficult to determine which situations or conditions requiring adaptation will actually be stressful to the individual's adaptive capacity. Stress is likely to occur because the adaptive capacity of the individual is limited or because the condition to which he is required to adapt is extreme. In other words, because adaptation is a learned process, the person's previously learned methods of adaptation may not be adequate to deal initially with a situation, and stress results. Psychological stresses place strain on the adaptive capacity of the organism by acting on the brain and mental apparatus.[33] Although other agents that place strain on the adaptive capacity of the organism may produce psychological stress, this action is secondary. Their primary effect is on biochemical processes, cells, organs, or system. Psychological stress may also, and often does, involve structures other than the mental apparatus, but its primary effect is on the mental apparatus. Whatever the cause of the disturbance, agents that act as stimuli result in the initiation of mechanisms of response that serve to reduce or relieve the discomfort. In general these mechanisms enable the individual to attack or to withdraw from the danger or to play dead (possum).

From the previous statements one can assume that adaptation is not a static condition. We have mentioned the individual's need to strive for emotional homeostasis, which requires continuing use of adaptive processes. It also would be well to mention *heterostasis,* or the concept that deals with the tendency of the organism to seek imbalance or new stimuli, which, in turn, lead to new levels of adaptation.[34] The latter concept is important in health care because it clearly implies that an individual can acquire new learning from a state of imbalance such as illness or disability. The positive or negative quality of this learning often depends on the kind of assistance the patient receives from health professionals and others in the course of his illness.

During illness the individual may lose or be threatened with the loss of something that has value to him. He is almost certain to suffer painful procedures or to fear that he will. The fear is often made worse by the fact that he

does not know what to expect and therefore fears the worst. In the process of growing up, the individual learns to master his drives so that his needs can be met in keeping with reality. Sometimes the manner in which he regards his drives is a source of conflict. During illness these conflicts may be intensified. Whatever the specific source of psychological stress in illness, it leads to unpleasant feelings such as anxiety, anger, helplessness, hopelessness, guilt, shame, and disgust. To counteract these feelings and to restore emotional homeostasis, psychological defense mechanisms that have been relatively effective in the past will be initiated. When defense mechanisms such as rationalization, projection, sublimation, displacement, or denial are ineffective or inadequate to restore emotional homeostasis, physiological and/or behavioral changes follow.

What actually will be disturbing to any patient during illness and how he will react are highly individual matters. There are, however, some causes of psychological stress that occur frequently enough that they should be considered when each patient's needs are assessed. Engel classifies the causes of psychological stress as (1) the loss of something that is of value to the person, (2) injury or threat of injury to the body, and (3) the frustration of drives. These, obviously, are interrelated. Contained within Engel's list of causes are other elements such as the altered concept of self, failure of the intellect to resolve the illness, threats to economic security, confusion in the definition of the sick role, and fears that needs will not be adequately met.

SELF-CONCEPT

The first of these subelements, self-concept, includes all the ideas, conscious and unconscious feelings, beliefs, and attitudes that the person has about himself and his possessions. In his concept of himself he answers the questions where am I, what am I, who am I. Among the many things that the person may or may not value about himself are his body image or picture of himself; his feeling of being intact or whole; his role and status in his family, community, and job; his adequacy and acceptability as a marriage partner; his success and sense of fulfillment; and his hope that tomorrow will be better than today. He may value his family, home, state, and country. Other values that may be threatened during illness include the way in which he regards financial, physical, or emotional dependence and independence; how he feels about relinquishing control over events that relate to his welfare; as well as the way in which he ordinarily relates to other people.

[32] George L. Engel: "A Unified Concept of Health and Disease," *Perspect. Biol. Med.,* 3:480 (Summer) 1960.

[33] *Ibid.,* p. 480.

[34] Helen D. Sargent and Martin Mayman: "Clinical Psychology," *American Handbook of Psychiatry,* Vol. II, Silvano Arieti, ed. (New York: Basic Books, Inc., 1959), p. 1717.

Because they threaten the self-concept of the individual in some way, certain types of disease are more likely to cause psychological stress than others. These include those that cause disfigurement, especially of the face, or the loss of a part that is easily identified, such as an extremity. Diseases or treatments that threaten the organs of reproduction are also sources of anxiety. Some diseases such as venereal diseases are regarded as bringing disgrace on the person and his family. In some groups tuberculosis and cancer are also perceived as a cause for shame. Mental illness and mental retardation fall in the same category. Other diseases such as heart disease or cancer are associated in the minds of many people with death. In addition cancer is generally equated with an extended and painful illness.

INTELLECTUAL RESPONSES TO ILLNESS

Failure of the intellect to resolve illness and all its consequences is also a source of psychological stress for many persons. In illness each individual reacts closely to the way he does in other crises in his life—at least initially. His reactions are often complex, involving both his intellect and his emotions. Through the use of his intelligence, man is often able to foresee the consequences of his actions and to plan to avert injury or correct the damage that has been done. Inasmuch as he is able to acquire knowledge and to grasp and identify the significant factors in his situation and to use his capacity to reason and think, to modify his behavior, or to adapt the environment to meet his needs, his intelligence is useful to him. However, what if intelligence fails? What if illness imposes such overwhelming changes on the physical functioning of the person that his intelligence fails in every way except to tell him that this time he cannot reason his way out of the mess he is in? Anxiety increases, and various defensive maneuvers are called into action to protect the individual from experiencing the full impact of what has happened.

How well a person uses his intelligence depends on numerous factors including educational background and emotional state. Hence, a highly intelligent and well-educated person (not excluding physicians or nurses) may act irrationally as well as rationally in a personal crisis such as illness. Intelligence is useful to the individual only as long as he can remain objective, identify the nature of the threat, and plan to protect himself from it or eliminate it. It fails him inasmuch as the knowledge on which he bases his decisions is inadequate, inaccurate, or not applicable or his emotional state is such that he is unable to use his knowledge. The theories of crisis intervention take these points into account. The significance of crisis intervention is in helping an individual utilize his intelligence to do problem solving in relation to the immediate critical situation in his life. If the person in crisis receives appropriate help—that is, help that allows him to think through the problem and come to some conclusions about acceptable solutions or alternatives—the experience can lead to new, more mature levels of adaptation.

This does not imply that education and intelligence are of no importance when a person is ill. However, the point that intelligence is not synonymous with years of schooling is worth making. Some people who are intelligent but who have had little opportunity to go to school are well educated. Because of the tendency to equate schooling with education and with intelligence, quite intelligent but unschooled people may be treated as if they were not capable of understanding or of participating in plans for their care.

When a patient's level of education is similar to that of the people responsible for his care, communication is facilitated. They are more likely to have similar vocabularies and values than when their backgrounds differ widely. When there are differences in background, the degree of success with which the needs of patients are met depends on the extent to which these differences are taken into account.

SICK ROLE

Another source of psychological stress to the patient and those who provide his care is the difference in their respective concepts about the appropriate role and behavior of each other in illness. The role of the sick person in the American culture has been studied and defined by sociologists. Parsons [35] defines illness as a "socially institutionalized role-type" characterized in the American culture by some incapacity to carry on the normally expected role and tasks. He summarizes the American culture view of illness as follows:

1. The person is exempted from his role obligations.
2. He is not held responsible for being ill.
3. This state is held to be legitimate, if
4. He accepts the need for help and cooperates with those who help him.

The meaning of each of these will be clarified later in this chapter.

Conflict, with its accompanying psychological

---

[35] Talcott Parsons: "Definitions of Health and Illness in the Light of American Values and Social Structure," *Patients, Physicians and Illness,* E. Gartly Jaco, ed. (New York: The Free Press, 1958), p. 176.

stress, arises between the patient and the people providing his health care when differences in interpretation of their respective roles arise. If the patient is interpreting his role in one way and the nurse is interpreting the patient's role differently, there is little or no communication taking place between them. Each has a set of values to which the other is expected to conform, but when conformity does not take place power struggles frequently occur. The patient will start behaving in ways that are intended to maintain his role image, and the nurse probably will react in a similar manner.

In general, when there is an increase in nonconformity, there is a counterincrease in rigidity. Thus, if a nurse does not conform to the patient's stereotype of "nurse," the patient may become more rigid and determined in his effort to make sure that the nurse does conform. For example, if the patient's stereotype is that all nurses are crabby, he may unconsciously behave in such a way that the nurse will eventually get angry at him. Then the patient has reinforcement for his view. These situations work both ways. In an instance where a patient is not able to accept his need for help and continues to be uncooperative with those who help him, the patient is demeaned, treated with suspicion, or discharged as a hopeless case. What may be operating in the latter example is that the patient and nurse are defining *help* in different ways and neither is able to communicate this difference to the other. Anxiety usually increases on both sides. After all, the nurse is taught that she is supposed to be helpful. Failing in this, she becomes anxious. The patient, at some level, must want help or he would cease being a patient. Failing to get the assistance he thinks would be useful to him, he too gets anxious. The breech between the helper and the one seeking help usually widens unless someone, usually the nurse, can stop and make a conscious effort to look at what is getting in the way of satisfactory and satisfying care.

Similar struggles frequently occur between the patient and his family, between the patient and the community, or between the patient and the hospital culture. The patient begins to sense that he is under pressure to conform to a stereotype that comes from a group and not just from an individual. Finding that behaving in accordance with his own feelings and standards gains him nothing, he may gradually fall into the system's stereotype of what he should be in order to get the attention he needs. The writer recently observed a situation where one norm of ward culture was to yell. The patients who yelled the loudest received the most favorable attention from the nursing staff. This usually made new patients and new staff members very uneasy, especially if they came from backgrounds where people spoke quietly, said what they meant, and were listened to. The new patient, for example, would expect that when he turned on his call light a nurse would respond, he would tell her what he wanted, and then she would take some appropriate action. However, this did not happen. Finally, even the most mild-mannered patients recognized that in this culture sick people were expected to yell. If you did not yell, apparently you were not considered to be sick enough to need attention.

The nurse does not have to search very far for examples of strained nurse-patient relationships that occur when a patient violates one of Parsons' norms for illness. Let us look at the one that says that a patient is not held responsible for his illness. What happens if a person is hospitalized because of self-inflicted wounds or because of blatant disregard for measures that might have maintained his health? What usually happens is that the staff will either help the patient deny that he is responsible for his illness, or treat the patient with contempt, or both. Another aspect of this norm is that the patient may be relieved of responsibility for his illness, but he is almost always judged as being responsible for his behavior. There is a tendency in the American culture to evaluate the expression of emotion in terms of good (desirable) or bad (undesirable). Thus anger, or the expression of anger, is bad, and people who express anger are treated as if they were bad. This view neglects the fact that emotions are the substance of life. They give it color and meaning. Emotions are useful when they are directed toward socially acceptable goals. Their usefulness is impaired when they are inappropriate to the situation or excessive or deficient in degree. Anger, when properly controlled and directed toward the accomplishment of goals, may serve as a spur to the correction of an injustice. When it is uncontrolled, or excessive in amount, it may be destructive. What is appropriate is in the eye of the beholder. For example, what the nurse may think is appropriate behavior for a patient in a given situation may not be what the patient feels is appropriate. When their views differ widely, conflict may result.

Regression is another part of illness that frequently leads to confusion in the definition of the sick role. Holmes and Werner write that "Not only is regression a necessary concomitant of an illness, but also it always accompanies and is fostered by hospitalization."[36] In other words, return to a less mature level of behavior is observable in any illness—even the common

[36] Marguerite J. Holmes and Jean A. Werner: *Psychiatric Nursing in a Therapeutic Community* (New York: The Macmillan Company, 1966), p. 66.

cold. People may become more dependent, insist that they be taken care of, become short-tempered, and engage in a variety of behaviors that were not common to their personality when they were well. In addition, the very nature of health care demands that a patient give up certain independent functions and rely instead on the judgment of those individuals from whom he seeks help. Conflict arises because the limits of the sick role and the helper role are difficult to define. There are double messages going from patient to staff and vice versa. The nurses may make it clear that patients must submit to all types of care and at the same time expect patients to behave as mature adults. Patients frequently behave as if they expect to be treated as mature, capable adults and at the same time insist that their "patient status" give them the right to have even the most unreasonable demands met.

The point was made previously that illness involves relinquishing, to a greater or lesser degree, the ability of the person to control events in relation to himself. This is not only related to actual need imposed by the physical inability to perform certain functions but again is related to the way we define the sick role. According to our perceptions, the person is exempted from his role obligation of making decisions for himself. Furthermore, because he is not held responsible for being ill, he is treated as if he cannot assume responsibility for anything. The patient is told when to go to bed, when to get out of bed, when and what he shall eat, and when to bathe. He may be asked to perform procedures that he does not feel able to do. For example, Mrs. Mel had a hysterectomy following several days of severe hemorrhage. On the day after surgery the nurse entered the room and said, "Now it is time for you to get up." Mrs. Mel asked, "How can I get up? I have all these tubes and I feel too weak." She had three tubes, one into her stomach, one into her urinary bladder, and another connected to a needle in a vein in her left arm. "Doctor's orders," said the nurse. "All patients get up the day after surgery. Just turn on your side and swing your feet over the edge of the bed and raise up as you do so." Mrs. Mel got up because she felt she was helpless to alter the situation. She also felt that the nurse was harsh and unfeeling. Mrs. Mel's feeling that she was called on to perform activities for which she was unprepared and without adequate physical and emotional support is all too common. The nurse could have assisted the patient better by acknowledging her question and her concern and by explaining why it was necessary for her to be out of bed so soon after surgery. Some expression from the nurse that indicated that she appreci-

ated how Mrs. Mel felt and that she would help her might have reduced Mrs. Mel's fear.

OTHER SOURCES OF STRESS TO THE PATIENT

There are many ways in which the performance of various aspects of patient care can be a source of psychological stress and unnecessary anxiety. Such instances occur because we are more oriented to the necessity for completing tasks than we are to the fact that we are caring for a person who, feeling-wise, has not abdicated his entire sense of responsibility for himself. Because we fail to take the psychological needs of the patient into account, the following omissions in care often occur: (1) failure to prepare the patient for what to expect and when to expect it; (2) failure to provide consistency in care; (3) lack of skill in handling the patient or the equipment—including awkwardness, roughness, uncertainty about how to proceed, and failure to give necessary emotional and physical support; (4) lack of needed supplies; (5) changing the performance of a procedure without explanation; (6) failure to observe the patient's modesty patterns by omitting such things as adequate covering and screening while performing procedures; and (7) making thoughtless or careless remarks in the presence of the patient that suggest dangers that may or may not exist.

Diagnostic and therapeutic procedures that are performed by as many strangers as there are procedures are sources of anxiety to patients. There is always the possibility that the patient knows or believes that a procedure may be harmful or painful as well as helpful. No list of situations in which the performance of a procedure may add to the patient's anxiety will ever be complete. However, awareness of some common ways in which anxiety is prevented or provoked should be helpful when planning patient care. To illustrate, Mrs. Taylor was to have a urea clearance test on Tuesday. On Monday the physician told her about the test and that she would be moved to the treatment room for it. Later the nurse found Mrs. Taylor weeping. As the nurse attempted to comfort Mrs. Taylor, she learned that the patient called the treatment room the "death room." This belief had its origin in the fact that the artificial kidney was in this room and that some of the patients who went into the room died. The nurse reported Mrs. Taylor's feelings to the physician, who replied, "That is the reason that she looked so forlorn when I told her about the test." He arranged to perform the procedure in Mrs. Taylor's room and, of course, talked with her about the change of plans. In this example it was possible to change a physical aspect of a procedure and, therefore, reduce the threat to the patient. This may not always be true. When it is not, the nurse can still be helpful to the patient by recognizing his feelings, by trying to understand the source of the anxiety, and by planning alternatives that might alleviate it.

The cost to the patient and his family because of pain and suffering, or the fear of pain and suffering, is a real part of any illness. Here nurses can do much through the use of appropriate measures to relieve and prevent unnecessary pain.

Although the psychological cost of pain and suffering is great, the actual expense of illness is also a source of anxiety to patients and their families. Here, too, patients are by cultural definition exempted from their role obligations but only to a degree. They are not exempted from the obligation of paying for their care or other debts. Direct costs are of great concern to those whose incomes are limited and who do not have hospital and medical insurance. This is especially true of people who have always been able to meet their financial obligations. Since the advent of Medicare, the burden of the cost of medical care for the elderly has been greatly reduced. However, care for this age group is still a costly matter. The costs of hospitalization and medical care are also the expenses that are the most obvious to the nurse. Patients may have insurance that pays their medical expenses and still be extremely concerned because illness is accompanied by loss of income, the inability to meet other obligations such as mortgage payment, or additional burdens such as payments for child care. Even relatively short illnesses may make serious demands on a limited income. Other costs of illness include the demands made on family members to visit the sick or to provide for his care if he is not hospitalized. Sometimes this means the expense of traveling long distances, of shifting home responsibilities to meet the patient's needs, and so forth.

The nurse is not responsible for the cost of illness, but she should be aware that it may be a problem for the patient. She can attempt to find out the nature of the patient's concern and alert the physician to the fact that the patient is worried. Depending on the nature of the situation, the problem may be referred to a social worker or a community agency. In communities where home-care plans are available, some patients may be able to receive the care they need at home. From the patient's point of view this may be more satisfactory as well as less expensive. Patients are not always aware of available community services. The nurse should be aware of community resources, or reference

points for community resources, so that she can bring these to the attention of the patient and his family.

To illustrate how differences in definition of the sick role may produce psychological stress, six patients will be presented.

First there is Mr. Tompkins, admitted to ward X. By the very act of admission to the hospital he was separated from his responsibilities as a husband, father, and executive. Hospitalization also established the fact that he was incapable of carrying on his normal role activities. Correct sick-room behavior for Mr. Tompkins and his visitors was interpreted to mean the avoidance of talking about his business or the problems that his son was having in school. In fact, visitors were expected to "cheer him up." Anyone who violated this code was immediately labeled as harmful to his welfare. His employer assured him that he was not being held responsible for his illness by providing him with sick leave and medical and hospital insurance and the assurance that his job would be waiting for him when he recovered. His co-workers took up a collection for flowers and set him cards to indicate their support and concern.

The diagnosis—peptic ulcer—afforded Mr. Tompkins a certain amount of status in the community. It was assumed to indicate that he was hard-working and successful. Therefore, he was allowed to be hospitalized without the loss of status. He could refuse to do certain things commonly expected of persons in his social or employment group. He could even refer to his ulcer with modest pride because it was considered, by some, to be one of the badges of success.

Mr. Tompkins was accepted as a sick person capable of being helped. He recognized that he was ill and placed himself in the hands of professional people. He was considered cooperative or uncooperative to the degree to which he did or did not question care, follow orders, and the like. If he was "cooperative" he won favor for himself, the title of "good patient," and the approval of the personnel concerned with his care. To the degree that he questioned his treatment and did not follow orders and suggestions he was labeled "uncooperative." Depending on the intensity of his behavior he was titled "demanding, unreasonable, stubborn, impossible, or neurotic." Under the latter circumstances he was held responsible for his behavior and care was withheld or given in such a way as to remind Mr. Tompkins of his role as a patient. This tactic seldom succeeds in doing anything except make the patient feel misunderstood. The patient often continues to exhibit the offending behavior or may increase the intensity of his efforts in order to be recognized as an individual. The staff, failing to recognize the defensive nature of Mr. Tompkins' behavior, accomplishes little by resorting to maneuvers that deprive him of care he needs until he acts in accordance with some mystical model for "good patient."

Next there is Mr. Helm, who was hospitalized following an acute myocardial infarction. His illness constituted a serious threat to his self-concept. He always had taken great pride in the fact that he was strong and healthy. He had boasted to his friends that he never lost a day of work because of illness. He always perceived being sick as a sign of weakness. The onset of the myocardial infarction was accompanied by severe substernal pain. Mr. Helm felt frightened, angry, and helpless. He tried to tell himself that the pain would go away—that it was probably indigestion. When the pain became very severe, he called his doctor.

After his admission to the hospital, Mr. Helm made many demands on the nursing staff for attention. When he turned on his light, he expected it to be answered immediately. Through his behavior he indicated that he wanted what he wanted when he wanted it. His behavior demonstrated his need to feel that he had some control over his situation. Though he vented his angry feelings on the nursing staff and his wife, he did not feel safe in attacking his physician. He covered his angry feelings by telling the doctor stories and making light of his situation. As Mr. Helm began to improve, and the physician was able to reassure him that his heart was healing, he began to press for changes in his medical regime and in the management of the nursing unit. In fact, he did this to some extent from the beginning by refusing to use a commode and insisting that he use the bathroom. Part of his reaction to illness was to deny its severity and also to deny the change from his role of a well person to that of a sick person.

It was evident that Mr. Helm's behavior did not conform to that expected in the American cultural pattern. If others did not recognize the true meaning of Mr. Helm's behavior they might have interpreted it to mean that Mr. Helm did not like them. With these feelings they would find it difficult to meet his needs. Conversely, if they were able to accept Mr. Helm as a sick man whose behavior was in keeping with his effort to cope with a critical situation in his life, they might have been able to identify his needs and provide a therapeutic environment for him. Even when the nurse recognizes that a patient's behavior has a cause and serves a purpose, acceptance of the patient who violates the "rules" may not be easy. Knowledge

of possible sources of conflict should facilitate their identification and serve as a basis for making appropriate adjustments in the patient's environment.

In the room next to Mr. Helm was Mr. Quinn. He, too, was in the hospital for the treatment of a myocardial infarction. At the onset of the pain under his sternum, Mr. Quinn also felt helpless and frightened. In contrast to Mr. Helm, however, he was described as a good patient because he conformed to the cultural definition of a sick person. After consulting his physician, Mr. Quinn went to the hospital where he cooperated with the prescribed care. That is, he followed orders exactly. He lay quietly, permitting himself to be fed and bathed. He seldom asked for anything and, when he did, he was both patient and polite. Instead of reacting with anger, he responded to his fears and feelings of helplessness by withdrawing from interactions. He became dependent on others for his care and allowed his dependency without murmur. Although nursing care provided well for his physical needs, his psychological needs were in danger of being overlooked. Mr. Quinn was worried not so much about whether he would die but about his ability to return to his job as a riveter in an automobile plant and about what would happen to his wife and five children if he were not able to work. He always had been able to provide for his family. He had hoped to send his sons to college. Because Mr. Quinn was quiet and undemanding, there was also danger of his being left alone for long periods of time. Elements in establishing a therapeutic environment for Mr. Quinn included instituting a pattern of regular visits and trying to set a climate in which he felt comfortable in expressing the thoughts that troubled him.

Each of the next two patients had an above-the-knee leg amputation. Though the surgical procedure was similar for both patients, their emotional reactions were quite different.

The first patient was Mrs. Oeski, an elderly Polish woman. She seemed to have little concern about the loss of her leg per se. She was, however, very fearful that she would no longer be able to go up and down stairs. This was serious, for though her home had a "company" kitchen and dining room on the first floor, these were seldom used. The kitchen that was used for everyday living was in the basement. Her concept of herself as a homemaker appeared to be more important than that of her physical self. She worked hard to learn to use her prosthesis so that she would be able to walk up and down stairs. Her family were also interested in what they could do to make it possible for her to go up and down stairs. Because of Mrs.

Oeski's personal resources and goals and the support given her by her family, she was able to be rehabilitated to the point where she could continue her homemaking role. The fact that she was highly motivated toward a goal was very helpful to her.

Down the corridor from Mrs. Oeski was Mr. Young. His amputation followed an accident in which a basket of ingots fell on his right leg and crushed it. For days afterward he lay with his face to the wall and refused to eat, be bathed, or perform any activity that was considered necessary to his welfare. Though he guarded against anyone seeing him weep, the nurses were sure that he did. He lacked interest in his children and in events that had interested him previously. His general appearance was that of a dejected, depressed person. It was assumed that he was mourning the loss of his leg.

If nurses are to provide a therapeutic environment for a patient reacting like Mr. Young, they must recognize the grief reaction that frequently follows the loss of a part or a function of the body. Nurses need to understand that each person views his body as part of his identity, his self-image. To some people their body represents almost their total self-image and is of extreme importance to them. Others may have their identity anchored in other aspects of their being such as their intellect, and although their body is important to them, it may not be as significantly important as it is for others. These factors have a bearing on the magnitude of the grieving that is present. The more importance the body has to identity, the greater the grief reaction and vice versa. However, everyone can be expected to grieve to some extent.

In cases such as Mr. Young's the nurses must also recognize that the behavior, although symptomatic of grief, violates two of the tenets of the accepted sick role in the American culture. Mr. Young did not cooperate with those responsible for his care nor did he make an effort to recover. His crying, although appropriate to his grief, is considered inappropriate for a man in this culture. If the nurses who provide Mr. Young's care are able to accept his behavior as having meaning, then they may be able to provide an environment in which he is able to express his grief and examine his feelings. With this help he may be able to move forward toward making plans for his rehabilitation.

Mary Belle Smith represents another manifestation of role confusion resulting from illness. She had rheumatic fever at ages 3 and 7 that was followed by mitral stenosis. As a consequence, she spent little time in school and was overprotected by her family. At age 23 she had a mitral commissurotomy, which, according to the surgeon, was a success. Mary Belle, however, continued to behave like an invalid and resisted all efforts at rehabilitation. Her self-concept remained unaltered and she continued to cope with life in the only way she knew. She only knew how to relate to others as an invalid and continued to do so. Mary Belle's reaction, though not the one desired, is not unique. It is representative of more deeply seated psychological problems than some of the acute reactions to crises that were cited in the previous examples. Therefore, Mary Belle will have greater difficulty changing her self-concept and may require professional psychiatric help to do so. Kaplan,[37] in a study of patients having cardiac surgery, found that some did not recover despite the correction of their physical disability. In some instances the patient continued to be a cardiac invalid; in others he developed other disabilities. According to Kaplan, the patient who uses heart disease as a means of adapting psychologically to the problems in his life is less likely to be benefited by surgery than one who does not. This reaction is not unique to patients with heart disease. Studies of patients with other diseases such as asthma, arthritis, and duodenal ulcer affirm the preceding.

Sometimes people make self-derogatory remarks in an attempt to get others to reaffirm their role perception and give reassurance that they really are acceptable. At times the person wants to be assured that what happened was interpreted in a favorable light. For example, Mrs. Terry had a hysterectomy. As she passed through the stage of excitement in her recovery from a general anesthetic, she cried, screamed, and thrashed about in bed. She was aware of her behavior but was unable to control it. Later, when the effects of the anesthetic had diminished, she said to the nurse, "I behaved very badly when I was under the anesthetic, didn't I?" The nurse replied, "You certainly did." Mrs. Terry burst into tears. She had not wanted to have her fears confirmed. What she wanted was to be reassured that her behavior was not unusual. Had the nurse stopped to examine the intent of Mrs. Terry's question, she could have responded in such a way that Mrs. Terry might have been relieved.

Through the examination of the manner in which some patients reacted to illness, a few of the causes of psychological stress related to role definition have been reviewed. Another way to learn about the psychological needs of patients during illness is to examine the reactions

[37] Stanley M. Kaplan: "Psychological Aspects of Cardiac Disease," *Psychosom. Med.,* **118:**233 (May–June) 1956.

of patients during the different stages of illness. These are the stage of onset, the stage of accepted illness, and the stage of convalescence. Some attention will be given to the ways in which patients are expected to react and how these expectations may affect the care they receive.

EMOTIONAL REACTIONS OF THE PERSON WHO RECOGNIZES HE IS ILL

The significant principle is that anxiety alerts the person to danger. The amount of anxiety provoked in any illness depends on the meaning the illness has to the individual. When the person recognizes that his illness does not respond to home remedies or that he cannot explain its cause or effects to his satisfaction, his anxiety may act as a stimulus for his seeking attention. In contrast, he may be so anxious that he denies that he is ill or attempts to avoid the fact that he is ill. He is too busy to see the doctor, or the doctor is too busy to see him, or he has an important meeting coming up, and so on. His denial may be so complete that he cannot recognize that he is ill even though it may be obvious to his family and associates. Denial in some degree is a common psychological defense against anxiety, and the degree of the denial usually serves as a clue to the degree of anxiety with which the individual is struggling.

Acceptance of illness requires that the individual place himself in the hands of others. To do this he must return to earlier modes of behaving, or regress. Inasmuch as he is able to allow himself to do this, he will be able to follow orders and allow others to attend to his personal, emotional, and physical needs.

According to Barker et al.,[38] if the patient can tolerate being dependent on others, he regresses to a more childlike state that is characterized by the following four features:

1. He becomes self-centered. He sees events and people in relation to himself and existing for his benefit. He becomes demanding and less able to wait to have his needs and wants satisfied. Where he was once considerate of the needs of others, he now is concerned only with his own. Experienced nurses are well aware of this characteristic. One of the criteria by which a patient is judged to be recovering is evidence that he is less self-centered. Perhaps he inquires about the patient in the next bed, or tells his wife to go home early because she looks

weary, or generally is more interested in things going on around him.

2. His interest becomes circumscribed; that is, he is interested in what is happening to him at the present time. Things that were of interest to him before he became ill may be of little concern to him now. For example, when he was well he was an avid baseball fan, but when he is ill he will not even watch the World Series games on television.

3. He is dependent emotionally on those who care for him. He often personalizes the actions of those who care for him as being a direct indication of their acceptance or rejection of him. When a new nurse is assigned to his care, he may interpret this to mean that the nurse who cared for him previously dislikes him. In addition, his feelings may be ambivalent—one minute he feels one way and just the opposite the next. Nurses, and others who care for sick people, should learn to recognize this tendency of the sick to be ambivalent. Thus recognized, the patient's expression of feelings can be viewed as one part of his total illness. This may help nurses, and others, avoid becoming overly elated or downcast by the patient's expression of feelings.

4. He becomes preoccupied with his bodily functions. He is concerned with what he eats or does not eat, with whether the food is suitable for an invalid, with his bowel functions, with the amount of time he sleeps, and so on.

Recognition of the value and characteristics of regression in illness should be helpful to the nurse in understanding the patient and his behavior. It is stated in *Social Interaction and Patient Care* [39] that "It is conceivable that through social and emotional regression the sick person re-distributes his energies to facilitate the healing process or possibly that the regressive integration is in itself an essential factor in the healing process." Regression helps the patient because it makes it possible for him to depend on others to do many things for him that, when well, he could and would do for himself. This includes activities that are of a personal nature. As he was growing up and became able to care for his personal needs, this was accepted as evidence of maturation. Therefore, activities such as bathing, feeding, enemas, and catheterizations have psychological significance that surpasses the actual procedure. Often these activities are not acceptable to the patient

[38] Roger G. Barker et al.: *Adjustment to Physical Handicap and Illness: A Survey of the Social Psychology of Physique and Disability,* rev. ed. (New York: Social Science Research Council, 1953), pp. 239–42.

[39] Henry D. Lederer: "How the Sick View Their World," *Social Interaction and Patient Care,* James K. Skipper, Jr., and Robert C. Leonard, eds. (Philadelphia: J. B. Lippincott Company, 1965), p. 162.

because they demand that he relinquish control over some of the first, and most basic, functions that he mastered in his life. When a patient is able to allow others to care for him, however, he can redirect the energy thus conserved toward the process of getting well.

As his condition improves the patient is expected to resume responsibility for himself. In general, the belief is held that the sooner the patient can resume his normal activities, the more rapid his recovery will be. However, he needs to understand that these activities are as much a part of his plan of therapy as are his medications and his diet. The patient too often interprets being asked to bathe himself as the nurse's shifting some of her work on him because she is too busy or unwilling to help him. Very often the nurse reinforces this feeling because she feels guilty about letting the patient care for himself or does not understand why this activity is important to the patient's recovery. The patient needs to know that the nurse is standing by to help him if and when he requires help.

The person with an illness or disability frequently feels angry. The anger is often associated with the feeling that being ill or hurt is an injustice. The person may be angry at what has happened to him, angry at his own helplessness, and so forth. What is even more difficult is that he does not know where to direct his anger or, in some instances, he does not even know why he is angry—only that he is. Because he cannot shout at the walls and gain satisfaction in the expression of his anger, the patient frequently displaces his anger onto people in the environment because they are real and will react. The patient may express his anger at those who care for him, including friends, family, nurses, and other health workers. If the nurse recognizes that the patient's behavior is part of his reaction to illness and knows that it serves a purpose, then she is better able to help the patient explore or examine the situation without herself becoming upset or hurt. Families frequently require some support in order to develop understanding of the situation. There is some evidence to support the observation that patients who are able to express their hostility during illness make more rapid recoveries than those who do not.

Some patients turn their anger inward and become depressed. Some degree of depression is probably associated with any serious illness and indeed may be a necessary stage in recovery. Inasmuch as depression enables the patient to withdraw and conserve his energy, it is protective. When it gets in the way of any movement toward health, depression is considered to be destructive. Sutherland [40] found that patients who had radical mastectomies almost always evidenced some depression during their first few days at home. In instances where the family accepted the patient's depression and increased dependency, the patient made more rapid recovery than those whose families did not accept this behavior.

The depression that accompanies the loss of a part or of an ability that has been important to the patient may be an expression of grief, as was seen in the case of Mr. Young. Acceptance by the nursing staff of the fact that a patient not only does but has the right to mourn the loss of part of himself and that he may need help in expressing his grief is fundamental to an adequate plan of care. The nurse may think that the patient should be glad to be rid of a gangrenous leg, but the patient views his situation differently. Because the leg was part of himself, part of his concept or image of himself, opportunities for the expression of sorrow in an understanding and accepting environment may lessen the need for feelings of self-pity or self-chastisement. People often find it easier to do what they have to do when they feel that others are trying to understand their point of view.

When illness is a serious threat to the individual's integrity, he is likely to become confused. Confusion may cover up other feelings such as anxiety, anger, or the fear of being dependent. Confusion makes people feel less responsible for their other feelings because these are hidden under the blanket of the confusion. For example, Mrs. Wilson found her husband dead in bed beside her. She went next door for help but could not remember going or how she got there. She kept repeating, "What did I do? How did I get to your house? I can't remember, I'm so confused. I do not know what to do." The thing she stated as being most helpful to her was that, after confirming the fact that her husband was dead, the neighbors assumed responsibility for calling the doctor, the relatives, and so on. They took the necessary responsibility and appeared to have the situation under control. Sometimes confusion is not as evident as in the instance of Mrs. Wilson. Confusion may show only when the patient is called on to remember or to learn. It is likely, however, that it is more common than is generally appreciated. This is one reason instructions and explanations given to patients need to be repeated, sometimes over and over. Nurses should not be surprised when patients forget or distort instructions given to them by themselves or physicians.

[40] Arthur Sutherland: "Psychological Impact of Cancer Surgery," *Public Health Rep.,* **67:**1139–43 (Nov.) 1952.

Confusion tends to limit the person's perception of reality in many situations.

As implied, patients may adapt to illness by attack or withdrawal. Each method has its advantages and disadvantages and implications for nursing. During illness the patient needs his energy to recover. The patient who adapts by attack should be protected from circumstances that increase his feeling that he has to use aggressive behavior to have his needs met. This is often difficult for nursing personnel (and others), because sick people are expected to follow orders and appreciate the care that is offered them. When the patient demands attention and does not seem to appreciate the efforts made in his behalf, the nurses may feel frustrated and ineffectual. If the nurse understands that the use of aggressive behavior is the patient's attempt at adapting to illness, she should feel less responsible for the behavior. She might then find it easier to understand the patient's motivation, plan his care so he can feel secure that he will receive the care he needs, and assist him in looking at other ways of getting his needs met without having to use attack.

The patient who withdraws during illness is also trying to adapt. Withdrawal serves the positive purpose of conserving his energy, but the patient does not gain insight into what his illness means to him or what he needs to do differently in order to adapt in a healthier way. The withdrawn patient is likely to be considered a "good patient" unless he becomes overly dependent on those who provide his care. The problems in his care derive from the ability of those who provide his care to accept the patient in his regressed state and also to prevent the withdrawal from going too far. This means that those who care for him must recognize when the patient no longer needs to conserve his energy and can assume responsibility for meeting some of his own needs and for making his own decisions. This transition may take considerable time, especially when the patient has been seriously ill. It also requires skillful assessment on the part of the staff and consistent messages about expectations so that the patient is not being asked to assume responsibility one minute and being told he cannot the next.

During the stage of convalescence the patient is expected to progress from illness to physical and emotional health. He must give up his dependent and self-centered behavior and fend for himself again. Lederer [41] states that there are many similarities between the dynamics of adolescence and illness. During the stages of illness the patient goes from dependence to independence and finally to interdependence. Some patients find it difficult to give up being the center of attention and to assume responsibility for themselves again. When a patient has been able to enjoy the legitimate claim to dependency that illness affords, and which he may deny himself when well, he may go through a rather difficult dependent-independent struggle on the road to recovery.

Recovery may also be delayed if illness provides more satisfactions than does health. The many factors that contribute to the development of a preference for illness to health will not be discussed in detail. They are, however, defined as the secondary gains of illness. For some reason illness provides more security and satisfaction than health for certain people. Mary Belle, who continued to be an invalid despite correction of her cardiac disability, was one example. There are techniques that may reduce the likelihood of this happening. The first is to encourage the patient to assume responsibility by including him in the decision-making process concerning his care. As this is done the patient should understand that, as he assumes responsibility, he helps himself recover and that assistance is available if and when he requires it. When and how to help the patient requires judgment so that the patient is not assisted unnecessarily and thus robbed of the feeling of accomplishment. Nor, on the other hand, should he be pushed beyond his capacity to perform. The nurse must be able to stand by and wait as the patient struggles, but she must also be alert enough to restructure the patient's learning experience when the struggle seems insurmountable and the same goal can be reached in another way. Through grappling with his problem and experiencing some successes as well as being able to look at the things that cause him frustration, the patient gains the strength to progress toward recovery.

A few practices that are useful in helping patients with long-term illnesses keep before them the objective of returning to the community and an active life are restricting visitors as little as possible, permitting overnight leaves from the hospital, encouraging family and friends to take patients to community events, having patients wear their own clothing when at all possible, encouraging self-expression and participation in activities that are of interest in the hospital, and moving the patient to home care as soon as the situation permits. During hospitalization a patient can be assisted to use time constructively by reviewing his home situation and thinking ahead about the kinds of physical adaptations that will help him live as normally as possible. If his house has stairs and he is in a wheelchair, what needs to be done so he can move about and not be confined to

41 *Op. cit.,* p. 164.

one area? Who, in the community, is available to help the patient maintain outside contacts after he goes home? What other professional assistance such as physical therapy and occupational therapy is available to help the patient learn useful diversional or self-maintaining activities? These are some of the questions nurses need to ask themselves when planning patient care. There are many social agencies and social clubs whose aim is to help people to help themselves. The patient should be familiarized with some of the available resources so he does not begin to feel that posthospitalization offers nothing but isolation and frustration. In addition to planning for his physical needs, the patient should be helped to look at how the nondisabled respond to the disabled and how he anticipated he might react in some situations where others are either oversolicitous or studiously ignore his limitations.

EMOTIONAL REACTIONS OF OTHERS TO AN INDIVIDUAL'S ILLNESS

Family and friends of handicapped persons or of those who have had a long illness and are being prepared to return to the community require instruction in what they should do for the patient, how they should do it, and what they should expect from the patient. Families tend to react either by doing too much for the person and overprotecting him or by rejecting him. Nurses should be alert for clues that indicate how significant family members feel about the patient's illness and be prepared to help the family talk about some of their responses. For example, a young male quadriplegic was preparing to go home on his first weekend pass since he was hospitalized. The nurse was teaching his wife how to care for her husband's bowel and bladder functions. The wife learned to irrigate the catheter, but the nurse noted that the wife recoiled every time she had to touch her husband's penis or the catheter. The nurse asked the wife about her reaction after they left the patient's room. The wife said that she was very distressed. Here was the man she married, whom she had expected to care for her, raise a family with, and so forth. Instead, he was completely helpless and needing care from her for the most basic functions. She was suddenly overwhelmed with her own feeling of being cheated of a husband, being angry at him for becoming an invalid, and then feeling guilty for having these feelings. In this situation, and in many like it, couples or families who face such prolonged stressful situations should be referred for joint counseling. The nurse is not necessarily prepared to deal with all these problems but, it is hoped that she will become astute enough

to recognize that problems exist and refer people to proper resources for help.

Families also need help and support the first few times they take the handicapped person out in public. They need to be prepared for the fact that people are made uncomfortable by seeing those who are disabled or deformed. Liss [42] explained this phenomenon as follows: "The ill, with their dysfunctions of body or mind, are reminders of the precariousness of health. We prefer not to be reminded, for it is not pleasant, it is threatening, and the inevitable dissolution of all living things is to be thrust aside and away." However, after the patient and his family get through the first painful adventures, they begin to be less sensitive and find that people are generally helpful and willing to listen to ways in which help can be given.

Nursing Care

Because illness, particularly that which produces some degree of incapacity or requires hospitalization, is a crisis situation in the life of the patient and his family, it produces psychological stress resulting in various feelings of discomfort, one of which is anxiety. Despite popular opinion to the contrary, not all anxiety is bad or undesirable, nor is it all preventable. However, much can be done in the practice of nursing to reduce the incidence of unnecessary anxiety and to provide the patient with needed support. To prevent and reduce unnecessary psychological stress the nurse needs to be aware of possible causes, and she must be able to recognize clues in the patient's behavior that indicate how the patient feels about himself and his illness.

How can the nurse identify the patient's emotional reaction to his illness?

According to Sartain,[43] emotion has four aspects. The first is the personal emotional experience. These are feelings that the person is conscious of and can describe verbally. The person, in describing his feelings, says, "I feel so happy that I could fly or cry" or "I feel so angry and disappointed that I want to cry." The words used to describe emotions and the ability to describe feelings verbally vary from person to person. The nurse must therefore be alert to the significance not only of what the person says but of how and why he says it.

[42] Edward Liss: "Conscious and Unconscious Factors in Rehabilitation," *Occup. Ther. Rehab.*, 27:20 (Feb.) 1948.
[43] Aaron Sartain *et al.: Psychology: Understanding Human Behavior,* 2nd ed. (New York: McGraw-Hill Book Company, Inc., 1962), pp. 103–16.

The second aspect of emotion is that it is also expressed through bodily changes. These changes are those associated with altering the person to meet danger and restore the body to a state of equilibrium. They result from activation of the autonomic nervous system and that part of the hormonal system that enables the organism to respond to emergency situations. Physiological changes that may accompany anxiety include trembling or shaking, restlessness, sleep disturbances (including insomnia), loss of appetite or anorexia, inability to concentrate, irritability, and the symptoms that indicate an imbalance in the autonomic nervous system. Increases in pulse, respiratory rate, and blood pressure are common, as are increased frequency of urination and disturbances in gastrointestinal activity. Peristalsis may be increased or decreased. As a result of anxiety the patient may be nauseated, vomit, have diarrhea, suffer abdominal distention, or be constipated.

The third aspect of emotion is behavior that can be observed by others. These behaviors are expressive and should be viewed as a significant part of nonverbal communication. These behaviors involve bodily changes, too, but usually ones that can be altered consciously if the person becomes aware of them or if his emotional state changes. Skeletal muscle tension or relaxation indicates something about the emotional state of the individual. The frightened or anxious individual tenses his muscles in preparation for flight or fight even when neither course is open to him. To illustrate, Tom was an active 18-year-old whose chest x-ray showed a well-defined lesion in the lower lobe of his right lung. Surgery was performed promptly and the diseased tissue removed. Both Tom and his parents were badly frightened. Tom did not talk about his fears but was seen lying against his pillows with his fists clenched and with obvious body tension. Deep-breathing, turning, and coughing were accompanied by more than the usual amout of pain and difficulty. His cough was unproductive and the lung on the operated side was slow in re-expanding. Attempts at reassurance were of little help until one morning when the surgeon told Tom, "The reports are back from the pathologist. Your lung had a harmless little tumor in it. You are cured." The change in Tom was remarkable. He relaxed, assumed responsibility for his own care, and in other ways demonstrated that he was no longer frightened.

Behavioral expressions are especially useful when trying to identify the emotional state of the individual who is unable to talk. The nurse should keep in mind that there is no single reason people do not talk about their feelings. Some may not understand their own feelings well enough to discuss them, or they may recognize the feeling and be reluctant to discuss it because they do not know how it will be received, or they may be physically unable to talk. Facial expression is one common source of information about a person's emotional state. We frequently hear comments such as, "He talks with his eyes," "The boss is in a good mood today; he was smiling when he came in," "She looks as if she just lost her best friend," and "Her face is peaceful as if she were a happy person." Though facial expression serves as a clue to the emotional state, more information is required in order to make an accurate assessment of how the individual really feels. A person may smile when he feels like crying, or he may pride himself on his "poker face." Cultural and environmental factors also play a part in how a person learns to use various body or facial gestures to express emotion. In some cultures individuals learn to keep their faces immobile, and they may suffer pain and other discomfort without any change of expression. When this is the case, other means of estimating the degree of discomfort must be used. The main point here is that the facial expression is only a signal that alerts the nurse to explore its meaning. The patient is really the only person who can say what his expression means. Too often nurses are guilty of making assumptions about the meaning of the patient's behavior without actually clarifying the situation with him.

Emotion may also be expressed through movements of the hands and body. In the instance of Tom, he expressed his fright by tensing his muscles and clenching his fists. Another patient may move about. In bed he twists and turns. Out of bed he paces the floor, wrings his hands, or shakes his fists. Other emotions are also expressed through body movement. Friendliness may be shown by shaking hands, joy by clapping the hands, and so forth. Posture and step also reveal the feelings of the individual. When a person's posture is erect and his step is firm, he creates the impression that he is healthy and feeling good about himself and others. Conversely, when his shoulders sag, his feet drag, and his movements are languid, he creates the impression of being dejected or depressed. Clarification is necessary here as well. For example, a patient is observed picking at the edge of his covers. At this point the nurse does not actually know if the patient is anxious and needs to talk about something, is trying to get a gravy stain off the blanket binding, or is anoxic and in dire need of attention. She can find the answer by obtaining more information and by closer inspection of the situation.

In the American culture, where high value is

placed on a healthy body and cleanliness, grooming and other evidence of cleanliness are clues to the emotional state of the individual. Uncombed and untidy hair, soiled and ragged clothing, dirty and poorly kept fingernails, or run-over shoes may be interpreted as meaning that the person has a low opinion of himself. Before arriving at any conclusions, one must know such things as (1) the type of work the person does, (2) the expectations of the group with whom he identifies, and (3) whether his appearance is a significant change associated with illness or a life-long pattern. For example, a man who spends his working days greasing automobiles is likely to have a problem keeping his fingernails clean. Another man may look as if he needs a shave not because he is neglecting his appearance but because he is growing a beard.

Vocal expressions of emotion may be through talking, crying, whistling, laughing, or screaming. In talking, the person's feeling is conveyed not only by what he says but by whether what he says is usual for him and by his tone of voice. It is also helpful to know how the person usually expresses satisfaction or dissatisfaction. Sometimes the words and tone used by a patient are offensive to the nurse. When this happens, the nurse should try to discover what the patient is trying to communicate rather than making judgments about the words themselves. When a patient is able to modify his behavior, limits can be set based on the patient's needs and the situation.

In general, laughter and humor are acceptable ways of expressing feeling in the American culture. This may be related to the fact that laughter is often associated with "good" feelings such as joy. The fact is that laughter and humor may hide feelings such as sorrow, anxiety, or hostility. The patient who is always laughing and joking may be admired at first, but this "bravado" type of behavior tends to wear thin and others become suspect of the patient's motives. A little thought given to the reasons behind his behavior might reveal that he is frightened, or angry, or both. The last example points out the fourth aspect of emotion, which is motivation. This term refers to the fact that people are goal-directed. Our laughing, joking patient may be frightened or angry—those are his feelings. Because it is natural for man to want to avoid pain, we can speculate that the goal this patient seeks is to avoid the pain of his own feelings. One way he has learned to do this is seen in the behavior he uses, namely laughing and joking. Laughter is often used to relieve tension. Playwrights use humor to break the tension in a serious drama, so it is not too sur-

prising that patients might use humor to break the tension in the serious drama of illness.

Although joy and gladness may be expressed by crying, the shedding of tears is usually associated with "bad" feelings such as pain, sorrow, helplessness, and anger. Though adults have these feelings, their expression by crying is disapproved of. Moreover, when men, who are expected to be strong, cry, their behavior is regarded as being particularly inappropriate. Crying is for babies who are still dependent on their mothers and not for grown men and women who have long since reached adulthood. Nurses who find themselves with a crying adult may feel uncomfortable because they do not understand the regressive phenomenon of illness, of which crying may be one part. The nurse may be embarrassed because the patient is unable to control his behavior. She may become uncomfortable because crying is viewed as a distress signal and yet she does not know what to do to intervene. Or she may feel uncomfortable because a crying patient is a reflection on the quality of nursing care—or so she thinks. Whatever the reason, or combination of reasons, for her discomfort, the nurse's first impulse is usually to get the patient to stop crying. Instead of concentrating her attention on trying to stop the crying, it would be more helpful for the nurse to understand what the patient is trying to express through crying. It is also important to know the individual. Does he come from a subculture where crying is a fairly common means of expression? Does this patient cry easily, or is this the first time that such behavior has been noted? These are just two of the questions the nurse can ask herself. Usually, an effective way to find out what is going on is for the nurse to wait until the patient stops crying. She can indicate that she is willing to listen when the patient is ready to talk about his feelings.

It may be helpful if the nurse makes an attempt to understand her attitudes about crying. How does she feel when she cries? Does she ever allow herself to cry, and if not, why not? Under what circumstances does she cry? What does she expect from others when she cries in their presence? This self-inspection does not preclude talking with the patient about why he cries, but it may make the situation more understandable and tolerable for the nurse. The nurse may come to understand that what the patient really wants is for someone to indicate that they care about his concerns. He may not be asking for solutions because he may know that there are no solutions available in terms of performing some technical procedure that will "cure all." On the other hand, if there is some physical comfort measure that is indicated, this should be used.

Other ways in which patients express their emotions vocally are by shouting, screaming, moaning, and sighing. These behaviors, for much the same reason as crying, may be upsetting to nurses. They are also disturbing to other patients. When this behavior is continued and is upsetting to other patients, it may be necessary to isolate the patient in a soundproof room. In one hospital the isolation of Puerto Rican women who were in labor was found to be necessary. When these women reached a certain point in labor they screamed, and their screaming was very frightening to other patients. Before placing a patient in isolation one should be certain that there is no other solution and that the isolation is for the good of the other patients or the patient himself. When isolation is necessary, the nurse has an obligation to try to identify and meet the needs of the patient. Someone should stay with the patient, or, if continuous supervision is not necessary, the patient should be told how to summon the nurse and his calls should be answered promptly. Though the welfare of others may make isolation of the patient necessary, this procedure increases his need for nursing. Studies of the effects of isolation on healthy young men indicate the importance of environmental stimulation to healthy mental functioning. Soon after the subjects were separated from external stimuli, they began to have hallucinations.[44]

Sometimes when the behavior of a patient is deemed unacceptable, he is isolated by neglect rather than by physical isolation. Mr. Jones was screaming as if he were in severe pain, but no one was paying attention to him. The reason given for the neglect was that he was "just a neurotic with a low tolerance for pain." On investigation he was found to be hemorrhaging into his urinary bladder at a spot where the bladder wall had been eroded by a bladder stone. Mr. Jones was a paraplegic and had what is called a neurogenic bladder; that is, it emptied spontaneously when it reached its capacity, which was very small. As the bladder filled, painful muscle contractions were initiated. Because blood clots blocked the urethra and prevented his bladder from emptying, the painful muscle spasms increased in frequency as the bladder wall stretched. Perhaps Mr. Jones' tolerance for pain was minimal. Be that as it may, he was suffering and needed relief. When the physician saw Mr. Jones, he scheduled him for emergency surgery. Following surgery, Mr. Jones was well-controlled. This is an excellent

example of the danger of categorizing patients according to their behavior without adequate investigation into its cause. That some of this man's care was inhumane should not require saying. Moreover, conclusions about the cause of a patient's behavior should not be reached without thorough knowledge of the patient and the situation.

There are many ways in which patients manifest their anxiety. A variety of behaviors characterized by action may be called "flight into activity." The patient makes jokes and is the life of the ward because, for him, talking relieves tension and serves much the same purpose as whistling in the dark. Pacing up and down the corridor or going from one activity to another serves a similar purpose. Careful listening may yield clues about the meaning of the patient's behavior that may make it possible to initiate action that will help allay his fears.

One of the problems in planning care directed toward minimizing anxiety is that despite identification of signs and symptoms these do not, in themselves, identify the cause of the anxiety. Nor does the relief of anxiety always take precedence over other necessary care. The patient who is bleeding excessively will be anxious, but the problem that takes priority is the hemorrhage. At the time the most reassuring thing that can be done is to initiate prompt action to stop the bleeding. In the words of a patient who experienced this situation, "I turned on my light and the student nurse came right away. She ran and got the head nurse who ran and got the doctor. The doctor came right away and I was in the operating room before I knew what was happening—and a good thing too. I owe my life to the fact that they were on their toes."

It has been mentioned that it is not always possible to determine all the factors contributing to anxiety. Nor is it possible to relieve anxiety entirely even if such a thing were desirable. There are times in patient care when anxiety is necessary to keep the patient motivated to work toward the achievement of healthier goals. Sometimes it is necessary to stimulate anxiety in patients so they will be less willing to accept the status quo of hospitalization. This must be done with careful planning and by personnel who have considerable skill in the area of human behavior.

There are also many factors in illness and its diagnosis and treatment that are anxiety-provoking but cannnot be avoided. One of the greatest fears in life is the unknown. Anytime the nurse can anticipate the unknown and interpret it for the patient, she is creating an environment that may make it easier for the

---

[44] Woodburn Heron: "The Pathology of Boredom," *Sci. Amer.*, **146:**52–56 (Jan.) 1957.

patient to participate more effectively in treatment. Reasonable explanations given to the patient, so he knows what is being done and why, usually help keep his anxiety within reasonable bounds.

In individualizing care it is helpful if the nurse can recognize the pattern the patient uses in establishing or avoiding relationships with others. The mature adult in American culture is thought to be one who can relate to others as an equal. He can work interdependently or cooperatively with others and can give and take as the situation demands. In actuality this is a myth. Some people form dependent relationships, some need to dominate others, some rebel against others (especially those in authority), and some avoid forming any lasting relationships. These patterns may not be as evident when the person is well as they are when he is sick. The aggressive executive, for example, may deny any dependent strivings when he is well but may deny them even more when he is threatened by illness.

Patients are expected to place themselves in a dependent relationship to those who provide their care. This dependency is considered "healthy" when the patient cooperates with getting the care he realistically needs. The trend in health care is toward encouraging patients to participate in the decision-making process rather than expecting them to submit to decisions that others make about their care. In this view, the patient is recognized as being an important element in his own recovery. That is, the recovery of the patient depends on the patient. The services of doctors, nurses, and other health workers only provide conditions under which the patient's recovery can be facilitated. Because all patients do not interact or react in the same manner, recognition of the patient's pattern should alert the nurse to some problems that may arise in his care. If the patient is one who characteristically rebels against others, he may need time to talk himself into doing what he knows he must do. For this patient, pressure from another person may only increase his resistance. If the pressure is too great, he may take a position from which he cannot retreat without considerable loss of self-esteem.

How may the nurse minimize psychological stress through nursing intervention?

Florence Nightingale,[45] in *Notes on Nursing,* emphasized the need for the nurse to recognize and relieve anxiety in the patient. She wrote the following:

Apprehension, uncertainty, waiting, expectation, fear of surprise, do a patient more harm than any exertion. Remember, he is face to face with his enemy all the time, internally wrestling with him, having long imaginary conversations with him. You are thinking of something else. "Rid him of his adversary quickly," is a first rule with the sick.

Wertham,[46] a psychiatrist, in discussing his experiences as a patient, made the following comments about how the sick person can be helped: "Medical and surgical patients need psychological advice about how they should act, what their experiences mean; they need psychological preparation for what to expect; they need guidance so that they can make the best of their possibilities." He also listed the kinds of remarks that were antitherapeutic for him. Sometimes these comments were made in jest and sometimes to give information. The intention of those who made the remarks was to reassure him. For example, he was told that thrombophlebitis, though fairly common in the legs, seldom affects the arms. Until that time he had not considered the possibility of the disease affecting his arms. For some time thereafter, he was sure that he was developing thrombophlebitis in his arms and would lie in bed mentally examining them for indications of disease.

Sometimes suggesting problems to the patient can be prevented by making certain you understand what he is asking or what he wants to know. This can be done by asking for clarification or by indicating that you do not understand what he wants. The principle here can be illustrated by the classic story about the little boy who asked his mother where his baby sister came from. The mother had been anxiously awaiting the day when her boy would raise this question, so she went into her detailed story about how his father planted the seed and so on. When she finished, she asked the boy if he understood. He said, "All I wanted to know was did she come from the hospital down the street or from the Sister's hospital?"

The question "What can we do to relieve the patient's anxiety and thus reassure him?" suggests other questions. How does one person reassure another? What does reassurance mean? Is it accomplished by telling the other person that everything will be all right? Does one person stop worrying when another says, "Leave the worrying to me"? Dictionaries define *reassure* as a transitive verb meaning to restore to courage or confidence, also to re-establish. Its synonyms include to encourage, which in turn means to inspire with courage, hope, con-

[45] Florence Nightingale: *Notes on Nursing: What It Is, and What It Is Not,* revised and enlarged ed. (London: Harrison and Sons, 1860), p. 53.

[46] Fredric Wertham: "A Psychosomatic Study of Myself," *When Doctors Are Patients,* Max Pinner and Benjamin F. Miller, eds. (New York: W. W. Norton and Company, Inc., 1952), p. 115.

fidence, or resolution; to help forward as well as to animate, cheer, hearten, and inspire. It is also interesting to note that synonyms of encourage include console, comfort, solace, and sympathize with. How can the nurse through the practice of nursing assist the patient to regain his courage or confidence? The emphasis here is on the patient's regaining hope and confidence, not on the nurse's giving this to him. However, the nurse contributes to this by what she does and how she does it. Wertham [47] states that during an operation two factors contributed to decreasing his general feeling of insecurity. One was the calm, deep, authoritative voice of the surgeon. The other was the soothing effect of the touch of a woman physician as she said something to him. Though he recognized that the friends who were with him were trying to reassure him by talking and joking, he did not find this behavior at all reassuring.

Barker et al.[48] talk of helping patients to think in terms of what they have left and what they can do rather than what they have lost and what they cannot do. This approach has great supportive value for those, for example, who suddenly become handicapped. On the other hand, nothing is more devastating to a patient than the thoughtless statements that suddenly confront him with his loss and the meaning this loss has to his total identity. The author (then a patient) experienced the latter when a physician introduced her to another physician and added, "Before her accident, she was a nurse." This does not mean that patients should never look at the readjustments they need to make as the result of illness. They do need to realistically assess their situation but not without help that enables them to look at what is possible for them, what they need to do differently, and what they may have to defer or give up entirely.

Reassurance of patient is frequently difficult. Sometimes it is not achieved until the patient knows the outcome of his treatment. In another situation, a patient who had undergone a bronchoscopy stated that he did not think he could have withstood the procedure had the nurse not given him instructions during the procedure about what he should do and about the progress of the procedure. Here the talking related directly to what the patient could expect from himself and from the situation and was not intended to distract his attention. Though what is reassuring differs from one person to another, confidence that the situation is under control is often helpful. For some patients that is all that is necessary.

One of the ways to learn what actions enhance the patient's confidence in his care is by listening to what he says. Some of the things that patients comment on as being reassuring and adding to their security include having nurses work with them who (1) have the ability to assess the situation quickly and initiate prompt action when required; (2) appear to know what to do; (3) take over when the patient is overwhelmed and know how to do the "right thing"; (4) will be there when needed —a group of patients requested that a nurse not be transferred from night to day duty because they could depend on her to be there when they needed her; (5) keep the patient informed about what they are doing and why, when they can be expected, how long they will be away, and how much time they will spend with him; (6) learn what the patient expects and helps correct his misunderstandings and misconceptions about what he can expect; (7) maintain uniformity in the performance of frequently repeated procedures and apprise him of changes that are planned; (8) encourage the patient to help himself in ways that he is able not because it helps the nurse per se but because in this way he can learn to do for himself; (9) help the patient become aware of even small gains; (10) can modify their behavior in such a manner that the patient knows they are sensitive to and concerned about his feelings; (11) take care of the patient's personal belongings and his physical environment; (12) give attention to those things that are important to the patient, such as respecting his right to some privacy; and (13) keep informed about changes in the therapeutic plan—even though this is not always easy—and can develop a plan for nursing care based on the therapeutic plan.

Both the person and the circumstances under which the need for reassurance arises are determining factors in the type of behavior that is to be effective. Though some suggestions can be made for the type of behavior that may be reassuring, no recipe can be given for what will always result in reassurance. Reassurance requires competence in the practice of nursing. By this is meant that the nurse knows what she is doing, why she does it, and how to do it or is reassuring in the fact that she will seek help if she does not know something. She gives appropriate attention to detail not for the sake of detail but because it is important to the outcome of what she is doing. She thinks about what she is doing, its effect on the patient, and about how it can be improved. This and much more is important to help the patient feel that he is valued as an individual, that his needs will be met, and that he is in safe hands. Acceptance involves the transmission of the feeling that the patient is important. This can be accomplished, in part, by doing for and with the patient those

[47] Ibid., p. 108.
[48] Barker et al., op. cit., p. 82.

things that are important to his welfare. Because his welfare includes both physical and psychological aspects, his care also includes both—bathing, feeding, listening, supporting, protecting, comforting, anticipating, and relieving. It also includes allowing, encouraging, and supporting him in assuming responsibility for his own care as soon as he is able. It also involves validating the meaning of his behavior and then acting appropriately.

To illustrate, a nurse answers Mr. Jason's call signal. She observes that he is irritable. She knows that irritability is common in sick people and that it indicates not what is wrong but that something is wrong. It is a warning signal. Instead of feeling personally attacked, the nurse asks herself why Mr. Jason may be irritable. Is he receiving insulin in the treatment of his diabetes? If so, is he suffering from hypoglycemia? Is he having difficulty with his oxygen intake? Does he have a low frustration tolerance as the result of brain damage? Is he cold? Is he disappointed because his wife and family have not been to visit him? Has he had too many visitors? Is he troubled about the nature of his illness, its cost, or what is going to happen in relation to his job? Is he lonely? Has he been accustomed to consuming large amounts of alcohol and is he now beginning to show signs of withdrawal? Did the patient in the next bed keep him awake all night? Is this usually the way he behaves under stress? The nurse tries to determine the cause of Mr. Jason's irritability and institutes action aimed at solving or relieving the identifiable problem. She may listen to his complaint, get him a glass of orange juice, call a social worker, or do any number of other meaningful things. What she does depends on her perception of what the patient needs at the time.

Another illustration is Mr. McGraw, who swears when he is in pain. The nurse notes the beads of perspiration on his brow and his clenched fists. She recognizes that his pain is severe and understands that swearing is his way of emphasizing its severity. The nurse lets Mr. McGraw know that she recognizes his suffering, talks with him about what he thinks will relieve it, and then does something to relieve it not because she approves of swearing but because she is concerned with what prompted it. Under other circumstances, Mr. McGraw's swearing may have other meanings. He may be in the habit of swearing. If his swearing really is offensive to others, the nurse may have to set limits by pointing out that his behavior disturbs others. She may ask him to try to use other, equally understandable words to convey his message.

The nurse also needs to be aware of what causes her to become anxious or uncomfortable. To return to Mr. McGraw, if the nurse becomes anxious, or feels that his swearing is a personal affront, she may leave him to "stew in his own juice until he can act like a gentleman." If, however, she is aware of her own discomfort and still can remain with Mr. McGraw, she may be able to take the next step, which is to find out why he is behaving this way. Her further action then can be directed toward the primary goal of meeting Mr. McGraw's needs. When she is successful in meeting the patient's needs, she also meets her own need for self-realization as a nurse.

Another skill needed in nursing is in the use of purposeful conversation. Though all conversation has purpose, the kind we are talking about is for the specific purpose of furthering communication that is so important to the improvement of patient care. Purposeful communication is an essential part of the nursing process because it makes possible the collection of information, the identification of the problem, the formulation of a plan of action, the implementation of that plan, and the evaluation of its effectiveness. What this means essentially is that the nurse becomes accustomed to thinking in a logical sequence and uses all her communication skills—including conversation—to help her do this.

The first step in purposeful conversation is the establishment of a goal that is valid and sincere. When a problem is known or suspected, the objective should be based on the desire to assist the patient rather than identifying the problem just for the sake of knowing what the problem is.

Second, purposeful conversation implies a dialogue. Hearing both the words and what they mean is important. Communication takes place only when the message sent is the same as the message that is received. Too often we assume that the listener understood exactly what we intended only to find that there was a major breakdown between what was intended and how it was interpreted. Listening only with the ears is perhaps too restrictive. The really skillful nurse usually has learned to listen with all her senses. One needs to hear what the speaker is saying, how he is saying it, and what his facial expression is. Attention should also be given to shifts in the person's conversation. What he does not say, or skips over, may be just as important as what he does say. Purposeful conversation also means that the responder may need to take time to think out his reply. To do this he must be able to keep the objective of the conversation in mind and to tolerate silence. Some of the world's most skillful conversationalists talk very little but listen much. This is illustrated by the taxi driver who, on discharging a passenger, said, "My, you are a good listener." During the hour's ride, the passenger had said little except "Mmm," "Not really", "You like your work," and a few other similar comments. The only purpose of the listener's responding at all was to indicate that she was following what the driver was saying and was interested in it.

In addition to listening, conversation may be facilitated by asking open-ended questions or by asking the patient to clarify what he has said. In the use of open-ended questions, the questioner tries to avoid asking the question in a way that suggests the answer. Statements such as, "I don't understand," "Could you clarify that?" or "You were saying . . . ?" or even "Oh," or "Mmm" when said with rising inflection can be used to indicate that one is interested, is following what is being said, and would like to hear more. The patient should also be given time to respond. This means that the nurse must be able to stay with the patient and wait for his response.

The nurse may suspect that something is worrying the patient and she may have clues as to the nature of what is troubling him. She must put these to the test. This can be done by repeating what the patient has said or what appears to be the intent of his comment. For example, Miss Tente, a patient in her teens, appeared to be upset when the student nurse tried to instruct her in how to inject her own insulin. The student was surprised because up to this time Miss Tente had seemed eager to learn. The student suspected that Miss Tente's hesitancy might be related to something other than inserting the needle. To test her hypothesis she said, "You are troubled this morning"; then she waited. In a few moments Miss Tente started to cry. Between her sobs she told the student nurse that when she told her boy friend about her diabetes he no longer wanted to "go steady."

The use of silence may give some people an opening to talk about their troubles or problems, and it has other uses as well. In the care of the seriously ill, conversation should be limited in order to conserve the patient's energy. Some seriously ill people are comforted by the closeness of having someone sit quietly by their bedside. This may give a relative or close friend an opportunity to make a substantial contribution to the patient's welfare. A relative may need some instruction in how to behave in the presence of the patient and support and recognition of their contribution to the welfare of the patient from nursing personnel. This is especially necessary when the patient is ill over a long period of time. For example, Mr. Clark was seriously ill in a hospital located some distance from his home. His wife was notified of his illness, and the suggestion was made that she arrange to come to the hospital as soon as possible. When she arrived, she was understandably distraught. The nurse, recognizing Mrs. Clark's emotional condition and that she had been riding on the bus all night, arranged for her to wash her face and hands and apply cosmetics. Then she suggested that after Mrs. Clark greeted her husband, she might sit quietly by his bed and, if she would like to do so, hold his hand. In this instance the nurse helped Mrs. Clark compose herself and then suggested how she might be helpful to her husband.

Another too frequently neglected practice of silence is what may be called friendly silence. Everyone feels good toward the other members of the group. All are comfortable and relaxed. This is the silence that says, "All is calm and serene. I am glad to be with you." With all the emphasis on togetherness and sociability, the fact that some people need and desire an opportunity to be by themselves may be overlooked. Over the course of history the value and pain of solitude have been expressed in prose and poetry. Of modern writers few have expressed this more beautifully than Anne Morrow Lindbergh in *Gift from the Sea*. In essence she says that for life to have its full meaning and purpose, time must be set aside for contemplation in peace and quiet. To quote Mrs. Lindbergh, "Here there is time; time to be quiet; time to work without pressure; time to think; time to watch the heron, watching with frozen patience for his prey. . . . Time, even, *not* to talk." [49]

A purposeful conversation is one of the tools used by the nurse to establish a therapeutic relationship with a patient. The goal of a particular conversation may be to identify what is troubling a patient so that, when possible, appropriate measures can be initiated to relieve him. Conversation may be used to gain or to impart information, to determine the patient's expectations, to determine what he knows and what he wants to know, or to learn something about his family, work, or living conditions, as a basis for planning future care. During recovery from acute illness or during chronic illness, conversation may also provide needed diversion and recreation. Loneliness is one of the difficult problems in long-term illness. This is equally true whether the person is cared for at home or in the hospital. He longs for conversation with a sympathetic friend. A friendly listener may be the one bright spot in the person's day or week. Here again, attention to what the patient is saying, to what his interests are, and to encour-

[49] Anne Morrow Lindbergh: *Gift from the Sea* (New York: Pantheon Books, Inc., 1955), p. 116.

aging him to expand his interest and to bring in a bit of outside world may be rewarding experience for patient and nurse alike. Whatever the purpose of the conversation, its goals should be known. As in the use of other techniques in the care of the patient, the goals should be defined in terms of the needs of the patient. Conversation, like other skills, is learned and can be improved. This requires practice and evaluation of each conversation. What went well? Where did I get off the track? Why? What could have been done to keep on the track? What are my real goals?

Summary of Steps in Establishing a Significant Relationship with a Patient

Throughout this chapter the goal of establishing a therapeutic or helping relationship with the patient has been emphasized. The steps in the establishment of a significant relationship, as they have been stated by Schmahl,[50] are as follows: (1) "Awareness of one's own anxiety." In addition to this, the nurse must be willing to cope with it by moving slowly, waiting, and staying with it. (2) "Sustained physical thereness." The nurse must remain with the patient when he needs her. This is easier to do when giving physical care. The nurse should eventually develop the ability to stay with the patient when no physical care is required. (3) "Critical listening" and (4) "open-ended questions." As emphasized earlier with regard to critical listening, attention is given not only to the obvious meanings of the words that the patient uses but to their hidden meanings. The use of open-ended questions has been discussed. (5) "Consensual validation." By consensual validation is meant that what one thinks something means is also what it actually does mean. This can be done by putting hunches to the test and getting feedback from the patient that validates the accuracy of the hunch.

In this chapter some of the knowledge required by the nurse to meet the psychosocial needs of patients has been presented. Because of the rapidity with which knowledge in this area is growing, no single chapter can do more than summarize the more pertinent information. The hope is that students will become interested in exploring further resources.

Throughout the chapter emphasis has been placed on the fact that human behavior is the product of multiple factors. Each individual's behavior results from his reactions to and his interaction with his culture. His biological inheritance and structure are also a significant element in his behavior, for they determine his

possibilities for development as well as his limits. A bird can fly. Man cannot, or could not until he invented the airplane. Sophia Moore is a grown woman, but she is less than 3 feet tall. She is deeply depressed. She says, "I am a nobody. How can anyone who is small like me be anybody when to be somebody one must be big?" Sophia's size is biologically based. Her self-concept is derived from the value placed on physical bigness in the culture into which she was born. In another culture she might have been made a queen or treated as a god. In another, where smallness was the rule, she would not have been the object of any special attention. Culture is both universal and unique to man. Though all men are of the same species and cultures have common characteristics, both men and culture run the gamut in relation to variety.

Illness is, however, a personal experience. How the person behaves during illness usually depends on how he behaves in other crisis situations in his life. But his reaction also depends on the psychological meaning that illness has for him. Other crisis situations may not have had the identical personal meaning, and therefore his reaction would be different. Studies of people who are ill reveal that not all persons react to illness in the same manner. This point is emphasized by the findings of Kaplan,[51] who studied the psychological aspects of heart disease. Some of the factors that he found to influence the reaction of the individual included (1) the personality of the patient before he became ill and his life situation, (2) the degree or extent of his physical incapacity, (3) the abruptness of the onset, (4) the degree of severity, (5) the duration of the illness, and (6) the relationship of the patient to his family and to his physician. Though the subjects for this study were people having mitral commissurotomies, recent literature indicates that these factors enter into the behavior of patients with other diseases. This supports the concept that it is the patient and not his diagnosis that is of first importance in his reaction to disease.

Failure to identify and interpret appropriately a patient's behavior may be a source of psychological stress to the patient and to the nurse. When the patient and the nurse have a common cultural heritage, their expectations and values will more likely be in agreement than when they are from dissimilar backgrounds. When the behavior of patients differs from that expected by the professional staff, the professional staff has a responsibility to accept the patient's behavior as having meaning and to adapt its own behavior accordingly. The burden

[50] Jane A. Schmahl: "The Price of Recovery," *Amer. J. Nurs.,* **58**:90 (Jan.) 1958.

[51] Kaplan, *op. cit.,* p. 233.

should be on the professional person rather than on the patient. Application of knowledge of the psychosocial aspects of patient care should enhance the patient's feeling that he is accepted as an individual human being with dignity and rights. He should further feel that he is safe and protected and that he can depend on those who are responsible for his care. Skillful use of the knowledge of the psychosocial needs of patients should add to the satisfaction the nurse derives from the practice of nursing. It is one of the marks of a truly professional nurse.

REFERENCES

BOOKS

Abdellah, Faye G., and Levine, Eugene: *Effect of Nurse Staffing on Satisfactions with Nursing Care* (Chicago: Hospital Monograph Series No. 4, American Hospital Association, 1958).

Allport, Floyd Henry: *Theories of Perception and the Concept of Structure* (New York: John Wiley & Sons, Inc., 1955).

Apple, Dorrian (ed.): *Sociological Studies of Health and Sickness* (New York: McGraw-Hill Book Company, Inc., 1960).

Bauer, Julius: *The Person Behind the Disease* (New York: Grune & Stratton, Inc., 1956).

Garrett, Annette: *Interviewing* (New York: Family Service Association of America, 1959).

Ingle, Dwight J. (ed.): *Life and Disease* (New York: Basic Books, Inc., 1963).

King, Stanley H.: *Perceptions of Illness and Medical Practice* (New York: Russell Sage Foundation, 1962).

Maslow, Abraham H.: *Toward a Psychology of Being,* 2nd ed. (Princeton, N.J.: D. Van Nostrand Company, Inc., 1962).

Paul, Benjamin D. (ed.): *Health, Culture and Community* (New York: Russell Sage Foundation, 1955).

Ruesch, Jurgen: *Therapeutic Communication* (New York: W. W. Norton & Company, Inc., 1961).

Schwartz, Doris, Henley, Barbara, and Zeitz, Leonard: *The Elderly Ambulatory Patient* (New York: The Macmillan Company, 1964).

Solomon, Philip, *et al.* (eds.): *Sensory Deprivation* (Cambridge, Mass.: Harvard University Press, 1965).

Walker, Virginia H.: *Nursing and Ritualistic Practice* (New York: The Macmillan Company, 1967).

PERIODICALS

Aasterud, Margaret: "Defenses Against Anxiety in the Nurse-Patient Relationship," *Nurs. Forum,* 1:35–38 (Summer) 1962.

Alfano, Genrose J.: "What Rapport Means to Me," *Nurs. Outlook,* 3:326–27 (June) 1955.

Ball, Geraldine: "Speaking Without Words," *Amer. J. Nurs.,* 60:692–93 (May) 1960.

Beecher, Henry K.: "Nonspecific Forces Surrounding Disease and the Treatment of Disease," *JAMA,* 79:437–40 (Feb. 10) 1962.

Bojar, Samuel: "The Psychotherapeutic Function of the General Hospital Nurse," *Nurs. Outlook,* 6:151–53 (Mar.) 1958.

Bowlby, John: "Disruption of Affectional Bonds and Its Effects on Behavior," *Canad. Ment. Health Suppl.,* 59:2–12 (Jan.–Feb.) 1969.

Cantril, Hadley: "A Study of Aspirations," *Sci. Amer.,* 208:41–45 (Feb.) 1963.

Cattell, Raymond B.: "The Nature and Measurement of Anxiety," *Sci. Amer.,* 208:96–104 (Mar.) 1963.

Davis, Anne J.: "The Skills of Communication," *Amer. J. Nurs.,* 63:66–70 (Jan.) 1963.

Eldred, Stanley H.: "Improving Nurse-Patient Communication," *Amer. J. Nurs.,* 60:1600–1602 (Nov.) 1960.

Engel, George L.: "A Life Setting Conducive to Illness: The Giving-Up–Given-Up Complex," *Ann. Intern. Med.,* 69:293–300 (Aug.) 1968.

Harrison, Cherie: "Deliberative Nursing Process Versus Automatic Nurse Action," *Nurs. Clin. N. Amer.,* 1:387–97 (Sept.) 1966.

Hart, Betty L., and Rohweder, Anne W.: "Support in Nursing," *Amer. J. Nurs.,* 59:1398–1401 (Oct.) 1959.

Hewitt, Helon E., and Peznecker, Betty L.: "Blocks to Communicating with Patients," *Amer. J. Nurs.,* 64:101–103 (July) 1964.

"Hospital Ward: The Social Order," *Atlantic Monthly,* 200:57–60 (Dec.) 1957.

Hulicka, Irene M.: "Fostering Self-Respect in Aged Patients," *Amer. J. Nurs.,* 64:84–89 (Mar.) 1964.

Hunter, John: "The Mark of Pain," *Amer. J. Nurs.,* 61:96 (Oct.) 1961.

Hyde, Robert W., and Coggan, Norma E.: "When Nurses Have Guilt Feelings," *Amer. J. Nurs.,* 58:233–36 (Feb.) 1958.

Jacobson, Gerald F., Strickler, Martin, and Morley, Wilbur E.: "Generic and Individual Approaches to Crisis Intervention," *Amer. J. Public Health,* 58:338–43 (Feb.) 1968.

Jourard, Sidney M.: "To Whom Can a Nurse Give Personalized Care?" *Amer. J. Nurs.,* 61:86–88 (Mar.) 1961.

Kaufmann, Margaret A., and Brown, Dorothy E.: "Pain Wears Many Faces," *Amer. J. Nurs.,* 61:48–51 (Jan.) 1961.

Kneisl, Carol Ren: "Thoughtful Care for the Dying," *Amer. J. Nurs.,* 68:550–53 (Mar.) 1968.

Ludemann, Ruth S.: "Empathy: A Component of Therapeutic Nursing," *Nurs. Forum,* 7:275–88 (No. 3) 1968.

McCaffery, Margo, and Moss, Fay: "Nursing Intervention for Bodily Pain," *Amer. J. Nurs., 67:* 1224–27 (June) 1967.

Macgregor, Frances C.: "Uncooperative Patients: Some Cultural Interpretations," *Amer. J. Nurs.,* 67:88–91 (Jan.) 1967.

Martin, Harry W., and Prange, Arthur J.: "The Stages of Illness—Psychosocial Approach," *Nurs. Outlook,* 10:168–71 (Mar.) 1962.

Mead, Margaret: "Understanding Cultural Patterns," *Nurs. Outlook,* 4:260–62 (May) 1956.

Minckley, Barbara Blake: "Space and Place in Patient Care," *Amer. J. Nurs.,* 68:510–16 (Mar.) 1968.

Monteiro, Lois: "The Patient Had Difficulty Communicating," *Amer. J. Nurs.,* 62:78–81 (Jan.) 1962.

Monteiro, Lois A.: "Hip Fracture: A Sociologist's Viewpoint," *Amer. J. Nurs.,* 67:1207–10 (June) 1967.

Norris, Catherine M. "The Nurse and the Crying Patient," *Amer. J. Nurs.,* 57:323–27 (Mar.) 1957.

Peplau, Hildegard: "Loneliness," *Amer. J. Nurs.,* 55:1476–81 (Dec.) 1955.

Peterson, Donald I.: "Developing the Difficult Patient," *Amer. J. Nurs.,* 67:522–25 (Mar.) 1967.

Rapoport, Lydia: "Motivation in the Struggle for Health," *Amer. J. Nurs.,* 57:1455–57 (Nov.) 1957.

Rubenstein, Vera M. (ed.): "Symposium on the Difficult Patient," *Nurs. Clin. N. Amer.,* 2: 691–796 (Dec.) 1967.

Schmitt, Madeline H.: "Role Conflict in Nursing: Is It Based on a Dubious Dichotomy?" *Amer. J. Nurs.,* 68:2348–50 (Nov.) 1968.

Skipper, James K., Jr., Mauksch, Hans O., and Tagliacozzo, Daisy: "Some Barriers to Communication Between Patients and Hospital Functionaries," *Nurs. Forum,* 2:14–23 (No. 1) 1963.

Skipper, James K., Jr., Tagliacozzo, Daisy L., and Mauksch, Hans O.: "What Communication Means to Patients," *Amer. J. Nurs.,* 64:101–103 (Apr.) 1964.

Sorensen, Gladys: "Dependency—A Factor in Nursing Care," *Amer. J. Nurs.,* 66:1762–63 (Aug.) 1966.

Strauss, Anselm: "The Intensive Care Unit: Its Characteristics and Social Relationships," *Nurs. Clin. N. Amer.,* 3:7–15 (Mar.) 1968.

Wittreich, Warren J.: "Visual Perception and Personality," *Sci. Amer.,* 200:56 (Apr.) 1959.

Wygant, W. E., Jr.: "Dying, But Not Alone," *Amer. J. Nurs.,* 67:574–77 (Mar.) 1967.

8

Nursing the Patient Having a Problem in Maintaining the Supply of Oxygen and/or in the Removal of Carbon Dioxide *

The only way of real advance in biology lies in taking as our starting point, not the separated parts of an organism and its environment, but the whole organism in its actual relation to environment, and defining the parts and activities in this whole in terms implying their existing relationships to the other parts and activities.[1]

Overview

What are some of the conditions in which oxygen supply may be threatened?

What are the implications to nursing?

Structure and Function of the Airway

What is a bronchoscopy? What are the requirements of the patient undergoing this procedure?

How may the nurse prevent airway obstruction?

What are the nursing responsibilities in caring for a patient with a tracheostomy?

Structure and Function of the Lung

What factors bring about a decrease in lung compliance?

What are the nurse's responsibilities in caring for a patient with an open pneumothorax?

Regulation of Respiration

What are some of the causes of failure of the respiratory center?

What are the ways of performing artificial respiration?

Conditions Essential to the Exchange of Gases in the Lung

What are some of the common causes of failure to transport oxygen?

What are the nurse's responsibilities in inhalation therapy?

Adequacy of Respiratory Function

IN common with other living organisms, the survival of man depends on a continued supply of energy for the performance of work by his cells. Every manifestation of life is dependent on the liberation and utilization of free energy. Every increase in energy requires an increase in the supply of materials that can be converted to energy. Energy is obtained through the combination of oxygen with a limited variety of compounds—carbohydrates, fats, and proteins by the so-called oxidation-reduction reaction.

[1] J. B. S. Haldane: *Respiration* (New Haven, Connecticut: Yale University Press, 1922).

This chapter is devoted to the processes involved in providing cells with oxygen and with the elimination of carbon dioxide. The factors in the maintenance of a supply of carbon-containing compounds and the processes involved in their use will be discussed in Chapter 12.

What are some of the conditions in which oxygen supply may be threatened?

At body temperatures, the natural rate of oxidation is exceedingly slow. Enzymes are therefore required to catalyze or speed oxida-

---

* This chapter has been revised by Roberta Adler, Instructor in Nursing, Rutgers University, Newark, New Jersey.

tion-reduction reactions. Survival is threatened by any condition interfering with the supply of oxygen or of carbon-containing compounds to the cells or with the processes involved in the release of energy by the cells. The child who is trapped in a discarded refrigerator dies because his supply of oxygen is limited. One of the reasons the child who drowns dies is because his air passages are blocked by water and ventilation is impeded. Since oxygen is required for the release of energy from its potential sources, cellular processes require not only oxygen but also compounds in which energy is stored. In shock death may be caused by failure to supply cells with the oxygen and to remove intermediary products of metabolism. In cyanide poisoning, oxidation-reduction reactions cease because cyanide poisons the enzymes, catalyzing oxidation-reduction reactions. In all the above disorders, death is caused by the failure of the oxidation-reduction reactions by which cells release energy for the maintenance of their activities.

Carbon dioxide is one of the products of oxidation-reduction reactions that is returned to the external environment. It participates in the regulation of the mechanisms for the supply of oxygen to cells and for its own elimination. All the processes involved in the delivery of oxygen to cells and the removal of carbon dioxide are known as respiration. Respiration is not complete until oxygen is combined in the cell with hydrogen to form water or with a compound containing carbon to form carbon dioxide. Respiration therefore includes

1. Breathing or ventilation—transport of air from the atmosphere to the alveoli and back to the atmosphere. Ventilation takes place in two phases—inspiration and expiration.
2. Diffusion of oxygen and carbon dioxide from the alveoli to the blood and from the blood to the alveoli.
3. Transportation of oxygen and carbon dioxide by means of the blood and other body fluids to and from cells.
4. Oxidation-reduction reactions in cells.
5. Regulation of all aspects of respiration—not only breathing, but also all processes involved in supplying cells with oxygen and including those by which priority needs are met.

What are the implications to nursing?

Knowledge of the importance of a continuous supply of oxygen to all cells has countless implications in the practice of nursing, which may be summarized as follows:

1. To prevent conditions in the external environment predisposing to a deficient supply of oxygen. For example, the nurse should support and promote community efforts to protect babies from smothering in plastic bags, and children from suffocating in discarded refrigerators.
2. To protect patients who are unable to protect themselves—for example, the unconscious patient who may be suffocated or drowned by his own secretions.
3. To protect patients from the effects of oxygen deficiency—local or general. The nurse must be able to recognize signs and symptoms indicating a lack of oxygen and to take appropriate steps to correct the situation.
4. To carry out measures to maintain ventilation or to increase the supply of oxygen available for absorption.

Oxygen Needs

To obtain energy stored in foodstuffs, cells of all organisms require a continuous supply of oxygen. In the absence of oxygen cells die, just as they do when they are deprived of food. There is, however, considerable variability in sensitivity to low oxygen tension [2] among species, individuals of the same species, and tissues of the same individual. A person requires more oxygen when he exercises, has a fever, or increases his metabolic rate. These additional demands are met by a corresponding increase in the heart rate and the degree of deoxygenation of oxyhemoglobin in the capillaries.

Certain factors appear to influence the ability of the organism to withstand low oxygen tension. It is better tolerated by the fetus than by the adult, by immature cells than by mature cells, and by females than by males. The structural and physiological status of an individual is also a factor. For example, an individual whose circulatory system is able to compensate for a decrease in oxygen supply by increasing blood flow is better able to tolerate hypoxia than the one whose circulatory response is defective or lacking. For instance, Mrs. White, who has had an extensive sympathectomy, tolerates hypoxia poorly because she is unable to constrict the arterioles in a large part of her body. This inability to respond to an increased need for oxygen prevents her from being able to redistribute blood from less vital to more vital areas. Despite differences in sensitivity to low oxygen tension,

[2] Oxygen tension is determined by the percentage composition of oxygen in the air and the pressure (usually atmospheric) under which it is confined. Low oxygen tension results from a reduction in the percentage composition of oxygen in the inspired air or a significant reduction in atmospheric pressure.

all individuals have limits to their ability to adapt to and to survive deficiencies in the supply of oxygen. Because oxygen is not stored in appreciable quantities, the effects of an acute failure of supply can be observed almost immediately.

Tissues most sensitive to oxygen lack are the cerebral cortex, the myocardium, and the kidney. Although the cerebral cortex is highly sensitive to oxygen deprivation, it is probably the best protected by the circulation. In hypoxia,[3] blood is rerouted to maintain flow to the cerebral cortex, sometimes at the expense of other organs. Irreparable damage to the cells of the cerebral cortex can result from failure to supply oxygen for as few as 4 or 5 minutes. Other parts of the central nervous system are better able to withstand hypoxia. The medulla can function for as long as 20 to 30 minutes without oxygen. It is not unusual to see a patient whose brain has been temporarily deprived of its oxygen supply retain his ability to regulate vegetative functions, but lose functions that are dependent on the cerebral cortex. For example, when the heart is started after prolonged cardiac arrest, cerebral cortical function may fail, or be markedly impaired, despite the return of vegetative functions. Mr. Peters experienced cardiac arrest associated with myocardial infarction. After some delay artificial respiration and cardiac massage were administered and approximately an hour elapsed before cardiac function was re-established. Although Mr. Peters was able to eat, digest food, and breathe, he suffered serious mental deterioration. He gave little evidence of recognizing his wife or children. Because he was unable to care for himself, he had to be cared for like a young child.

The myocardium is also sensitive to a lack of oxygen. According to Guyton,[4] it begins to die within one hour of total ischemia. Exercise or activity decreases the length of time the heart will survive in the absence of oxygen. Unlike skeletal muscle, the myocardium is unable to accumulate more than a small oxygen debt before it ceases to function.

Like the brain and the myocardium, the kidney is sensitive to hypoxia. Renal shutdown is always a possibility in any condition associated with prolonged or severe hypoxia. That is why an accurate record of urinary output is essential for patients in shock.

Other tissues, such as bone and cartilage, are able to withstand oxygen deprivation for longer periods of time. Because skeletal muscle is able to accumulate an oxygen debt, it can contract for a time despite a deficiency of oxygen. For muscle contraction to continue or for the muscle to be restored to its resting condition, oxygen must be provided to remove the lactate accumulated in the tissue during anaerobic catabolism. In biological systems, lactic acid appears to have only one possible fate: reoxidation to pyruvic acid. All tissues, including those that are relatively insensitive to hypoxia and those that are able to function for a time anaerobically, must have oxygen to obtain the free energy from foodstuffs required to carry on their activities. Without it, they die.

Oxygen Supply

Man's cells are similar to those of most other organisms inasmuch as they obtain oxygen from their fluid environment. Single-cell organisms and those consisting of relatively few cells obtain oxygen from the pool of fluid in which they are suspended. The fluid is in direct contact with the external environment or atmosphere. In man, the fluid bathing his cells is separated from the external environment by semipermeable membranes. Special structures are necessary to cleanse, warm, humidify, and bring air in contact with these membranes, as well as to distribute oxygen to the fluid environment of the cells. The process is finally complete when oxygen penetrates the cell and enters into an oxidation-reduction reaction. The products of this reaction are heat, carbon dioxide, and water. Some of the heat is used as energy to perform the work of the cell. Most of the excess heat is eliminated by the skin. A small amount is lost through expired air. Most excess water is eliminated by the kidney. Carbon dioxide is eliminated by way of the same semipermeable membranes in the alveoli that serve as a site for the entrance of oxygen.

The source of oxygen is air. Inspired air is composed of approximately 20.95 per cent oxygen, 79 per cent nitrogen, and 0.04 per cent carbon dioxide. Though the percentage composition of air is the same at all altitudes below 80,000 ft, the pressure under which air is confined decreases as elevation increases. At sea level atmospheric pressure is 760 mm of mercury, or 1 atmosphere. As elevation increases, atmospheric pressure decreases or becomes less than 760 mm of mercury. Atmospheric pressure is one of the significant factors in the exchange of gases in the lung.

Knowledge of the gas laws is essential to understanding the importance of atmospheric pressure in the exchange of gases in the lung.

---

[3] Hypoxia is a better term than anoxia because it implies varying degrees of oxygen lack. Anoxia literally means an absolute lack of oxygen.

[4] Arthur C. Guyton: *Textbook of Medical Physiology* (Philadelphia: W. B. Saunders Company, 1969), p. 317.

BOYLE'S LAW

When the temperature of a gas remains constant, its pressure varies inversely with its volume. In other words, with increasing elevation above sea level, the volume or space in which the air is contained is enlarged, and as a result, pressure decreases. Movement of air into and out of the lung also illustrates Boyle's law. As the size (volume) of the lung is increased during inspiration, pressure within the lung decreases and air enters. Gases tend to move by diffusion from areas of greater concentration or pressure to areas of lesser concentration or pressure; the reverse happens during expiration.

LAW OF SOLUBILITY OF GASES

As with other states of matter, gases vary in their solubility. Carbon dioxide is 20 times as soluble as oxygen. Other things being equal, however, gases go into solution in proportion to their partial pressures. If a mixture of gases is placed in contact with a liquid in a closed flask, each gas goes into solution until equilibrium is reached.

DALTON'S LAW OF PARTIAL PRESSURES

In a mixture of gases, each gas exerts its own pressure independently of the others, behaving as if it were alone. The total pressure of a mixture of gases is equal to the sum of the pressures of its components. For example, the pressure of air at sea level is 760 mm of mercury. The percentage composition of oxygen in dry air at sea level is 20.93. Its partial pressure is therefore 20.93 multiplied by 760, or about 159 mm of mercury. Air is approximately 79 per cent nitrogen. Its partial pressure is therefore about 600 mm of mercury. Together they add up to 759 mm of mercury.

The direction and rate of the movement of gases across the respiratory membranes are explained by Dalton's law of partial pressures and the law of solubility of gases. Because gases diffuse from areas of greater to lesser pressure, and the partial pressure of oxygen is higher in the alveoli than it is in the blood, oxygen moves from the alveoli to the blood. The reverse is true for carbon dioxide. Moreover, the rate at which carbon dioxide is removed from the blood can be increased by increasing the rate and depth of respiration. When the alveoli are enlarged by deep breathing, their volume or capacity to hold air is increased. With an increase in volume, the partial pressure of carbon dioxide in the alveoli decreases—another illustration of Boyle's law. The difference in pressure or gradient between the partial pressure of carbon dioxide in the blood and that in the alveoli is raised. The capacity to alter the partial pressure of carbon dioxide in the alveolar air is of importance in the regulation of acid-base balance of the body fluids and is discussed in Chapter 9.

Because atmospheric pressure varies inversely with the distance above sea level, it affects the exchange of gases between the lung and the blood. The higher the elevation, the lower the atmospheric pressure, and the lower the partial pressure of each of its component gases. Despite a similar percentage composition of oxygen at sea level and at 18,000 ft, less oxygen is transferred across the alveolar membrane because its partial pressure is significantly lowered by elevation. Atmospheric pressure not only is important in maintaining oxygen supply but is also a source of difficulty when a person rapidly changes from an atmosphere of high pressure to one markedly lower. Though people differ, a decrease of approximately 2 atmospheres is usually required to cause difficulty; that is, when the atmosphere to which an individual is exposed is rapidly halved, he is likely to experience a disorder variously known as Caisson disease, decompression sickness, or "the bends." For the manifestations of decompression sickness to appear, the person must have been in a region of relatively high atmospheric pressure long enough for the gases to attain equilibrium between the air and his blood. The rapid reduction in the atmospheric pressure has two effects. The first results from the tendency of the volume of a gas to expand with a decrease in pressure—an illustration of Boyle's law. The air in the lung expands rapidly as the atmospheric pressure falls and first distends and then ruptures the lungs with the result that the air is drawn into the heart and large arteries. The second effect of a rapid drop in atmospheric pressure results from its effect on the solubility of gases. Because a gas, nitrogen, for example, goes into and out of solution in proportion to its partial pressure, a decrease in atmospheric pressure causes a decrease in the solubility of the nitrogen in the blood. If the fall is precipitous, nitrogen comes out of solution in the form of bubbles. This is because nitrogen is only physically dissolved and not buffered by chemical combination as are oxygen and carbon dioxide. The effect is similar to that observed following the removal of a cap from a bottle of carbonated beverage such as ginger ale. The carbon dioxide that is confined in the liquid under pressure escapes from the liquid in the form of bubbles. The difference between the partial pressure of carbon dioxide in the ginger ale and in the air is so great that it escapes very rapidly from the liquid. On a hot day, if the bottle is shaken before it is opened, the gas and solution form foam and overflow. Were the gas to be released in a confined space, such as a blood vessel, the bubbles would fill the vessel and obstruct blood flow.

Mr. Gold, a miner, illustrates the effects of decompression sickness. Decompression sickness is not limited to miners, however, and it can develop during high-altitude flying, following deep-sea diving, among submarine crews, or even in the hospital situation when hyperbaric oxygenation is employed. Pilots of planes can prepare themselves for high-altitude flying by inhaling pure oxygen to remove nitrogen from their blood. Crew and passengers in planes are protected by the pressurizing of airplane cabins. Miners and others who work below the surface of the earth are protected by returning to the surface in decompression chambers. After working all day in a mine located well below the surface of the earth, nitrogen and oxygen dissolved in the blood of Mr. Gold are in equilibrium with the greater than sea level partial pressure of nitrogen and oxygen in the air. When he returns to the surface of the earth quickly, the air in his lungs will expand rapidly causing distention of his lungs and possibly their rupture. The nitrogen dissolved in his blood will come out of solution quickly and may cause aeroemboli.

To prevent decompression sickness, Mr. Gold and his fellow miners are moved slowly to the surface in a decompression chamber where the atmospheric pressure is slowly reduced to sea level; they also breathe a mixture of oxygen and helium that contributes to clearing out the nitrogen. Persons who develop decompression sickness are treated by being placed in a decompression chamber and subjected to higher than atmospheric pressure. After their symptoms are relieved, they are gradually decompressed; that is, they are exposed to a gradually decreasing atmospheric pressure, and the nitrogen is removed from their blood without bubbles forming.

The signs and symptoms manifested by the person who experiences decompression sickness depend on which of his tissues are deprived of their blood supply. Nitrogen emboli can cause serious or even fatal damage when vessels supplying the brain or heart are obstructed. Pain in the bones and joints is common and accounts for the term *the bends*. There are many other possible effects.

Another problem of importance to an ever-increasing number of people has its origin in the fact that atmospheric pressure diminishes as altitude increases. Despite differences in individuals, an altitude above sea level is finally reached where the partial pressure of oxygen is no longer adequate to maintain life. At one time this problem was largely confined to high, mountainous areas of the world. With high altitude and space travel, it is now frequently encountered. The effects of both acute and chronic oxygen deprivation are discussed later in this chapter. Much can be learned about the effects of continued oxygen deprivation and man's adaptation to it by reading the accounts of mountain climbers such as William O. Douglas.[5]

Under certain conditions the percentage of oxygen in the air may be reduced because it is utilized and not replaced or because of the dilution of oxygen with another gas. Two different types of situations may be responsible for the depletion of oxygen in the air. In one, an individual enters an airtight space. Examples include the child who is trapped in an old refrigerator or who pulls a lightweight plastic bag over his head or a person who enters a room in which the oxygen content has been exhausted by a flame. In the above instances a person is trapped in an oxygenless space. As soon as the oxygen supply is exhausted, he dies of suffocation. The second type of situation in which suffocation is possible is the administration of oxygen, either by itself or in a mixture of gases in a closed system. When the supply of oxygen is exhausted or its concentration is inadequate, hypoxia develops. This possibility should be anticipated when inert gases such as helium or certain general anesthetics are administered. The use of some general anesthetics is limited by the fact that effective concentrations of the anesthetic limit oxygen supply too greatly. For example, for nitrous oxide to produce an adequate degree of relaxation for an abdominal operation, it must be present in a concentration of 90 per cent. Obviously, an oxygen concentration of 10 per cent is inadequate to the needs of the organism, and signs and symptoms of hypoxia follow if the percentage composition of oxygen in the air is reduced to this extent.

Oxygen Lack

Lack of oxygen may be either acute or chronic. The signs and symptoms accompanying the acute deprivation of oxygen resemble those of acute alcoholic intoxication, whereas those of chronic hypoxia are similar to those of fatigue. Symptoms that result from the effects of hypoxia on the nervous system include headache, depression, apathy, slowness of thought, excitement that borders on panic, irritability, restlessness, loss of memory, defective judg-

[5] William O. Douglas: *Beyond the High Himalayas* (Garden City, New York: Doubleday & Company, Inc., 1952), pp. 121–28.

ment, emotional disturbances, poor muscular coordination, fatigue, stupor, and insomnia. When hypoxia is prolonged or of marked degree, the person may suffer disturbances in seeing and hearing or experience pain. Because numerous conditions may be responsible for a lack of oxygen, nurses should be alert to the possibility of hypoxia when a patient exhibits one or more of the above signs and symptoms. Prompt action should be taken to correct the cause.

Hypoxia is accompanied by changes in the functioning of the nervous, circulatory, respiratory, and gastrointestinal systems. Because the nervous system regulates the activity of other organs, the effects of hypoxia can be either directly on the other organs, or indirectly through its effect on the nervous system. Inasmuch as alterations in function increase the supply of oxygen to cells, they are adaptive. In some instances they are maladaptive, as they increase the need for oxygen by increasing the activity of cells. For example, when a person panics and fights to escape from a space in which he is trapped, he uses more oxygen than he would if he were quiet. If he cannot escape quickly, the struggle is maladaptive, because it decreases his chances of survival.

Changes in the function of the circulatory system in hypoxia include tachycardia, which may be the earliest sign, especially in an anesthetized patient, a slight rise in blood pressure, and epistaxis. In advanced stages of hypoxia, the heart rate and blood pressure fall and loss of consciousness occurs. When the latter signs and symptoms appear, prognosis is grave.

As is to be expected in hypoxia, an attempt is made to increase pulmonary ventilation. There is also a tendency toward periodic respiration, especially during sleep.

CYANOSIS

Despite the importance of cyanosis, a sign in which the skin and mucous membranes are a dark blue or purplish color, a patient may be suffering from a severe degree of hypoxia and not be cyanotic. For cyanosis to be present, blood in the surface capillaries must contain a certain proportion of nonoxygenated hemoglobin or hemoglobin compounds such as methemoglobin or sulfhemoglobin. Some hemoglobin compounds such as carboxyhemoglobin (hemoglobin and carbon monoxide) do not cause cyanosis. Because carboxyhemoglobin is cherry-red in color, it gives the skin a pink tint. The patient is hypoxic, however, because the hemoglobin that is combined with carbon monoxide is not available to carry oxygen. With the exception of those conditions wherein abnormal

hemoglobin or its products are responsible for cyanosis, two conditions are required for it to be evident. Capillary blood must contain approximately 5 g per 100 ml or more of unoxygenated hemoglobin, and the surface capillaries must be dilated and have blood circulating through them.

According to Houssay,[6] four elements enter into the production of cyanosis. They are (1) the level of hemoglobin in the blood; (2) the extent to which hemoglobin in the blood leaving the lungs is oxygenated; (3) the proportion of oxygenated arterial to venous blood when they are mixed, as when there is a right-to-left shunt in cardiac malformations; and (4) the extent to which oxygen is removed from the blood as it moves through the capillaries.

To illustrate, Mrs. Ash, who has a hemoglobin of 6 g per 100 ml of blood (normal range for women is 12 to 15 g per 100 ml), is not likely to be cyanotic, because her hemoglobin is fully oxygenated, but she is hypoxic. Cyanosis may also be present in the absence of hypoxia. Cyanosis without hypoxia occurs in persons with abnormally high hemoglobin levels, such as those who are adapted to a high altitude. Persons may be hypoxic despite a high level of hemoglobin and a normal volume of oxygen per 100 ml of blood. Patients with polycythemia vera are, in effect, hypoxic even though the total quantity of oxygen carried per 100 ml of blood may be normal or high because arterial pO_2 is low and oxygen available to tissues is decreased. Under these conditions, blood leaving the lung is not fully oxygenated. In disorders where large portions of the lung are inactivated, poorly oxygenated hemoglobin will result in both cyanosis and hypoxia. The significance of cyanosis, therefore, depends on knowledge of the factors contributing to its development. In the care of sick people, other signs and symptoms indicating hypoxia should not be neglected because cyanosis is absent. Because of the sensitivity of the gastrointestinal tract to conditions in the body, nausea and vomiting frequently occur in hypoxia.

From the preceding discussion, it should be clear that hypoxia has widespread effects. The most serious threat associated with a rapidly developing and acute hypoxia is to the central nervous system, particularly to the cerebral cortex.

There are circumstances under which an individual may feel that he is not receiving enough oxygen although the supply is adequate. Certain conditions in the external environment predispose to sensations interpreted as a lack of

[6] Bernardo A. Houssay *et al.: Human Physiology,* 2nd ed. (New York: McGraw-Hill Book Company, Inc., 1955), p. 309.

oxygen. Probably the most common causes of discomfort are associated with the temperature, the humidity, and the movement of air. When the air is overheated and still, a person may feel that he is not obtaining sufficient oxygen. A feeling of suffocation is often a problem in a closed room ventilated by a poorly functioning air-conditioning system. Adding a fan may do much to improve comfort. Too great a movement of air, however, may cause chilling and should be avoided. When nothing can be done to lessen the movement of air, a properly placed screen may correct the condition by altering its flow.

ADAPTATIONS TO SLOWLY DEVELOPING HYPOXIA

When hypoxia develops slowly, the organism makes certain adaptations that enable it to survive, grow, and be productive. These adaptations have been studied in relation to acclimatization to high altitudes. As previously indicated, atmospheric pressure decreases as altitude increases, with the result that the partial pressure of oxygen and other gases in the air falls. At an altitude somewhere between 9,000 and 10,000 ft most persons who are not acclimatized begin to show signs and symptoms of mountain sickness. Much higher altitudes can be tolerated by those who are adapted to high altitudes than by those who are not. Individuals differ in their susceptibility to mountain sickness so that signs and symptoms develop at a lower level for some than for others. Physical exercise or any other condition increasing oxygen requirements lowers the level at which signs and symptoms are manifested. Visitors to high mountains are advised to delay active sightseeing for a day or so, in order to avoid mountain sickness. Even then acclimatization will not be complete and may take days or weeks.

Signs and symptoms of mountain sickness are the result of oxygen want. Lack of oxygen to the centers in the brain leads to loss of memory, errors in judgment, headache, and dizziness. Nausea and vomiting occur as the oxygen tension falls. These, as well as other previously listed manifestations of oxygen deprivation, can be prevented by supplying oxygen under pressure. Within limits, and given time, man can adapt to altitudes of 10,000 ft and higher.

Individuals who were born in, or have lived at, high altitudes for an extended period of time have made physiological adaptations which enable them to be more active than those not acclimatized. For example, there is an increase in their erythrocyte count and hemoglobin. Rises in the levels of hemoglobin and erythrocyte counts that occur soon after entering a region of high altitude are probably due to the contraction of the spleen. Elevation of the reticulocyte count indicates that the activity of the blood-producing elements in the bone marrow is stimulated, directly or indirectly, by the low oxygen tension in the blood. Persons living at high altitudes normally have higher hemoglobin levels than those living at sea level.

In addition to the increase in the capacity of the blood to carry oxygen, changes in the composition of the alveolar gases and in the shape of the chest facilitate adaptation. According to Houssay,[7] partial pressure of carbon dioxide in the alveoli falls at high altitudes. This permits an increase in the alveolar oxygen tension and partly compensates for the low tension of oxygen in the atmosphere.

In individuals whose ancestors have lived at high altitudes for several generations, there is some evidence that the shape of the chest changes. For example, Indians living on the high plateaus of Peru have large chests in which the anteroposterior diameter is greater than it is in persons living at lower levels. The visitor to this area cannot escape being impressed with two things. One is his own feeling of being short of breath from physical exertion; the other is the ease with which the natives perform heavy physical work.

Structure and Function of the Airway

As stated earlier, the first phase of respiration is ventilation, or breathing. During ventilation, air containing about 20 per cent oxygen is taken from the atmosphere, cleansed, warmed, humidified, and delivered to the alveoli, where it is exchanged for air containing a high concentration of carbon dioxide, some oxygen, and water which is returned to the atmosphere. This cycle takes place some 14 to 18 times per minute throughout the lifetime of the individual. As with other vital functions, the rate varies with age, exercise, and other factors. Ventilation is the means by which air in the alveoli is renewed regularly making a constant supply of oxygen available and protecting the blood and cells from an overaccumulation of carbon dioxide and from contaminants in the external environment.

To achieve this regular interchange of air in the alveoli, structures are required to do the following:

1. Cleanse, warm, and moisten the air.
2. Provide a passageway for the air, that is, an airway.
3. Move the air through the airway and into and out of the alveoli.

[7] *Ibid.,* p. 308.

There are many factors in illness and its treatment that decrease the efficiency of mechanisms utilized by the healthy individual to protect ventilation. Bed rest decreases ventilatory capacity. Narcotics, analgesics, and general anesthetics depress the mechanisms by which the patency of the tracheobronchial tree is maintained. They are also depressed in the unconscious state, whatever its cause. Most patients for whom bed rest is prescribed require some attention to ventilation. Although problems related to maintaining or re-establishing the patency of the airway are more frequent, disturbances in the mechanisms whereby air is moved into and out of the lung are not rare.

An understanding of the mechanisms that serve to protect the patency of the airway in health is necessary to the anticipation of conditions that are likely to threaten or disrupt them. It should also provide a basis for care directed toward the support or replacement of inefficient mechanisms until such time as the patient recovers sufficiently to meet his own need for oxygen.

The structures that form the airway can be seen in Figures 8-1 and 8-2. They are arbitrarily divided into the upper and lower respiratory tract. The upper division includes the larynx and the parts above it. The structures below the larynx form the lower respiratory tract. There is no barrier between the divisions. Ventilation of the alveoli depends on all these structures being patent or unobstructed. The lower airway can be obstructed from within by foreign bodies, fluid, pus, or a tumor. It can be obstructed from within its wall by swelling, paralysis, or spasm of the vocal cords, and from the outside by hemorrhage, edema, or abscess.

The respiratory tract serves not only as a passageway for air but also to condition it, so that the internal environment is protected from too rapid change in its constituents and from potentially harmful agents. The structure of the airway favors both these purposes. Figure 8-1 shows that the passageway is somewhat tortuous. Changes in the direction of the airway contribute to the cleansing of the air. As the air comes in contact with an obstruction, the direction of its flow is changed. Because the weight of air is less than that of particulate matter, its flow is impeded less than that of the heavier bodies. With deceleration, energy keeping the particles suspended is lost and the particles fall out of the moving stream of air. As

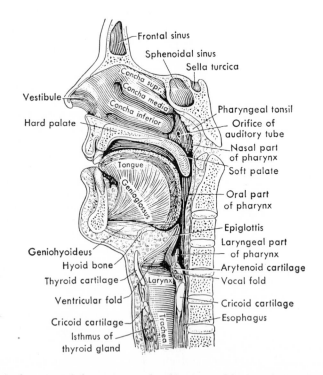

Figure 8-1. Sagittal section of the nose, mouth, pharynx, and larynx. (After *Gray's Anatomy.*) (Adapted with permission of The Macmillan Company from *Anatomy and Physiology*, 15th ed., Fig. 18-2, p. 517, by Diana Clifford Kimber, Carolyn E. Gray, Caroline E. Stackpole, and Lutie C. Leavell. Copyright © The Macmillan Company, 1966.)

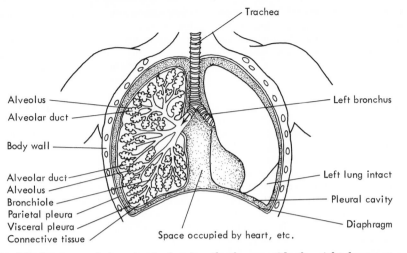

FIGURE 8-2. Lower respiratory tract, showing the lungs, with the right lung cut open to show the internal structure. (Adapted with permission of The Macmillan Company from *College Zoology*, 7th ed., Fig. 389, p. 537, by Robert W. Hegner and Karl A. Stiles. Copyright © The Macmillan Company, 1959.)

a result, dusts and other contaminants in the air are caught by the sticky surface with which they come in contact. The structure of the nose and glottis is particularly adapted to cleansing the air. In both, air moves through a narrow passageway and the direction of its flow is somewhat deflected. Hair in the anterior nares is helpful in moving particulate matter. The most important factor in the cleansing of the air by the nose is what Guyton calls turbulent precipitation.[8] As the air passes through the nares it comes in contact with and is deflected by the turbinates and the septum. As indicated previously, the movement of larger particles is slowed more than that of the air, and they are caught by the sticky mucous membranes.

The nose also contributes to the warming of the air. The mucous membrane covering the middle and inferior turbinates is richly supplied with blood vessels that dilate and increase the surface for warming the air. Some physicians discourage sleeping in a room with excessively low temperatures because this favors chronic engorgement of the nasal mucosa and predisposes to respiratory infections. Swelling of this tissue is responsible for obstruction of the nares in rhinitis. Irritation of the nasal mucosa initiates the reflex for sneezing and forcefully clears the nostrils of irritating materials. The mucosa lining the nares contains the receptor cells for the sense of smell and, as such, further adds to the ability of the organism to evaluate conditions in its external environment.

[8] *Op. cit.,* p. 555.

Although the mouth can serve as the site where air is taken from and returned to the atmosphere, it is not nearly as well suited to this function as the nose. The reasons are obvious. As a passageway, the mouth is satisfactory, but it is a poor conditioner of air. In addition, the mouth suffers readily from drying. Prolonged and unrelieved mouth breathing predisposes to parotitis. Patients who breathe entirely through their mouths lose pure water and are subject to dehydration. This is why it is necessary for a patient who is a mouth breather to receive thorough mouth care, and to be encouraged to drink sufficient fluids.

Like other body cavities in contact with the external environment, the respiratory tract is lined with mucous membrane. Two characteristics of this membrane are of particular importance in the protection of the patency of the respiratory tract. With the exception of the vocal cords, the mucous membrane lining the respiratory tract contains goblet cells that secrete mucus. The mucus forms a continuous sheet throughout the respiratory tract. It is constantly being renewed and serves to catch any particulate matter coming in contact with it. The mucous membrane is also ciliated. The cilia sweep in the direction of the pharynx and, in so doing, move the sheet of mucus into the pharynx, where it is swallowed or expectorated. This is true in the nares as well as in lower structures. The mucous membrane of the nose and pharynx may secrete as much as a quart of mucus a day. This accounts for much of the postnasal drip experienced by people who live in cold climates. In cold climates and in areas where the air is filled with soot or dust, secretion is likely to be increased. As long as the mucus is clear, the condition is probably physiological.

One of the most important mechanisms for the maintenance of the patency of the tracheobronchial tree is the cough reflex. Afferent nerve endings in the larynx, trachea, and bronchi are highly sensitive to irritants. Afferent impulses pass from these nerve endings by way of the vagus nerve to the medulla. Cough results from an integrated set of activities. These actions include (1) the inspiration of a moderate amount of air, (2) closure of the glottis, and (3) the forceful expiration of air against the closed glottis. The expiration that produces the cough is accomplished by contracting the abdominal muscles and pushing against the diaphragm and other expiratory muscles so that they contract forcefully. The cough occurs when the glottis opens and the air that has been confined under pressure is expelled explosively, carrying with it mucus or other materials. Although the cough is generally beneficial, there are times when it may not be. A patient may be exhausted by a dry, nonproductive cough that continues over a period of time. Cough has also been implicated in the spread of infection throughout the lung. When coughing is an essential part of the patient's treatment, he should be instructed and helped to cough effectively.

In illness or as a result of some overwhelming condition in the external environment, the capacity of the natural mechanisms to maintain the patency of the airway may be threatened or disrupted. Some of the conditions under which this is most likely to occur have previously been indicated. They include bed rest, drugs depressing to respiration, and unconsciousness. In general, conditions that predispose to obstruction of the tracheobronchial tree do so by inactivating or making ineffective one or more of the mechanisms by which it is cleansed, or by increasing the quantity or tenacity of mucus so that it is difficult to remove. Often a combination of factors contribute to the problem. To illustrate, Mrs. Fair, aged 45, underwent a cholecystectomy. In preparation for the operation she was given morphine sulfate, 10 mg (⅙ grains), and atropine sulfate, 0.4 mg (1/150 grains). The expected physiological responses to these drugs are:

1. Depression of the respiratory center by the morphine, which results in lessened respiratory excursion and may decrease the rate of respiration. Ventilation is, however, decreased without a decrease in rate.
2. Depression of the secretions of the glands in

the respiratory tract caused by the anticholinergic effects of atropine. This results in the formation of thick, tenacious mucus.

Both morphine and the anesthetic that Mrs. Fair received depress the action of cilia. Mrs. Fair's incision was high on the abdominal wall. To prevent pain, the area around the incision was splinted, and this resulted in shallow respirations. All these factors predispose to obstruction of the tracheobronchial tree and to the following effects and complications.

Obstruction of a duct or tube leading to, or draining, an organ has three effects: *stasis* of secretions behind the obstruction, which predisposes to *infection* and *loss of function* of the part or organ. Which of these predominates depends on the organ and the extent of the obstruction. If the trachea is obstructed, air cannot reach the alveoli and asphyxia occurs rapidly. If, on the other hand, a main bronchus or one or more of its branches are obstructed, then the air is absorbed into the circulation from the affected lung or the portion of the lung that is collapsed. The condition resulting from the collapse of a lung or a portion thereof is known as *atelectasis*. Bacteria present in the area multiply and the patient develops pneumonia. Atelectasis is a possibility in any seriously ill patient including the postoperative patient. Fever of 104°F or higher, with a corresponding increase in pulse and respiration in a patient who has recently experienced a general anesthetic or major surgery, suggests the possibility of atelectasis. In addition, the patient usually has a productive cough with thick, tenacious sputum. Dyspnea and cyanosis are prominent when a large area of lung has collapsed. To prevent atelectasis, Mrs. Fair was turned from one side to her other and encouraged to deep-breathe and to cough every two hours. Despite preoperative instruction Mrs. Fair required considerable encouragement to cough effectively. In order to lessen the pain of coughing, the nurse supported Mrs. Fair's incision. As soon as she was able Mrs. Fair was taught to support her incision herself by placing her hands and arms across her upper abdomen. Because standing and walking increase the depth of respiration and encourage productive coughing, Mrs. Fair was ambulated as soon as her surgeon prescribed it. The evening of the day she was operated on, she sat up with her feet hanging over the edge of the bed. The next day she was up and walking. Surgeons vary in the exact time they prescribe ambulation after various surgical procedures. There is seldom any delay, however, in mobilizing the patient in bed. One of the important aspects in nursing all patients who are confined to bed is attention to maintaining a clear airway.

In the preoperative period Mrs. Fair was instructed in how to deep-breathe and cough and why these were important to her convalescence. Instructions included explanation, diagrams, demonstrations, and supervised practice. Content selected to teach Mrs. Fair to cough was based on knowledge of coughing as an automatic act, which was previously described.

In addition to the mechanisms for clearing the tracheobronchial tree, the elasticity of the lung is a factor in the removal of secretions, particularly at the periphery. Any condition that is accompanied by a loss of elastic tissue favors the accumulation of secretions in the lung proper.

Despite the number and effectiveness of the mechanisms utilized to protect the alveoli from substances contaminating the air, particles less than 10 μ in diameter do pass through and line the alveolar walls. Ridding the alveoli of particulate matter depends on the action of macrophages. To be effective, phagocytosis must be accomplished quickly.

Coordination of Swallowing and Breathing

To this point the discussion has centered on the protection of the alveoli from contaminants in the inspired air. They are also protected from foods and fluids that are ingested. They are protected despite the fact that the pharynx provides a common opening into both the esophagus and the larynx. In the healthy person, and barring some accident, inspiration and swallowing are so regulated and integrated that neither is air swallowed nor is food or fluid inhaled. Both breathing and swallowing are under the control of the nervous system. As food enters the pharynx, receptors are stimulated and impulses are transmitted to the medulla and lower pons. Centers in the brain stem initiate a series of automatic actions that progress in an orderly sequence, with the result that one swallow differs very little from another. During swallowing, the respiratory center is briefly inhibited so that swallowing may progress. The vocal folds are approximated so that the aperture in the larynx (glottis) is closed. The larynx is moved forward and the tongue moves back so that the epiglottis shields the glottis and food enters the esophagus rather than the larynx.

Obstruction of the Airway

Injury to, or pressure on, the medulla, the pons, or the cranial nerves, 5 through 12, may disrupt the swallowing reflex and predispose to the aspiration of food or fluids into the tracheobronchial tree unless appropriate measures are taken. The aspiration of a large volume of fluid causes death by drowning. Lesser amounts may block a small unit in the lung and act as a focus for infection or aspiration pneumonia. Aspiration pneumonia is also a possibility when a patient is forced to ingest food or medications and he resists by struggling. Under these circumstances the swallowing reflex may be inhibited and the material may be aspirated into the larynx rather than the esophagus. Hedden et al.[9] state that fluid aspiration can also occur as a result of prolonged intubation of the trachea. The constant pressure of the tracheal tube on the submucosal neuronal plexuses causes analgesia of the larynx to develop, thereby causing difficulty in swallowing and consequently possible aspiration. Therefore, prior to beginning oral feedings on these patients, the protective airway reflexes should be tested. This can be done by having the patient drink a weak solution of methylene blue and then doing tracheal suction; dye should not appear in the aspirate.

Prevention of suffocation by aspiration of fluid or food by the patient who has partial or complete disruption in his swallowing reflex may be difficult. The patient who chokes when he is given food or fluids should be suspected of having difficulty in swallowing. If, when he attempts to swallow, fluids come back through his nose, he is having a problem and fluids should be discontinued until the swallowing reflex is re-established. Whenever there is any doubt about the ability of a patient to swallow, the physician should be notified promptly. When a patient has a problem with swallowing he should be placed in a position that favors fluid entering the esophagus or draining from the mouth. The back lying position, particularly when the head falls back, should be avoided. Depending on the extent of the difficulty the patient has with swallowing and other factors, he may be placed in a position with his head elevated and turned to one side; he may be horizontal, but lying on one side; he may be lying on his side with his head lower than the rest of his body; or he may be placed in a prone position with his head lower than his trunk and his head turned to the side. When secretions are abundant, regular suctioning of the mouth and pharynx may be necessary.

Obstruction to the flow of air may occur at any level of the respiratory tract. The consequences depend on the degree of obstruction and whether or not there is an alternate route through which air can pass. The causes of obstruction vary somewhat at different levels of

[9] Michael Hedden, et al.: "Laryngotracheal Damage After Prolonged Use of Orotracheal Tubes in Adults," *JAMA,* **207**:703–708 (Jan. 27) 1969.

the airway. For example, obstruction of the nares does not interfere with the flow of air, because there is an alternate pathway, the mouth. It does lessen the extent to which the air is properly conditioned. Because of the richness of the blood supply of the middle and inferior turbinates and the narrowness of the passageway, vascular congestion quickly causes interference with breathing. Inflammations caused by viral and bacterial infections and allergic responses of the mucous membranes are always accompanied by vascular congestion. Congestion is sometimes aggravated by the overuse of nose drops containing a drug acting as a vasoconstrictor when it is applied locally. Constriction is followed by overdilatation and passive congestion of the nasal mucosa. Patients using drugs such as Neo-synephrine Hydrochloride [10] should be cautioned against their overuse, because it is likely to lead to a rebound congestion that is more severe than the original condition. The nares may also be obstructed by polyps or foreign bodies. Polyps are frequently associated with allergic rhinitis. The latter are more likely to be a problem in young children who introduce small objects such as peas, beans, or buttons into one or both nares. See Figure 8-3.

The nurse has a responsibility to educate the

[10] Trade name for phenylephrine hydrochloride, U.S.P.

public concerning ingestion of foreign bodies into the tracheobronchial tree. Many times these accidents are preventable. Patients should be instructed to chew their food properly and to avoid eating at a rapid pace, as well as to exercise caution in preparing food so as to prevent small bones, eggshell fragments, and other materials from contaminating it. Haugen [11] reported that nine deaths initially attributed to heart attacks were found to be caused by obstruction of the airway caused by unchewed food. Parents should also be cautioned to avoid giving nuts and other similar foods to children with unerupted molars.

OBSTRUCTION OF THE GLOTTIS

Strictures or lesions in the pharynx most frequently obstruct the airway by blocking the glottis. One of the causes of death in diphtheria is obstruction of the airway by a pseudomembrane formed in the pharynx and/or larynx. Obstruction of the glottis is an ever-present danger to the unconscious patient whose reflexes are depressed and whose musculature is relaxed. If he is placed in bed on his back, there is danger that the base of his tongue and the other structures in his pharynx will sag against the

[11] R. K. Haugen: "The Cafe Coronary; Sudden Death in Restaurants," *JAMA,* **186**:142–43 (Oct. 12) 1963.

FIGURE 8-3. Nasal polyps, which obstruct the nasal passage. The drawing shows the appearance of the polyps when seen from the anterior view of the nose with retractors. (Adapted from "Anatomy of the Nose and Sinuses in Health and Diseases." Courtesy of the *Pfizer Spectrum.*)

glottis and block the opening. This can be prevented by a properly placed airway and/or by placing the unconscious patient on his side and maintaining him in this position until his reflexes and muscle tone have been restored. This simple precaution would have saved the life of Charles Brown, a healthy young man of 22. He had been given Pentothal Sodium [12] in preparation for a circumcision. After this minor procedure, he was returned to his room in an unconscious state. He was placed in bed on his back. Twenty minutes later, he was found dead from suffocation. The contents of his pharynx had obstructed his glottis. Any space-occupying mass in the pharynx may obstruct the glottis.

The glottis is the narrowest passageway in the upper airway. As such, it offers some resistance to the flow of air during inspiration. As indicated previously, the sudden slowing of the flow of air contributes to the removal of particles by creating turbulence. The glottis offers even more resistance to the flow of air during expiration than it does during inspiration. The resulting turbulence is an important factor in the mixing of air in the respiratory tract and alveoli.

There are a variety of sources of obstruction of the glottis. Some are extrinsic while others are intrinsic to the larynx. Any space-occupying mass in the neck or involving the vocal folds or other parts of the larynx may block the glottis. Neoplasms or hemorrhage into the neck usually do this by interrupting the passage of impulses over the recurrent laryngeal nerves. Passage of nerve impulses may be interrupted by injury to or severing of the recurrent laryngeal nerves during operation on the neck, such as thyroidectomy. The recurrent laryngeal nerves are motor to all the muscles of the larynx except the cricothyroid. Severance of one nerve causes a paralysis of the vocal folds on one side with the result that the voice becomes bitonal. Disruption of both nerves results in suppression of phonation and causes serious disturbances in respiration. Hoarseness and respiratory stridor (high-pitched, noisy respirations) accompany weakness or paralysis of the vocal folds. The voice may have a nasal quality caused by paralysis of the soft palate. The appearance of any of the above in a patient in whom there is a possibility of disease or injury of peripheral nerves or medullary centers controlling speech should be reported to a physician immediately.

Acute obstruction of the glottis, larynx, or trachea is a grave emergency. Not only does it prevent air from gaining access to the alveoli, but it predisposes to pulmonary edema, which

is the accumulation of serous or serosanguineous fluid in the alveoli, bronchioles, and bronchi. The accumulation of fluid in the alveoli and air passages further impairs oxygenation. The factors in the development of pulmonary edema are similar to those causing edema in other areas of the body. Following obstruction of the airway, pulmonary edema results from both chemical and mechanical disturbances. As hypoxia develops, the capillaries in the lung increase in permeability, thus allowing fluid to escape therefrom into the alveoli. Among the mechanical factors that may contribute to pulmonary edema after severe obstruction of the airway is a suction effect created on capillaries during inspiration. As a patient attempts to inhale, pressure within the alveoli is lowered by the expansion of the thoracic cavity. When the airway is patent, air flows into the alveoli, thus maintaining pressure relationships between the alveoli and capillaries. When inspiration is blocked to a greater extent than expiration, pressure is lowered in the alveoli during inspiration and fluid exudes from the capillaries to the alveoli. The situation may be further aggravated by interference with the outflow of blood from the left ventricle. Because blood flow to the right heart increases during inspiration, failure of the left ventricle to move blood into the circulation at as rapid a rate as it is presented to it results in a progressive accumulation of blood in the lungs. Pulmonary edema, whatever the cause or causes, is always a dangerous complication. A tracheotomy tray should be in readiness so that no time will be lost if a tracheostomy becomes necessary. Food and fluids should be withheld until the ability of the patient to swallow has been established.

When afferent fibers supplying the larynx are sectioned or there is a disturbance in their ability to transmit impulses, the larynx is insensitive to irritating particles that adhere to it. One unfortunate effect is the failure to initiate the cough reflex automatically when irritating materials come into contact with the larynx.

On occasion the nurse cares for a patient who has a weakness or paralysis of one vocal fold that was caused by disease or injury to the centers in the brain that integrate breathing and swallowing. One such patient was Mrs. Oakson, who had been admitted to the hospital for a mitral commissurotomy—a procedure by which a narrowed mitral valve is enlarged. Some months earlier, she had a cerebrovascular accident, which was believed to have been caused by an embolus that originated from a thrombus in her left atrium. According to Mrs. Oakson, despite good recovery her voice continued to be hoarse and nasal in quality. In addition, she noticed that she could not cough effectively

[12] Trade name for thiopental sodium.

because she was unable to close her glottis tightly and build up pressure behind it. She was therefore deprived of one of the most effective mechanisms for cleansing the tracheobronchial tree. After the mitral commissurotomy was performed, and despite real effort on her part, she was unable to clear her tracheobronchial tree of secretions. Bronchoscopy was required in order to remove secretions and to prevent atelectasis.

Tumors or edema of the vocal folds blocks the glottis. Hoarseness is common in both conditions. When a tumor is involved, the hoarseness is likely to be intermittent. With edema, hoarseness is likely to be progressive and, if the edema is marked, to be associated with respiratory obstruction.

OBSTRUCTION OF THE BRONCHI

The larynx narrows to form the trachea, which branches into the two bronchi. Each bronchus forms a series of branching tubes that finally terminate in the alveoli. Collectively these tubular structures form the airway. They may be obstructed at any level by accumulated secretions, blood, foreign bodies, or fluid. The effects of obstruction will depend on the nature of the obstructing agent, the level at which blocking occurs, and whether it is partial or complete. Obstruction of the trachea or larynx promptly causes asphyxia. Obstruction of a bronchus or one of its branches, when partial, may trap air in the lung and interfere with the drainage of secretions. When it is complete, the lung collapses as the air is absorbed. The major danger of a small airless region is that it is predisposed to infection because drainage is blocked. The consequences of a collapse of an entire lung are immediate, because the pressure relationships among the various structures in the thoracic cavity are disrupted. When a lung collapses because air cannot enter, the contents of the thoracic cavity may shift toward the side of decreased pressure (mediastinal shift) and the flow of air into the other lung is impaired. Furthermore the venous return to the heart is impaired by the alterations in pressure within the thoracic cavity. Prompt action to remove the obstructing body is imperative.

Comparison of Structures

The walls of the larynx, trachea, and the bronchi, and its larger branches are strengthened with cartilage. In the trachea and bronchial tubes the rings of cartilage are incomplete dorsally, which permits some alteration in their size and shape during the various phases of breathing. At the point where the tubes are 1 mm or less in diameter, the cartilage disappears. These small subes without cartilage in the walls are the bronchioles. As the cartilage decreases in the tubes, the smooth muscle and elastic tissue increase.

The smooth muscle in the tracheobronchial tree is innervated by the autonomic nervous system. Increased activity of the parasympathetic nervous system causes the muscles of the bronchioles to constrict. The sympathoadrenal system has the opposite effect. It causes the bronchioles to dilate. The capacity to regulate the diameter of the bronchioles is a factor in regulation of the flow of air to the alveoli.

Constriction of the bronchioles, when appropriate in degree, is part of the system for the protection of the alveoli from noxious agents. For example, smoke reaching the bronchioles stimulates them to contract, thus limiting the quantity of smoke reaching the alveoli. When the response of the broncheolar musculature is appropriate to the stimulus, and appropriate in degree, it protects the alveoli from harmful contaminants in the air.

In contrast, when the bronchiolar musculature is hyperreactive, it may be the source of pathology. When, for example, hyperresponsive muscle contracts in response to inappropriate stimuli, its degree of contraction is too great, and/or the contraction is sustained for too long a period of time, there is likely to be some interference with ventilation. For example, in asthma and asthmalike diseases, obstruction of the bronchioles interferes with ventilation. One of the factors in their obstruction is smooth-muscle spasm. Other elements increasing resistance to the flow of air in these disorders are edema of the mucosa due to increased capillary permeability and an increase in the secretion of mucus. All these factors are in response to the release of serotonin and histamine by the injured cells. Because they interfere with expiration to a greater extent than with inspiration, air is trapped in the lungs and they are maintained in an inflated state. Irritation by highly irritating substances such as smoke provokes a similar type of inflammatory reaction.

THE RESPIRATORY TRACT AS AN AIR CONDITIONER

The respiratory tract serves not only to deliver air to the respiratory alveoli, but to condition it so that it is protected from drying and other noxious conditions. Air, as it enters the airway, may be relatively clean or it may be laden with dust or microorganisms, or both. Despite the efficiency of the mechanisms for cleansing the air, particles may get beyond the glottis. If they are very small, they may even reach the alveoli.

Thus bacteria or viruses may gain entrance to the body through the respiratory tract where they may set up an infectious process or enter the internal environment. The respiratory tract serves as the portal of entry for a large number of microorganisms. Microorganisms also escape into the atmosphere in discharges from the respiratory tract. Elements to be considered in the control of respiratory infections are treated in Chapter 5. The point should be made here, however, that appropriate measures should be utilized by the nurse to protect herself and others from respiratory discharges. The simplest measure is always to turn her head when someone coughs. She should never allow anyone to cough in her face. Adequate ventilation so that fresh air dilutes the ward air is also helpful. Acute infections of the respiratory tract are by far the most frequent cause of acute disabling illness lasting only a few days.

EFFECTS OF RESPIRATORY TRACT IRRITATION

Many of the manifestations resulting from the exposure of the respiratory tract to noxious agents are caused by hyper- or hypoactivity of a protective mechanism. For example, the mucosa responds to irritation by an increase in the secretion of mucus. This reaction is beneficial inasmuch as it serves to dilute the irritant and to remove it from the body. It may, however, cause harm when the character or quantity of mucus is such that the mechanisms for its removal are overwhelmed. As mucus collects in the tubes forming the airway or in ducts draining into it, water is absorbed from the mucus and it becomes more difficult to remove. Unless drainage is maintained, a mucus plug obstructs the tube. With obstruction of the tube, the improperly drained area is liable to infection, and among other effects, the character of the drainage is altered. In infectious diseases of the lung, such as pneumonia, the exudate formed in the alveoli is discharged into the airway. Blood in the sputum, hemoptysis, results from bleeding into the alveoli or from the mucosa of the airway. The character of the discharge from the respiratory tract provides significant clues as to the nature of a patient's illness. Its color, odor, consistency, and amount should be observed and recorded.

Cough, as previously emphasized, is a valuable mechanism for cleansing the lower respiratory tract. In disorders in which there is continued irritation of the larynx, trachea, and bronchi, its frequency is increased so that the person becomes aware that he is coughing. Like other symptoms, the circumstances under which the cough occurs modify the importance the individual attaches to it. For example, many people who smoke dismiss a chronic cough as caused by smoking. In contrast, most people perceive themselves to be ill when they have a cough that raises blood or purulent sputum, or when the cough is accompanied by evidence of an acute respiratory infection. Some of the observations to be made about cough include the circumstances accompanying its occurrence, its timing, whether or not it is productive, and its sound, that is, either wet or dry.

Other observations that provide information about the airway include the presence or absence of noticeable sound during breathing, changes in the voice, and laryngeal stridor. As air passes through fluids accumulated in the tracheobronchial tree, breath sounds are altered. They may or may not be audible to the ordinary listener. When they are heard on auscultation of the chest, they are known as râles. Air passing through fluid in the tracheobronchial tree produces what is known as a moist râle. Râles can sometimes be felt through the chest wall. The usual method of detecting râles is by listening through a stethoscope placed on the chest wall. Changes in the voice such as a nasal quality or hoarseness have been previously discussed. Since the character of the voice differs in healthy people, an observer who has not known a patient previously may have to depend on the judgment of the patient or a member of his family that his voice is or is not normal. Laryngeal stridor is always abnormal because it results from laryngeal spasm. It is characterized by a crowing or high-pitched sound on inspiration. The sound is sometimes compared to the blowing of the wind. Laryngeal stridor is usually accompanied by cyanosis. The most common condition in which laryngeal stridor occurs is croup in children but it may also occur in tetany.

EFFECTS OF OBSTRUCTION OF THE AIRWAY

When an obstruction of the part of the airway for which there is no alternate route occurs suddenly, as in drowning or the blocking of the trachea or glottis by a foreign body, asphyxia develops in a matter of minutes. When it develops more slowly, as in an acute infectious process, signs and symptoms of oxygen want develop over a period of time. The urgency of the situation depends on the extent to which the patient is able to meet his own needs for oxygen. Accumulated secretions or any foreign body, whatever its size or source, must be removed. Even when they do not seriously interfere with ventilation, they block the ducts distal to the obstruction and predispose to infection.

The usual method by which foreign bodies or secretions are extracted from the tracheobronchial tree is by bronchoscopy accompanied by bronchial aspiration.

What is a bronchoscopy? What are the requirements of the patient undergoing this procedure?

Bronchoscopy is a procedure in which a lighted tube is introduced into the trachea by way of the mouth, pharynx, glottis, and larynx. Like other scopes used in medicine, the bronchoscope contains a series of mirrors which are so located in the tube that the interior of the tracheobronchial tree can be directly visualized. The bronchoscope is used in diagnosis as well as in treatment. In diagnosis, the bronchoscope is useful in the examination of the larynx, trachea, and bronchi. Secretions and/or cells may be removed for study. In therapy it is used to remove foreign bodies, excessive secretions or those that the patient cannot expel by his own efforts.

Bronchoscopy may therefore be performed as an emergency procedure or after a period of preparation. When relief of an acute obstruction is required to save the life of the individual, preparation is limited to the bare essentials. When bronchoscopy is planned for, the patient should be prepared for what to expect and for what will be expected of him. He should have answers to his questions. Bronchoscopy is not a pleasant procedure, nor is it without danger. The patient may fear the implications of the procedure to diagnosis, most particularly to a diagnosis of cancer. Questions by the patient about the dangers of bronchoscopy or the possibility of cancer should be referred to the physician. Recognition by the nurse of the fact that the patient is worried may in itself be helpful. The patient should know that he will receive a medication, such as codeine and/phenobarbital, which will help him to relax and to be less aware of his surroundings. Barbiturates also decrease the danger of a toxic reaction to the local anesthetic, because the barbiturates are antidotes to certain types of reaction to cocaine and its relatives. To lessen the concentration of bacteria in the mouth, special attention should be given to the care of the mouth on the evening preceding and the morning of the day of bronchoscopy. Removable bridges and dentures should be removed in preparation for the procedure.

In order to facilitate the passage of the bronchoscope, the patient is positioned so that the pharynx is brought into line with the glottis and trachea. A small, hard pillow is placed under the shoulders of the patient and the head is allowed to drop back. The eyes of the patient are covered with a folded towel, so that he will not have to watch the proceedings.

Before the bronchoscope is passed, the physician anesthetizes the pharynx and larynx with cocaine or one of its relatives. Since a topical anesthetic depresses the swallowing reflex, food and fluids are withheld for about eight hours before bronchoscopy is performed and for two or three hours after it is completed. It usually takes about this long for the swallowing reflex to return. When the patient is able to swallow his own saliva, he can safely be given fluids. Until then he should be encouraged to lie on his side and let it drain into an emesis basin.

During the performance of bronchoscopy, the nurse assists the physician as needed. She also directs her attention to the patient. Unless the physician acquaints the patient with the progress of the procedure, the nurse should do so. Mr. Roberts stated at the completion of bronchoscopy that he did not think he could have tolerated it if the nurse had not kept him informed about the progress of the procedure from start to finish.

Following bronchoscopy, the patient should be observed for indications that the swallowing reflex is re-established and for signs and symptoms signifying that cocaine has been absorbed. Cocaine stimulates the nervous system from above downward. Signs and symptoms associated with a moderate degree of absorption include an increase in the strength and rate of the pulse, elevation in blood pressure, an increase in the rate and depth of respirations, and an increase in mental activities. The patient is active, talkative, and euphoric; that is, he has an exaggerated and often unrealistic sense of well-being. If the amount of drug absorbed is excessive, overstimulation is followed by depression of the nervous system, beginning with the higher centers and proceeding downward. Should symptoms of overactivity develop, the nurse should promptly administer a rapidly acting barbiturate, such as Seconal Sodium,[13] intramuscularly. In an extreme emergency the drug must be given intravenously by the physician. If there is no order, the nurse should obtain one promptly. The patient will also probably need some type of artificial respiration. Time is limited; unless prompt and appropriate action is taken, the patient dies from respiratory failure.

OTHER HAZARDS OF BRONCHOSCOPY

Although infrequent in occurrence, the trachea or a bronchus may be perforated during

[13] Trade name for secobarbital sodium.

bronchoscopy. When this happens air and secretions escape into the mediastinum. Signs and symptoms depend on the size of the tear. They include minor to marked dyspnea, crepitus (crackling on pressure or palpation) of tissues, and a puffing of the face and neck. The latter two are referred to as subcutaneous emphysema and are caused by air escaping from the lung into the tissue. Any of these signs or symptoms should be reported promptly because this is a serious complication.

Another serious though infrequent complication is severe laryngeal edema, which blocks the airway and leads to respiratory embarrassment. The patient should always be observed for difficulty in breathing. Should it occur, the physician should be promptly notified. Preparation should be made for a tracheotomy, should one be required.

Following bronchoscopy, the patient is likely to have a sore throat and to be hoarse. Administration of warm or cold liquid by mouth may lessen the degree of soreness. Some physicians prescribe warm saline gargles. As long as hoarseness continues, talking and smoking should be discouraged because they increase the irritation of the larynx. The patient may be given a pad of paper or a slate and pencil with which to write. The call light or bell should be within easy reach, and the patient should be instructed to call for the nurse when he needs her. The nurse should try to look in on the patient from time to time, and the call light or bell should be answered promptly.

POSTURAL DRAINAGE

In chronic conditions such as bronchiectasis or emphysema, the mechanisms for cleaning the tracheobronchial tree may be ineffective. Collections of secretions may then be removed by postural drainage. In postural drainage the patient is placed in a position so that the region to be drained is higher than the ducts through which the fluid is to pass to the outlet. Application is made of the well-known fact that, as a result of gravity, water runs downhill. For the postural drainage to accomplish its purpose, the area to be drained must be known and the patient must be placed in (or assume) the appropriate position. Usually, the disorders in which secretions accumulate are accompanied by bronchiolar spasm and thickening of secretions. In preparation for postural drainage a bronchiolar-dilating drug such as isoproterenol (Isuprel), and a medical detergent such as Alevaire [14] may be inhaled about 10 to 15 minutes

before postural drainage is initiated. When inhaled, Alevaire liquefies secretions and thereby facilitates their removal. Both types of drugs are converted to a fine mist in a nebulizer and inhaled. (See Figure 8-4.)

After suitable preparation, the patient assumes the appropriate position, which is determined by the area of the lung to be drained. In the past, postural drainage was utilized to drain the posterior and lower lobes of the lung. Recently its use has been extended to include all parts of the lung. To increase the effectiveness of postural drainage, the patient is instructed to perform two other procedures. One is to cough, a series of little rapid-fire coughs similar to clearing of the throat. The other is to tap the chest with the fingers of both hands beginning with the bottom of the ribs and continuing to the collarbone and back again. A member of the family can be taught the chest-tapping routine and can tap the posterior wall of the chest when the patient is in the prone or sitting position. Coughing and the chest-tapping techniques aid in loosening secretions by vibration.[15]

When postural drainage is prescribed, the patient assumes the appropriate position or series of positions. Postural drainage is frequently prescribed to drain posterior portions of the lower lobes. There are several methods that can be used in order to have the chest lower than the rest of the body. One method is to assist the patient to lie face down and crosswise on the bed. He is then assisted so that he hangs over the side of the bed at a 45-degree angle. Only his legs and thighs rest on the bed. His head and trunk are over the side. His arms rest on a pillow or low footstool on the floor. A basin should be placed at the patient's head to catch the drainage. From the nature of the position, it is obvious that it is unsuitable for very sick patients. All patients should be given assistance in attaining the position until they are able to get into the proper position and can do so without excessive fear. Some patients refuse to do postural drainage, because they are fearful of falling. In the beginning, the time should be limited to three minutes or even less. As the patient gains strength and confidence, he will be able to remain in the position for 20 to 30 minutes. Another method is to raise the knee gatch of the patient's bed and have him lie with his head and chest lower than the rest of the body. This position is particularly advantageous for elderly

[14] Trade name for tylaxapol.

[15] See Albert Haas: *Essentials of Living with Pulmonary Emphysema*, Patient Publication No. 4 (New York: The Institute of Physical Medicine and Rehabilitation, New York University Medical Center, 1963).

1. Postural drainage in supine position over pillow to drain anterior
    segments and middle lobe.

2. Prone position over pillows to drain basal segments and superior segments.

3. Left lateral decubitus position over pillow to drain left lateral segments.

4. Right lateral decubitus position over pillow to drain right lateral segments.

FIGURE 8-4. Positions assumed to drain various areas of the lung. [Adapted from "Patient
Education and Emphysema Care," *Medical Times*, 97:123 (Feb.), 1969, by Thomas L. Petty
and Louise M. Nett.]

or debilitated patients who cannot tolerate lying over the side of the bed.

OTHER CAUSES OF INADEQUATE LUNG VENTILATION

As emphasized, one of the essential factors in the maintenance of a supply of oxygen is a clear airway. In health the mechanisms for keeping it patent and for warming, moistening, and cleansing the air are usually adequate. In illness, they often are not. Any patient who is treated by bed rest is predisposed to obstruction of the tracheobronchial tree, primarily because of a reduction in the expansion of the chest. Expansion is limited by the resistance offered to the chest wall by the bed and by the loss of muscle power accompanying any decrease in activity. Distention of the abdomen either by gas or fluid exerts pressure on the diaphragm and prevents its descent during inspiration. Diseases involving areas in the nervous system regulating respiration or the muscles of respiration are also accompanied by a loss of muscle power. Drugs that depress the central nervous system—sedatives, narcotics, and general anesthetics—interfere with normal cleansing mechanisms by depressing the respiratory and cough centers and by paralyzing the cilia in the trachea and bronchi. In the unconscious state secretions are increased and the mechanisms for their removal are inhibited. Pain associated with breathing, whether caused by disease involving the pleura or by surgical procedures in which the route of approach is through the chest wall or the upper abdomen, is accompanied by a protective inhibition of breathing. This is why the judicious use of narcotics in such patients is necessary in order to improve respiratory excursions. By prevention and relief of pain the patient can be encouraged to voluntarily increase the depth of inspiration and to cough. Infections, chemical irritants such as smoke, and allergic responses such as in asthma may increase secretions to such an extent that the normal physiological mechanisms for their removal are inadequate. There may be, in addition, some reduction in the adequacy of one or more mechanisms themselves. For example, spasm of the muscles of the bronchioles narrows their lumen and therefore increases the resistance to the removal of the secretions. The glottis may be blocked by soft tissues or foreign bodies including food in the hypopharynx, paralysis of the vocal folds, neoplasms, and swelling of the area that surrounds it.

How may the nurse prevent airway obstruction?

There are few areas where the nurse can do

more to protect and to assist the patient. To prevent airway obstruction, patients who are likely to have some problem in maintaining a clean airway must be identified. This requires that the nurse know which patients can be anticipated to have difficulty and that she recognize signs and symptoms indicating that pathology is developing—such as cough, wet-sounding respirations, and pain on breathing. When the signs and symptoms indicate that the patient is receiving an inadequate supply of oxygen, obstruction is either acute or extensive or both.

Prevention is the most desirable objective. In the care of the bedfast and sick individual, attention to a regular schedule of turning the patient from side to side, deep-breathing, and coughing will usually do much to protect him from obstruction by secretions. When the patient can be up and walking this is of further assistance. When the patient has pain on coughing, splinting the affected area of the chest by supporting it with the hands or a binder may enable him to cough more deeply. Although pain-relieving medications do have an adverse effect when they are overused, they may also be a help when given about 15 minutes before the patient coughs or deep-breathes.

A patient may require assistance in removing secretions from his airway when (1) one or more of the mechanisms for their removal is inactivated or (2) the quantity or character of the secretions makes their removal difficult or impossible. Often both factors play a part. For example, when in disease or its treatment swallowing mechanisms are inactivated, saliva collects in the hypopharynx. The patient should be placed in a position in which gravity facilitates drainage. The side-lying, prone, and Trendelenburg positions all facilitate drainage by gravity. When the patient lies on his back, his head should be turned to the side and his jaw moved forward and up. When the swallowing reflex continues to be depressed and secretions are abundant, they may have to be removed by suctioning. For the procedure to be effective, secretions must be removed from the hypopharynx and suctioning must also be performed frequently enough to prevent a large collection of fluid from accumulating.

When secretions accumulate in the tracheobronchial tree and natural methods are not successful in removing them, a catheter may be used to irritate the nerve endings in the larynx and stimulate coughing. This procedure is usually performed by the physician, and should not be done by the nurse unless she has received specialized instructions. Neither should the nurse who has not been instructed introduce a catheter into the tracheobronchial tree by way of the glottis for purposes of aspirating secretions. Either procedure is accompanied by the possibility of inducing laryngeal spasm and, with it, obstruction of the airway. Unless laryngeal spasm is promptly relieved, the patient will suffocate. The precautions to be observed will be discussed together with those that should be taken when tracheostomy is suctioned.

TRACHEOSTOMY OR ENDOTRACHEAL INTUBATION

When the measures just described are insufficient to protect the patency of the airway, a tracheostomy may be performed or an endotracheal tube may be inserted. The method chosen depends on several factors: (1) the length of time the artificial airway must be maintained, (2) the condition for which the artificial airway is being established, (3) whether or not there are profuse secretions, and (4) whether or not it is an elective procedure.

In tracheostomy a vertical slit is made in the anterior portion of the neck and a double-cannula airway is introduced into the trachea. The incision in the trachea is usually below the first or second tracheal cartilage. The outer cannula is held in place by ties around the neck of the patient and the inner cannula is locked into the outer cannula. At one time tracheostomy was performed almost entirely as an emergency measure to relieve obstructions of the airway located in the pharynx and larynx. Particularly in the days when diphtheria was common, a crude kind of tracheostomy was part of the folk medicine of certain groups.[16] It is now employed to prevent or relieve hypoxia caused by the accumulation of secretions in the lower tracheobronchial tree and to lessen the work of breathing as well as to bypass the naso-oral passage or the larynx.

Tracheostomy is utilized to prevent or to relieve hypoxia due to the accumulation of secretions in the tracheobronchial tree in patients suffering a wide variety of disorders. Among these are the weak and feeble, the critically ill, and those whose brains are injured or diseased. Among the latter are persons who have suffered head injuries, bulbar poliomyelitis, cerebrovascular accidents, or overdosage of drugs that depress the respiratory and cough centers in the brain. In these and other similar conditions secretions are formed more rapidly than they can be removed by natural mechanisms. When secretions are unusually profuse, a tracheostomy is superior to the endotracheal tube because the inner tube can be cleaned and it is easier to handle the excess secretions. The imbalance between the formation and removal of secretions may be caused by an actual in-

crease in secretion, or by a depression or failure of the cleansing mechanisms, or by both factors. In any event, secretions remain to block the airway and to prevent the passage of air to and from the alveoli. In the lung this predisposes to tracheobronchitis, atelectasis, and bronchopneumonia. The general and more immediately serious effect of one or more of these disturbances is hypoxia. When hypoxia is caused by failure of the service facility to present adequate amounts of oxygen to the blood, the condition resulting from airway obstruction is sometimes called arterial hypoxia. In patients who have suffered head injury or some other disorder involving the brain, hypoxia is particularly dangerous because it worsens cerebral edema. Furthermore, obstruction of the airway not only causes hypoxia, but it interferes with the elimination of carbon dioxide and predisposes to respiratory acidosis. (See Chapter 9.)

In weak and feeble patients a tracheostomy may be instituted to reduce the work of breathing. A tracheostomy is slightly more effective in accomplishing this purpose than the endotracheal tube. However, to be effective it must be cuffed, thereby preventing any leakage about and above the tube. The decrease in the work of breathing is accomplished primarily by lessening the volume of the anatomical dead-air space by as much as 60 per cent. The anatomical dead-air space extends from the nose and nasopharynx to the level in the respiratory tree where exchanges of oxygen and carbon dioxide take place. It holds a volume of approximately 150 ml of air. Although the air in the dead-air space does not participate directly in the exchange of gases, it performs a valuable function. It dilutes the air entering and leaving the lung and thereby protects the alveoli from sudden change. It does, however, add to the work of breathing. The reduction in volume of air that is secured by the tracheostomy is therefore of considerable value. In the patient with an unstable chest wall ("flail chest" caused by multiple fractures of the ribs), tracheostomy may also improve ventilation by reducing the work of breathing.

Tracheostomy is also performed to relieve obstruction of the larynx and upper trachea of either extrinsic or intrinsic origin. Although some of these obstructions were indicated previously, they will be summarized here. The soft tissues in the pharynx are a frequent and often preventable cause of obstruction of the glottis. Hemorrhage into the pharynx or the soft tissues of the neck may be responsible for obstruction of the airway. In the first instance blood is aspirated into the airway. In the second, blood in the soft tissues exerts pressure on the trachea. Hemorrhage into the soft tissues causing pres-

[16] Harriette Arnow: *The Dollmaker* (New York: The Macmillan Company, 1954), pp. 10–17.

sure on the trachea is most frequently a complication following thyroidectomy and radical neck resection. Either surgical procedure may be responsible for obstruction of the glottis by paralyzing the vocal folds. Trauma to or severing of both recurrent laryngeal nerves may also be responsible. Collapse of one vocal fold does not cause complete obstruction of the glottis. It does, however, increase resistance to the passage of air. Edema involving the tissues of the neck or the larynx may also obstruct breathing.

A neoplasm having its origin in tissues within the respiratory tract may cause obstruction. Tumors may be located in the larynx, bronchi or in the mediastinum.

A tracheostomy may be temporary or permanent. If an artificial airway must be maintained for over 48 hours, a tracheostomy is usually preferable to an endotracheal tube because of the decreased chance of damage to the larynx. In adults the most frequent reason for establishing a permanent tracheostomy is to maintain an airway after the removal of the larynx in the treatment of laryngeal cancer. With the loss of the larynx, the person loses, forever, his ability to speak normally. In conversations with patients who have experienced laryngectomy or are about to do so, the most terrifying aspect is the loss of the ability ever to speak again.

REASONS FOR TRACHEOSTOMY

The reasons for the performance of a tracheostomy are summarized as follows:

1. It lessens the tracheopharyngeal dead-air space and thereby reduces the work of breathing.
2. It bypasses the naso-oral passage and the larynx, establishing a new airway.
3. It provides easy access to the tracheobronchial tree and makes it easier to remove secretions.[17]
4. It may also be utilized with one of the various mechanical types of respirators now on the market to provide partial or total respiratory assistance to the patient. Nurses who are going to work with any type of mechanical respirator should learn how to operate the apparatus before they attempt to take care of the patient. Unless this equipment is properly used, the respirator is of no advantage to the patient and may actually be harmful.

What are the nurse's responsibilities in caring for a patient with a tracheostomy?

The plan for the preparation of the patient

who is facing a tracheostomy will depend on many factors. When the patient is conscious and time permits, the patient should know why it is required and what to expect, as well as what is expected of him. As with other surgical procedures, the physician has the responsibility for informing the patient about the nature of the procedure to be performed and why it is necessary. The nurse must work closely with the physician in order to reinforce and supplement the information he has given the patient. Often when a laryngectomy is to be performed, a person who has recovered from the procedure and has mastered esophageal speech will be asked to visit the patient preoperatively. Most cities have clubs made up of laryngectomized individuals who donate their time to helping others faced with this type of surgery. Esophageal speech can be learned providing the person has a strong desire and is willing to devote time and effort to it. Many persons who have had laryngectomy are able to return to their former employment, and some very prominent positions are held by people who have recovered from this type of surgery.

The nurse has multiple responsibilities. These responsibilities differ somewhat in detail, but not in principle, from those involved in the care of the patient who has any operative procedure. These are discussed in some detail in Chapter 17.

In both preoperative preparation and postoperative care the nurse should take into account the reason the tracheostomy is performed and the way in which the physiology of the patient is altered. As stated earlier, the patient is unable to speak. In the patient who has an associated laryngectomy, loss of natural speech is permanent. The one who has a temporary tracheostomy can speak by placing a finger over the opening in the tube. Sometimes when the patient is being prepared for the removal of the tracheostomy tube, the tube will be plugged for short periods of time before it is permanently removed, to test the ability of the patient to breathe normally. When the patient is critically ill or he has a problem maintaining ventilation, closure of the tracheostomy tube is not recommended.

PSYCHOLOGICAL PROBLEMS

Inability to speak or to cry out adds to the emotional stress of the patient. He fears that he will not be able to get help when he needs it. Particularly when the patient has a permanent loss of voice, he is likely to grieve because he will never be able to speak again. As a result of the loss of his voice he may fear that he will not be able to carry on his work or, equally as important, that he will become unacceptable to

[17] "Emergency Tracheotomy," *Med. Times,* **86**:1587 (Dec.), 1958.

his family, friends, or co-workers. For the first few days after tracheostomy someone ought to be with the patient continuously.

To illustrate some of the problems experienced by the patient who is to have a tracheostomy, Mr. Frederickson will be described. Mr. Frederickson, who was in the process of making a decision about whether to have a laryngectomy for the removal of a malignant neoplasm, was able to express to his nurse the inner turmoil he felt at having to make this decision. Mr. Frederickson was 60 years old. Although he was nearly illiterate, he had a remarkable knowledge of the Bible, which he quoted frequently. He worked with his brother, who was a minister, as a lay minister. His nurse was a sensitive and perceptive woman who spent an entire morning listening to Mr. Frederickson debating with himself whether or not he should keep his voice and continue to do God's work as long as he lived or give up his voice and his work so that he might continue to live. At the end of the morning, he agreed to wait to make his decision until a visitor from the laryngectomy club would come in the afternoon to talk to him. Mr. Frederickson finally decided to have the laryngectomy. The decision was truly his.

PHYSIOLOGICAL PROBLEMS

Besides being unable to speak, the patient is deprived of his mechanisms for conditioning environmental air. The air enters the tracheobronchial tree without having been filtered, warmed, and moistened. Moreover, objects (catheters) are introduced into the respiratory tract. The two problems that are most difficult to cope with in the care of the airway are achievement of an adequate degree of humidity of the air and maintenance of cleanliness of catheters introduced into the tracheostomy tube. Lack of moisture in the inspired air has two adverse effects. It dries the delicate mucous membrane lining of the respiratory tract, and the secretions become thick and viscous. Drying predisposes to the formation of encrustations of the trachea, which may be large enough to obstruct the trachea and to increase the difficulty of removing secretions. The most common site of tracheal encrustation is just beneath the tip of the tracheostomy tube and at the level of the coryna. Various methods are used to increase the humidity of the air. Cold steam or hot steam is added to the air to try to increase moisture content. Cold steam is formed by converting a liquid such as water into a fine mist by mechanical means. It has the advantage over hot steam of neither heating the air nor being a source of burns. To effectively elevate the moisture content of the air, the doors and windows should be kept closed. It is impossible

to significantly elevate the moisture content of the air when windows and doors are open. Another method sometimes prescribed by the physician to combat the drying effect of the inspired air is to introduce 0.5 to 1 ml of sterile physiological saline solution into the tracheostomy tube at regular intervals. By this method water lost to the air by evaporation is replaced. Attention should also be paid to maintaining the fluid intake of the patient.

CARE OF THE TRACHEOSTOMY

To limit the introduction of microorganisms into the tracheostomy tube, a few elementary precautions should be taken. First, separate trays should be set up and plainly marked so that different catheters and rinsing solutions are available and *used* for suctioning the nose, mouth, and oropharynx and for suctioning the tracheostomy tube. The all-too-common practice of using the same catheter for suctioning the nose and oral cavities and the tracheostomy violates the most basic principles of microbiology.

Another grave omission often observed is failure of the person performing the suctioning of the tracheostomy to wash his hands. Although this procedure can never be a sterile one, utmost cleanliness is important. Thorough hand washing (sometimes with special solutions such as pHisoHex),[18] the wearing of rubber gloves, and the use of forceps in carrying out the procedure may be employed. The technique employed is probably not as important as the recognition of the principle involved and consistency in carrying out a clean technique by those involved in the care of the patient.

Second, the procedure that is used should provide for keeping the equipment clean. A fresh sterile setup should be provided at least every eight hours. After suctioning, water or physiological saline should be drawn through the catheter to remove the secretions. Then the catheter should be wiped clean with a sterile four-by-four sponge. Marchetta,[19] *et al.* recommend that the catheter be wiped, with a sponge soaked in a small amount of Zephiran Chloride [20] and that it be detached from the suction apparatus and placed in a 1:10,000 dilution of benzalkonium solution. The reason for detaching the catheter is to prevent the tubing from being dragged out of the container. According to Marchetta, benzalkonium in the suggested dilution is effective in destroying bacteria and is at the same time nonirritating to the tracheal

---

[18] Hexachlorophene soap.
[19] Frank C. Marchetta, Sidney Anthone, and Anna Aungst: "A Method of Tracheotomy Care," *Arch. Otolaryng.* (Chicago), **65**:296–99 (Mar.) 1957.
[20] Trade name for benzalkonium chloride.

lining. In some hospitals, after use the catheter is rinsed, wiped dry, and stored in a bag or in a folded towel. The important point is that it not be draped on the suction machine or placed on a table top or some unclean surface. In an ideal technique, a clean catheter would be used each time the trachea was suctioned. With the introduction of inexpensive plastic catheters, the practice of discarding catheters may be feasible. Whatever the details of the method of handling the equipment used in suctioning, they should be based on the knowledge that the patient has been deprived of his own mechanisms for cleaning the air before it enters the tracheobronchial tree. The catheter is introduced into a region that in health is sterile. The lining of the trachea is not adapted to direct exposure to unconditioned air and can be injured by the catheter or the suctioning procedure.

Knowledge of the physiology of the trachea is also of significance in the care of the tracheostomy tubes. The physician is usually responsible for the changing of the outer cannula. The frequency with which the outer cannula is changed varies; it is usually dependent on the condition of the patient and whether or not the tube is patent. It may not be changed more frequently than every four to five days. The nurse is responsible for checking the ties on the outer cannula to be sure that they fit snugly around the neck of the patient and for having the necessary equipment ready for the physician. Although the nurse should check the ties, she should not remove them unless she has received instruction and the physician has delegated the responsibility to her. Should the cannula slip out of the trachea, the nurse may keep the trachea open with forceps or another dilating instrument to prevent suffocation.

CARE OF THE CANNULAS

In contrast to the outer cannula, the nurse removes the inner cannula as necessary in order to clean it. When secretions are voluminous this may have to be done as often as every one-half to one hour. Procedures for cleaning the inner cannula vary. The procedure suggested by Marchetta [21] and his co-workers is based on the following: (1) the inner cannula is coated with protein-containing mucus; (2) it is of silver or other metal; [22] and (3) it is to be inserted into the outer cannula. They suggest the following:

1. The cannula should be placed in hydrogen peroxide and water to soften the mucus.
2. A soft brush and green soap and water should be used to cleanse the inside of the cannula. Some authorities suggest that pipe cleaners be used rather than a brush. When a brush is used, there is a possibility that a bristle may remain in the cannula. As a precaution the cannula should be checked after it is cleansed for extraneous material.
3. The cannula should be scoured with silver polish.
4. The cannula should be rinsed thoroughly.
5. The cannula should be boiled for two minutes.
6. The cannula should be cooled.
7. The cannula should be reinserted.

Because the two parts of a tracheostomy tube are matched, one inner cannula cannot be substituted for another.

Another factor in the physiology of the respiratory tree having relevance in nursing is that secretions increase markedly during the first few hours after tracheostomy. The cilia are likely to be overwhelmed by the volume of secretion. The situation is aggravated by the fact that the newly tracheotomized patient is unable to cough efficiently. When the patient is able, he should be encouraged to cough. Before the patient attempts to cough, the suction apparatus should be in readiness. In preparation for coughing, the patient is instructed to take a deep breath, and the tracheostomy tube is occluded as expiration begins. As secretions are raised, they should be removed by wiping the end of the tube with gauze and by suctioning the tube. Aspiration of secretions into the airway should, when possible, be avoided. Excessive coughing should be prevented, as this damages the ciliated epithelium of the respiratory tree. The combination of an increase in secretions and the failure of mechanisms for ridding the tracheobronchial tree of them predisposes the patient to two dangers, encrustation of the trachea and tracheobronchitis. Tracheobronchitis further increases secretion and intensifies the destruction of the ciliated mucous membrane. Thus, a vicious circle is initiated. Increased secretion overwhelms the cleansing mechanisms of the tracheobronchial tree and predisposes to encrustation and tracheobronchitis, which in turn further increase secretions. As indicated previously, whenever secretions accumulate in the tracheobronchial tree, the patient is predisposed to atelectasis and pneumonia.

To prevent the accumulation of secretions, suctioning is required. Whether the nurse does shallow or deep suctioning depends on the policy of the institution and of the physician attending the patient and on the skill and confidence of the nurse. To achieve the greatest benefit to the patient, the secretions in deeper

21 *Op. cit.*, p. 298.
22 New materials such as plastic are now being used.

structures must be regularly removed. When deep suctioning is performed, maximum consideration must be given to the fragility of the respiratory membrane. As emphasized earlier, attention must be paid to asepsis so that the patient is protected from the introduction of pathogenic microorganisms into the airway. Aspiration of the tracheobronchial tree must also take into consideration the fact that the airway is obstructed during suctioning and that hypoxia is intensified if the catheter is left in place too long.

After studying the respiratory tree of tracheotomized persons who died and of rabbits that had been subjected to tracheotomy and suctioning, Plum and Dunning [23] devised a technique of deep suctioning that they state minimizes trauma to the mucous membrane. At the same time, it is effective in removing secretions. They state that suctioning, as it is all too frequently performed, serves as a crude biopsy technique. As do other authorities, they emphasize the importance of scrupulous cleanliness. They suggest that number 12 firm-rubber whistle-tip catheters be used and that 5 per cent sodium bicarbonate solution be employed as a lubricant. To prevent trauma to the wall of the trachea or bronchi as a result of the catheter's adhering to it, they place a Y tube in the suction line. The Y tube makes it possible to release the vacuum immediately by fingertip control. During insertion, the Y valve is left open. It is directed into the right or left bronchus by having the patient turn his head to the opposite side. The catheter is then withdrawn 1 to 2 cm to remove the tip from the mucous membrane before the suction is started by putting the finger over the Y valve. At any sign that the mucous membrane has been suctioned into the tube, the finger should be immediately removed from the Y valve to release the suction. As the tube is removed, it should be slowly rotated. When a Cuday catheter is used, it should not be rotated, as the hook on the end of the catheter traumatizes the mucosa. No aspiration should be longer than 15 seconds and the patient should be allowed to rest at least three minutes, unless secretions are so abundant that there is no choice but to remove them. A warning emphasized by Plum and Dunning is *not* to pinch the tube while suctioning, as this increases the negative pressure and the possibility of sucking the mucous membrane into the catheter.

In the words of John M. Lore,[24] the care of

[23] Fred Plum and Marcella F. Dunning: "Technics for Minimizing Trauma to the Tracheobronchial Tree After Tracheotomy," *New Eng. J. Med.,* **254:**193–200 (Feb. 2) 1956.
[24] John M. Lore: "Tracheostomy," *Arch. Otolaryng.* (Chicago), **68:**727–36 (Dec.) 1958.

the patient following a tracheostomy is based on three principles: (1) "Keep moist." (2). Use "deep suction." (3) "Keep clean." Throughout this discussion, these three principles and ways of achieving them have been emphasized. These three principles take priority in achieving the purposes of the procedure. Unless the airway is kept open, the life of the patient is endangered from hypoxia. The patency of the airway is threatened by secretions, encrustations, and infection, which is predisposed to by the first two and intensifies both.

As indicated earlier, in the patient who is conscious, tracheostomy is a frightening procedure. Hypoxia, from whatever cause, is attended by feelings of anxiety which may be so great as to cause panic and intensify the degree of hypoxia by increasing activity. When the airway is kept clean, ventilation is improved and the feelings of anxiety are thereby reduced. Anxiety will be increased when the patient has reason to fear that he will not be able to get help when he needs it and therefore runs the risk of suffocation. Survival depends on a patent airway.

As soon as the patient *is able,* he should be taught to suction himself. Some patients ask to be taught. Others are reluctant to learn. Even when there is a policy to instruct patients as soon as possible, timing should take into account the readiness of the patient to learn and his physiological status. For example, Mrs. Cardinal, who had had a laryngectomy the day previously, asked to be taught to suction her own tracheostomy. The day following the operation she found the noise of the air passing through mucus in her airway most irritating and frightening.

The nurse demonstrated the procedure and then helped Mrs. Cardinal suction herself. After several supervised practice periods, Mrs. Cardinal expressed confidence that she was able to carry on by herself. The nurse checked from time to time to be sure that Mrs. Cardinal was managing successfully and that the suction apparatus was in satisfactory working condition. Mrs. Cardinal learned to care for her tracheostomy very quickly. She was relieved by being able to control her own situation and expressed satisfaction with her ability to care for herself.

By way of contrast, Mr. Quill, an elderly and feeble man, refused to try to suction himself. In a conference with his physician, the decision was made not to insist that he try. Tracheostomy had been performed on Mr. Quill to lessen the work of breathing and to facilitate the removal of secretions. Because of widespread emphysema and his inability to clear his tracheobronchial tree of secretions, Mr. Quill was in a continuous state of hypoxia. He could not be expected to improve until the hypoxia was corrected. Nurses were to suction the airway for a few days with hope that, as the physical status of Mr. Quill improved, he would possibly be able to assume some responsibility for himself. Because he had extensive emphysema and lack of motivation to learn, efforts to teach him were not successful. His wife had recently died. Grief over the loss of his wife and changes in his living arrangements contributed to his lack of interest in living and in caring for himself. Therefore, it was decided that Mr. Quill required help with suctioning and that he should not be expected to perform the procedure for himself. His life situation was too overwhelming to permit him to act independently, and some degree of dependency was necessary for his recovery.

ENDOTRACHEAL INTUBATION

Provided prolonged airway assistance is not anticipated, endotracheal intubation is often the procedure of choice. When this is the case the endotracheal tube is inserted via the laryngoscope. With special attachments it, too, like the tracheostomy tube, can be utilized with the mechanical respirator. The biggest drawback to the endotracheal tube is that with prolonged use laryngeal damage, possibly leading to stenosis, may result. Probably the biggest advantage of endotracheal intubation is that surgery is avoided.

Structure and Function of the Lung

In addition to a patent airway, two other interrelated structures, the lung and the thoracic cavity, enter into ventilation. The lungs are elastic distensible bodies that stretch as air enters and deflate as it leaves. They contain no muscles and are not attached at any point to the chest wall, yet they adhere to it closely and follow its motions faithfully. A number of factors account for this. Because of their elasticity, the lung and the chest wall act like springs. When they are expanded, their tendency to collapse is greater than their tendency to remain expanded. After expansion, the lung and thorax tend to return to their resting state. Expansion is always opposed by the tendency to collapse. The characteristic of the lung enabling it to return to its resting state after it is stretched is known as elastic recoil, and the characteristic enabling it to expand is known as compliance. The wall of the thorax also exhibits these properties.

Emphysema

A diminution of elastic recoil or of compliance interferes with ventilation. With a loss of elastic recoil, the lung remains partly expanded during expiration. The retained air adds to the volume of air that does not participate in ventilation; therefore, it adds to the dead-space air by increasing the amount of residual air. It also adds to the difficulty of mixing inspired air with residual air. The disorder in which the air sacs in the lung are overinflated with air and their walls are disrupted is known as chronic emphysema. Walkup [25] defines emphysema as "an anatomic alteration of the lung characterized by an abnormal enlargement of the air space distal to the terminal, nonrespiratory bronchiole accompanied by destruction of the alveolar walls." As with other chronic progressive diseases, the progress of emphysema can frequently be delayed if it is detected early, and proper treatment is instituted. The frequency with which the diagnosis of emphysema is made has increased greatly in the last decade, and it can be expected to increase even more as the number of aged persons in our society increases.

Because of the loss of elastic tissue and changes in posture that accompany aging, emphysema is common in the aged. Though it reduces their respiratory reserve somewhat, when it is uncomplicated emphysema in the aged is not of serious import.[26] When they are ill and bedfast, it does predispose them to respiratory complications. Moving and turning from side to side on a regular schedule of no less often than every two hours is imperative.

Compensatory emphysema is a physiological process following some conditions such as a lobectomy that reduce the lung parenchyma. Remaining or functioning portions of the lung tend to expand after a portion of the lung is removed by resection of the lung or destroyed by fibrosis. To a degree, this type of emphysema is adaptive.

The most serious form of emphysema results from obstruction of the smaller bronchioles. Common etiological factors include bronchial asthma, chronic bronchitis, bronchiectasis, tu-

[25] Harry E. Walkup and Eleanor C. Connolly: "The Dimensions of the Chronic Respiratory Disease Problem," *Amer. J. Public Health, Suppl.,* Part II, **53**:1–6 (March), 1963.

[26] John H. Killough: "Protective Mechanisms of the Lungs; Pulmonary Disease; Pleural Disease," *Pathologic Physiology,* 4th ed., William A. Sodeman and William A. Sodeman, Jr., eds. (Philadelphia: W. B. Saunders Company, 1967), p. 545.

berculosis and other infections of the lungs, sarcoidosis, and pneumoconiosis.[27] The basic pathological change predisposing to emphysema is a narrowing of the airway, particularly of the smaller bronchioles, which may be caused by edema with exudate or by spasm of the bronchiolar musculature. Both are frequently factors. Because airways are wider during inspiration than expiration and the inspiratory muscles are more powerful than the expiratory muscles, air is trapped in the alveoli behind the partly obstructed bronchioles. Air is pulled into the alveoli during inspiration, but the forces of expiration are insufficient to drive it out. Because of small pores in alveolar walls, an alveolus whose bronchiole is blocked may receive air. The air trapped in the alveoli raises the intra-alveolar pressure, and with the rise, septa break down and the alveoli collapse. Dilated air sacs that do not collapse, that is, remain distended, during the entire respiratory cycle are called blebs. They reduce the surface available for the exchange of gases as well as decrease the area of the capillary bed in the lung. Blebs at the surface of the lung may rupture into the pleural space and establish a connection between the atmosphere and the pleural space which, if sufficient in size, can result in a spontaneous pneumothorax. In spontaneous pneumothorax there is a collapse of lung tissue due to the presence of atmospheric positive pressure in the pleural space where normally the pressure is subatmospheric or negative.

As a consequence of the physiological changes in obstructive emphysema the patient is predisposed to hypoxia, and shortness of breath is the earliest manifestation. Because emphysema interferes with the elimination of carbon dioxide as well as with the intake of oxygen, respiratory acidosis develops sooner or later. When the acidosis is severe, the medullary centers may be relatively insensitive to carbon dioxide, and the low oxygen tension in the blood serves as the stimulus to respiration. Unless the respiratory acidosis can be corrected, oxygen should be administered with extreme caution, because it may precipitate respiratory failure and result in the death of the patient. The correction of respiratory acidosis depends on improving ventilation, particularly the expiratory phase. This can be done by administering oxygen with intermittent positive pressure breathing (IPPB) whereby pressure is increased on inspiration causing ventilation to occur and carbon dioxide to be eliminated more effectively. The percentage of oxygen should not exceed 40 per cent.

Patients with emphysema who are receiving

oxygen should be watched closely for signs of carbon dioxide narcosis. Patients who exhibit shallow respirations, confusion, or drowsiness should be removed from oxygen and watched closely. If their signs improve without oxygen, this tends to support the conclusion that they are experiencing carbon dioxide narcosis. Above all, it is important for the nurse to understand that the patient's color will remain good, and if he is not removed from oxygen, he will go into progressive coma and die pink. He will not be cyanotic. The general objectives of therapy in emphysema are (1) to eliminate insofar as is possible existing infection and (2) to improve ventilation. To accomplish the first objective, to eliminate infection, antimicrobial drugs are administered orally or by intramuscular injection.

Accomplishment of the second objective, to improve ventilation, will be facilitated by the first. Removal of retained secretions and prevention of further accumulation are essential factors in the improvement of ventilation. Some of the measures utilized to remove secretions have previously been described. They are postural drainage, bronchiolar dilating drugs, medical detergents or wetting agents, and humidified air. In addition, attention should be paid to the intake of fluid by the patient. Dehydration aggravates the tendency to thick, tenacious secretions. Liquefying expectorants such as potassium iodide or ammonium chloride may be prescribed.

In the earlier stages of emphysema and before severe respiratory acidosis develops, oxygen or air may be administered under intermittent positive pressure. Helming [28] states that to be successful, IPPB [29] must be administered at eight to ten respirations per minute over a 20- to 30-minute period several times a day until the desired effect is produced; bronchodilator aerosol also should be utilized. The administration of oxygen may improve the feeling of well-being of the patient by lessening the degree of hypoxia. When a positive pressure room is available, air, rather than oxygen, is used to ventilate the lungs. The patient may be taught to keep the bronchioles open by maintaining positive pressure during expiration by expiring against closed lips. Any method preventing the trapping of air in the lung at the end of expiration will improve ventilation.

As indicated previously, tracheostomy may be instituted to lessen the size of the dead-air space and to facilitate the removal of secretions. In weak and tired patients, a respirator may be

[27] Ibid.

[28] Mary G. Helming: "Nursing Care of Patients with Chronic Obstructive Lung Disease," Nurs. Clin. North Amer., 3:418 (Sept.) 1968.

[29] Intermittent positive pressure breathing.

prescribed to improve the adequacy of ventilation.

What factors bring about a decrease in lung compliance?

Compliance or expansibility of the lung is decreased by a variety of disorders of the lung and of the structures of the chest wall. Diseases of the lung that reduce compliance are accompanied by one or more of the following changes: (1) destruction of lung tissue, as in tuberculosis with caseation necrosis and cavity formation; (2) fibrosis of the lung, as in tuberculosis with fibrosis; (3) pulmonary edema, as in congestive heart failure or associated with overloading a patient having a limited renal reserve with fluids; and (4) blocking of the alveoli with exudate, as in pneumococcic pneumonia. Although the pathology in each of the above is different, they all interfere with respiration by limiting the expansion of the lung.

Diseases or effects of disease limiting the expansion of the thoracic cage also have the effect of limiting the expansion of the lung. Kyphosis, severe scoliosis, fibrotic pleurisy, hydrothorax, paralyzed or fibrotic muscles—all limit in some manner the expansion of the lung and therefore decrease compliance. Some forms of therapy such as tight binders and bed rest decrease compliance; a person who lies in bed has a reduction in compliance on the side of his chest that lies next to the bed, which can and should be relieved by moving him or encouraging him to move from side to side.

In addition to a patent airway and the expansibility of the lung, the flow of air into and out of the lung is dependent on changes in the capacity of the thoracic cavity during breathing. Intrapleural pressure is normally less than atmospheric pressure; that is, intrapleural pressure is negative in relation to atmospheric pressure. Negative pressure is greatest during inspiration and least during expiration. Changes in intrapleural pressure are possible because the lungs are contained in a space or box that is too large for them. During growth the thoracic cage grows more rapidly than the lungs, with the result that the space containing the lungs is larger than the lungs. The greater size of the thoracic cavity in relation to the size of the lung increases the elastic pull on the lung as well as the negative intrapleural pressure. Expansion of the lung during inspiration puts pulmonary tissue, including the elastic tissue of the bronchial tree, the blood vessels, and the air sacs, on a stretch. As the lung is stretched, the elastic tissue offers resistance to further stretching and prevents the lung from being overexpanded.

Another necessary condition in the maintenance of subatmospheric or negative pressure is that the intrapleural cavity be closed to the external environment. The chest wall is lined by serous membrane, the pleura, which continues and is reflected over the lung on the same side. Each pleura is similar to a sealed envelope with one side lining the chest and the other side reflected over the lung. The layer lining the chest is the parietal pleura. The layer covering the lung is the visceral pleura. The space between the two layers is comparable to the inside of the envelope and is known as the intrapleural space. It is actually a potential space as the pleura is separated only by a thin layer of fluid, which also holds the two layers together. The effect of the fluid can be demonstrated by placing the wet sides of two glass slides together. The water causes the slides to adhere to each other, and it takes considerable force to separate them. Without this fluid the lung would not follow the chest wall in breathing. The intrapleural fluid lessens the friction between the two layers and allows one layer to glide smoothly over the other.

During inspiration the chest is expanded in all directions. The length or vertical diameter is increased by the contraction and flattening of the diaphragm. Because the vertebrae are relatively fixed, most of the vertical increase is due to the elevation of the ribs and sternum and is in the anterior direction. Not all parts of the lung are expanded equally. Parts lying next to relatively fixed structures cannot expand unless other parts of the lung get out of the way. This effect can be demonstrated by inhaling while in a supine position and holding the breath while assuming the upright position. Breathing starts with inspiration. The same phenomenon can be observed when a patient who has been lying in bed is ambulated. As he assumes the upright position, he takes a deep breath and, incidentally, often coughs.

In quiet breathing, expiration is largely passive. As the contraction of inspiratory muscles ceases, the chest wall and lung through their own weight and inherent elasticity tend to resume their former position. Air is forced out of the lungs by a lessening of the intrapleural negative pressure; that is, the pressure in the intrapleural space approaches that of the atmospheric pressure.

During inspiration, negative pressure may reach 10 to 15 mm of mercury less than atmospheric pressure. During expiration, muscles of expiration return the thorax to its resting position with a corresponding decrease in its size and a decrease in negative pressure. Intrapleural pressure is from 5 to 8 mm of mercury during expiration. Although the intrathoracic or intrapleural pressure is always less than atmospheric pressure, it approaches atmospheric pressure at the end of expiration.[30] As a result of lowering of intrathoracic pressure during inspiration, air is sucked into the airway to the alveoli. During expiration, air is forced out of the lung. Expiration is largely due to the elastic rebound of the lungs.

Any disruption of the pleural membrane establishing a communication with the outside environment destroys the negative intrapleural pressure with the result that the lung collapses. Collapse should be expected, since the tendency of the lung to collapse is greater than the tendency for it to remain expanded. Collapse of the lung due to a collection of air in the intrapleural space is called pneumothorax. Collapse of the lung due to air entering the intrapleural space from the lung or large air passages is known as closed pneumothorax. The rupture of an emphysematous bleb or bulla is a common cause. Openings through the chest wall into the intrapleural space cause an open pneumothorax. Stab wounds of the chest extending through the chest wall and parietal pleura cause an open type of pneumothorax. In some types of injuries, air entering the pleural space during inspiration remains. This increases intrapleural pressure (decreases negative pressure) and leads to the development of tension pneumothorax, a dangerous condition which must be corrected if the life of the patient is to be saved.

Motor vehicle accidents are becoming increasingly common. According to Loh,[31] one out of every two Americans can expect to be injured by a car in his lifetime. Thoracic injuries frequently occur because the thorax is vulnerable to injury from the steering wheel, dashboard, or side of the car. These injuries can range in severity from a simple fracture of a rib to severe crushing injuries of the chest. Crushing injuries of the chest occur in 15 per cent of all automobile accidents [32] and may result in hypoxia and shock because of the altered physiology of the thoracic cage and diaphragm. Patients with pre-existing chronic respiratory diseases have a poor prognosis if thoracic trauma occurs because of their decreased pulmonary and cardiac reserves and their retained secretions.

[30] The intrathoracic or intrapleural pressure should be distinguished from the intrapulmonary pressure. The first is the pressure within the space between the parietal and visceral pleurae. The latter is the pressure in the alveoli. It is difficult to measure, but it varies rhythmically between being above and below atmospheric pressure.

[31] W. P. Loh and A. S. Williams: "Traffic Deaths in Lake County Indiana: A Two-Year Study," *Med. Times*, **96**:982 (Oct.) 1968.

[32] Lyman A. Brewer and Lyle E. Steiner: "The Management of Crushing Injuries of the Chest," *Surg. Clin. North Amer.*, **48**:1279 (Oct.) 1968.

Penetrating chest injuries also influence respiratory function. This type of injury is often the result of bullet or stab wounds. Figure 8-5 illustrates the consequence of such a wound.

When the chest wall becomes unstable, as after removal of ribs in thoracoplasty or in traumatic injuries causing fractured ribs, the patient may exhibit a type of breathing which

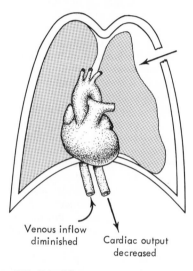

Venous inflow diminished   Cardiac output decreased

FIGURE 8-5. Possible consequence of penetrating chest injuries. The sequence of physiological effects of an open wound is (1) collapse of the homolateral lung, (2) shift of mediastinum to opposite side with impaired ventilation of contralateral lung, and (3) diminished cardiac output caused by reduced venous return. [Adapted from "Initial and Late Management of Penetrating Chest Wounds," *Medical Times*, 96:982 (Oct.), 1968, Fig. 1, by Richard J. Prather *et al.*]

is the opposite of normal and is therefore referred to as paradoxical. In paradoxical breathing the portion of the lung underlying the unstable area moves opposite to what is normally expected. Therefore, the involved area of the lung sucks in on inspiration and balloons out on expiration. If a large area of the lung is involved, a pool of unoxygenated air will be pushed from one lung to another by the abnormal respiratory movements.

An illustration of this type of breathing was demonstrated by Mrs. Anna Tree, who had three ribs removed prior to a pulmonary resection. When she returned to the recovery room she was awake, restless, and attempting to sit up in bed. When Miss Sutherland, the nursing student, took her vital signs, she noticed that Mrs. Tree's breathing was unusual, but she was not sure why. The surgeon came into the room at this point and Miss Sutherland mentioned her concern about the unusual breathing to him. He told her to place one hand on each side of Mrs. Tree's chest and to watch their movement. She noted that the operative side tended to move opposite to the unoperated side; that is, when the hand on the operated side was elevated by the chest wall, the hand on the unoperated side was lowered. She asked if this was paradoxical breathing. (See Figure 8-6 for illustration of the difference between normal and paradoxical respiration.) The surgeon said it was, and reviewed with her what the treatment should be. Because the principle of treatment is to stabilize the chest wall, one of the following measures can be taken: (1) apply weights such as sandbags to the chest, or (2) apply a pres-

sure binder to the chest. The latter is usually the more convenient because it allows the patient to move about more freely. In the absence of the physician, the nurse should turn the patient onto his operative side so that the mattress can offer some resistance to the unstable chest wall. The surgeon also called Miss Sutherland's attention to other characteristics of Mrs. Tree's respirations. They were short and rapid —40 per minute. He then suggested that she give Mrs. Tree morphine sulfate, 10 mg (gr 1/6), as needed. Fifteen minutes later Mrs. Tree's respirations were 28 and she was resting quietly. The pressure bandage had reduced the paradoxical motion considerably.

Although emphasis has been on the effects of openings into the intrapleural cavity on the

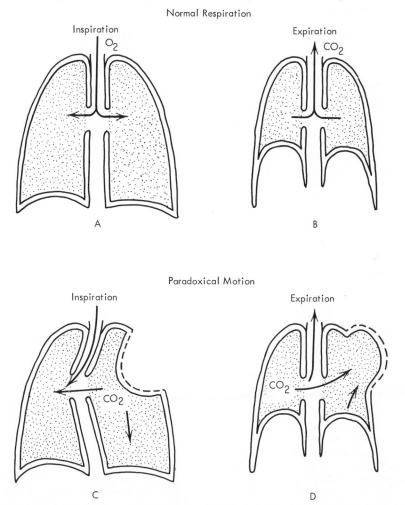

Figure 8-6. Normal respiration and paradoxical motion. (Adapted with permission of Year Book Medical Publishers, Inc., from *Surgery of the Chest*, 1954, p. 21, by Julian Johnson and Charles K. Kirby; Edna Hill, illustrator.)

mechanics of respiration, circulatory function is likely to be severely disturbed as well. One of the factors determining the seriousness of the situation is the size of the opening into the thoracic cavity. Small openings may cause little difficulty when a patient is at rest. Large or multiple openings may very quickly cause asphyxia.

What are the nurse's responsibilities in caring for a patient with an open pneumothorax?

Treatment of the patient who has suffered an open pneumothorax is directed toward the re-establishment of negative intrapleural pressure so that the lung can be re-expanded and the expansion maintained. The opening in the chest wall must be closed, and the blood, fluid, or air remaining in or entering the pleural cavity after closure must be removed. To facilitate their removal, one or more tubes are inserted at the time the chest wall is closed. One tube is placed in the lower part of the cavity to remove blood and other fluids and a second tube may be, but is not always, placed in the upper intrapleural space to remove air. The tube or tubes are then attached to waterseal bottles. Suction may or may not be applied to facilitate the removal of the contents of the intrapleural cavity. The number and types of bottles and the devices used to obtain and regulate the degree of suction vary from one institution to another. The important point is that the purpose of these tubes and equipment is to *remove* foreign elements from the intrapleural space. Because intrapleural pressure is less than atmospheric pressure, precautions must be taken to prevent fluids or air in the tubing from being introduced into the intrapleural space. Unless certain precautions are observed, the tubing will act like the trachea when the pressure within the thoracic cavity is reduced. The first precaution taken is to place the tubing, connected to the catheter entering the chest, under water to prevent air from being aspirated into the pleural cavity. The second precaution is always to keep the bottle containing the water and draining the intrapleural space at a level lower than the chest, to prevent the water from running into the chest cavity. Should the bottle be elevated to or about the level of the chest, water will be suctioned into the intrapleural space. As long as the end of a chest tube is covered with water and the bottle into which it drains is kept below the level of the chest, and the system is intact and patent, air and fluid will be forced out of the intrapleural space with each inspiration. When the lung is fully expanded, no air or fluid remains.

To prevent the introduction of fluid or air into the pleural cavity, by raising the drainage bottles to or above the level of the chest, they may be taped to the floor. Taping the bottle to the floor should not be necessary if everyone, including the patient and his visitors, knows why the bottles are to be kept at a level lower than the chest. When the chest bottles are of glass they may inadvertently be broken. Plastic bottles that are less easily broken are now available. One or two hemostats should be pinned or otherwise fastened to the top of the patient's bed or mattress where they are readily seen and are not likely to be removed. The patient, his relatives, and all personnel should be instructed to clamp the tube or tubes in case a bottle is broken or the tubing is disconnected.

In addition to making sure that the system draining the intrapleural space is intact and working, attention must be given to maintaining the patency of the tracheobronchial tree. Obstruction of the tracheobronchial tree is always possible because conditions interfering with the expansion of the lung also disturb the mechanisms for cleansing the tracheobronchial tree. All the previously discussed measures aiding in the cleansing of the airway should be instituted and carried out regularly at hourly or no less than two-hour intervals. When the patient is in the hospital for a day or more before the chest cavity is opened, he should be instructed in the how and why of the various procedures that will be utilized to promote the re-expansion of the lung. The patient who is admitted with a stab wound in his chest usually is treated as an emergency, and instruction is usually delayed until after closure of the wound.

Throughout the period of recovery, the patient should be observed for signs of hypoxia, dyspnea, and infection. The drainage system should also be observed to be sure that all connections are tight and the system is in working order. The level of water in the bottle should be marked at the time the bottle is attached to the tubing connected with the catheter inserted into the intrapleural space, so that the quantity of drainage can be measured. Until the lung is fully re-expanded, the fluid in glass tubing connected to the chest tube whose end is submerged in water can be expected to fluctuate with respiration. When the fluid ceases to fluctuate, blood clotted in the tube may be responsible or the lung may be fully expanded. To prevent a blood clot from occluding the tube and interfering with drainage, the tubing may be milked or stripped at least every two hours. Before doing this the nurse should, however, check with the physician. When the nurse performs this procedure and it is not successful, the surgeon should be notified. The extent to which the lung is expanded is checked by x-ray. In some hospitals only physicians change the drainage bottles. In others, this responsibility is delegated to nursing. Some surgeons prefer that the drainage bottles not be changed unless the volume of drainage is unusually great and demands a new setup in order to (1) determine the amount of new drainage (i.e., bleeding), or (2) reduce the amount of negative pressure in the drainage bottle. When drainage bottles are changed, tubes should be clamped so that air cannot enter the pleural space, and all equipment including the water should be sterile. Blood-containing fluids offer a fine medium for the growth of bacteria.

The quality of nursing that a patient who has had an opening into his thoracic cavity receives influences for good or ill the rate at which he recovers and even whether he recovers. This nursing should, inasmuch as the circumstances allow, do the following:

1. Prepare the patient for what to expect and for what is expected of him.
2. Maintain the integrity of the system for the removal of fluids and air from the intrapleural space.
3. Support the mechanisms for cleansing the tracheobronchial tree and for promoting the re-expansion of the lung.

In addition to air, collapse of the lung may be induced by collections of serous fluid (hydrothorax), blood (hemothorax), or pus (pyothorax, or empyema). Accumulation of serous fluids is commonly associated with pleural effusion due to infections involving the pleura. A frequent cause of pleurisy with effusion is tuberculosis, but it may also accompany neoplasms involving the lung or structures in the mediastinum. Whether or not accumulated fluid is removed from the pleural space will depend on the likelihood of its being absorbed and the degree to which the fluid causes respiratory embarrassment. Some surgeons are very reluctant to remove fluid unless it is causing respiratory embarrassment, because of the danger of introducing pathogenic organisms during the procedure. An initial tap is done, however, to obtain specimens for culture and determination of sensitivity of microorganisms to antimicrobial agents so that proper drugs may be ordered when necessary. Purulent material is usually removed, because it delays healing. Pus acts as a foreign body and must be removed before healing can take place. When possible, the fluid is aspirated through a needle introduced into the thoracic cavity. The procedure is known as thoracentesis. Precautions are taken to prevent the introduction of air.[33]

TREATMENT OF CHRONIC EMPYEMA

Chronic empyema may require surgical intervention; that is, a thoracotomy may be performed. In this procedure a section of a rib is removed and a tube is inserted into the space containing pus. Often the tube is connected to a water-seal bottle and the pus drains into the drainage bottle. This type of water seal must be changed at least daily and sometimes more often if the amount of drainage is copious. If the chest wall is fixed and there is no danger of a pneumothorax developing, the drainage tube is often allowed to drain directly into a large chest dressing which is usually changed two to three times daily. Occasionally, antimicrobial agents as well as enzymes that dissolve fibrinous and purulent materials are introduced into the empyema space, either through a needle or through the drainage tube.[34] If the drainage tube is used, it is clamped for a few hours after instillation of the drugs.

Movement of the Chest Wall

The power by which the size of the chest is altered is provided by skeletal muscles. The most important muscles of respiration are the diaphragm and the intercostals. The nervous system initiates muscular activity and coordinates the various movements involved in breathing with circulation so that some degree of failure of one is compensated for by an increase in activity of the other. The effect of failure of respiratory function is illustrated by John Blue, who was dependent on a mechanical respirator to maintain ventilation. His pulse rate was consistently between 90 and 100 beats per minute. As his ventilation improved, his pulse rate fell toward normal. The integration of respiratory and circulatory function is protective, inasmuch as the effect of failure in one can to some extent be compensated for by increased activity of the other. These functions are dependent on the nervous system for stimulation as well as for the integration of breathing with the needs of the entire organism. When the need for oxygen is increased by exercise, fever, or a fail-

---

[33] Bertha Harmer and Virginia Henderson: *Textbook of the Principles and Practice of Nursing*, 5th ed. (New York: The Macmillan Company, 1955) pp. 805–10.

[34] Streptokinase-streptodornase (Varidase) is one preparation used for this purpose. It is available in forms suitable for buccal and topical application as well as for intramuscular administration and injection into tubes.

ure to maintain the supply of oxygen, the pulse rate rises.

There are a number of conditions which result in a reduction in muscle power. These include aging, debility and disease, and undernutrition. Of diseases of muscle, muscular dystrophy is the most common. In myasthenia gravis, as the name implies, there is grave or serious weakness of muscles. This results not from a failure of muscles, but from a defect in their stimulation. The transmission of impulses from the nerve ending to the muscle is defective. In poliomyelitis involving the respiratory centers in the brain, or the upper portion of the spinal cord, muscles fail from lack of stimulation. In poliomyelitis motor nerve cells are injured or destroyed, thus depriving skeletal muscles of necessary stimulation.

Regulation of Respiration

The regulation and integration of the activities that are involved in breathing are highly complex and only partly understood. The rate of respiration is regulated so that there is a rhythmical change in the capacity of the thorax 15 to 16 times per minute. The depth is also regulated. At rest man breathes about 7 liters of air per minute. During strenuous exercise rate and depth can be increased to as much as 20 liters per minute.[35] In the healthy person oxygen supply is determined by the rate and depth of respiration.

The neural regulation of any activity and at any level can be described very simply as the action of a receptor and an effector with something in between. In breathing the effectors are the muscles of respiration. Receptors are primarily proprioceptors and interoceptors located in the alveoli, in the carotid and aortic bodies, and in centers in the brain stem. Exteroceptors sensitive to cold and pain also initiate impulses that cause alteration in breathing. The something in between the receptors and effectors includes afferent and efferent nerve pathways carrying impulses from receptors to centers in the brain stem and to the muscles of respiration. Afferent fibers arise primarily from the vagus nerve, though some sensory fibers in the phrenic nerve are involved.

The medulla has a predominant role in the regulation of respiration. Here are located the "respiratory centers" consisting of two groups of neurons, one expiratory and the other inspiratory. There are no discrete loci that are devoted to expiration and inspiration but rather

[35] Wallace O. Fenn: "The Mechanism of Breathing," *Sci. Amer.*, **202**:138 (Jan.) 1960.

the two types of neurons overlap anatomically.[36] In addition to the medulla the pons also regulates respiration. (See Figure 8-7.)

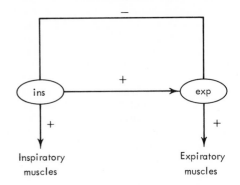

FIGURE 8-7. Postulated relationship between medullary inspiratory (*ins*) and expiratory (*exp*) activity. + = Excitation, − = inhibition. (Adapted with permission of The Macmillan Company from *Animal Function: Principles and Adaptations*, 1968, p. 143, by Malcolm S. Gordon.)

Respiratory Centers

There is no one center for respiration, but a group of interconnected centers. Although they have connections with the cerebral cortex, rhythmical breathing continues when these connections are destroyed. Animals decerebrated (connections between the cerebrum and lower centers destroyed) through the upper part of the pons maintain a normal type of respiration. Those in whom the structures in the brain stem are injured or seriously damaged by disease cannot maintain breathing without mechanical help. For example, the patient with the ascending spinal or bulbar type of poliomyelitis, or who has suffered trauma to those areas in the nervous system, requires mechanical help to continue breathing. According to Hardy,[37] there is a subsidiary respiratory center in the spinal cord which includes the motor cells located in the anterior horn of the cord. Anterior horn cells coordinate the action of respiratory muscles, but they do not coordinate respiration as a whole. Although higher centers can and do at times modify breathing, for the most part they have a minor effect.

Two principal types of stimuli play a role in initiating impulses resulting in breathing. The

[36] M. S. Gordon: *Animal Function: Principles and Adaptions* (New York: The Macmillan Company, 1968), p. 143.
[37] James D. Hardy: *Pathophysiology in Surgery* (Baltimore: The Williams & Wilkins Company, 1958), p. 470.

first of these is chemical. The second is the direct effect of stretching tissue of the lung. Stretching or tugging on other tissues, particularly the viscera, also causes changes in the rate and depth of respiration. Pain and emotional states such as fear are also accompanied by changes in breathing.

Chemical Control

Three chemicals are natural stimulants to respiration. They are carbon dioxide, the hydrogen ion, and oxygen. Carbon dioxide and the hydrogen ion act by their presence in the respiratory center to stimulate the rate and depth of respiration. Oxygen acts, not by its presence, but by its absence. Minor deficits of oxygen are not believed to have an appreciable

effect on breathing. Hypoxia has a depressing effect on respiratory centers. Authorities are not agreed as to whether severe hypoxia can be stimulating to the respiratory centers. Chemoreceptors in the aortic and carotid bodies are, however, sensitive to low oxygen tensions and initiate impulses resulting in the stimulation of respiration. Disagreement also exists as to whether carbon dioxide directly stimulates cells in the respiratory center or produces its effect by raising their hydrogen ion concentration. In any event, an elevation in the level of carbon dioxide or of hydrogen ions in the plasma is accompanied by an increase in the rate and depth of respiration. Conversely, a drop in the level of carbon dioxide or hydrogen ions in the blood plasma is accompanied by a decrease in respirations. See Figure 8-8.

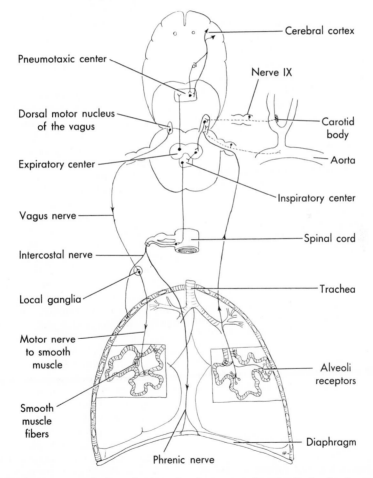

FIGURE 8-8. Nervous control of respiration, showing connections in the brain. Arrows indicate the direction of the nerve impulse. (Adapted with permission of The Macmillan Company from *Anatomy and Physiology*, 15th ed., Fig. 18-15, p. 533, by Diana Clifford Kimber, Carolyn E. Gray, Caroline E. Stackpole, and Lutie C. Leavell. Copyright © The Macmillan Company, 1966.)

Reflex Control

Breathing not only involves rate and depth and their integration with other bodily activities, but the coordination of inspiration and expiration so that the act of breathing is in itself coordinated. The latter activity is what is usually referred to as the reflex control of breathing. Stretch receptors in the alveoli and the aortic and carotid bodies initiate impulses that are carried over vagal fibers to the inspiratory and expiratory centers in the brain stem and result in inhibition of inspiration. In other words, they prevent either inspiration or expiration from going too far. As tissues are stretched during inspiration, impulses are initiated that result in the reflex inhibition of inspiration. Expiration is controlled in essentially the same manner. These reflexes are known as the stretch reflexes or the Hering-Breuer reflexes.

By a combination of chemical and reflex control, rate and depth of respiration are regulated in relation to the needs of the cells for oxygen. Equally important, the pattern of breathing is modified in a variety of activities such as coughing and sneezing. Fear and other emotions may greatly modify breathing. Sudden exposure of the skin to cold such as in a cold shower is accompanied by a gasp and a holding of the breath. For short periods breathing can be controlled voluntarily.

In the regulation of respiration a number of activities are involved. In terms of the objectives of this chapter, the first activity is to regulate the act of breathing so that fresh air is brought to the respiratory membrane in the quantities required to supply the cells with oxygen and to remove carbon dioxide. The second, related to the first, is the coordination and integration of activities that protect the respiratory tree and the alveoli from foreign materials. The third is the coordination of the act of breathing with the metabolic needs of cells and with the circulation. Failure to accomplish one or more of these functions predisposes to hypoxia and to carbon dioxide retention. The most common sites of disturbances in regulation of breathing are the centers in the brain stem and at the myoneural junction (the site where nerve impulses are transmitted to the muscles).

What are some of the causes of failure of the respiratory center?

Causes of depression and failure of the respiratory center include edema of the brain, pressure conus, depressant drugs, and infectious diseases such as poliomyelitis. An injury or disease that interferes with the function of, but does not inactivate, the cells of the medullary centers produces irregularity in the rhythm, depth, and rate of breathing. With inactivation of the cells, breathing ceases.

Edema of the brain occurs in a variety of conditions. Concussion of the brain as the result of a blow to the head is often followed by some edema. Any disorder markedly diminishing the flow of blood to the brain predisposes to brain edema. In hypertensive encephalopathy, edema results from the limitations on blood flow by markedly constricted arterioles. Capillary permeability is increased by hypoxia. Any disorder causing hypoxia sets into motion a vicious circle which, unless corrected, leads to death from depression of the respiratory and other vital centers.

PRESSURE CONUS

In addition to edema of the brain, respiratory failure may be due to pressure conus. In pressure conus, the brain is pressed downward into the foramen magnum. Since the medulla oblongata is directly over the foramen magnum, pressure is exerted on the medulla and partly or completely cuts off its blood supply. Death as a consequence of respiratory failure occurs almost immediately. Pressure conus is one of the causes of death in the patient who has a head injury or a brain tumor causing a rise in intracranial pressure. In the patient who has increased intracranial pressure, removal of the cerebrospinal fluid can precipitate pressure conus. With the reduction of the pressure in the spinal canal, the fluid in the cranial cavity rushes toward the area of reduced pressure, carrying the medulla with it, and causes the death of the patient. Patients who are predisposed to pressure conus should be regularly observed for signs of increasing intracranial pressure. The length of the interval between observations varies depending on the degree of increasing intracranial pressure and the possibility of its rising rapidly. The patient who is newly admitted after a head injury may be observed every 15 minutes for from four to eight hours. If, at the end of the designated time, he has no abnormal findings, the interval may be extended to one, two, or four hours. The observations, which include noting the character and rate of respiration, are listed in more detail in Chapter 15, Part B.

To prevent pressure conus, the patient who is predisposed is usually placed in the supine position. Because muscular activity causes some increase in intracranial pressure, the conscious patient should be instructed to lie quietly and to avoid sudden movements. He may be allowed one thin pillow, but he should not raise his head, nor should he feed himself. Activities that involve holding the breath after a deep inspiration, such as coughing and straining during defecation or urination, are particularly dangerous. Elevation of the intrathoracic pressure interferes with the venous return from the brain and thereby increases intracranial pressure. The importance of conscientious observation and the above regime in the prevention of respiratory failure in susceptible patients cannot be overemphasized.

RESPIRATORY DEPRESSION

One of the most common causes of depression of the respiratory centers in hospitalized patients is depressant drugs. These include general anesthetics, sedatives such as the barbiturates, and narcotics. In the therapeutic use of these agents, excessive respiratory depression can usually be prevented by limiting their dosage and by observing their effects. When depressant drugs such as the barbiturates are ingested for purposes of self-destruction, the patient may be in serious respiratory depression at the time he is admitted to the hospital; death, if it results, is due to respiratory arrest.

Although the depression of respiration is initiated by the effects of the drug on the respiratory center, it is intensified by two other related factors. With depression of the respiratory centers, ventilation becomes less adequate and some degree of hypoxia develops.[38] As the hypoxia of the brain increases, ventilation is further impaired and oxygenation of the blood becomes less and less effective. Moreover, the depression of the breathing centers is accompanied by inhibition of the cough centers, as well as by the inactivation of cilia in the airway. Consequently, secretions accumulate in the airway and obstruct the passage of air, further decreasing ventilation. Therapy is based on two objectives, that is, to remove or decrease the concentration of the depressant drug, and to sustain breathing in order to improve the supply of oxygen to the brain and other tissues. To accomplish the first objective, drugs causing respiratory depression are discontinued, and an attempt is made to remove the accumulated drug from the body. When an artificial kidney is available, the drug may be removed by dialyzing the blood of the patient, or peritoneal dialysis may be employed.

The second objective is accomplished by the administration of oxygen, often under pressure, and by the use of mechanical devices which perform artificial respiration. Secretions must be removed from the tracheobronchial tree. The measures required will depend on the degree of depression. In the deeply depressed patient tracheobronchial suction may be required.

[38] The effects of hypoxia have been previously discussed.

Any drug or disorder capable of lessening the effectiveness of ventilation by depressing the respiratory centers in the brain can also cause sufficient depression to stop breathing. In addition to the drugs listed above, curare causes respiratory failure by preventing the transmission of nerve impulses across the myoneural junction. Curare was originally utilized as a poison on the tips of arrows. It is utilized in modern medicine to increase muscular relaxation during some types of operative procedure. Other causes of respiratory failure not mentioned above are drowning and electric shock. Whatever its cause, cessation of breathing should always be treated as an emergency, and action should be taken immediately to re-establish breathing.

What are the ways of performing artificial respiration?

When breathing fails, life depends on the promptness with which ventilation is re-established. In fact, if resuscitation is to be successful, it must take precedence over all other procedures. Artificial respiration has as its goal the maintenance of breathing until the patient can perform this function himself. It should, therefore, be continued until natural breathing is re-established or until there is clear evidence that it cannot be.

Although there are a variety of methods used in artificial respiration, they all have three common objectives. These are (1) to oxygenate the blood, (2) to remove carbon dioxide, and (3) to maintain the circulation. Three different types of artificial respiration are available to ventilate the lungs. They are classified as manual, mechanical, and mouth-to-mouth breathing. The method selected will depend on where the emergency occurs and the length of time that the patient can be expected to have a problem with breathing. For example, John Francis is rescued from a lake after being submerged for five minutes. Artificial respiration either by mouth-to-mouth breathing or by the manual method should be initiated as rapidly as possible. There is no time to wait and obtain special equipment. In contrast, Robin George, who is hospitalized with acute poliomyelitis, can be observed for manifestations of respiratory failure. A respirator may be in readiness outside his room to be used should his physician decide that it is necessary. Equipment is also available in the operating room to sustain respiratory function in Mr. Coombs, who stopped breathing during an operative procedure.

MANUAL METHODS

The manual methods of artificial respiration are of two types, the Schafer prone pressure method and the push-pull methods, one of which was introduced by a Danish physician, Dr. Holger. Although the Schafer method was in vogue for a number of years, it has been found to be the least effective of all the manual methods of artificial respiration.

In all the push-pull methods of artificial respiration the chest is compressed to cause expiration and then the body is lifted to increase the size of the chest and thus aid inspiration. Gordon et al.[39] found in all their studies that the hip-lift-back-pressure method provides the greatest degree of ventilation of the lungs. Furthermore, it has the advantage of being easy to teach. It may, however, be difficult for small adults or children to perform. Gordon and his associates state that the air-lift-back-pressure method is most applicable for general use. Because one method is not suitable in all instances, they emphasize that medical and other trained personnel should be competent in several methods. References describing the performance of the various methods are included at the end of the chapter.

MOUTH-TO-MOUTH METHOD

The method that is said to be most efficient of all is mouth-to-mouth breathing. Despite the impression that mouth-to-mouth breathing is new, it is in fact very old. In movies and novels references are made to a doctor or midwife blowing "the breath of life" into the lungs of a newborn baby who fails to start to breathe. Mouth-to-mouth breathing fell from favor because of the belief that expired air would not contain enough oxygen to be of any value to the recipient. This is now known to be false. Another factor probably influencing the rejection of mouth-to-mouth breathing was the acceptance of the germ theory in the causation of disease. According to the germ theory the secretions of one person are considered to be a potential source of danger to other persons. Because ideas are bases for action, a number of sanitary and hygienic measures are instilled in us to protect one person from the secretions of others. For example, children are taught not to put anything in their mouths that has been in the mouth of another. Mothers teach their children not to allow casual acquaintances, or even close relatives, to kiss them on the lips. Thus, by precept and by practice, the individual learns to avoid situations by which he may come in contact with the secretions of others. As a result, it is not unusual for a person to find it difficult, if not impossible, to place his mouth

directly over that of another. For the person who finds it difficult to place his mouth over the mouth or nose of another person, some measure of protection, as well as a feeling of being protected, can be afforded by placing a handkerchief or gauze over the face of the victim. When one is available, an S-shaped airway may be introduced into the mouth of the patient, over the tongue and back into the pharynx. Air is then expired by the operator into this tube. Such a tube should be kept with the emergency equipment on each hospital unit.

A number of points apply to all methods of artificial respiration. The first is that time is a critical factor and delay can be fatal. Second, no method can be expected to be successful unless a clear airway is established and the procedure is performed properly. Before starting any procedure, foreign bodies and secretions in the mouth of the patient should be removed by inserting the fingers into the mouth and grasping the foreign body or wiping the secretions away. If materials are available and time allows, the fingers may be covered with gauze or a handkerchief. Suction can be used when it is available. Gravity may be utilized by placing the patient in a head-down position or turning the head to the side.

After foreign bodies and secretions have been removed, the airway should be established by fully extending the head of the patient and supporting the chin. Halfway measures are useless. The head may be turned from side to side to find the most favorable position. If these maneuvers are unsuccessful, the fingers should be flexed and placed behind the angles of the patient's mandible, and the patient's jaw should be moved forward as far as possible. Another method that may be used to move the mandible forward is to place the fingers under the chin of the patient and, with the thumb in his mouth, move the jaw forward.[40] After an open airway is established, the next step is to start ventilating the lungs.

In mouth-to-mouth respiration, the operator inhales deeply and blows the air forcibly into the nose or mouth of the patient. When air is blown into the mouth, the victim's nose must be closed, or vice versa. If an airway is used, be sure that it is in the posterior pharynx. As air is exhaled into the victim, his chest should rise. If it does not, or there are rumblings of air in the stomach, the support to the jaw which holds the airway open should be improved. If this does not help, blow more forcefully. Placing a hand over the abdomen and pressing down slightly also seems to help. Unless the chest expands well, air is not being introduced into

[39] Archer S. Gordon, Max S. Sadove, Frank Raymon, and A. C. Ivy: "Critical Survey of Manual Artificial Respiration," *JAMA*, 147:1444–53 (Dec. 8), 1951.

[40] Jay Jacoby et al.: "Treatment of Respiratory Emergencies," *Postgrad. Med.*, 25:373–75 (Apr.) 1959.

the lung in a sufficient amount. Expiration is allowed to take place naturally. Fishbein [41] recommends approximately 20 cycles per minute, but other authorities state that although as many as 20 may be required for optimum ventilation, 10 to 12 are probably adequate. When only one person is present, he should modify the rate so that he will be able to continue the procedure for an extended period of time.

To summarize the essentials of mouth-to-mouth respiration, the airway should be cleared and the lungs rhythmically inflated. Ventilation of the lungs must be continued for as long as the possibility of life exists. The nurse should support community efforts to teach the public at least one method of resuscitation, preferably mouth-to-mouth respiration.

In the hospital, equipment is available to blow air or oxygen into the lungs by way of a face mask or an endotracheal or tracheostomy tube. Although there are special machines for this purpose, an anesthesia machine with bag is often employed. When working on a hospital unit, the nurse must familiarize herself with where this emergency equipment is kept and also check that it is in good working order, ready for use when required.

RESPIRATORS

When there is a prolonged failure in breathing, other methods are used to maintain ventilatory function. After the airway is established, often by insertion of an endotracheal tube or by a tracheostomy, breathing is restored and maintained by means of a mechanical cycling respirator. These respirators can be adjusted for either intermittent positive pressure breathing (IPPB) or for intermittent positive pressure ventilation (IPPV). The selection is based on ventilation and arterial blood gases. These readings must be done frequently and appropriate changes made on the respirator in order to maintain normal blood gas exchange. Muscle relaxants may be utilized to synchronize rapid respirations with the respirator, and morphine may be ordered to decrease the metabolic rate.

The correlation of the mechanical respirator with the ventilation and arterial blood gas readings is the physician's responsibility. However, it is the nurse who is constantly with the patient. She must observe the patient closely, keep a close check on his vital signs, check that the respirator is functioning properly, and give physical care and emotional support as indicated by her assessment of the patient. If the patient is conscious, an explanation of the equipment should be given. He should be told that the clicking sounds of the respirator are normal

and that it is working properly. He also needs to be assured that in his type of case it is standard to take frequent blood samples because this gives the physician an indication of how the patient is progressing.

In many patients who require assistance in maintaining breathing, secretions tend to accumulate in the airway. The methods used in this situation are similar to those previously described. The specific measures will depend on the severity of the problem. The patient on the respirator requires all of the care needed by any seriously ill patient. He must be moved, turned, and bathed, and his extremities put through the range of motion exercises.

Many patients who require respirator care recover sufficiently to maintain respiratory function independently. McAlpine [42] states that the weaning of the patient is based on three factors: "(1) role of the work of breathing—noting the degree of dyspnea and respiratory effort, (2) the level of consciousness and adequacy of neuromuscular function, and (3) the stability and integrity of the cardiovascular system." The weaning process is never abrupt. The patient is put on a trial period of spontaneous breathing during which time he is given an air and oxygen mixture. Ventilation and blood gas readings are taken frequently and evaluated and the patient is observed closely for tachycardia, tachypnea, or dyspnea.

The period during which the patient is learning to breathe without the respirator may be a time of stress for him and for his attendants. If the patient has become very dependent on the respirator, he may lack confidence in his ability to maintain breathing without it. The nurse should encourage the patient to stay off the respirator for increasing periods of time and she should try to bolster his confidence in himself. At the same time, the patient should be protected from overfatigue. He should be observed for signs of developing hypoxia. In the past, some persons who were believed to be psychologically dependent on the respirator were in fact physiologically dependent on it. Nurses should make careful observations of the behavior of the patient, so that nursing care and medical therapy can be planned to meet the needs of the patient. Moreover, the patient who is learning to breathe for himself should be confident that when he needs help he will get it.

Patients who require respirator care to maintain breathing usually have other serious threats to their lives and health. Because this chapter is devoted to the maintenance of oxygen sup-

[41] Morris Fishbein: "Medical Progress 1958," *Postgrad. Med.*, **25**:111 (Jan.) 1959.

[42] Frederick S. McAlpine: "Cardiopulmonary Resuscitation: The Anesthesiologist's Role," *Med. Clin. N. Amer.*, **53**:393 (Mar.) 1969.

ply to cells, these threats will not be discussed here.

In summary, the maintenance of breathing is essential in the total respiratory process. Breathing may fail temporarily or permanently. In any event death ensues unless ventilation is promptly re-established and maintained. The essential features of any method include (1) prompt action, (2) clearing of the airway, and (3) the use of the method that gets the air into and out of the lungs in sufficient volume to adequately ventilate the lungs.

Conditions Essential to the Exchange of Gases in the Lung

As previously described, air must be regularly delivered to and removed from the respiratory membrane. The direction of movement of a gas across the respiratory membrane is determined by the difference in its partial pressure on the two sides of the membrane. Gases move from an area of higher to an area of lower pressure. Because the partial pressure of oxygen in the inspired air is higher than in the venous blood in the lung, oxygen moves from the alveoli into the blood. Since the tension of carbon dioxide in the blood is higher than in the inspired air, it moves from the blood to the alveoli.

The Respiratory Membrane

Whereas the partial pressure of a gas on the two sides of a semipermeable membrane determines the rate and direction of movement, the permeability of the membrane regulates what is transferred across it. The respiratory membrane consists of the respiratory bronchiole, the alveolar ducts, and the alveoli, as well as the corresponding capillaries, lymphatics, and connective tissues. The latter structures are included because of their intimate relationship with pulmonary membrane. The structure of the respiratory membrane is well suited to permit the free diffusion of gases between the air and the blood. It consists of an extremely thin layer of epithelium in the alveoli and of endothelium in the capillary. The total surface is enormous, as the alveolar membrane is variously estimated to present a surface of from 50 to 90 sq m, and the capillaries' surface area is estimated to be from 38 to 60 sq m. The total alveolar surface is one half the size of a tennis court. The alveolar walls are lined with a lipoprotein substance, pulmonary surfactant, which reduces the surface tension and thereby prevents their inherent tendency to collapse. This surfactant is being continuously replaced and is

dependent on sufficient pulmonary blood flow.

Aeration of the blood is protected by the fact that only a fraction of the pulmonary membrane is required to support most activities. Hypoxia caused by failure of diffusion does not occur unless there is an appreciable decrease in available pulmonary membrane or it is thickened; that is, the permeability of the membrane is diminished. Some of the disorders that are associated with a decrease in the area of pulmonary membrane have already been mentioned. They include emphysema, atelectasis, and pneumothorax. By thickening the membrane, pulmonary edema lessens its efficiency or permeability. In pneumonia consolidation of one or more lobes or of scattered areas reduces the area available for diffusion. Diseases such as tuberculosis predispose to tissue destruction and fibrosis. Surgical removal of a part or all of a lung lessens respiratory reserve, by diminishing the surface area available for the diffusion of gases. Decreased pulmonary circulation due to hypoventilation can interfere with the replacement of surfactant and can lead to atelectasis.

Ventilation of the alveoli is protected and regulated by a number of conditions and elements. Dead-space air prevents too rapid dilution of the alveolar air. Although all parts of the lung are not ventilated equally, the distribution of the air is facilitated by both structure and function. According to Fenn,[43] when the distance from the trachea to the alveoli is short, the tubes are narrower in diameter than they are when the distance is greater. The bronchioles contain muscle fibers which enable them to regulate air flow to the alveoli. Pores in the walls of the alveoli allow for the aeration of alveoli whose ducts are obstructed.

Pulmonary Circulation

Because of the relationship of the alveoli to the pulmonary circulation, alveolar pressure is believed to have important effects on the circulation of the blood through the lung. Unlike the systemic circulation, the pulmonary circulation is a low-pressure system. Whereas in the systemic circulation the capillaries are supported and surrounded by the tissue they supply, pulmonary capillaries are surrounded by air and are supported by a thin network of elastic and reticulum cells. The pulmonary circulation carries all the blood from the right to the left ventricle. It is a highly distensible system capable of holding the entire blood volume. It is affected not only by the beating of the heart, but by

---

[43] *Op. cit.*, pp. 138–48.

changes in the pressure within the thoracic cavity.

Pulmonary circulation differs from systemic circulation in another way. In the systemic circulation, the hydrostatic pressure at the arteriolar end of the capillary is considerably higher than that of the colloid osmotic pressure of the blood proteins. This results in the transudation of fluid, that is, water and the substances dissolved in it into the interstitial space. (See Chapter 9.)

Transudation in the pulmonary capillaries is avoided because the hydrostatic pressure of the blood is within a few millimeters of mercury of atmospheric pressure and is at least 20 to 25 mm lower than the colloid osmotic pressure (oncotic pressure) of the blood proteins. When the lungs are normally ventilated, air surrounding the capillaries creates a pressure that serves to counteract the effect of the hydrostatic pressure of the blood. Failure to aerate a lung or a portion thereof upsets the balance between the atmospheric pressure and the hydrostatic pressure in favor of the hydrostatic pressure and increases the possibility of pulmonary edema. The seriousness of the situation is increased by the fact that an increase in transudation is not followed by a comparable increase in tissue pressure. Hydrostatic pressure may be increased by any condition interfering with the flow of blood into the left atrium or increasing blood volume. It is an ever-present possibility in mitral valve disease, in failure of the left ventricle, and in high-volume anemias. It may occur in kidney failure, especially when there is sodium retention. Dyspnea is a common symptom in pulmonary edema, and orthopnea is not uncommon. The responsibilities of the nurse in the prevention and treatment of pulmonary edema are discussed in Chapters 9, 10, and 11.

As emphasized, one of the significant factors in the diffusion of oxygen from the alveoli to the blood is difference in the pressure gradient between the atmosphere and the blood. One of the factors in maintaining this gradient is the regular renewal of alveolar air. Another is the high affinity of hemoglobin for oxygen. As venous blood circulates through the pulmonary capillaries, hemoglobin rapidly combines with oxygen in the plasma. Carbon dioxide passes through the respiratory membrane even more rapidly, because its rate is about 20 times that of oxygen. Despite the brief time that the blood remains in the pulmonary capillaries, the hemoglobin picks up a full complement of oxygen.[44]

The uptake of oxygen by hemoglobin is facilitated by the sudden drop in level of carbon dioxide which increases the alkalinity of the blood. A decrease in hydrogen ion concentration increases the affinity of hemoglobin for oxygen, and a rise decreases it.

Transport of Oxygen

Oxyhemoglobin is carried through the arteries to the capillaries virtually unchanged. In the tissues conditions change so that the dissociation of oxyhemoglobin is facilitated. The partial pressure of oxygen in the tissues is low, and oxygen moves from the plasma by way of the interstitial fluid to the cell. The equilibrium between the oxygen dissolved in the plasma and the oxyhemoglobin is upset, and oxygen is released by the hemoglobin to restore the balance. The decomposition of oxyhemoglobin is increased by elevation in the temperature of the tissue and in the presence of carbon dioxide and acid metabolites such as lactic acid. Depending on the degree of activity of a tissue, the blood may lose from 20 per cent to almost all its oxygen as it passes through the capillaries.[45] The capacity to release oxygen from hemoglobin in relation to conditions in the tissue is adaptive, inasmuch as it reduces the burden on the circulatory system during exercise.

What are some of the common causes of failure to transport oxygen?

ANEMIA

Since hemoglobin is required for the transport of oxygen, any reduction in its level or availability is accompanied by a decrease in the quantity of oxygen delivered to the cells. Although there are some exceptions, 3 g of hemoglobin per 100 ml of blood is generally required to sustain life.[46] The most common cause of a deficiency of hemoglobin is anemia. In anemia there is a decrease in the number of circulating erythrocytes as well as in the amount of hemoglobin. Depending on the cause of the anemia, there may be a greater decrease in one than in the other, but both are reduced. The principal effect of anemia is a loss in the oxygen-carrying capacity of the blood. Most of the signs and symptoms are caused by hypoxia. For example, Scott Giles, a 16-year-old high school student, was admitted to the hospital with lethargy and poor muscular coordination.

[44] George W. Wright: "Dyspnea and Allied Manifestations," *Principles of Internal Medicine*, 5th ed., T. R. Harrison, ed. (New York: McGraw-Hill Book Company, 1966), p. 66.

[45] Charles Herbert Best and Norman Burke Taylor (eds.): *The Physiological Basis of Medical Practice*, 8th ed. (Baltimore: The Williams & Wilkins Company, 1966), p. 977.

[46] Harry A. Davis: *Principles of Surgical Physiology* (New York: Paul B. Hoeber, Inc., 1957), p. 76.

Initial laboratory tests revealed a low hemoglobin. Upon investigation it was discovered that Scott had been sniffing glue and that this had affected his bone marrow production of red blood cells. Scott was informed of the dangers inherent in glue sniffing, and he made an uneventful recovery. Other young people have not been as fortunate as Scott; glue sniffing has so impaired their oxygen-carrying capacity that permanent brain damage has resulted.

CARBON MONOXIDE POISONING

In addition to a deficient quantity of hemoglobin, hemoglobin though present in adequate quantities may be unavailable to carry oxygen. In carbon monoxide poisoning, the level of hemoglobin is satisfactory, but carbon monoxide has an affinity for hemoglobin approximately 210 times greater than oxygen. Although carbon monoxide can be displaced from hemoglobin, carboxyhemoglobin is a more stable compound than oxyhemoglobin. When carbon monoxide is inhaled, it is absorbed into the blood, where it combines with the hemoglobin. The source of carbon monoxide is incompletely oxidized carbon compounds. Poisoning, either accidental or intentional, occurs when a person is exposed to gases formed in combustion. For example, the Oriole family lived in a small house heated by a space heater. The weather was cold and the house was cold, so they kept a fire in the stove through the night. The windows were closed and insufficient oxygen was available for the complete combustion of the fuel. Therefore, carbon monoxide was formed rather than carbon dioxide. As it was formed, it was released into the surrounding air. Because carbon monoxide is odorless, the Oriole family had no warning that the air was poisoned. When the neighbors noticed that no one was about, they called the police, who discovered the family dead in their beds. Although the details differ, death that results from remaining in a closed automobile in which the motor has been left running has the same cause—carbon monoxide poisoning.

If one of the members of the Oriole family had awakened in time, their lives might have been saved by treatment with oxygen. This is one of the few situations in which oxygen may be administered in concentrations up to 100 per cent. The treatment of carbon monoxide poisoning with 100 per cent oxygen is based on the law of mass action. According to this law, the speed of a chemical reaction is proportional to the molecular concentrations of the reacting agents. The molecules of carbon monoxide and of oxygen both compete for hemoglobin molecules. The chances of oxygen combining with hemoglobin can be increased by increasing the amount of available oxygen.

DECREASED BLOOD FLOW

At the tissue level, the availability of oxygen to the cells also depends on the adequacy of the blood flow. Therefore, any condition that decreases the output of blood by the heart or that increases resistance to the flow of blood will lessen the quantity of oxygen available to the tissue, that is, cause ischemia. The harmful effect of diseases, such as atherosclerosis, that narrow the diameter of blood vessels is due to the fact that they interfere with the supply of blood to the tissues. Edema, either temporary or chronic, lessens blood supply by causing pressure on capillaries. Edema also interferes with the diffusion of oxygen delivered to the tissues. Any disturbance in oxygen supply to the tissue lessens the capacity to adapt to increased demands. The causes and effects of ischemia are discussed in more detail in Chapter 4.

ENZYME IMPAIRMENT

Finally, for oxidation-reduction reactions to take place at body temperature, enzymes are required to catalyze the necessary chemical reactions. These enzymes are sensitive to conditions in body tissues and are inactivated by certain poisons. Loss of homeostatic conditions —temperature, pH, water, and electrolytes— may inhibit the action of cellular enzymes. Poisons such as cyanide cause rapid and irreversible changes in cells because they inactivate the enzymes that enable the cells to utilize oxygen.

Whether or not cells receive enough oxygen depends on the degree to which the oxygen delivered to the cells meets the demands of the tissues. When the needs of the cells are in excess of the capacity to deliver oxygen, a condition of relative hypoxia exists. One of the limiting factors on strenuous exercise is the development of relative hypoxia. The needs of tissues for oxygen can be diminished by rest or by lowering of the body temperature. For patients who have some defect in their oxygen delivery mechanism, rest may be prescribed. Whether or not the patient actually achieves a state of rest depends in part on the skill of the nurse in modifying his social, psychological, and physical environment toward that end.

To recapitulate, the survival of all living organisms including man depends on a continuous supply of oxygen to the cells of the body and the removal of carbon dioxide which is formed in metabolism. In man, oxygen is supplied to, and carbon dioxide removed from, the tissue by the coordinated functioning of the respiratory and circulatory systems. All cells require oxygen. Some cells, such as those in the nervous system, are highly sensitive to hypoxia.

Failure to supply oxygen in quantities required by the cells can have its origin in the atmosphere, or in a failure in the respiratory, circulatory, or nervous systems. The causes of failure of oxygen supply may be summarized as follows:

1. Atmospheric
2. Failure of ventilation

   a. Obstruction of the airway
      { Mechanical
      { Infections
      { Allergy
      { Neoplasms

   b. Paralysis of the muscles of respiration
      { Poliomyelitis
      { Myasthenia gravis
      { Injuries of the brain stem
      { Muscle relaxants during anesthesia

   c. Loss of muscle tissue—muscular dystrophy
   d. Decreased compliance of lung
   e. Pneumothorax, hemothorax, pleural effusion
3. Loss of aerating surface in the lung
   a. Pulmonary edema
   b. Emphysema
   c. Pneumonia and other infections involving the lung
   d. Surgical removal of the lung
   e. Pneumothorax
   f. Atelectasis
4. Loss of oxygen-carrying power of the blood
   a. Anemia
   b. Carbon monoxide poisoning
   c. Methemoglobinemia, sulfhemoglobinemia
   d. Other defects in hemoglobin
5. Insufficient blood delivered to the tissues—ischemia
   a. Generalized decrease in the output of the heart
   b. Localized ischemia
      (1) Atherosclerosis
      (2) Infarcts
      (3) Edema
6. Cellular utilization, anoxia
   a. Poisoning of respiratory enzymes
   b. Excessive demands of the tissues for oxygen [47]

---

[47] The formation of carbon dioxide and its elimination are intimately related to oxygen supply and use. Because of effects of carbon dioxide on cation-anion balance in the body, it is discussed in the following chapter.

The conditions and processes whereby oxygen is obtained from the atmosphere and made available to the cells have also been presented. The capacity to provide oxygen to the cells may be threatened at any point by the failure of one or more of these processes. When the condition develops slowly and is of long-standing, the individual may be able to adapt by increasing the effectiveness of one of the processes or by decreasing his need for oxygen, or both. When the condition develops rapidly and is of marked degree, however, his survival is jeopardized. When the lack of oxygen is due to a failure of diffusion across the respiratory membrane, the addition of oxygen to the respired air may be life-saving.

Inhalation Therapy

Inhalation therapy is prescribed by the physician in order to increase the supply of oxygen available to the cells. The prescription should include the method by which it is to be administered, the concentration to be maintained, the duration of treatment, and the medications to be added if aerosol therapy is employed. Medications commonly used in aerosol therapy include antibiotics, bronchodilators, detergents, and antifoaming agents. Normal saline is frequently added for increased humidity.

More and more frequently, inhalation therapists are assuming increased responsibility for this phase of the patient's treatment. Not only do they deliver and maintain the necessary equipment, but also they usually administer the treatment to the patient. The nurse must work closely with the inhalation therapist. It is her responsibility to prepare the patient physically and psychologically and to make sure that his needs are being met throughout the procedure. She also instructs the patient, his visitors, and personnel in safety precautions and in the essential aspects of the treatment. The nurse and inhalation therapist work together to instruct the patient and his family in the performance of oxygen therapy at home.

What are the nurse's responsibilities in inhalation therapy?

To fulfill her obligations, the nurse should have knowledge of the principles basic to effective and safe inhalation therapy and information about the different methods used to administer oxygen, as well as an understanding of the reasons for oxygen therapy.

Inhalation therapy is frequently prescribed to combat arterial hypoxia in pneumonia, pulmonary edema, or obstruction of the airway. It is also often prescribed for patients in congestive heart failure and after myocardial infarctions, because these patients usually have some degree of pulmonary edema as well as failure of the peripheral circulation. In hot and humid weather, an oxygen tent has the additional value of providing a comfortable environment. Because of its availability oxygen is also utilized as a carrier gas in aerosol therapy.

As indicated earlier, the diffusion of oxygen and carbon dioxide across the respiratory membrane into the blood depends on (1) the partial pressures of these gases in the respired air, (2) a patent airway, (3) the cyclical expansion and contraction of the chest, and (4) a diffusing surface adequate in extent and permeability. A deficiency in the supply of oxygen can therefore be the consequence of a low atmospheric or partial pressure of oxygen in the respired air, an obstructed airway, inadequate breathing, or a decrease in the quantity or permeability of the diffusing surface in the lung. Obviously, increasing the percentage composition of oxygen in the respired air will be of more value in some of these conditions than in others. For example, the addition of oxygen to the air is essential in the prevention of hypoxia in nonacclimatized persons at altitudes above 10,000 or 12,000 ft. A higher than normal concentration of oxygen is of little or no value unless the airway is patent and the patient is breathing. Increased concentrations of oxygen have their greatest value in the therapy of disorders in which the permeability of the diffusing membrane is decreased or the surface area is diminished. In the use of oxygen in therapy, the enrichment of the air with oxygen does not usually correct the cause of hypoxia, but it prevents its injurious effects.

Oxygen is administered by mask, catheter, cannula, tent, or canopy, or in a chamber or room. Each method has its advantages and disadvantages. The method chosen depends on the patient's condition, the concentration desired, and, of course, the facilities available. High concentrations of oxygen are most easily maintained by mask. Because the mask fits the face snugly, oxygen can also be administered under positive pressure by this means. Both the mask and the catheter require relatively simple equipment and allow the patient considerable freedom of movement. They offer little interference with personal care. The tent or canopy provides not only a satisfactory concentration of oxygen, but an air conditioner. The temperature and humidity of the air surrounding the patient can be maintained at comfortable levels. In hot and humid weather, control of temperature and humidity may make a valuable contribution to the well-being of the patient. Special rooms into which oxygen is piped are ideal inasmuch as the patient can be cared for in the same manner as he is in an ordinary room. The concentration of oxygen can be maintained at the desired level. Concentrations prescribed by the physician range from 45 to 100 per cent.

Some of the disadvantages of the different methods of administering oxygen can be minimized by appropriate nursing measures. The mask can cause irritation of the skin of the face, which can be minimized by adjusting the mask to the contours of the face and adjusting the straps so that the patient is comfortable. The straps should not be so loose that the mask moves about or so tight that the edges cut into the face. The mask should be removed every one and one-half to two hours and the face of the patient should be washed, dried, and dusted lightly with powder. Each time the mask is removed, necessary nursing procedures such as mouth care and administration of fluids should be carried out. The mask should be applied during exhalation. Some patients are very frightened about having anything applied over their face, and some are never able to adjust to the mask.

One of the methods most frequently selected for the administration of oxygen is the nasal catheter. The catheter is introduced by way of the nares into the naso- or oropharynx. Except for the level to which the catheter is introduced, the performance of the procedure is essentially the same. The nasal catheter has several disadvantages. Concentrations of oxygen above 50 per cent are difficult to secure. To achieve the highest concentration possible, the patient must be instructed not to breathe through his mouth. The catheter can be irritating to the nasal mucosa. To prevent injury to the mucosa, the catheter selected should fit comfortably and be lubricated with saline solution or a water-soluble lubricant before it is introduced. To maintain the patency of the catheter, it must be changed no less frequently than every eight hours. If nasal secretions are abundant, the catheter may have to be changed more frequently to maintain its patency. When it is reinserted after removal, the other nostril should be used. Occasionally, because of structural defect in the septum, only one nostril can be used.

After as large a catheter as can be introduced comfortably into the nares of the patient has been selected, it should be attached to the oxygen source and checked by placing the tip in a glass of water. Bubbling in the water indicates that the system is open. To determine the length of catheter to be introduced, using the catheter, measure the distance between the tip of the nose and the lobe of the ear. Mark the length of the catheter to be introduced with a small piece of tape. The direction of the natural droop of the catheter is then determined, by holding the taped portion of the catheter between the thumb and forefinger. The catheter is held in this position and slowly and gently inserted until the measured point reaches the entrance to the nostril. The position of the catheter should be observed through the mouth. The tip should lie just behind the uvula. The catheter should be taped firmly at the end of the nose and then carried across the cheek and taped at the temple. The catheter should be adjusted so that it lies on the inner floor of the nose, but does not loop in the nostril. It should not press against the skin of the nose, or obstruct the vision of the patient. Because oxygen is dry, humidification of the air is essential.

Nasal inhalers or cannulas are also used to administer oxygen. These are metal or plastic tubes of various sizes with tips that fit into the nostrils. Approximately a 30 to 35 per cent oxygen concentration is possible with this means. As with the nasal catheter, the patient must breathe with his mouth closed and humidification of the air must be provided.

The oxygen tent is another method frequently utilized for the administration of oxygen. The tent provides for a closed system in which the temperature, humidity, and oxygen concentration can be well controlled. It has several disadvantages. The patient is confined in the relatively small space of the tent. Unless the canopy is tucked in and the openings closed promptly after use, the oxygen concentration falls very rapidly.

Oxygen can also be administered under slight positive pressure or pressure greater than atmospheric pressure. This permits more oxygen to be pushed into the lungs. One method of providing this is a mask that builds up pressure when the patient exhales. Another method, more commonly used, is intermittent positive pressure breathing (IPPB). With this type, positive pressure is exerted during inhalation. As the patient inhales, oxygen is forced into his lungs. Pressure is then decreased and the patient exhales. The patient is able to control both the rate and depth of breathing. IPPB can be administered by mask or mouthpiece. If a mask is used, it must fit snugly over the face to prevent leakage of oxygen and a consequent reduction in pressure. If the mouthpiece is used, it also must be secured so that oxygen leakage does not occur. The patient must be instructed to breathe entirely through his mouth. A nose clip may be used if necessary.

IPPB is usually used to promote adequate ventilation and thereby to increase the oxygen tension in the arterial blood. It is also utilized for the administration of certain medications. It is commonly employed in such diseases as emphysema, bronchiectasis, asthma, and pulmonary edema. It is also frequently used pre- and postoperatively to prevent atelectasis.

The hyperbaric oxygen chamber is gaining in popularity as a means of supplying large amounts of oxygen quickly. It has been found to be effective in such conditions as gas gangrene, carbon monoxide poisoning, and tumor therapy. These units consist of steel chambers in which it is possible to deliver up to 4 atmospheres of oxygen or 4 times as much oxygen as can be provided by breathing 100 per cent oxygen at atmospheric pressure.

Handbooks [48] are available that present in greater detail methods and types of equipment used in oxygen therapy, and the nurse may refer to these when questions arise. When she has access to a trained inhalation therapist, she can usually obtain desired information.

When oxygen is administered to the patient, it cannot be expected to be of benefit unless it reaches his alveoli in the desired concentration. All the equipment must be in working order, and a supply of oxygen must be available at all times. Appropriate measures must be instituted to maintain the concentration of oxygen in the respired air. Since oxygen therapy benefits the patient only if the oxygen can reach his alveoli, attention must be given to cleansing his airway. The patient should be moved, turned, and encouraged to deep-breathe and to cough. When these measures are ineffective, secretions have to be removed by suctioning. Tubing connecting the source of oxygen supply to the device by which oxygen is delivered to the patient should be checked to be sure that it is free from kinks and attached properly and tightly.

In many of the modern and well-equipped hospitals, nurses do not have to be concerned with the supply of oxygen, because it is piped in from a central supply tank. In hospitals where oxygen is supplied in tanks and for patients receiving oxygen at home, the nurse carries a number of responsibilities. The nurse must check the pressure gauge to make certain that the tank contains oxygen under sufficient pressure to supply the patient with oxygen. Should the tank be allowed to empty, the concentration of oxygen in the inspired air will fall rapidly below that in the surrounding atmosphere. Precautions should also be taken to protect personnel and visitors from a falling tank. Tanks containing oxygen or other gases tend to be unstable, because they have a relatively narrow base in relation to their height. The danger of upsetting a tank can be lessened by placing it on a rack with a wide base or strapping it to the bed.

[48] *Linde Oxygen Therapy Handbook* (New York: Linde Company, Division of Union Carbide Corporation. July, 1967).

The maintenance of an adequate supply of oxygen and the safety of the patient depend on the application of knowledge of the physical and chemical characteristics of oxygen. It is a colorless, odorless, tasteless gas that is slightly heavier than air. It does not burn, but it supports combustion. The fact that it is colorless, odorless, and tasteless enables it to escape unnoticed into the surrounding atmosphere. Since oxygen is heavier than air, it tends to settle toward the bed or floor. This characteristic is most significant in the care of the patient in an oxygen tent. If the concentration of oxygen in the tent is to be maintained, the canopy must be smoothly tucked under the mattress. The part that goes over the thighs should be pulled toward the foot of the bed and tucked in at the sides and around the patient. Although instructions frequently state that a draw sheet should be utilized to secure the canopy over the thighs of the patient, according to the findings of a study made by Eileen Cronicun [49] this is not necessary. In fact, lower concentrations of oxygen were usually observed when a draw sheet was utilized to secure the canopy. When the draw sheet was tucked in tightly, patients felt restrained. They then raised their knees and dislodged not only the draw sheet, but the sides of the canopy. The most important point in maintaining oxygen concentration was found to be keeping the canopy well tucked under the mattress. In fact, an effective concentration of oxygen can be maintained at the floor of a tent that has an open top.

Oxygen, as a gas, diffuses readily. Openings in the tent allow oxygen to escape and lower its concentration. Vents in the wall of the tent should be opened only when necessary to give care, and they should be closed completely after care is completed. The lower the opening, the more rapidly oxygen escapes.

Regardless of the method of application, the fact that oxygen supports combustion is an important consideration in the safety of the patient. Oxygen does not burn, but it lowers the kindling point of combustible materials so that they burn, often with almost explosive rapidity. To illustrate, Frank Jay, a 58-year-old former carpenter, was in severe congestive heart failure. At the time he was placed in the oxygen tent, both he and the members of his family were instructed not to smoke. One evening when Mr. Jay's son came to visit him, Mr. Jay asked for a cigarette, which his son gave to him. Despite the fact that the canopy was made of rubber, it burned in a matter of moments. Although his face, hands, and scalp were burned, Mr. Jay was saved from death by an orderly who smothered the flames with a

[49] Unpublished master's thesis.

woolen blanket. To prevent this sort of accident, *No Smoking* signs should be prominently displayed. Relatives and friends, as well as the patient, should be helped to understand the importance of this prohibition. No open flame, whatever its source, is permissible. Patients such as Mr. Jay may be allowed to smoke once or twice daily, provided the supply of oxygen is discontinued for the duration of the period of smoking.

Sources of electric sparks, whether static electricity or faulty equipment, should be avoided. The call light of the patient should be replaced with one having a shockproof switch or with a hand bell. Because woolen blankets may be a source of static electricity, they should be replaced with cotton blankets. Static electricity is a particular problem in regions in which the humidity of the environment is low. Another precaution generally advised is to avoid the use of oil or alcohol when rubbing the back of the patient in an oxygen tent.

Should a procedure be performed that requires the use of electrical or thermal energy, the oxygen supply should be discontinued while it is in progress. For example, the oxygen supply should be discontinued during the taking of x-rays at the bedside, and during the use of cautery and suction machines. Sometimes suctioning must be continued to keep the airway patent.

Because of the implications oxygen therapy has for many people, the patient may experience increased fear and anxiety as a result of his feeling unsafe, at the time the therapy is started. Furthermore most patients who are acutely hypoxic have some degree of anxiety. Before oxygen therapy is instituted, a simple statement to the effect that oxygen will improve his breathing should be made. While the equipment is being brought from the storeroom, the patient should be prepared by placing him in the desired position and making him as comfortable as possible. When oxygen is administered by tent, the motor should be turned on and the oxygen flow started before placing the patient in the tent. The flow of oxygen should be started before any device for administering oxygen is directly applied. Care should be taken to get the tent over the head and face of the patient without touching him. After oxygen therapy is instituted, the nurse should stay with the patient until she is sure that the equipment is operating properly and the patient is comfortable. Fifteen or twenty minutes spent with the patient at this time can do much to add to his feeling of safety. As with any seriously ill patient, he should be visited regularly for observation and care.

When oxygen is used more or less routinely

in therapy, the patient should be prepared to expect it. For example, it often is prescribed in the postoperative treatment of patients undergoing a surgical procedure in which the route of approach is through the chest wall. Part of the preoperative preparation of the patient should be to inform him that oxygen therapy not only is possible, but is usual. Then, if he wakes up in the oxygen tent, he will be less likely to be frightened.

Patients who are seriously ill at the time oxygen therapy is started may become dependent on it and be afraid to have it discontinued. The patient who is treated in a tent is more likely to have difficulty than patients treated by other techniques. Return to breathing ordinary air can usually be accomplished by gradually extending the time that the patient remains outside the canopy. The capacity of the patient to tolerate ordinary concentrations of oxygen can be checked by removing the canopy while he eats his meals or is bathed. The patient is returned to the tent if signs or symptoms indicating hypoxia appear. Some patients take very little time to become readjusted to breathing air; others require time and considerable support to make the transition. Among the advantages of discontinuing oxygen therapy during a period when the patient is receiving care is that it facilitates the giving of care. Furthermore, the patient is reassured by the presence of the nurse. He does not have to fear that he will have to wait to have the canopy replaced promptly should he require oxygen. The fact that the patient has been through a frightening experience should not be forgotten. He may require time, patience, and encouragement to regain confidence in his ability to maintain his own oxygen supply.

Oxygen administered by methods other than the oxygen tent threatens the safety of the patient by its effect on mucous membranes. Oxygen gas is dry, and when it comes in contact with the mucous membranes of the respiratory tract, it takes on moisture. Water is added to the oxygen gas by bubbling it through water. Although the oxygen gas introduced into the oxygen tent is dry, it is circulated in a closed system that contains the expired air of the patient. Therefore, moisture is readily available to moisturize the air. In fact, expired air contains more water than is required to maintain a suitable degree of humidity. Excess water is removed by circulating the air over ice or through a refrigeration unit. Steaming of the tent on the *inside* indicates some failure in this mechanism. Condensation on the *outside* occurs for the same reason that moisture accumulates on a pitcher of ice water on a hot, humid day. Cold air holds less moisture than hot air. When hot air is chilled rapidly, water precipitates as rain or as drops on a water glass.

OXYGEN POISONING

Although oxygen poisoning does not occur very often in adults, it can occur when the patient inhales a high concentration for 24 hours or longer. Concentrations of 100 per cent can be inhaled for up to 24 hours without observable effects. With prolonged inhalation of high concentrations of oxygen, changes characteristic of irritation take place in the lung. Lung tissue becomes swollen. Treatment is given to lessen the percentage concentration of oxygen inhaled. The condition can be prevented by reducing the percentage concentration of oxygen inhaled after 12 to 24 hours.

A point relating to the safety of the patient, though not directly affecting the effectiveness of oxygen therapy, is that all equipment should be clean when it is brought to the bedside. At the completion of oxygen therapy, all equipment that has been in contact with the patient, his secretions, or expired air should either be discarded or thoroughly washed and disinfected. For example, when disposable canopies are used, they should be removed and discarded. If they are saved, they should be washed in a detergent solution and dried. Although nurses are not always directly responsible for the cleanliness of the equipment, they should refuse to use it when it is unclean.

Whatever method is used for the administration of oxygen, attention to the comfort as well as the survival of the patient is essential. The care of the patient should be planned so that his hygienic needs are met. He should be bathed, moved, and turned, and have mouth and back care. An extra effort may have to be made to ensure an adequate fluid and food intake. Attention should be paid to the body alignment and the position of the patient in bed. A footboard serves not only to support the feet, but to lessen the weight of bed covering on the feet. Care directed toward increasing the comfort and relaxation of the patient is important, not only for the usual reasons, but because relaxation decreases the need for oxygen and thereby increases the effectiveness of oxygen therapy.

Finally, as in the care of any sick patient, observation is an important facet of care. Among the pertinent observations are included: (1) observations related to the degree to which the needs of the patient for oxygen are being met, (2) observation of the equipment, and (3) observation of safety precautions and identification of threats to the safety of the patient.

The nurse, therefore, has many responsibilities in the care of the patient under oxygen therapy. They include (1) the preparation of the patient for what to expect; (2) care throughout the treatment that encourages his cooperation, lessens his fears, increases comfort and relaxation, and contributes to the benefits of the procedure; (3) attention to the details in the performance of oxygen therapy that increase the likelihood of the desired concentration of oxygen reaching the alveoli; (4) observations of the respiratory status of the patient, his reactions to oxygen therapy, and his general condition; (5) observation of the equipment and its functioning; (6) attention to the details that reduce the threats to the safety of the patient; (7) care directed toward keeping the airway clean and promoting the expansion of the lung; and (8) coordination of the care of the patient, so that his care is individualized.

Adequacy of Respiratory Function

For the purposes of discussion, respiratory function can be considered as involving four general types of processes: (1) the movement of air to and from the respiratory membrane, (2) its diffusion across the respiratory membrane, (3) the transport of oxygen and carbon dioxide to and from the pulmonary circulation and the tissues, and (4) the utilization of oxygen by the cells.

With the development of thoracic surgery and the discoveries of the space age, interest in pulmonary function and ways of measuring it have been greatly stimulated. At one time, tests were limited to a determination of the vital capacity and to the clinical judgment of the physician. Methods are now available whereby function at the different levels can be measured with some degree of accuracy.

Some of the terms used to describe pulmonary function are defined as follows:

The **tidal volume** represents the volume of air moved in or out during one respiratory cycle. In the adult at rest, the tidal volume is approximately 500 cc of air. The **minute ventilation** can be obtained by multiplying the tidal volume by the number of times the person breathes per minute. If the patient can and does cooperate, a decrease in tidal volume is clinically significant. A normal volume may be found in patients with certain diseases of the lung, such as emphysema.

Inspiratory reserve volume is the maximum amount of air that can be inspired at the end of a tidal inspiration, usually about 3,000 cc.

Expiratory reserve volume is the maximum quantity of air that can be expelled at the end of a tidal expiration; this amount is about 1,500 cc.

The **residual volume** is the quantity of air remaining in the lung at the end of a maximum expiration, and is approximately 1,500 cc.

The **vital capacity** is the largest volume of air that can be expelled after a maximum inspiration, about 4,800 cc. At one time this was the only test of breathing that was available. Present knowledge indicates that, by itself, a normal vital capacity is not a very dependable indicator of pulmonary function. Its value can be increased by timing the length of expiration. This is known by the term **timed vital capacity.** The normal young person can expel at least 95 per cent of his vital capacity in three seconds. The findings in this test relate well with the maximum breathing capacity.[50] Patients with emphysema frequently have a normal untimed vital capacity, but an abnormal timed vital capacity.

The **total lung capacity** is the total volume of air found in the lung after a maximum inspiration. It equals the sum of the vital capacity and the residual air and is about 6 liters.

The **maximum breathing capacity** is the largest volume of air that can be breathed on command during a specified interval of time. The patient is instructed to breathe as rapidly and deeply as he can into a system that offers little resistance for a period of 15 seconds. The rate of breathing usually varies from 50 to 70 per minute. Whatever the unit of time, the result is converted to liters per minute. The normal value for men is from 80 to 120 liters per minute. For women it is somewhat less. This test gives more accurate information about an individual's pulmonary function than any single test. In some disorders of the lung the vital capacity is normal, but the maximum breathing capacity is markedly diminished. The reverse may also be true. Although the accuracy of all the tests is influenced by the understanding and cooperation of the patient, cooperation is imperative to the performance of maximum breathing capacity.

Although tests of ventilation may be determined under any degree of activity, they are usually obtained with the patient at rest. Physical activity, excitement, emotional upsets, or any condition increasing the need for oxygen will be accompanied by changes in ventilation. The patient who is to have his maximum breathing capacity measured should be prepared as if he were to have a test of basal metabolic rate.

[50] Eli H. Rubin and Morris Rubin: *Thoracic Diseases* (Philadelphia: W. B. Saunders Company, 1961), p. 173.

Details for the preparation of the patient vary somewhat in different institutions, but they are essentially as follows:

1. No food is eaten after dinner or, at the latest, 9:00 P.M.
2. Breakfast and medications are withheld until after the test.
3. The patient is expected to retire early.
4. The patient is to stay in bed until after the test. Activities—morning care, shaving, showering, smoking, gum chewing—are prohibited.
5. Height, sex, and age are recorded.
6. Temperature, pulse, and respiration are then recorded before the test. An elevation in body temperature should be reported.
7. The patient should be transported to the respiratory laboratory in a wheel chair.
8. After the test has been completed, the patient should be served his breakfast and his usual schedule of activities should be restored.

The objective of the preparation of the patient is to send him to the laboratory in a relaxed state, so that the findings will have value. One of the reasons for performing the maximum breathing capacity is to determine whether or not the patient's respiratory reserve is sufficient for him to tolerate and benefit from the removal of a portion of his lung tissue. The patient requires information about what to expect and what is expected of him. The test may be performed with the patient in the sitting or standing position. He breathes into an instrument known as a spirometer. As the patient breathes into and out of the mouthpiece, changes in pressure in the floating drum cause it to move up and down. These excursions are recorded on the writing drum. From measurements of the size and number of respiratory cycles, the quantity of gas moved in each excursion or over a period of time can be calculated.

The nurse is usually responsible for the physical preparation of the patient for breathing tests. She is often responsible for explaining to the patient what to expect and what is expected of him.

A second type of test of pulmonary functional reserve is the exercise tolerance test. This test is performed in a variety of ways. The purpose is to determine the amount of exercise that the patient can take before he develops dyspnea. For example, if he can walk the length of a hallway or up one or two flights of stairs without experiencing dyspnea, he has a satisfactory respiratory reserve. If, on the other hand, he becomes dyspneic on walking a short distance

or at rest, his reserve is probably unsatisfactory. His exercise tolerance can be measured more exactly by having him walk on a treadmill, pedal a stationary bicycle, or step up and down from a stair step. Ordinary exercise serves very well, however. Various methods are available to measure the volume of residual air. The test is usually performed by having the patient inhale a gas such as helium and measuring its dilution in the expired air.

Methods are available for determining the adequacy of diffusion of oxygen and carbon dioxide through the respiratory membrane as well as the degree of oxygen saturation of the blood. Carbon dioxide content can also be determined. The level of hemoglobin and the hematocrit provide information about the oxygen-carrying power of the blood. In chronic hypoxia, not caused by anemia, both are likely to be elevated. With a significant decrease in the level of hemoglobin in the blood, all the tissues are deprived of an adequate supply of oxygen.

The determination of the utilization of oxygen by the tissues is known as the basal metabolic rate. It is decreased in any condition in which the tissues are deprived of adequate supplies of oxygen- or calorie-containing compounds or of substances that regulate the rate of metabolism. Because temperature influences the rate of chemical reactions, the rate of metabolism is increased by fever and decreased by lowering the body temperature. The metabolic rate is elevated by exercise, ingestion of food, hyperthyroidism, and hyperthermia. It is also elevated in leukemia. Some examples of conditions in which the metabolic rate is diminished include starvation, inactivity, chronic hypoxia, hypothyroidism, and hypothermia.

The most common method used to determine the structural condition of the lung and its relationship to the other organs is x-ray and/or fluoroscopy. X-ray provides information about vital capacity as well. Chest x-ray and photofluoroscopy are indispensable tools not only in diagnosis of diseases involving structures in the thoracic cavity, but in case finding. Although their most extensive use is in case finding, that is, in identifying persons who have lesions indicative of tuberculosis, they are proving to be of value in discovering other disease processes in the lung as well as in the heart and other structures in the mediastinum. When an abnormality is found, the patient is encouraged to see his physician for further study and diagnosis.

Despite the value of the various methods used to measure respiratory processes, the day-by-day evaluation of the status of the patient depends on the observation of the patient. Among these observations are included the characteristics of breathing. Normal breathing has certain characteristics that can be described. The breathing cycle occurs at regular intervals of from 14 to 16 per minute. During and immediately following strenuous exercise it may rise to as high as 24 cycles per minute, but it does not normally rise much beyond that. The depth of respiration is sufficient to move about 500 cc of air during quiet respirations, but the quantity is increased during activity. One of the features of normal respiration is its effortless character. The individual is not consciously aware that he is breathing, and except when he has been exercising strenuously, the onlooker is not aware that he is making an effort. A simple description of normal breathing, then, is that it is rhythmical and effortless, and though the rate and depth do change, changes are within limits and are in response to a stimulus placing known extra demands on the individual.

Disturbances in Breathing

Similar to other bodily functions, breathing may deviate from the normal. The rate and depth may be greater or less than normal. The rhythm may be abnormal, or breathing may become difficult or labored. Sources of disturbances in breathing include any condition that increases the need for oxygen or for the elimination of carbon dioxide. Because the functioning of respiratory and circulatory systems is integrated, disturbance in the function of either may cause alteration in breathing. Because the action of the muscles of respiration depends on stimulation from the nervous system, abnormalities of breathing may have their origin in the nervous system.

The same prefixes are used to indicate changes in the direction from normal as are used to describe deviations from the normal of other body functions. They include *a-, olig-, brady-, hypo-, hyper-, poly-, tachy-,* and *dys.* The prefix is added to the suffix, *-pnea,* which means to breathe. The term for normal or easy breathing is eupnea.

Tachypnea, hyperpnea, and polypnea are all terms that are loosely defined as rapid breathing. Tachypnea should be used when the rate of breathing is above 24 per minute, but the depth of respiration is not changed appreciably. In contrast, hyperpnea should be used when the depth of respiration is increased. The breathing of a well-trained athlete is a good example of the proper use of the term "hyperpnea." When he exercises, the depth of his respiration increases, but the rate rises very little. Polypnea should be used when the minute volume of

breathing is markedly increased. The term "hyperventilation" is sometimes used as a synonym.

At the other end of the breathing range, apnea means a cessation of respiration. Continued apnea is, of course, incompatible with life. Apnea does occur in certain types of periodic breathing.

Bradypnea is used to characterize an excessively slow rate of breathing in which the rate is less than 10 cycles per minute. There is no appreciable change in the depth of respiration. A common cause of bradypnea is respiratory depression from excessive dosages of narcotics or sedatives.

Hypopnea is used to indicate a decrease in the depth of respiration that is out of proportion to the decrease in rate. Sleep is a condition in which hypopnea is physiological. Sedatives and narcotics may also be responsible for hypopnea.

PERIODIC BREATHING

Two disturbances in breathing will be discussed in detail. They are periodic breathing and dyspnea. Periodic breathing occurs in a number of disease conditions. It is characterized by repeated cycles in which a person breathes deeply for a period of time and then breathes only slightly or not at all.

The most common type of periodic breathing is Cheyne-Stokes breathing. In Cheyne-Stokes respiration there is a slow waxing and waning of respirations with the cycle lasting from 45 seconds to three minutes. Although all the mechanisms for the development of Cheyne-Stokes respirations have not been explained, according to Guyton,[51] the condition must be initiated by some condition that under- or overstimulates respiration. For example, for some reason Mr. Oaks' breathing becomes more rapid and deeper than usual. With the increased rate and depth of respiration, the level of carbon dioxide in his blood falls. When, a few seconds later, arterial blood with a low tension of carbon dioxide reaches his brain, there is insufficient carbon dioxide to stimulate respiration, and his breathing wanes or ceases. During the period of hypopnea or apnea, the concentration of carbon dioxide in the blood plasma rises. When the level of plasma carbon dioxide is sufficiently elevated, breathing is reinitiated.

Although the mechanisms have not been clarified, Cheyne-Stokes respirations have been observed in aviators and mountain climbers at high altitudes and in patients with heart failure. Although the reasons for their occurrence have not been elucidated, their cause is probably re-

[51] *Op. cit.,* p. 601.

lated to a decrease in the sensitivity of the respiratory center to carbon dioxide.[52]

Another type of periodic breathing is known as Biot's breathing. According to Guyton,[53] this type of breathing is frequently confused with Cheyne-Stokes breathing. Rather than waxing and waning, breaths come in couples, triples, quadruples, or some other number of cycles, with periods of apnea between cycles of breathing. This type of breathing is characteristically associated with a disorder of the brain. It is seen in patients with very great increases in intracranial pressure, with contusion or compression of the brain tissues, or with destructive diseases of the brain. It is indicative of a very poor prognosis. Death usually follows soon after it appears.

The basic mechanism in the development of Biot's breathing is quite different from that of Cheyne-Stokes respiration, as the former is related to oscillations in the blood flow to the brain. High intracranial pressure compresses the arteries and cuts off the flow of blood to the brain. Lack of blood flow to the brain is followed by the initiation of reflexes which, if successful, elevate the pressure of the blood above the intracranial pressure. As the nutrition of the vasomotor center improves, impulses to maintain the high blood pressure diminish and the blood pressure falls. During the period when the blood pressure is rising, the individual breathes deeply. During the phase when it is falling, he stops breathing or is apneic.

DYSPNEA

A second commonly observed disturbance in breathing is dyspnea. Dyspnea is defined as difficult or painful breathing and as such is a subjective sensation. The patient who is dyspneic has a desire or hunger for air and is conscious of the need for increased respiratory effort. Some authorities do not exclude labored breathing from the definition, however. Rubin[54] quotes Christie as defining dyspnea as "a conscious or visible increase in respiratory effort." The latter definition covers the person who, though dyspneic when awake, is typically not conscious of having to make an increased respiratory effort when he is asleep. A person such as a well-trained athlete may be hyperpneic and yet not be dyspneic, as breathing, though increased in depth, is effortless. A person who

is dyspneic may or may not have labored breathing which is obvious to the observer. To illustrate, Mary Willow flew from Lima to Cusco, Peru, which is at an elevation of about 12,000 ft. The hotel where Mary stayed had no elevator, and her room was on the second floor. Although she did not experience any difficulty as she walked up the stairs, after she arrived at her room, she felt short of breath. She did not have obviously labored breathing; but she felt short of breath, or dyspneic.

Mrs. Bird, who is described in the next chapter, has true dyspnea. She has congestive heart failure with marked edema of her lungs. She is conscious of the necessity for breathing, and her breathing appears labored. She has been experiencing air hunger and she makes an obvious effort to breathe.

MECHANISMS UNDERLYING DYSPNEA

According to Rubin,[55] whatever the nature of the disorder that predisposes to dyspnea, the immediate cause of increased effort in breathing is stimulation of the centers in the nervous system controlling respiration. Inasmuch as the respiratory centers are interconnected with the cerebral cortex, dyspnea may be initiated by impulses having their origin in the cerebral cortex or from the muscles of respiration. Because cells in the respiratory centers are sensitive to carbon dioxide and to hydrogen ions as well as to severe deficiencies in oxygen supply, a rise in the level of the first two or a fall in the latter may act as a stimulus in the development of dyspnea.

Guyton[56] summarizes the factors in the development of dyspnea as (1) "an actual abnormality of the respiratory gases in body fluids, especially hypercapnia,[57] and to a much lesser extent hypoxia, (2) the amount of work that must be performed by the respiratory muscles to provide adequate ventilation, and (3) the state of the mind itself."

To relate the above to Engel's *Unified Concept of Disease,* previously discussed in Chapter 7, dyspnea may arise from a disturbance in the mental apparatus or from the direct effect of an injurious or potentially injurious agent on cells. In any given individual any one or all of the above factors may be operating.

Dyspnea is found in patients with a variety of disturbances in the pulmonary, circulatory, and nervous systems. Conditions associated with dyspnea include:

---

[52] Norman Brachfeld and John S. La Due: "Congestive Heart Failure, Coronary Insufficiency and Myocardial Infarction," *Pathologic Physiology,* 4th ed. William A. Sodeman and William A. Sodeman, Jr., eds. (Philadelphia: W. B. Saunders Company, 1967), p. 479.

[53] *Op. cit.,* p. 602.

[54] *Op. cit.,* p. 189.

[55] *Ibid.,* p. 190.

[56] *Op. cit.,* p. 613.

[57] Hypercapnia is the technical term for an elevated carbon dioxide in plasma.

1. Pulmonary—conditions increasing the work of breathing or predisposing to carbon dioxide retention, hypoxia, or to both
   a. Obstruction of the trachea and bronchi
   b. Loss of compliance of the lung, as in pulmonary edema from congestion, inflammation, or fibrosis of the lungs as seen in persons with far-advanced tuberculosis
   c. Following resection of the lung, particularly after pneumonectomy
   d. Limited movement of the chest and diaphragm
      (1) Emphysema—chest is almost fully expanded at end of expiration
      (2) Weakness or paralysis of muscles of respiration
      (3) Pneumothorax
2. Abnormalities in circulation
   a. Inadequate oxygenation of blood in lungs
   b. Increased blood in the pulmonary vascular tree
   c. Insufficient transport of oxygen
      (1) Severe anemia
      (2) Cardiac failure
3. Acidosis
   a. Respiratory acidosis (interference with elimination of carbon dioxide)
   b. Metabolic acidosis (accumulation of hydrogen ion)
4. State of mind—fear, anxiety

Persons differ greatly in their susceptibility to dyspnea. This is true even among those who have a serious reduction in their vital capacities. Persons whose dyspnea is on a psychic basis become short of breath when they are exposed to an anxiety-inducing situation. For one person dyspnea occurs only when he is in a crowd, or a closed room; for another, it develops when he enters an automobile or when he has to see his boss. The individual may or may not associate the anxiety-producing event with his dyspnea.

Most, if not all, dyspneic persons who are conscious and alert suffer some psychic stress, for they know that breathing is essential to life. The diseases with which shortness of breath occurs are frequently of a serious nature. Most, if not all, patients are conscious of the implications of dyspnea. Moreover, dyspnea is accompanied by highly unpleasant sensations which in turn intensify the awareness of the patient of his precarious state. The degree to which altered biochemical conditions, that is, hypercapnia and hypoxia, and the psychic state influence the development of dyspnea in a given individual varies, but both are often present.

Despite some differences in the details, the following incident illustrates the influence of biochemical and psychic factors in dyspnea. Jim Warbler, aged 25, was acutely ill. His diagnosis was ascending spinal poliomyelitis. As the hours passed, his muscles of respiration became progressively weaker. To pull air into his lungs, he used his accessory muscles of respiration. As breathing became more difficult, Jim felt short of breath, and he could be seen to be using the muscles of his neck and upper thorax to breathe. Although he was placed in a tank-type respirator, he continued to complain of feeling that he was about to smother. Each time the portholes in the tank were open, he became frantic, and remained so until they were tightly closed. At times Jim's behavior suggested that he was in a state of panic. The reasons underlying his behavior were physiological as well as psychological. Compared to normal respiration, the tank respirator is an inefficient instrument. Jim undoubtedly suffered from hypercapnia and relative hypoxia. He was acutely ill with a disease that deprived him of his capacity to meet his own need for oxygen and would probably leave him seriously handicapped. He had been discharged from the Army only a few months earlier and had just completed arrangements for his lifework. Because the occupation that he had chosen was one requiring a strong and healthy body, the likelihood of his being able to carry out his plans seemed remote. Was it any wonder that in the first days after he was placed in the respirator, he was terrified? As Jim recovered, function returned to his muscles of respiration, and he was eventually able to maintain his own breathing without difficulty. During the period of acute illness, Jim's survival was threatened by his inability to ventilate his own lungs. His behavior was undoubtedly influenced by the meanings the entire situation had for him.

In patients whose dyspnea is associated with congestive heart failure, or emphysema, shortness of breath usually appears first in response to exercise. Mrs. Bird complained for some weeks that each time she walked upstairs, she had to stop and "catch her breath" on the landing before climbing to the top. She noticed that when she walked against the wind she became short of breath before she had walked very far. In individuals such as Mrs. Bird, dyspnea is protective, inasmuch as it decreases activity to the degree to which the pulmonary and circulatory system can supply oxygen to the tissues.

In planning the nursing of the patient who is dyspneic, several factors should be known. Certainly, the nature of the disorder responsible for the dyspnea influences the care required by the patient. When there is a significant defect in the ability of the patient to obtain oxygen or to eliminate carbon dioxide, his need for oxygen and for the elimination of carbon dioxide can be reduced by rest. The degree of rest required will vary with the nature and seriousness of the condition of the patient. In patients with congestive heart failure, such as Mrs. Bird, the sitting position often provides some relief, since the vital capacity is greater in the sitting than in the supine position. Although the reasons for the improved vital capacity are not completely known, it is probably because the blood is pooled in the splanchnic areas and lower extremities.

In patients in whom dyspnea appears to be associated with an increase in a sensitivity of the vagal receptor mechanism, morphine sulfate may give relief by depressing this mechanism. Morphine sulfate is often prescribed for patients who are dyspneic in association with heart disease, because it not only lessens the dyspnea, but decreases awareness of the situation. Mrs. Bird's physician prescribed 10 mg (⅙ grain) of morphine sulfate for the relief of her dyspnea. Not only was her dyspnea improved, but she appeared to be less apprehensive. In contrast, morphine sulfate is contraindicated in patients whose dyspnea is associated with a depression of the respiratory center. For example, Jim Warbler was not given morphine. Neither was Mrs. Pine, who had asthma and an associated emphysema.

ORTHOPNEA

Orthopnea, which is usually associated with long-standing dyspnea, is made more difficult by the recumbent position. Orthopnea is usually associated with heart disease. Elevation of the diaphragm is believed to aggravate pre-existing pulmonary congestion and further decrease the vital capacity. Although the sitting position does not always completely relieve orthopnea, it is the position assumed by the patient, if he has a choice. Moreover, when orthopnea is severe, maximum relief is afforded by sitting forward slightly. The position can be attained by supporting the patient in the upright position and placing a tray table to rest on over his thighs. When a cardiac bed is available, the foot of the bed can be dropped, so that the bed essentially becomes a chair. A comfortable chair can be used in the same way. The chair or cardiac bed has at least two advantages. The legs and feet are in the dependent position, and a certain amount of fluid is in effect removed from the circulation and the position is more natural. Whatever type of bed or chair is utilized, the trunk and extremities of the patient should be well supported. When a patient is placed in a cardiac bed or chair, the feet should be supported on a footboard or footstool and should not be permitted to dangle. The objective of the position is to provide for the comfort of the patient and to ensure maximum rest.

PAROXYSMAL DYSPNEA

In addition to orthopnea, another form of dyspnea is paroxysmal dyspnea. Although it is not a form of asthma, this condition is sometimes called cardiac asthma. Because of its tendency to occur at night, it is sometimes called paroxysmal nocturnal dyspnea. Although paroxysmal dyspnea develops in much the same manner as orthopnea, it differs from orthopnea inasmuch as it is accompanied by bronchiolar spasm. There is a wheezing type of respiration, which is probably caused by an accumulation of exudate in the airway associated with a swelling of its mucous lining and bronchiolar spasm.

The circumstances under which an attack occurs are similar to the following. When Mr. Whipple, who has some degree of congestive heart failure, goes to bed at night, he lowers his headrest somewhat. Later he awakens, acutely short of breath and wheezing. He sits up, hanging his feet over the edge of the bed. After a short time his breathing improves and he coughs and removes the accumulated secretions.

HYPERVENTILATION

One final alteration in breathing will be discussed, that is, hyperventilation, a condition in which both the depth and rate of breathing are increased. As is to be anticipated, hyperventilation increases the loss of carbon dioxide, and as a consequence respiratory alkalosis develops. The effects of hyperventilation can be corrected by holding the breath for a few moments or by rebreathing air in a paper bag. Hyperventilation occurs in healthy persons who are under stress or in a state of exhaustion and in the emotionally unstable, as well as in persons who have disorders in which the hydrogen ion content of the blood is raised. Hyperventilation, which occurs in metabolic acidosis, is known as Kussmaul breathing. It is physiological or compensatory inasmuch as the increase in the rate and depth of respiration is caused by stimulation of the respiratory center by the hydrogen ion and for a time, at least, it facilitates cation-anion balance in the blood by increasing the elimination of carbon dioxide. (See Chapter 9 for a fuller discussion.)

As emphasized throughout this chapter, cell function depends on the continuous delivery of oxygen to the cells and the prompt removal of carbon dioxide. Carbon dioxide is not only a product of metabolism, but it regulates respiratory processes, both at the site of respiratory exchange in the lung and at the tissue level as well as by its effects on the respiratory center in the brain. The respiratory system is the site at which exchange of gases takes place between the internal and external environment. The two environments are separated by a semipermeable membrane, through which oxygen and carbon dioxide diffuse with great rapidity. In this chapter the importance of the exchange of gases —oxygen and carbon dioxide—to cell function has been stressed. The structure of the respiratory system is such that as air passes through it, the air is warmed, cleansed, and humidified. The organism is further protected from foreign material by an active phagocytic system that destroys particulate matter that reaches the alveoli.

Diseases of the Respiratory System

The respiratory system is subject to a great variety of diseases. The general nature of these is no different from those found in other regions of the body. Their specific effects result from the nature of the function of the respiratory system and the part of the respiratory system that is involved. They are of infectious, chemical, hypersensitivity, neoplastic, degenerative, or traumatic origin. The upper and, to a lesser extent, the lower respiratory tracts are exposed to contaminants in the surrounding atmosphere. Recently, increased attention has been given to the problem of air pollution. Such agents as sulfur dioxide, particulates (for instance, dust, fumes, and mist), photochemicals (including nitrogen oxides, hydrocarbons, and oxidants), and the carbon oxides are potentially hazardous to the maintenance of an adequate oxygen supply, particularly to a person with chronic lung disease. Some of these air pollutants act by irritating the air-exposed membranes of the upper respiratory tract. Others act at the alveolar level. However, it is usually only during periods of meteorologic inversions that these agents are considered to be especially harmful.

Exposure may be continuous or single, large or small. For example, exposure to smoke may be continuous or it may be an isolated event. The respiratory systems of persons who smoke heavily and who live in large cities are more or less continuously exposed to smoke and its products. Single or isolated exposures occur when individuals are in a smoke-filled room.

The correlation between smoking and respiratory disease has become the focus of considerable attention. It is a well-established fact that tobacco smoke paralyzes ciliary action. Lung cancer is primarily a disease of smokers. It is estimated that approximately 80 per cent of epidermoid and undifferentiated carcinomas

are caused by cigarette smoking.[58] One reason patients with chronic lung disease are instructed not to smoke is that this is a source of respiratory irritation and consequently increased bronchial secretions. The nurse should make every effort to educate her patients about the risks involved in smoking.

Disorders of the respiratory system may be acute or chronic. According to reports by the U.S. National Health Survey, acute disorders of the respiratory system rank at the top as a cause of disabling illness involving one or more days in bed. Although the incidence of respiratory diseases changes from year to year, it remains the most frequent cause of morbidity.

Within the last ten years increasing emphasis has been placed on chronic respiratory diseases as causes of morbidity and mortality. In the past, tuberculosis was the only major chronic disease of the respiratory system to receive much attention. Presently, tuberculosis is again on the increase but malignant neoplasms of the respiratory system, chronic bronchitis, emphysema, bronchiectasis, and asthma–hay fever are also known to be responsible for an increasing incidence of disability and mortality. According to Scott,[59] emphysema is second only to heart disease as a disabler. Petty and Nett [60] estimate that 50 per cent of men over 50 years have some degree of emphysema. Approximately 30,000 patients surrender their jobs each year as a result of disability from emphysema and at least 30,000 people die from directly related causes. Emphysema and chronic bronchitis constitute what is known as CAO or chronic airway obstruction. CAO is a contributing cause of death in an additional 80,000 people and it is doubling every five years. It is the nation's most rapidly growing health problem. All of these disorders decrease respiratory reserve and, as such, limit the capacity of the individual to obtain oxygen from the air and to return carbon dioxide to it.

One aspect of respiratory disease that has not been discussed, because it does not have a direct bearing on respiratory function, is the fact that ducts from the paranasal sinuses and from the middle ear open into the nasal passages and nasopharynx. Furthermore, the mucous membrane lining these ducts and their

[58] *Smoking and Health: Report of the Advisory Committee to the Surgeon General of the Public Health Service* (Washington, D.C.: U.S. Public Health Service), Publication No. 1103.

[59] Bertha A. Scott: "Tensions Linked with Emphysema," *Amer. J. Nurs.,* **69:**538 (Mar.) 1969.

[60] Thomas Petty and Louise M. Nett: *For Those Who Live and Breathe with Emphysema and Chronic Bronchitis* (Springfield, Ill.: Charles C Thomas, 1967), p. 117.

related cavities is continuous with the mucous membrane lining the airway. Infections with swelling of the respiratory mucous membrane can interfere with drainage of the paranasal sinuses or middle ear by obstructing their respective ducts, or an infectious process can spread by way of a duct to one or more of the above structures. With the extension of an infection to the paranasal sinuses or to the middle ear, microorganisms multiply and abscess formation is likely. In addition to the signs and symptoms associated with a pyogenic process, there is pain in the area of the affected structure. Because of its proximity to the mastoid cells, infections of the middle ear may spread to the mastoid cells. Because of the proximity of the mastoid cells and the paranasal sinuses to the brain, infections in these structures predispose to meningitis and brain abscess. Middle-ear infections (otitis media) may also impair hearing. The drum membrane may rupture as a consequence of increased pressure. Subsequent scarring reduces its ability to respond to sound waves. The general factors in the therapy of infections are discussed in Chapter 5.

The focus of this chapter has been the importance to survival of supplying cells with oxygen, so that energy can be released to support the activities of the cell. Although oxygen is continuously present in the air, its partial pressure depends not only on its percentage composition but on atmospheric pressure. In the presence of an adequate partial pressure of oxygen in the air, delivery of oxygen to the cells depends on the coordinated functioning of the respiratory and circulatory systems. Integration and coordination of the functions of these two systems is effected by the nervous system. A number of activities are regulated: the act of breathing; modifications of breathing during swallowing, coughing, and sneezing; the rate and depth of respiration; the rate of circulation in relation to respiratory function; and the integration of respiratory and circulatory function in relation to the needs of the entire individual.

Disturbances in the function of respiration can occur at any level. Acute and chronic diseases that threaten respiratory function are common causes of disability and mortality. In the care of the acutely ill, one of the aspects of nursing care having a high priority is maintaining the supply of oxygen to the alveoli. Often the survival of the patient depends on the achievement of this objective.

Table 8-1 summarizes the diseases and/or conditions involving the respiratory system, supplementing the discussion in the text.

TABLE 8-1

Summary of Diseases and/or Conditions Involving the Respiratory System

Diagnostic Category	Etiological Factors	Incubation Period and Nature of Onset	Severity of Illness and Course	Part of Respiratory Tract Involved and Response	Effect on Adequacy of Respiratory Function	Focus of Nursing	Major Medical Treatment
Infections Common cold Acute rhinitis	Variety of viruses 1. Virus of Andrewes 2. Enteroviruses 3. Adenoviruses 4. Myxoviruses	18–48 hr Gradual onset with irritation, dryness, rawness, or tickling in the nasopharynx or nose. Highly contagious	Mild Too sick to work but not enough to stay in bed	Nasal passages and related structures Coryza, sneezing, nasal obstruction: thin, watery discharge becomes thick and purulent and lasts for several days or weeks	Nasal congestion interferes with conditioning air	Isolation Rest Fluids Adequate diet Teach protection, prevention, and purpose and methods of treatment	Rest Medication for headache, nasal congestion, and elevated temperature Isolation Antibiotics have no effect on viruses and should not be used in primary infection Individual may be sensitized to the antibiotic
Sinusitis Paranasal	Bacterial infection secondary to allergic or viral rhinitis, obstruction that follows smoking, use of alcohol, and damp weather	Local pain and tenderness Headache in morning when exudate has collected overnight Sometimes have edema of overlying facial skin	Sinusitis usually subsides as primary infection runs its course Can become serious with frank suppuration and abscess formation that can lead to osteomyelitis and spread of infection to the orbit, meninges, and brain	Related sinuses— frontal, maxillary, ethmoid and sphenoid and nasal passages Nasal swelling and congestion Drainage from sinuses into nasal pharynx With repeated attacks there may be thickening of the sinus mucosa, continuous partial obstruction, and		Position—semi-Fowler's Control of pain Mouth care, especially if surgery with nasal packing Fluids encouraged	Re-establish drainage channels Surgery to correct structural defects, for example, deviated septa Antibiotic therapy after causative organism has been identified Mucosa- and vessel-constricting medications Irrigation of sinuses

Condition	Etiology	Symptoms	Complications / Course	Pathology	Effect on Air	Nursing Care	Treatment
Tonsillitis Acute Chronic	Hemolytic 1. Streptococci 2. Staphylococci	Mild to severe sore throat If chronic infection, becomes disseminated to other parts of the body, such as the joints, muscles, bursae, ear, and eye	Acute tonsillitis usually does not warrant hospitalization unless complications arise, such as pneumonia Surgery is usually indicated in chronic tonsillitis	Tonsils and crypts Adenoids usually affected also Tonsils are inflamed and enlarged Ulcerations may be found in crypts	Obstruction to flow of air through the pharynx, usually not serious	Bed rest Control of sore throat Throat irrigations Ice collar Control temperature Fluids encouraged Sponge bath	chronic inflammation Tonsillitis usually treated by a tonsillectomy, after attack subsides Medication for pain, sore throat, and causative agent Antibiotics usually ordered after or organism is identified and sensitivity studies are carried out

Chronic pharyngitis	1. Sinusitis
	2. Adenoiditis
	3. Allergic response to
	  a. Food
	  b. Inhalants, smoke, house dust
		Dryness, scratchiness, sense of irritation with mild to severe soreness on swallowing	Can become severe infection extending either upward to cause acute otitis media, rhinitis, or sinusitis or downward to cause laryngitis, tracheitis, bronchitis, or pneumonia	Mucous membranes of the pharynx without infiltration or ulceration
				Mucosa becomes red with hypertrophy of superficial lymphoid nodules
				Dryness and crusting in nasopharynx
				May have hacking cough
					May have mild disturbances in transportation of incoming air	Alertness for streptococcal infections in those with a history of rheumatic fever
						Throat irrigations
						Easily swallowed diet
						Fluids encouraged
							Antibiotics
							Prevent superimposed infection
							Throat irrigations
							Discovery and removal of etiological factor
							When lateral bands affected, 10% silver nitrate applied to reduce inflammation
							Nasal spray for dryness and crusting

Laryngitis inflammation	1. Filtrable viruses, sequelae of acute rhinitis 2. Pneumococci 3. Hemolytic streptococci 4. Hemolytic staphylococci 5. Other inflammation of the upper	First and most important symptom is hoarseness Cough and aching pain in larynx accompanied by hoarseness Fever usually the first day or two	May have epidemic character Edema of the larynx might necessitate tracheotomy Pharyngitis a common complication Cough may	Hyperemia of laryngeal mucosa Hoarseness, sore throat, sputum can become purulent Cough	Can lead to severe obstruction to incoming air—asphyxia	Isolation (not strict) Rest—especially to voice Anticipate needs Provide means of communication Fluids encouraged No opiates Diet limited to	Isolation Rest—limited use of voice Medication for causative agent Local treatment—silence Promote elimination—fluids Aspirin for ele-

TABLE 8-1

Summary of Diseases and/or Conditions Involving the Respiratory System (*cont.*)

Diagnostic Category	Etiological Factors	Incubation Period and Nature of Onset	Severity of Illness and Course	Part of Respiratory Tract Involved and Response	Effect on Adequacy of Respiratory Function	Focus of Nursing	Major Medical Treatment
	respiratory tract 6. Mouth breathing 7. Trauma— chronic a. Smoke b. Dust c. Voice abuse		become choking and strangling Usually self-limiting within 10 days; however, without proper treatment and disuse of voice may lead to chronic situation			fluids in acute stages Room well ventilated, temperature 72°F., and humidity 50%	vated temperature Elixir of terpin hydrate or ammonium carbonate for cough— NO OPIATES Throat sprays
Acute undifferentiated respiratory disease (includes *grippe* or *flu*— not influenza)	Adenoviruses in military populations	4–7 days Gradual onset	More severe than common cold Patient frequently goes to bed voluntarily	Pharynx and associated structures Lungs usually clear Sore throat, discomfort in chest Nasal discharge infrequent		Same as common cold	Symptomatic therapy Aspirin for relief of feverishness, headache, and malaise
Primary atypical pneumonia	Adenoviruses Eaton agent	12–14 days Insidious onset, may have minor respiratory symptoms for several days	Acute illness usually lasts 1 week Convalescence prolonged—6 weeks or more Return of strength slow	Lung—lower lobes most frequent Pulmonary lesions and infiltrates Cough, sputum (can become mucopurulent) Substernal discomfort Râles are audible	Impairment of exchange of gases	See Pneumonia	See Pneumonia

Influenza (A used as example)	Viruses: 1. Influenza A, B, and C 2. Sendai virus	18–36 hours to 3 days Sudden onset usually See last column	Sporadic infections are relatively mild; however, in epidemics some may be serious to critical Recovery ranges from 2–3 days to weeks depending on complications such as bacterial infections The most serious complication is staphylococcal pneumonia	Respiratory epithelium Response is often less than in common respiratory disease Sneezing, watery nasal discharge, or stuffy nose Productive cough frequently occurs usually develops along with substernal chest pain	Interference with conditioning of air	See common cold and care to minimize: Fever and chills Onset accompanied by severe frontal headache usually followed by fever and chills Stabbing retro-orbital pain Widespread myalgia especially in the legs Spasm of abdominal muscles, also periarticular pain Prostration to some degree Most common secondary symptoms are anorexia, nausea, and constipation	Vaccine for prevention (influenza A, A_2, and B) Chemotherapy reserved for secondary infections Bed rest Codeine for cough
Chronic bronchitis	1. Irritants: smoke and other air pollutants 2. Pneumococcus 3. Staphylococcus	Insidious or may follow other respiratory diseases such as pneumonia and bronchial asthma Persistent cough and expectoration	Mild to severe depending on the development of other respiratory diseases, such as emphysema	Mucus-secreting glands in mucosa of trachea and bronchi Hypersecretion of mucus, bronchial spasm, and bronchiolar fibrosis Chronic productive cough Sputum is ropy, white, and elastic Postnasal drip is frequent, choked-up feeling to dyspnea	Ventilation difficult because of the narrowing of the bronchial tree	Rest—isolation (limited exposure to others) Fluids encouraged Control of cough and expectoration	Promote cleansing airway with expectorants, steam inhalations, and proteolytic enzymes Antimicrobial therapy Intermittent positive pressure breathing may be necessary

TABLE 8-1

Summary of Diseases and/or Conditions Involving the Respiratory System (*cont.*)

Diagnostic Category	Etiological Factors	Incubation Period and Nature of Onset	Severity of Illness and Course	Part of Respiratory Tract Involved and Response	Effect on Adequacy of Respiratory Function	Focus of Nursing	Major Medical Treatment
Bronchiectasis	1. Bronchial obstruction 2. Infections such as bronchopneumonia that cause stagnant exudate 3. Atelectasis causes traction on bronchi	Symptoms can be intermittent or chronic depending on respiratory infection Usually seen in lower lobes of the lung	Depends on superimposed infection and not necessarily degree of bronchial dilatation Can become irreversible	Smooth muscle and elastic tissue of bronchial tubes Tubular or saccular dilatation of bronchial tube system Patchy distribution or local May lose ciliated epithelium, which is then replaced by fibrous tissue Cough, mucopurulent sputum—large amounts in the morning and hemoptysis dyspnea Postnasal drip, sinusitis	Loss of protective mechanisms Difficulty in transportation of gases	Collection of sputum, postural drainage Teach postural drainage Protection from other respiratory diseases Control atmosphere (moist air) Position—ease of ventilation Much emotional support—chronic recurring disease Teach patient to avoid infections by staying out of crowds, etc., especially in cold, damp weather	Antibacterial medication to control infection, which is common diagnosis Postural drainage Bronchograph—extent of dilatation Tracheostomy—keep bronchial tree patent Aerosol to promote cough and expectoration Moist air—help liquefy tenacious sputum Resection of damaged segments of the lung if disease is discovered early enough Chronic forms—treatment is mainly symptomatic and supportive, as outlined above
Pneumonia	Infectious agents (70 types):	Descending infection	Usually lasts 2 or 3 weeks with	Entire lobe of lung (lobar) or patchy	Decrease in surface area of lung for	Bed rest—respiratory	Bed rest—respiratory isolation

1. Pneumococcus 2. Staphylococcus 3. Hemolytic streptococcus 4. Friedlander's bacillus 5. Other viruses, fungi, and parasites	Coryza may precede the onset of pneumonia for several days. Onset is usually abrupt with shaking, chills, fever, tachycardia, and the development of pleuritic pain and productive cough. Sputum is "rusty" or pinkish	complete resolution. Fatality with treatment is rare today in the middle-aged group. Severe complications can arise: 1. Atelectasis 2. Pleural effusion (empyema)	area throughout lung tissue (lobular or bronchopneumonia). Lung consolidation in stages: 1. Red hepatization (blood serum and cells pour into alveoli) 2. Gray hepatization, alveoli are packed with rbc's and fibrinous exudate 3. Resolution—by phagocytosis. Some signs and symptoms: Dyspnea, pleuritic pain, cough, sputum, rāles	the exchange of gases	isolation. Fluid encouraged. Collection of sputum. Deep breathing and coughing. Vital signs. Mouth care. Oxygen therapy. Teach protection, prevention, and methods of treatment	Antimicrobial therapy, depending on causative agent. Medication for elevated temperature. Sputum examined—gram stain, culture, and sensitivity. Blood studies and culture. Oxygen therapy if necessary. X-rays—determine extent of lung consolidation and effects of treatment. Fluid therapy. Analgesics for chest pain—no morphine (Cecil-Loeb states it is used).
Pleural effusion	Usually secondary to some lesion outside the pleura. Examples: (1) Inflammatory pleural effusion (pleurisy) is secondary to an inflammatory process of the lung. (2) Noninflammatory hydrothorax—clear, pale, straw-colored serous fluid—associated with	Inflammatory transudate can become an exudate and progress to empyema (frank pus), severe constitutional symptoms—fever, night sweats, chills, anorexia	Pleura—clear transudate or exudate within the *pleural cavity*. Dyspnea develops from compression. Chest pain produced—varies from dull to stabbing. Dry cough. Shift of mediastinum to unaffected side	Increase in negative pressure. Decrease in distensibility of lung. Decreased vital capacity	95% of pleural effusion is tuberculous. Use proper precautions. Bed rest. Fluids	1. Antimicrobial therapy if underlying cause is infection. Many treat as primary tuberculous lesion for 3–6 months. Frequent x-ray follow-up. Antimicrobials may be instilled in the pleural cavity if nontuberculous. 2. Removal of fluid if necessary by instituting

TABLE 8-1

Summary of Diseases and/or Conditions Involving the Respiratory System (*cont.*)

Diagnostic Category	Etiological Factors	Incubation Period of Onset and Nature	Severity of Illness and Course	Part of Respiratory Tract Involved and Response	Effect on Adequacy of Respiratory Function	Focus of Nursing	Major Medical Treatment
		healthy pleura. (3) Hemorrhagic, hemothorax—frank blood—traumatic penetration of chest wall					water-sealed drainage or aspiration 3. With empyema usually surgical evacuation of abscess is necessary 4. Analgesics for chest pain
Asthma	Bronchial obstruction caused by (1) allergic reaction to inhaled antigens, (2) respiratory infection, and/or (1) and (2) together Emotional disturbances Some individuals have atopic tendency which is inherited They should be protected from becoming sensitized to environmental and seasonal inhalants not harmful to nonatopic	Episode may begin suddenly without warning and may last from minutes to several hours Shortness of breath is usually accompanied by wheezing, and respiratory effort The person feels as if he were suffocating and exhibits fear	Episodes may be mild and controlled with medication or may persist with status asthmaticus, which is resistant to treatment	Bronchial tubes: Response 1. Edema of mucosa 2. Hypertrophy of walls 3. Contraction of smooth muscle 4. Dilatation of blood vessels 5. Increase in secretion by mucous glands Signs and symptoms: 1. Expiratory dyspnea and wheezing 2. Cough 3. Overinflation of the lungs, which can lead to emphysema	Disturbances in exchange of gases (ventilation) To maintain air exchange, great effort is required, leading to fatigue	1. Observe situation and/or circumstances of episode 2. Position—ease of respiration 3. Medication given promptly for relief of attack 4. Rest 5. Oxygen therapy 6. Nonstimulating environment 7. No matter what the cause of the attack, treatment is necessary to neutralize the histamine release which is causing the symptoms	1. Bronchodilators —relief of bronchospasm by drugs such as aminophylline, ephedrine, and epinephrine Acute attack— epinephrine, 0.3 ml subcutaneous. May be followed by ephedrine, aminophylline, etc. 2. Postural drainage 3. Expectorants— iodide compounds 4. Study of allergies—skin test, sensitivity, and psychogenic causes

	Causes	Onset and Symptoms	Course	Signs	Pathology and Effects	Nursing Care	Treatment
(continued from previous entry)							5. Oxygen therapy with intermittent positive pressure breathing 6. Antibiotics if superimposed infection 7. Limited use of sedation 8. Support general health 9. Adrenocortical steroids—chronic episodes
Emphysema	1. Partial bronchial obstruction, e.g., chronic bronchitis; also atmospheric irritants—dusts and fumes 2. Loss of elasticity of pulmonary tissue—degenerative 3. Loss of pulmonary tissue (decrease in mass)	Insidious Shortness of breath upon arising, without cough Shortness of breath progresses to a point where a steady effort is required to ventilate the lungs during waking hours	Course of the disease may be rapid with ensuing death within a few years or the duration may be as long as 20–30 years depending on other superimposed respiratory diseases	Air sacs become overdistended with air Productive cough Dyspnea Hyperinflation of chest—"barrel chest"	Poor distribution of gases throughout the lung Difficulty in expelling air Increase in residual lung volume and decrease in maximum breathing capacity Decrease in arterial oxyhemoglobin saturation Respiratory failure may occur when normal gas exchange cannot be provided, resulting in carbon dioxide retention and unsaturated arterial blood Respiratory acidosis	1. Rest—conservation of energy 2. Teach breathing exercises, energy savers 3. Position—ease ventilation 4. Vital signs	1. Elimination of bronchial irritants—no smoking 2. Antibiotics to control infection 3. Bronchodilator drugs 4. Oxygen therapy should be used with caution as patients with severe emphysema may have CO_2 narcosis and it is their lack of O_2 which is keeping them alive. Oxygen may be ordered at only 1–2 liters per minute. Should not be over 40% oxygen when using intermittent positive pressure de-

TABLE 8-1

Summary of Diseases and/or Conditions Involving the Respiratory System (*cont.*)

Diagnostic Category	Etiological Factors	Incubation Period of Onset and Nature	Severity of Illness and Course	Part of Respiratory Tract Involved and Response	Effect on Adequacy of Respiratory Function	Focus of Nursing	Major Medical Treatment
							vices. Watch patient for signs of CO_2 narcosis 5. Breathing exercises—economy of ventilation 6. Treatment of cardiac complications 7. Tracheostomy may be necessary with bronchial obstruction 8. Need some form of artificial respiration to help them eliminate CO_2 Also may need intermittent positive pressure devices, which will increase the inspiratory phase and deliver more oxygen across the alveolar membrane
Pneumothorax Open communication between pleural space and atmos-	1. Bronchopleural fistula, tuberculosis, malignant disease, postoperative compli-	Sudden large pneumothorax can be very serious, causing collapse of the	Absorption of the gases depends on the state of health of the pleura	Gas in the pleural space shifts to the unaffected side Collapse of lung	Vital capacity decreases proportionately with amount of air in pleural	1. Observe stability of blood pressure, productive character of respiration, chest	1. Medical emergency—air must be removed from pleural space to prevent

302

phere Closed—not in communication with atmosphere cation of lung resection, emphysema 2. Opening in thoracic wall (trauma) 3. Rupture of subpleural bleb 4. Artificial pneumothorax as therapy	lung on the affected side with exquisite chest pain and respiratory distress A small pneumothorax may be asymptomatic If spontaneous, usually sudden sharp pain followed by dyspnea	Re-expansion of the lung may be prevented by fibrosed lung tissue or thickened visceral pleura	space Hypoxic hypercapnia may develop because of disturbances in exchange of gases	tissue depending on amount of gas within pleural space, and this is dependent on the size of the pleural leak	pain, increase in temperature 2. Care of patient with chest tubes and water-sealed drainage 3. Teach patient necessity for safety with tubes and purposes of treatment	mediastinal shift and collapse of other lung, which would cause death 2. Removal of air from pleural cavity if necessary by instituting water-sealed drainage 3. Removal of fluid from pleural cavity if present, by aspiration 4. Activity restricted until lung expands 5. Surgery may be indicated in the presence of a ruptured bulla that fails to close 6. Immediate closure of open wound 7. Expansion of lung followed by x-ray, clear airway
Atelectasis 1. Bronchial obstruction 2. External compression * 3. Failure of lung to expand at birth 4. Mucus, foreign body in airway	May be sudden and/or gradual If a lobe or entire lung collapses, person experiences anxiety, dyspnea, and tachypnea	Seen postoperatively caused by mucus plugs Mild to severe Can lead to death from asphyxia Also can lead to emphysema, spontaneous pneumothorax	Pulmonary alveoli Collapse of alveoli Dyspnea and tachypnea Difficulty raising sputum	Prevents adequate exchange of respiratory gases	Coughing and deep-breathing bedfast patients Ambulation	If massive, bronchoscopy Pulmonary toilet If infection present, antibiotics

* Reduced tone of respiratory muscles.

REFERENCES

BOOKS

American Red Cross: *First Aid Textbook, Prepared by The American National Red Cross for the Instruction of First Aid Classes,* 4th ed. (New York: Doubleday & Company, Inc., 1957).

Baum, G. L.: *A Textbook of Pulmonary Diseases* (Boston: Little, Brown and Company, 1965).

Beal, John M.: *Manual of Recovery Room Care* (New York: The Macmillan Company, 1962).

Boies, L. R.: *Fundamentals of Otolaryngology,* 3rd ed. (Philadelphia: W. B. Saunders Company, 1959).

Cherniack, R. M., and Cherniack, L.: *Respiration in Health and Disease* (Philadelphia: W. B. Saunders Company, 1961).

Cumming, Gordon, and Hunt, L. B.: *Form and Function in the Human Lung* (Baltimore: The Williams & Wilkins Company, 1968).

Flitter, Hessel H.: *An Introduction to Physics in Nursing,* 4th ed. (St. Louis: The C. V. Mosby Company, 1962).

Fundamentals of Hyperbaric Medicine, Publication No. 1298, Prepared by the Committee on Hyperbaric Oxygenation (Washington, D.C.: National Academy of Sciences, National Research Council, 1966).

Introduction to Respiratory Diseases (National Tuberculosis Association, 1961).

Jenson, J. Trygve: *Introduction to Medical Physics* (Philadelphia: J. B. Lippincott Company, 1960).

Liebow, Averill, and Smith, David E. (eds.): *The Lung: International Academy of Pathology Monograph* (Baltimore: The Williams & Wilkins Company, 1968).

Major, Ralph H.: *Classic Descriptions of Disease* (Springfield, Ill.: Charles C Thomas, Publisher, 1939), pp. 597–630, 635–40.

Manhattan Eye, Ear and Throat Hospital: *Nursing in Diseases of the Eye, Ear, Nose and Throat,* 10th ed. (Philadelphia: W. B. Saunders Company, 1958).

Riley, Richard L., and O'Grady, Francis: *Airborne Infection* (New York: The Macmillan Company, 1961).

Safar, Peter (ed.): *Respiration Therapy* (Philadelphia: F. A. Davis Company, 1965).

Seedor, Marie M.: *Therapy with Oxygen and Other Gases* (New York: Teachers College Press, 1966).

Van Liere, Edward J., and Stickney, J. Clifford: *Hypoxia* (Chicago: University of Chicago Press, 1963).

West, Edward Staunton, *et al.: Textbook of Biochemistry,* 4th ed. (New York: The Macmillan Company, 1966).

PERIODICALS

American Thoracic Society: "Principles of Respiratory Care," *Amer. Rev. Resp. Dis.,* **95**:327–37 (Feb.) 1967.

Andrewes, Christopher Howard: "The Viruses of the Common Cold," *Sci. Amer.,* **203**:88–102 (Dec.) 1960.

Ashenburg, Norman J.: "The Effects of Air Pollution on Health," *Nurs. Outlook,* **16**:22–25 (Feb.) 1968.

Banyai, Andrew: "Chronic Bronchitis," *Geriatrics,* **17**:5–14 (Jan.) 1962.

Bates, D. V.: "Chronic Bronchitis and Emphysema," *New Eng. J. Med.,* **278**:546 (Mar. 7) 1968.

Baum, Gerald L., *et al.:* "Pulmonary Sporotrichosis," *New Eng. J. Med.,* **280**:410–13 (Feb. 20) 1969.

Baum, Gerald L., and Schwarz, Jan: "Pulmonary Histoplasmosis," *New Eng. J. Med.,* **258**:677–84 (Apr. 3) 1958.

Bedell, George N.: "Chronic Bronchitis and Pulmonary Emphysema," *Curr. Med. Dig.,* **35**:1203–1206 (Dec.) 1968.

Betson, Carol: "Blood Gases," *Amer. J. Nurs.,* **68**:1010–12 (May) 1968.

Bickerman, Hylan A.: "Antitussives," *Amer. J. Nurs.,* **63**:61–64 (Apr.) 1963.

Blalock, John B., and Ochsner, John L.: "Management of Thoracic Trauma," *Surg. Clin. N. Amer.,* **46**:1513–24 (Dec.) 1966.

Bloch, Virginia C.: "Helping the Patient To Ventilate," *Nurs. Outlook,* **17**:31–33 (Oct.) 1969.

Bradford, Joseph K., and DeCamp, Paul T.: "Bronchiectasis," *Surg. Clin. N. Amer.,* **46**:1485–92 (Dec.) 1966.

Burch, G. E., *et al.:* "Influence of Temperature and Oxygen Concentrations in Oxygen Tents," *JAMA,* **176**:1017–25 (June 24) 1961.

Burrows, Benjamin, and Earle, Richard H.: "Course and Prognosis of Chronic Obstructive Lung Disease," *New Eng. J. Med.,* **280**:397–404 (Feb. 20) 1969.

Chapel, James L., and Taylor, Daniel W.: "Glue Sniffing," *Missouri Med.,* **65**:288–92 (Apr.) 1968.

Creighton, Helen, and Coulter, William: "The Whys of a Pulmonary Function Test," *Amer. J. Nurs.,* **60**:1771–74 (Dec.) 1960.

Dantzig, Senge M., *et al.:* "A Mathematical Model of the Human External Respiratory System," *Perspect. Biol. Med.,* **4**:324–76 (Spring) 1961.

Davies, D. F., and Davies, A. H.: "Lung Cancer—Cigarette Smoking as a Cause," *Amer. J. Nurs.,* **61**:64–69 (Apr.) 1961.

Filley, G. F.: "Emphysema and Chronic Bronchitis: Clinical Manifestations and Their Physiologic Significance," *Med. Clin. N. Amer.,* **51**:283–92 (Mar.) 1967.

Gardner, Warren: "Problems of Laryngectomies," *J. Chronic Dis.,* **13**:253–60 (Mar.) 1961.

Gilmore, Stuart I.: "Rehabilitation After Laryngectomy," *Amer. J. Nurs.,* **61**:87–89 (Jan.) 1961.

Hall, Wendell H.: "The Specific Diagnosis and

Treatment of the Pneumonias," *Med. Clin. N. Amer.*, 43:191–207 (Jan.) 1959.

Hammarsten, James F., and Wolf, Stewart: "The Role of Emotions in Respiratory Disease," *Med. Clin. N. Amer.*, 43:113–26 (Jan.) 1959.

Hargreaves, Anne G.: "Emotional Problems of Patients with Respiratory Disease," *Nurs. Clin. N. Amer.*, 3:479–87 (Sept.) 1968.

Harris, H. Williams: "What Do You Know About Coughing," *Amer. J. Nurs.*, 53:162–63 (Feb.) 1953.

Hasenfus, Joseph L.: "Report of the World Conference on Smoking and Health," *J. Maine Med. Ass.*, 58:234–40 (Nov.) 1967.

Hatch, Hurst B.: "Preoperative Evaluation and Management of Patients with Pulmonary Insufficiency," *Surg. Clin. N. Amer.*, 46:1377–80 (Dec.) 1966.

Hopkins, William A., and Turk, L. Newton: "The Current Treatment of Severe Chest Injuries," *Southern Med. J.*, 62:243–48 (Mar.) 1969.

Hunter, Samuel: "Traumatic Hemopneumothorax," *Postgrad. Med.*, 29:374–79 (Apr.) 1961.

Jackson, G. G., *et al.:* "Susceptibility and Immunity to Common Upper Respiratory Viral Infections—The Common Cold," *Ann. Intern. Med.*, 53:719–37 (Oct.) 1960.

Jimison, Carmin: "Nursing Care After Laryngectomy," *Amer. J. Nurs.*, 57:741–43 (June) 1957.

Kurihara, Marie: "Assessment and Maintenance of Adequate Respiration," *Nurs. Clin. N. Amer.*, 3:65–75 (Mar.) 1968.

LeJeune, Francis E., Jr.: "Foreign Bodies in the Tracheobronchial Tree and Esophagus," *Surg. Clin. N. Amer.*, 46:1501–12 (Dec.) 1966.

Levine, E. R.: "Inhalation Therapy: Aerosols and Intermittent Positive Pressure Breathing," *Med. Clin. N. Amer.*, 51:307–21 (Mar.) 1967.

Linden, Maurice E.: "Some Psychological Aspects of Rescue Breathing," *Amer. J. Nurs.*, 60:971–74 (July) 1960.

McCallum, Helen P.: "The Nurse and the Respirator," *Nurs. Clin. N. Amer.*, 1:597–619 (Dec.) 1966.

McGrath, Dorothy, and Kruger, Betty K.: "Chest Suction," *Amer. J. Nurs.*, 62:72–73 (June) 1962.

MacVicer, Jean: "Exercises Before and After Thoracic Surgery," *Amer. J. Nurs.*, 62:61–62 (Jan.) 1962.

Marple, Charles D.: "Cyanosis," *Amer. J. Nurs.*, 58:222–25 (Feb.) 1958.

"Mouth-to-Mouth Artificial Respiration," *Nurs. Outlook*, 7:520 (Sept.) 1959.

Murphy, Eleanor R.: "Intensive Nursing Care in a Respiratory Unit," *Nurs. Clin. N. Amer.*, 3:423–36 (Sept.) 1968.

Nelson, T. G., *et al.:* "Cricothyroidectomy," *Amer. J. Nurs.*, 61:74–76 (Nov.) 1961.

Ochsner, Alton,, Jr., and Ochsner, Alton: "Cancer of the Lung: Recognition and Management," *Surg. Clin. N. Amer.*, 46:1411–25 (Dec.) 1966.

Overholt, Richard: "Resection of Carotid Body for Asthma," *JAMA*, 153:809–12 (June 9) 1962.

Petty, T. L., *et al.:* "A Comprehensive Care Program for Chronic Airway Obstruction," *Ann. Intern. Med.*, 70:1109–20 (June) 1969.

Pitorak, Elizabeth Ford: "Laryngectomy," *Amer. J. Nurs.*, 68:780–86 (Apr.) 1968.

Prather, J. Richard, *et al.:* "Initial and Late Management of Penetrating Chest Wounds," *Med. Times*, 96:1013–1021 (Oct.) 1968.

Pratt, Loring W.: "Tracheostomy or Peroral Endotracheal Intubation?" *J. Maine Med. Ass.*, 59:23–25 (Feb.) 1968.

Rackemann, Francis M.: "The Natural History of Hay Fever and Asthma," *New Eng. J. Med.*, 268:415–19 (Feb. 21) 1963.

Reimann, Hobart: "Current Problems of the Pneumonias," *Med. Clin. N. Amer.*, 56:144–54 (Jan.) 1962.

"Risk of Lung Cancer in Filter Cigarettes," *Current Med. Dig.*, 36:228 (Mar.) 1969.

Sheffer, Albert L., and Valentine, Martin D.: "The Treatment of Bronchial Asthma," *Med. Clin. N. Amer.*, 53:239–48 (Mar.) 1969.

"Symposium on the Major Pulmonary Diseases," *Med. Clin. N. Amer.*, 43:1–333 (Jan.) 1959.

Thomas, John M., and Ulpis, Elza B.: "A Seasonal Hazard—Laryngotracheobronchitis," *Amer. J. Nurs.*, 61:52–54 (Mar.) 1961.

Totman, Laurence E., and Lehman, Roger H.: "Tracheostomy Care," *Amer. J. Nurs.*, 64:96–98 (Mar.) 1964.

"Tracheostomy in Acute Respiratory Failure," *Current Med. Dig.*, 35:1157–69 (Nov.) 1968.

Turner, Howard G., Jr.: "The Anatomy and Physiology of Normal Respiration," *Nurs. Clin. N. Amer.*, 3:383–441 (Sept.) 1968.

Valdivia, Enrique: "Mountain Sickness," *Amer. J. Nurs.*, 61:77 (Aug.) 1961.

Weiss, Earle B., *et al.:* "Acute Respiratory Failure in Chronic Obstructive Pulmonary Disease. Part II: Treatment," *DM*, (Nov.) 1969, pp. 3–58.

Wilson, Rodger H. L., and Farber, Seymour M.: "Concepts and Misconceptions about Oxygen Therapy," *Postgrad. Med.*, 27:158–64 (Feb.) 1960.

Zellos, S.: "The Diagnosis and Treatment of Bronchial Adenoma," *Geriatrics*, 18:107–20 (Feb.) 1963.

9

Nursing the Patient with a Disturbance in Fluid and Electrolyte Balance

When they went ashore the animals that took up land life carried with them a part of the sea in their bodies, a heritage which they passed on to their children and which even today links each land animal with its origin in the ancient sea. Fish, amphibian, and reptile, warm-blooded bird and mammal—each of us carries in our veins a salty stream in which the elements sodium, potassium, and calcium are combined in almost the same proportions as in sea water. This is our inheritance from the day, untold millions of years ago, when a remote ancestor, having progressed from the one-celled to the many-celled stage, first developed a circulatory system in which the fluid was merely the water of the sea. In the same way, our lime-hardened skeletons are the heritage from the calcium-rich ocean of Cambrian time. Even the protoplasm that streams within each cell of our bodies has the chemical structure impressed upon all living matter when the first simple creatures were brought forth in the ancient sea. And as life itself began in the sea, so each of us begins his individual life in a miniature ocean within his mother's womb, and in the stages of his embryonic development repeats the steps by which his race evolved, from gill-breathing inhabitants of a water world to creatures able to live on land.[1]

Overview

The Kidney

How does the kidney regulate the constancy of the internal environment?

Fluid Compartments

What factors influence the volume and distribution of water in the body?

How do electrolytes function within the body?

Disturbances in Body Fluid and Electrolyte Balance

How does illness affect fluid and electrolyte equilibrium?

Acid-Base Equilibrium

What are the clinical manifestations of acid-base imbalance?

Signs and Symptoms of Alterations in Volume, Osmolality, and Hydrogen Ion Concentration

What tests are useful in determining fluid and electrolyte balance and renal function?

What are the objectives of therapy?

Overview

JUST as a continuous supply of oxygen is necessary to life, maintenance of the composition and distribution of body fluids is also essential.

These fluids not only form the environment of the cells but also enter into their structure. In health, exchange between the internal and external environment is so regulated that (1) conditions favorable to the functioning of enzymes and hormones in cellular activities are preserved within the internal environment, (2) materials needed by the cells are supplied, and (3) products of metabolism are removed from the cells.

In this chapter the discussion will be centered on (1) the constituents of the body fluids, (2) the function of each constituent, (3) the distribution and concentration of each con-

[1] Rachel Carson: *The Sea Around Us* (New York: Oxford University Press, 1950), pp. 13–14.

stituent in the various fluid compartments, and
(4) the effects of each on the volume, osmotic
pressure, and hydrogen ion concentration in the
body fluids. Most disturbances in fluid balance
in the body are related to its volume, osmolality,
and hydrogen ion concentration. Most illnesses,
acute or chronic, are accompanied by some
local or general disturbance in the body fluids.
One of the factors in recovery is the ability of
the individual to maintain or to restore the normal distribution and composition of body fluids.
In order to anticipate and meet the needs of
patients with understanding, the nurse requires
some knowledge of the normal mechanisms for
maintaining the constancy of the internal environment and the manner in which these
mechanisms are disrupted in disease.

Body fluids are composed of water with electrolytes and nonelectrolytes suspended or dissolved in it. The types and concentrations of
electrolytes in body fluids resemble those of sea
water. According to one popular theory of the
origin of life, the first living creatures developed
in the sea. Those that were successful in making the adaptation to living on land took some
of the sea with them in the form of extracellular
fluid. Land animals, including man, continue to
surround their cells with fluids like those that
were present in the primeval seas.

Undue loss of fluid is prevented by a water-
tight jacket—the skin. A special structure, the
gastrointestinal tract, enables the organism to
take from the external environment the materials required to replenish fluid constituents
utilized by, or lost from, the body. The kidney,
lung, and skin remove waste products and excesses in supply. All of these are regulated so
that they function with remarkable accuracy
in maintaining the composition and concentration of this fluid. The seas have no such means
for protecting their composition and concentration. In the eons of their existence, water laden
with minerals has been emptied into them by
the rivers of the earth. Water is evaporated by
the sun and wind with the result that minerals,
especially salt, have become concentrated in the
sea water.

In the hospital the physician is usually responsible for the prescription of the amount,
character, and route of administration of the
patient's fluid intake. He shares with the nurse
the responsibility for making observations on
which to base decisions about the fluid needs
of the patient. The nurse is usually responsible
for the administration of the fluids and for determining and meeting the related needs of
patients.

This chapter will be limited to knowledge
essential for nurses to (1) administer fluids in
a safe and effective manner, (2) observe and

report with clarity the signs and symptoms and
the deviations from normal behavior that the
patient presents, (3) interpret the signs and
symptoms indicating a deviation from health
and constitute nursing problems, and (4) select
the course of action which will help the patient
attain the goal that is realistic for him, as she
plans for total care.[2]

In the past, understanding of fluid and electrolyte balance has often been difficult. One of
the reasons for this has been the confusing use
of terminology. To prevent unnecessary confusion, a number of terms will be defined and,
in some instances, discussed.

Electrolyte is a substance which, when dissolved
in water, conducts an electric current. When
an electrolyte is dissolved in water, it dissociates into its component ions. The degree to
which a dilute solution of a given electrolyte
dissociates is constant, but it differs for each
electrolyte. Strong electrolytes dissociate almost completely. They include most soluble
salts and inorganic acids and bases.

Acids were once defined as compounds yielding
hydrogen ions. They are now defined as *pro-
ton donors*. Though they exist in solution as
H_3O^+ (hydronium ion), they are generally
referred to as H^+.

Bases were once defined as compounds yielding
hydroxyl ions. They are now defined as *pro-
ton acceptors*.

Ion is an electrically charged particle in solution. Examples are the hydrogen ion (H^+)
and the chloride ion (Cl^-).

Ionization is the process whereby an electrolyte
in solution dissociates into its component
ions, i.e., an atom of one element donates
an electron from its outer shell to complete
the outer valence shell of an atom of another
element.

Cations are positively charged ions, that is, they
are electron donors.

Anions are negatively charged ions, that is, they
are electron recipients.

Milliequivalent is one one-thousandth of an
equivalent weight. An equivalent weight is
the number of grams of an element that will
combine with 8 g or parts of oxygen or 1.008
g of hydrogen. The equivalent weight of an
element is obtained by dividing its atomic
weight by its valence. For example, the
atomic weight of oxygen is 16. It has a valence of 2. Its equivalent weight is therefore
8. In forming water, 2 atoms (parts) of hydrogen combine with 1 atom (part) of oxygen. In terms of equivalent weights, 2.016 g

[2] Faye G. Abdellah *et al.: Patient-Centered Approaches to Nursing* (New York: The Macmillan
Company, 1960), p. 26.

of hydrogen combines with 16 g of oxygen to yield 18.016 g of water. To cite another example, 1 equivalent of potassium weighs 39.1 g. This is the amount of potassium that will combine with 8 g of oxygen. One equivalent of potassium (39.1 g) combines with 1 equivalent of chlorine, which weighs 35.5 g, to yield 74.6 g of potassium chloride. Because the quantity of electrolytes found in a liter of body fluids is small, milliequivalents rather than equivalents are used to express the concentration of electrolytes in body fluids.

Formerly, electrolytes in the blood were measured in milligrams per 100 ml of serum or plasma. The current trend is toward reporting them in milliequivalents per liter. The reason for this change is that the milliequivalent provides information about the number of anions or cations available to combine with cations and anions. To illustrate, the level of sodium cations in the blood serum ranges from 137 to 147 (average 142) mEq per liter. This means there are approximately 142 sodium cations available to combine with 142 anions. The average level of chloride ions in blood serum is 103 mEq per liter. Therefore, approximately 39 mEq of sodium are available to combine with other anions.

Buffer is a substance that protects a solution from changes in pH when an acid or base is added. It is sometimes referred to as a chemical sponge.

Buffer system is composed of a weak acid and a salt formed by neutralizing the weak acid with a strong base. There are a number of buffer systems in the blood—*oxyhemoglobin, and reduced hemoglobin; sodium acid phosphate* and *bisodium phosphate; acid protein and B protein*. A weak base and a salt formed by neutralizing the base with a strong acid functions similarly.

Alkali reserve is a term used to refer to the sodium in the blood that is in combination with bicarbonate. It is called the alkali reserve because the sodium can combine with other anions. The term is really a misnomer.

Osmotic pressure may be defined as the force created by particles in solution that attracts water across a membrane that is fully permeable to water, but impermeable to the particles, ions, or molecules. The direction of flow of the water is always from the less concentrated toward the more concentrated solution. Flow continues until the solution on the two sides of the membrane is of equal concentration. An increase in the osmotic pressure of the fluid in one fluid compartment in the body results in the movement of water into that compartment.

Hydrostatic pressure may be defined as the force exerted by a fluid against the wall of the chamber in which it is contained. Literally, it means the pressure created by the standing weight of water. Applied to the blood, it includes not only the pressure created by the weight of blood against the wall of the capillary, but the force with which the blood is propelled.

Osmol is one gram molecular weight of an unionized solute. One osmol of glucose is the molecular weight of the glucose expressed in grams. One gram molecular weight of sodium chloride yields two osmols because each molecule of sodium chloride breaks up into one sodium ion and one chloride ion.

Osmolality is the number of osmotically active particles per kilogram of water.

Osmolarity is the number of osmoles per liter of solution.

Filtration may be defined as the separation of a liquid from a solid by passing the liquid through a semipermeable membrane. The force responsible is gravity or weight.

Diffusion may be defined as the distribution of one substance throughout another by the movement of molecules.

Hyponatremia is a condition characterized by too little sodium in the blood plasma.

Hypernatremia is a condition in which there is too much sodium in the blood plasma.

Hypokalemia is a condition in which there is too little potassium in the blood plasma.

Hyperkalemia is a condition in which there is too much potassium in the blood plasma.

The Kidney

Because the kidney is essential to the maintenance of the internal environment, its functions are discussed here. The consequences of renal failure are considered at the end of the chapter.

How does the kidney regulate the constancy of the internal environment?

In health, the kidney functions to maintain within limits (1) the volume of water in the extracellular fluid, (2) the concentration of electrolytes in extracellular fluid, (3) the osmolality of the extracellular fluid, and (4) the concentration of hydrogen ion in the extracellular fluid. The kidney is the site for the excretion of the wastes of metabolism, particularly those of protein catabolism. Under certain abnormal conditions, the kidney produces vasoexcitatory substances or their precursors. At the present time this is thought to revolve around the juxtaglomerular apparatus and the renin-angiotensin system. The kidneys secrete a substance that influences the maturation of red blood cells.

Although the kidneys are frequently referred to as organs of excretion, the above list of their functions indicates the inadequacy of this concept of renal function. The primary function of the kidneys is to regulate the volume and composition of the extracellular fluid; their excretory function is incidental to this regulatory function.

Blood Supply to the Kidney

Blood is supplied to the kidney by the renal arteries, which are branches of the abdominal aorta. Occlusions of the aorta, whether due to thrombi or emboli located above the origin of the renal artery may deprive the kidney of adequate blood flow and predispose to renal failure. Just before or after the renal artery enters the hilus of the kidney, it divides into a series of branches. Abnormalities in the branching of a renal artery may obstruct a ureter and impede the drainage of urine from the renal pelvis. In general, the veins draining the kidney follow a pattern similar to that of the arteries. One of the most important points about the renal blood supply is that in health it receives about 25 per cent, or one quarter, of the cardiac output. This is despite the fact that the kidneys constitute only approximately 0.4 per cent of the total body weight.[3]

One of the special features of the blood vessels in the kidney is that the nephron is supplied by two capillary beds: the glomerulus and the peritubular capillaries. Unlike most capillaries, the glomerulus has an arteriole at its exit as well as its entrance. The quantity of blood entering the glomerulus is regulated by the afferent arteriole. Dilation results in increased blood flow into the kidney and constriction results in a decrease. The efferent arteriole regulates the pressure of the blood in the glomerulus. With dilation, resistance to the outflow of blood from the glomerulus diminishes the glomerular filtration and pressure drops. With constriction, resistance to the flow of blood out of the glomerulus increases resulting in an increased filtration pressure in the glomerulus. The vessels supplying the glomerular bed are short and have a wide lumen, allowing the glomerular capillary bed to act as a high pressure system. This can be contrasted with the peritubular capillary bed which is a low pressure system. As a con-

sequence of this arrangement, the kidney is able to closely adapt blood flow to its own and the body's needs.

The Nephron

The work of the kidney is performed by the nephron. In man there are a million or more nephrons in each kidney. They are all basically similar in structure and each one is presumed to be grossly similar to all others in function. See Figure 9-1. Nephrons are located in the cortex. Those situated near the periphery of the kidney are called cortical nephrons. Nephrons situated in the cortex adjacent to the medulla are called juxtamedullary nephrons. Classically, a nephron is described as consisting of a renal or malpighian corpuscle (glomerulus and Bowman's capsule), proximal convoluted tubule, loop of Henle, and a distal convoluted tubule. Finally, many nephrons empty into a collecting tubule. Although the glomeruli are found in the cortex, the proximal and distal renal tubules and especially the loop of Henle dip far down into the medulla of the kidney.

FILTRATION BY THE GLOMERULI

Of the processes involved in the formation of urine, the first is filtration by the glomeruli. Filtration depends on the hydrostatic pressure created by the pumping action of the heart, the volume of blood circulating through the glomeruli, and the resistance offered by the afferent and efferent arterioles. The glomerular filtrate is an ultrafiltrate of the blood and as such it does not contain red cells or colloid materials such as protein. It does contain water and crystalloidal solutes such as electrolytes, glucose, and urea, as well as other wastes of protein metabolism. In other words, the glomerular filtrate contains water and almost all of the substances dissolved in plasma water. The rate of glomerular filtration averages about 125 ml per minute in men and 110 ml per minute in women.

TUBULAR FUNCTION

As the glomerular filtrate passes through the tubules, it is converted to urine by selective reabsorption and the secretion of certain substances. Of the 180 liters of glomerular filtrate all except one or one and one-half liters are reabsorbed. Within the limits of its renal threshold, all glucose and amino acids are reabsorbed.

THE PROXIMAL TUBULES

In the proximal tubules approximately 60 to 80 per cent of the water and almost all of the

---

[3] More detailed discussions of the gross structure of the kidney may be found in any one of a number of anatomy textbooks.

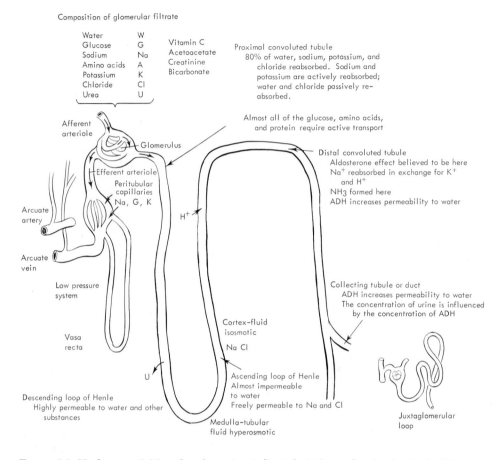

Composition of glomerular filtrate

Water	W
Glucose	G
Sodium	Na
Amino acids	A
Potassium	K
Chloride	Cl
Urea	U

Vitamin C
Acetoacetate
Creatinine
Bicarbonate

Proximal convoluted tubule
80% of water, sodium, potassium, and
chloride reabsorbed. Sodium and
potassium are actively reabsorbed;
water and chloride passively reabsorbed.

Almost all of the glucose, amino acids,
and protein require active transport

Afferent
arteriole

—Glomerulus

—Efferent arteriole

Peritubular
capillaries
Na, G, K

H⁺

Arcuate
artery

Arcuate
vein

Low pressure
system

Vasa
recta

Descending loop of Henle
Highly permeable to water and other
substances

Cortex–fluid
isosmotic

Na Cl

U

Ascending loop of Henle
Almost impermeable
to water
Freely permeable to Na and Cl

Medulla–tubular
fluid hyperosmotic

Distal convoluted tubule
Aldosterone effect believed to be here
Na⁺ reabsorbed in exchange for K⁺
and H⁺
NH₃ formed here
ADH increases permeability to water

Collecting tubule or duct
ADH increases permeability to water
The concentration of urine is influenced
by the concentration of ADH

Juxtaglomerular
loop

FIGURE 9-1. Nephron; activities of each portion indicated. (After a drawing by Leola Hogan.)

glucose, amino acids, bicarbonate ions, and vitamins are normally reabsorbed. The water is absorbed isotonically so that the osmotic pressure of the fluid in the proximal tubule is about the same as in plasma. The return of water to the blood is largely by diffusion and is believed to be determined by the number of ions reabsorbed; therefore, water reabsorption is obligatory. Glucose requires an active transport mechanism. When the level of glucose in the glomerular filtrate exceeds the capacity of the transport mechanism, glucose is lost in the urine.

LOOP OF HENLE

The loop of Henle connects the proximal and distal tubules and is the portion of the nephron that extends farthest down into the medulla of the kidney. It consists of two basic parts, the descending and the ascending loop. In the descending loop, sodium is pumped out of the tubular fluid and about 6 per cent of the water in the glomerular filtrate is reabsorbed. The ascending loop is almost impermeable to water.

DISTAL TUBULES AND COLLECTING TUBULES

The work of the kidney is completed in the distal and collecting tubules. As the urine leaves the collecting tubules, it contains only about 1 per cent of the original fluid that was filtered. Depending upon the level of the antidiuretic hormone which increases the permeability of this portion of the tubule to water, water is or is not reabsorbed. As much as 10 to 15 per cent of the filtered load of sodium is reabsorbed in this area. Aldosterone is the main hormone influencing the rate of sodium reabsorption in the distal and proximal tubules.

SECRETION BY THE TUBULES

In addition to selective reabsorption of certain substances, the tubules also secrete a variety of substances, including penicillin, phenol red, and Diodrast. The distal tubules and collecting ducts also secrete potassium and hydrogen ions. The proximal and distal tubules and collecting ducts can secrete hydrogen ions and ammonia.

Summary

The kidney is a remarkable organ. With each heartbeat approximately one fourth of the blood pumped by the heart circulates through the kidney. Each day 180 liters of glomerular filtrate are formed. In health 99 per cent of the water in the glomerular filtrate is returned to the extracellular fluid. Other substances are either absorbed or secreted as needed to maintain the constancy of the fluid environment of the cells. Depending on intake and losses from the body, the quantity of sodium excreted in the urine varies from negligible to considerable amounts. The volume of extracellular fluid is directly related to this renal control of sodium balance.[4]

Except for a certain amount returned by diffusion, urea is largely concentrated and excreted in the urine. In general, substances useful to the body are reabsorbed, while those of no use or in excess are eliminated.

The kidney closely regulates the volume and concentration of urine in relation to the quantity of water and solutes added to extracellular fluid from exogenous and endogenous sources.

With a large fluid intake, the kidney excretes a large volume of dilute urine; with a small fluid intake, it excretes a small volume of concentrated urine. When both salt and water intake are limited, the minimum volume of urine depends on the volume of nitrogenous wastes, principally urea, presented to the kidney for excretion, and the kidney's capacity to concentrate urea. About 500 ml of water are required for this purpose. The capacity of the kidney to alter the concentration and volume of urine is adaptive. Within limits, it enables the body to survive water deprivation and/or loss and to rapidly eliminate excesses of intake. The extent to which the kidney is able to concentrate or dilute urine or specific substances

in it is a useful test of renal function. The daily requirements, sources, organs of excretion, daily average excretion, and sources of excessive loss for water and electrolytes are summarized in Table 9-1. Because all losses require replacement, accurate observation and reporting of the quantity lost by any avenue are important to the welfare of the patient.

Fluid Compartments

The largest component of the body is water. In multicellular organisms body fluids are divided into two large compartments, the intracellular and the extracellular fluids. These two compartments are separated from each other by the cell membrane. Water diffuses more or less freely across this semipermeable membrane. The movement of solutes across the cell membrane is regulated so that the concentration of each component is maintained within a limited range. Extracellular fluid is further divided into two compartments—the intravascular and the interstitial. Intravascular fluid is the fluid component of the blood. Interstitial fluid is that found in the spaces between blood vessels and surrounding cells. Most of the interstitial fluid is a transudate formed by the filtration of blood plasma through the capillary membrane. There are collections of extracellular fluids that are not simple transudates. They are formed by the secretory activity of cells. Examples include the cerebrospinal fluid, gastrointestinal secretions, bile, and pancreatic secretions. In health, potential spaces such as the peritoneal and pleural cavities contain only small amounts of fluid; however, in certain diseases the quantity of peritoneal and/or pleural fluid may be large enough to interfere with body functions. Recent studies have, however, demonstrated that water and electrolytes do not move as freely from some tissues as they do from others. Bone, cartilage, and other dense connective tissues contain large quantities of water and electrolytes. Bone, for example, holds a volume of water about equal to the blood plasma. This water and its electrolytes are not freely exchangeable with other body compartments. Fluid in the interstitial spaces does not appear to be a simple solution of water and the electrolytes dissolved in it. It is held in the tissue spaces by collagen fibers and hyaluronic acid. Hyaluronic acid does not interfere with the capacity of the water to dissolve electrolytes or nonelectrolytes. It enters into the cement substance that binds cells together.

In the extracellular fluid, sodium is the most abundant cation, although it also contains calcium, magnesium, potassium, and trace ele-

[4] Howard S. Frazier: "Renal Regulation of Sodium Balance," *New Eng. J. Med.*, 279:868–75 (Oct. 17) 1968.

TABLE 9-1

Summary of Sources of and Factors Relating to Water and Electrolytes

Substance	Symbols	Normal Concentration in Plasma in mEq/L	Daily Requirement	Source of Intake	Organ of Excretion	Daily Average Excretion	Sources of Excessive Loss
Water	H·HO		1,500–3,000 ml	Fluids, 1000 ml Food, free water 1,000 ml Water of oxidation, 300 ml	Skin Kidney Lung Intestine	1,000–1,500 ml 600–1,000 ml 350 ml 100 ml	Up to 8,000 ml of gastrointestinal secretions per day Burn fluid Renal failure Sweating Mouth breathing Polyuria
Sodium	Na^+	138–145 mEq/L	2–4 g	Food and fluids	Kidney Skin	2–4 g	May be lost when excess loss of fluid from GI tract, or by kidney
Potassium	K^+	3.5–5.5 mEq/L	3–4 g	Abundant in food, especially fruit juices	Kidney		Polyuria, excessive catabolism of cells, catharsis, diarrhea, enemas
Calcium	Ca^{++}	4.5–5.5 mEq/L	800 mg	Milk, dairy products, egg yolks	Intestine, e.g., insoluble soaps Kidney		Renal failure Inadequate intake of vitamin D Hyperparathyroidism
Magnesium	Mg^{++}	1.5–2.5 mEq/L	1.0 mEq/L		Intestine Kidney	200 mg	
Chloride	Cl^-	92–108 mEq/L		With sodium as sodium chloride	Kidney Skin		Losses may be excessive when vomiting, or if gastrointestinal tract suctioning continues
Bicarbonate	$HCO_3^=$	24–31 mEq/L		End product of metabolism	Lung		
Phosphate	$HPO_4^=$			With calcium	Kidney Possibly intestinal tract		See Calcium
Sulfate	$SO_4^=$				Kidney		
Protein+		6–8 g/ 100 ml	40–80 g	Meat, milk, dairy products, eggs, lentils, legumes, etc.	End products of protein metabolism excreted by kidney but not as protein		May be lost via kidney, draining wounds, ulcers, burns
Hydrogen	H^+			Metabolism	Kidney		

ments. In the intracellular fluid the most abundant cation is potassium with other cations present in lesser amounts. Whatever the amount, however, each cation and anion has an important function. For the electrolyte components of each fluid compartment see Figure 9-2.

What factors influence the volume and distribution of water in the body?

The volume and distribution of water in the body vary with the age, sex, and amount of adipose tissue. These differences are illustrated by the Martin family in Figure 9-3. The family

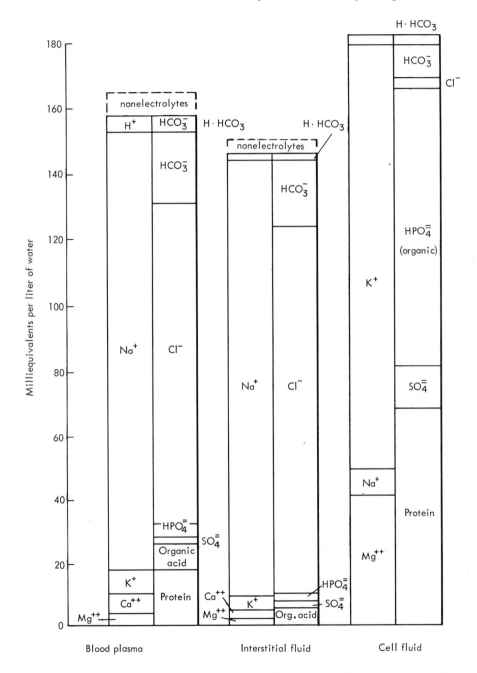

FIGURE 9-2. A comparison of the electrolyte composition of body fluids. (Adapted with permission of Stanford University Press from *Companionship of Water and Electrolytes in the Organization of Body Fluids*, 1951, p. 13, by James L. Gamble.)

is composed of five members—John Martin, aged 30; Mary Martin, aged 28; Billy, aged 9; Suzy, aged 8 weeks; and Mary Martin's mother, Mrs. Bird, aged 68. Because at all ages the intravascular fluid comprises about 5 per cent of the total body weight, the extracellular fluid, as shown in Figure 9-3, has not been divided into interstitial and intravascular compartments. The most marked difference in the distribution of water at the different age levels is in the amount of interstitial fluid. In the newborn baby, the proportion of body water in the interstitial fluid compartment is larger than at any period in life. From Figure 9-3 the reader will note that with advancing age there is a progressive decrease in the proportion of water in the interstitial space, as well as in the total volume of water in the body. Interstitial fluid accounts for 40 per cent of eight-week-old Suzy's weight, 30 per cent of Billy's weight, and only 20 per cent of the weight of the adults. Although not shown in Figure 9-3, the water content of the body falls sharply from birth to about four years of age and then levels off. Maturity, in respect to water and electrolytes, is reached at about 20 years of age. Thenceforth throughout life there is a slow decline in body water. This change is also demonstrated in Figure 9-3. Although water is responsible for 75 per cent of Suzy's weight, it accounts for only 45 per cent of her grandmother's weight. Objective evidence of the loss of water in older age groups is seen in the dry skin and hair of the aged. It is also seen in their flabby muscles and wrinkled skin.

The degree of dryness of the skin should be taken into consideration when planning the number and type of baths for elderly people. Men, in particular, may be troubled by dry and itching skin. For the comfort of the patient, full baths may have to be limited to one or two per week. A mild soap should be selected. Rather than alcohol, a hand cream or lotion, or other emollient should be used for back rubs and applied to other skin areas to reduce dryness. Mrs. Bird finds that her skin is excessively dry and applies an oily lotion to the skin of her legs and arms each day.

Tissues also vary in their water content. Enamel of the teeth is about 3 per cent water. Fat and bone are about 25 per cent water, while active tissues such as muscles, nerves, liver, and skin have a much higher water content. They vary from 70 to 85 per cent water.

SOURCES OF WATER

The maintenance of any homeostatic mechanism depends on a supply of required materials. Water is replenished in the body in two ways: by the ingestion of fluids and preformed water in food and by water of oxidation, or water that is formed while carbohydrate fat, or protein is metabolized. Even solid foods such as meat and vegetables contain from 60 to 97 per cent water. Over 500 ml of water may be derived from these metabolic reactions (oxidation-reduction reactions). (See Chapter 12.) This water is an important consideration in acute renal shut-

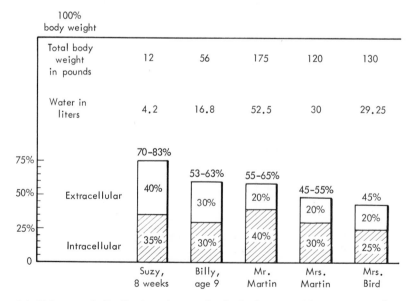

FIGURE 9-3. Volume and distribution of water in the body vary with age, sex, and amount of adipose tissue, as seen in the Martin family.

down. The amount of water from metabolism must be calculated if water intoxication is to be avoided.

The point at which water is normally taken from the external environment into the internal environment is the gastrointestinal tract. Any condition disturbing the function of the gastrointestinal tract may interfere with the patient's intake of fluid. Accurate measurement and recording of the patient's fluid intake, as well as losses by vomiting or diarrhea are essential. Rapid loss of weight is usually indicative of insufficient water intake. As a matter of fact, any gain or loss of weight greater than 0.5 kg per day can be assumed to be due to fluid gain or loss.

LOSSES OF WATER

Water is lost from the body in urine, feces, sweat, and expired air. The quantity lost in feces, by evaporation, and by expired air is obligatory; that is, fluid is lost regardless of the fluid intake. This is not true of urine; the kidney plays a primary role in the homeostasis of water and electrolytes in the body and may greatly increase or decrease the amount of water lost in the urine.

FACTORS INFLUENCING ABILITY TO TOLERATE WATER LOSS

Because some water is stored and because there are effective mechanisms for its renewal and conservation, the need for a continuous intake is not as urgent as is the need for intake of oxygen. Under favorable conditions an adult can live as long as ten days without water. The person who finds himself in a situation where there is an inadequate supply of fresh water can reduce water loss by shading himself from the sun and the wind, thereby reducing evaporation from the skin. He can reduce the amount of urea formed from the oxidation of tissue protein by remaining inactive. Under extreme conditions, such as those found in the desert, survival without water is limited to about two days. Children are more sensitive to water deprivation than are adults. They can survive only about five days without water. The younger the child, the more sensitive he is to water deprivation. Suzy Martin is much more sensitive to water deprivation than the other members of the family. This is true because infants have a relatively greater surface area, a higher metabolic rate, and their kidneys are less efficient in concentrating urine than they are in older children and adults. Suzy loses about twice as much fluid per gram of body weight through her skin as her father does. Any condition that interferes

with Suzy's fluid intake, particularly when this is combined with an excessive loss of fluids, can produce serious effects within a few hours. With a relatively high metabolic rate, water is required to take up the heat produced in oxidation-reduction reactions and carry it to the surface of the body where it is eliminated. With the excessive loss of water, Suzy's temperature can be expected to rise. Because she is unable adequately to retain the volume of her blood by concentrating urine, the electrolytes become concentrated in the blood. Unless treatment is quickly instituted, the circulation may fail, and death may occur.

WATER: ITS PROPERTIES AND FUNCTIONS

Water has a number of properties that make it well suited to its role in the body. It is chemically stable. It is a so-called universal solvent. This does not mean that all substances dissolve in it, but more do than in any other liquid. It has a high ionizing power. It also has a number of properties that make it well suited to its role in temperature regulation; these include its high specific heat, its high latent heat of evaporation, and its great capacity to conduct heat. Its specific heat is the highest for all liquids.

Water functions in the body in many ways. As has been stated, it functions in temperature regulation by taking up large quantities of heat produced by cells and distributing it throughout the body. At the surface of the body, heat is lost to the atmosphere by evaporation of water and the blood is cooled. Because of the large number of substances that are soluble in water, it serves as a vehicle for the transportation of substances to and from cells. In the lung, oxygen goes into solution as it enters the blood. Carbon dioxide is in solution in the blood before it escapes into the alveoli. The volume of blood is dependent on water. Products of metabolism are diluted by water and are thus prevented from injuring cells. End products of metabolism and excesses of intake dissolved in water are excreted by the kidney. Water is necessary to the physiochemical activities of the body. Digestion of food is at least partly accomplished by hydrolysis—the breakdown of molecules through the addition of water. The chemical processes within the cell take place in water. Storage of nutrients depends on water. For each gram of protein deposited in the body, 4 g of water are needed. Growing children therefore require proportionately more water than do adults. Fat requires only 0.2 g of water to store each gram.

Water, as the principal solvent in the body, regulates the osmolality of body fluids. When water is lost from the body in excess of that ingested, body fluids become concentrated and their osmolality is increased. Since the body does not tolerate differences in osmotic pressure between the fluid compartments, water is then shifted from the compartment in which the concentration of water is greatest to the one in which the concentration of electrolyte is greatest. For example, when extracellular fluid is hypertonic in relation to intracellular fluid, water moves from the cell into the interstitial fluid, thereby dehydrating the cell. Conversely, when the interstitial fluid is hypotonic in relation to the cellular fluid, water moves into the cell, causing it to swell. Responses of the body to increased concentration of body fluids or electrolytes, as well as the role of water in the regulation of hydrogen ions, will be discussed later.

Water is essential to all body functions. It is the medium in which the physiochemical activities of the cell take place. In some bodily processes, such as hydrolysis, it is one of the reacting agents. In others, as in oxidation-reduction reactions, it may be a product. It is an essential element in the internal environment of the cell. It is the medium through which or by which all substances are transported to and from the cell and external environment. Without it, life is impossible.

REGULATION OF WATER

As water is removed from the cells, the cells become dehydrated. This causes drying of the mouth and pharynx and may result in the sensation of thirst. Satisfaction of the thirst by ingestion of water may correct the deficit. The kidney can also function to conserve water and protect the concentration of electrolytes in the body fluids. The chain of events leading to the correction of increase in osmotic pressure by the kidney increasing the reabsorption of water is described as follows: Osmoreceptors, especially in the supraoptic nuclei, are sensitive to increased osmotic pressure. They initiate impulses which bring about the release of the antidiuretic hormone (ADH) from the posterior pituitary gland. The antidiuretic hormone increases the permeability of the distal and collecting tubules to water and thereby facilitates and increases the reabsorption of water. A decrease in the osmolality in the extracellular fluid tends to produce the opposite effect. As the extracellular fluid becomes hypotonic in relation to the intracellular fluid, water moves from the extracellular space into the cells in the supraoptic nuclei; special cells in this area act like tiny osmometers, swelling when the extracellular fluid becomes hypotonic and shrinking when it becomes hypertonic. Swelling of the cells is

thought to inhibit the secretion of the antidiuretic hormone and shrinking is presumed to stimulate its secretion. With a decrease in the level of ADH, the quantity of water reabsorbed in the distal and collecting tubules is reduced and the volume excreted in the urine is increased. Conversely, augmentation of the secretion of ADH increases the reabsorption of water by the distal and collecting tubules and decreases the volume of water excreted in the urine.

TABLE 9-2

Factors Influencing the Amount of Water in the Body

Water Balance	
Increase Water In the Body	Decrease Water In the Body
Thirst	Satiety
Retention by the kidney (ADH)	Dilution of ADH
↑ Sodium intake Aldosterone	Decreased secretion of aldosterone
	Decreased sodium intake
↓ Thyroid hormones	Increased loss of sodium
Heart failure	Increased metabolic rate
Edema	Lack of insulin, resulting in glycosuria
	Acidosis
	Vomiting
	Diarrhea
	Gastric suction
	Mouth breathing
	Tracheostomy
	Sweating
	Blistering of skin
	Large draining wounds
	Obesity

As was stated earlier, body fluids are separated into compartments by the semipermeable membranes surrounding cells and capillaries. These membranes serve as the points where exchange takes place between each cell and its fluid environment (the interstitial fluid) and between the interstitial fluid and the plasma within the circulatory system. Five factors influence the movement of fluids across the capillary membrane. They are (1) capillary permeability, (2) diffusion, (3) filtration pressure, (4) the colloid osmotic pressure of the blood, and (5) interstitial fluid pressure. More fluid moves from the intravascular to the interstitial compartment than returns by way of the capillary membrane. This excess fluid is restored to the blood by the lymphatic system.

In general, capillaries are freely permeable to low molecular weight electrolytes and nonelectrolytes, and they are much less permeable to blood proteins or other high molecular weight substances. The degree to which capillaries are permeable to proteins differs in various parts of the body. Those in the sinusoids of the liver, the heart, the lungs, and the gastrointestinal tract are quite permeable to protein. Those in the skin and skeletal muscles are much less permeable. Capillaries forming the glomeruli of the kidney are nearly impermeable to protein. The degree of capillary permeability influences the volume of water and the size of the molecules that can escape into the interstitial fluid compartment. For example, Mrs. Bird complains that on warm days her feet swell. One of the contributing factors is that, with an increase in the environmental temperature, peripheral blood vessels dilate to increase heat loss. As the capillaries dilate, permeability is increased and with it the volume of interstitial fluid is enlarged. Just as, or perhaps more, important, the filtration pressure at the arterial end of the capillary may increase, forcing more fluid out of the capillaries. A variety of physical and chemical agents increase capillary permeability. Some common examples include anoxia, some of the products of inflammation, bacterial toxins, and carbon dioxide. In any condition in which capillary membrane permeability is increased, the volume of fluid and the size of the molecules that move from the intravascular to the interstitial space can be expected to be increased.

Water and solutes move across the capillary membrane by diffusion, filtration, and osmosis. Each of these forces affects the transfer of fluid into and out of the capillary. In general, diffusion of substances to which the capillary is freely permeable occurs along the entire length of the capillary and takes place in both directions. An increase in the concentration of a solute in either the blood plasma or the interstitial fluids can be anticipated to be followed by an increase in the rate at which it diffuses through the capillary membrane.

Whereas substances move into and out of the capillary by diffusion, the primary effect of filtration is to transfer fluid from the capillary to the interstitial space. The filtration pressure of the blood in the capillary is determined by (1) the arterial blood pressure, (2) the rate of the flow of blood through the capillary, and (3) the venous pressure. Arterial blood pressure is affected by the volume of blood, the force of the heart beat, the resistance of the arteries and arterioles to the blood flow, and the viscosity of the blood. At the tissue level, capillary blood flow is regulated primarily by arteriolar constriction or dilatation. Constriction of arterioles decreases blood flow into the capillaries, thereby decreasing filtration pressure. Conversely dilatation of the arterioles increases blood flow into the capillary and thereby increases the filtration pressure. Because the circulatory system is a closed system, the effect of arteriolar constriction is an increase in blood pressure behind the constriction and a fall in pressure distal to it.

Normally the hydrostatic pressure of the blood is much higher in the arteriolar end of the capillary than it is in the venous end. This results in a corresponding decrease in filtration at the venous end. The primary reason for the drop in hydrostatic pressure of the blood is that considerable energy is required to overcome the resistance offered by the capillary to the flow of blood. The effect of increasing resistance to the flow of a fluid on its movement can be demonstrated by placing water in a tuberculin syringe and in a 50-ml syringe. Water escapes from the tuberculin syringe very slowly because much of it comes in contact with the wall of the syringe and the wall offers resistance to the movement of the water. Water escapes very rapidly from the larger syringe because little of the water comes in contact with its wall. In general, the smaller the lumen of a tube, the greater the surface that comes in contact with the fluid contained in the tube and the greater the resistance to its movement.

Any condition that interferes with the flow of blood through a vein will increase the hydrostatic pressure of the blood in the capillary by increasing the volume of blood in the capillary. The effect is similar to that produced by placing a dam in a stream. The volume and pressure of fluid behind the dam are increased. This increases filtration of fluid out of the capillary. The quantity of fluid that actually leaves the capillary by filtration is determined by the relationship of the filtration or hydrostatic pressure of the blood to the interstitial fluid pressure. The greater the hydrostatic pressure of the blood in relation to that of the interstitial fluid, the greater the net filtration pressure.

The main force responsible for the transfer of fluids from the interstitial space into the capillary is created by the colloid osmotic pressure of the blood. Normally the concentration of protein is greater in the blood plasma than it is in interstitial fluid. In health, the level of protein in the blood plasma ranges from 6.5 to 8 g per 100 ml. Of this, albumin comprises the largest fraction, with an average range of from 4.0 to 5.2 g per 100 ml. Because it has the smallest molecules of the blood proteins, the effect of albumin on the colloid osmotic pressure of the blood is greater than can be accounted for by its weight. The critical factor in osmotic pressure is the number of particles per unit of water and not the size of each particle. For example, if a particle the size of a grain of sand exerts approximately the same osmotic effect as one the size of a marble, then a cupful of osmotically active particles the size of a grain of sand will have many times the effect of a cupful of particles the size of marbles.

The extent to which osmotic pressure is effective in returning fluid to the capillary depends on a number of factors. One is the difference between the colloid osmotic pressure of the blood and that of the interstitial fluid. Anything that decreases the colloid osmotic pressure of the blood or increases that of the interstitial fluid will reduce the return of fluid to the capillary. The relationship of the hydrostatic pressure of the blood to its colloid osmotic pressure will also affect the rate of exchange between the capillary and the interstitial fluid. A rise in the hydrostatic pressure in relation to the colloid osmotic pressure of the blood will increase the quantity of fluid in the interstitial compartment.

Any condition that results in a serious loss of protein from the blood can be expected to interfere with the return from the interstitial fluid compartment to the blood. Examples of conditions in which blood protein levels fall include severe and prolonged starvation and continued loss of body fluids containing protein, such as in severe burns and in kidney disorders in which protein is lost in the urine. A blood albumin level of 2.0 g or less is usually associated with an increase in the volume of interstitial fluid, that is, with edema. Restoration of the normal distribution of water depends on reducing the loss of protein from the body and raising the level of osmotically active substances in the blood. This is sometimes difficult to do. When the condition is severe, the patient may require intravenous infusions of blood, plasma, of plasma expanders. If the patient is able to take food by mouth, he should be given appropriate assistance and encouraged to eat.

LYMPHATIC DRAINAGE

The return of interstitial fluid back into the capillaries is usually not complete. The lymphatic capillaries take up excess tissue fluid and return it to the blood stream via the lymphatic and thoracic ducts. Any obstruction to the flow of fluid in the lymphatics leads to the accumulation of interstitial fluid in the tissues. Following extensive injury to the soft tissues, scar tissue formed during the healing process may obstruct the lymph channels draining the area. In tropical regions, lymph channels may be obstructed by parasites; the resulting edema can cause various parts of the body to swell so enormously that one of these diseases has been called elephantiasis. Lymphedema can also be a troublesome problem after extensive radical mastectomy. In this operation, the axillary lymph nodes are removed, thereby interfering with the flow of lymph. This can result in swelling of the hand and arm on the affected side.

FACTORS IN MOVEMENT OF FLUID BETWEEN INTRACELLULAR AND INTERSTITIAL COMPARTMENTS

As stated earlier, sodium ions have about the same concentration in plasma and interstitial fluid. Therefore they have little effect on the movement of fluids into and out of the capillary. Sodium, however, is responsible for about one half of the osmotic pressure of extracellular fluid. Because it is present in relatively small amounts in the intracellular fluid, it is an important factor in the movement of fluid between the intracellular and extracellular compartments. Any condition that results in the retention of sodium in the body will generally be accompanied by the retention of water. Whatever the specific factor, any disorder that causes a retention of sodium in the extracellular fluids is usually accompanied by the retention of water and an expansion of the extracellular fluid volume. In persons whose mechanisms for eliminating sodium are defective or persons treated with drugs that increase the effectiveness of sodium-saving mechanisms, limitation of sodium intake can be expected to reduce water retention. For these reasons, sodium is often restricted in patients with heart and liver disorders, especially if there is edema formation. Sodium is also often restricted in patients who are treated with adrenal steroids. All salts containing sodium are interdicted, not just sodium chloride. Patients and those preparing their food should be taught to read the labels on prepared foods and medicines to see if sodium-containing salts are present. Foods, such as cured meats, to which salt has been added in preparation should ordinarily be avoided.

In health, a balance is maintained between the amount of fluid leaving and returning to the intravascular fluid compartment. The main mechanisms involved in this exchange are summarized in Figure 9-4.

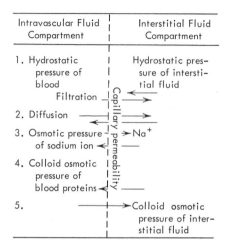

FIGURE 9-4. The mechanisms by which fluids are exchanged between the intravascular and interstitial fluid compartments. Arrows indicate direction of flow. Lymphatic drainage is not indicated.

In most discussions of fluid and electrolyte balance, more attention is given to the mechanisms that regulate the volume and concentration of extracellular fluid than to those that control the intracellular fluid. (See Figure 9-4.) This is partly because intracellular fluid is so difficult to obtain for study. Because all body fluids are interrelated, the state of the intracellular fluid compartment can be assumed from the studies of extracellular fluids.

Electrolytes

Body fluids are composed of water, electrolytes, and nonelectrolytes. The electrolyte structure, which is described in Figure 9-2, has been modified from Gamble.[5] In each diagram, cations are to the left and anions to the right. The total number of cations is equal to the total number of anions. Extracellular fluid also contains small amounts of nonelectrolytes. Unless they are greatly increased, they do not affect the behavior of extracellular fluid.[6] Concentra-

[5] James L. Gamble: *Lane Medical Lectures: Companionship of Water and Electrolytes in the Organization of Body Fluids* (Stanford, Calif.: Stanford University Press, 1951), p. 13.
[6] Gamble, *op. cit.*, p. 12.

tions of each electrolyte are expressed in milliequivalents per liter.

Gamble was the first to draw attention to the similarities between the composition of sea water and extracellular fluid. Although there are marked similarities, there are also significant differences. One is that sea water contains a higher concentration of most of the electrolytes. Some reasons for the changes in the electrolyte concentration of sea water are discussed previously. Other differences derive from the fact that extracellular fluid is part of a living system. As a result, it has a higher concentration of bicarbonate anion and contains protein. The latter is not found in sea water.

How do electrolytes function within the body?

Comparison of the composition of the fluids contained in the extracellular and intracellular compartments shows that the principal cation in extracellular fluid is sodium while that of the intracellular fluid is potassium. At one time scientists thought that sodium was not able to enter the cell or potassium to leave it. Evidence now indicates that sodium does enter the cell and energy is expended in preventing sodium from accumulating in the cell. The mechanism for preventing its accumulation is not clear. In conditions accompanied by starvation or semistarvation, sodium tends to replace potassium to the detriment of cellular activities. Improvement in a patient's condition may require an increase in the intake of food. The principal anions in the intracellular and extracellular fluid can also be seen to differ. The principal anion in extracellular fluid is the chloride ion, while that in intracellular fluid is the phosphate ion. With the exception of the red blood cell, the quantity of chloride ion found within cells is believed to be small.

All the cations and anions entering into the composition of body fluids have important functions in the body. Healthy functioning of cells depends on the maintenance of the level of each electrolyte within its so-called normal range. Deviations outside this range in either a downward or upward direction can be anticipated to have adverse effects on bodily function. Some electrolytes, such as sodium, are present in relatively large amounts. Others, such as chromium, are found only in traces. Whether the quantity is large or small, they are all essential to cell activity.

The daily average requirements, the sources of intake, and the organs of excretion for water and the more important electrolytes are summarized in Table 9-1. Iron and the trace elements have not been included in the table. Although they are indispensable for normal function, they are not pertinent to this discussion of fluid and electrolyte balance. They will therefore be discussed in Chapters 10 and 12.

Electrolytes participate in at least four basic physiological processes. These are (1) the distribution of water, (2) the osmolality of body fluids, (3) neuromuscular irritability, and (4) acid-base balance. The volume and distribution of water depend primarily on the presence of dissociated electrolytes and proteins. The volume of extracellular water is regulated primarily by sodium. When the concentration of sodium in the extracellular fluid rises, water moves across the semipermeable membrane of the cell in the direction of the interstitial fluid. Water thus serves to correct the increased osmolality of the extracellular fluid, thereby reducing the number of ions per unit of fluid.

SODIUM REGULATION

The regulation of the level of the sodium ion is complex, involving hormonal and nervous factors. Although all the hormones of the adrenal cortex increase the reabsorption of sodium, the mineralocorticoid with the most potent effect is aldosterone. Although ACTH from the anterior pituitary gland directly and profoundly affects the secretion of most adrenocortical hormones, it is not a primary factor in aldosterone production. Under appropriate circumstances, ACTH can cause aldosterone to be secreted, so that ACTH can be described as a sufficient but not necessary factor for its release. Aldosterone secretion is stimulated by many factors including decreased sodium, increased potassium, and increased angiotensin II in the blood flowing through the adrenal cortex.

A volume receptor may lie in the juxtaglomerular apparatus.[7] A drop in the blood pressure or blood flow through this area may stimulate the local release of renin. Renin acts on angiotensinogen converting it to angiotensin I which is then converted to angiotensin II. Angiotensin II then increases the release of aldosterone. With the increase in aldosterone, sodium and water are conserved and potassium is excreted. Water conservation increases blood volume and thus blood flow through the kidney. Control of sodium excretion by aldosterone is not rapid and it is not complete. Experimentally, there is a time lag between the administration of aldosterone and its effect. Further, sodium loading brings about an increase in sodium excretion that is independent of glomerular filtration rate and aldosterone secretion.[8]

Williams [9] states that the kidney is innervated by both the sympathetic and parasympathetic parts of the autonomic nervous system. Until recently the function of the autonomic nervous system has been thought to be limited to regulating blood flow through the kidney. Williams postulates that the autonomic nervous system may well have other functions as acetylcholine (parasympathetic) increases the excretion of sodium chloride and stimulation of the sympathetic nervous system is accompanied by sodium chloride retention.

Frazier [10] relates the effect of the nervous system to blood supply of the kidney by saying that a variety of neural stimuli and circulatory stresses have a similar effect: they cause a reduction in the perfusion of the outer cortex of the kidney. With ischemia of the outer cortex of the kidney, excretion of sodium is decreased. With increased conservation of sodium, water is also saved and the blood volume is maintained or increased. Whether or not the patient is protected by this mechanism depends on the degree of renal ischemia, how long it lasts, and what caused it.

Summary

The regulation of water and electrolytes provides an excellent example of the functioning of a homeostatic mechanism. To summarize the processes involved in the homeostasis of water and electrolytes, we will return to Mr. Martin. On a hot, sunny Saturday afternoon he mowed the lawn. Because he was exercising and the day was warm, he perspired freely. Every now and then he stopped to mop his brow. By the time he had finished, his shirt and underwear were saturated. Evaporation of sweat, because of its cooling effect, prevented a building of heat in Mr. Martin's body. He was thereby able to keep his body temperature within physiological limits, despite an increase in heat production that accompanied his activity and the warmth of the day. His sweat was a hypotonic solution of water and electrolytes. Let us suppose that Mr. Martin lost a liter of water in the hour he spent in mowing the lawn. As water was taken from the blood for the secretion of sweat, his blood plasma became concentrated, and developed a greater osmolality than the fluid in his interstitial space. Water was attracted across his semipermeable capillary membranes from the interstitial fluid by the increase in the osmolality of the blood.

[7] Frazier, *op. cit.*, p. 870.
[8] *Ibid.*, p. 871.

[9] Ronald L. Williams: "A Re-Evaluation of the Role of the Autonomic Nervous System upon Renal Function from the View of a Pharmacologist," *Perspect. Biol. Med.*, **10**:257 (Winter) 1967.
[10] *Op. cit.*, p. 872.

If the quantity of fluid added to the blood was not sufficient to restore its normal dilution, osmoreceptors in the internal carotid arteries and the supraoptic nuclei were stimulated. Stimulation of the osmoreceptors resulted in an increase in secretion of antidiuretic hormone (ADH). Because of the effect of ADH, Mr. Martin's kidney increased the reabsorption of water and the concentration of his urine.

If the loss of water and sodium in the sweat decreased blood volume enough to reduce the flow or pressure of the blood in the adrenal cortex, increased amounts of aldosterone would be secreted. The aldosterone in turn would cause increased absorption of sodium and water in the kidney. As fluid moved from Mr. Martin's interstitial fluid into his blood, its osmotic pressure increased. Water was then attracted from the cells to correct the situation, creating a sensation of thirst. Mr. Martin then entered the house and told his wife, "I'm thirsty. How about a pitcher of lemonade?" Later he sat on the patio and drank lemonade and ate some potato chips. The water in the lemonade helped restore his blood volume to normal and probably increased it to above normal temporarily. The salt on the potato chips helped replace the sodium chloride lost in sweating. After the volume, concentration, and distribution of his body fluids were restored to preexercise levels, the excess water and electrolytes were excreted by his kidneys. When blood volume was restored and the osmolality of his cells returned to normal, his thirst was quenched.

Disturbances in Body Fluid and Electrolyte Balance

The capacity to maintain the stability of body fluids is greatest during youth and early middle life and is least at the extremes of life. Many illnesses are accompanied by some disturbance in water and electrolyte balance. In some illnesses the disturbances are minor. In others, the recovery of the patient may depend on the ability to correct disturbances and to restore and maintain the normal regulatory mechanisms. In these patients the regulation of fluid and electrolyte balance may be a major objective of the therapy. The constancy of the fluid environment of cells, as well as of the intracellular fluid, depends on (1) the supply of required materials; (2) the regulation of intake, transportation, and storage; and (3) the excretion of excessive wastes and/or excess of required materials.

Disturbances in fluid and electrolyte balance may result from hypo-, hyper-, or disorganized function. A disturbance in the capacity of one organ to regulate one mechanism may set into action a chain of events leading to widespread and complicated disturbances.

Disturbances in body fluids are usually characterized by some change in volume, concentration, osmotic pressure, or hydrogen ion concentration. The specific effects on the patient will depend on factors such as whether the disturbance is local or general, how severe it is, and its effects on other components of the body fluid. Disturbances in a single component seldom occur. They are usually multiple and often complicated. Each substance entering into the composition of one of the fluid compartments has a significant function. Alterations in the level of any one component of body fluids outside the so-called normal range is likely to be attended by adverse effects and changes in other compartments.

The most frequent disturbances in fluid and electrolyte balance are those resulting from an excess or deficit of water or of sodium, potassium, calcium, or hydrogen ions. The effects of a disturbance on a particular person or patient will depend on (1) the direction and degree of change, (2) the effects the disturbance has on the other components of the system, and (3) the effectiveness of the body's mechanisms for correcting or adapting to the disturbance. For example, as Mr. Martin mowed his lawn, he lost increased amounts of water and electrolytes in sweat, which is a hypotonic solution of sodium chloride. His mechanisms for adapting to these losses were efficient and he was able to maintain the stability of his extracellular fluids.

How does illness affect fluid and electrolyte equilibrium?

In illness there are many causes of disturbances in fluid and electrolyte equilibrium. They fall into the following categories: (1) a simple deficit or excess in the supply of water and/or electrolytes; (2) inability to ingest or to absorb water or electrolytes; (3) failure of the kidney to eliminate excesses of exogenous or endogenous origin; (4) excessive losses through the skin, gastrointestinal tract, lung, or kidney; (5) loss of fluids through abnormal avenues or as the result of injury to tissues, as in surgery and other trauma, fistulae, burned tissues, blood loss, or inflamed serous membranes; (6) disturbances in the transportation system; and (7) shifts of fluid from one compartment to another, as in ascites, edema, burns, or acute gastric dilatation. The ultimate effect on the individual patient will be determined by how these changes affect the volume, distribution, osmolality, and concentration of fluid and electrolytes in each compartment.

Water Deficit

Probably the most frequent disturbance in water and electrolyte balance is a simple deficit of water, with output of water exceeding its intake. This may simply be the result of an inadequate intake or an excessive output. This leads to an increase in the concentration and osmolality of the extracellular fluid. Water may be lost alone or in combination with electrolytes. Sweating causes proportionately greater loss of water than of sodium chloride. Diarrhea in the early stages has the same effect. In breathing, water with little or no electrolyte content is lost. Patients who breathe rapidly and deeply lose more water from the lungs than those who breathe normally. Water losses can be expected to be further increased in patients who breathe through their mouths. Often, patients who have increased loss of water through respiration are those who have difficulty in replacing water by their own efforts. Lethargic, comatose, or confused patients are especially likely to develop water deficits unless attention is paid to keeping up their fluid intake. Patients with fever also lose increased amounts of water. Loss of water from the skin is of two types: insensible water loss and sweat (sensible water loss). Insensible water loss refers to loss of water directly from the skin or other body surfaces without our being aware of its presence. This water loss results in little or no electrolyte loss. In contrast, sweat can be seen and felt and has a sodium and chloride content which is about one third or one fourth of that which is found in the plasma. Thus, increased insensible water loss caused by excessive respiration or fever without sweat, is pure water loss. Increased loss of sweat, on the other hand, can result in significant deficits of both water and salt. Maintenance of adequate fluid intake under these circumstances is essential and may require careful planning, patience, and effort.

PHYSIOLOGICAL EFFECTS OF LOSS OF WATER

In any condition in which the loss of water from the body exceeds that of intake, water is lost from the extracellular fluid. As a result, the remaining extracellular fluid becomes hypertonic in relation to the intracellular fluid. Water can then be expected to move from within the cell to the more concentrated extracellular fluid. This results in cellular dehydration. In the person who is conscious and competent, the most prominent and reliable symptom is thirst. When water is available and the patient is able to ingest and absorb it, the condition is easily corrected by drinking water.

When the loss of water continues without a comparable loss of electrolytes, the amount of available intracellular fluid may be insufficient to correct the water deficit in the extracellular fluid. This results in an increase in the level of hemoglobin, nonprotein nitrogen, sodium, and other electrolytes in the blood. The hematocrit, that is, the proportion of red blood cells to the blood plasma, also rises. The kidney adapts by excreting a small volume of concentrated urine. In patients with normal kidneys, a urine output of less than 500 to 800 ml per 24 hours is usually indicative of an insufficient intake of water. As dehydration increases, skin and mucous membranes become dry and parched. The tongue becomes wrinkled and furry. Sordes, collections of dried secretions and other debris, are formed in the mouth and on the lips. When fluid losses are great, water may even be taken from extracellular spaces, such as the eyes, with the result that the eyeballs become soft. In infants and young children, fever may result from dehydration alone. Irritability, muscle twitching, and eventually drowsiness and coma result as the brain becomes progressively dehydrated.

When any condition disturbs the balance between the intake and output of water so that more water is lost from the body than is replaced, the extracellular fluid is decreased in volume and becomes hypertonic in relation to the intracellular fluid. Since the body does not tolerate differences in osmotic pressure, intracellular fluid moves from the cell to the extracellular fluid. The increase in osmotic pressure in certain cells stimulates the sensation of thirst. As a result of decreased blood flow through the kidney and increased secretion of the antidiuretic hormone, the kidney secretes a small volume of concentrated urine. When the condition is allowed to persist for a long period, the body's mechanisms for adaptation fail. Circulatory collapse followed by death is the result.

PREVENTION OF WATER DEFICIT

For many patients, the prevention of a deficit of water involves little more than providing adequate amounts of water in a clean and palatable form. From a study reported by Walter,[11] the water offered to patients in carafes does not always meet the latter criteria. The water provided to patients was often grossly contaminated with microorganisms, unpalatable, and possibly unsafe for drinking. Two practices contributed

[11] Carl W. Walter et al.: "Bacteriology of the Bedside Carafe," New Eng. J. Med., 259:1198–1202 (Dec. 18) 1958.

to the contamination of the water. The carafes in which the water was served had narrow necks. This made thorough cleaning difficult. Ice used to chill the water was handled by hand rather than with the tongs provided for this purpose. The net result was that patients were served foul-smelling, potentially unsafe water.

Some patients require assistance with meeting their need for water. The nurse may have to help patients who, because of their age or the nature or degree of their illness, are unable to meet their own need for water. The amount and type of assistance needed by patients varies greatly. The apathetic, the confused, or the very ill patient will require more attention than the patient who is alert and thirsty. The patient may be completely dependent on the nurse. When the patient is unable to drink unless water is placed in his mouth, a cup with a spout, a teaspoon, or a drinking tube filled with water may be used. When water is placed in the mouth, care should be taken to adjust the patient's position so swallowing is favored and the danger of aspiration of fluid is minimized. The sitting position is most satisfactory. When a patient is in the supine position, his head should, if possible, be turned to the side. Those on mechanical respirators should be instructed to swallow during expiration. Another patient may only require that fluids be placed within easy reaching distance and an explanation of why a given fluid intake is desirable. Some patients will more willingly drink water that is iced. Others refuse to drink water, but will take other types of fluids such as ginger ale, broth, or tea. Whatever the problem, the nurse has a responsibility not only to identify it, but also, within the limits of the situation, to try to find a solution.

Attention should be given to the distribution of the patient's fluid intake over the ordinary waking hours. The patient should be observed for signs and symptoms indicating that his need for water is being met. In addition to the absence of thirst, a urine output of at least 500 to 800 ml in 24 hours, lack of irritability, and moist, clean mucous membranes are all indications that the patient's fluid intake is adequate. Conversely, a urine output of less than 500 ml, irritability, and dry, cracked mucous membranes, with sordes on the lips and in the mouth are indicative of an inadequate fluid intake. Day-to-day loss of more than a pound of weight indicates an insufficient intake of water or an excessive loss of fluid.

PARENTERAL FLUID ADMINISTRATION

Following surgical procedures involving the gastrointestinal tract and related structures, and in acute illness, the patient may not tolerate fluids by mouth. Fluids must then be administered parenterally, usually by intravenous infusion. The dangers to which the patient is exposed are more numerous than when fluids are taken by mouth. Precautions should be taken to make certain the patient gets the correct solution, in the proper amounts, and at the rate prescribed. Attention should also be given to maintaining the sterility of the solution and equipment. Although all patients should be observed regularly throughout the period when fluids are being administered, observation is of special importance in those whose homeostatic mechanisms are inadequate or defective. When the rate at which fluids are to be administered is prescribed, some method should be used to simplify checking. For example, a marker may be placed on the bottle of solution, indicating the number of drops per minute or milliliters per hour. Devices are available that can be set to regulate the rate of flow automatically.

The patient who receives a blood transfusion is exposed to all the risks of patients receiving intravenous fluids. In addition, care must be taken to ensure that the patient is given blood that has been properly cross-matched for him, and to prevent air embolism. Most hospitals have policies for the identification of blood which, when followed, reduce to a minimum the danger of giving the patient the wrong type of blood. These policies should always be followed.

According to Tarail,[12] the possibility of air embolism during blood transfusion is not sufficiently appreciated. Although air embolism is possible in the administration of any intravenous injection, it is greatest when a Y setup is used. The point in the administration of blood when air embolism is most likely to occur is after the blood transfusion has been completed and the stopcock on the tubing leading to the saline bottle has been opened. The effect of this is illustrated in Figure 9-5. When clamps one and two are fully open and clamp three is only partly open, the pressure above clamp three is greater than atmospheric pressure. Below clamp three, the pressure is less than atmospheric pressure. Fluid can be expected to move from the area of greater to that of lesser pressure. As the pressure above clamp three is lessened, air is sucked through the blood bottle and into the tubing below clamp three, that is, air replaces the blood. To prevent air embolism, Tarail[13] suggests that when clamp three is opened, it should be opened wide, and clamp two closed. This prevents air from entering the system via the blood bottle. Last, the rate of flow of fluid

[12] Robert Tarail: "Practice of Fluid Therapy," *JAMA*, 171:45–46 (Sept. 5) 1959.
[13] *Ibid.*, p. 46.

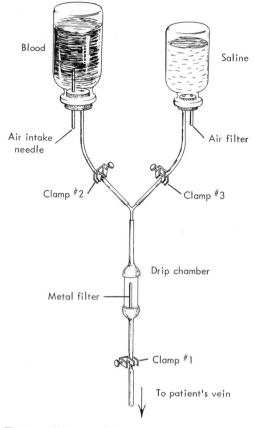

Blood

Saline

Air intake needle

Air filter

Clamp #2

Clamp #3

Drip chamber

Metal filter

Clamp #1

To patient's vein

FIGURE 9-5. Y-type blood transfusion administration set.

to the patient's comfort and to the stability of his fluid and electrolyte balance than do fluids administered in a 6-hour period. Patients had less thirst when fluids were distributed over a longer period. Talbot also found that fluid balance was the same whether fluids were given by mouth or by intraveous infusion.

The rate at which fluids can and should be administered varies with the condition of the patient and the concentration of the solution. As much as 600 ml of an isotonic solution can be safely administered in an hour. Under emergency situations the rate may be increased so that the patient receives as much as 2,000 ml per hour. The patient must, however, be under constant supervision. Should the urinary output exceed 50 ml per hour, the rate of infusion should be decreased, because the amount of solution the patient would be receiving is too great. In elderly patients the rate of flow should be slower than in younger ones. The concentration and the composition of the fluid also affect the rate at which it can be safely administered. Hypotonic solutions should not be given. Solutions with less than 5 per cent glucose or with a concentration of cations or anions less than 150 mEq per liter can be considered hypotonic. Hypertonic solutions should not be administered at a rate faster than 200 ml per hour. The maximum rate of flow for glucose solutions is 0.5 g per kilogram of body weight per hour. A more rapid rate results in glycosuria and the loss of potassium. When there is a question about the rate at which a solution should be administered, the nurse who is responsible for the care of the patient should consult with the patient's physician.

Except in serious emergencies, blood is usually transfused at a rate of about 500 ml, each 2 to 4 hours. In dire emergencies, however, it may have to be given under pressure at rates up to 100 ml per minute. Care must be taken not to introduce air or fibrin clots. If at all avoidable, drugs should never be administered with blood or injected into blood transfusions or the intravenous tubing used for the transfusion. If this must be done, one should be certain that the drug is compatible with the blood and its constituents. Calcium should never be given in blood or in the same tubing with the blood because it neutralizes sodium citrate used as an anticoagulant, and causes clotting.

In the regulation of the flow of the solution, both the number of drops per minute and the size of each drop are significant in the determination of the number of milliliters delivered per hour. Most intravenous sets have tubing in the drip chambers that deliver 10 to 20 drops per milliliter. Microdrip tubing sets usually deliver 45 to 60 per milliliter. Individual manu-

should be regulated by placing clamp one as close to the patient as is possible.

Another risk to the patient receiving parenteral fluids or blood transfusions is pulmonary edema. This danger is greatest in those receiving repeated blood transfusions, in elderly patients, and in persons who have a limited cardiac or renal reserve. This hazard can be reduced by maintaining a slow rate of flow of blood or solution. Patients receiving parenteral fluids or blood transfusions require regular and frequent observation. Should the patient become short of breath, the flow of the blood or fluid should be discontinued and the physician notified.

Not only is the rate of flow of parenteral solutions a factor in the safety of the patient, but it affects his comfort and the stability of his fluid and the electrolyte balance as well. Studies reported by Talbot,[14] indicate that fluids given over a 12- to 24-hour period contribute more

[14] Nathan B. Talbot *et al.:* "Application of Homeostatic Principles to the Management of Nephritic Patients," *New Eng. J. Med.,* **255:**655–62 (Oct. 4) 1956.

facturers should provide this data on the package. No matter how carefully the rate is set, it can be expected to change, especially if the patient changes the position of his hand or arm.

Although parenteral injections are everyday procedures to hospital personnel, this is not necessarily true for patients. Patients receiving them are often very ill. Patients who receive intravenous injections present special problems not only because they are often seriously ill, but also because intravenous injections carry special risks. Patients with marginal renal or cardiac reserve can easily be put into pulmonary edema or congestive heart failure, especially if the infusion rate is too rapid. In some hospitals, patients are instructed to call the nurse when the solution stops running or when the bottle becomes nearly empty. Before a patient is asked to do this, however, the nurse should be sure the patient is emotionally and physically well enough to assume this responsibility. Moreover, the nurse should not rely on the patient and should continue to observe him closely. Calls for help should be answered promptly. If there is any evidence of increased anxiety, the nurse should resume full responsibility for observing the fluid level. The importance of this to the sick patient is illustrated by an excerpt from a letter written by Mrs. Blonde, who wrote to a friend concerning her experience in a hospital after a cholecystectomy: "to have to supervise every step of your own care when you feel rotten is, to say the very least, very disturbing. I had to be sure that I stayed awake to watch the I.V.'s, blood, etc., because, sure as anything, if I dropped off to sleep they would run dry, etc., etc. This happened even after I had discussed it with the head nurse and she had assured me that I could relax because they would watch it very closely." Whether Mrs. Blonde's physical safety was threatened is not known; certainly, she felt unsafe and neglected. Energy and rest she should have been using for recovery were expended in protecting herself against possible injury.

Attention should also be given to the patient's general comfort. When the needle or cannula is inserted over a joint, the part should be supported by a padded board or splint. When necessary, the patient should be assisted in moving and turning. When a patient receiving intravenous fluids is ambulated, enough assistance should be available to give the patient the help he requires. He should be told what to expect and what is expected of him. This may be an everyday procedure to the nurse, but this is not true for the patient.

As stated earlier, a deficit of water in the body is reflected in a decrease in the volume of extracellular fluid and a corresponding increase in its concentration. Unless the loss of fluid, including whole blood, is great or continued, the condition is corrected by an increased fluid intake and/or by dehydration of cells. The body's mechanisms for adapting to changes in the volume of extracellular fluid are such that the blood volume is kept relatively constant. When, however, the loss of water from the body is excessive, blood volume cannot be adequately maintained. The seriousness of the situation depends on the extent to which the decrease in the volume of blood interferes with the nutrition of vital structures. (See Chapter 11.)

Water Excess

Water may be found in the body in excess as well as in deficit. With an excess of water there is an increase in the volume of water in one or more of the fluid compartments. This then alters the osmotic pressure relationship between the intracellular and the extracellular fluid compartments. Since materials from the external environment enter and leave the body by way of the extracellular fluid, an excess of water is usually first reflected in a change in the extracellular fluid volume. Neither the healthy nor the sick will ordinarily drink themselves into water intoxication, but they may occasionally be persuaded to do so. In the sick, the usual source is water administered by intravenous infusion. Water of oxidation may contribute to the total quantity of water in the body. Water intoxication need not develop if attention is given to the fact that the patient's fluid intake is in excess of his total fluid output. The patient's weight also provides evidence for or against the storage of water. A gain in weight by a patient who is ingesting a limited amount of food should create more than a suspicion that water intake is exceeding its loss. For each pound of weight gained, about a pint of fluid is retained. Tarail [15] states that, in the absence of food intake, a patient should be expected to lose about 14 oz per day.

To obtain an accurate weight, the patient should be weighed at the same time each day and with the same amount of clothing. When at all possible, the patient should be weighed in the morning before breakfast, after having emptied his bladder. If he is able to stand on a scale, the simplest way is to remove all clothing except a hospital gown, and have the patient step onto a paper towel that has been placed on the scale. If he is weighed on a bed scale, the same amount of covering can be used each day, or it can be weighed each time and subtracted from the total. The scale should be balanced before the weight is taken. Accurate weighing of the

[15] *Op. cit.,* p. 48.

patient contributes data which, when added to other facts, can be used to judge the patient's response to therapy. It is probably the best single measure of the state of the patient's fluid intake. Improperly done, the weight obtained is worthless. It may even be the basis for making harmful changes in therapy. To state this another way, the value of the information obtained by weighing a patient depends, as do the data in any scientific investigation, on the care with which the variables are controlled.

REDUCED SERUM OSMOLALITY

An excess of water dilutes the sodium (hyponatremia) and other osmotically active substances in the extracellular fluid. This dilution results in hypotonicity and a decrease in the osmolality of the extracellular fluid. As a consequence of the loss of osmotic activity, water moves from the extracellular fluid into the cell, causing it to swell. The symptoms presented by the patient have their origin in disturbed cerebral function. Initially, these symptoms are probably caused by the swelling of neurons. They include disturbed thought and behavior. If the condition is allowed to progress, coma and death may follow. In general, the severity of the symptoms is related to the rapidity of change and not to the extent of the hyponatremia or the dilution. For example, slow development of hyponatremia from the use of diuretics is generally fairly well tolerated. Rapid development of hyponatremia with excess water infusions may cause convulsions and death.

As has been previously emphasized, thirst is a reliable indicator of the need for water. For a variety of reasons, the quantity of water ingested may be insufficient or in excess of the needs of the individual. In health, the kidney does a remarkably efficient job of removing or conserving water. Under most circumstances, water intoxication is not likely unless the renal mechanisms for the elimination of water fail. The fault may be in the kidney itself, in the overproduction of the antidiuretic hormone, or the result of an impairment in the circulation of blood through the kidney. The first few days after surgical procedure,[16] or following a serious injury, patients are susceptible to overloading with water. As stated earlier, overloading is dangerous because it predisposes to circulatory failure with pulmonary edema and disturbed cerebral function. This is the reason accurate recording of intake, output, and weight is important during this period.

Prevention and treatment of water intoxica-

---

[16] D. A. K. Black: "Symptoms and Signs in Disorders of Body Fluid," *J. Chronic Dis.*, 11:341 (Mar.) 1960.

tion include the limitation of the patient's water intake, so that water is not allowed to accumulate in the body. In patients with acute renal failure, this may mean the patient receives as little as 300 to 500 ml of fluid in 24 hours. Careful observation and recording of the patient's intake, output, and weight provide information about the patient on which his needs for fluid can be based. Urine may be collected and measured hourly as well as every 24 hours. Because specific gravity of urine is determined by the capacity of the kidney to concentrate urine, each specimen of urine may be tested for specific gravity.

Hyponatremia or Sodium Deficit

Hyponatremia (less than 135 mEq per liter) may be associated with a contracted or expanded extracellular fluid volume and with an adequate or inadequate circulation. One classification of these conditions is as follows:

1. Inadequate circulation and reduced extracellular fluid volume, including
   a. Excessive losses from the gastrointestinal tract—severe diarrhea, vomiting, gastrointestinal fistula, or ileostomy
   b. Excessive sweating
   c. Adrenal insufficiency
   d. Diabetic acidosis
   e. Salt-losing kidney disease
   f. Excessive use of diuretics usually combined with overconscientious restriction of sodium intake
   g. Burns
2. Inadequate circulation and excessive extracellular fluid volume, including
   a. Congestive heart failure
   b. Liver disease
   c. Nephrotic syndrome
3. Adequate circulation and excessive extracellular fluid volume, including
   a. Inappropriate secretion of antidiuretic hormone associated with decreased aldosterone secretion, increased urine osmolality, and excessive loss of sodium in the urine
   b. Excessive administration of water with inadequate salt

SIGNS AND SYMPTOMS

Hyponatremia is usually associated with an increased blood volume and is generally the result of excessive intake of water and inadequate intake of salt. The syndrome of hyponatremia with hypovolemia is quite uncommon, but very serious. When this syndrome develops acutely, the symptoms are those of circulatory collapse. There is a low plasma volume, a high hematocrit, hypotension, oliguria, thready pulse, tachycardia, and collapsed neck veins. In advanced cases, the eyeballs become soft and the eyes appear to be set deep in their sockets.

When sodium deficits develop slowly, as might be the case in the patient on a restricted diet, particularly during hot weather, manifestations are less dramatic. They may include cramps, fainting on assuming the upright position as the result of postural hypotension, or simply general lethargy. The onset of hot weather, with the attendant increase in perspiration, may precipitate a sodium deficit in patients who have been on a prolonged regime of diuretics and salt restriction. The nurse supervising the care of these patients, in either the hospital or the home, should be alert to this possibility and should not too quickly dismiss the patient's complaints of fatigue or loss of energy, or of feeling faint on arising in the morning, as being due to spring fever. What the patient needs is not sulfur and molasses, but an increase in his salt intake. His symptoms should be reported to his physician.

These combined deficits require replacement of both sodium and water. It should be remembered always that most patients with hyponatremia actually have increased amounts of body and plasma water. Treatment in these instances requires hypertonic solutions. Fluids may be administered by mouth or by intravenous injection. The salt content of oral fluids may be increased by giving them in the form of bouillon or soup. If fruit juices are administered, they should have salt added to them. When the loss of sodium is proportionately greater than the loss of chloride, sodium bicarbonate or lactate may be administered. Intravenous fluids containing sodium bicarbonate and sometimes sodium lactate may also be used. Control of the rate of administration is important. Too rapid administration leads to an increased loss of electrolytes, and thus defeats the purpose of the treatment. In patients who undergo prolonged gastric or intestinal suction, physiological saline solution should be used to irrigate the tube to prevent the loss of sodium and chloride ions that can occur if water alone is used as an irrigating fluid.

Sodium Excess

As is to be expected, an increase in the retention of sodium in the body results in the retention of water and an increase in the extracellular fluid volume. Sodium concentration in such patients is often low in spite of an increased total body content of sodium because body water is generally increased. This pro-

duces a generalized edema. The most immediate and serious results are edema of the lung and an overloading of the circulatory system. Generalized edema occurs when the body's homeostatic mechanisms for eliminating excess sodium break down. As stated previously, the kidney regulates the level of the sodium ion in extracellular fluid. Kidney function depends on an adequate blood flow and the presence of aldosterone. The level of aldosterone depends on the relationship of the quantity secreted by the adrenal cortex to the rate at which it is destroyed by the liver, and other regulatory mechanisms may be involved as well. Therefore, sodium excess becomes a problem in (1) renal failure accompanied by salt retention, (2) disorders in which circulation of blood through the kidney is inadequate, such as congestive heart failure, (3) cirrhosis of the liver, (4) disorders characterized by overproduction of aldosterone by the adrenal cortex, and (5) patients who are treated with large doses of adrenal corticoids. In all these conditions there is sodium retention and with it an increase in the volume of extracellular fluid. It should be stressed that the increase in body water often exceeds the increase in sodium, thereby producing hyponatremia.

Prevention and treatment of sodium excess are directed toward correction of the condition causing sodium retention, combined with the restriction of sodium intake. The degree to which salt intake is reduced varies. In some patients, all that is required is to eliminate the use of salt in cooking. In others, all salts of sodium are prohibited. This includes sodium as bicarbonate, lactate, or benzoate. These patients should be taught to read the labels on foods and medicines and to reject those to which any sodium salt has been added. In the patient with congestive heart failure, restoration of the normal force of the heartbeat by digitalis, together with a restricted salt intake and diuretics to increase water and salt elimination, may be accompanied by remarkable changes in the patient. For example, Mrs. Martin, who suffered from a severe degree of cardiac insufficiency, lost 50 lb or 25 liters of fluid during her first week in the hospital. She entered the hospital short of breath to the point of orthopnea. She was also cyanotic and nauseated. Within a week she was no longer orthopneic at rest. Her color and appetite were also improved.

Although an excess of sodium ion in the extracellular fluid predisposes to edema by holding water, it is not the only factor in edema (edema is the abnormal retention of fluid in the interstitial spaces or in serous cavities). It results when the balance between the quantity of fluid entering the interstitial space is greater

PHYSIOLOGICAL FACTORS	INCREASE IN INTERSTITIAL FLUID VOLUME (EDEMA)
1. Capillary permeability ↑	a. Inflammation—increases capillary permeability b. Acute nephritis c. Burns
2. Hydrostatic pressure in the capillary ↑	a. Local venous obstruction, as in the use of constricting bandages or casts pressing on vein, swelling, varicose veins, etc. b. Generalized increase in venous pressure, as in congestive heart failure
3. Colloid osmotic pressure ↓ (decrease in blood proteins)	a. Nephrosis b. Starvation c. Burns d. Chronic diarrhea e. Acute nephritis, but not a usual cause
4. Sodium retention ↑	a. Congestive heart failure b. Salt-saving nephritis c. Increase in level of adrenocortical hormones (endogenous) (exogenous) (1) Aldosterone (2) Desoxycorticosterone (3) Cortisone, hydrocortisone, etc. d. Following trauma (1) Surgical procedures (2) Burns (3) Fractures
5. Lymphatic drainage ↓	Lymphatic obstruction Cancerous lymph nodes, removal of lymph nodes, elephantiasis such as follows parasitic invasion of lymph channels

than that leaving it. The physiological factors having a role in the movement of fluids across the capillary membrane are listed at the left. It should be remembered that more than one mechanism is frequently involved.

LOCATION OF EDEMA

The location of edema depends on the nature of the cause and whether it is localized or generalized. Generally, edema appears first in tissues that are poorly protected against the effects of hydrostatic pressure, such as the skin and subcutaneous tissues, and in dependent parts of the body. As a consequence, edema is found in the feet and ankles of those who are up and about and in the buttocks and sacrum of the bedridden. The influence of gravity on the distribution of edema fluid can sometimes be observed in the patient who has marked generalized edema. In the morning, after the patient spends the night on a lowered headrest, the eyelids may be so swollen that the patient has difficulty in opening his eyes, but there may be little or no pedal edema. Later in the day, and after he has been sitting upright, the swelling around the eyes is much less marked but the feet may be greatly swollen again.

Edema of the lungs is a possibility in patients with limited cardiac or renal reserve, or in conditions accompanied by capillary injury such as infections involving the lung. When the hydrostatic pressure of the blood in the pulmonary capillaries rises so it is equal to, or exceeds, the colloid osmotic pressure of the blood, transudation of fluid into the lung tissue takes place. Pulmonary edema is always a serious condition. Manifestations depend on the extent to which the hydrostatic pressure is increased and the rapidity with which the condition develops. In milder cases, the patient can be expected to have moist râles and shortness of breath. In severe cases, the alveoli may fill with so much fluid that adequate ventilation is difficult or impossible. Essentially, the patient drowns in his own fluid. In patients who are predisposed to pulmonary edema, the possibility of this catastrophe can be reduced by modifying the fluid intake in relation to output. Intravenous infusions and blood transfusions should be slow enough to prevent blood volume from suddenly increasing. Throughout the procedure, the patient should be observed for shortness of breath and an increase in pulse or respiratory rate. The urine output should also be measured hourly so that the status of the patient's output in relation to his intake will be known. Should there be any indication that excessive fluid is being retained or that pulmonary edema is developing, the infusion should be stopped or slowed to a minimum rate and the physician called immediately.

Edema in tissues other than the lung interferes with their nutrition by limiting the flow of blood to them. This renders the tissue more vulnerable to injury. In the bedfast patient with edema of the sacrum and buttocks, special attention to these areas is required to prevent the development of decubiti. Prevention of decubiti is especially difficult when the patient is orthopneic as a result of pulmonary edema. In orthopnea, the patient's breathing is so difficult that he is comfortable only when he sits leaning forward. Because he is short of breath and miserable, he resists changes in position; this continued pressure on edematous tissue leads to tissue breakdown. Prevention taxes the best efforts of the nurse. Small shifts in position, the use of an alternating pressure mattress, a flotation pad, or a water bed may be helpful in the prevention of decubiti.

Patients with generalized edema are often undernourished. When measures are initiated that are successful in eliminating edema fluid, the patient generally becomes thin or even emaciated. Improvement of the patient, therefore, depends not only on the elimination of edematous fluid, but also on improvement of his nutritional state. In some patients, edema lessens as the patient's nutrition is rectified. This is especially true if the serum albumin is less than 3 per cent. The feeding of the patient is therefore an important aspect of his nursing care.

The edema or swelling following injury is discussed elsewhere. This is also true for the effects of edema in specialized organs such as the brain. The effect of edema fluid in any structure that is enclosed in a limited space is that it reduces the blood flow to the part, thereby interfering with its nutrition.

A variety of terms are used to describe the location of edema fluid. A severe and generalized edema is called anasarca. Accumulation of fluid in the peritoneal cavity is called ascites. In the pleural cavity, it is called hydrothorax, and an accumulation in the pericardial sac is known as hydropericardium. In all these conditions, the fluid takes up space normally occupied by an organ or system, thereby interfering with its function. The clinical effects depend on the site and quantity of the edema fluid.

SUMMARY

The factors that enter into the development of edema and its effects will be reviewed in relation to Mrs. Bird, who was admitted to the hospital in congestive heart failure. Mrs. Bird has been selected because multiple factors appeared to play a role in the development of edema in her case. For many years, Mrs. Bird had essential hypertension. For the last few months she noticed that her ankles were swelling and that she became short of breath when she walked up a flight of stairs or simply walked rapidly. On medical examination, she was found to have cardiac insufficiency on the basis of longstanding essential hypertension.

All the factors responsible for the development of edema in the patient with cardiac insufficiency are not understood. Authorities appear to agree that, as a result of a decrease in the force of the heartbeat, blood flow to the kidney is diminished. Mrs. Bird's heart was unable to pump all the blood brought to it. This increased venous hydrostatic pressure, and fluid tended to accumulate, especially in her feet, when she was standing. When the heart failure is severe, fluid with a low protein content (transudate) tends to accumulate in the peritoneal and pleural cavities. Mrs. Bird's condition may have been aggravated by an increase in the production of aldosterone by the adrenal cortex. Aldosterone secretion tends to increase in any condition associated with decreased blood flow through the kidney. As a consequence, the volume of her extracellular fluid rose. As the blood volume enlarged, the hydrostatic pressure of the blood rose further. With the elevation in hydrostatic pressure, filtration of fluid from the capillary to the interstitial space exceeded that removed from it. This, combined with the inability of the kidney to remove the necessary amount of water and salt, resulted in edema.

In the treatment of Mrs. Bird, the physician had two principal objectives. One was to improve the function of the heart. The other was to support the body's physiological mechanisms for the elimination of salt and water. The first objective was achieved by treating Mrs. Bird with digitalis. To support her physiological mechanisms for the regulation of sodium and water, she was placed on a low-sodium diet, and a diuretic to increase her renal excretion of salt and water was also given.

OBJECTIVES OF NURSING CARE

The objectives on which the nursing care of Mrs. Bird was based included (1) making pertinent observations as the basis for modifications in the medical regime and the nursing care of Mrs. Bird, (2) reducing the work of the heart by meeting her physical and emotional needs, (3) preventing the breakdown of edematous tissue, (4) carrying out those aspects of the medical regime that are the responsibility of the nurse so that the therapy is effective, and (5) as Mrs. Bird recovers, participating in a program to prepare her to return home and to activity.

The observation of Mrs. Bird was directed toward gathering information about how she was responding to her illness and to the therapy, and how she regarded her illness. Her nurse was interested in what Mrs. Bird expected in relation to her illness, hospitalization, nursing, and medical care. Because Mrs. Bird was obviously ill and apprehensive when she was admitted, she was given complete physical care. Every effort was made to reassure Mrs. Bird that her needs would be met promptly and to prepare her for what to expect. Her environment was controlled so that all unnecessary stimuli were eliminated. Planned periods of rest were provided. Visitors were restricted to the members of her immediate family. Arrangements were made for the hospital chaplain to visit her every day. As her general condition improved, a number of effects were noted: (1) she felt better, (2) she had a marked diuresis and lost 50 lb during the first week of hospitalization, (3) she could breathe comfortably in a recumbent position, and (4) her appetite improved and her activity was increased. After each increase in activity, the nurse checked her pulse and noted her respirations. Had her pulse rate risen more than ten beats per minute, or continued to rise, the nurse would have reduced her activity during that time. She also explained to Mrs. Bird that the reason for her increased activity was that she was improving. As Mrs. Bird improved, her daughter was also included in discussions of planning for Mrs. Bird's convalescence after her discharge from the hospital. Further and more detailed discussion of the care of the patient in congestive heart failure may be found in Chapter 10.

Other Electrolyte Imbalances

In addition to affecting the distribution of body fluids, certain ions regulate neuromuscular irritability. According to Weisberg,[17] elevated levels of sodium and potassium increase neuromuscular irritability and responsiveness, while decreased concentrations of them decrease it. The irritability of the myoneural junction is decreased by increased concentrations of calcium, magnesium, and hydrogen ions. It is increased by decreased levels of calcium. Potassium affects the functioning of cardiac and skeletal muscle, and possibly smooth muscle.

THE FUNCTIONS OF POTASSIUM IN THE BODY

Potassium, as the most abundant cation in the intracellular fluid, plays an important role in the maintenance of the volume of fluid within the cell. It participates in the regulation of

[17] Harry F. Weisberg: *Water, Electrolyte and Acid-Base Balance*, 2nd ed. (Baltimore: The Williams & Wilkins Company, 1962), p. 67.

neuromuscular irritability and in the maintenance of the hydrogen ion concentration in the blood. Because of the difficulties involved in measuring the level of potassium in the cell, the state of potassium balance is inferred from its level in the blood potassium. The blood plasma level may or may not give an accurate picture. It may be normal or even elevated in the presence of a deficiency of potassium in the body. This is most likely to be true in conditions in which the cells are deprived of an adequate supply of oxygen or when fluids and electrolytes are lost in excessive quantities. Common examples include diabetic ketoacidosis and gastrointestinal disorders associated with the continued loss of secretions. Prolonged or severe gastrointestinal distention after surgery is occasionally due to poor motility caused by hypokalemia. Alterations in the level of potassium in the blood in either direction have an adverse effect on the function of the heart with the result that the patient may die suddenly from heart failure. It should also be remembered that electrolyte concentrations affect the activity of certain drugs. For example, digitalis is more likely to be toxic in patients with low potassium and/or high calcium levels in the blood.

Mary Kay illustrates some of the causes and effects of low potassium levels in the body. She was admitted to the emergency room with a tentative diagnosis of acute appendicitis. On examination, her urine was found to contain glucose, acetone, and diacetic acid. Further investigation revealed that she was in diabetic acidosis. For some time she had been drinking large amounts of water (polydipsia) and voiding large quantities of urine (polyuria). Her blood sugar was 700 mg per 100 ml of blood plasma, and her carbon dioxide content was 10 mEq per liter. The level of potassium in her blood was 4.0 mEq per liter. To correct severe dehydration she was given 10,000 ml of fluid intravenously in a period of about ten hours. Despite the fact that metabolism of glucose was re-established by insulin therapy and her hypovolemia corrected, she was not given adequate potassium. As acidosis is corrected, blood potassium levels tend to fall. Also, as glucose enters the cells with the help of insulin, potassium also enters the cells, causing further hypokalemia. Her respirations became shallow, her pulse weak and rapid, and her color ashen. When adequate amounts of potassium were added to her intravenous fluids, her condition rapidly improved.

The body's mechanisms for conserving potassium are not as effective as they are for sodium. Some potassium continues to be lost in the urine, even with a low intake and low blood and tissue levels. Further, potassium loss is accentuated in metabolic alkalosis, which may be induced by excessive loss of hydrochloric acid caused by vomiting or nasogastric suction. Certain types of treatment aggravate potassium loss. These include enemas, mercurial diuretics, sodium bicarbonate, and the adrenocortical steroids. Patients who have been in the habit of taking drastic cathartics or enemas may also suffer from a deficiency of potassium.

Low levels of potassium may cause failure of cardiac, skeletal, and possibly smooth muscle. The sensitivity of the heart muscle to digitalis [18] is increased when there is hypokalemia, and symptoms of toxicity may occur at dosages of digitalis that are ordinarily therapeutic. For this reason, a major part of the treatment for digitalis toxicity is a salt of potassium such as potassium chloride. Symptoms and signs of potassium deficiency include tachycardia, cardiac arrhythmias, altered ECG patterns, hypotension, muscle weakness, tetany, and paralytic ileus. In severe potassium deficiency the contractility of the heart muscle may be so impaired that the heart stops in diastole.

TREATMENT OF POTASSIUM DEFICIENCY

The treatment is to replace the potassium that has been lost. Fruit juices, especially unstrained orange juice, bouillon, and meat broths, are rich in potassium. As soon as the patient eats a varied diet, potassium is promptly restored. When the patient is unable to take fluids by mouth, potassium may be given by intravenous infusion. Care should be taken to limit the rate of infusion of potassium in patients who have a limited renal reserve, so that blood levels do not become excessive. Intravenous infusions containing potassium require extremely careful supervision. The patient should also be observed for any signs or symptoms indicating hyperkalemia. The symptoms include paresthesias, which may be of the scalp rather than of the extremities, muscle weakness, and cardiac arrhythmias. Death may result from cardiac failure, with the heart stopping in systole.

Disorders in which hyperkalemia most commonly occurs are acute or chronic renal failure, too rapid administration of potassium, and adrenal insufficiency. Careful attention to the rate at which potassium salts are administered by intravenous injection cannot be overstressed. In adrenal insufficiency, hyperkalemia can usually be controlled by the administration of the adrenocortical hormones.

In patients with renal failure, the blood level of potassium may be more difficult to control. When the failure is of short duration, this may be accomplished by eliminating all potassium intake and maintaining the patient at complete bed rest. Since most foods contain some potassium, the diet may be limited to glucose and vegetable oil, neither of which contains potassium. Elimination of potassium by the gastrointestinal tract may be increased by the ingestion of cation exchange resins, which have no potassium. Unfortunately, many patients do not tolerate these very well.

Schwartz and Kassirer [19] state that a potassium level of 6.5 mEq per liter and abnormalities in the ECG constitute an emergency. They recommend that it be treated by the administration of 100 g of glucose and 50 units of insulin to induce potassium to enter the cells. Sodium bicarbonate may be administered to buffer the hydrogen ion and allow the potassium ion to return to the cell. They also recommend that calcium gluconate be given intravenously because calcium antagonizes the effect of potassium on the heart.

Some patients, such as Mrs. Murray, respond to conservative therapy. She suffered an acute renal shutdown as the result of transfusion with about 400 ml of incompatible blood. At the time she was admitted to Hospital X for possible hemodialysis, she had been severely oliguric for two days. It is well to remember that even in severe renal failure, a few milliliters of urine are excreted. If there is absolutely no urine, one wonders if the renal vessels, ureters, or urethra are blocked. Blood studies and electrocardiogram indicated that Mrs. Murray had some elevation of potassium, but was not in any immediate danger. She was placed on strict bed rest; ice chips not to exceed 200 ml in 24 hours; a diet composed of glucose and Crisco; and daily weight, electrocardiogram, and blood specimens for potassium, sodium, and urea. A polyethylene catheter was introduced into the saphenous vein. It was to be kept patent with a 10 per cent solution of glucose. A micro set was used in order to minimize the quantity of solution required. An indwelling catheter was introduced, so that all urine excreted could be collected. Her total fluid intake was kept at about 500 ml plus additional volume equal to her urine output. Fortunately for Mrs. Murray, on the fifth day following the onset of oliguria, she started to excrete increasing amounts of urine. Since the ability to concentrate urine does not return as rapidly as the ability to excrete water, the urine had a low specific gravity. Despite a marked increase in the volume of urine, Mrs. Murray's blood potassium and urea did not begin to fall for a few days. During the

[18] Louis S. Goodman and Alfred Gilman (eds.): *The Pharmacological Basis of Therapeutics,* 3rd ed. (New York: The Macmillan Company, 1965), p. 684.

[19] William B. Schwartz and Jerome P. Kassirer: "Medical Management of Chronic Renal Failure," *Amer. J. Med.,* 44:794 (May) 1968.

initial period of diuresis, Mrs. Murray was carefully observed for any indication of electrolyte imbalance. Either hypo- or hypernatremia could have occurred. Neither developed. Sometimes diuresis is so extreme that the patient requires a large fluid intake. Fortunately for Mrs. Murray, her kidney function was restored rapidly enough so that hemodialysis was not required.

Mrs. Murray's nursing care was directed toward trying to make it possible for her to achieve a maximum amount of rest. Since activity increases the rate of metabolism, she was given complete care. She was turned and rubbed every two hours and encouraged to lie quietly. Because of the nature of her diet and limitations on her fluid intake, she was given special mouth care every four hours. The ice chips were divided over the 24-hour period. Because the rate of flow of the intravenous solution was important, this was noted at hourly or more frequent intervals. Strict control of fluid intake so that it does not exceed output by more than 500 ml is one of the most important aspects of the patient's care. Unless this is done, the patient may die from the effects of overhydration. Because Mrs. Murray was from out of town, she had no visitors except her husband and the hospital chaplain. Both Mr. and Mrs. Murray were concerned about the possible outcome of her illness. Nurses and doctors were aware of their concern. They encouraged Mrs. Murray's hopes and were sympathetic to her feelings of uncertainty. Through attention to meeting her immediate needs, they were able to minimize her discomfort and to convey to her that everyone was concerned about her welfare.

Not all patients in acute renal failure are as fortunate as Mrs. Murray. Recovery of the kidney may be slow and the levels of potassium in the blood may be elevated to the point of toxicity. In this event, the level of potassium and the nonprotein nitrogenous wastes in the blood may be lowered by the methods previously indicated or by hemo- or peritoneal dialysis. These procedures have other uses as well. One or the other may be utilized to remove ingested poisons such as barbiturates, salicylates, bromides, and other drugs. These procedures will be described in this chapter.

FUNCTIONS OF CALCIUM IN THE BODY

Although calcium has little effect on the shift of fluids in the body, it has many important functions. About 99 per cent of it is found in the bone. In addition to the formation of bone, it functions in the (1) regulation of neuromuscular irritability, (2) coagulation of the blood, (3) regulation of the irritability of the heart muscle, and (4) formation of milk.

Calcium exists in the blood in two forms. About 45 per cent is bound to the serum protein and is nondiffusible. About 55 per cent is ionized and is diffusible. The level of calcium in the blood serum is regulated in relation to the level of the phosphate ion, and the product of the two is often kept relatively constant. With an increase in one, the level of the other can be expected to decrease. The level of calcium in the blood is regulated by the parathyroid hormone, which increases the absorption of calcium from bone. The parathyroid hormone acts on the kidney to decrease the reabsorption of phosphate by the tubules. It also increases absorption of calcium from the intestine. A hormone called thyrocalcitonin also regulates the blood level of calcium; one of its effects is to reduce the breakdown of bone, especially if hypercalcemia is present.

As with other elements of body fluids, calcium may be present in deficit or in excess. Deficits of calcium may be in the total quantity or in the proportion that is in ionized form. In alkalosis, the proportion of calcium in the ionized form diminishes; in acidosis, it rises. Tetany results when the amount of ionized calcium in the blood is low. This in turn may be caused by alkalosis, excessive loss of calcium, or inadequate calcium intake. For example, tetany develops in susceptible persons who induce respiratory alkalosis by overbreathing. It is seen in infants and very young children with rickets, as a result of a lack of calcium and/or vitamin D. In adults, tetany may follow injury or removal of the parathyroid glands during thyroid surgery or following the removal of an adenoma of the parathyroid gland. In the absence of the parathyroid hormone, the level of calcium in the serum falls. In advanced renal disease, the kidney loses its ability to conserve calcium. As a consequence, it is lost from the blood. Whatever the cause, a decrease in the level of calcium in the blood is followed by a heightening in neuromuscular irritability.

Often the first symptoms of impending tetany are paresthesias about the mouth or in the fingers or toes. With an increase in muscular irritability, the hands and feet assume a characteristic position which is referred to as carpopedal spasm. In infants, spasms of the glottis may interfere with breathing. In patients whose blood level of calcium remains just above the critical point, tapping over the facial nerve in front of the ear causes a twitching of the muscles of the face. If the face muscles twitch, this is called a positive Chvostek sign. Muscle spasm is accompanied by considerable pain and discomfort which can be relieved by the intravenous administration of calcium gluconate or calcium chloride. Calcium solutions should be given very slowly and are very dangerous in patients who are getting digitalis-like drugs.

Though the function of the calcium ion on muscle irritability and excitability has been stressed, irritability is the function of the relationship of several ions. This relationship is expressed by:

$$\frac{Na+ \quad OH- \quad K+}{Ca++ \quad Mg++ \quad H+}$$

Thus muscle irritability is increased as the levels of sodium, hydroxyl, and potassium ions are increased in relationship to calcium, magnesium, and hydrogen ions. Relationships as well as particular levels are significant. Occasionally, tetany occurs in patients with normal calcium levels. In such instances, hypomagnesemia may be the cause of the symptoms and should be treated accordingly.

FUNCTIONS OF MAGNESIUM IN THE BODY

Although magnesium has been known to be present in extracellular fluid for some time, its functions are still not well understood. Its concentration inside cells is second in amount to potassium. It activates many enzyme systems such as the phosphatase enzymes, and is a cofactor with thiamine in intermediate carbohydrate metabolism. It functions in calcium and phosphorous metabolism and in the regeneration of protein. Magnesium deficiencies may be important in the development of delirium tremens and should be watched for in patients with severe burns or excessive gastrointestinal fluid loss.

Acid-Base Equilibrium

Regulation of the Hydrogen Ion Concentration

One of the truly remarkable features of the body is that, despite continuous additions of metabolites from cells and from food, its pH is maintained at relatively constant levels. The mechanisms for regulating the concentration of hydrogen ions include (1) the dilution of the products of metabolism by a large volume of fluid; (2) the elimination of hydrogen ions, as well as other cations and anions, by the lung and kidney; and (3) the removal of hydrogen ions by buffering.

The **dilution** of strong acids and alkalies by a large volume of water is one of the most effective means of diminishing their effect. The principle is utilized in first aid to minimize the effects of a strong acid or alkali on tissue, by flooding the tissue or structure with a large volume of running water. In other words, a teaspoonful of concentrated sulfuric acid in contact with the skin or mucous membrane produces serious tissue injury. Diluted by 10 gal of water, it has little, if any, effect. In the living organism, the extracellular fluid dilutes the strong acids produced by the cells in the process of metabolism and thereby prevents them from injuring tissues.

A second mechanism utilized by the body to control the level of the hydrogen ion is the **elimination of carbon dioxide** by the lung. This serves two purposes. In addition to helping to regulate the level of the hydrogen ion, it also serves to keep the level of cations equal to anions without the loss of water. This mechanism is, in fact, the most rapid method the body has for adjusting the level of anions in the blood plasma. It will be described in detail in the discussion of buffering.

A third mechanism for the protection of a solution against changes in hydrogen ion concentration is **buffering**. A buffer can be described as a chemical sponge. It can take up or release hydrogen or hydroxyl ions as the circumstances demand and thereby protect the fluid against changes in pH. Each buffer system for controlling hydrogen ion concentration consists of a solution of a weak acid and one of its salts, formed by neutralizing the acid with a strong base. The acid and salt are maintained in a definite relationship to each other. There are a number of so-called buffer systems in the body. They include (1) carbonic acid and sodium bicarbonate, (2) monosodium or potassium phosphate and disodium or dipotassium phosphate, (3) oxyhemoglobin and reduced hemoglobin, and (4) acid proteinate and neutral protein. They all function in essentially the same manner. As in nature, the strong take from the weak. In the presence of a strong acid, the following events take place:

1. The cation from the salt of the weak acid and the strong base (sodium or potassium, for example) combines with
2. The anion (chloride, sulfate, phosphate, acetate, etc.) from the strong acid to form a salt, and
3. The hydrogen ion from the strong acid (hydrochloric, phosphoric, lactic, acetoacetic) combines with
4. The anion from salt of the weak acid to form
5. A weak acid

The weak acid ionizes less completely than the strong acid that it replaces, that is, it does not release hydrogen ions as readily as the stronger acid. Hydrogen ions are therefore removed from the solution. Stated simply, as the result of buffering, the strong acid is replaced by a weak acid and a neutral salt. In a weak acid, a larger proportion of the substance remains in the molecular form and fewer hydrogen ions are released than in a strong acid.

To clarify further, and to apply the manner in which buffer systems function in the body, the carbonic acid–sodium bicarbonate system is described below. This system plays an important role in the protection of the extracellular fluid from changes in the hydrogen ion concentration. Carbonic acid is a weak acid. Sodium bicarbonate ($NaHCo_3$) is a salt formed by the neutralization of carbonic acid (H_2CO_3) with sodium hydroxide ($NaOH$), a strong base. In health, one molecule of carbonic acid is maintained in the blood for every 20 bicarbonate ions.

When an acid stronger than carbonic acid is formed in, or ingested into, the body, it ionizes to the hydrogen ion and the appropriate anion. The anion combines with the sodium ion to form a salt. The hydrogen ion unites with the bicarbonate anion to form the weak carbonic acid. For example, if hydrochloric acid (HCl) is added, the following reaction takes place:

$$HCl + NaHCO_3 \rightleftarrows NaCl + H_2CO_3$$

Regulation of the Bicarbonate Anion

The level of the bicarbonate anion in the blood plasma is regulated by the excretion of carbon dioxide by the lung, which in turn regulates the quantity of carbon dioxide dissolved in the blood. The more carbon dioxide dissolved in the blood, the higher the level of the bicarbonate anion and carbonic acid, and vice versa.

When the level of chloride, sulfate, phosphate, or organic acid anions increases, they combine with sodium ions, thereby reducing the number of sodium cations (alkali reserve) available to combine with bicarbonate anions. The bicarbonate ion then combines with hydrogen ions to form carbonic acid, which in turn can break down into water and carbon dioxide. As the amount of carbon dioxide increases, the depth and rate of respiration also increase.[20] With an increase in the depth and rate of respiration, the carbon dioxide in the alveolar air decreases, and carbon dioxide moves from the blood to the alveoli. As the level of carbon dioxide in the blood plasma drops, more carbonic acid in the presence of carbonic anhydrase decomposes to carbon dioxide and water.[21] This

results in a lowering of the level of the bicarbonate and the hydrogen ions in the blood plasma.

As the carbon dioxide and the hydrogen ion concentrations decrease, the respiratory center is depressed and the process is reversed. Respiration diminishes in rate and depth. The partial pressure of carbon dioxide in the alveoli increases. This is followed by an increase in the level of carbon dioxide in the blood. Finally, this is reflected by an increase in the bicarbonate ion in the blood.

As previously stated, the immediate source of the bicarbonate ion in the blood plasma is sodium bicarbonate ($NaHCO_3$) and hydrogen carbonate or carbonic acid (H_2CO_3). The quantity present in the molecular form, that is, as hydrogen carbonate, can be increased by adding more of the bicarbonate ion in the form of sodium bicarbonate. Conversely, the amount of hydrogen carbonate that ionizes can be increased by decreasing the level of sodium bicarbonate in the blood. This results from what is known as the common ion effect. Additions of sodium bicarbonate to the blood decrease the number of free hydrogen ions in the blood by decreasing the ionization of hydrogen carbonate. The same effect can be produced by inhaling carbon dioxide or by holding one's breath.

Just as increases in the level of other anions result in a lowering of the level of the bicarbonate ion, a depression in the level of other anions is compensated for by an increase in the bicarbonate ion. Thus, a fall in the level of the chloride ion in the blood is compensated for by an increase in the bicarbonate ion. Although the levels of the chloride and other anions in the blood plasma are subject to change, there do not appear to be as active mechanisms for their upward or downward adjustment as there are with bicarbonate.

To return to Mr. Martin for a moment, though the day was hot, he hurried as he mowed the lawn. This required a considerable expenditure of energy. In the process of obtaining the energy, he formed and released into his extracellular fluid a considerable volume of organic and inorganic acids. More specifically, hydrogen ions and the corresponding anions were added to his extracellular fluid. To adjust the level of anions to that of the cations, principally sodium, in his blood, some of the bicarbonate anion in his blood was eliminated by the lungs as carbon dioxide. In the process, hydrogen ions were converted to water and therefore had no effect on his acid-base equilibrium. The anions from the acids that were stronger than carbonic acid combined with sodium to form salts. This resulted in a reduction in Mr.

---

[20] The pressure of a gas within a container is inversely proportional to the size of the chamber.

[21] $CO_2 + H_2O \rightleftarrows H_2CO_3(H^+ + HCO_2^-)$—reaction catalyzed by carbonic anhydrase.

Martin's alkali reserve, that is, in the quantity of sodium ion in the form of sodium bicarbonate in the blood. With a reduction in the bicarbonate in the blood, the capacity of the blood to carry carbon dioxide was diminished. Carbon dioxide and hydrogen ions accumulated in Mr. Martin's body, including the area of his respiratory center. His respiration increased in rate and depth, and the partial pressure of carbon dioxide in his alveolar air fell. The tension of carbon dioxide in the blood then became higher than in the alveolar air, and carbon dioxide therefore diffused from the blood to the alveoli to equalize the pressure on the two sides of the membrane. With a lowering of the tension of carbon dioxide in the blood, the depth and rate of his respirations diminished. As a result, the partial pressure of carbon dioxide in his alveolar air again rose and, as a consequence,

the level of carbon dioxide and the carbonic acid in his blood plasma also rose.

Role of the Kidney in Maintaining the Acid-Base Equilibrium

By regulating the level of carbon dioxide in the blood plasma, the lung plays an important role in acid-base equilibrium. However, neither the buffer system nor the lung is able to control completely the hydrogen ion concentration. The kidney plays a significant part in this by selectively reabsorbing or rejecting both cations and anions. Its role in the maintenance of the concentration of sodium and potassium in body fluids has previously been discussed. The kidney tubules utilize three mechanisms to control the hydrogen ion. They reabsorb the bicarbonate ion from the glomerular filtrate, acidify urinary

FIGURE 9-6. Mechanism by which urine becomes acidified by changing the dibasic phosphate to monobasic or dihydrogen phosphate. (Modified from Davenport and adapted with permission of The Macmillan Company from *Anatomy and Physiology,* 15th ed., p. 683, by Diana Clifford Kimber, Carolyn E. Gray, Caroline E. Stackpole, and Lutie C. Leavell. Copyright © The Macmillan Company, 1966.)

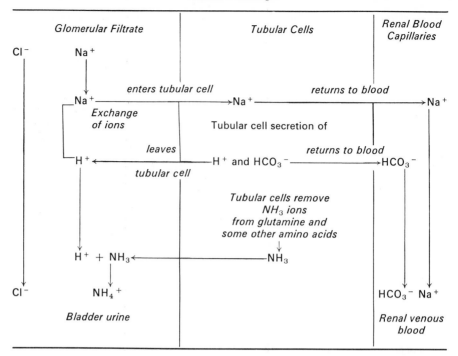

FIGURE 9-7. Formation of ammonia by the kidney. (Modified from Davenport and adapted with permission of The Macmillan Company from *Anatomy and Physiology*, 15th ed., p. 684, by Diana Clifford Kimber, Carolyn E. Gray, Caroline E. Stackpole, and Lutie C. Leavell. Copyright © The Macmillan Company, 1966.)

buffers, and secrete ammonia. Because ammonium ions can replace sodium or other cations in the urine, they are part of the mechanism for the excretion of "strong" anions without losing necessary cations. The kidney reduces hydrogen ions by combining them with bisodium phosphate to form monosodium phosphate. By these mechanisms, the kidney eliminates the hydrogen ion and conserves sodium and potassium ions as well. The functions of the various parts of the nephron and the processes utilized by the kidney in the excretion of the hydrogen ion and the conservation of the sodium ion are summarized in Figures 9-6 and 9-7.

Though the kidney is able to excrete either an alkaline or an acid urine, the urine is usually acid. The lowest pH at which urine is excreted is 4.5. Only weak acids are found to any extent in the urine. Strong acids, such as hydrochloric and sulfuric acids, are not present in the urine as free acids. They are excreted as sodium or ammonium salts. The acid buffers are responsible for much of the acidity of the urine.

Failure to control the hydrogen ion concentration so that the pH is maintained between 7.35 and 7.45 results in acidema or alkalemia. The condition is said to be compensated as long as the ratio of bicarbonate to carbonic acid is maintained at about 20:1. As can be seen in Figure 9-8 in acidosis the ratio of bicarbonate to carbonic acid is less than 20:1; in alkalosis the ratio is greater than 20:1. In the presence of an increase or decrease in hydrogen ion concentration, mechanisms for its control act to produce changes that restore the ratio of carbonic acid to bicarbonate.

Summary

The mechanisms for maintaining a normal pH include the taking up or release of hydrogen ions by the buffer systems, increase or decrease in ventilation by the lung, and elimination or conservation of hydrogen and bicarbonate ions by the kidney. A decrease in ventilation reduces the elimination of carbon dioxide and favors the formation of carbonic acid. An increase in the rate and depth of respiration has the reverse effect.

When the level of the bicarbonate ion in the blood is excessive, reabsorption of bicarbonate by the kidney is decreased and the quantity of

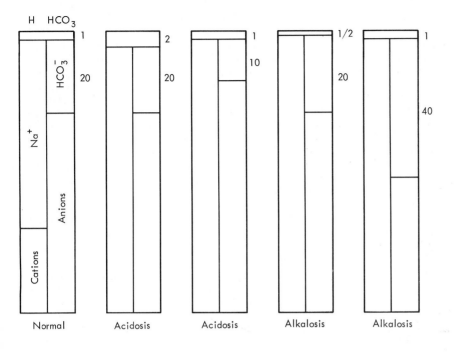

H   HCO₃

HCO₃⁻

Na⁺

Anions

Cations

1   2   1   1/2   1
20   20   10   20   40

Normal   Acidosis   Acidosis   Alkalosis   Alkalosis

FIGURE 9-8. Possible changes in H—HCO₃ to HCO₃ in acidosis and alkalosis.

bicarbonate in the urine is increased. An increase in the production of hydrogen ions is followed by a rise in the rate at which tubular cells secrete them. The kidney also excretes monosodium phosphate and the hydrogen ion, and conserves sodium by eliminating the phosphate ion in the monosodium form and excreting other anions as ammonium salts. All these mechanisms serve to restore the hydrogen ion concentration so that the pH of the blood is maintained within normal levels.

What are the clinical manifestations of acid-base imbalance?

Depending on their origin, deviations in the concentration of the hydrogen ion are classified as metabolic or respiratory.

METABOLIC ACIDOSIS

In metabolic acidosis, the ratio of bicarbonate to carbonic acid is decreased by a reduction in the quantity of sodium available to combine with bicarbonate; the quantity of sodium in combination with anions other than bicarbonate is increased. A characteristic feature of metabolic acidosis is therefore a decrease in the alkali reserve. One of the common causes of metabolic acidosis is inadequately controlled diabetes

mellitus. As a consequence of failure to metabolize adequate quantities of glucose, the liver increases the metabolism of fatty acids. This results in the production of ketonic acids at a rate more rapid than the muscles can handle. As a consequence, they accumulate in the blood. Since beta hydroxybutyric and diacetic acids are stronger than carbonic acid, they displace the bicarbonate ion in sodium bicarbonate. The body defends itself by increasing the rate and depth of respiration, thereby increasing the elimination of carbon dioxide. The kidney responds by converting glutamic and other acids to ammonia. In the presence of the hydrogen ion, ammonia is converted to the ammonium ion. ($NH_3 + H^+ \rightleftharpoons NH_4^+$). As the production of ammonia increases, the loss of sodium and potassium decreases. Although the secretion of ammonia is a relatively slow adaptive response, it is an effective one.

Although the rate of formation of ketone acids is slower, some degree of metabolic acidosis develops when the patient has not eaten and adequate amounts of glucose are not present. Other conditions with which metabolic acidosis occurs include

1. Renal failure—phosphate and sulfate anions are retained

2. The administration of large doses of acidifying salts such as ammonium chloride
3. Excessive exercise
4. Anoxia or hypoxia
5. Severe diarrhea in which the loss of sodium ions exceeds that of chloride ions

Whatever the underlying cause, hyperpnea of the type known as Kussmaul breathing is the outstanding symptom; this hyperventilation eliminates carbon dioxide and counteracts the metabolic acidosis by producing a respiratory alkalosis. In severe or prolonged acidosis, the kidney mechanisms for conserving sodium and water and for excreting the hydrogen ion fail. As a result, water, sodium, and potassium are lost in excess of intake with a resultant increase in the acidosis. The situation is frequently aggravated by further dehydration from vomiting. As a consequence, the skin and mucous membrane becomes dry and tissue turgor diminishes. Even the eyeballs may lose fluid with a reduction in their tension. With the loss of fluid and the decrease in pH, restlessness, abdominal pain, and eventually coma develop. Unless the condition is corrected, death can occur.

TREATMENT OF METABOLIC ACIDOSIS

Treatment of metabolic acidosis is directed toward two objectives. The first is to correct the underlying cause. The second is to restore the water, electrolytes, and nutrients that have been lost from the body. In the instance of Mary Kay, she was given insulin and glucose to enable her to metabolize glucose and to decrease the formation of ketone acids. In this way the underlying cause of her acidosis was attacked. At the same time, she received fluids containing sodium chloride and sodium lactate. Because the lactate ion is metabolized, the sodium ion becomes available to combine with the bicarbonate ion. The sodium ion thus enlarges the alkali reserve. In the beginning, the fluids are likely to be administered parenterally. It was also important to give Mary Kay some form of potassium. After the patient is able to tolerate fluids by mouth, they may be given in the form of bouillon, orange juice, or other fluids containing the necessary electrolytes.´

The functions of the nurse include making pertinent observations, protecting the patient from injury, performing therapeutic procedures, and providing for the comfort and well-being of the patient. Significant observations include his general behavior. Is he conscious, drowsy, or stuporous? Is he quiet or restless? What is the character of his breathing? His color? Is his skin dry or moist? Examination of the urine in metabolic acidosis is extremely important.

Because the urine should be analyzed frequently, an indwelling catheter is sometimes inserted so that urine can be obtained for regular half-hourly or hourly analyses. In addition to recording the rate of urine formation, it is also important to have it examined for glucose, acetone, diacetic acid, specific gravity, and pH. Samples of blood should also be checked at regular intervals for glucose, sodium, potassium, chlorides, carbon dioxide content or carbon dioxide–combining power, and acetone. Hemoconcentration of the blood is reflected by an elevated hematocrit or hemoglobin in the blood. Because these diagnostic tests require repeated venipuncture, the patient should be told why repeated venipuncture is necessary.

The common therapeutic measures have been indicated. The nurse's responsibilities in each of these have been previously discussed. After fluids are started by mouth, attention should be given to make certain the patient gets and ingests the required amounts. The patient in acidosis has a tendency to have gastric dilatation. When this occurs, the fluid ingested remains in the stomach. Later, the patient may vomit a large quantity of fluid. A feeling of fullness in the epigastric region is the common warning symptom accompanying gastric retention.

When the patient is restless and not fully conscious, more than usual attention to his safety is required. Side rails may be placed on the bed to lessen the danger of his falling out of bed. If he is very restless, they should be padded. Other precautions in his care do not differ materially from those for any patient who is not fully aware of his actions.

As in the care of any other patient, the nurse should be alert to the need of the patient for comfort and support. During the period when the patient is not fully conscious, the nurse should assume responsibility for reminding everyone involved in the care of the patient that he may be able to hear and comprehend what is said in his presence.

RESPIRATORY ACIDOSIS

In addition to acidosis of metabolic origin, acidosis may result from a failure of the body to ventilate adequately and remove carbon dioxide from the body. This type is known as respiratory acidosis. In respiratory acidosis, the level of carbon dioxide and carbonic acid in the blood plasma is increased, and the ratio of carbonic acid to bicarbonate is increased. This results in an increase in the hydrogen ion concentration in the blood. Respiratory acidosis occurs in a wide range of conditions in which there is an inadequate exchange of gases in the lungs resulting in retention of carbon dioxide in the blood. Inadequate exchange of gases in the lung may be caused by anything that depresses the respiratory center in the medulla or decreases the areating surface in the lung. Narcotics such as morphine and meperidine hydrochloride, general anesthetics, and barbiturates all predispose to respiratory acidosis because they depress the respiratory center. Diseases such as poliomyelitis and injuries that involve the respiratory center can also be expected to do so. Emphysema, bronchiectasis, and pneumonia predispose to respiratory acidosis by decreasing the aerating surface in the lung.

As in metabolic acidosis, the kidney's mechanisms for maintaining the level of the hydrogen ions are utilized. The buffers also help. As the blood level of carbonic acid rises, some chloride moves into the red cell, leaving more sodium available to form sodium bicarbonate. The increased bicarbonate helps to restore the bicarbonate-to-carbonic acid ratio of 20:1. Thus the body attempts to compensate for respiratory acidosis by producing a metabolic alkalosis, and vice versa.

PREVENTION OF RESPIRATORY ACIDOSIS

In the prevention and treatment of respiratory acidosis, therapy is directed toward correcting the cause. Narcotics should be given infrequently and then only in the smallest amounts required to relieve pain. When a patient is receiving narcotic drugs, he should be encouraged to perform deep-breathing at regular intervals. In the patient with emphysema, a tracheostomy is sometimes performed to reduce the dead-air space, to facilitate the removal of secretions, or to allow him to be put on a respirator. Ordinarily, however, a tracheostomy allows more expiratory bronchiolar collapse, thereby causing more air trapping; this may be very detrimental to a patient with emphysema. The patient who is suffering from respiratory paralysis is placed on respirator. Because hypoxia increases the degree of acidosis, the administration of increased oxygen would appear to be indicated, especially if the hemoglobin saturation is less than 90 per cent or the pO_2 is less than 60 mm of mercury. However, it may have disastrous effects in the patient with severe emphysema. The emphysema patient may have severe depression of his respiratory center because of a chronic hypercarbia. When this occurs, the only stimulus to respiration is the effect of hypoxia on the chemoreceptors, such as the carotid and aortic bodies. If such a patient is given oxygen, the oxygen content of his blood rises and the stimulus to respiration

is lost. The reduced ventilation causes further hypercarbia which may be enough to kill the patient by respiratory acidosis.

ALKALOSIS

In certain disorders the level of the hydrogen ion may be decreased to below normal. This results in alkalosis. Like acidosis, alkalosis may be of metabolic or respiratory origin. In metabolic alkalosis, the bicarbonate anion is increased in relation to carbonic acid. This results in an increase in the ratio of bicarbonate to carbonic acid, so that there are more than 20 parts of bicarbonate ions to 1 part of carbonic acid. Another way this is stated is that there is a relative increase of fixed cations in relation to fixed anions. Metabolic alkalosis is most commonly associated with disorders in which there is an undue loss of the chloride ion or excessive intake of sodium bicarbonate. Continued vomiting from pyloric stenosis and gastric suction are the most frequent causes of chloride depletion. Loss of chlorides from the patient on gastric suction is intensified by vigorous irrigation of the nasogastric tube. For this reason, some physicians limit irrigation or ask that isotonic saline solution be used as the irrigating fluid. Fluid intake is generally limited for the same reason in the patient having gastric suction. Chloride depletion also occurs in patients who are given mercurial diuretics frequently. Loss of potassium from the body can also cause metabolic alkalosis.

The ingestion of excessive quantities of sodium bicarbonate is most likely to be observed in persons who treat themselves for indigestion and who have a limited renal reserve. Everyone, especially persons in older age groups, should be cautioned against this practice.

A characteristic sign of alkalosis is shallow breathing. This results from the body's attempt to raise the level of carbonic acid in the blood. In shallow breathing, the concentration of carbon dioxide in the alveolar air is raised. This serves to raise the level of carbonic acid in the blood. The kidney also responds by excreting sodium bicarbonate in the urine and by depressing the mechanisms for the excretion of the hydrogen ion. Less hydrogen ion is secreted by the tubules. The formation of ammonia is suppressed. Phosphates are excreted as disodium rather than monosodium salts. Lactic acid and ketone acid anions are reabsorbed. They help to displace the bicarbonate ion in the plasma. The urine excreted is alkaline in reaction. Thus, the body, through the initiation of compensatory mechanisms, attempts to maintain the pH of the blood within normal limits.

Occasionally, a patient with alkalosis tends to excrete an acid urine. This is referred to as a *paradoxical aciduria* and is usually caused by hypokalemia.

Treatment in alkalosis is based on the same general principles as in acidosis. It is directed toward the correction of the cause and the support of the body's compensatory mechanisms. Several authorities emphasize that in alkalosis, potassium is lost and the condition cannot be treated sucessfully without repairing the deficit of potassium, especially if there is paradoxical aciduria. In addition to replacement of chlorides, attention should be given to improving the patient's nutrition.

Respiratory alkalosis occurs less frequently than other disturbances in hydrogen ion concentration. It results when the concentration of carbonic acid in the blood is decreased in proportion to the bicarbonate anion. The most common cause is an increase in the rate and depth of respirations in the absence of an increase in the hydrogen ion or carbon dioxide. Respiratory alkalosis is an example of a disorder arising from the inappropriate use of a physiological mechanism. This condition is most commonly seen in the nervous patient who overbreathes but may also be an early sign of sepsis or a pulmonary embolism. Because the hydrogen ion concentration of the blood plasma is diminished, the level of ionized calcium in the blood is also decreased. As a consequence, these persons frequently have symptoms and signs of tetany. Treatment is directed toward correcting the underlying cause of the condition. Respiratory alkalosis can be corrected by any measure that elevates the level of carbon dioxide in the alveoli and blood. This can be done by holding the breath or by inhaling carbon dioxide. Sedatives may be used to slow down the patient's respirations. A simple method of treatment for this is to have the patient breathe into a paper bag. As the patient breathes into the paper bag, the partial pressure of carbon dioxide rises in the bag and then the pCO_2 in the alveoli and blood also rises.

SUMMARY

Disturbances in the acid-base balance or in the hydrogen ion concentration of extracellular fluids produce alterations in the ratio of carbonic acid to the bicarbonate ion in the blood plasma. In disorders of metabolic origin, the change is primarily in the level of the bicarbonate anion. In metabolic acidosis the bicarbonate anion is decreased. In metabolic alkalosis it is increased. In disorders of respiratory origin, the site of the disorder is in the carbonic acid fraction. In respiratory acidosis it is increased. In respiratory alkalosis it is decreased in relation to the bicarbonate ion.

The manifestations observed in these conditions result from (1) the compensatory responses to the condition, (2) the loss of water and electrolytes, and (3) the nature of the cause. The characteristic compensatory response is a change in the rate and depth of respiration. In metabolic acidosis, ventilation is increased by an increase in the rate and depth of respiration. In metabolic alkalosis, breathing becomes shallow. Alterations in breathing bring about rapid adjustments to changes in hydrogen ion concentration. When the disturbance continues for more than a few minutes, the kidney also participates in correcting the condition.

OBJECTIVES OF TREATMENT

Treatment is directed toward removing the cause and supporting the body's mechanisms for correcting the disturbance. This includes not only restoring any water and electrolytes that have been lost, but also maintaining an adequate nutritional state.

The essential factors in the regulation of water and electrolytes are summarized below. The volume, distribution, and concentration of water and electrolytes in the various fluid compartments result from a carefully regulated balance between intake and output. An increase in intake or output results in the initiation of mechanisms that very quickly correct any change from normal. Continued deficits in supply or failure in any of the regulatory mechanisms results in a loss of homeostasis and disturbed cellular function.

From the preceding discussion, it should be apparent that disturbances in fluid and electrolyte balance result in disturbances in volume, osmolality, and the hydrogen ion concentration of body fluids. Fluid and electrolyte balance may become a serious problem in any sick person. It becomes a more serious problem when the illness persists or when the patient's mechanisms for adjusting to the situation are inadequate.

The physician has the responsibility for making the medical diagnosis and for establishing the plan of therapy. The nurse assists in the collection of the data on which the diagnosis is based, participates in and supervises therapeutic measures, and provides comfort and support for the patient. For all patients, and most particularly those who have a chronic condition, she assists in their instruction. She may carry more or less responsibility for assisting them in their adjustment after dismissal from the hospital.

Signs and Symptoms of Alterations in Volume, Osmolality, and Hydrogen Ion Concentration

The characteristic signs and symptoms of alterations in volume, osmolality, and hydrogen ion concentration have been previously discussed. They are summarized here, not in relation to a specific condition, but in general terms. They include changes in (1) the patient's mental state and behavior, particularly increasing apathy, lethargy, and weakness, or restlessness and occasionally convulsions; (2) the skin —either increasing or decreasing turgor or dryness; (3) the mucous membranes—dryness in the mouth and sordes; (4) the urine output— polyuria or oliguria; (5) the concentration of urine, specific gravity—lowered, elevated, or fixed in the region of 1.010; (6) respiration— increased or decreased in rate or depth; (7) thirst—increased or absent; and (8) the blood —increased or decreased level of electrolytes and the nonprotein nitrogenous wastes as expressed by the blood urea, urea nitrogen, nonprotein nitrogen, or hematocrit. Any or all elements in the blood may be increased when additions to the blood exceed losses or when the intake or addition of water is below its output. The level of any substance in the blood will be decreased when the loss of that substance exceeds supply or when the addition of water is greater than its loss. For example, in renal failure, the nitrogenous wastes as well as electrolytes such as potassium and sodium tend to rise in the blood. In salt-wasting nephritis, the level of sodium cations may fall because the kidney's mechanisms for conserving sodium are defective. When water intake is insufficient, the hematocrit, hemoglobin, blood proteins, and electrolytes, as well as nitrogenous wastes, tend to rise.

In conditions in which the body mechanisms are likely to need assistance in maintaining or restoring the normal character of the extracellular fluids, the blood and urine may be examined to determine the level of the various constituents. In disorders of the kidney, renal function tests are performed. In complicated cases where the results may give misleading information, other body fluids such as gastric juice may also be analyzed.

What tests are useful in determining fluid and electrolyte balance and renal function?

Blood Tests

1. The most useful tests of renal function include the *blood urea nitrogen* (BUN) and *creatinine;* elevations above the normal values, especially for creatinine, usually imply impaired renal function. Absorption of blood from the intestinal tract may raise the BUN, but seldom affects the creatinine levels in the blood.

2. *Hematocrit.* The blood is treated with an anticoagulant and centrifuged until the cells are packed in the bottom of the tube. The average range for packed cells is from 41 to 48 per cent. Increases in the hematocrit are associated with a loss of extracellular fluid. In severe burns, the hematocrit may be as high as 75 per cent. Hematocrits above 55 per cent increase the viscosity of blood enough to interfere with blood flow.

3. *Hemoglobin.* With a loss of extracellular fluid, the hemoglobin is increased in concentration. In patients whose hemoglobin is usually within the average range of 14 to 16 g per 100 ml of blood, the level may rise to 18 or 20 g.

4. *Levels of electrolytes in the blood plasma.* These may rise or fall.

5. *Carbon dioxide content.* The measurement of carbon dioxide, carbonic acid, and bicarbonate of the plasma collected under oil is called carbon dioxide content. It is reported in volumes per cent or milligrams per liter.

6. *Carbon dioxide-combining power.* Plasma is equilibrated with air and then the carbon dioxide content is determined.

7. *The pH of arterial blood* may be determined to differentiate between respiratory acidosis and metabolic alkalosis.

Urine Tests

The urine should also be examined routinely in all patients.

1. The presence of increased quantities of red blood cells, white blood cells, protein, or sugar also may indicate renal impairment or disease. Casts of any type usually indicate some renal disease.

2. *Volume*

3. *The urine specific gravity* may be very useful to know, especially in the patient with oliguria. A decreased volume of urine with a high specific gravity usually implies dehydration or inadequate perfusion of the kidney. With a healthy kidney the specific gravity decreases as the fluid intake increases. A fixed specific gravity of about 1.010 even when there is oliguria or hypovolemia indicates severe renal failure. So-called concentration tests may be performed to determine the capacity of the kidney to alter the specific gravity of the urine.

4. *pH of the urine.* Normally acid, but its pH may vary from 4.5 to 8.5 depending on the

nature of the food and chemicals ingested by or administered to the patient.

5. *Presence of electrolytes in abnormal amounts or types.* For example, an absence of the sodium ion in the urine usually indicates a deficit of sodium in the body. The presence of the ketonic acids in appreciable amounts is indicative of acidosis in which the metabolism of fat is excessive.

Tests for Specific Renal Functions

1. *Measurement of filtration rate.* Glomerular filtration rate can be measured by injecting a solute which is filtered by the glomeruli and which is not metabolized in the body or secreted or reabsorbed by the renal tubules. One such substance is inulin, a polysaccharide obtained from dahlia roots. Because inulin is neither reabsorbed nor secreted by the renal tubule, the quantity found in the urine is equal to the amount filtered by the glomeruli. If one knows both the quantity of urine excreted or collected per minute and the concentration of inulin in the urine and the plasma, then one can calculate the volume of plasma filtered. The result is known as the glomerular filtration rate. Because no single milliliter of plasma loses its entire complement of inulin (urea, creatinine) as it passes through the glomeruli, the results represent the volume of plasma required to provide the amount of a particular substance excreted by the kidney per minute. Metabolites such as urea and creatinine are also employed in clearance tests to estimate glomerular filtration rate. Because they are products of protein metabolism, the patient should be kept quiet during the performance of the test. In calculating the results of the test, the fact that some urea diffuses back into the blood has to be taken into account.

   The creatinine clearance test is not as accurate a measure of glomerular filtration as the inulin clearance test, but is more easily performed. If the patient puts out 1,440 ml of urine per day, and his serum creatinine is 2 mg per cent and the urine creatinine concentration is 120 mg per cent, then the creatinine clearance rate is 60 ml per minute. (See Table 9-3.)

2. *Tests to determine the concentration and dilution powers* of the kidney. When water intake is restricted the specific gravity of the urine should rise. When combined with a high intake of sodium and protein, it should rise above 1.025 or 1.030 and may rise as high as 1.048.

3. *Tests of the ability of the kidneys to excrete dyes and other substances such as phenolsulfonphthalein.*

Table 9-3

$$C = \frac{UV}{P}$$

C = clearance rate (ml/min)
U = urine concentration (mg%)
V = urine volume (ml/min)
P = plasma (or serum) concentration (mg%)
V = 1 ml/min (1,440 ml in 1,440 min)

$$C = \frac{(120)(1)}{2} = 60 \text{ ml/min}$$

Some of the data required to evaluate the status of the patient's fluid and electrolyte balance have been presented. In short-term illnesses in patients whose health is essentially good, attention to the patient's desire for water may provide a satisfactory guide to his fluid intake. In patients who are suffering from serious or long-term illness or whose capacity to adapt is limited, the problem of evaluating fluid and electrolyte status may be difficult and require many tests or procedures.

What are the objectives of therapy?

The objectives of medical therapy will depend on the nature of the patient's disturbance. In general they will be

1. To maintain the volume of blood.
   a. Too little endangers the nutrition of the brain, kidney, and heart (all tissues).
   b. Too much overburdens the heart and circulation and predisposes to pulmonary edema.
2. To replace past and current losses of water and electrolytes.
3. To provide an intake of water of sufficient volume for the kidney to excrete the nitrogenous wastes brought to it.
4. To supply water and electrolytes in such amounts that dehydration or waterlogging of tissues and acidosis or alkalosis are prevented or corrected.

The nursing objectives include

1. To observe each patient for signs and symptoms indicating his physiological status.
2. To carry out in a safe and effective manner the procedures that have been ordered.
3. To care for the patient in such a manner that he is protected from unnecessary discomfort and feels safe, protected, and cared for.

In the preceding pages emphasis has been placed on the regulation of water and electrolytes. In the section that follows, disorders of the kidney that are likely to lead to renal failure are summarized.

[Text continued on p. 348.]

TABLE 9-4

Disorders of the Kidney that Are Common Causes of Renal Failure

Classification	Etiology	Nature of Onset	Severity and Course of Illness	Structures Involved, Primary Disease	Major Manifestations	Major Medical or Surgical Therapy
I. Bilateral inflammatory diseases of the kidney A. Glomerulonephritis 1. Acute	Most frequently associated with preceding infections caused by group A beta-hemolytic streptococcus. Not a bacterial infection but an antigen-antibody reaction damaging the glomeruli. Most common in childhood and young adults but may occur at any age	Classically, an abrupt onset occurring 1–4 weeks after an attack of pharyngitis or scarlatina	Evidence of healing occurs within 3 weeks. Most patients go on to complete recovery. A few die during the acute phase of the disease or progress into the subacute or chronic phase	Diffuse exudation and proliferative inflammation of the kidney glomeruli	1. Puffy eyes, swelling of feet and ankles, shortness of breath 2. Signs of congestive heart failure often prominent 3. Albuminuria 4. Hematuria. Urine may be smoky 5. Oliguria which may progress to anuria 6. Hypertension. Some degree is a common occurrence. When severe, may precipitate cardiac failure or cerebral manifestations 7. Headache 8. Malaise—abdominal pain may be colicky or steady 9. Anorexia, nausea, and vomiting 10. May be moderate to severe aching in lumbar regions 11. About one half of hospitalized patients have normal renal function. Others have some degree of retention of nitrogenous wastes	1. Treatment of infection with group A streptococci by penicillin. Penicillin is of no value unless streptococci are present 2. Bed rest until gross hematuria, edema, and hypertension have disappeared 3. Nutrition. With evidence of impaired renal function and oliguria, edema, or heart failure, intake of protein, sodium, and potassium is restricted 4. Fluid intake. In presence of oliguria, intake may be restricted. If nausea and vomiting, intake may be more liberal 5. Antihypertensive therapy. When hypertension and headaches are severe, drugs such as hydralazine hydrochloride, reserpine, or a combination of the two may be administered parenterally 6. Antiuremia therapy

TABLE 9-4 (cont.)

Disorders of the Kidney that Are Common Causes of Renal Failure

Classification	Etiology	Nature of Onset	Severity and Course of Illness	Structures Involved, Primary Disease	Major Manifestations	Major Medical or Surgical Therapy
2. Chronic	Failure of kidneys to heal following an attack of acute glomerulonephritis. An occasional strong familial predisposition is found	Following a latent phase which may persist for as long as 20–30 years or even longer. Patient develops evidence of renal failure		Few signs and symptoms of renal insufficiency until renal function falls below 20% or less of normal. Inflammatory changes and scarring of the glomerular tufts	12. In renal failure, hyperkalemia (elevated blood potassium) 13. Mild anemia frequently occurs	*Latent phase*—none
					Onset of renal failure 1. Oliguria 2. Elevated blood urea nitrogen 3. Anemia 4. Weakness, nausea, and somnolence if oliguria persists 5. Hypertension and cardiovascular complications 6. Electrolyte abnormalities	
					Nephrotic syndrome or phase—occurs sometime before death in one half of patients 1. Heavy loss of protein in urine—exceeding 5 g daily 2. Hypoalbuminemia 3. Hypercholesterolemia 4. Edema	
					Advanced and terminal glomerulonephritis See discussion of renal failure	See discussion of chronic renal failure

Table 9-4 (cont.)

Disorders of the Kidney that Are Common Causes of Renal Failure

Classification	Etiology	Nature of Onset	Severity and Course of Illness	Structures Involved, Primary Disease	Major Manifestations	Major Medical or Surgical Therapy
B. Pyelonephritis: Disease resulting from the immediate or late effects of bacterial infections of the kidney.						
1. Acute	Usually caused by the coliform group of gram-negative enteric bacilli. Frequently follows urinary tract infections. A small number caused by gram-positive streptococcus, Proteus, Pseudomonas, enterococcus, and staphylococcus. Infection may reach the kidney via the blood or by way of the urinary tract Predisposing factors: 1. About one half of cases not known 2. Obstruction—prostatic hypertrophy, cicatricial tissue anomalies	Sudden		Lesion(s)—diffuse 1. Inflammation of the renal pelvis and calyces 2. Infection of renal substance, medulla, and cortex with the formation of minute abscesses 3. Healing with the formation of scar tissue	1. Sudden rise of body temperature 37.3° to 40.5°C (102° to 105°F) 2. Shaking chills 3. Aching pains in one of costovertebral areas or flanks 4. Symptoms of inflammation of the bladder: (a) frequency of urination, (b) burning pain on urination (dysuria), (c) passage of cloudy and occasionally blood-tinged urine 5. Tenderness in region of the kidney 6. Nausea, vomiting, diarrhea, and occasionally constipation 7. Laboratory tests: (a) polymorphonuclear leukocytosis, (b) many leukocytes in the urine, (c) bacteria in the urine	1. Attempt to sterilize the urine (difficult to do). Drugs employed a. Methenamine mandelate (Mandelamine) b. Nitrofuratoin (suppresses infection) c. Urotropin (suppresses infection) d. Methionine (an acidifying agent that inhibits the growth of bacteria) e. Mandelic acid f. Antibiotics such as tetracycline, chloramphenicol g. Sulfanilamides (bacteriostatic effect) h. Streptomycin (not used alone because streptomycin-resistant bacteria emerge rapidly) 2. Maintain water intake to keep urine dilute 3. Relieve or remove obstructing lesions

TABLE 9-4 (cont.)

Disorders of the Kidney that Are Common Causes of Renal Failure

Classification	Etiology	Nature of Onset	Severity and Course of Illness	Structures Involved, Primary Disease	Major Manifestations	Major Medical or Surgical Therapy
	3. Age and sex a. A comparatively high incidence before 18 months of age. More common in female than in male infants b. Much more common at 18–40 yr in women than in men 4. Instrumentation of the urinary tract including catheterization 5. Autonomic disturbances of bladder function 6. Diabetes mellitus 7. Pregnancy 8. Indwelling (Foley) catheter					
2. Chronic (one of the most common forms of chronic renal disease)	Results from the effects of scar tissue formed in the healing of an earlier bacterial infection of the kidney or from some other agent	Over half of the persons with chronic pyelonephritis have a history of attacks of acute urinary tract infection Usually onset is insidious and the progress of the	Fatigue, lassitude associated with anemia Signs of hypertension and congestive heart failure		1. Usually no symptoms of infection 2. Symptoms common to chronic illness Fatigue Headache (may be related to hypertension) Poor appetite Weight loss 3. Symptoms associated with failing renal function	1. Eliminate urinary tract infections by drug therapy and by the removal of obstructing lesions

TABLE 9-4 (cont.)

Disorders of the Kidney that Are Common Causes of Renal Failure

Classification	Etiology	Nature of Onset	Severity and Course of Illness	Structures Involved, Primary Disease	Major Manifestations	Major Medical or Surgical Therapy
		disease is often slow			Polyuria Thirst 4. Signs of renal failure Impaired capacity to concentrate urine Elevated blood urea nitrogen	
II. *The nephrotic syndrome*	1. Idiopathic 2. A phase of glomerulonephritis			In some textbooks of pathology this disease is referred to as a disease of the tubules. It is a disease in which the glomeruli are affected in such a manner that massive quantities of protein are lost in the urine	1. Profuse proteinuria secondary to loss of proteins 2. Hyperlipemia 3. Hypoalbuminemia 4. Generalized edema Other signs and symptoms depend on the cause	Idiopathic 1. ACTH and adrenal steroids. Treatment continued for six months or longer 2. A nutritious diet containing adequate amounts of protein. Should be sufficient to cover amounts lost in urine
III. *Diseases of the arterioles (nephroscleroses)* A. Benign B. Malignant	Hypertensive vascular disease	Hypertension antedates proteinuria by many years. Hematuria may occur		Intimal thickening of the small arteries and arterioles of the kidney. Eosinophilic hyaline thickening of entire walls of arterioles and prearterioles which may progress to generalized atrophy of the cortex with focal scars	Increased proteinuria and hematuria mark onset of malignant phase. Very high blood pressure, retinal hemorrhages, papilledema, heart failure, and hypertensive encephalopathy	

Disturbances in water and electrolyte balance can result from disorders in gastrointestinal, respiratory, circulatory, or renal function. The first three are discussed in detail in other chapters and will not be further considered here. As are other organs, the kidney is subject to a variety of diseases that, depending on their extent and nature, reduce renal reserve or result in renal failure. Because one half of one kidney contains enough tissue to perform the ordinary functions of the kidney, there may be considerable kidney damage before evidence of renal failure develops. When one kidney is healthy, the other one can be safely removed. The manifestations accompanying renal disease depend on the nature of the cause and the extent to which renal function is impaired. For example, bacterial infections of the kidney are accompanied by signs and symptoms of infection. Whether or not renal failure occurs depends on the extent to which nephrons are destroyed by the infectious process or by the healing process. Disorders of the glomeruli usually render them more permeable to constituents of the blood. In nephroses, profuse amounts of protein are lost into the urine because the glomerular capillaries become permeable to protein. Because large quantities of protein are lost in the urine, blood protein level may fall. Many of the other manifestations observed in the nephrotic patient are due to the effects of the low blood protein. In acute glomerular nephritis, the kidney is hyperemic; some glomeruli rupture, and blood escapes into the urine. Prolonged ischemia of the kidneys or agents toxic to the kidneys may cause tubular necrosis. Whatever the cause, tubular necrosis usually results in acute renal failure and is manifested by oliguria or anuria and rapidly developing azotemia. (See Table 9-4.)

Many of the details about the disorders listed in Table 9-4 have not been included in the summary. Among them are the particular hazards to which each exposes the patient. In the essay that follows, the role of the nurse in anticipating and identifying evidence of developing cardiac failure or of hypertensive encephalopathy in the child or young adult with acute glomerular nephritis is outlined. Although acute glomerular nephritis is more common among children, it can and does occur in young adults.

Acute Glomerular Nephritis *

Every year, especially in the springtime, nurses who are serving in medical units of children's hospitals or in the pediatric departments of general hospitals care for patients suffering from acute glomerular nephritis. Some years, there are more children than in other years, but always there are several. Usually, they are from four to seven years old. Although sometimes a child is very sick, often the patients are not much bothered by their symptoms. More than 95 times out of 100 they recover completely, often after little in the way of specific treatment. But of the four or five for whom this is not the happy outcome, two or three may die quite promptly. These children usually die of heart failure or hypertensive encephalopathy, which develops rapidly indeed, but not as a rule without a few signs to herald its coming. Lack of treatment that was available but not instituted because the approaching demand for it was not recognized in time by those present, may be the cause for much sadness, as well as for resentment, anger, and guilt—and the child's life is lost to society.

The significant point may be found in the inference that the progression of symptoms in the child usually gives some clues to the prepared observer. The observer who is prepared both to recognize and comprehend their meaning may use these clues to the patient's advantage. A hospital unit which admits acutely sick children may be expected to have one or more professional nurses there at all hours, even though physicians may not always be at hand. These nurses should be the prepared observers, able to evaluate what they see in the sick child on the basis, not just of their general knowledge of children, but of an understanding of what changes are induced in the body by acute glomerular nephritis and in what manner these changes may quickly embarrass the essential welfare of the patient. Nurses who can go this far will not often fail to take the next steps to benefit the child—those of acting on the orders already available and procuring the physician promptly to meet the critical medical needs of the child.

Although most children recover from acute glomerular nephritis without evident permanent injury to the kidneys, the changes that occur incident to the damaging inflammation are considerable, and the effects at the time may be severe. The sequence often starts a week or two after sore throat caused by infection with group A beta-hemolytic streptococcus type 12. Toxin from the streptococcus provokes pathological changes that have been revealed by the electron microscope in recent years. Briefly, they are these: The host produces antibody capable of reacting with this toxin (antigen), and immune complexes that are globulins result. These are laid down as nodular deposits on the epithelial

---

* This portion of the chapter was contributed by Esther R. Read, R.N.

side of the basement membrane of the glomerular capillary. Complement attracts leukocytes that curl up the endothelium and increase its permeability. In the inflamed capillaries there is a proliferation of endothelial cells, the main pathology of acute glomerular nephritis. Disturbances of filtration result. Increased permeability means that medium-sized and large molecules will not be held back as heretofore, so that hemoglobin, and eventually even albumin, will get through the inflamed capillary endothelium; hematuria and proteinuria will appear and set the stage for the familiar symptomatology of the children.[22,23,24]

Generalized vasospasm is a characteristic of this type of nephritis, and awareness of this fact contributes to understanding of some of the symptoms. When the vessels are all in spasm, the blood delivered to the kidney may be reduced in amount. Vasospasm increases peripheral resistance. Even the amount of blood that enters comes at the expense of increased effort by the heart. The arterial pressure rises, and unless the child already has a weakened heart, the pulse rate may be expected to slow somewhat because of pressure on the receptors in the carotid sinus, with resultant discharge of impulses to vasomotor centers. If the vasospasm is extremely severe, the heart muscle itself may suffer hypoxia and fail under the strain of the effort in a weakened state of pumping a large volume of blood, increased as a result of sodium and water retention, out into vessels narrowed by spasm. Cerebral anemia may result from inadequate supply to the brain as a result of the vascular spasm alone or assisted by heart failure. The child may be drowsy, or have headache, dimness of vision, or convulsions.

Children with acute glomerular nephritis do not usually look very edematous, but, if weighed, show an increase which suggests that there is a good deal of water retention consequent to the sodium reabsorption that occurs. If the child is in heart failure, not only will the edema be more marked than otherwise, but the failure further jeopardizes his welfare, because no organ, the heart included, is receiving the nutrition it needs.

Much of the pathophysiology is revealed by physical examination and laboratory tests, but

22 Alfred F. Michael *et al.:* "Acute Poststreptococcal Glomerulonephritis: Immune Deposit Disease," *J. Clin. Invest.,* 45:237–18 (Feb.) 1966.
23 John R. Hoyer *et al.:* "Acute Poststreptococcal Glomerulonephritis Presenting as Hypertensive Encephalopathy with Minimal Urinary Abnormalities," *Pediatrics,* 39:412–17 (Mar.) 1967.
24 Thomas S. Edgington, Richard J. Glassock and Frank J. Dixon: "Autologous Immune Complex Pathogenesis of Experimental Allergic Glomerulonephritis," *Science,* 155:1432–34 (Mar. 17) 1967.

the reports of these come late to the child's record. Concern here is for comprehension of what the sick child himself can demonstrate to his nurse of his needs for her attention and understanding care.

Usually he is of an age to talk readily. Children of four, five, and six years suffer severely in hospital from homesickness, and especially from conscious, expressed need for their mothers. Nurses cannot by any means satisfy this, but they can mitigate suffering a little by expressing sympathy for the child in his unhappiness and by showing their readiness to let him talk about his mother. With a little skill they can help him to build verbal bridges to his home. It is not, as a rule, helpful to a sick child to try to divert him when he is mournful, even though one can do it. He is put in the position of having to do his mourning alone, which is sad for him and lessens, rather than strengthens, his nurse's relationship with him.

In pediatric nursing one has often to do without verbal communication because the patients are too young to talk. When, however, a nurse has an acutely sick child who is old enough to be articulate, she is unwise indeed if she does not use every opportunity to demonstrate to him both by word and action her interest, her liking, and her desire to know all about him. The child should learn that his nurse wants to know about him and to take care of him however he feels—sick, lonely, or, as he invariably replies to the casual inquirer, "fine." The relentless amuser, who cannot see a child sitting forlornly in bed without feeling constrained to try to cheer him up and play with him, may not be his most helpful nurse. He may not confide in her the things she would like to know, for she has not shown him that she likes him when he is unhappy; she seems always to want to change him.

The prepared nurse, faced with the responsibility for care and professional nursing observation of a child newly sick with acute glomerular nephritis, will value her understanding of children for many reasons, one of which is that it contributes to the excellence of her nursing care. This is, however, but a part of all she needs to know, and she may do well to review whatever relevant knowledge she has from all fields and consider the application of it to her patient.

With inflammation present in the glomeruli, she expects to see evidence of blood in the urine. Because of sodium retention she expects the amount passed daily to be diminished. To become aware of whether or not the oliguria is becoming more severe, signaling less efficient glomerular filtration and increased water retention, she realizes the need for accuracy and completeness in the recording of fluid intake and output, and not only sees that this is accomplished, but keeps herself informed of the relationships. If the blood pressure is elevated or the child is gaining weight, or if he looks paler or more puffy than before, she stops and observes his breathing. Two checks may be necessary before she can assure herself that this ever-useful indicator of cardiac embarrassment (increase in respiratory rate without increase in patient activity) is not a source of concern for her about the patient at this time. She has been led to make this observation by knowing that vasospasm has increased the peripheral load of the heart and may be severe enough to result in some hypoxia to the myocardium, which, emptying the chambers of the heart incompletely with each stroke, initiates the whole sequence of adjustments made by the body to compensate for the lessening efficiency of the heart muscle. Increasing respiratory rate is one such adjustment.

When, however, she does observe that the child is breathing faster, she has something to do. First, it is to help the patient to the position of comfort and provide him with the pillow support he needs so that he requires no exertion to maintain it. Then she will count the pulse, note the quality, measure the blood pressure, and procure the means of administering oxygen to assist the failing efforts of the heart. It may be that the blood pressure is rising and that she already has orders provided for medication. In this event, she is prepared to treat the child further at once. But when there is no medical order to act upon, the nurse will do well to gain a little more information from her patient in the next two or three minutes before calling his physician. The prepared nurse will have this sequence pass through her mind: vasospasm → hypertension → cerebral anemia → cerebral hypoxia → cerebral symptoms. Then, she will ask herself: Does he have any of these? Here is the place where one *does* try to capture the attention of the child, whatever his mood, but with an objective more serious than that of simple diversion. By showing him a small picture of a familiar object, or reviewing the illustrations of a picture book he knows well, a fair guess can be made as to whether the child's vision is still clear. A far better judgment can be made at the same time concerning his mental alertness, for if the child and his nurse are already good friends, he will try to respond to her, however ill he feels. By his response he will reveal the absence or extent of his drowsiness. It may be that after a sudden light tap or from a moment's close observation she will see muscle twitching that may presage a convulsion soon to follow. So, within a minute or two, his nurse will have additional useful information

to give the doctor when she proceeds immediately to notify him of the changes in the condition of the patient, and to request his presence.

If, in the absence of a physician to note rapidly advancing symptoms, there is no nurse prepared to recognize and act upon significant changes, the child who goes quickly into heart failure may die. When his needs are promptly recognized and successfully treated, his recovery from this emergency is quick and complete. The same is essentially true of hypertensive encephalopathy, although there is no one who would like to say that convulsions and cerebral hypoxia are conditions that one wants to see occurring often in any child.

Sometimes, when everyone has been alert, and all have given their best knowledge and skill to care and treatment, a child with acute glomerular nephritis will die. At the present time, this cannot be avoided. An effort has been made here to indicate some, though not by any means all, of the pathological changes that take place in this disease. These are changes producing symptoms with accompanying physical signs that a nurse can recognize. Recognizing the signs and relating them to a disease process of which she has an understanding permits her to make judgments that are useful. It is at this point that she becomes free to do professional nursing.

The sick child whose parents have loaned him to the hospital for care has been entrusted by them to the doctors and nurses only because they believe that specialized care may, for a brief time, be better for him than their own. If their confidence is not to have been falsely placed, not only the doctor but also the nurses, with whom the child surely will find less comfort than with his mother when he is sick, must be able to offer something that is even more important for him at the moment than his mother's presence. This is, for nurses, intelligent vigilance based on a knowledge of emergencies that can arise because of the stress of the child's disease on his body. Confidence that they are fulfilling their entire responsibility can be felt by nurses only when they (as well as doctors, for whom this is to be assumed) accept the thesis that all aspects of the care of the sick child are subjects for their attention and concern: "No Trespassing" signs have no proper place in pediatrics. All that each nurse knows about children, including normal growth and development, normal or pathophysiology, techniques and skills of bedside nursing, and psychology, will be of value only when integrated and used to further the objective of all who are devoted to the hospital care of sick children. This objective is fairly met when a child is returned home well on the road to health with, as far as can be managed, few lasting scars sustained from his hazardous journey.

Renal Failure

Although many of the consequences of renal failure have been included in the discussion of water and electrolyte balance, they merit discussion and emphasis here. Renal failure may develop suddenly from prolonged ischemia of the kidney or from the effect of nephrotoxic agents. More commonly, it develops slowly over the course of months and years from the effects of ischemia secondary to disease of the arterioles or arteries supplying them, from infection of kidney tissue, or from other causes. Whatever the cause or causative factors of renal failure in a given patient, the presenting signs and symptoms are due to the effect on all the organ systems of the body of the *inability of the kidney to maintain the composition and volume of body fluids*. The eventual prognosis of the patient depends on the cause of the renal failure as well as his ability to prevent hyperkalemia, hypertensive encephalopathy, and congestive heart failure, all of which may complicate renal failure. When the degree of injury to the kidney is such that too little renal tissue remains to perform the functions of the kidney, many patients can still be helped to lead a reasonably comfortable existence for a time by proper medical management.

The syndrome resulting from functional failure of the kidney is known as uremia or azotemia. The term *uremia* is the older and means, literally, urine in the blood. The term *azotemia* has a more limited meaning inasmuch as it refers to the presence of excessive quantities of nitrogenous compounds in the blood. The manifestations of uremia are due to the effects of the failure of the kidney to regulate the volume and composition of body fluids in total bodily functioning. As in other chronic diseases, much can now be done by appropriate medical management to extend the length of the patient's useful life.

In contrast to the rapidly developing threat to life that characterizes nonspecific acute renal failure, the manifestations accompanying chronic renal failure are that the patient may be aware only of tiring more easily than formerly and having some degree of muscular weakness. He seeks medical attention because he does not feel well, and he may not have felt healthy or energetic for some time. Other systemic effects of chronic renal failure include increased susceptibility to infection and delayed wound healing. In children, growth and development may be retarded.

Among the most disagreeable effects of the uremic syndrome are those on the alimentary tract, as the patient experiences anorexia, nausea, and vomiting. These symptoms may be so severe that they are precipitated by the smell, sight, or even thought of food. When they are marked, they lead to marked emaciation as a consequence of failure to ingest sufficient food to meet the caloric needs of the tissues.

Nausea and vomiting can be controlled by antiemetic drugs such as chlorpromazine or one of the other phenothalazines. Every effort should be made to encourage the patient to try to eat. Some patients desire special foods and will try to eat if they are provided with them. Particularly in advanced stages of the uremic syndrome, the breath has an ammoniacal or uriniferous odor that limits the ability of the patient to taste food. Some patients find foods with a definite taste more acceptable than bland ones. For example, Mr. Thomas, who was in the terminal phase of the uremic syndrome, requested canned clams. He could taste them because they have a strong and pungent taste.

In the later stages of uremia, ulcerations along the gastrointestinal tract are common. In the mouth they are associated with stomatitis (inflammation of the soft tissues of the mouth). Ulcerations in the stomach or more distal portions of the alimentary canal may lead to gastrointestinal bleeding. Although mouth care should be given regularly, the tissues should be treated with gentleness. Vomitus as well as feces should be observed for blood.

As the uremic syndrome develops, functioning of the nervous system is altered. In the early stages, the patient may be irritable. Later as the disorder progresses, he becomes apathetic, drowsy, and eventually comatose. Long-acting barbiturates and other drugs excreted by the kidney should be avoided. Muscular weakness and twitching, neuralgic or neuritic pains, headache and dizziness may be observed. In patients in whom there is some degree of hypertensive encephalopathy, failing vision or even blindness occurs.

Effects on the respiratory system are due to congestive heart failure as well as to metabolic acidosis. Dyspnea occurs as a result of the congestive heart failure, and Kussmaul breathing as a result of the acidosis.

Many of the manifestations referable to the circulatory system are caused by the hypertension accompanying renal disease. Some are, however, due to the effects of the failure of the kidney to regulate the composition and volume of the blood. The effects of hyperkalemia on the contractility of the myocardium have been previously discussed. In addition, purpura develops as a result of increased capillary fragility and alteration in the clotting mechanism. A marked and progressive anemia develops as a consequence of hemolysis and failure of hematopoiesis. Uremic pericarditis may cause precordial pain and a friction rub, or tamponade.

Changes in the skeleton include osteomalacia in the adult and rickets in the child.

The skin is also affected. One of the earliest symptoms is pruritus. The pruritus may be intense, leading to extensive self-inflected excoriation of the skin. Later after the level of nonprotein nitrogenous substances in the blood becomes very high, uremic frost can be seen on the skin. The white crystals are more easily seen in areas where perspiration is most abundant, such as around the mouth. They can and should be removed by bathing.

Because the composition and volume of body fluids depend on adequate renal function, the uremic patient often presents many problems, including (1) malnutrition, (2) anemia, (3) water and electrolyte imbalance, (4) hypertensive vascular disease, and (5) circulatory failure.

In nursing the patient who is in some phase of renal failure, attention should be given to the maintenance of his physiological status as well as to his general comfort. Inasmuch as his physiological status can be supported, his feelings of well-being will be improved. Eventually the patient becomes dependent on others to meet most if not all of his needs. He should be observed for evidence of changes in his condition, and his care should be modified accordingly.

In addition to measures specifically directed toward the alleviation of specific symptoms of renal failure, two other types of procedures may be of benefit to the patient. The first is a low-protein diet. The second is either hemodialysis or peritoneal dialysis.

LOW-PROTEIN DIET

According to Schwartz and Kassirer,[25] patients may be maintained in a comfortable and useful condition for long periods of time by appropriate medical care. One of the most important features is a low-protein diet. The objective is to maintain positive nitrogen balance, but not to exceed the amount necessary to maintain it. Although the minimum quantity believed to be required has been 40 g, it is now known that as little as 20 g of high-quality proteins will suffice. By using eggs and milk rather than meat and vegetable proteins, azotemia can be controlled. It is not known whether the length of the patient's life is actually increased, but the quality of his life is.

[25] Op. cit., p. 797.

HEMODIALYSIS

During the past ten years the outlook for some patients in renal failure has changed. Remarkable progress has been made in the transplantation of whole organs, especially the kidney. Significant progress has also been made in regulating the composition and volume of extracellular fluids by hemo- and peritoneal dialysis. Not only has hemodialysis equipment been simplified, but machines are also available for use by the patient in his home. Most machines no longer need to be primed with bank blood, which can be the source of many complications, including hepatitis. Although costs have been reduced, they still remain a serious consideration. For home dialysis the patient must remain in the hospital for several weeks of training. The cost of the machine and its installation may be as much as $6,000. The cost for supplies range from $1,500 to $7,500 each year.[26]

Bluemle,[27] in his review of chronic hemodialysis, states that there are many questions to be asked about the procedure. These include: How long can a person survive? What is the quality of his useful life? Who can be successfully treated? How much does it cost? The cost ranges from $8,400 to $19,000 per year. There are insufficient well-trained personnel available for this job. The number of personnel can be reduced by one third when the patient is treated at home. Home treatment has a further advantage because a patient can be treated three times instead of twice in a week. The success of home treatment depends on thorough training of the patient and appropriate supervision by the physician. Successful care of the patient also includes the nurse who prepares the patient to go home and the one who follows his progress at home.

Currently hemodialysis is being used to (1) tide the patient over a period of acute renal failure, (2) remove toxic substances normally excreted by the kidney, (3) prepare the patient for a renal transplant, (4) maintain the composition of the blood following renal transplant until the new kidney functions well, and (5) prolong the life of the patient in chronic renal failure. Some patients have been dialyzed for more than seven years because of poor or no renal function and are still alive.[28]

The general principles and facts on which hemo- and peritoneal dialysis are based and the main problems associated with each will be presented. No attempt will be made to describe

[26] "Home Hemodialysis," Med. Lett., 10:53–54 (July 12) 1968.
[27] Lewis W. Bluemle, Jr.: "Current Status of Chronic Hemodialysis," Amer. J. Med., 44:749–66 (May) 1968.
[28] "Home Hemodialysis," op. cit., p. 53.

either in detail. When hemodialysis was first introduced the procedure was performed by, and under continuous supervision of, a physician. With experience and improved equipment, more and more responsibility has been delegated to nurses and technicians and finally to patients and/or the members of their families.

THE SHUNT

One advance which has made repeated hemodialysis practical is the Teflon tube or shunt connecting an artery and vein in an extremity; this is often referred to as a Scribner Shunt. It is U-shaped; one arm of the shunt is implanted in an artery and the other in a vein, in an arm or leg. The center portion can be removed. The arterial tube is attached to a tube leading into the dialysis machine. The venous tube is attached to a tube carrying blood back from the machine to the patient. At the completion of the procedure the central portion of the tube is replaced and the blood again flows through the shunt from the artery directly to the vein.

The principal problems associated with the shunt are infection and blood clotting. Either may make repeated cannulation necessary. To lessen the possibility of infection, aseptic technique should be used when the shunt is implanted. Following its implantation the area around it should be kept clean and dry. As a preliminary step in the prevention of clotting, heparin may be placed in the tubing near its insertion in the artery. Attention should be given to prevention of kinking of the tubing.

THE DIALYZING MEMBRANE

Both hemo- and peritoneal dialysis are based on the principle that a substance present in different concentrations on two sides of a semipermeable membrane moves from the side of the greater to that of the lesser concentration. If the process is continued, the concentration of the substance will eventually be equalized on the two sides of the membrane. Either procedure can perform most of the kidney's functions. They can remove the wastes of protein metabolism and restore acid-base and electrolyte balance.[29]

In hemodialysis, blood is circulated through cellophane tubing similar to that used for sausage casing. It is permeable to ions and molecules of small size, usually molecules with a molecular weight less than 15,000, and impermeable to large molecules such as protein, some viruses, and bacteria. These characteristics of the tubing simplify the procedure, because they allow ordinary nonsterile tap water to be used to bathe the tubing through which the

[29] John P. Merrill: "The Artificial Kidney," *Sci. Amer.*, **205**:56–64 (July) 1961.

blood is circulated. The tubing is placed on a device suspended in a tank of water to which is added sufficient glucose and electrolytes to make it isotonic with normal blood plasma. When the purpose is to reduce the level of potassium or magnesium or some other constituent in the blood, none or limited quantities of the substances to be removed are added to the water bath. The dialysis is usually continued for four to eight hours or until the constituents in the blood are restored to normal or near-normal levels.

NURSING RESPONSIBILITIES

In the performance of her role, the nurse should be guided by the fact that all material and equipment with which the blood comes in contact must be kept sterile. Provisions should be made for the taking of blood samples. The patient should be prepared for what to expect and what is expected of him. Exactly what is taught to the patient depends on whether hemodialysis is used to relieve an acute or a chronic condition and whether or not he has previously experienced dialysis. Under all circumstances the patient should be included in any conversation carried on in his presence. Both he and his family should be kept informed of his progress. This is particularly important when the procedure is being performed for the first time. Because the procedure usually takes from four to eight hours, attention should be given to the patient's comfort. If the patient is required to lie on his back throughout the procedure, the backrest may be elevated slightly. Passive exercises should be instituted and performed regularly. With the use of the shunt, the patient is usually free to move about as long as the arm or leg with the shunt does not move excessively.

PERITONEAL DIALYSIS

The general principles, objectives, and uses of peritoneal dialysis are similar to those of hemodialysis. Isotonic solutions of electrolytes are introduced into and removed from the peritoneal cavity. As the fluid bathes the peritoneal membrane, substances to which the membrane is permeable diffuse into the fluid. Although they diffuse in both directions, the net transfer is in the direction of lower concentration. Peritoneal dialysis has the advantage of not requiring any blood. Peritoneal dialysis can be carried on intermittently or continuously to maintain the concentration of substances normally removed by the kidney at physiological levels. Because the peritoneal cavity is entered, there is danger of peritonitis and adhesions.

Patients treated by peritoneal dialysis require

competent nursing care with careful attention given to their physiological and emotional needs. The patients should be allowed to turn or move carefully to prevent pulmonary complications and decubiti. As much as is possible, the extremities should be put through their normal range of motion at least once a day. Muscle strain should be relieved by shifting the patient's position and by raising and lowering the headrest of the bed. If the patient is conscious, he should be encouraged to cough and deep-

breathe. Special mouth care is required because oral intake is limited. When monitoring devices are applied, such as continuous recordings of the blood pressure and the electrocardiogram, the nurse should check to see that they are properly applied and working. She should also report any significant changes in the patient's condition.

See Chapter 6 for special problems of patients having organ transplants. References are included at the end of this chapter as well.

REFERENCES

BOOKS

Black, Douglas A. K.: *Essentials of Fluid Balance,* 4th ed. (Philadelphia: F. A. Davis Company, 1967).

Black, Douglas A. K.: *Renal Disease,* 2nd ed. (Philadelphia: F. A. Davis Company, 1967).

Bland, John H.: *Clinical Metabolism of Body Water and Electrolytes* (Philadelphia: W. B. Saunders Company, 1963).

Brest, Albert N., and Moyer, John H. (eds.): *Renal Failure: A Symposium Sponsored by Hahnemann Medical College* (Philadelphia: J. B. Lippincott Company, 1967).

Calne, Roy: *Renal Transplantation,* 2nd ed. (London: Edward Arnold & Company, 1967).

Colby, Fletcher H.: *Essential Urology,* 4th ed. (Baltimore: The Williams & Wilkins Company, 1961).

Deane, Norman: *Kidney and Electrolytes* (Englewood Cliffs, N.J.: Prentice-Hall, Inc., 1966).

Dutcher, Isabel E., and Fielo, Sandra B.: *Water and Electrolytes: Implications for Nursing Practice* (New York: The Macmillan Company, 1967).

Fearing, Margery O., Freeman, Richard M., and Lawton, Richard L.: *Nursing Implications of Caring for Patients on Long-Term Intermittent Hemodialysis,* ANA Regional Clinical Conferences, 1967, Philadelphia/Kansas City (New York: Appleton-Century-Crofts, 1967).

Fellows, Barbara, Blagg, Christopher R., and Scribner, Belding H.: "Acute Renal Failure and Renal Dialysis," in *Concepts and Practices of Intensive Care for Nurse Specialists,* Lawrence E. Meltzer, Faye G. Abdellah and J. Roderick Kitchell, eds. (Philadelphia: The Charles Press Publishers, Inc., 1969), pp. 395–424.

Frisell, Wilhelm: *Acid-Base Chemistry in Medicine* (New York: The Macmillan Company, 1968).

Merrill, John P.: *The Treatment of Renal Failure,* 2nd ed. (New York: Grune & Stratton, Inc., 1965).

Metheny, Norma M., and Snively, William D.: *Nurses' Handbook of Fluid Balance* (Philadelphia: J. B. Lippincott Company, 1967).

Mikal, Stanley: *Homeostasis in Man* (Boston: Little, Brown & Company, 1967).

Mostofi, F. K., and Smith, David E. (eds.): *The Kidney* (Baltimore: The Williams & Wilkins Company, 1966).

Pitts, Robert F.: *Physiology of the Kidney and Body Fluids,* 2nd ed. (Chicago: Year Book Medical Publishers, 1968).

Robinson, James R.: *Fundamentals of Acid-Base Regulation,* 3rd ed. (Philadelphia: F. A. Davis Company, 1967).

Smith, Donald R.: *General Urology,* 5th ed. (Los Altos: Lange Medical Publications, 1966).

Strauss, Maurice B., and Welt, Louis G. (eds.): *Diseases of the Kidney* (Boston: Little, Brown & Company, 1963).

Woolf, L. I.: *Renal Tubular Dysfunction* (Springfield, Ill.: Charles C Thomas, Publisher, 1966).

PERIODICALS

Structure and Function of the Kidney

Briggs, J. D., *et al.:* "Renal Function After Acute Tubular Necrosis," *Brit. Med. J.,* 3:513–16 (Aug. 26) 1967.

Haber, Edgar: "Recent Developments in Pathophysiologic Studies of the Renin-Angiotensin System," *New Eng. J. Med.,* 280:148–54 (Jan. 16) 1969.

Lauler, David P., and Thorn, George W.: "Aldosterone in Clinical Medicine," *Heart Bull.,* 15:81–86 (Sept.–Oct.) 1966.

Strong, Cameron G.: "Hormonal Influence on Renal Function," *Med. Clin. N. Amer.,* 50:985–95 (July) 1966.

Fluid and Electrolyte Balance

Abbey, June C.: "Nursing Observations of Fluid Imbalance," *Nurs. Clin. N. Amer.,* 3:77–86 (Mar.) 1968.

Albert, Morris S., *et al.:* "Quantitative Displacement of Acid-Base Equilibrium in Metabolic Acidosis," *Ann. Intern. Med.,* 66:312–21 (Feb.) 1967.

Aliapoulios, Menelaos A., Bernstein, Daniel S.,

and Balodimos, Marios C.: "Thyrocalcitonin," *Arch. Intern. Med.,* **123**:88–94 (Jan.) 1969.

Crandell, Walter B.: "Parenteral Fluid Therapy," *Surg. Clin. N. Amer.,* **48**:707–21 (Aug.) 1968.

De Veber, George A.: "Fluid and Electrolyte Problems in the Postoperative Period," *Nurs. Clin. N. Amer.,* **1**:275–84 (June) 1966.

Donnelly, William J. (ed.): "Hypercalcemia and Lethargy," *Postgrad. Med.,* **41**:623–29 (June) 1967.

Epstein, F. H.: "Calcium and the Kidney," *Amer. J. Med.,* **45**:700–14 (Nov.) 1968.

Gillies, J. C.: "Fluid Balance," *Nurs. Times,* **62**:1493–94 (Nov. 11) 1966.

Hubel, Kenneth A.: "The Ins and Outs of Bicarbonate in the Alimentary Tract," *Gastroenterology,* **54**:647–51 (Apr.) 1968.

Liberman, Bernardo, Wajchenberg, Bernardo L., and Pieroni, Romulo Ribeiro: "Water and Electrolyte Metabolism in Adrenal and Pituitary Insufficiency. II. Effect of Gluco- and Mineralocorticoid Adrenal Steroids on Sodium Metabolism, with Special Reference to Exchangeable Sodium," *Metabolism,* **15**:992–1001 (Nov.) 1966.

"Magnesium Deficiency—A Clinical Entity?" *Postgrad. Med.,* **41**:650 (June) 1967.

Moore, Francis D.: "Blood Transfusions: Rates, Routes, and Hazards," *Nurs. Clin. N. Amer.,* **1**:285–94 (June) 1966.

Peirce, E. Converse, II: "Is Acid-Base Balance Important?" *Med. Times,* **95**:1231–56 (Dec.) 1967.

"Potassium Imbalance," *Amer. J. Nurs.,* **67**:343–66 (Feb.) 1967.

Steinmetz, Philip R.: "Excretion of Acid by the Kidney—Functional Organization and Cellular Aspects of Acidification," *New Eng. J. Med.,* **278**:1102–09 (May 16) 1968.

Thompson, David D. (ed.): "Symposium on the Treatment of Fluid and Electrolyte Imbalance," *Mod. Treatm.,* **5**:617–726 (July) 1968.

Vorburger, C.: "Pathogenesis of Edema," *Angiology,* **19**:362–71 (June) 1968.

Wacker, Warren E. C., and Parisi, Alfred F.: "Magnesium Metabolism," *New Eng. J. Med.,* **278**:712–17 (Mar. 28) 1968.

Whang, Robert: "Some Aspects of the Interrelationship of Magnesium and Potassium," *J. Chronic Dis.,* **21**:207–10 (July) 1968.

Renal Disease

Hunt, James C., and Johnson, William J. (eds.): "Symposium on Diseases of the Kidney," *Med. Clin. N. Amer.,* **50**:925–1196 (July) 1966.

Platts, Margaret M.: "Renal Disease in Women," *Nurs. Times,* **64**:1009–11 (July 26) 1968.

Waterlow, J. C.: "Observation on the Mechanism of Adaptation to Low Protein Intakes," *Lancet,* **2**:1091–97 (Nov. 23) 1968.

Nephrotic Conditions

Cameron, J. S.: "Nephritis and the Nephrotic Syndrome," *Nurs. Times,* **63**:442–44 (Apr. 7) 1967.

Monroe, Jewel M., and Komorita, Nori I.: "Problems with Nephrosis in Adolescence," *Amer. J. Nurs.,* **67**:336–40 (Feb.) 1967.

Acute Glomerulonephritis

Adamson, J. W., Eschbach, J., and Finch, C. A.: "The Kidney and Erythropoiesis," *Amer. J. Med.,* **44**:725–33 (May) 1968.

Cotran, Ramzi S.: "Delayed and Prolonged Vascular Leakage in Inflammation," *Exp. Molec. Path.,* **6**:143–55 (Apr.) 1967.

Dixon, Frank J.: "The Pathogenesis of Glomerulonephritis," *Amer. J. Med.,* **44**:493–98 (Apr.) 1968.

Epstein, Franklin H.: "Acute Glomerulonephritis," *Hosp. Med.,* **4**:30–42 (Nov.) 1968.

Germuth, Frederick, Senterfit, Laurence, and Pollack, Abou: "Immune Complex Disease. I. Experimental Acute and Chronic Glomerulonephritis," and "II. The Role of Circulatory Dynamics and Glomerular Filtration in the Development of Experimental Glomerulonephritis," *Johns Hopkins Med. J.,* **120**:225–57 (Apr.) 1967.

Lerner, R. A., Glassock, R. J., and Dixon, Frank J.: "The Role of Anti-Glomerular Basement Membrane Antibody in the Pathogenesis of Human Glomerulonephritis," *J. Exp. Med.,* **126**:989–1004 (Dec.) 1967.

Renal Failure

Austen, George: "Management of Postoperative Acute Renal Failure," *Amer. J. Surg.,* **116**:346–61 (Sept.) 1968.

Cramond, W. A., *et al.:* "Psychological Aspects of the Management of Chronic Renal Failure," *Brit. Med. J.,* **1**:539–43 (Mar. 2) 1968.

Franklin, Stanley S., *et al.:* "Use of a Balanced Low Protein in Diet in Chronic Renal Failure," *JAMA,* **202**:477–84 (Nov.) 1967.

Kuba, Anna: "The Nursing Needs of Patients with Renal Failure," *ANA Clinical Sessions* (New York: American Nurses Association, 1964).

Levin, Sidney, and Winkelstein, Jerry A.: "Diet and Infrequent Peritoneal Dialysis in Chronic Anuric Uremia," *New Eng. J. Med.,* **277**:619–24 (Sept. 21) 1967.

Levinsky, Norman G.: "Management of Chronic Renal Failure," *New Eng. J. Med.,* **271**:358–60 (Aug. 13), **271**:460–63 (Aug. 27) 1964.

Lewis, Edmund J., and Magill, John M.: "Symposium: Proceedings of the Conference on the Nutritional Aspects of Uremia," *Amer. J. Clin. Nutr.,* **21**:547–643 (June) 1968.

Maddock, Robert K., Bloomer, H. A., and De St. Jeor, Sachiko W.: "Low Protein Diets in the Management of Renal Failure," *Ann. Intern. Med.,* **69**:1003–1008 (Nov.) 1968.

Merrill, John P.: "Management of Chronic Renal Failure," *Amer. J. Med.,* **36**:763–77 (May) 1964.

Montgomerie, John Z., Kalmanson, George M., and Guze, Lucien B.: "Renal Failure and Infection," *Medicine,* **47**:1–32 (Jan.) 1968.

Parets, Albert D.: "Emotional Reactions to Chronic Physical Illness: Implications for the

Internist," *Med. Clin. N. Amer.*, **51**:1399–1408 (Nov.) 1967.

Schwartz, Franklin D., and Dunea, George: "Acute Renal Failure," *Med. Times,* **95**:1287–94 (Dec.) 1967.

Vertel, Capt. Robert M., and Knochel, Lt. Col. James P.: "Nonoliguric Acute Renal Failure," *JAMA*, **200**:598–602 (May 15) 1967.

Welt, L. G.: "Symposium on Uremia," *Amer. J. Med.*, **44**:653–802 (May) 1968.

Wills, M. R.: "Biochemical Consequences of Chronic Renal Failure: A Review," *J. Clin. Path.*, **21**:541–54 (Sept.) 1968.

Diagnostic Tests

Dunea, George, and Freedman, Philip: "Renal Clearance Studies," *JAMA*, **205**:120–21 (July 15) 1968.

Gault, M. H., and Dossetor, J. B.: "Evaluation of Renal Function Without Collection of Urine," *Ann. Intern. Med.*, **69**:1326–28 (Dec.) 1968.

Kelly, Ann E., and Gensini, Goffredo G.: "Renal Arteriography," *Amer. J. Nurs.*, **64**:97–99 (Feb.) 1964.

"Tests of Renal Function," *Nurs. Clin. N. Amer.*, **2**:800–802 (Dec.) 1967.

"Voiding Cystourethrogram," *Ther. Notes,* **75**:53 (Fall) 1968.

Hemodialysis

Albers, Joann: "Evaluation of Blood Volume in Patients on Hemodialysis," *Amer. J. Nurs.*, **68**:1677–79 (Aug.) 1968.

Blumentals, Ausma S., Eichenholz, Alfred, and Mulhausen, Robert O.: "Acid-Base Balance Changes During Hemodialysis," *Metabolism*, **14**:667–73 (June) 1965.

Brand, Lucy, and Komorita, Nori I.: "Adapting to Long-Term Hemodialysis," *Amer. J. Nurs.*, **66**:1778–81 (Aug.) 1966.

Curtis, J. R., *et al.:* "Maintenance Haemodialysis," *Quart. J. Med.*, **38**:49–88 (Jan.) 1969.

Eastwood, John B., *et al.:* "Hepatitis in a Maintenance Hemodialysis Unit," *Ann. Intern. Med.*, **69**:59–72 (July) 1968.

Fellows, Barbara J.: "Hemodialysis at Home," *Amer. J. Nurs.*, **66**:1775–78 (Aug.) 1966.

Fellows, Barbara Jo: "The Role of the Nurse in a Chronic Dialysis Unit," *Nurs. Clin. N. Amer.*, **1**:577–86 (Dec.) 1966.

Goodey, Josephine, and Kelly, Josephine: "Social and Economic Effects of Regular Dialysis," *Lancet,* **2**:147–48 (July 15) 1967.

Hampers, Constantine L., and Merrill, John P.: "Hemodialysis in the Home—13 Months' Experience," *Ann. Intern. Med.*, **64**:276–83 (Feb.) 1966.

"Home Dialysis for Chronic Renal Failure," *Canad. Med. Ass. J.*, **98**:366–67 (Feb. 17) 1968.

Lewis, Edmund J., *et al.:* "Survival Data for Patients Undergoing Chronic Intermittent Hemodialysis," *Ann. Intern. Med.*, **70**:311–15 (Feb.) 1969.

Meldrum, W., Wolfram, J. G., and Rubini, M. E.: "The Impact upon the Socio-economics of a Veteran Patient Group," *Chronic Dis.*, **21**:37–52 (Jan.) 1968.

Menzies, I. C., *et al.:* "Psychiatric Observations on Patients Receiving Regular Dialysis Treatment," *Brit. Med. J.*, **1**:544–47 (Mar. 2) 1968.

Rae, Angus I., *et al.:* "Hemodialysis in the Home," *JAMA,* **206**:92–96 (Sept. 30) 1968.

Shaldon, Stanley, and Abrahams, Carole: "Independence Concept of Haemodialysis," *Nurs. Times,* **64**:1329–31 (Oct. 4) 1968.

Shea, Eileen J., *et al.:* "Hemodialysis for Chronic Renal Failure: IV. Psychological Considerations," *Ann. Intern. Med.*, **62**:558–63 (Mar.) 1965.

Smith, E. K. M., *et al.:* "Haemodialysis in the Home—Problems and Frustrations," *Lancet,* **1**:614–17 (Mar. 22) 1969.

U.S. Department of Health, Education, and Welfare, Public Health Service: "A Dialysis Symposium for Nurses" (Washington, D.C.: Government Printing Office, 1968).

Whitehead, V. M.: "Homeostasis of Folic Acid in Patients Undergoing Maintenance Hemodialysis," *New Eng. J. Med.*, **279**:970–74 (Oct.) 1968.

Peritoneal Dialysis

Berlyne, G. M., *et al.:* "Aminoacid Loss in Peritoneal Dialysis," *Lancet,* **1**:1339–41 (June 24) 1967.

Cohen, S. L., and Percival, A.: "Prolonged Peritoneal Dialysis in Patients Awaiting Renal Transplantation," *Brit. Med. J.*, **1**:409–13 (Feb. 17) 1968.

Downing, Shirley R.: "The Patient Who Has Peritoneal Dialysis: Care During the Exchange," *Amer. J. Nurs.*, **66**:1572–77 (July) 1966.

O'Neill, Mary: "Peritoneal Dialysis," *Nurs. Clin. N. Amer.*, **1**:309–23 (June) 1966.

Shea, Eileen J.: "Peritoneal Dialysis," *Nurs. Forum,* **4**:33–39 (No. 3), 1965.

Kidney Transplantation

Bois, Marna S., *et al.:* "Nursing Care of Patients Having Kidney Transplants," *Amer. J. Nurs.*, **68**:1238–39, 1242–47 (June) 1968.

Hager, Edward B.: "Current Status of Renal Transplantation," *Postgrad. Med.*, **41**:585–91 (June) 1967.

Hume, David M.: "Renal Homotransplantation in Man," *Ann. Rev. Med.*, **18**:229–68, 1967.

Kincaid-Smith, Priscilla, *et al.:* "Cadaveric Renal Transplantation," *Lancet,* **2**:59–62 (July 8) 1967.

Martin, Alfred J.: "Renal Transplantation: Surgical Technique and Complications," *Amer. J. Nurs.*, **68**:1240–41 (June) 1968.

Merrill, John P.: "Present Status of Kidney Transplantation," *Med. Times,* **95**:403–15 (Apr.) 1967.

Russel, P. S.: "Kidney Transplantation," *Amer. J. Med.*, **44**:776–85 (May) 1968.

Shebelski, Dorothy I.: "Nursing Patients Who Have Renal Homotransplants," *Amer. J. Nurs.*, **66**:2425–28 (Nov.) 1966.

Diuretics

Bank, Norman: "Physiological Basis of Diuretic Action," *Ann. Rev. Med.,* **19**:130–18, 1968.

Blenkiron, C. H.: "Diuresis and Diuretics," *Nurs. Times,* **63**:755–57 (June 9) 1967.

Cafruny, Edward J.: "The Site and Mechanism of Action of Mercurial Diuretics," *Pharmacol. Rev.,* **20**:89–116 (June) 1968.

Schneider, William J., and Boyce, Barbara A.: "Complications of Diuretic Therapy," *Amer. J. Nurs.,* **68**:1903–1907 (Sept.) 1968.

Wilson, G. M.: "Diuretics," *Practitioner,* **200**:39–44 (Jan.) 1968.

10

Nursing the Patient Having a Problem with Some Aspects of Transporting Material to and from Cells *

It is proved by the structure of the heart that the blood is continuously transferred through the lungs into the aorta, as by two clacks of a water bellows to raise water. It is proved by the ligature that there is a passage of blood from the arteries to the veins. It is therefore demonstrated that the continuous movement of the blood in a circle is brought about by the beat of the heart. Is this for the sake of nutrition, or the better preservation of the blood and members by the infusion of heat, the blood in turn being cooled by heating the members and heated by the heart? [1]

Overview

EMPHASIS has been placed on the fact that survival, growth, reproduction, and productivity

[1] William Harvey: quoted in "Lives in Science," *A Scientific American Book* (New York: Simon and Schuster, Inc., 1953), p. 189.

depend on a continued supply of the materials required by cells to support their chemical activities. Waste products must be removed from the cells and eliminated so the physical and chemical conditions of the fluid environment of cells are maintained within limits favorable to cell processes. Excesses of supply must

* This chapter revised by Elizabeth Ford Pitorak, Associate Professor of Nursing, Case Western Reserve University, Frances Payne Bolton School of Nursing, Cleveland, Ohio.

be stored or eliminated. Products produced by one group of cells, such as hormones, require some means of distribution if they are to influence the activity of other cells. In previous chapters, discussion has centered around how the organism acquires needed materials from its external environment and around the mechanisms involved in maintaining the constancy of the internal environment within limits.

References have been made to the importance of transportation to each of the preceding. Unless required substances can be taken into the internal environment and distributed to the cells, life ceases. This chapter is devoted to the factors important to the transportation of materials from one part of the body to another and to the causes and consequences of failure of transportation.

In man, cells are bathed in a fluid that is separated from the external environment by semipermeable membranes. To meet the needs of the cells, materials must be transported to and from these membranes. This is accomplished by a system of tubes arranged in what is essentially a closed circuit. Some of these tubes are thick-walled structures serving as distensible and elastic conduits conveying blood from the heart to the tissues or from the tissues back to the heart. After tubes (arteries) leave the heart and approach the tissues, they branch into smaller and smaller vessels. Finally, they form microscopic structures (capillaries) that are only one endothelial cell in thickness. It is in the capillary that the function of transportation is accomplished. In the capillary, materials are taken into the internal environment or returned to the external environment. Materials are exchanged between the internal and external environment, as well as between the blood and the interstitial fluid.

The circuit is filled with a modifiable medium of exchange, the blood. Some of the substances transported in the blood are in solution. Others are as formed elements. Still others are in chemical or physical combination with formed elements.

How is blood transported throughout the body?

The major factor in the movement of blood is the force of contraction of the heart. Other factors that contribute to keeping the circuit filled and to a continuous flow of blood to tissues include (1) the distensibility and elasticity of the arteries; (2) the resistance offered by the walls of arteries, particularly small arteries, to the flow of blood; and (3) the viscosity of the blood. Return flow of blood through the veins is supported by the contraction of skeletal muscles and valves that prevent backflow in veins carrying blood against gravity. Because of

their contribution to the forward movement of blood in veins, skeletal muscles are sometimes referred to as secondary hearts. Alpha receptors in the walls of veins respond to the release of norepinephrine by causing the veins to constrict.[2] Lessening of pressure in the thoracic cavity during inspiration as well as reduction of pressure within the heart following systole also aids in the return of blood to the heart.

One of the remarkable features of circulatory function is that, in health, blood is moved into and out of all of the tissues of the body, so the needs of cells in varying states of activity are met.[3] Moreover, function can be adapted in relation to the activity of the entire organism or to a localized area of tissue. At the same time, blood flow is regulated so that vital structures, such as the brain, heart, and kidney, are nourished despite greatly increased demands by other parts of the body. Respiration and circulatory functions are regulated in relation to each other, so that their function is complementary.

Like other tissues in the body, the structures comprising the transportation system are susceptible to conditions in the internal environment. They are dependent for continued function on the quantity and quality of blood circulated through them. They are also subject to disease and injury. Malfunction may result from disturbances in the mental apparatus (see Chapter 7) or from direct injury to cells. Injury, beyond that induced by the initiating factor, may result from excessive response of damaged tissues. For example, deformations of the heart valves as a result of rheumatic fever can be increased by the formation of excessive quantities of scar tissue. Conversely, scarring and its undesirable sequelae can be reduced if the severity of the exudative and proliferative phases of the disease can be lessened.

Causes of Failure of Transportation

Although the effects of failure in function will be discussed later in this chapter, the causes of failure of transportation may generally be summarized as (1) inadequate quantity or quality of the blood; (2) insufficient power to move blood into the arteries; (3) failure to return blood to the heart; (4) obstruction, intrinsic or extrinsic, to the flow of blood; (5) overdilatation of the tubular structures—local or general; (6) disturbances in the volume of circulating fluid; and (7) disturbances arising from defects in regulation of one or more parts of the transportation system.

---

[2] J. Edwin Wood: "The Venous System," *Sci. Amer.*, **218:**86 (Jan.) 1968.

[3] Factors in the movement of substances to and from the blood and the cell are discussed in Chapter 9.

Manifestations resulting from disease or injury to the transportation system depend on the degree to which the needs of the tissues are met and the specific tissues affected. As long as an activity of a person is within the adaptive capacity of his circulatory system, there may be no symptoms and few, if any, observable signs indicating failure of transportation. The affected tissues may receive sufficient blood of high enough quality to function at rest or during mild or even moderate activity. Examples include the instance of Frank Sparrow, who has arteriosclerosis obliterans of the arteries of his lower extremities. Blood flow is impeded but not completely obstructed. He can walk from his house to the corner—about a short city block—without discomfort. When he tries to walk farther, he develops a cramplike pain in the calf of his leg. For some weeks, Mrs. Bird (the grandmother in Chapter 9), who had a diagnosis of congestive heart failure, found she became short of breath when she walked up a flight of stairs or walked against the wind. Enid Elm's hemoglobin was 7 g per 100 ml of blood. She was comfortable only when resting. She became short of breath when climbing stairs or running for a bus. Although each of these individuals had a disorder limiting the functional capacity of some part of their circulatory system, the blood supplied to the tissues of each of them was adequate in quantity and quality when they were at rest or exercising moderately. It was not sufficient, however, to enable them to increase their activity.

Many of the manifestations of failure in transportation result from a lack in the supply of oxygen and nutrients and from an accumulation of carbon dioxide and other metabolites in the affected tissues. Effects of failure will also be influenced by whether the disturbance involves the entire individual or is limited to a localized area of tissue. Disorders involving the heart or blood frequently affect the function of the body as a whole. Signs and symptoms are likely to be the result of disturbances in the functions of organs particularly sensitive to oxygen want or carbon dioxide excess. Sooner or later all tissues—organs and systems—will be affected. Lesions involving blood vessels may have either local or general effects. In some diseases of blood vessels, such as atherosclerosis, the disorder may be more or less generalized, but its effects are more marked in some organs than in others, as in the brain, kidney, heart, and lower extremities. Whatever the causative factor or factors, the effects of failure in transportation result from inadequate nourishment of cells. Survival of the affected cells is possible when the failure is relative, but death of cells or of the entire organism quickly follows complete failure. It is important to note that any disturbance, whatever its origin, involving circulatory function can be expected to arouse some degree of anxiety in the patient. This anxiety is often a factor in the magnitude of the response of the patient to his illness.

Knowledge of the factors necessary for the maintenance of a satisfactory blood supply to all tissues of the body, as well as of some of the causes and effects of failure, is essential in the practice of nursing. Some of the causes of failure are the result of the general effect of illness or its therapy on the circulatory system. Others are the consequence of disease or injury of some part of the circulatory system itself. Often the manifestations are caused by multiple factors. As an illustration, Mr. Frank has generalized atherosclerosis. Because neither his heart nor his arteries are able to adapt to an increase in activity, bed rest has been prescribed. A decrease in activity is accompanied by venous stasis, thus predisposing to the formation of thrombi in the veins. Pressure, particularly over bony prominences, impedes arterial circulation and leads to tissue injury because it limits the blood supply to the affected part.

Diseases involving the cardiovascular system rank first as a cause of death. They are also important causes of morbidity and disability. They are found among people in all age groups and in all walks of life. With the exception of the second decade of life, their incidence rises from birth to death. From the community point of view, the most serious form of disease is the one that kills or maims persons in the productive years of life.

What are some of the objectives of nursing care?

Because of differences in the function of the various structures in transportation, each will be presented separately. No part, however, functions alone. Each part is dependent on all others if tissues are to be adequately nourished. Nursing care as it relates to a disturbance in transportation should be planned to achieve one or more of the following objectives:

1. To lessen the activity of a part or of the whole individual so the discrepancy between supply and demand is minimized
2. To strengthen or improve the functioning capacity of the diseased organ or organs
3. To supply needed materials for cellular activity
4. To assist the patient to as full a recovery as his condition permits
5. To provide an environment that affords the patient physical and emotional comfort and support
6. To protect the patient from disturbances

or conditions in his internal or external environment that will place added stress on his already defective transportation system

In the following pages, the consequences of failure of the heart, arteries, veins, capillaries, and blood to function within physiological limits will be discussed. Implications for nursing care will be indicated.

The Healthy Heart

Anyone who reads the daily newspaper knows the heart is an important source of mortality, morbidity, and disability. What may not be sufficiently appreciated is that, in health, the heart is a powerful organ with a considerable degree of reserve power. According to authorities such as Paul Dudley White, the heart, rather than being injured by, benefits from physical exercise. This is apparently true of the diseased heart as well as the healthy heart. In health, the heart is capable of adapting the quantity of its output of blood to the quantity of blood delivered to it by the veins. Stated simply and directly, cardiac output equals cardiac intake. The ultimate test of cardiac function is the capacity or power of the heart to move as much blood into the arteries as is delivered to it by the veins. This implies that when the volume of blood delivered to the heart is increased, cardiac output is also increased. After a stroke or two, a new balance is struck between intake and output and there is no gain in the quantity of blood remaining in the heart at the end of systole.

The remarkable power of the heart is illustrated by the fact that the heart of an adult weighing 70 kg pumps about 60 ml per stroke, or about 5 liters of blood, each minute, at rest, and up to 120 to 150 ml per stroke, or 20 or 25 liters each minute, during exercise. In a well-trained athlete, the cardiac output may be as high as 35 liters per minute.[4] An important characteristic of a healthy heart is its ability to adjust its output to the needs of the tissues.

Structure and Function

In structure, the heart is a double pump, each side of which has two chambers—an atrium and a ventricle. The two sides of the heart are separated from each other by a muscular septum that prevents the mixing of arterial and venous blood. Openings in the septum may be caused

[4] Carl J. Wiggers: "The Heart," *Sci. Amer.,* **196:**75 (May) 1957.

by failure to close the foramen ovale [5] or by failure to close either the interventricular or interatrial septum in the developing embryo. Septal defects, especially those in the ventricular septum that allow for mixing of arterial and venous blood, are one of the more serious congenital anomalies of the heart. Interseptal defects, when combined with other anomalies such as pulmonic stenosis or right ventricular hypertrophy, are a cause of cyanotic heart disease, as in the so-called "blue baby."

The right side of the heart receives blood from the systemic circulation and ejects blood into the pulmonary or lesser circulation. The left side of the heart receives blood from the pulmonary circulation and pumps blood into the systemic circulation. With the exception of the small amount of blood circulated through the bronchial arteries, the right side pumps the same quantity of blood as the left. The bronchial veins empty into the pulmonary veins and thus drain into the left rather than the right atrium. The myocardium of the right ventricle is not as thick as the left ventricle because it pumps blood into a relatively low-pressure system while the left ventricle pumps blood into a high-pressure system. In health, the ventricle provides the main force in the movement of blood, and the atrium acts primarily as a reservoir. In disease of the heart, the atria may account for as much as 30 per cent of the propulsive power of the heart.

As indicated, the heart is a rhythmically contracting organ that regularly ejects the blood received from the venous circulation into the arteries. In Figures 10-1 and 10-2 the layers and other essential structures of the heart are depicted. The essential structures of the heart include the endocardium, the myocardium, the pericardium, the blood and lymphatic vessels, the nerve supply, and the supporting structures. All these structures are subject to disease and injury. An injury or disease in one part may directly or indirectly affect the function of other parts, including the pumping mechanism.

The Endocardium

The heart is lined by the endocardium. The inner layer of the endocardium is made up of a single layer of simple squamous epithelium that is continuous with the lining or intima of blood vessels. The endothelial cells lie over a layer of connective tissues. The endocardium lines the chambers of the heart and is reflected over the heart valves. It serves the same function as the

[5] The foramen ovale is an opening in the interatrial septum that connects the right and left atria in the fetal heart.

intima of the blood vessels; that is, it provides a smooth surface for contact with blood. It lessens friction between the blood and the walls of the heart and lessens danger of clotting of blood.

What are some of the causes and results of injury of the endocardium?

When, as a result of infection, stasis, trauma, aging, infarction, or the collagen diseases,[6] the

[6] The collagen diseases are a group of disorders or syndromes involving connective tissue. They are grouped together because they have certain histological features in common, such as widespread inflammatory injury of the connective tissue and the deposition of a fibrinoid material in the ground substance. Each collagen disease presents a distinct clinical picture, but they have general manifestations as well as local lesions in a variety of organs including the joints, heart, blood vessels, skin, muscle, and supporting reticulum of other organs. The involvement of one or more organs should be expected, because some type of connective tissue is found in all parts of the body. The specific clinical manifestations of the collagen diseases will depend on the location of lesions and the rate at which they develop. Many of these disorders respond favorably for a time to therapy with the adrenal corticosteroids. Included among the collagen diseases are systemic lupus erythematosus, dermatomyositis, and polyarteritis. (A. McGehee Harvey: "Diseases of Connective Tissue," *Cecil-Loeb: Textbook of Medicine,* 12th ed., Paul B. Beeson and Walsh McDermott, eds. (Philadelphia: W. B. Saunders Company, 1967), pp. 447–67.

endocardium is damaged and no longer presents a nearly frictionless surface, it may serve as a site for the formation of intracardiac thrombosis. As an example, Mary Olive has atrial fibrillation and stenosis [7] of the mitral valve. Stasis of blood in the left atrium predisposes to the clotting of blood. Thrombi have been formed in the auricular appendages of her left atrium. As another example, Mr. Frank Carp has a serious myocardial infarction.[8] The area of ischemia extends through the myocardium and into the endocardium of his left ventricle. Necrosis of endothelial cells roughened the endocardium and predisposed to the formation of a thrombus.[9] Whenever a thrombus is present in any part of the vascular system, there is always a possibility that before the thrombus is organized a piece will be dislodged and become an embolus and be carried forward in the circulation until it obstructs an artery. The site of obstruction will depend on whether the embolus originates in the right or left side of the heart

[7] Stenosis is a condition in which an opening or tubular structure is narrowed or constricted.
[8] Death of an area of heart muscle as a result of obstruction of the blood supply to it.
[9] Because the thrombus is attached to the wall of the heart, it is called a mural (wall) thrombus.

HEAD & ARMS

RIGHT LUNG

LEFT LUNG

AORTA

to all parts of the body

PULMONARY VEIN

PULMONARY ARTERY

ATRIUM   PULMONARY VEIN

mitral valve

aortic valve

ATRIUM

pulmonary valve

VENTRICLE

inside lining of heart (endocardium)

RIGHT HEART

receives blood from the body and pumps it through the pulmonary artery to the lungs where it picks up fresh oxygen.

tricuspid valve

VENTRICLE

heart muscle (myocardium)

LEFT HEART

receives oxygen-full blood from the lungs and pumps it through the aorta to the body.

bag of tissue surrounding heart (pericardium)

TRUNK & LEGS

FIGURE 10-1. Diagram of the human heart, the veins and arteries entering and leaving it, and the route of the blood through it and to parts of the body, indicated by arrows. (Information adapted with permission of the American Heart Association from *Your Heart and How It Works,* 1963.)

Superior vena cava

Ascending aorta

Right auricular appendix

Corpus arantii

Membranous septum

Tricuspid valve
- Anterior cusp
- Posterior cusp
- Internal cusp

Papillary muscles

Trabeculae carneae

Reflection of pericardium on to pulmonary artery and pulmonary veins

Left coronary artery

Left auricular appendix

Left semilunar flap of aortic valve

Posterior semilunar flap of aortic valve

Anterior cusp of bicuspid valve

Posterior cusp of bicuspid valve

Papillary muscles

Myocardium

FIGURE 10-2. The heart seen from the front. (Modified from Toldt.) What is the function of the right heart? The left heart? Why are valves needed? (Information adapted with permission of The Macmillan Company from *Anatomy and Physiology,* 15th ed., Fig. 13-6, p. 389, by Diana Clifford Kimber, Carolyn E. Gray, Caroline E. Stackpole, and Lutie C. Leavell. Copyright © The Macmillan Company, 1966.)

and on the size of the clot. An embolus originating in the left side of the heart will block an artery in the systemic circulation. The blood supply to any organ supplied by the systemic circulation may be partly or entirely obstructed. Emboli originating in the right side obstruct the pulmonary circulation. Besides obstructing arterial blood flow, thrombi or emboli may serve as sites of infection.

Valvular Function

In addition to predisposing to intracardiac thromboses, disease or injury of the endocardium often results in deformity of one or more of the valves of the heart and, as a consequence, interference with valvular function. The effects of injury to the valves can best be understood in the light of their structure and function. Valves in the heart help to keep the blood moving in one direction through the vascular circuit. They and their attachments are so shaped and arranged that pressure in one (forward) direction causes the valve to open, and pressure in the

other or (backward) direction causes the valve to close. The valves between the atria and ventricles are prevented from inverting during systole by the chordae tendineae and the papillary muscles. See Figures 10-1, 10-2, 10-3, and 10-4. During closure there is a considerable degree of overlapping of the valve leaflets, which helps prevent the backward flow of blood. The semilunar valves, which lie between the ventricles and the pulmonary arteries and the aorta, are cup-shaped, with the bowl of the cup toward the pulmonary artery or aorta. As the artery fills so do the cusps (cups). The filling of the cusps brings the edges of the valve into contact. Unlike the atrioventricular valves, there is no overlapping of the edges of the valvular cusps. During diastole the pressure of blood in the artery and the cusps is greater than the pressure within the heart; the valves are maintained in a closed position. During systole, the pressure within the heart is greater than the pressure in the arteries and the valves are opened. Briefly, the opening and closing of these valves are determined by blood pressure.

Front

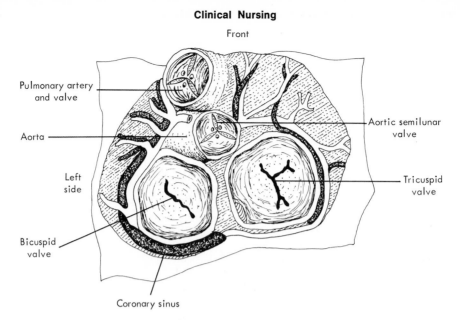

Pulmonary artery
and valve

Aorta

Aortic semilunar
valve

Left
side

Tricuspid
valve

Bicuspid
valve

Coronary sinus

Figure 10-3. Valves of the heart as seen from above, atria removed. (Information adapted with permission of The Macmillan Company from *Anatomy and Physiology*, 15th ed., Fig. 13-8, p. 391, by Diana Clifford Kimber, Carolyn E. Gray, Caroline E. Stackpole, and Lutie C. Leavell. Copyright © The Macmillan Company, 1966.)

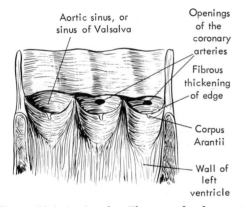

Aortic sinus, or
sinus of Valsalva

Openings
of the
coronary
arteries

Fibrous
thickening
of edge

Corpus
Arantii

Wall of
left
ventricle

Figure 10-4. Aortic valve. The artery has been cut open to show the aortic semilunar valve. The sinuses of Valsalva are three pouches or slight dilations that are located between the semilunar valves and the wall of the aorta. These sinuses are also found on the pulmonary artery between the semilunar valves and the wall of the artery. Note the openings of the coronary arteries and the cup shape of the aortic semilunar valves. (Information adapted with permission of The Macmillan Company from *Anatomy and Physiology*, 14th ed., Fig. 225, p. 314, by Diana Clifford Kimber, Carolyn E. Gray, Caroline E. Stackpole, and Lutie C. Leavell. Copyright © The Macmillan Company, 1961.)

VALVULAR DYSFUNCTION

When, as a result of injury or disease, the valve leaflets, or cusps, are damaged, the valve may no longer close tightly or open fully. Failure of the valve to close an opening between the atrium and ventricle or the ventricle and its artery allows blood to flow in a backward direction. Failure of a valve to open normally impedes the forward movement of blood. When a valve does not close properly, it is said to be insufficient or incompetent. In lay terms, the valve "leaks." When it does not open fully, because it is narrowed or constricted, it is said to be stenosed. Valves may be both insufficient and stenosed. The seriousness of deformities of a heart valve depends on the degree of "leakiness" or obstruction and on its location. For example, when the aortic semilunar valve is incompetent, blood leaks back into the heart during diastole. The return of arterial blood to the left ventricle has two serious effects. The heart has to move "leaked blood" back into the aorta, as well as the blood delivered to the heart by the veins, and it has difficulty in meeting its own nutritional needs. Maximum blood flow through the coronary arteries takes place at the end of systole and beginning of diastole. Coronary artery blood flow, especially to the left ventricle, depends on the pressure of the blood in the ascending aorta at the beginning of diastole. The contracting ventricle obstructs the lumen of its own blood vessels and limits the flow of blood to the myocardium during systole. Therefore, any condition resulting in a lowering of the pressure of the blood in the ascending aorta during diastole lessens the quantity of blood circulated to the myocardium. To recapitulate, a leaking aortic valve allows blood to fall back into the heart as soon as diastole begins. Blood, therefore, moves not only forward into the circulation but backward into the ventricle, with the result that the pressure of the blood in the ascending aorta falls abruptly. As a consequence, there is a loss in the force required to move blood through the coronary arteries. Each time the heart contracts, it is called on to move the blood that returns to it from the aorta during diastole as well as the blood that continues in the normal circuit. Despite the increase in the demands made on it for work, the capacity of the heart to nourish itself is diminished rather than increased. The heart is called on to perform increased work despite a decrease in supply of oxygen and nutrients.

MURMURS

In addition to the effect of stenosis or insufficiency on the forward movement of the blood, deformation of the valves increases the turbulence of the blood as it passes through the opening guarded by the heart valve. These changes in turbulence result in alterations in the heart sounds caused by the flow of blood from one chamber to another in the heart. These abnormal sounds are called murmurs. Contrary to popular opinion, murmurs do not always indicate serious disease of the heart. Factors such as the time they occur in the cardiac cycle and the conditions under which they are heard aid the physician in making a decision about their significance. Unfortunately, after learning of the presence of a heart murmur people have become invalids by themselves or because they were overprotected by their parents. When a patient or a parent appears to be concerned about a heart murmur, this information should be brought to the attention of the physician.

VALVULAR DEFORMITIES

Valvular deformity may be the direct result of a developmental defect or the effect of the injury caused by hypersensitivity reactions, infections, or other types of inflammatory processes that cause cellular necrosis and stimulate fibrous tissue proliferation. Frequently the degree of deformity is increased by the scar tissue formed in the process of healing. The latter illustrates Claude Bernard's thesis and more recently Selye's that processes set in motion by disease or injury may cause further and sometimes greater damage than the initiating factor. As an example, in rheumatic fever, scar tissue formed in healing the affected valves may increase the degree of valvular deformity. Damage to cells stimulates the formation of scar tissue. The scar tissue that is formed contracts as it

matures and deforms the affected valves so the opening is narrowed (stenosed), or does not close properly (incompetent), or both. In addition to the above, over a period of years calcium may be deposited in the already deformed valve, thus adding to its rigidity.

Finally, valvular or other cardiac deformities involving the endocardium predispose to infection of the abnormal tissues. The most common organism infecting the defective heart valves is the *Streptococcus viridans,* which causes subacute bacterial endocarditis. The major manifestations of this condition result from (1) infection, (2) embolic phenomena, and (3) failure of the heart as a pump. Minor surgical procedures such as dental extraction or tonsillectomy may be followed by subacute bacterial endocarditis in persons who have old rheumatic or congenital heart lesions. Persons with valvular heart lesions should be advised to see their physicians for a course of antibiotic or chemotherapy before undergoing any form of surgical therapy.

The effects of injury to the endocardium and valves that have been discussed can be summarized as

1. Predisposition to intracardiac thrombosis
2. Obstruction to the movement of blood from one chamber to another or from a ventricle to the great arteries
3. Regurgitation of blood into the chamber from which it came
4. Predisposition to infection of the deformed valve

These conditions predispose to failure of the heart as a pump chiefly by increasing the work performed by the heart and/or by decreasing cardiac nutrition. In general, stenosis leads to failure of the chamber behind the narrowed valve and insufficiency leads to failure of the chamber both preceding and following the insufficient valve. Some disorders, such as rheumatic fever, not only injure the endocardium but also cause direct injury to the muscle and pericardial layers as well.

How can deformities of the heart valves be prevented?

Fundamentally, the prevention of valvular deformity depends on the prevention of a number of disorders, including rheumatic fever, developmental cardiac defects, atherosclerosis, syphilis, bacterial endocarditis, and trauma. With the exception of trauma and possibly of congenital anomalies, prevention of valvular deformities depends on the prevention of some other disorder. Whatever the nature of the cause, deformities of the heart valve place an added burden on the pumping mechanism of the heart by their mechanical effects. Because rheumatic fever is relatively common and is the most frequent cause of heart disease among the young, it will be discussed here in some detail. The elements in the prevention of rheumatic fever as well as of heart damage after the disease is in progress will be presented.

To illustrate the factors in the development of, as well as the problems accompanying, rheumatic fever, Henry Crabtree will be presented. At this time Henry is a 16-year-old boy. He is tall and slender. He lives with his mother and five siblings in a four-room flat in Northeastern Central City. His father is living but lives apart from the family. He maintains some contact with the children, though he does not see them regularly. The family is supported by Aid to Dependent Children (ADC). When Henry completed the eighth grade at 15 years of age he dropped out of school. Henry has only two interests, sports and automobiles. He hopes to become, as is an older brother, a professional basketball player. A year previous to his present admission he was hospitalized for eight weeks and treated for rheumatic fever. Two or three weeks previous to his first attack of rheumatic fever, Henry had a sore throat and fever from which he appeared to recover completely. The day before his first admission to the hospital he had a fever of 38.9°C (102°F) and severe pain in his knee joints. When he was discharged, he was instructed to return to the clinic at monthly intervals to have his progress checked and to receive a supply of oral penicillin. He kept his clinic appointments each month for three months, after which he failed to return. A year after his initial attack he was readmitted to the hospital for the treatment of an acute attack of rheumatic fever. This time there was noticeable damage to his heart.

RHEUMATIC FEVER

The name *rheumatic fever* is derived from the manifestations resulting from inflammation of the joints. Pathology is neither limited to the joints nor is inflammation of the joints its most serious effect, for multiple areas of focal inflammation are found in the heart and blood vessels as well. The most serious effects are those on the heart. The areas of focal inflammation are widely scattered throughout the body and have a special predilection for connective tissues. Small blood vessels are extensively involved. Lesions found in the myocardium of the heart are known as Aschoff bodies or nodules. Actually, lesions similar to Aschoff bodies occur wherever the connective-tissue components are found. Moreover, similar lesions are found in other diseases in which there is injury to the collagen fibers.

Although authorities are not certain of the specific etiology of rheumatic fever, they are generally agreed that it follows infections by the group A hemolytic streptococci. Recent evidence indicates that the myocardium and the streptococcus contain a common antigen. Antibody formed in response to the streptococcal antigen also reacts against the myocardial antigen. It has been demonstrated that the streptococci are not in the lesions of rheumatic fever and may or may not be recoverable from the nose and throat at the time of the onset of the disease. Even when streptococci are found and eradicated by antimicrobial therapy, the course of rheumatic fever is not altered.

The exact incidence is not known and estimates vary. However, about 3 per cent of individuals having streptococcal infections develop rheumatic fever. From 30 to 50 per cent of individuals experiencing one attack of rheumatic fever have one or more recurrences of the disease. Although the incidence of both streptococcal disease and rheumatic fever is believed to be declining, rheumatic fever remains an important disease among children and adolescents.

As inferred, Henry Crabtree illustrates a number of factors that appear to affect the incidence of rheumatic fever. He falls within the age group in which it is most common. Though rheumatic fever may occur at any age, its onset is highest between the ages of 5 and 15. Henry was 15 at the time of his first known attack. Socioeconomic conditions appear to influence the likelihood of developing rheumatic fever, as the incidence seems to be higher among those who live under overcrowded conditions. Overcrowding is important because it increases the opportunities for the transmission of infectious agents. Henry shares a small bedroom with three brothers. Because they sleep in the same room, the intensity and duration of exposure to any infection acquired by one person to others is increased. Because several people live in four rooms, there is little possibility of isolating the sick from the well. When income is limited, the nutritional status of the children may be less good than when more money is available. Susceptibility to rheumatic fever may possibly be increased by inadequate nutrition during early life.[10] Though Henry is slender, he was thought to be reasonably well nourished at the time of his admission. Heredity appears to be another factor predisposing to rheumatic fever, as several siblings in the same family sometimes develop the disease. A history of rheumatic fever in the family of the affected child is not

[10] Alvin F. Coburn: "The Pathogenesis of Rheumatic Fever—A Concept," *Perspect. Biol. Med.,* **6**:495 (Summer) 1963.

uncommon. The nature of the hereditary factor is not known, but it is believed to be related to the tendency to develop rheumatic fever and not to susceptibility to streptococcal disease. There was no known history of rheumatic fever in Henry's family. One further factor appearing to predispose to rheumatic fever is climate. The incidence of the disease is believed to be higher in colder than in warmer climates. A variety of factors, therefore, predispose to rheumatic fever. Some, such as age, overcrowding, a diet deficient in essential nutrients, and climate, probably do so by increasing the possibility of streptococcal infections. Infection by the group A hemolytic streptococci is directly or indirectly required to trigger the response. Second, there must be some type of genetic defect that makes the child susceptible. Third, a diet deficient in essential nutrients early in life may increase the likelihood of the susceptible child developing rheumatic fever.

What are the clinical manifestations of rheumatic fever?

The following points about the nature of rheumatic fever are useful in anticipating its clinical manifestations. It is a febrile disease. Furthermore, rheumatic fever is not limited to a single organ. Rather, focal inflammatory lesions are distributed throughout the body in the mesenchymal connective tissues. According to Coburn,[11] one of the earliest lesions in rheumatic fever is swelling of the vascular endothelium. With each attack the lining of the arterial tree suffers physical and chemical injury. Signs and symptoms vary in intensity and range. Some individuals who have heart damage characteristic of rheumatic fever have not had a known attack of the disease, and others experience a classic picture of the disease.

Henry experienced an almost textbook picture of the disease in both attacks. He had several of the so-called major manifestations, which included fever, pain in his joints, and evidence of cardiac involvement. He did not have abdominal pain nor did he have skin manifestations, chorea, or epistaxis (nose bleeds). As in most febrile disorders he had anorexia, weight loss, fatigability, and weakness. His erythrocyte sedimentation rate was markedly elevated. Elevation of the sedimentation rate, indicative of a systemic inflammatory process, is characteristic of rheumatic fever, as it occurs in almost all instances. The degree to which it is elevated is an index of the activity of the disease. The leukocyte count is usually elevated to from 15,000 to 30,000 during the acute phase of the disease, but it may be normal. Henry's

11 Corburn, *ibid.*, p. 507.

leukocyte count was elevated. As he improved, his sedimentation rate fell toward normal and his leukocyte count became normal.

As is not infrequently observed, particularly among older children and adults. Henry had polyarthritis. Joint pain is less common among young children, though it may occur in a mild form and be dismissed as growing pains. The degree of pain varies from a vague pain to the exquisite pain associated with acutely inflamed and swollen joints. Although the degree of pain experienced by Henry was moderate, in some patients it is so severe that actions resulting in jarring of the bed or any movement of the bed are unbearable. Among the characteristic features of the arthritis associated with rheumatic fever is that it tends to involve one joint or area at a time and to be migratory, that is, to move from one joint to another. It involves large and small joints and heals without causing crippling of the joints.

When the joints are painful, measures should be instituted to protect the patient from unnecessary discomfort. Jarring of the patient should be avoided. Bed coverings should be supported, so that the joints are protected from their weight. Because the joints are not likely to be deformed by the disease process, the extremities should be supported in the position the patient finds to be most comfortable. When handling the affected extremity, care should be taken to minimize movement of the joint. To do this, the extremity should be supported both above and below the joint. Measures prescribed by the physician such as local applications of heat may give the patient a measure of relief. They should be carried out conscientiously. Other measures prescribed to modify the inflammatory response minimize the discomfort to the patient.

As should be expected in view of the widespread involvement of connective and vascular tissues, lesions of the skin and subcutaneous tissues develop in some patients with rheumatic fever. About 25 per cent of children have a skin lesion known as erythema marginatum or circinatum. The lesions are red and roughly circular in shape. Because adjacent lesions tend to coalesce, they form larger lesions with an irregular outline. They are usually flat (macular), though some may be slightly raised (papular). They are not usually the cause of discomfort, though they may occasionally be accompanied by itching.

Another skin lesion, erythema nodosum, is believed to be a manifestation of acute rheumatic fever. It does not occur as frequently as erythema marginatum, and it sometimes develops when other rheumatic manifestations are minimal or lacking. The lesions are dull red nodules occurring most frequently on the extensor surfaces of the extremities. Unlike the lesions of erythema marginatum, those of erythema nodosum are exquisitely tender to touch and discomfort is increased with movement. Affected extremities should be protected from the weight of the bedding by the use of cradles. Gentleness should be an outstanding characteristic when extremities are moved.

Subcutaneous nodules are firm, insensitive lesions occurring over bony prominences of the various joints and tendons of the extremities. They are more frequently observed in patients with a serious form of rheumatic fever and who have severe heart damage.

Chorea, or, as it is frequently called by lay persons, St. Vitus's dance, is a disorder characterized by marked involuntary contractions of the skeletal muscles. Though it is not easily described, one of the outstanding features of movement in chorea is its purposelessness. At the onset of chorea, the child may appear to be awkward and careless. He spills his food when he tries to eat and drops his schoolbooks and other objects. As the manifestations become more severe, the purposeless movements made by the child may be ascribed to nervousness. Later they may become so severe as to be incapacitating. Chorea results from the involvement of the nervous system. It may be the sole manifestation of rheumatic fever. It generally occurs late.

Just as the degree and range of the possible manifestations in rheumatic fever are highly variable, the nature of the course and the outcome of an attack are also variable. Though few die during the first attack, some have a fulminating form of the disease and die within a few days or weeks. Some recover in as few as three or four weeks, whereas others, such as Henry (he was ill for eight weeks), are ill for more extended periods of time. Some individuals improve, but some degree of activity persists for weeks or months, or for the lifetime of the individual. Although some recover fully from the first attack and never have another, one attack predisposes to recurrences of the disease. As in the instance of Henry, the extent of cardiac damage during the first attack of rheumatic fever is frequently minimal, but with each subsequent attack the degree and permanence of cardiac damage increases. At the time Henry was discharged from the hospital after his second attack of rheumatic fever he had mitral and aortic stenosis.

A statement of prognosis is a prediction of probable outcome that is based on past experience. Fundamentally, Henry's prognosis depends on the nature and degree of involvement of his heart. Certainly his prognosis was better after his first attack of rheumatic fever and

becomes poorer with each subsequent attack, inasmuch as the extent and degree of cardiac damage are likely to be increased. Most of the patients who have severe cardiac involvement die within ten years in congestive heart failure. In addition, patients with deformed heart valves are predisposed to the formation of intracardiac thrombosis and to bacterial endocarditis—usually of the subacute type.

Treatment of Rheumatic Fever

Rheumatic fever is an acute febrile disease that may cause a period of extended illness. Though focal inflammatory lesions can and do occur throughout the body and may be responsible for discomfort or even temporary disability, the lesions in the heart are the ones most likely to cause permanent injury and death. Treatment is therefore directed toward the alleviation of the symptoms and the prevention of cardiac damage. An important aspect of prevention is the prevention of recurrences.

In the traditional and conservative management of rheumatic fever the physician prescribes bed rest for as long as the disease is active. Currently some clinicians are modifying this practice and allowing greater amounts of activity than in the past. When rest is prescribed, as it often is, the nurse has the responsibility for creating an environment in which the patient can rest. To achieve rest for the patient, the cooperation of the patient and his family is essential.

Henry was treated by bed rest. During the first two weeks of his illness he was encouraged to lie quietly and to have all activities of daily living performed for him. He was fed, given mouth care, turned, and bathed. He was allowed to be up once a day to go to the bathroom. Otherwise he was to remain quietly in bed. Because his knees and later his wrists and elbows were acutely inflamed, he was glad to lie still. Later, as he recovered, the maintenance of bed rest became more difficult to achieve.

As soon as Henry began to improve, recreational activities were planned to occupy his time. Because Henry was interested only in sports and in automobiles, this was taken into consideration in planning. Provisions were made for him to listen to football and hockey games on the radio. Because his intellectual achievements and interests were limited, reading material was selected with his interests in mind. His nurse tried to encourage him to consider returning to school in order to obtain specialized training, but his real interest was in becoming a professional basketball player. Although a visiting teacher was available and arrangements were made for her to visit Henry, he was unwilling to consider a study program at this time. Because of the prospects for an extended period of illness, recreational, occupational, and educational facilities should be available to the patient with rheumatic fever. Through their appropriate use, the morale of the patient can be maintained and the child or adolescent prevented from falling too far behind in school. When indicated, they may also help the patient to select a new or modified occupation.

In addition to bed rest (or modified activity) drugs are prescribed to eradicate the streptococcus and to relieve the symptoms and effects of the disease. The drug employed to eliminate the streptococcus is penicillin. The preparation and dosage of penicillin are prescribed by the physician. The drug should be administered as prescribed in order to maintain a satisfactory level at all times. In addition to therapy to eliminate the streptococcus, the patient should be protected against exposure to persons with respiratory infections.

Two different types of drugs, the salicylates and corticosteroids, are prescribed singly or in combination to relieve the symptoms of rheumatic fever and to decrease the tissue response. Again the physician makes the decision as to the drug to be employed. The corticosteroids bring about the relief of signs and symptoms more quickly than the salicylates; they are more likely to be prescribed when there is a significant degree of carditis.

Exactly how the salicylates or the corticosteroids act is not known, but they are believed to alter the tissue response to the abnormal process. They do not, however, accelerate the rate at which the patient recovers from rheumatic fever. When the preceding drugs are administered in adequate dosages, not only do the signs and symptoms associated with the disease disappear but the blood changes tend to return to normal. The erythrocyte sedimentation rate and the leukocyte count drop. If, however, treatment is prematurely discontinued, signs and symptoms and the changes in the blood characteristic of rheumatic fever reappear. Because the length of the course of the disease is unpredictable, the physician sometimes has difficulty in being certain as to whether the improvement of the patient is caused by the suppressive therapy or by the elimination of the cause of the inflammatory reaction. Therefore, at the time drug therapy is being discontinued, the patient should be under observation so that therapy can be re-established if indications of rheumatic activity reappear.

A problem may arise following the relief of the patient's symptoms because the patient feels well. As Henry improved, he rejected the idea that he was ill. He felt well and therefore he was certain that he must be well. He interpreted the taking of medicine and continued attendance at the clinic as a sign of weakness. Henry's feelings are not unusual. In some instances, it is possible through education of the patient and his parents to make and ensure a plan for continued treatment.

As in other long-term illnesses, the education of the patient and/or family members in the nature and effects of rheumatic fever is imperative if they are to assume responsibility for treatment of the current attack and prevent recurrences. When the home situation allows, patients may be discharged from the hospital after the acute manifestations are relieved. Even when the patient is "cured," antimicrobial therapy in the form of penicillin is prescribed. This therapy may be continued for from one to five years or as long as the child is in school. Responsibility for the continuance of treatment is borne by the patient or a family member. Regular medical supervision is also necessary, not only for renewal of the required prescriptions but to maintain the interest of the patient in continuing his therapy.

In addition to caring for the patient during the acute phase of his illness, the nurse has many opportunities to serve the patient. Often it is a nurse who instructs the parents and/or the patient in the reasons continued medical supervision is necessary and in the need for his medication. The nurse may also uncover areas of misunderstanding or reasons for the failure of the patient to follow instructions. The visiting or public health nurse may visit the patient's home to determine whether home care is a reasonable possibility and to help the person who is responsible to carry out the prescribed regime. She may act as a liaison between the patient and his physician.

According to the American Heart Association,[12] most patients will be on prophylactic doses of penicillin or the sulfonamides throughout life. The most reliable method is intramuscular injections of penicillin, 1,200,000 units per month; however, patients will usually prefer the oral medications, 200,000 or 250,000 units of penicillin twice a day or sulfadiazine, 1 g per day. Because the continued use of penicillin and other drugs is expensive, the patient may be able to obtain them from the state or city health department. The nurse should know what the resources are in the area where she is practicing and know how to assist the patient in securing aid when this is necessary. Because the physician is responsible for prescribing the extent of the patient's activity, the nurse should know what his plans are for the patient. There is usu-

12 "Prevention of Rheumatic Fever" (New York: American Heart Association, 1968), pp. 1–3.

ally no reason, however, for her not to discuss with the physician the possibility of a service such as a visiting teacher if the condition of the patient seems to warrant it. The physician, as well as the nurse, is desirous not only of preventing recurrences of the disease but of minimizing as much as possible undesirable effects of the disease.

HEART SURGERY

Until recently, after the valves of a patient's heart were deformed nothing could be done to restore normal or nearly normal function. During the last decade or two, surgical procedures have been developed by which stenosed and incompetent valves are opened and repaired or valvular prostheses are introduced to replace damaged ones. In some patients these operations are highly successful. In others they are less so. Some of the factors appearing to influence the outcome of surgery include the extent of damage to the heart muscle, whether or not the disease process is inactive, and how early in life and the extent to which the person was made an invalid by his disease. Some individuals who are "cured" by surgical correction of defects in the heart remain invalids because for them invalidism is a way of life. Individuals whose cardiac disability occurred early in life and continued for many years are more likely to have a problem in adjusting to the responsibilities of a healthy life than those whose defect is corrected early or whose cardiac disability developed later in life. In some persons, heart damage is so great that the operation comes too late to be of real benefit. In others, the disease appears to be quiescent but is reactivated following surgical therapy. The expectation that surgical treatment of cardiac defects will benefit the patient is realized in many patients.

What are the needs of patients undergoing heart surgery?

Patients undergoing cardiac surgery have needs relating to the following:

1. The fact of a surgical procedure
2. The fact that the route of approach is through the chest wall
3. The fact that the heart is the organ involved and it has suffered previous injury

The first two points are discussed in Chapter 17. The care of the patient undergoing cardiac surgery will not be discussed in detail. The remarks that follow apply to patients who have surgery on the heart and are not limited to those who have surgery to correct a defective heart valve. The author believes that patients undergoing cardiac surgery require care by nurses who are experienced and who have specialized

preparation. In the words of Thung and Dammann,[13] "The best postoperative care requires that the patient be placed in a special unit, equipped with the necessary instruments for monitoring, a complete supply of the needed medications and well-trained, experienced, and well-motivated personnel." Books and journal articles devoted to the problems of patients undergoing cardiac surgery are included in the References.

As in other types of surgery, the preoperative preparation of the patient for cardiac surgery is as important to his recovery as other aspects of therapy. The patient is usually admitted to the hospital a few days previous to the date of operation for the purpose of performing diagnostic procedures requiring hospitalization and for improving his health status. Attention is paid to

1. Acquainting the patient with the personnel who are to be responsible for his care and hopefully enhancing his confidence in their competence and interest in his welfare. They prepare him for what to expect and for what is expected of him.
2. Improving his nutritional status. Patients who have been in chronic heart failure and have been eating poorly and/or have impaired liver function require improvement in their intake of protein, glucose, and vitamins, including vitamin K.
3. Correcting fluid and electrolyte imbalances, including elimination of edema. Because diuretics may cause electrolyte imbalances, they are usually discontinued about two days before surgery is anticipated.
4. Eliminating infections in the respiratory tract. Because respiratory infections increase the risk of cardiac surgery, the patient should be protected from persons who have infections.
5. Improving cardiac functioning, when this is required.

During the postoperative period the patient is exposed to all the possible surgical complications. Though the patient is often able to tolerate one or more complications, the poorer his condition, the more severe the complications, and the more numerous they are, the greater will be the hazard to the patient. To state it positively, the patient who is in good physical condition, who develops few complications that, when they do occur, are spaced at intervals, and in whom complications are not allowed to become severe is not likely to be seriously affected by one or more complications. Therefore, one

[13] Nalda Thung and J. Francis Dammann: "Postoperative Care After Cardiac Surgery," *Heart Bull.,* **12:**87 (Sept.–Oct.) 1963.

of the most important aspects of the postoperative care of the patient who has undergone cardiac surgery is observation of vital functions by means of monitoring devices as well as the more usual methods.

Action taken in the care of the patient who has undergone cardiac surgery should be based on observations tempered by knowledge of the causes and effects of complications. Because monitoring equipment is not infallible, clinical judgment developed by study and thoughtful experience is indispensable. The earlier any threats to the well-being of the patient are discovered, the greater are his chances for survival.

The complications of cardiac surgery are similar to those associated with other types of surgery but their import is more immediately serious. Among the most common and important complications is respiratory insufficiency, that is, the inability to transport the quantity of oxygen required by the cells and/or to remove the carbon dioxide formed in metabolism. Unless respiratory insufficiency is detected early and the resulting hypoxia and hypercapnia are corrected promptly, there will be a deterioration in essential body functions, leading to the death of the patient. Respiratory insufficiency may be caused by impaired ventilation, pulmonary or cardiac failure, or an increase in the demands made by the cells for oxygen. The causes of impaired ventilation and pulmonary failure are discussed in Chapter 8. The causes and effects of cardiac failure are considered in this chapter. Any condition leading to the increased use of oxygen by the cells, such as exercise or elevated body temperature, will increase their need for oxygen and predispose to or intensify hypercapnia and hypoxia. Hypoxia can predispose to cardiac arrhythmias. Frequently the etiology of premature ventricular contractions is hypoxia. In the immediate postoperative period following cardiac surgery, much of the care provided for the patient is directed toward the prevention of respiratory insufficiency and the earliest possible detection of evidence that it is developing.

The general principles applying to the care of any patient undergoing surgical therapy apply to the patient having heart surgery. Because the heart is directly involved, the need for attention to the details of care during all phases of surgery cannot, however, be overemphasized. Certainly the patient undergoing heart surgery deserves to have his chances for recovery improved by being cared for by nurses who as a result of education and experience are prepared to meet his needs. Just as surgeons who perform cardiac surgery undergo a period of specialized training, it is no less important that nurses do likewise.

The Pericardium

The outer covering of the heart, or pericardium, may also be a source of interference with the action of the heart as a pump. The pericardium is an inelastic sac or envelope reflected over the heart and lining the cavity. The layer lying next to the heart, the visceral layer, adheres closely to the heart. The outer portion of the sac is known as the parietal layer. The inner and outer surfaces of the pericardial sac are separated by serous fluid. The pericardium has a number of important functions. It helps to anchor the heart and to lessen the friction between the heart and its environment. Because the pericardium does not stretch, it prevents overdilatation of the heart during diastole.

How can the pericardium be injured?

The pericardium can be injured by trauma, infection, or neoplasms with the result that fluid, blood, or pus collects in the pericardial sac. As the fluid accumulates, it occupies space in the pericardial sac and reduces the capacity of the heart during diastole. Because the blood is circulated in a closed system, the lessening of the capacity of the heart to receive blood has at least two detrimental effects on the entire system. Because the heart can deliver into the arterial system only the blood that it receives during diastole, cardiac output falls. Tissues throughout the body suffer from the effects of undernutrition. When cardiac output is markedly diminished, the coronary circulation cannot be maintained, and the heart dies in fibrillation.[14] A second major effect is caused by interference with the venous return. Because of the limitations on the quantity of blood that the heart can accommodate during diastole, blood tends to accumulate in the veins, causing passive congestion of organs such as the liver. The situation is similar to that resulting from placing a dam in a river. The dam or obstruction impedes the forward flow of water. When water is added to the channel behind the dam, it floods the land in the surrounding area. Similarly, the limitations on the capacity of the heart during diastole act to impede the forward movement of blood from the veins into the heart with the result that it accumulates in the veins. The effects of venous congestion are discussed later in this chapter.

Because of the location of the pericardium, disease of other organs in the thoracic cavity may spread to it. For example, the pericardium may be infected by tubercle bacilli as well as

[14] Multiple and ineffective contractions of individual muscle fibers rather than the more or less synchronous contraction of the entire myocardium.

pneumococci. Disease of the pericardium may also extend to and injure the myocardium, coronary vessels, and the nerves supplying the heart. In the process of healing, bands or sheets of fibrous tissue, with or without calcification, may encompass the heart and lead to slow cardiac failure. Because they act as a splint, they limit the degree to which the heart can expand or dilate, just as a splint or cast encasing a limb limits the degree to which blood can enter it. The effects are similar to those produced by the distention of the pericardial sac with fluid, but they are likely to develop more slowly. Furthermore, the myocardium and other structures of the heart may be damaged by the infectious process causing the pericarditis, as well as by lack of use. The myocardium is similar to other muscles. It responds to a decrease in work by atrophy and to an increase by hypertrophy. The fact that the myocardium atrophies in the presence of constrictive pericarditis is an important consideration in its surgical treatment. Sometimes the constrictive bands can be removed successfully by cardiac decortication. The procedure may have to be discontinued because the myocardium may have been so weakened by disease and the consequent scarring, and by lack of use, that on the removal of the fibrous tissue splint the heart dilates excessively. When damage to the heart muscle is not too great, the patient may be greatly benefited by resection of the pericardium. Treatment of constrictive pericarditis is also directed toward relieving venous congestion and improving the general status of the patient.

The Myocardium

From the standpoint of function, the essential part of the heart is the myocardium. This is true because it provides the power that keeps blood moving through the circuit. Like all other tissues, the myocardium is dependent on a continuous blood supply. Because it does not tolerate an oxygen debt to the same extent skeletal muscle does, the myocardium is more susceptible to hypoxia than skeletal muscle. Death of cells occurs when oxygen deprivation continues longer than 30 minutes.

Functions

The function of the myocardium can be simply stated as the ejection into the arteries of the blood delivered to it by the venous circulation. A number of factors contribute to effectiveness of the myocardium as a pump. One is the arrangement of the muscle fibers. Layers of muscle fibers are wrapped around the heart in spiral and circular directions. This arrangement has a number of mechanical advantages. As the ventricles contract, blood is not only pushed but is literally wrung out of the heart, much as water is wrung out of a cloth. Because the muscle fibers extend around the heart, both ventricles contract at the same time and move the same quantity of blood. The effectiveness of ventricular contraction is further increased by the fact that during contraction the septum stiffens and acts as a fulcrum to which muscle fibers are attached.

Any disorder that deprives the myocardium of its blood supply, either in whole or in part, or injures it, may decrease its efficiency as a pump. Before discussing the possible consequences of failure of the myocardium as a pump, however, some of the structural and functional characteristics of myocardial cells will be reviewed. Two developments have contributed much to an understanding of the structure of myocardial cells. They are the electron microscope and a technique for separating individual living mammalian myocardial cells. In the past the myocardium was usually described as a single multinucleated cell. As a result of his studies with individual heart cells, Harary [15] confirmed earlier reports that nuclei in the myocardium are surrounded by a membrane. The myocardium is, therefore, composed of many cells.

Like other muscle cells, those of the myocardium are contractile. When stimulated, they shorten and thicken. Following contraction they lengthen. They are also similar to skeletal muscle in that they obey the all-or-none law; that is, when they contract they do so to the fullest extent possible. Although this might be interpreted to mean the force of cardiac contraction should always be the same, it does not, as another factor also influences the force of myocardial contraction. The force of contration is a function of the length of the fiber at the end of diastole. Within physiological limits, the longer the muscle fiber is at the end of diastole (or at the beginning of systole), the more forceful the contraction of the heart (Starling's law of the heart). It can be demonstrated by stretching a rubber or elastic band. When the band is stretched and released, the force with which it returns to its original form depends on the degree to which it was stretched. Within the limits of its extensibility, the more it is stretched, the more forcibly it contracts. With a small amount of stretching, the contraction of the band is weak. When the degree of stretching approaches the limits of its extensibility, the force of contraction is great. It too demonstrates the all-or-

15 Isaac Harary: "Heart Cells in Vitro," *Sci. Amer.,* 206:144 (May) 1962.

none law inasmuch as the rubber band contracts fully or not all.

A healthy heart can adapt to an increase in venous return without much increase in the diastolic fiber length. Within a stroke or two the heart is able to eject as much blood into the circulation as is delivered to it by the veins. When, as a result of disease, this is no longer possible, muscle fibers lengthen. For a time this lengthening, and with it dilatation of the chambers of the heart, may enable the heart to meet the needs of all cells, including its own, without signs of embarrassment. The healthy, and often the diseased, heart has a reserve power that enables it to maintain an appropriate balance between intake and output. This reserve power lies in the difference between the degree to which the muscle fiber must lengthen to eject as much blood into the circulation as is delivered to it and the extent to which it can lengthen and function physiologically. The longer the diastolic fiber length, the more forceful the contraction but the less the cardiac reserve. When the point is reached that further lengthening of the muscle fibers during diastole results in inefficient function, cardiac reserve has been lost. At this point the heart is no longer able to adapt to an increase in venous return or to increase output in relation to the requirements of cells. The individual is no longer able to increase his activity above resting levels without manifestations associated with failure of the heart as a pump. Eventually he may be unable to meet the needs of his cells at rest.

The capacity of the heart muscle to lengthen (dilate) is one of the ways in which the heart adapts to an increase in work. This, combined with an increase in heart rate, enables the heart to move the increased volume of blood delivered to it as a result of an increase in activity. Adaptation fails, sooner or later, as do other adaptive mechanisms when a condition exists that makes continued adaptation necessary or directly injures the myocardium.

As might be expected, the size of an individual's heart is roughly proportional to the size of his body. Contrary to popular opinion, physical exercise is necessary to a healthy heart. As stated earlier, the heart responds to "lack of use" by atrophy, as do other tissues. Likewise, the heart muscle adapts to a continued increase in work load by hypertrophy. Associated with hypertrophy of the myocardium is dilatation of one or more chambers of the heart. Authorities are not agreed as to whether hypertrophy precedes dilatation of the heart or dilatation precedes hypertrophy. The hypertrophied heart is larger than the healthy heart. Hypertrophy is physiological inasmuch as it occurs in response to an increased work load. Hypertrophy enables the heart to move blood against an increased resistance and at the same time to maintain the normal equilibrium between intake and output. Like other adaptive mechanisms, hypertrophy has certain limitations. One important limitation is that as muscle mass increases the blood supply does not increase to a comparable degree. In the healthy heart a capillary is said to be available to supply each muscle fiber. Even when this ratio is maintained in the hypertrophied heart, the quantity of blood delivered to the tissue is reduced in relation to its mass. A larger fiber receives no more blood than the former smaller fiber. Blood supply is therefore not increased in proportion to the quantity of tissue to be nourished. Undernutrition may be further aggravated by vascular disease that limits blood flow to the myocardium.

For the most part, the healthy heart adapts to changes in the demands made on it by altering its rate of contraction and by adapting the force of contraction to the quantity of venous blood returned to it. Essentially the function of the heart as a pump is satisfactory as long as (1) the myocardium is able to eject as much blood into the circulation as is delivered to it without a gain in residual blood at the end of systole and (2) it can meet the needs of the tissues under different degrees of activity. When activity is increased, there should be no increase of residual blood in the heart. Neither should there be evidence of marked or unexpected increase in the heart or respiratory rate. Although some rise in the pulse and respiratory rates does occur during physical activity, this should not be out of proportion to the degree of activity and should be within physiological limits. The pulse rate should also return to normal within a reasonable period of time. The return to normal usually occurs in two stages. Within a short period of time after exercise ceases, the pulse rate drops sharply toward, but not to, pre-exercise level. It then declines slowly. The healthy heart can also adapt to a regular program of physical exercise. In well-trained athletes, the resting pulse rates are lower than average, but the output per beat is greater.[16]

Failures in Myocardial Function

Pruitt [17] summarizes the causes of failure in the pumping mechanism under three general headings: (1) failure to fill, (2) overloading,

---

[16] Arthur C. Guyton: *Textbook of Medical Physiology*, 3rd ed. (Philadelphia: W. S. Saunders Company, 1966), p. 225.

[17] Raymond D. Pruitt: "The Origins of Cardiac Failure," *Heart Bull.* 7:18–20 (Jan.–Feb.) 1958.

and (3) deterioration in functional capacity. Each of these will be discussed briefly.

Failure of the heart to fill depends on three factors. There must be a sufficient volume of blood in the circulation in relation to the size of the vascular chamber to provide for an adequate venous return. For the heart to move blood into the arteries, it must receive blood from the veins, and it can only eject the quantity of blood that is delivered to it. The most common cause of an inadequate venous return is shock. Shock results from any disorder causing a disproportion between the circulating blood volume and the capacity of the vascular chamber. The blood volume may fall as a result of hemorrhage or from the excessive loss of fluid into the tissues such as occurs in burns —or the volume of blood may be within physiological limits, but generalized dilatation of the blood vessels may enlarge the capacity of the vascular system so much that the quantity of blood returned to the heart is insufficient to maintain an adequate output. The result in either instance is ischemia of the tissues. If it is severe or continued, death may result. The reader is referred to Chapter 11 for a more detailed discussion of shock.

A second cause of inadequate ventricular filling is obstruction to the inflow of blood. The most common cause is mitral stenosis. Sometimes the stenosis is so severe that the opening is no larger than a broom straw. Such marked narrowing of the mitral valve seriously limits the quantity of blood that can enter the left ventricle. As previously indicated, constrictive pericarditis, by limiting diastole, interferes with the filling of the heart. Like any other pump, the heart can eject into the arteries only the quantity of blood that enters into it.

A third factor that may limit the intake of blood is a reduction in the length of diastole or of the interval during which the heart fills. Blood enters the heart only during diastole. When ventricular rates are excessively high, the length of diastole is shortened to a greater extent than systole. Consequently, the period for filling is relatively shorter than the period for the ejection of blood. An extreme example may be seen in auricular fibrillation when the volume of blood entering the heart during diastole may be so little that, despite ventricular contraction, there is no pulse. Excessively high ventricular rates may, when continued, lead to heart failure.

In contrast to failure caused by inadequate ventricular filling, the myocardium may fail because too much blood is delivered to it or the resistance that it must overcome in moving the blood into the arteries is excessive. When the myocardium fails because too much blood is

returned to it, the condition is called high-output failure. According to Pruitt,[18] high-output failure is of two types. In the first, a large volume of blood is received by the heart and is ejected into the circulation. Common examples include thyrotoxicosis, fever, and anemia. In these disorders the organism adapts to an increased need for oxygen and nutrients or to failure to carry oxygen by increasing the blood volume. Because an elevation in the blood volume increases the work performed by the heart, disorders accompanied by increased blood volume will, if continued, and particularly in the presence of pre-existing disease of the heart, precipitate failure of the heart.

In the second type of high-output failure, the heart also expels an increased volume of blood into the arteries, but some of the blood returns to the heart during diastole. The increased volume of blood ejected by the heart results from a failure to maintain the forward movement of blood in the circuit. Common causes of regurgitation of blood include mitral and aortic insufficiency, uncomplicated patent ductus arteriosus,[19] and arteriovenous shunts.[20] The effects of aortic regurgitation can be felt in the pulse. During systole the pulse is full and bounding. As diastole begins the artery collapses quickly. The pulse associated with aortic regurgitation is the so-called water-hammer or Corrigan's pulse.

The second type of ventricular overloading Pruitt[21] calls high-resistance failure. The site of the resistance may be any place between the outlet of the ventricle and the peripheral arterioles. An example of the first is aortic stenosis, and of the latter, the arteriolar sclerosis associated with hypertension, or aortic stenosis, such as is seen in coarctation of the aorta.[22] In all the preceding and similar conditions, the ventricle must move the blood with sufficient force to overcome the resistance offered by the narrowed channels. The amount of energy required is well illustrated by coarctation of the aorta. Above the point of narrowing, the systolic blood pressure may be 200 mm of mercury or more. Below, it may be 100 mm or less.

The third general cause of heart failure is incompetence of the ventricle as a result of dis-

---

[18] *Ibid.*, p. 19.

[19] In the fetal circulation, the pulmonary artery and the aorta are connected by the ductus arteriosus. Shortly after birth the ductus closes and becomes a fibrous cord or band. Occasionally the ductus arteriosus remains open or patent, thus the term *patent ductus.*

[20] In an arteriovenous shunt there is a direct connection between an artery and a vein.

[21] *Op. cit.*, p. 18.

[22] In contraction of the aorta, the aorta is markedly narrowed at some point after it leaves the heart. The condition is usually of congenital origin.

ease of the myocardium. Pruitt[23] classifies myocardial diseases as (1) degenerative diseases, (2) inflammatory diseases, (3) metabolic diseases of the myocardium, and (4) disturbances in the rhythm of the heart.

The most common cause of failure of the heart because of degeneration of the heart muscle is coronary sclerosis complicated by myocardial infarction. Because of the importance of this disorder, it will be discussed in more detail later in this chapter.

Inflammatory diseases affecting the myocardium include rheumatic carditis, diphtheria, infectious mononucleosis, and lupus erythematosus. Diphtheritic myocarditis is infrequent in the United States and could be eliminated by immunization.

A number of metabolic disorders are accompanied by weakening of the myocardium. These disorders cause biochemical or biophysical changes that interfere with the utilization of nutrients. These include thyrotoxicosis, hypothyroidism, beriberi, anemia, and shock. Most of the preceding can be prevented or cured by early and effective treatment of the precipitating abnormality. Some, such as hypothyroidism (myxedema heart), require therapy throughout the lifetime of the individual. In hypothyroidism the thyroid hormone is required for the remainder of the life of the individual.

Disturbances in the rhythm of the heart, either by excessively high or low heart rates, predispose to myocardial weakening by interfering with the capacity of the heart to maintain its own nutrition. These are discussed later in this chapter.

With advancing years, even in the absence of demonstrable lesions in the heart, there is a reduction in the myocardial reserve and with it a decrease in the capacity of the myocardium to cope with the various handicaps placed on it. For example, one of the reasons that elderly persons tolerate a rapid or large increase in blood volume less well than younger persons is that their cardiac reserve is less adequate. Although the degree to which myocardial reserve is diminished differs among elderly persons, any elderly person who is receiving a blood transfusion or one or more intravenous infusions should be observed for evidence indicating that his heart is or is not tolerating the increase in blood volume. (See Chapters 9 and 11.) The patient should be observed for evidence of circulatory distress or developing pulmonary edema.

Should either occur, the rate of flow of the fluid should be reduced to the minimum required to keep the needle open and the physi-

cian should be called immediately. According to Resnik and Harrison,[24] occasionally an elderly person who dies in congestive heart failure is seen at autopsy with no significant cardiac lesions other than hypertrophy and dilatation. Apparently, the hearts of these patients become so weakened as a result of senile changes that they die of senile heart disease.

In the preceding paragraphs the causes of heart failure have been summarized in relation to the effect the causative factor has on the pumping action of the heart. According to this classification, the heart may fail because it receives too little or too much blood or must pump the blood against too great resistance. It may also fail because the muscle degenerates as the result of injury caused by a variety of diseases. Although not the result of disease, the adaptive capacity of the heart diminishes with advancing age. This lessens the capacity of the heart to cope with any additional burden. Eventually, when the heart fails, it is unable to supply the tissues with the blood required to support their activities. What happens then depends on the completeness of failure and the rate at which failure develops. Like other chronic illnesses, heart failure is frequently, though not invariably, the result of the interaction of multiple factors.

In the patient whose cardiac reserve is seriously reduced, any condition making demands on the heart for increased circulation of blood may precipitate heart failure. Thus infection, particularly when it is accompanied by a fever or a cough, may precipitate congestive heart failure. Emotional stress, excessive activity, the ingestion of excessive amounts of salt, anemia, and the onset of hyperthyroidism may do likewise. The list is not exhaustive. Any disorder that increases the demands made on the heart can be responsible.

The estimated deaths from specific diseases of the heart and blood vessels are summarized in the following graph. In this graph diseases are categorized according to structures involved. It can be noted that coronary artery disease far exceeds other diseases of the heart as a cause of death. (See Figure 10-5.)

To what degree may the pumping mechanism of the heart fail?

Terminology used to describe the degree of heart failure includes cardiac arrest or standstill, acute heart failure, and chronic heart failure or cardiac decompensation. In cardiac arrest or

[23] *Op. cit.,* p. 19.

[24] William H. Resnik and T. R. Harrison: "The Approach to the Patient with Heart Disease," *Principles of Internal Medicine,* 5th ed., T. R. Harrison *et al.,* eds. (New York: The Blakiston Division, McGraw-Hill Book Company, Inc., 1966), p. 734.

Coronary heart disease 524,550

Strokes 197,590

Hypertension and hypertensive heart disease 75,200

Non-rheumatic endocarditis and myocardial degeneration 54,920

General arteriosclerosis 36,730

Rheumatic fever and rheumatic heart disease 17,280

All other CV diseases * 48,600

TOTAL 954,870

* Cardiovascular diseases

FIGURE 10-5. Estimated number of deaths caused by specific diseases of the cardiovascular system (heart and blood vessels). (Information adapted from the National Office of Vital Statistics, 1962.)

standstill, the heart stops beating with the result that the circulation of blood ceases. In acute and chronic heart failure, the myocardium contracts, but the mechanical efficiency of the heart as a pump is below that required to meet the oxygen and nutritional requirements of the tissues under varying degrees of activity and to prevent an increase of residual blood in the ventricle at the end of systole. Acute and chronic heart failure differ in the suddenness with which failure develops. There are also differences in the manifestations that the patient exhibits.

CARDIAC ARREST

As the term *cardiac arrest* implies, myocardial contraction ceases and with it circulation of blood. Unless the heart beat is restarted in approximately four minutes, permanent damage to the higher centers in the brain will occur. As emphasized in other chapters, time is therefore of the essence. The patient can arrest in either asystole (cardiac standstill) or ventricular fibrillation. In ventricular fibrillation the muscle fibers of the heart are contracting in an erratic manner. Without the aid of an electrocardiogram it is impossible to establish whether the heart is in standstill or ventricular fibrillation as the patient will be without a pulse in both instances. Prior to standstill the heart usually goes into a progressive bradycardia, whereas tachycardia usually precedes ventricular fibrillation.

Cardiac arrest may result from any condition causing airway obstruction (aspiration of vomitus, excessive secretions, bronchospasm), hypoxia (shock, cardiac failure), overstimulation of some of the vagal fibers (nasotracheal suctioning), electrolyte imbalances (acidosis, low potassium in combination with digitalis), or dangerous arrhythmias (heart block secondary to disease of the bundle of His, ventricular fibrillation secondary to myocardial infarction). Another not infrequent cause of ventricular fibrillation is electrocution. An example of this was a child who went to explore the damage done by a windstorm and stepped on a broken high-tension wire. The high-voltage electric current caused his ventricles to fibrillate. Because the fibrillating ventricle was unable to eject the blood from the heart with sufficient force to maintain its own blood supply, the myocardium quickly deteriorated, resulting in death. Cardiac arrest occasionally occurs in the anesthetized patient. To illustrate, a patient was undergoing a cholecystectomy. As a result of the handling of the abdominal organs and stretching of the peritoneum or mesentery, vagal reflexes were initiated putting the heart into standstill. In this situation the patient could be resuscitated by closed chest resuscitation.

Depending on the circumstances, the chest may be opened and the heart massaged directly or external cardiac massage may be initiated. If the patient is attached to a monitor and cardiac standstill is confirmed by a straight line, a thump of the chest wall with a fist may be beneficial in helping to restart the heart before initiating closed chest massage. In those cases where fibrillation occurs, the heart is defibrillated by applying electrical current to it so that the muscles will contract simultaeously. When the current is broken they should relax simultaneously. Thus the heart muscles will contract in a synchronous rather than erratic manner. It is rare that a fibrillating heart can be resuscitated without first defibrillating it.

HEART FAILURE (CHRONIC)

When injury to the heart takes place slowly, the manifestations of heart failure develop gradually over a period of days, weeks, or months. Blood flow to tissues is diminished and congestion of fluid in the tissues is an outstanding feature.

Some of the signs and symptoms evidenced are caused by lack of nutrition of the tissues, whereas others result from congestion of blood in the lungs or extrapulmonary tissues or both. The latter interferes with function by occupying space and by limiting blood flow through the affected tissues. Although all tissues are affected when the heart fails, the effects on the function of vital organs such as the kidney, lung, brain, liver, and the heart itself are for obvious reasons the most serious.

Mrs. Bird, who was introduced in Chapter 9, illustrates the course of events in chronic heart failure. Multiple factors contributed to her loss of myocardial reserve. Aging, with its attendant loss of muscle tissue, essential hypertension, and atherosclerosis, of which the last two increased the resistance against which the blood had to be moved, contributed to a loss of cardiac reserve. The hypertension, accompanied by atherosclerosis, diminished the quantity of blood circulated to the heart muscle. Over a period of time, hypertrophy and dilatation of the heart occurred. The growth of new capillaries lagged behind the increase in the mass of myocardium. This further added to the discrepancy between the quantity of blood delivered to the myocardium and its nutritional requirements. Mrs. Bird was unable to augment the supply of blood to her myocardium in proportion to the increase in work load. Eventually her heart was not able to adapt the quantity of blood delivered into her circulation to the needs of her tissues during activity. In fact, stimuli, such as exercise or excitement, that call forth an increase in cardiac output in persons with a healthy heart actually were followed by a decrease in output of Mrs. Bird's heart. A fall in cardiac output when activity is increased is frequent in patients with congestive heart failure.[25] At rest Mrs. Bird's heart was able to eject as much blood into her circulation as was delivered to it. When she exercised, her heart was no longer strong enough to eject as much blood as was returned to it, and the quantity of blood remaining in the heart at the end of systole increased. As time passed, she found she required several pillows at night to avoid feeling short of breath. Activities such as walking to the corner store or up a flight of stairs caused her heart to pound (palpitation) and shortness of breath. At night she noted her feet were swollen and in the morning she had difficulty in putting on her shoes. Despite a loss in appetite, or anorexia, she also had a marked gain in weight. Eventually, shortness of breath was present at rest, even when she was in the sitting position. By this time, blood flow to all of Mrs. Bird's tissues was diminished.

There are different ways to describe heart failure; however, basic to all failure is the fact that the atria and ventricles are unable to pump as much blood into the circulation as is delivered to them. Perhaps one of the easiest ways to think of heart failure is left- and right-sided failure. Left- and right-sided failure can occur as isolated entities or in combination. With left-sided failure the pumping ability of the left side of the heart fails, whereas the pumping ability of the right side fails with right-sided failure. In heart failure either the atria or ventricles or both can fail.

LEFT-SIDED FAILURE

In left-sided failure blood returning from the

[25] Eugene A. Stead, Jr.: "Pathologic Physiology of Heart Failure," *Cecil-Loeb: Textbook of Medicine,* 12th ed., Paul B. Beeson and Walsh McDermott, eds. (Philadelphia: W. B. Saunders Company, 1967), p. 578.

lungs meets increased resistance in either the left atrium or ventricle. Because of the increased resistance, the amount of blood that the left side can accept will be decreased with a resulting engorgement of the pulmonary vascular bed. With this engorgement there is an increase in the pressure at the capillary level causing fluid to exude into the interstitial space. Some of the underlying causes of left-sided failure are structural abnormalities of the heart (mitral and aortic stenosis or insufficiency), myocardial disease (myocarditis or myocardial infarction), and cardiac arrhythmias (tachycardias).

An example of left atrial failure is mitral stenosis. With stenosis there is an impediment to the forward flow of blood. With each atrial contraction a small volume of blood remains in the left atrial appendage. Eventually hypertrophy and failure of the left atrium occur. A classic example of left ventricular failure is that following a myocardial infarction. Because of the necrosis of part of the left ventricle, pumping is less effective.

RIGHT-SIDED FAILURE

In right-sided failure venous blood returning to the right side of the heart meets increased resistance in either the right atrium or ventricle. A damming up of blood occurs in the peripheral blood vessels. With the increased pressure at the capillary level, fluid is forced into the interstitial spaces, causing systemic edema.

Right-sided failure probably occurs most frequently secondary to left-sided failure. Because the circulatory system is a closed circuit, there cannot be any discrepancy in the amount of blood returned to a chamber and the output of that chamber.

As the heart fails, its output falls and causes a relative ischemia of the tissues. According to Guyton,[26] this low cardiac output has a profound effect on renal function. The kidney responds to diminished blood flow by a reduction in glomerular filtration. Renal blood flow is further decreased by the activation of sympathetic reflexes, which cause a marked constriction of afferent renal arterioles. Although it has been suggested that one of the factors in edema formation in congestive heart failure is an increase in the secretion of aldosterone, chronically elevated levels of aldosterone do not lead to edema, even though the total circulating blood volume may be increased. There is recent evidence that a humoral extra-adrenal, extra-renal factor may be implicated in the development of edema in heart failure. Its source and

type are unknown.[27] The increase in the blood volume and the congestion of tissues result primarily from the inability of the heart to eject as much blood into the circulation as needed by the tissues to maintain their function. A number of hypotheses have been proposed to explain the increase in the volume of extracellular fluid and congestion of tissues accompanying chronic heart failure. Currently more factors than the response of the kidney and its regulatory agencies to ischemia are thought to be involved.

Congestion of the tissues is primarily caused by a failure of the ventricles to eject as much blood into the circulation as is delivered to them. Output may or may not be reduced below normal limits. Because output is less than input, blood accumulates in the heart. The increase of residual blood in the heart causes the myocardial fibers to stretch. For a time the increase in residual blood may stimulate the myocardium to contract more forcibly. This is to be expected unless some condition, such as dilatation, exists that weakens the heart muscle. According to the law of the heart, lengthening of the myocardial fibers results in increased force of contraction. Eventually, however, the residual blood in the ventricles becomes so great that the heart is overdilated. Despite an increased expenditure of energy, the heart is no longer effective as a pump. As blood accumulates in the heart, the intra-atrial pressure rises and offers resistance to the incoming or venous blood. The increase in venous pressure is reflected by elevation of pressure in the great veins as well as in the venous tributaries. As the pressure of blood within the veins, that is, the venous hydrostatic pressure, rises, the tissues drained by these veins become congested with blood and fluid.

What changes are responsible for the signs and symptoms in congestive heart failure?

Signs and symptoms in congestive heart failure arise from the failure of the heart to adequately nourish and oxygenate the tissues and from the accumulation of blood and fluid in the various tissues and organs in the body. In the early stages of congestive (chronic) heart failure, the most outstanding symptom is shortness of breath during ordinary activities. The reader will remember that Mrs. Bird's first symptom was shortness of breath when she walked to the store or up a flight of stairs. With the elapse of time the amount of activity re-

---

26 *Op. cit.*, pp. 373–74.

27 James O. Davis *et al.:* "An Extra-Adrenal Factor Essential for Chronic Renal Sodium Retention in Presence of Increased Sodium-Retaining Hormone," *Circ. Res.*, 14:17–31 (Jan.) 1964.

quired to precipitate the sensation of breathlessness becomes less and less. Apprehension usually accompanies shortness of breath because anything interfering with respiration threatens survival. Despite the presence of fatigue and lack of energy, patients seldom complain of these effects.

The signs and symptoms accompanying pulmonary congestion caused by left-sided heart failure are similar to those resulting from congestion of the lung from any cause. With the congestion of blood in the lung, pulmonary edema develops. Both the slowing of the flow of blood through the lung and the pulmonary edema predispose to hypoxia and hypercarbia. Many of the manifestations observed in congestive heart failure are caused by failure to adequately oxygenate the blood and to remove carbon dioxide from it. Some of the manifestations commonly observed are caused by the congestion of the lung tissue itself.

As indicated, one of the early and most distressing symptoms in congestive heart failure is dyspnea. Although the symptom dyspnea was discussed in some detail in Chapter 8, it, along with other disturbances in breathing, will be reviewed in relation to heart disease. Although dyspnea in heart disease is associated with pulmonary congestion, its severity is not always in direct proportion to the degree of congestion. Why this is true has not been explained to the satisfaction of all who are interested in this problem.

Because dyspnea can be induced in a healthy person by a variety of physical (strenuous exercise) and emotional factors (fear, excitement, or other strong emotions), some believe it results when one or a number of factors in combination are sufficiently powerful. As a result of a series of experiments Wasserman and his associates,[28] concluded that dyspnea results from the "summated effects of a number of physiologic stimuli to respiration." (See Chapter 8.) Further, a single stimulus may be so great that dyspnea occurs. Under other circumstances, a number of less powerful stimuli may combine to produce it. In the healthy or non-dyspneic person, a balance is maintained between the impulses stimulating respiration and those inhibiting it. According to Wasserman et al.,[29] in dyspnea there is a powerful stimulus to inspiration and in some instances an accompanying reduction in respiratory inhibition.

In the patient in congestive heart failure, the lungs become engorged with blood with the

[28] A. J. Wasserman, H. P. Mauck, Jr., and J. L. Patterson, Jr.: "The Nature and Pathogenesis of Dyspnea," *Heart Bull.,* **11**:2 (Jan.–Feb.) 1962.
[29] *Ibid.,* p. 3.

result that the lung becomes inelastic and edematous. This causes a reduction of the vital capacity. The patient may, however, be relatively free of dyspnea at rest. During activity, because his ventilatory minute volume of air rises, he becomes dyspneic. The activity may be physical exercise, but it may also be excitement or anger. As previously emphasized, some patients experience dyspnea with less engorgement of their lungs than others do. Dyspnea is made worse by conditions that reduce vital capacity or the effective ventilating surface of the lung such as hydrothorax, pulmonary infarcts, and ascites.

When dyspnea or breathlessness becomes so severe that the patient cannot lie in a recumbent position, the patient is said to be orthopneic. Orthopnea can often be relieved by elevating the trunk in relation to the rest of the body. Though there is some increase in the vital capacity when the trunk is raised, some authorities do not feel this completely explains the beneficial effect of the upright position. A variety of methods may be used to secure the desired result. The patient may sit in Fowler's position in bed, the head of the bed may be elevated, or he may be more comfortable sitting in a chair. Whether he sits in bed or in a chair, the patient often seeks relief by sitting forward. When the most comfortable position is found, the patient should be adequately supported with pillows. An over-the-bed table may be placed so the patient can rest on it as he leans forward. As previously emphasized, the patient should be supported in a comfortable position and in good alignment by the supports. Also, his position should be changed regularly.

Both dyspnea and orthopnea are causes of and result from apprehension. For this reason every effort should be made to assure the patient that his needs will be met and that he can trust his safety to those responsible for his care. Because morphine sulfate depresses the higher centers in the brain, it is sometimes prescribed to alleviate anxiety. This is one of the few instances in which morphine sulfate is administered for relief of a symptom other than pain.

The importance of the relief of dyspnea and orthopnea is illustrated by Mrs. Oriole, a young woman in severe congestive failure associated with mitral stenosis and rheumatic heart disease. She was markedly orthopneic. Relief was not achieved by the orthopneic position. Her basal metabolic rate was found to be +100 per cent. This young woman, whose heart was unable to perform as an efficient pump, was actually "working hard." The pathophysiology in the instance of Mrs. Oriole is an illustration of a positive feedback (a vicious circle). One event—failure of her myocardium—led to congestion of her lungs and the development of orthopnea. As her need for breathing increased, she required more energy to maintain breathing. As the work required to breathe increased, strain on her weakened myocardium was increased. One event initiated a second that either directly or indirectly intensified the first. Unless the chain is broken, or successful medical treatment and/or rest, which help the heart maintain the body's demands is instituted, death results.

Another form of dyspnea is known as paroxysmal nocturnal dyspnea or cardiac asthma. It is most frequently observed in patients who have a disorder that places a burden on the left ventricle. Because it usually occurs after the patient has been asleep and is therefore seen most frequently at night, it is referred to as nocturnal. Nocturnal dyspnea may develop in patients who do not have dyspnea when they are up and about and who may even be able to work. The recumbent position predisposes to or precipitates dyspnea because blood tends to accumulate in the lungs in this position. In the patient who already has some impingement on his vital capacity, a few hundred milliliters of blood added to that already present in the lung may be sufficient to cause dyspnea. During an attack of paroxysmal dyspnea the patient is awakened from sleep. He either sits upright, hangs his feet over the edge of the bed, or stands upright. He may be ashen in color and sweating profusely. Because there is often some bronchial constriction, he may be wheezing. He is usually frightened.

Other signs and symptoms that occur include periodic or Cheyne-Stokes respiration and cyanosis. They are both discussed in Chapter 8.

Cough with clear or blood-tinged sputum may accompany pulmonary edema. Though cough is an important mechanism in maintaining a clear airway, it requires a considerable expenditure of energy and may interfere with sleep.

Although blood-tinged sputum is not uncommon in left heart failure, larger amounts may appear. Hemoptysis may result from a sudden increase in pulmonary venous pressure, which leads to the rupture of a pulmonary vessel or to an infarction in the lung. Although it is not usually dangerous, *it may be,* and any quantity of blood in the sputum is likely to frighten the patient.

Needless to say, appreciable amounts of blood in the sputum are likely to terrify the patient as well as other persons in his environment. Blood issuing from the lung is bright pink or red and foamy in appearance. Foaming is caused by air passing through it. When blood appears in the sputum for the first time or is present in considerable quantity, the physician should be notified. The quantity of blood should be estimated or measured and described accurately. The patient should be encouraged to lie quietly in whatever position he finds is comfortable. Because morphine sulfate allays apprehension, the physician may prescribe it. When at all possible the nurse should remain with the patient in order to increase his feeling of safety and to determine the extent of his bleeding.

To recapitulate, besides interfering with the oxygenation of the blood and the removal of carbon dioxide, pulmonary congestion is responsible for a number of other effects. It causes several disturbances in breathing, the most common of which are dyspnea and orthopnea. Cough with clear or blood-tinged sputum is not infrequent.

In addition to disturbances in breathing, pulmonary congestion places an added burden on the right ventricle by increasing the resistance against which it has to move the blood. Eventually, unless the left-sided heart failure is corrected, the right heart fails. Failure of the right side of the heart may be secondary to diseases of the lung that cause an increase in resistance to the flow of blood through the lung. Diseases such as emphysema, therefore, predispose to failure of the right heart.

What are some of the possible factors in the development of generalized edema in congestive heart failure?

Sooner or later patients in chronic congestive heart failure develop generalized systemic edema. In the beginning the principal evidence of edema may be a gain in weight as a patient can be expected to store at least 10 to 20 lb (5 to 10 liters) of fluid before pitting edema occurs. Usually by the time a patient has dyspnea at rest he has stored at least 30 lb of fluid.

The cause of edema in heart failure has never been adequately explained. As stated earlier, one factor is thought to be the elevation of the hydrostatic pressure of the blood in the capillaries as a result of increased venous pressure. Factors in this increase include augmented tone of veins and resistance to incoming blood by an overdilated ventricle. A second factor is the retention of salt and water by the kidney. An extra-adrenal and extrarenal humoral agent may be implicated. Why edema occurs has not been agreed on. With the retention of salt and water, the blood volume increases and the quantity of protein in the blood is also elevated. During the day, the fluid is deposited in tissues below the level of the heart. At night it tends to be more generally distributed. The patient notices that his ankles swell during the day and that his shoes are tight. By morning the swelling disappears. As the disorder progresses, the edema is continuous. The patient may also complain of a feeling of heaviness but not of pain. In general, edema appears where capillary pressure is high and tissue pressure is low. Later, when the patient becomes bedfast, sacral edema as well as edema of the genitalia may be manifested. When edema is severe, the skin becomes tightly stretched and shiny in appearance. Because it has difficulty in maintaining its nutrition, it breaks down and fluids drain from it. Cellulitis may result from infection. When the legs are very distended with fluid, needles or small tubes may be introduced into the subcutaneous tissue to drain off some of the fluid.

Although accumulation of fluid in the parts below the heart is less dangerous to the patient than pulmonary edema, it does create problems for the patient. For the reasons cited, a patient in congestive failure is a candidate for decubiti unless special care is given. In the severely orthopneic patient the problem is commonly aggravated by resistance to moving and turning. Mr. Ash illustrates how quickly and extensively the skin may break down. He was severely orthopneic. About 7 o'clock in the evening, when back care was given, the skin of his buttocks was edematous but intact. In the morning, 12 hours later, the skin on the cheeks of both buttocks was denuded and bleeding. See Chapter 4.

Generalized edema may mask a serious state of undernourishment. In children physical and even mental development may be seriously retarded. Undernutrition and edema go hand in hand with chronic illness whatever the cause. When the patient responds to therapy, the true state of his nutrition becomes evident. It is not uncommon for these patients to appear to be nothing more than skin and bones following the removal of edema fluid. In some patients improvement of their nutritional status may be required before efforts to relieve their edema are successful.

Symptoms indicating involvement of the gastrointestinal tract are common. Anorexia, nausea, and vomiting are common. The patient frequently complains of indigestion. Especially in acute heart failure, these may be the predominant symptoms. The reasons for the symptoms have not been completely identified. The gastrointestinal tract is highly sensitive to disturbances in homeostasis. Both the heart and the gastrointestinal tract are supplied by branches of the vagus nerve. Reflexes arising in one organ may affect the function of the other through intermedullary connections between the heart and the stomach. Congestion of the viscera is also a possibility. In advanced heart failure, metabolism of the brain may be sufficiently disturbed to cause reflex vomiting. At times the origin of the gastrointestinal symptoms may create a problem in differential diagnosis for the physician. Mr. Sparrow illustrates this point. He sought medical attention with complaints suggestive of cholecystitis. The diagnosis of cholecystitis was confirmed and he was admitted to the hospital. A nurse noted and reported to his physician that at times his pulse was irregular. An electrocardiogram indicated some myocardial injury. In this instance the patient had both cholecystitis and heart damage. Knowledge of the status of his heart was an important consideration in making the decision about whether surgical therapy was to be undertaken. Furthermore, it influenced the selection of the surgical procedure to be performed as well as his care before, during, and after surgery.

Swelling of the liver (hepatomegaly) and abdominal pain are frequent. Because only about a fourth of the blood supply of the liver is arterial, under the most favorable circumstances it borders on hypoxia. In congestive heart failure, hypoxia leads to necrosis of the hepatic cells surrounding central veins. There may also be swelling of the liver because of edema. In addition to abdominal pain, some patients experience jaundice.

Hypoglycemia occurs in severe congestive heart failure. This may be caused by inadequate storage of glycogen in the liver and increased breakdown of glucose to lactic acid in the presence of hypoxia.

Distention and pulsation of the neck veins may be observed. Distention is especially marked when the patient is in the recumbent position.

Cerebral symptoms do not usually become marked until the patient has dyspnea at rest. Although the principal factor in their development may be insufficient oxygenation and nutrition of the brain, other elements enter into their development. Early symptoms are irritability, restlessness, and difficulty in fixing attention. They may also include personality changes, mild delirium, and mental depression. In terminal stages stupor and coma occur.

One symptom specific to the heart is palpitation—consciousness of the beating of the heart. The two common physiological changes predisposing to palpitation are an increase in cardiac output and a change in the rhythm of the heart. The causes may be physiological or pathological. For example, Mrs. Oaks, a middle-aged and somewhat obese housewife, ran around the block, or tried to. By the time she returned to her home, she was dyspneic and her heart was pounding. A few nights later, she had difficulty in going to sleep. One of the factors making sleep difficult was the pounding of her heart.

She had had a stimulating evening playing bridge and an argument with her husband over how the last hand should have been bid. In both instances the response was physiological. In the first the stimulus was exercise. In the second it was a psychological incident.

Mrs. Oaks' neighbor, Mrs. Maple, was severely anemic. Because increase in blood volume is one of the mechanisms of adaptation to anemia, one of her most worrisome symptoms was palpitation. Correction of the anemia eliminated the cause and relieved the palpitation. Palpitation may also be observed in thyrotoxicosis and fever as well as in psychological disorders. Consciousness of the heart beating may also be associated with changes in rhythm.

Patients in longstanding and chronic heart failure differ from those with acute heart failure inasmuch as they have disturbances in the concentrations of electrolytes, whereas the latter do not. Characteristically, whenever edema develops, there is sodium retention. The level of sodium per unit of blood plasma will depend on whether water and sodium are equally retained or water is retained in excess of sodium. In the latter event, the concentration of sodium in the plasma will be low. In longstanding and intractable heart failure, diuretics become ineffective.

The making of a medical diagnosis of heart disease is the responsibility of the physician. The symptoms usually observed in patients with congestive heart failure have already been described in some detail. In the early stages of failure, the physician must evaluate each symptom in light of the age of the individual, his weight in relation to height, and his emotional status, as well as the presence of some other disease that may account for a symptom or group of symptoms. Through objective observation and reporting, the nurse can often add to the information obtained by the physician. For example, she can note any conditions seeming to precipitate or relieve a given symptom and the patient's reaction to it.

DIAGNOSIS

Diagnostic procedures specific to the heart include the electrocardiogram, x-ray of the heart, and the circulation time. The electrocardiogram is discussed in another section of this chapter. From x-ray or fluoroscopy of the heart and chest, the physician obtains information about the size and position of the heart and the great vessels. Evidence of congestion of the lungs can also be obtained.

The circulation time can be defined as the time it takes one particle to travel from one point in the circulation to another. Circulation time can be estimated by injecting a substance and then measuring the time required for it to reach a specific receptor. In one method either dehydrocholic acid (Decholin [30]) or ether is injected into a vein in the arm. When dehydrocholic acid is injected, the time elapsing after administration until the person can taste it—it has a bitter taste—is measured. The normal time is from 8 to 17 seconds. This is known as the arm-to-tongue circulation time. The arm-to-tongue circulation time is increased in left heart failure. Both Mrs. Bird and Mrs. Oriole had an increase in arm-to-tongue circulation time. When ether is used, the patient smells it when it reaches the lung. Normally the arm-to-lung time is from 4 to 8 seconds. Arm-to-lung time is increased in right heart failure. For experimental work more accurate measures are now available in the form of dyes and radioisotopes.

Most patients in congestive heart failure have some elevation of the venous pressure. Venous pressure measures the relationship between blood entering the right side of the heart and leaving the right ventricle. Factors altering the venous pressure are changes in intrathoracic pressure (coughing, respirators, forced breathing, and pneumothorax), intra-abdominal pressure (abdominal distention), viscosity or volume of blood, muscle contraction, and body posture.

The procedure used to determine the venous pressure is essentially a venipuncture with a needle into the anticubital vein followed by the attachment of a glass tube or manometer. To obtain an accurate result, the arm should be elevated to the level of the right atrium. A second method can be used when pressure readings have to be taken at frequent intervals. With this method an intracath is threaded through the jugular or antecubital vein to the level of the right atrium to measure central venous pressure. The catheter is attached to an intravenous setup with a manometer and three-way stopcock. Thus the stopcock can be regulated so that intravenous fluids can be infused between pressure readings. To obtain accurate readings, the stopcock of the manometer must be at the level of the right atrium, which is approximately midway between the anterior and posterior chest. Harrison [31] states that the normal venous pressure in the antecubital vein is from 70 to 140 mm of water. Expressed in centimeters, this is 7 to 14.

As in all medical diagnosis, the history and physical examination are important. Sometimes

[30] Trade name.
[31] "Laboratory Values of Clinical Importance," *Principles of Internal Medicine,* 5th ed., T. R. Harrison et al., eds. (New York: The Blakiston Division, McGraw-Hill Book Company, Inc., 1966), p. 1812.

the patient fails to give the physician pertinent information. The nurse, as she gains information, is responsible for relaying it to the proper persons.

Patients in full-blown congestive heart failure offer few problems in the diagnosis of a failing heart. Early diagnosis of impending failure may be more difficult, but it may make it possible to institute a regime to protect the heart from added injury. As a case finder, the nurse should encourage patients to seek medical advice early.

To summarize, when the heart fails as a pump, the manifestations of failure depend on the degree of failure and the rate at which it fails. In all degrees of heart failure many of the effects are directly or indirectly caused by supply of oxygen or by the accumulation of carbon dioxide. In cardiac arrest death or incapacitating brain damage occurs unless the circulation is re-established within approximately four minutes. In acute heart failure the manifestations depend on the efficiency of the person's mechanisms for adapting to cardiac inefficiency and in many instances they are adequate. When adaptation is inadequate, the manifestations of heart failure are caused by the effects of failure of the heart to meet the needs of the tissues for oxygen and nutrition and by the retention of salt and water. In acute heart failure generalized edema is not usually marked. Pulmonary engorgement and edema are likely, however. When severe, they are life threatening.

In chronic heart failure, signs and symptoms develop gradually over a period of time. They, too, result from failure of the heart to adequately nourish and oxygenate the tissues and from the increase in the volume of extracellular fluid. Generalized edema is marked and many of the accompanying signs and symptoms are caused by it. There is also some degree of pulmonary congestion.

What are the therapeutic objectives in chronic heart failure?

Therapy of the patient in heart failure depends on the degree and suddenness with which his heart fails. Because the most common cause of acute heart failure is myocardial infarction, the treatment of the patient in acute heart failure will be discussed with this most important disorder. The objective of treatment of the patient in chronic or congestive heart failure is to restore the capacity of the heart to adapt or respond efficiently to the demands placed on it, that is, to restore the pumping mechanism of the heart so that as much blood is propelled into the circulation as enters the heart during diastole and there is no increase in residual blood at the end of systole. The re-establishment of the efficiency of the heart as a pump requires a two-pronged attack. One is to increase the force or strength of contraction of the myocardium. The other is to reduce the demands made on the myocardium until the efficiency of the pumping mechanism has been restored. Later the reserve power of the heart muscle will have to be evaluated and plans made with the patient and his family regarding any modifications of his living and working habits.

TREATMENT

At the time a patient, such as Mrs. Bird or Mrs. Oriole, seeks medical attention, he is often seriously, if not critically, ill. Health and life depend on restoring the pumping mechanism to as full efficiency as possible. Both aspects of treatment are carried out simultaneously. The physician prescribes a cardiac glucoside—usually a preparation of digitalis—to strengthen the force of cardiac contraction, a regime of rest and activity to limit the demands made on the failing heart, and diuretics combined with sodium restriction to reduce the volume of fluid in the body and thus lessen the burden on the weakened heart.

Digitalis

Digitalis contains an active principle in the form of a glucoside that has a number of important effects on the heart muscle. In congestive heart failure it increases the strength of ventricular contraction with the result that the volume of residual blood is reduced at the end of systole, that is, it increases the efficiency of the pumping mechanism of the heart. It has a second action that is modified by the level of potassium in the body. In the presence of normal amounts of potassium, it lessens the responsiveness of the conduction system of the heart. This has its greatest value in the patient who has atrial fibrillation. In atrial fibrillation the ventricle is bombarded by numerous impulses. Despite its failure to respond to all of them, diastole is sometimes so short that the heart receives little blood. Energy expended in the succeeding systole is largely wasted. Reduction in the number of impulses reaching the ventricles has the obvious advantage of reducing the number of wasteful contractions. Although digitalis occasionally restores the normal atrial contraction, it does not usually do so. For example, when Mrs. Bird was admitted to the hospital, her atria were fibrillating. Her pulse rate was completely irregular and averaged about 100 beats per minute. Her ventricular rate when counted by stethoscope was about 140; she had a pulse deficit of about 40. (The pulse deficit is defined as the difference between the number of ventricular contractions and pulse beat.) After

Mrs. Bird was digitalized, her atria continued to fibrillate, but her pulse rate averaged between 65 and 75 beats per minute. The pulse deficit disappeared.

Digitalis increases the irritability of the heart muscle whether the level of potassium is normal or low, but the effect is more marked in the presence of low potassium levels. The mechanism seems to be related to the effect on intracardiac calcium concentration. Potassium levels can also be effectively lowered by intravenous administration of glucose in water. Increased myocardial irritability may be manifested by premature beats and an increase in the pulse rate. The latter condition is known as pulsus bigeminus. Because there is an extra contraction interspersed between the normal contraction, the pulse rate is increased and irregular. Although all alterations in the rate and rhythm of the pulse are important and should be reported, this is particularly important for the patient taking digitalis. To prevent the possibility of digitalis-induced arrhythmias, potassium chloride is frequently administered to patients who are under regular and prolonged therapy with diuretics, as they predispose to potassium depletion.

An untoward effect of potassium chloride can be irritation of the gastric mucosa resulting in ulceration of the small bowel and stricture. Inadequate food intake, whether caused by anorexia or by poor food habits, also adds to the likelihood of potassium deficiency. Patients on diuretic therapy should have a daily intake of foods high in potassium, such as fresh fruits (a large glass of orange juice or two bananas), meats, or tea.

The specific preparation of digitalis prescribed by the physician will depend on his personal preference and the acuteness of the patient's symptoms. When the patient's life is endangered by marked pulmonary edema, the physician is likely to prescribe a rapidly acting preparation to be administered intravenously. For example, when Mrs. Oriole was admitted to the hospital, her lungs were engorged and her vital capacity was seriously reduced. Her physician prescribed and administered intravenously lanatoside C, 1.6 mg N.F. (Cedilanid [32]). Later she was placed on digitoxin U.S.P., administered orally.

At the time Mrs. Bird sought medical attention her condition was less urgent. Her physician, therefore, digitalized her slowly. Many physicians prefer this method as there is less likelihood of digitalis intoxication. He ordered digitoxin U.S.P., 0.6 mg, to be followed in six hours by another 0.6 mg. The dosage was then

reduced to 0.2 mg every six hours, to be continued until beneficial effects or early toxic effects were observed. Thereafter, 0.1 mg was sufficient to maintain the digitalis effect.

Both patients were given a relatively large initial dosage of digitalis. A smaller dosage was required to maintain its effect. Because digitalis is absorbed more rapidly than it is destroyed and excreted from the body, it tends to accumulate. Consequently sufficient digitalis is administered over a period of 24 to 48 hours to produce the desired action. This procedure is known as digitalization. Thereafter, only enough digitalis is administered to replace that which is destroyed or eliminated. The quantity of drug required is referred to as the maintenance dosage.

Among the responsibilities of the nurse in the care of patients under digitalis therapy is the administration of the drug at the times and in the quantities prescribed by the physician. Perhaps even more important is the observation of the effects—desired as well as undesired—on the patient and the reporting and/or possible adjustment of the dosage according to pertinent observations. There is a common misconception that all patients require the same dosage, but this is not true. Moreover, a given patient may vary from time to time in his susceptibility to digitalis.

Few descriptions of the effects of digitalis have improved on the one left by William Withering, who first introduced the drug about the time of the American Revolution. He said, "Let the medicine . . . be continued until it either acts on the kidneys, the stomach, the pulse, or the bowels; let it be stopped upon the first appearance of any of these effects."

In the past literature of nursing and in its practice, great emphasis has been and is being placed on a pulse rate of 60 as an absolute criterion for the administration of digitalis. There has been a tendency to neglect other and more significant observations of developing toxicity. The pulse rate is a good guide to adequacy of digitalization *only* in patients with atrial fibrillation. In patients with sinus rhythm, a slowing pulse indicates either restoration of cardiac compensation or complete heart block. Harrison, Reeves, and Hefner [33] state the gastrointestinal symptoms—anorexia, nausea, and vomiting developing in this order—are most common evidence of digitalis toxicity. Diarrhea is not common, although it can occur. These are followed by cardiac arrhythmias, premature

[32] Trade name.

[33] T. R. Harrison, T. J. Reeves, and L. L. Hefner: "The Congestive Syndromes: Chronic Heart Failure," 5th ed., T. R. Harrison *et al.*, eds. (New York: The Blakiston Division, McGraw-Hill Book Company, Inc., 1966), p. 798.

beat, bigeminal rhythm, and atrial tachycardia. Excessive slowing of the pulse is not even mentioned. A less common toxic effect is a disturbance in color vision. Visual abnormalities can include all types of color vision disturbances (yellow is most common). Central nervous system excitation is an unusual but possible effect (digitalis madness).

Observations indicating that the heart is responding favorably to digitalis are slowing of the pulse to 75 or 80 beats per minute, diminishing pulse deficit, greater force of cardiac contraction, and increase in the output of urine. As the mechanical efficiency of the heart improves, the patient's general status usually improves (however, even with digitalization some patients with heart disease may not improve). He is less dyspneic and apprehensive. The backrest can be lowered. His appetite is better. His morale is improved. He sleeps better. With the loss of fluid he loses weight. In some patients loss of edema fluid may be so great that the skin hangs in loose folds and they appear emaciated. The safety of the patient often depends on the accuracy of observation of the effects of digitalis on the patient. Adjustments in dosage depend on the effects of the drug. Most of these observations can be made by an informed and interested nurse.

The nurse has another responsibility to the patient who is treated with digitalis. All patients who are receiving digitalis must take it for prolonged periods of time, and most of them must take it for as long as they live. As in other situations where the patient and his family are responsible for continued treatment, the nurse can be helpful to him by ascertaining what he knows and what he wants to know. Certainly the patient should know how and where to obtain the drug he needs and how many tablets or pills he should take each day. He should be instructed about the meaning of, and what to do about, loss of appetite, nausea, or vomiting. Patients on a regime of diuretics are usually instructed to take potassium replacement daily. Because carbohydrate increases the loss of potassium, the patient should be advised to avoid carbohydrate "binges," that is, the eating of excessive amounts of candies or pastries. In elderly patients living alone and with a limited income, carbohydrate in the form of bread may form the basic part of the diet. Patients do not always follow directions. In one instance observed by the writer, 77-year-old Mr. Henry adjusted his dosage of digitalis according to how he felt. When he felt well, he omitted it. When he had a bad day, he took an extra tablet or two. The reasons for this behavior were not explored. Superficially they may relate to the fact that many people judge the state of their health by how they feel; medicines are to be taken when they do not feel well. Because the effects of omitting a dose or two of digitalis are not felt immediately, some time may elapse before the patient feels sick. By that time, he may be in serious trouble.

Diuretics

As indicated, diuretics are widely used in the therapy of congestive heart failure. They may increase the effectiveness of digitalis and, by increasing the elimination of salt and water, reduce the burden on the weakened heart. Digitalis has a diuretic effect inasmuch as it improves the circulation of the kidneys and thereby improves their function.

The true diuretics used in the treatment of congestive heart failure are those that suppress the reabsorption of salt and water by the kidney. In the past the mercurial diuretics were used for this purpose. Today their use is generally limited to patients with massive edema or those who fail to respond to newer diuretics. One disadvantage of most preparations of mercurial diuretics is that they must be administered intramuscularly.

According to Harrison, Reeves, and Hefner,[34] the most generally useful group of diuretics is the chlorothiazide group. They, like the mercurials, block the reabsorption of the chloride, sodium, and potassium ions in the proximal tubules. Continued and frequent use of these drugs may lead to the previously mentioned potassium depletion. When combined with a low-sodium intake, they may also cause a sodium deficiency. See Chapter 9 for further details.

Harrison *et al.*[35] suggest chlorothiazide (Diuril[36]) be administered in dosages of from 250 to 300 mg two to four times daily for five consecutive days each week. Potassium chloride is administered at the same time to prevent potassium deficiency.

One of the mechanisms implicated in the retention of salt and water is the oversecretion of aldosterone. It is believed to act principally in the distal tubule. To counteract the action of aldosterone, an antagonist, spironolactone (Aldactone), has been developed. So far the results of its use in cardiac failure have been disappointing.

The nurse has the usual responsibilities when administering drugs with a diuretic effect. Not only should the urine output be measured, but the weight of the patient should be accurately checked. Particularly pertinent to nurses working with patients in outpatient clinics and at

[34] *Ibid.,* p. 798.
[35] *Ibid.,* p. 799.
[36] Trade name.

home is the observation of patients for signs and symptoms of electrolyte depletion.

In addition to measures utilized to facilitate the excretion of sodium, its retention can be further diminished by decreasing its intake. In areas where the drinking water has a high sodium content bottled water may be necessary. The quantity of salt allowed in the diet varies greatly. At one extreme is the limitation of intake to from 200 to 400 mg of sodium. At the other the patient is instructed not to add any salt to his food at the table. A very low sodium intake is usually prescribed for the patient who has marked edema and is continued only during the acute phase of the illness. Mrs. Oriole is a good example. To achieve a sodium content of between 200 and 400 mg, all medicines containing sodium salts and foods naturally high in sodium, as well as those prepared with sodium salts, are restricted. Sodium is the offending agent and not the chloride anion. Therefore, Mrs. Oriole should not be given sodium bicarbonate or breads, cakes, or pastries leavened with it. There is at least one brand of baking powder prepared with a potassium rather than a sodium salt. Foods prepared with salts of sodium should be avoided. The patient should be taught to look at the label on food. If it contains a sodium salt, it should not be used. Other foods limited during a period when sodium intake is markedly restricted include milk and celery. Continued marked reduction in sodium is not the rule.

At one time water intake was markedly restricted. Presently, the trend is toward moderate or no restriction. Some physicians allow the patient as much water as he wishes. Others limit intake to as little as 800 ml a day. A prescription of from 1,500 to 2,000 ml is common. Whatever the prescription, the nurse has the responsibility for carrying it out and for bringing problems to the attention of the physician. When fluid intake is markedly restricted, a plan should be made to distribute it over the 24-hour period. The use of a small glass filled with chipped ice and just enough water to fill the spaces makes it easier to extend a limited quantity of water over the day.

When a patient has acute pulmonary edema, blood volume and consequently pulmonary engorgement may be reduced by venesection. Usually about 300 or 400 ml of blood can be removed without causing a fall in blood pressure. The patient and his family may require reassurance about why the removal of blood is therapeutic.

Tourniquets

The volume of blood circulating through the lungs can be temporarily reduced by applying tourniquets to the extremities so that blood enters but does not leave the area below the tourniquet. The blood pressure cuff is safer than ordinary tourniquets as the degree of pressure can be controlled. Ordinary tourniquets are frequently applied too tightly with the result that the tissues become ischemic.

Another method available is the automatic rotating tourniquet machine. With this method blood pressure cuffs are applied to all four extremities and attached to the machine. The machine is designed so that the pressure within the cuffs can be controlled and do a complete rotation of the pressure in the cuffs in 45 minutes. Tourniquets should be inflated to a level between the diastolic and systolic blood pressure. The pulses in the arteries should be palpated regularly to be sure that blood is gaining access to the parts below the tourniquets. Tourniquets may be applied to all four extremities or to three extremities with the fourth free. In the latter instance, they are rotated according to a regular pattern, so each extremity is free one fourth of the time. The pattern should be established when the treatment is initiated so that the circulation to each extremity is regularly released. Usually tourniquets are applied to three extremities and then rotated every 10 to 15 minutes. With this pattern, the tourniquet remains on each extremity about 30 to 45 minutes. When the tourniquets are discontinued, they should be removed, one at a time. Otherwise a large amount of fluid may gain entry into the circulation with a recurrence of pulmonary congestion. Following the removal of tourniquets, the patient may show some transient hyperpnea because of the release of carbon dioxide into the blood. During the period in which the tourniquets are in place, the patient should be observed for manifestations of shock. The sudden reduction of venous return to the lung predisposes to shock by lessening the volume of blood delivered to the left ventricle. Because cardiac output depends on cardiac intake, circulation cannot be maintained unless intake is adequate. Evidence indicating the development of shock should, of course, be brought immediately to the attention of the physician.

Other measures utilized to reduce the demands placed on the heart include the administration of oxygen, sedatives, and bed or chair rest. When oxygenation of the blood is impaired, oxygen therapy may also improve the quality of blood circulated to the heart muscle. In hot weather, oxygen administered by tent has the further advantage of providing an air-conditioned unit.

During the period in which the patient is acutely ill, sedatives may add greatly to the patient's comfort. Morphine sulfate or Pantopium (Pantopon) may be prescribed by the physician to allay the apprehension and to relieve dyspnea. When narcotics are used, they may be prescribed for bedtime in order to help the patient sleep well. Overuse with its attendant danger of habituation should be avoided. One of the meprobamate tranquilizing drugs or small doses of phenobarbital may be ordered for the daytime. Care must be taken not to oversedate the patient as this renders him less able to cooperate with measures required to prevent thrombophlebitis.

Although the discussion of rest and its antithesis, activity, is included here, much of the discussion applies equally well to any situation in which rest and activity are modified. Despite the fact that rest is probably one of the oldest forms of medical therapy, its use in the treatment of heart disease is of relatively modern origin. For the last 10 to 20 years, there has been some critical examination of the effects of bed rest and a considerable change in thought about the value of bed rest in the treatment of diseases of the heart as well as of other diseases.

Bed Rest

Despite the frequency with which *rest* and *bed rest* are prescribed, there is little agreement about what either term means. Sometimes little or no thought is given to whether rest in the true sense is likely to be achieved or is even possible. For example, about a year previous to her admission Mrs. Oriole's physician told her that she must get "more rest." Mrs. Oriole had three healthy preschool children. The oldest was four and the youngest was about a year old. Her husband worked long hours in a gas station to enable him to support his family and to pay his wife's medical bills. Neither Mr. nor Mrs. Oriole had any near relatives. Mrs. Oriole needed some help to analyze her situation and to find ways to get the rest she needed. Another example is that of Franz Timothy. When he visited his physician, the suggestion was made that he "get some rest." He went home and told his wife he needed a rest and that they would start for California (or Maine) the next morning. Mr. Timothy interpreted the term rest as a change in activity. Another patient, Mrs. Clover, informed her family after she received the same general prescription that her doctor wanted her to go to bed for a week. In the last two instances, both persons interpreted the term *rest* differently. In one instance rest was a change. In the other it meant a withdrawal from most, if not all, activity.

Interpretation of the term *bed rest* by physicians and nurses varies just as greatly. At one extreme, it means the patient is to be as completely immobilized as is possible. At the other, it means he is merely confined to his bed and can do anything in or from his bed. In the first instance the patient is fed, bathed, turned, and given any other care he requires. He may be instructed that the only voluntary activity he may perform is to turn on his light signal. In the latter instance, the patient may be responsible for much of his own personal care and may actually expend as much or more energy as he would were he up and about. Although the physician has the responsibility for prescribing the amount of activity for a patient, the nurse interprets the prescription to the patient and tries to provide the kind of environment that makes its achievement possible.

According to Roose,[37] as the physician's order progressed more toward ambulation, there tended to be a greater discrepancy in the interpretation between nurses and doctors. The doctors tended to permit more activity than the nurses interpreted. Therefore, the nurse has a responsibility to determine how much activity the physician's prescription actually allows. To ensure consistency in interpretation of prescriptions for rest and activity, some hospital, medical, and nursing staffs have defined or classified degrees of activity. This is often done in hospitals where patients are treated for tuberculosis or heart disease. For example, patients in class I are to be maintained on complete bed rest. They are to be fed, bathed twice a week, shaved, turned, and have all possible activities performed for them. They are allowed to use a bedside commode once daily. Patients in class II may in addition to the activities in class I feed themselves, wash their own face and hands, and go to the bathroom twice a day. Patients in higher classes are permitted more and more activity. Exactly what is allowed in a particular class is not important. What is important is that patient and personnel alike understand the limitation and the reason for it. Reasonable consistency in practice should increase the security of the patient and the likelihood of his receiving care suited to his needs.

In addition to widely differing interpretations of what bed rest means, true rest is more than a matter of limited physical activity. This is implied by the common definition of rest, that is, to take repose by lying down, particularly by going to sleep. Synonyms for the noun *rest* include calm, calmness, ease, pause, peace, peacefulness, repose, and tranquility. There are others, but these words convey the broad meaning of the term. What rest is not is clarified by some of its antonyms: agitation, commotion,

[37] Jeanine A. Roose: "Interpretation of Rest by Doctors and Nurses," *Nurs. Res.*, **12**:111–13 (Spring) 1963.

disquiet, disturbance, excitement, restlessness, tumult, unrest, and work. Bed rest does not necessarily include or exclude any of the preceding states. All the states indicated by the antonyms involve more than the expenditure of physical energy.

A prescription for rest therefore involves more than limitation of physical activity. There are many elements in sickness and all it entails that interfere with true rest, or a tranquil or peaceful state. Though many of these have been indicated in earlier chapters, a few will be repeated here. Boredom, loneliness, and worry about the possible outcome of the illness and the effect this will have on family, job, and future plans probably plague most patients. A high percentage of patients who suffer myocardial infarctions are in the prime of life when job and family obligations are great. In some patients, the dependent state precipitates intense anxiety. Anxiety may be aggravated by the insistence that the patient's life depends on immediate and complete conformity to the medical regime. Physical discomfort, resulting from pain and unpleasant diagnostic procedures, adds its bit to the failure to achieve repose. Even when a patient lies still in bed, he may not be in a state of rest. Tension may be betrayed by a worried or uneasy expression on his face, evidence of muscle tension, a higher than normal pulse rate or blood pressure, or an irritable reaction. True rest implies a state in which the individual is physically, emotionally, mentally, and socially at ease.

The elements that are necessary in assisting the patient to rest have been indicated in earlier chapters. The acceptance of the patient as a human being having dignity and worth is basic. Attention to his physical comfort and personal needs and wishes makes a significant contribution. Regulation of his environment, both social and physical, so he is protected from unnecessary stresses is essential. Answering his questions or providing him with the assistance he requires to get them answered will help to remove one important source of disquiet among patients.

The objective toward which rest is directed in the therapy of the patient in heart failure is to reduce the need for the heart to adapt to varying volumes of venous return. In general the dorsal recumbent position is most restful. Immediately after one goes to bed, the blood pressure falls slightly and the work performed by skeletal muscles is diminished. With a reduction in the activity of skeletal muscles venous return to the heart is decreased. Obviously a reduction in blood presented to the heart lessens its work. The dorsal recumbent position has a serious disadvantage for the patient in, or in danger of, congestive heart failure. When he assumes the recumbent position, fluid in tissues below the level of the heart returns to the blood and increases the blood volume. This, in turn, increases the quantity of blood returned to the heart and with it the need to increase the cardiac output. Should the output of the right ventricle exceed that of the left by even a very small amount, this results in pulmonary congestion.[38] With pulmonary congestion there is a decrease in vital capacity.

Continued bed rest in the recumbent position has other adverse effects on pulmonary and circulatory function. After a week or so in the recumbent position the capacity to adapt circulation to the erect position is limited. In the healthy person a change from the prone to the upright position is accompanied by peripheral vasoconstriction and a slight rise in blood pressure. These changes protect the brain from an inadequate blood supply as a consequence of the effect of gravity on the blood in vessels below the heart. In the person who has been inactive in bed for a period of time, assumption of the upright position is accompanied by orthostatic (standing) hypotension, tachycardia, and possibly syncope (fainting). The usual explanation is that these effects are largely caused by a loss of tone in the muscles and veins of the legs. To prevent fainting, the patient should assume the upright position gradually. First the head of the bed is raised. After the patient has had an opportunity to adapt to this position he can shift his legs over the edge of the bed and "dangle." During this time he should be encouraged to flex and extend his ankles and swing his legs back and forth. At this time his pulse should be checked. If there is a marked tachycardia, this is a sign to go slow. Before finally assisting the patient to his feet, the nurse should be sure she has enough help to support him should it be needed. After the patient gains his balance, he should be assisted to walk or be returned to bed. Unnecessary motionless standing should be avoided. Contraction of the muscles of the legs is essential to maintaining the venous return against gravity.

In addition to the wasting of muscle with the accompanying loss of nitrogen, bed rest and inactivity have other adverse effects. Calcium is absorbed from the bones and thereby predisposes to osteoporosis and renal lithiasis. Stasis of blood in the veins combined with chemical changes in the blood predisposes to thrombophlebitis. Gastrointestinal function is impaired. Few if any physiological and metabolic functions escape adverse effects. Altered psycho-

[38] S. A. Levine: "The Myth of Strict Bed Rest in the Treatment of Heart Disease," *Amer. Heart J.,* **42**:406 (Sept.) 1951.

logical functioning as well as mental depression is the rule.

The recumbent position is associated with a low expenditure of energy, but many routine activities require more work when performed in bed. Moreover, when these activities are performed in bed, they are more likely to be accompanied by what is known as the Valsalva maneuver. To perform the Valsalva maneuver, the person takes a deep breath, closes his glottis, and expires forcibly against the closed glottis, using both the muscles of expiration and the abdominal muscles. This exercise markedly raises the intrathoracic pressure. From the description, the reader will recognize the similarity between the Valsalva maneuver and straining or bearing down at stool. In addition to requiring a considerable expenditure of energy, the Valsalva maneuver places an additional burden on the heart. During the period of forced expiration, pressure within the thoracic cavity is elevated,[39] and this interferes with blood entering the large veins. At the termination of the procedure, a large volume of blood rushes in and is delivered to the heart. In the already failing heart, cardiac arrest may be precipitated. To prevent the Valsalva maneuver, patients should be cautioned against holding their breath and straining. When they are active, they should make a conscious effort to breath normally.

To reduce the hazards of bed rest, many physicians modify it to some extent. Patients are generally kept in bed only as long as absolutely necessary. During the time the patient is confined to bed, the extremities should be put through the normal range of motion several times a day. Elastic bandages may be applied from the toes to the groin to support the veins and to prevent the pooling of blood in them. They should be applied with firm, even pressure so that they give support without obstructing the venous circulation. They should be removed and reapplied at least every 24 hours and when they become loose or are creating uneven pressure at any point. Active exercises, especially of the legs, should be encouraged. A footboard should be placed in position to support the patient's feet and extremities in good alignment. The patient should be encouraged to press his feet against the board. This exercise is of value in preventing loss of muscle tone and in promoting the circulation in the lower extremities.

Because less energy is required to use a commode or bathroom stool than a bedpan, most physicians prefer to have the patient assisted out of bed for defecation. When the patient goes to the bathroom, he should be taken in a wheelchair until such time as he is up and walking.

Despite studies demonstrating the superiority of chair rest to bed rest, the practice is not widespread. It minimizes most of the adverse effects of bed rest including the common post-myocardial infarction depression. Perhaps chair rest would be prescribed more frequently if physicians were sure everyone—nurses, patients, family, and friends—understood and acted on the knowledge that these patients are seriously ill. Chair rest does not mean they are not ill. They require all the care needed by any sick patient. The chair should be comfortable and provide adequate support for the back, head, and extremities. Ideally it should allow for changes in position.

In some hospitals so-called cardiac beds are available. They are designed in such a manner that a bed can be converted to a chair. The head of the bed becomes the back of the chair, the center the seat, and the foot is dropped down so that the lower legs and feet hang over the edge. Unless care is taken to adjust the bed properly, the seat may slant downward, causing the patient to slip forward. An adjustable footboard is also required to provide a firm surface for the support of the feet. Pillows and an overbed table are required to support the arms. Because the depth of the seat may be too great for the patient, supports at the back may be required to keep the patient in a comfortable position.

In the immediately preceding paragraphs, discussion has been centered on the values and limitations of rest in the therapy of the patient with an impairment of cardiac function. As indicated, activity is also important to recovery. Although the physician prescribes the degree of activity, the nurse will be better able to interpret the prescription to the patient if she understands the reason for it. One of the factors regulating metabolism in cells is the physical stress placed on them. Physical inactivity is accompanied by wastage of cellular substance and loss of strength.

In popular as well as professional literature, Dr. Paul Dudley White is frequently quoted as stating that physical exercise is important not only to the healthy heart but to the diseased one as well. The critical aspect in the patient with a diseased heart is to avoid those activities placing an excessive strain on the heart. The most dangerous are those characterized by a sudden and great increase in work, as increased muscular activity is followed by a marked increase in volume of the venous return. For example, the patient should avoid running for a bus or assisting with pushing a car out of the mud or snow. Extremes of heat and cold should also be avoided as they place an extra burden on the

[39] "Bed Rest and Chair Rest in Cardiovascular Disease," *Heart Bull.*, 3:99 (Sept.–Oct.) 1954.

heart. As patients are recovering from congestive heart failure or a myocardial infarction, they should be taught not only what they should not do but even more important what they will be able to do. As the value of activity to the health of the heart is coming to be appreciated, more emphasis is being placed on what the patient can do rather than what he cannot do.

When a person with heart disease is obese, weight reduction is usually advised. The importance of loss of weight can be interpreted in graphic terms. A person who is 50 lb overweight is carrying the equivalent of a 50-lb sack of flour around with him all the time. Moreover, his already impaired heart must move blood through the adipose tissue. One figure cited is that each pound of fat contains seven tenths of a mile of capillaries. In 50 lb, there are, therefore, 35 miles of capillaries.

Therapeutic Classifications

Because the degree to which the functional capacity of the heart is impaired varies among individuals, various systems of classification have been developed. The one cited below was developed by *The Criteria Committee of the New York Heart Association*, fifth edition. The classifications listed below are therapeutic classes. Functional classes (I-I) have been defined. They reflect the patient's ability; therapeutic classes are an indication of what he should do.

Class A. Patients with cardiac disease whose physical activity need not be restricted.

Class B. Patients with cardiac disease whose ordinary physical activity need not be restricted but who should be advised against severe or competitive physical sports.

Class C. Patients with cardiac disease whose ordinary physical activity should be moderately restricted and whose strenuous efforts should be discontinued.

Class D. Patients with cardiac disease whose ordinary physical activity should be markedly restricted.

Class E. Patients with cardiac disease who should be at complete rest, confined to bed or chair.

Rehabilitation

Over the last 15 or 20 years, studies, such as the one performed in the work classification unit at Bellevue Hospital, have demonstrated that many patients with heart disease can continue to be productive.[40] Studies have also been made of the energy requirements for various activities.[41] Whether or not a person who has recovered from acute cardiovascular disease will be able to perform a particular job depends on many factors other than the amount of energy it requires. These include his work experience, emotional status, temperament, and dexterity. Some patients do not require any change in work. Sometimes the patient can continue in the same job, but he needs to alter the way in which he approaches his work or the manner in which it is performed.

An example of the latter is the housewife who suffers from heart disease. Considerable work has been done in recent years by the American Heart Association to help the housewife with heart disease evaluate her methods of housekeeping and to plan her house and work so that unnecessary work is eliminated and the work she does is performed as easily as possible. In some communities, classes sponsored by the local heart association are taught for housewives. They and their husbands can learn how to evaluate and improve housekeeping methods.

Rehabilitation services are available to patients with heart disease through the Office of Vocational Rehabilitation or the American Heart Association. The first can usually be contacted through the state health department and the latter through the local heart association. At least as important as the rehabilitation of adults is that of children with heart disease. Career planning considering the limitations of the child is important. Emphasis on what the child may do is an essential aspect of helping him realize a productive life.

Exactly what each person who has heart disease will be able to do is related to him as an individual. The consensus at the present time is that many patients can do something worthwhile. Perhaps the greatest deterrent is fear and misinformation about the effects of exercise on the heart. The first step with each patient is to help him to develop a healthy and optimistic attitude. Most people in the American society want to be productive and want an opportunity to do something constructive. One of the standards by which they judge their productiveness is that they are economically self-supporting. The stress arising from continued inactivity and dependency may be as great as or greater than that involved in useful work.

Families also need help in interpreting both the patient's limitations and his strengths. Nurses can often reinforce the recommendations of the physician and assist the patient and his family members to make reasonably realistic plans. This is as important when the family tends to overprotect the patient as when they

[40] "Cardiac Work Classification Unit," *Heart Bull.*, 2:99–100 (Sept.–Oct.) 1953.

[41] Edward E. Gordon: "Rehabilitation of the Cardiac Patient," *Heart Bull.*, 7:108–10 (Nov.–Dec.) 1958.

push him too hard. It is difficult to remember when the life of a loved one appears to be threatened "that there is a breadth to life as well as a length. There is no area in a straight line."

The patient in congestive heart failure is subject to certain hazards, some of which can be prevented, minimized, or at least delayed. Eventually, most patients who have experienced heart failure no longer respond to therapeutic measures; congestive failure becomes intractable and the patient dies. Death may be caused by the failure of the heart as a pump or by a complication arising from the effects of heart disease and/or its treatment. For example, pulmonary infarction is not an infrequent complication in both acute and chronic heart disease. The source of the embolus is usually a thrombus in the veins of the legs. As stated earlier, passive and active leg exercises, regularly performed, supporting bandages, and footboards are preventive measures.

The heart may also be the source of emboli, particularly when the congestive heart failure is secondary to a myocardial infarction or mitral stenosis with atrial fibrillation. Thrombi in the left heart may form emboli that occlude cerebral or renal arteries or arteries supplying the lower extremities. Signs and symptoms depend on the structures deprived of their blood supply.

Summary

In the preceding pages some of the causes, effects, and types of failure of the heart as a pump have been reviewed. Congestive heart failure is a common medical problem. It can result from any disorder that places an abnormal burden on the heart, lessens its nutrition, or interferes with the metabolic machinery of the myocardium. When the pumping mechanism of the heart is unable to adapt its output to the needs of the tissues, all tissues suffer. In the beginning the patient experiences symptoms when he performs activities that he was formerly able to do easily. Eventually the manifestations of disturbed cerebral, respiratory, renal, gastrointestinal, and liver function as well as disturbances of other structures become evident. One of the important objectives of therapy is to reduce the load placed on the pumping mechanism of the heart until the myocardium recovers some degree of cardiac reserve.

CARDIAC ARRHYTHMIAS

Heart muscle is similar to other muscle in that it is irritable or excitable; it is capable of responding to stimuli. It differs from skeletal muscle inasmuch as its refractory period (the period of recovery following contraction when it will not respond to stimuli) is relatively long. The prolonged refractory period protects the heart muscle from remaining in a continuous state of contraction and thereby interrupting the circulation.

REGULATION OF CARDIAC FUNCTION

One of the most important characteristics of heart muscle is its capacity to contract independently from the nervous system. Unlike the muscles of respiration and other skeletal muscles, the heart continues to contract even when it is removed from the body. The mammalian heart does not continue to function for more than 30 minutes unless provisions are made to supply it with oxygen. When oxygen is supplied, the heart can be kept contracting for several hours. In vitro studies (made in a test tube) using mammalian myocardial cells show that they contract in the tissue culture fluid. Amphibian hearts beat for 24 or more hours provided they are perfused with frog Ringer's solution. In the past the property of automaticity, that is, the capacity to initiate their own contraction, was thought to be the property of all myocardial cells. Recent studies made by Harary [42] indicate that there are two types of heart cells. One type, which he calls leading cells, beats spontaneously. The other type, or following cells, beats only on contact with a leading cell.

The property of automaticity and rhythmicity facilitates survival when there is a failure of conduction of impulses from regulatory centers to the muscle of the ventricle. Normally the lead cells scattered throughout the myocardium follow the lead of higher regulatory centers. When for some reason one or more groups of cells become abnormally irritable, they may initiate ectopic beats and create abnormalities of rhythm. Whether or not these are of a minor or serious import depends on the cause and the effect they have on the heart rate. When the connection between the higher and lower lead cells is disrupted, the latter may take over and maintain the heart beat. The resulting rate is slower than the normal rate.

Before presenting disorders in the rate and rhythm of the heart, however, the system for the regulation of the heart will be discussed. The function of the heart is regulated in relation to the activity of the body as a whole. Circulatory and respiratory functioning are also synchronized. The various components of the circulatory system are regulated in relation to each other. Heart rate and blood pressure are adjusted in relation to each other. The coordination of heart rate and blood pressure is

---

[42] *Op. cit.,* p. 148.

stated in Marey's law: As the heart rate rises, reflexes are initiated to decrease the blood pressure. As the blood pressure rises, the heart rate slows. When either the pulse rate or the blood pressure rises, the other falls. Integration of the activity of the heart with the activity of the body as a whole is under the control of the autonomic nervous system. Stimulation of the sympathoadrenal system increases the rate of the heart and also dilates the coronary arteries. Stimulation of the vagus nerve slows the heart. The heart is also responsive to the hormonal and chemical conditions in the body.

Within the heart itself are specialized cells that have as their function the conduction of impulses over the entire heart. (See Figures 10-6 and 10-7.) Because atria and ventricles are separated by fibrous connective tissue, impulses do not spread directly from one to another as

they do in smaller animals such as the frog. In the healthy heart the contraction is initiated in the sinoatrial node. In Figure 10-6 it can be seen to lie just under the superior vena cava. From the sinoatrial node the impulse spreads over the atria and the atrioventricular node. As the impulse passes over the atria, contraction begins. After a slight delay, the impulse passes from the atrioventricular node over the bundle of His and the branching Purkinje system to the muscle fibers of the ventricles. Although all the cells in the conducting system including the lead cells in the myocardium are capable of initiating myocardial contraction, in health they do not. The gradient or irritability of cells of the regulating system diminishes from the sinoatrial node downward. To be more specific, in health the cells of the sinoatrial node initiate from 70 80 impulses per minute, whereas the lead cells

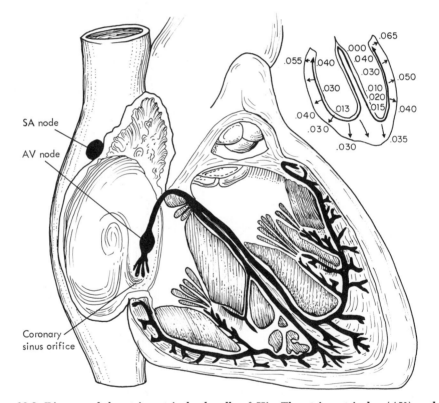

FIGURE 10-6. Diagram of the atrioventricular bundle of His. The atrioventricular (AV) node can be seen near the opening of the coronary sinus in the right atrium. At the upper end of the ventricular septum the bundle divides. The two branches run down in the ventricular septum and give off many smaller branches to the papillary muscles and to the muscular walls of the ventricles. Bundle indicated in black part of the sinoatrial node between the base of the superior vena cava and the right atrial appendix. The tip of the left ventricular chamber is not shown. The figures in the small inset indicate the time in seconds taken for the nerve impulses to reach the areas indicated. (Information adapted with permission of The Macmillan Company from *Anatomy and Physiology*, 15th ed., Fig. 15-3, p. 446, by Diana Clifford Kimber, Carolyn E. Gray, Caroline E. Stackpole, and Lutie C. Leavell. Copyright © The Macmillan Company, 1966.)

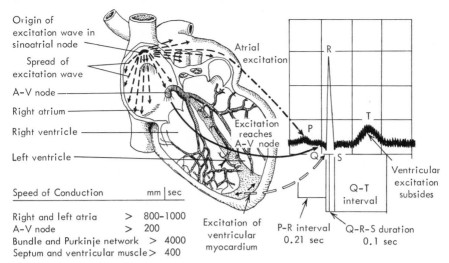

Speed of Conduction	mm	sec
Right and left atria	>	800–1000
A–V node	>	200
Bundle and Purkinje network	>	4000
Septum and ventricular muscle	>	400

FIGURE 10-7. Diagram showing the conduction system of the heart. Impulses are initiated at the SA node. As the wave of excitation travels through the conduction system, its relation to a tracing of a normal electrocardiogram is shown. (Information adapted with permission of The Macmillan Company from *Textbook of Physiology*, Fig. 73, p. 187, by Caroline E. Stackpole and Lutie C. Leavell. Copyright © The Macmillan Company, 1953.)

in the ventricles initiate about 35 impulses per minute. Because the higher leading cells initiate impulses more rapidly than those in the myocardium and the refractory period of the myocardium is relatively long, the impulses arising from the sinoatrial node control rate and rhythm.

HEART BLOCK

As a result of disease, the passage of impulses over the conduction system may be impeded or completely blocked or obstructed. The most frequent causes of complete heart block are coronary atherosclerosis and carditis (inflammation of the heart) associated with rheumatic fever and diphtheria. Digitalis poisoning may also be responsible. Hyperkalemia (excessive level of potassium in the blood) may precipitate heart block. When complete heart block is associated with hyperkalemia, myocardial irritability is decreased, the rate is usually slow, the duration of systole is prolonged, and the heart is in imminent danger of stopping in diastole.

Heart block may be induced by powerful stimulation of the vagus nerve. The parasympathetic nervous system, by way of the vagi, provides few fibers to the ventricles. It sends most of its fibers to the atria. The effect of stimulation of the vagi is to slow the heart by decreasing the rhythm of the sinoatrial node and by decreasing the excitability of the fibers lying between the atria and the Purkinje system. Powerful stimulation of the vagi may depress the sinoatrial node or the transmission of impulses

over the Purkinje system so powerfully that the ventricles stop contracting for from 4 to 10 seconds. Then the ventricles take over at their inherent rate of from 10 to 35 beats per minute. This action is known as vagal escape. The preceding and other disorders cause heart block by one of the following mechanisms:

1. Permanent structural damage or transitory inflammation of the conducting system
2. The toxic effect of chemicals such as digitalis or hyperkalemia
3. Deprivation of the tissues of nutrition, including oxygen
4. Intense stimulation of the vagus nerve [43]

The effect of heart block on the pulse and cardiac output varies with the location of the offending lesion and whether the block is complete or partial. For example, the report of an electrocardiogram made on Mr. Thompson states he has a left bundle branch block. This means there is an obstruction to the flow of impulses over the left bundle of His. (See Figure 10-6.) The blocking was caused by a myocardial infarction. The underlying disorder is coronary atherosclerosis and is not uncommon among the elderly. Because only one branch of the bundle of His is interrupted and the muscle fibers are in continuous sheets around the heart, the major way bundle branch block can be de-

[43] Calvin F. Kay: "Clinical Principles," *Cecil-Loeb, Textbook of Medicine,* 12th ed., Paul B. Beeson and Walsh McDermott, eds. (Philadelphia: W. B. Saunders Company, 1967), p. 682.

tected is by electrocardiogram. Left bundle branch block can, however, be detected by auscultation. (There is a paradoxical splitting of the second heart sound.) There is no detectable alteration of the pulse rate or rhythm of the pulse.

In partial heart block, the effect on the pulse rate and rhythm depends on the rate at which impulses are initiated by the sinoatrial node (and other irritable sites) and the extent to which impulses reach the ventricles. For example, if every other impulse fails to reach the ventricles, then the atria will contract twice for every contraction of the ventricles. This is known as a two-to-one block. The pulse will be regular in rate and rhythm. In other instances, the atria may contract three times to every time the ventricles beat—a three-to-one block —the rhythm is regular inasmuch as the same pattern recurs. It is abnormal, as the length of time elapsing between the contractions following the blocked impulse or preceding the next regular contraction is greater than normal. The force of each contraction varies with the length of the interval between beats. The greater the interval, the more time the heart has to fill during diastole and the more forceful the contraction during systole. When the patient is aware of the forceful contraction, he may interpret this as the heart skipping a beat. He is not likely to be aware of the missed beats.

In instances of complete heart block in which the flow of impulses from the atrioventricular node through the conduction system is interrupted, the ventricles will beat at their own natural rate, approximately 35 beats per minute. It may, however, be as low as 15 or 20. Cardiac arrest can occur after complete heart block if the ventricles fail to establish their own spontaneous rhythm promptly. The patient's life can be saved if effective closed chest massage is performed and the patient's heart is paced with a pacemaker. Each nurse has the responsibility to apprise herself of the laws and policies governing the practice of the nurse performing closed chest massage within her state and institution. References on external cardiac massage are in the References.

For patients who are unable to maintain a heart rate that is rapid enough to have an effective cardiac output, it may be necessary to insert an artificial pacemaker. There are two methods that can be used, either the transvenous (endocardial) or transpericardial (epicardial). For temporary pacing (days or weeks) the transvenous method is used. With this method a catheter electrode is threaded through a vein (jugular or brachial) into the vena cava to the right ventricle where it is wedged against the wall. The catheter is attached to an external pacemaker. The transvenous method may also be used for permanent pacing, in which case the catheter electrode is inserted through the jugular vein into the superior vena cava to the right ventricular wall. The electrode is attached to a generator, which is placed under the skin in a pocket in the chest wall. The second method, transpericardial, is used only for permanent pacing. The electrodes are applied to the epicardium of the apex of the left ventricle with the wires threaded through a tunnel to a pocket in the abdominal or chest wall where the pacemaker generator is placed. The disadvantage to this method is that it is necessary to perform a thoracotomy.

The most common types of pacing used are *set rate, asynchronous,* and *demand* or *standby.* The set rate units stimulate the ventricles at a constant preset rate regardless of the physiological needs of the patient or the cardiac rhythm. With a demand pacemaker the ventricular R wave is detected and the pacemaker fires only when a preset time interval has elapsed without the R wave (ventricular contraction) occurring.

Some of the more common complications associated with pacemakers are infections, thrombosis, arrhythmias, phlebitis, power failure, wire breakage, and electrode problems. Patients must be taught to count their pulse for a full minute at least daily as changes in the rate may be the first sign of malfunction of the pacemaker. An artificial pacemaker may relieve the patient's symptoms; however, the underlying pathology will still be present.

Some patients with complete heart block will be asymptomatic and will lead active lives. Others, particularly those with excessively slow rates, will be symptomatic. They experience dizziness and dyspnea on exertion and have attacks of syncope (fainting). Until the heart rate becomes established at a sufficiently rapid rate, they may also have convulsive seizures. The point should be emphasized, however, that complete heart block by itself may be completely asymptomatic and require no treatment (e.g., congenital or postdiphtheritic chronic heart block) and the patient may lead a normal, active life. Symptoms occur and treatment is indicated when (1) the rhythm is irregular (asystole or runs or irregular rhythm) or (2) the rate is excessively slow.

When the patient continues to have frequent attacks of syncope, drugs increasing the irritability of the heart muscle may be injected subcutaneously. One such drug is epinephrine, 0.5 to 1 ml of epinephrine, 1:1,000 solution. Because its effects last only one to two hours, its action can be prolonged by giving it in oil. Other drugs that may be useful in the treatment of the patient with chronic heart block include ephedrine sulfate, 20 to 30 mg three times daily. It has the advantage of oral administration. Isoproteronal glossets given sublingually are also effective as they increase the cardiac output, the force of contraction, the cardiac rate, and the coronary blood flow. In general, sympathomimetic agents are useful. Atropine is useful in some patients as it lessens the effect of the vagus nerve by depressing the effector substance responding to vagal stimulation. The nurse has the obvious responsibility of making certain that the patient gets his medications regularly, that his questions about them are answered by herself or his physician, and that he and his family understand why they should be continued—if they are to be—after his discharge from the hospital.

As with all patients, the nurse has a responsibility for the safety of the patient. Until heart block is stabilized, he is subject to syncope. To help lessen its likelihood, he should be taught to avoid sudden and rapid movement and straining. Changes in position, especially from the prone to upright, should be made slowly. Both to reassure the patient and to protect him from injury, the nurse should plan to have someone present when he gets out of bed.

Because any disorder in which the heart is involved carries with it the implication of the possibility of sudden death, most patients will also experience feelings of being unsafe. Attention should therefore be directed toward trying to increase the patient's feeling that, inasmuch as is possible, his needs will be met.

In addition to heart block, what are other disturbances in the rate and rhythm of the heart?

In addition to the obstruction of impulses over the conduction system, other disturbances in the rhythm of the heart may arise because of hyperirritability of leading cells some place in the heart. According to Harary,[44] the cells that control and regulate the contraction of the myocardium are those that are initiating impulses at the most rapid rate. When cells other than those in the sinoatrial node become hyperirritable, they regulate the rate and rhythm of the heart. Theoretically, any group of cells can, therefore, regulate the beating of the heart. The site at which impulses originate can be identified by an electrocardiogram.

TACHYCARDIA

The most frequent change in the rate of the heart is an increase, or tachycardia (any rate over 100). Although an irritable focus in any part of the heart may be responsible for an acceleration in rate, the usual site is the sinoatrial node. When an increase in rate is initiated by the sinoatrial node, the condition is called sinus tachycardia. An acceleration of the heart rate is a normal response to any condition in which the metabolic needs of cells are increased or in which there is some defect in the processes involved in supplying cells with needed substances. Conversely, the pulse rate tends to fall when the condition initiating the rise is relieved. Like other homeostatic responses, a rise in the pulse rate is physiological as long as it is initiated by an appropriate stimulus, is maintained within limits, and continues only as long as needed. The pulse rate can be expected to rise during exercise, with the ingestion of food, and as a result of excitement, fear, or anxiety. Tachycardia usually accompanies diseases in which there is fever or a rise in the metabolic rate, such as hyperthyroidism. In patients who have been ill for some time, particularly when they have been on bed rest, tachycardia associated with exercise may be excessive and the pulse rate slow to return to resting levels. Nurses should, therefore, check the pulse rate of patients whose activity is being increased. Should tachycardia occur or be sustained, the activity of the patient should be decreased and then increased more slowly.

As stated, the heart rate may be accelerated by fear and anxiety. Conversely, an increase in the heart rate may also be responsible for anxiety, particularly when the patient is conscious of the increase in rate and when it is accompanied by pounding. For example, Mrs. Almond is a tense woman who suffers from periodic attacks of tachycardia accompanied by palpitation and a "smothery" feeling. As far as she knows there is no relationship betwen the onset of an attack and any particular activity. Despite repeated reassurance on the part of her physician that she has a healthy heart, she continues to have what she calls "spells." During an attack she responds well to kindly and firm reassurance that she is not having a heart attack and to recognition of her obvious discomfort. Mrs. Almond's heart is believed to be responding to an impulse originating in her mental apparatus and affecting her heart by way of the accelerator nerves of the sympathetic nervous system. Her physician explains Mrs. Almond's symptoms to her by saying her nervous system is playing tricks on her. It is behaving as if she were in danger despite the lack of any obvious danger in her external environment. Because Mrs. Almond's attacks are infrequent and are of short duration, she is treated by supportive reassurance. In patients who are incapacitated, psychotherapy may be advised.

Although there are a number of disturbances

[44] *Op. cit.,* p. 150.

in the rhythm of the heart, only three types are of common occurrence. These are sinus arrhythmia, premature beat, and atrial fibrillation. Sinus arrhythmia occurs in most healthy children and adolescents. During inspiration the pulse rate speeds up; during expiration it slows down. In a healthy young person, these changes in the rhythm of the pulse are of no significance. Knowledge of this fact should be useful to nurses working in schools. When a child's pulse speeds up as he inhales and slows during exhalation, there is no cause for concern.

Premature beats are also a common phenomenon. They may arise from an irritable focus in the atria, in junctional tissues, or in the ventricles. Though they are more common in persons who have structural disease of the heart, they are not infrequent in healthy persons. Why they occur in the healthy heart frequently cannot be determined. Sometimes they can be shown to be related to such factors as emotional stress, or the excessive use of coffee, tea, or tobacco. Some individuals have attacks of premature beats during minor infections, such as the common cold.

As indicated by its name, a premature beat is one that occurs before the next contraction is due. It is ordinarily followed by an abnormally long interval. The normal contraction does not occur because the heart is in the refractory period at the time the normal impulse is initiated. The contraction following the premature beat is stronger than those occurring at normal intervals. The patient may be conscious of the disturbance in rhythm.

PREMATURE BEATS

Sometimes the premature beats come in groups. Coupled beats or a premature beat occurring with each regular beat is known as a bigeminal rhythm. In this situation the rhythm would be irregular. Ventricular bigeminy, a premature ventricular contraction occurring with each normal ventricular beat, is a classic sign of digitalis toxicity.

The treatment of premature contractions depends on their cause. When they occur infrequently and there is no evidence of organic heart disease, no treatment is usually necessary. When the physician believes excessive use of coffee, tea, or tobacco may be a contributing factor, their influence can be tested by eliminating them temporarily. In tense and anxious patients premature beats can sometimes be abolished by a mild sedative or tranquilizer. For patients with organic heart disease it may be necessary to treat with antiarrhythmic drugs. When they occur in patients receiving digitalis, the digitalis should be discontinued for a few days. According to Eddleman, Resnik, and Har-

rison,[45] a meal high in carbohydrate may precipitate premature beats in patients receiving digitalis. This is apparently related to a low level of potassium in the blood. When this is true, the premature beats disappear when the patient is given potassium replacement daily in divided doses. When patients being treated with digitalis develop irregularities in pulse, they should be recorded and reported to the patient's physician before another dose is administered. As stated previously, the carbohydrate content of the diet should also be reviewed. Particularly around holidays such as Thanksgiving and Christmas, patients should be cautioned to avoid eating a large quantity of sweets.

To recapitulate, premature beats are contractions of the heart arising from an abnormal focus in the heart that initiates a contraction before a normal one is due. The condition, though more frequently associated with structural changes in the heart, also occurs in persons who have no evidence of heart disease. The effects on the individual depend on the frequency with which premature beats occur and the extent to which they interfere with his capacity to function. In persons with organic heart disease, an increase in the heart rate because of premature beats may lead to a decrease in cardiac efficiency and predispose to failure. The needs of the patient will depend on the causative factors as well as his cardiac status.

ATRIAL FIBRILLATION

A common cardiac arrhythmia to require therapy is atrial fibrillation. In this condition the muscle fibers of the atria contract independently of each other with the result that the surface of the atria appears to quiver. Authorities do not agree as to what causes fibrillation. An old theory states that fibrillation is caused by the circular movement of contraction over the muscle of the atria. An impulse starts at one point and continues in a circular fashion over the same tissue. A newer theory gaining acceptance is that atrial fibrillation, like other cardiac arrhythmias, arises from areas of abnormal irritability.

Whatever mechanism is responsible, atrial fibrillation has a number of adverse effects on cardiac function. Fibrillation of muscle renders it ineffective as a source of power. The most serious effect is that the conduction system is bombarded with impulses. They are both frequent and irregular. Not all these impulses result in myocardial contraction. Many of them

---

[45] E. E. Eddleman, Jr., William H. Resnik, and T. R. Harrison: "Disorders of Rate, Rhythm, and Conduction," *Principles of Internal Medicine,* 5th ed., T. R. Harrison *et al.,* eds. (New York: The Blakiston Division, McGraw-Hill Book Company, Inc., 1966), p. 771.

fail to stimulate contraction because the conducting system or the myocardium is in the absolute refractory period at the time of their arrival. Even so, the myocardium does respond to many of them with the result that the pulse is rapid and totally irregular. Both the strength of contraction and distance between beats vary from one beat to another. There is no predictable pattern of rhythm.

When the interval between beats is very short, ventricular contraction may be too feeble to force open the aortic semilunar valves and drive blood into the arteries. The energy expended in each ineffective contraction is wasted. This places an additional burden on the heart. One measure of the extent to which ventricular contractions are ineffective is the pulse deficit. The pulse deficit is most accurately determined by the simultaneous counting of the ventricular and pulse rates. One person counts the ventricular rate using a stethoscope. Another counts the pulse at the wrist. When two people are not available, it can be approximated by counting first one and then another. Because of the highly irregular pulse, the pulse and the apical rate should be counted for at least a minute. The determination of the pulse deficit is often delegated to the nurse. The results are used to evaluate the extent to which the heart is wasteful of its energy and, perhaps most significantly, to evaluate the effectiveness of treatment.

When atrial fibrillation continues over a period of time, congestive heart failure is likely to be precipitated. Treatment is therefore usually instituted to restore the normal rhythm or to lessen the effect of the abnormal one. Despite the seeming appropriateness of directing therapy toward correcting the fibrillation, this is not always possible or even desirable. Sluggish flow of blood in fibrillating atria predisposes to mural thrombosis, which may be dislodged if effective contraction is restored. When atrial fibrillation is newly established, the likelihood of mural thrombosis is minimal. Quinidine may be prescribed because it lengthens the effective refractory period of cardiac muscle. It is not used when the patient is in congestive heart failure, because it decreases the force of cardiac contraction.

When quinidine is prescribed for a patient, the directions left by the physician should be followed explicitly. It is a potentially dangerous drug,[46] because a considerable number of individuals are hypersensitive to it. Because it is an alkaloid of cinchona, it may also cause symptoms of cinchonism, or quinine poisoning. Because of the possibility of a dangerous hyper-

sensitivity, the patient is given a test dose to determine his reactions to quinidine sulfate. He should be observed for tinnitus, vertigo, disturbances in vision, headache, confusion, skin rashes, nausea and vomiting, diarrhea, and abdominal cramps. The more severe manifestations of hypersensitivity are similar to those described earlier under acute anaphylactic reactions (see Chapter 6). Attacks of fainting as a result of ventricular standstill may also occur in patients taking quinidine. Any patient being treated with quinidine should, therefore, be subject to careful and regular observation. Should any manifestation of hypersensitivity or toxicity be evidenced or an adverse change in the rhythm of the heart appear, the drug should be discontinued and the physician notified. The use of quinidine sulfate is not limited to the treatment of atrial fibrillation. It may be prescribed for patients with other disorders, in which there is hyperriritability of the heart muscle such as premature systole.

Cardioversion may be necessary to convert atrial fibrillation to a normal sinus rhythm when there has been failure to control the rate or when angina pectoris or congestive heart failure is present. In doing cardioversion alternating current is discharged across the chest wall over the area of the heart to terminate the arrhythmia. The machine is synchronized so that the electrical discharge occurs during the R wave, the ventricular contraction, and not during the T wave, the vulnerable period, as this could cause the heart to go into ventricular fibrillation rather than terminating an arrhythmia.

Digitalis is a common drug employed in the therapy of atrial fibrillation. It does not usually abolish the fibrillation, but it slows the heart and lessens the pulse deficit. Its action and use are discussed with congestive heart failure.

VENTRICULAR FIBRILLATION

One cardiac arrhythmia, ventricular fibrillation, is incompatible with life because the ventricles are incapable of maintaining the circulation. Unless action is taken immediately and is effective in restoring ventricular contraction, death follows within a few minutes. Some of the causes of ventricular fibrillation are myocardial infarction, electrocution, and chilling of the heart. Ventricular fibrillation is one of the hazards of hypothermia. At a certain point in the warming or cooling of the heart, approximately 29°C, the myocardium becomes hyperirritable and there is danger of fibrillation. Because of the possibility of ventricular fibrillation, patients must be continuously observed during hypothermia. These patients should have a cardiac monitor attached so that any signs of impending ventricular fibrillation such as pre-

---

[46] Louis S. Goodman and Alfred Gilman (eds.): *The Pharmacological Basis of Therapeutics*, 3rd ed. (New York: The Macmillan Company, 1965), p. 705.

mature ventricular contractions can be detected.

In addition to conditions previously mentioned, such as alterations in the level of potassium ions, a number of disorders predispose to alterations in the rate and rhythm of the heart. In hyperthyroidism, the heart rate is increased as is the irritability of the myocardium. Output is increased and, when hyperthyroidism continues over a period of time, predisposes to high-output failure of the heart. These patients are sensitive to epinephrine, and ventricular fibrillation can result from its use.

The heart muscle is also very sensitive to the physical and chemical conditions of extracellular fluids. As stated, myocardial function cannot be maintained for more than 30 minutes in the absence of oxygen. Sodium and calcium ions have marked effects on the action of the myocardium. See Chapter 9 for a discussion of the effects of the various electrolytes on function.

There are a number of other arrhythmias having their origin in hyperirritable foci in the lead cells of the heart. Because they are of less frequent occurrence, they are not discussed here. Essentially disturbances in conduction and in the function of pacemakers have one or more of the following effects. They alter the rate and/or rhythm of the heart. Serious disturbances in rate and rhythm of the heart may decrease the mechanical efficiency of the heart and lead eventually to a loss in cardiac reserve. When a patient has a mild type of arrhythmia, he may suffer needlessly unless he can be helped to understand there is no objective cause for concern.

DIAGNOSIS OF ARRHYTHMIA

A physician can often establish the nature and significance of an arrhythmia from a study of the patient and the character of his heart beat and pulse. When he wishes to have additional information, he has an electrocardiogram (ECG) performed. An electrocardiogram is a graphic record of the electrical activity of the heart. An electrocardiograph is a device that receives the electrical impulses as they vary during the cardiac cycle and transforms them into a graphic record.[47] This machine not only records changes in electrical activity, but it also makes the film so a given distance on it is equal to a known time interval. From the information obtained during an electrocardiogram it is possible to determine not only alterations in electrical activity but changes in the timing of each phase in the cardiac cycle.

[47] Albert A. Kattus, Jr., and E. Raymond Borun: "Electrocardiography," *The Physiological Basis of Medical Practice,* 8th ed. C. Best and N. Taylor, eds. (Baltimore: The Williams & Wilkins Company, 1966), p. 658.

Similar to other diagnostic devices, an electrocardiogram has uses and limitations. It is useful in detecting alterations in irritability or excitability of the various parts of the heart, interference with conduction of electrical impulses over the heart, and areas of injury to the heart muscle. In the absence of some change in electrical activity, the electrocardiogram can be expected to be normal. A patient may have a normal electrocardiogram in the presence of heart disease. A patient might develop a myocardial infarction two days after a normal electrocardiogram.

A physician who has special training usually reads or interprets electrocardiograms. Nurses are, however, often interested in knowing what the record means. The electrocardiogram is made up of three components or waves. These are the P wave, the QRS wave, and the T wave (see Figure 10-7). The QRS wave really consists of three waves, the Q wave, the R wave, and the S wave. The P wave is caused by the electrical activity as the wave of contraction passes over the atria. The QRS wave or complex is the result of the electrical changes that take place in the ventricle during contraction. Both the P wave and the QRS waves result from depolarization of cells. The T wave occurs during the period in which the ventricles relax and recover from contraction, and the electrical activity of the heart is repolarized. Factors such as the height, shape, and timing of each wave are considered in the interpretation of an electrocardiogram. For example, in atrial fibrillation, the P wave is usually absent and F waves or fibrillatory waves are present. As the result of toxicity from digitalis, the T wave becomes negative (inverted).

Although the nurse does not have the specialized knowledge required to interpret an electrocardiogram, she is frequently called on to prepare the patient who has not experienced the procedure before. The unknown is a common source of anxiety. In addition, any possibility of disease of the heart is anxiety-provoking in most people. Persons unfamiliar with electrocardiograms sometimes interpret the procedure as involving the passage of electrical currents from the machine to themselves rather than the reverse. When the patient is conscious and able to communicate, the nurse has a responsibility to find out what the patient knows and thinks he knows and to correct frightening misconceptions.

To do this the nurse must know that the electrical activity is generated by the heart and transmitted to the surface of the body by blood and other tissues. Electrodes are applied to the patient and connected to wires or leads attached to the positive and negative terminals of the electrocardiograph. Leads I, II, and III are bipolar leads that measure the difference in electrical potential between two points. Lead I is recorded by connecting the negative terminal of the electrocardiograph to the right wrist and the positive terminal to the left arm. Lead II is attached so the electrode on the left leg connects with the positive terminal and the right wrist is connected to the negative lead. Lead III is recorded with the left ankle attached to the positive terminal and the left wrist is attached to the negative terminal of the machine. The unipolar leads measure the actual potential from one point. These leads are measured on three extremities—the right arm, left arm, and left leg. In addition precordial leads may be taken. There are six precordial leads positioned on the anterior chest wall around the heart. Unipolar leads can be equated to viewing a picture from different directions. Because the electrodes must adhere tightly to the skin, they are applied with a kind of jelly. This may cause a smarting sensation, but it does not damage the skin. Because the jelly is irritating, the nurse must remember to wash the patient's skin at the termination of the procedure.

CORONARY CIRCULATION FAILURE

Another way in which the heart may break down or fail is in its ability to maintain its own nutrition and oxygenation. Although the quantity varies with activity, an average of about 225 ml of blood flows through the coronary arteries each minute. The blood is carried to the myocardium by the right and left coronary arteries. Despite some individual differences, the left coronary artery supplies mainly the left ventricle, and the right coronary artery supplies the right ventricle. There are relatively few connections between the main coronary arteries. There are, however, many among the smaller branches.

As in other organs in the body, blood flow depends on the level of the blood pressure and the patency of the arteries. Although obstruction is by far the most frequent cause of ischemia of the heart muscle, any disorder resulting in a pathologically low blood pressure will be followed by myocardial ischemia. One of the threats to life in the patient in peripheral circulatory failure or shock is myocardial ischemia. As discussed earlier, a second, though less common, cause of failure to maintain the blood under a sufficient head of pressure is incompetency of the aortic semilunar valves. Aortic insufficiency may be the result of injury to the valves as the result of rheumatic fever or syphilis. An aneurysm of the ascending aorta may also be responsible. At one time all aneurysms of the aorta were believed to be caused by syphilis. Arteriosclerosis may, however, also be responsible.

ATHEROSCLEROSIS

The most frequent cause of myocardial ischemia is disease of the coronary artery, caused by coronary atherosclerosis. The importance of coronary artery disease as a cause of morbidity and mortality is emphasized by Dawber and Kannel,[48] who state that it accounts for two thirds of all heart disease in the United States. According to Wright,[49] a million or more persons per year suffer myocardial infarctions. The exact number is not known because many cases are not recognized. Myocardial infarction is also the leading cause of death as well as a major cause of disability among those between the ages of 45 and 60 years of age. Some authorities now describe coronary heart disease as reaching near epidemic proportions.

Throughout the United States the estimated mortality for patients with acute myocardial infarctions admitted to a general hospital is between 30 and 35 per cent, whereas the total mortality in coronary care units is approximately 20 per cent.[50] In general, coronary care units are designed to admit patients who could potentially have a sudden cardiac arrest. The units are not intended to have the extremely ill patient with complications such as acute pulmonary edema or shock admitted to them. Perhaps one of the greatest problems is screening the patient admitted to these units.

Among the misconceptions about coronary atherosclerosis is that it is a new disease. It is not, as evidence of it has been identified in the arteries of Egyptian mummies. Neither is this disorder confined to human beings. It occurs in dogs and other animals as well.

What causes atherosclerosis?

The simplest answer is that the cause is not known. From what has been learned about it, atherosclerosis will probably be demonstrated to be caused by the interaction of diverse genetic and environmental factors when together their total effect is sufficient to produce the disease. At the present time a number of factors have been identified as being frequently associated with coronary atherosclerosis. For some of these it is not known whether they are coincidental,

[48] Thomas R. Dawber and William B. Kannel: "Susceptibility to Coronary Artery Disease," *Mod. Conc. Cardiovasc. Dis.,* **30:**671 (July) 1961.

[49] Irving S. Wright: "Summary, Prevention and Control of Heart Disease," *Amer. J. Public Health,* **50:** 31–34 (Mar.) 1960.

[50] Lawrence Meltzer and J. Roderick Kitchell: *The Current Status of Intensive Coronary Care* (New York: The Charles Press, 1966), p. 67.

causative, or dependent on other conditions within the individual. As with other chronic diseases, no single causative factor is likely to be identified as the sole necessary element. Some of these etiological agents may be controlled so that the onset of the disease is delayed. Currently a large amount of money, effort, and time is being spent in an effort to learn more about the causes and, hopefully, the prevention of coronary artery disease as well as the other effects attributable to atherosclerosis. Theories about etiological agents are being extensively and intensively explored. These studies range from those in which normally herbivorous animals such as the rabbit are fed diets high in fat to those in which the effect of the saturated and unsaturated fatty acids on blood fats in man is determined. Not only are individuals studied, but entire populations are studied to determine the nature of their living habits. The value of comparisons between two groups of people depends on accurate knowledge and evaluation of the ways in which the population of the two groups are alike and different. The fact that the incidence of atherosclerosis is low in one group and high in another may be easy to establish. The significance of any one factor in its development is much more difficult to estimate.

When discussing the many factors contributing to the development of atherosclerosis, scientists sometimes say, somewhat facetiously, that the best protection against atherosclerosis is to have parents and grandparents who were resistant to it and to be a female. Both heredity and the female sex hormones offer protection. A number of environmental factors are also believed to influence its occurrence. Knowledge of these is important because they are subject to modification or control. These include emotional stress, insufficient exercise, smoking, excess carbohydrates and fats in the diet, and protein deficiency. There is a body of epidemiological and experimental evidence to support the theory that a high intake of fat accelerates the development of atherosclerosis. Some authorities believe fats composed of saturated fatty acids are the most serious offenders. Some unsaturated fatty acids, at least for a period of time, have the effect of lowering blood lipid. In persons who have diseases such as diabetes mellitus, hypothyroidism, and essential hypertension, atherosclerosis develops at an earlier age than in those who are free of these conditions. From these findings the conclusion that atherosclerosis develops as the consequence of the interaction of a number of factors seems sound.

Because the incidence of atherosclerosis including that occurring in the coronary arteries tends to rise with age, some authorities have in the past related it to the aging process. Evidence against this theory is that the disorder occurs in all age groups. It has been observed in the arteries of newborn infants. Atheromatous plaques have been demonstrated in the coronary arteries of young men dying in battle or as the result of an accident. Some persons who die in their eighties and nineties do not have any evidence of it. According to a *Special Research Report* of the American Heart Association, however, by middle age most Americans have some degree of coronary atherosclerosis.

Problems in the prevention of atherosclerosis and its sequelae relate to a number of factors. Atherosclerotic changes may be present for a long period of time without causing any demonstrable effect. Despite the presence of pathology individuals are frequently free of signs and symptoms of coronary disease. They are believed to be healthy by themselves and by others. Presently no method is available to identify those who have coronary artery disease, but who are apparently healthy, until blood flow is sufficiently impeded to impair the nutrition to the myocardium. Coronary angiocardiography is one diagnostic test that can be used to evaluate the coronary circulation and its collaterals. The tip of a catheter is introduced into the ostium of the right and left coronary arteries. A small amount of contrast media is injected into the arteries, thus outlining the coronary circulation and collaterals. At this time, photographs are taken.

CORONARY ARTERY DISEASE

Not until the characteristic clinical manifestations of coronary artery atherosclerosis appear are affected individuals aware of it. Clinical evidence may occur in the twenties and thirties, though this is not common. After age 40 in men and approximately 45 in women, the incidence of overt coronary heart diseases rises. With the exception of women who are diabetic or hypertensive, coronary artery disease is unusual in women before the menopause. Following menopause women lose their protection.

Because the etiology of atherosclerosis is uncertain, prevention consists of controlling the factors that are associated with it. According to the current hypothesis, control of atherosclerosis is predicated on long-term change in food, exercise, smoking, working, and living habits. If one word were to be used to summarize all the above, it would be moderation. There is not at this time, and may possibly never be, any magic substance that will prevent the formation of atheroma in the coronary or other arteries of all people. There are, however, measures known to be effective in preventing some heart attacks.

Possibly, the prevention of heart attacks is even more important than their cure, because a sizable proportion die during their first attack.

The Framingham Heart Study,[51] a prospective study, showed that the risk of heart attacks was twice as great among persons who smoked over a package of cigarettes per day as compared to non-smokers. The number smoked per day, not the duration of the smoking habit, was the influencing factor in the development of coronary heart disease.

It has been demonstrated that a heavy smoker who stops smoking can decrease the risk of having a heart attack. The possibility of a heart attack is also lessened by weight reduction in the obese. The maintenance of a desirable weight by diet and exercise is necessary. Hypertension, which predisposes to both congestive heart failure and to atherosclerosis, can sometimes be controlled by drugs. Thus through the control of conditions contributing to the development of coronary artery disease, its incidence can be reduced.

Because the incidence of atherosclerosis is higher in populations in which the level of cholesterol in the blood is high than it is in populations where the average level is low, some authorities suggest that the total intake of lipids in the diet should be controlled. Dale[52] recommends that fats comprise no more than 25 to 30 per cent of the food intake. Because this quantity exceeds that ingested by some groups such as the Italians and Spanish, it is judged to be compatible with health.

There is some disagreement about the relative importance of the type of fat ingested to the development of atherosclerosis. Some authorities are of the opinion that more than half of the fat should be in the form of unsaturated fatty acids. Others are of the opinion that the most important consideration is the total consumption of fats. Because the liver synthesizes cholesterol, there will always be some cholesterol in the blood, whatever the intake of fat or cholesterol-containing substances. Although agents such as the estrogens have a cholesterol-lowering effect on the blood, and heparin lowers the total blood lipids, their use is limited to those who have a greater than average predisposition to atherosclerosis. Many men find estrogens unacceptable because of their feminizing effect. New chemicals are being developed with the hope that they will depress the level of lipids in the blood, without, at the same time, causing feminization.

To recapitulate, factors in the development of coronary heart disease are being studied intensively at the present time. Studies are also under way to try to develop tests whereby persons who are predisposed to the disease or who are in its early stages may be identified. These persons may then be advised to undertake a regime designed to prevent or delay the onset of coronary heart disease. Though an individual cannot alter his heredity or body build, he can control the amount and type of food that he eats, the amount of exercise that he takes, whether or not he smokes, and the way he approaches the problems in his life.

Not only is there uncertainty about etiology and prevention of atherosclerosis but not very much is known about the formation of atheromatous plaques. According to Mann,[53] three hypotheses are currently suggested to explain their development. He summarizes them as

1. Diet
   Stress
   High blood pressure $\Big\}$ Lipemia → Atherosclerosis → Clinical event
2. Thrombosis → Atherosclerosis → Clinical event
3. Ground substance damage → Atherosclerosis → Clinical event

He states that the first is by far the most popular. According to the second hypothesis, the first event is the formation of a thrombus on the wall of the artery. This is followed by the formation of the atheromatous plaque and eventually the clinical event. The third hypothesis postulates some injury in the wall of the artery. Although the focal nature of atherosclerosis supports this theory, there is little other evidence in its favor.

In keeping with the first hypothesis, the formation of atheromatous plaques progresses somewhat as follows. After an indefinite period of lipemia plaques form in the subintimal tissue of one or more arteries. These plaques, which are a yellowish color, are formed of cholesterol, other liqids, and macrophages. Authorities are not agreed as to how the cholesterol gets into the intima. One theory is that it enters the intima directly from the blood. The other is that it is formed in the intima itself. According to the infiltration theory,[54] fatty particles flow

---

[51] "The Framingham Heart Study," *Public Health Service Publication* No. 1515, U.S. Department of Health, Education, and Welfare (Washington D.C.: U.S. Government Printing Office, 1966).

[52] Sebron C. Dale: "Dietary Fat, Blood Cholesterol, and Atherogenesis," *Heart Bull.,* **10**:88 (Sept.–Oct) 1961.

[53] George V. Mann: "Current Trends in the Study of Atherosclerosis," *Heart Bull.,* **9**:22 (Mar.–Apr.) 1960.

[54] Harry Kruse, Chairman: "Committee on Cultural, Societal, Familial, Psychological, and Genetic Influences," *Amer. J. Public Health Suppl.,* **50**:97 (Oct.) 1960.

constantly to and from the tissues forming the walls of the blood vessels. For some reason the rate of outflow does not keep up with the rate of inflow. Fatty particles accumulate at the junction of the media and the intima of the coronary arteries. One hypothesis offered to explain the site at which lipids are deposited is that the structures are congenitally defective. In the beginning, the accumulated lipids resemble those of the blood. As time goes on their character changes, and the proportion of cholesterol to other substances changes. The lipids, especially cholesterol and fatty acids, act as irritants or foreign bodies. They cause degeneration of the wall of the artery. This is accompanied by low-grade inflammation, and eventually the area may undergo calcification. The entire process results in the formation of raised areas (plaques) in the lumen of the artery, which in small arteries may be sufficient to cause obstruction. A second source of obstruction is that a roughened area may serve as a focus for the formation of a thrombus that then obstructs the artery. Hemorrhage into the atheroma may also precipitate formation.

In addition to patchy changes in the walls of the blood vessels themselves, there is evidence that the factors contributing to their development also increase the coagulability of the blood and decrease fibrinolysis.[55] As a consequence of atherosclerosis, tissues may be partially or completely deprived of their blood supply. When the walls of arteries are weakened, aneurysms may form. In those vessels where thinning of the arterial wall is marked, the vessel may rupture and hemorrhage occur. Depending on whether or not the blood supply to the tissue is gradually or suddenly decreased, the resulting ischemia that follows may not be accompanied by necrosis of the tissue supplied by the diseased artery. When the ischemia comes about slowly, the tissue atrophies and is accompanied by a decrease in its ability to function. For example, as a consequence of atherosclerosis of the coronary arteries, the blood supply to the heart muscle may decrease. As a result of a gradually diminishing blood supply, the capacity of the heart to move as much blood into the circulation as the tissues require diminishes. Relative ischemia of the lower extremities renders them vulnerable to trauma or other injuries that would normally be of little or no consequence. Atrophy of the brain is accompanied by a variety of changes including alterations in personality. The consequences may be serious

when it occurs in individuals in responsible positions. The implications of ischemia were discussed previously in Chapter 4.

Sudden obstruction of an artery is accompanied by tissue necrosis, such as occurs in myocardial infarction. The specific manifestations presented by the patient will, of course, depend on the organ that is deprived of its blood supply and the extent of the collateral circulation in the region. The heart, the brain, and the lower extremities are the most commonly affected organs.

In atherosclerosis, the abdominal aorta is the common site for the formation of aneurysms (an outward bulging of the wall). They are often small and are of no significance. When they are large, they may serve as a site for the formation of a thrombus or of rupture. With the occlusion of the abdominal aorta, the supply of blood to the lower extremities is diminished or shut off. If the occlusion occurs at the level of the renal arteries, renal failure develops rapidly. When occlusion develops gradually, the patient, usually a man, complains of cramping pains in the calf of his leg or in his feet on walking, which is relieved with rest. Over a period of time, the distance that he is able to walk becomes shorter.

The majority of infarcts in the brain are caused by a thrombus that develops on an atherosclerotic plaque. However, arteries in the brain are thinner-walled than those in other parts of the body and are therefore susceptible to rupture when they become atherosclerotic. This is especially true when hypertension is also present. According to Hopps,[56] hemorrhage into the brain is more serious than thrombosis. Not only is a part of the brain deprived of its blood supply, but the blood escaping from the blood vessel damages the brain tissue. It also increases intracranial pressure directly or by increasing the osmotic particles in the area. The needs of patients experiencing these effects for nursing will be discussed in Chapter 15, Part B.

Although authorities do not agree as to how the changes that lead to the development of atherosclerosis come about, two factors seem to be of importance. One relates to the changes taking place in the walls of arteries and the other to the tendency of blood to form clots or thrombi within blood vessels. The arteries in which atherosclerosis develops early or produces a serious degree of dysfunction are known. Atherosclerosis is found most frequently in the vessels in which there is a large amount of elastic tissue in the media. These include the aorta and its major branches, the larger arteries

[55] William Dock: "Atherosclerosis and Other Forms of Arteriosclerosis," *Principles of Internal Medicine*, 5th ed., T. R. Harrison *et al.*, eds. (New York: The Blakiston Division, McGraw-Hill Book Company, Inc., 1966), p. 699.

[56] H. C. Hopps: *Principles of Pathology*, 2nd ed. (New York: Appleton-Century-Crofts, 1964) p. 136.

of the brain, and the coronary arteries. The changes developing in the proximal aorta occur relatively early in life and rarely cause any serious difficulty. The changes in the branches of the aorta, or in its distal portions, as well as those that occur in the arteries supplying the brain and heart, may have serious effects.

The preceding discussion applies equally well to atherosclerosis in any important artery in the body. Because the coronary arteries supply the heart muscle, atherosclerosis in these vessels creates problems related to the heart. Coronary artery disease carries with it the possibility of three complications: sudden death caused by cardiac arrest or ventricular fibrillation, myocardial infarction, and angina pectoris. Not by any means do all persons who have atheroma in their coronary arteries develop any of these. These conditions all result from the effects on the heart muscle of an inadequate supply of blood, that is, ischemia of the heart muscle. When there is death of myocardial cells and the person survives, healing by fibrosis occurs. Ischemia of myocardial cells followed by fibrosis probably occurs more frequently than is generally appreciated, as hearts examined at autopsy of persons who have not had heart attacks are found to have areas of scarring. In addition to the possible loss of myocardial cells, ischemia of some parts of the heart may set up abnormal electrical changes that may be responsible in part for some of its effects.

The major manifestation of ischemic heart disease is pain caused by a deficiency of oxygen to the myocardium. Blood supply may be impaired or it may be completely blocked so that no blood reaches the muscle. Either partial or total blocking of the coronary arteries may be the cause of sudden death. The clinical picture differs depending on whether or not the heart muscle is partially or permanently and completely deprived of its blood supply and the extent to which it is ischemic. The condition in which blood supply is deficient, but not entirely lacking, is known as angina pectoris. Because in angina pectoris the capacity of the coronary arteries to adapt the supply of oxygen to the needs of the myocardium under varying degrees of activity is deficient, signs and symptoms are precipitated by physical or emotional stress. In contrast, when the blood supply is blocked, signs and symptoms may or may not be precipitated by activity, but they are not relieved by rest. Though coronary atherosclerosis is the usual cause of these conditions, there are others. Furthermore, coronary atheroma may be present in the absence of either. Neither condition develops until the blood supply is sufficiently compromised to cause hypoxia of the heart muscle.

ANGINA PECTORIS

The term *angina pectoris* when translated literally means sore throat of the chest. Sprague [57] calls it the cry of the myocardium suffering from anoxia. Doyle [58] describes it as "A discomfort or pain, occurring across both sides of the anterior chest wall or located centrally in the sternal region, brought on by effort, e.g., exercise, emotion, exposure to cold and wind. It may radiate to the left arm or both arms, the shoulders, the neck or jaw." The words used by different patients to describe the pain vary, for example, tight, heavy, pressing, burning, crushing, and numbing. This pain is usually promptly relieved by rest or nitroglycerine. Because of the severity of the pain most patients try to avoid activities that precipitate it.

With progressive occlusion of the coronary arteries, the blood supply is further impaired and angina is precipitated with less and less activity, or myocardial infarction occurs. The results are not always unfavorable, however. In many individuals, despite marked impingement on the lumen of coronary arteries, the blood supply to the heart muscle may be protected by the development of the collateral blood vessels as well as the recanalization of obstructed ones.

The medical management of the patient who experiences angina pectoris is directed toward two objectives. One is to help the patient learn to regulate his life so that his heart is protected from periods of anoxia. The other is to improve the blood supply to the myocardium. The patient who is obese is encouraged to reduce his weight. Circumstances causing nervous tension or emotional stress should be identified and avoided when possible. Although many physicians advise patients who smoke to stop, and some refuse to treat them if they will not, others encourage them to smoke sparingly, if they must smoke. Studies indicate that the death rate from coronary artery disease is significantly higher among those who smoke than among those who do not.[59]

The most frequently prescribed drug in the treatment of angina pectoris is nitroglycerine. It is equally useful in the prevention of pain induced by exercise or emotion. One patient wrote a newspaper columnist physician to thank him for making this fact known to her. She commented that she found the use of nitroglycerine to prevent pain even more beneficial than

[57] Howard B. Sprague: "Coronary Heart Disease." *Heart Bull.,* **1**:74 (Sept.–Oct.) 1952.

[58] Joseph T. Doyle: "Committee on Criteria for Diagnosis of Disease and Clinical Evaluation." *Amer. J. Public Health Suppl.,* **50**:21 (Oct.) 1960.

[59] Howard B. Sprague: "What I Tell My Patients About Smoking," *Mod. Conc. Cardiovasc. Dis.,* **33**:882 (Oct.) 1964.

to provide relief. By relaxing the blood vessels, alcoholic beverages in small amounts are often helpful in the prevention of anginal attacks. Alcohol is particularly useful when taken at night to prevent nocturnal angina.[60]

The nurse can frequently be helpful to the patient in identifying those aspects of his life that require modification and in learning to follow the medical regime. The combination of a diagnosis of disease of the heart, the pain, and the knowledge that sudden death is a possibility is frightening to even the most stoic. Some patients fear taking any medication lest they become habituated to it. The modification of important aspects of life is not easy. Someone to talk to and to suggest possible alternatives may be helpful.

MYOCARDIAL INFARCTION

When blood flow is obstructed by coronary atherosclerosis so that no blood reaches the myocardium, myocardial infarction occurs. Mr. Anderson illustrates many of the characteristics of this disorder.

One morning shortly after 8 o'clock, Mr. Anderson, a 60-year-old, native-born American, was admitted to Community Hospital. After arriving at work, he had collapsed. He stated that he had severe crushing pain in his chest radiating to his left shoulder. He might have employed any of the terms used to describe the pain of angina to characterize his pain. The pain differs from that of angina, however, inasmuch as it is a steady pain and is not relieved by rest or nitroglycerine. It frequently develops when the patient is at rest or some time following a meal or an activity. Mr. Anderson located the pain by placing his hand over his sternum and then moving it over his upper chest. The location of his pain is identical with that observed in angina pectoris. It might have radiated to the right shoulder and down either arm. The ancients noted the frequency with which pain radiated from the region of the heart down the left arm to the ring finger. According to legend, they believed that the left ring finger was directly connected to the heart, and this belief is said to be the reason for placing the wedding ring on the left ring finger, thus securing constancy of affections.

As a male between the ages of 45 and 64, Mr. Anderson is in the age group in which the incidence of coronary arteriosclerotic heart disease is highest. With increasing age there is a progressive rise in the number of deaths from this disease entity.

In addition to being predisposed by age to

myocardial infarction, Mr. Anderson was also hypertensive. For a number of years his blood pressure had fluctuated betwen 150/90 and 200/100. He had taken medications to lower his blood pressure for the past two years. Two of his brothers died following myocardial infarction. Whether this was a coincidence or indicated a common genetic defect or the effect of a common environment is not known. Any of the preceding could be true. Certainly knowledge that his brothers had died after "heart attacks" could be expected to increase Mr. Anderson's anxiety during his illness.

Mr. Anderson was of average height, large-boned, and muscular. Though he was a big man he did not appear to be fat. His body type was that described by the term *mesomorph*. Some authorities claim that the incidence of coronary heart disease is highest among this group.

Mr. Anderson's food intake was similar to that of other Americans of modest income. His wife stated that despite a preference for meat, he ate some of most other foods. His preference in meat was for beef that was well marbled with fat. For the past two or three years, his salt intake had been restricted. He had smoked up to two packages of cigarettes a day until his high blood pressure had been discovered. For a time he stopped smoking entirely. Recently, he had been seen smoking occasionally.

At one time his work required quite a bit of physical exercise. For the past ten years he had a sedentary job. Mr. Anderson's supervisor described him as a good and careful worker who arrived at work on time and did a full day's work. Though he bowled occasionally in the wintertime, and mowed the lawn in the summer, he got very little physical exercise. Despite his intentions to exercise regularly, he seldom walked when he could ride. He was too tired or there was not time to walk.

From this superficial survey of the life of Mr. Anderson, many of the factors that appear to be associated with coronary heart disease are seen to be a part of his life. They include a possible genetic predisposition to the disease, body build, food and working habits, hypertension, lack of physical exercise, and smoking. These and other factors are presumed to have acted over time to lead to changes in his coronary arteries that were eventually manifested as a myocardial infarction.

Despite the fact that the onset appeared to be sudden, Mr. Anderson had had previous attacks of discomfort and mild pain in his chest. He had dismissed them by ascribing them to indigestion or to something that he had eaten. His reaction was by no means unusual. Neither is it unusual for patients to have attacks of pain

---

[60] Sprague, *Op. cit.*, p. 74.

before a myocardial infarction. According to Beamish and Storrie,[61] the reported incidence of warning symptoms is from 30 to 50 per cent. They also indicate that evidence is accumulating indicating that the incidence of sudden death and myocardial infarction can be prevented by the prompt administration of anticoagulant drugs. If this is true, it becomes important for men and women who have premonitory pain to report this pain to their physicians immediately. Characteristically, this warning pain occurs in a person who has been in good or relatively good health. He finds that he cannot walk very far before he has pain. He also has chest pain at night when he is at rest. If he takes nitroglycerine, the pain is relieved, but it takes increasingly larger doses to be effective. Nurses who are working in industry or elsewhere in the community are not infrequently consulted by patients or their families. When an apparently healthy man or woman recites the above history, he should be encouraged to see his physician promptly for diagnosis. Should a myocardial infarction be impending, there is a possibility that it can be prevented. Should future studies demonstrate that myocardial infarction can be prevented, then the role of the nurse as a case finder and in public education will become increasingly important.

To return to Mr. Anderson, immediately after he collapsed in severe pain, the plant physician was called and Mr. Anderson was moved in a wheelchair to the plant infirmary. The physician prescribed morphine sulfate, ¼ grain (15 mg), to be given subcutaneously. Practice varies as to which particular analgesic is prescribed and the route selected for administration. Prompt relief of pain is important, as pain intensifies shock, which is always present in some degree in clinical myocardial infarction. Many physicians prefer that the drug be administered intravenously as no time is lost during the absorption of the drug and the full dosage can be expected to be effective. As a consequence of peripheral circulatory failure in shock, absorption from subcutaneous tissues may be so poor that the patient gets little or no relief. Later, as the circulation improves, the drug is absorbed. When repeated, but poorly absorbed, dosages are given, the patient may suffer from toxic effects. Although morphine was administered subcutaneously to Mr. Anderson, he experienced relief from his pain.

Besides pain, which was the predominant symptom at the onset of Mr. Anderson's illness, he also felt weak. Beads of perspiration stood out on his brow and his skin was an ashen gray. He complained of feeling short of breath. Shortly after his admission to the infirmary, his blood pressure dropped to 110/70. Some drop in blood pressure is common. Though Mr. Anderson was nauseated, he did not vomit. Both nausea and vomiting are also frequent symptoms. After an electrocardiogram confirmed the plant physician's diagnosis that Mr. Anderson had suffered a myocardial infarction, preparations were made to transfer him by ambulance to Community Hospital. Some physicians advise against moving seriously ill patients or those who are in profound shock.[62] During the period that follows the onset of clinical manifestations of myocardial infarction the patient is in danger of ventricular fibrillation and shock. Neither the heart nor the peripheral circulation can be depended on to respond favorably to increased demands made by moving or being transported to another location. Even minor stimuli can and often do worsen the patient's condition. The patient should therefore be protected insofar as possible from all emotional and physical stimuli. Despite the seeming importance of getting the patient to the hospital where he can be treated, the transfer should be made without hurry or a feeling of great urgency. There should be no fast driving over rough roads with the siren screaming. The atmosphere surrounding the patient should insofar as possible be one of calm and gentleness. Many modern ambulances are now equipped with oxygen and other life-saving devices. These can be used as indicated. Attention should be directed to the patient and his responses.

To prepare Mr. Anderson for the move, the plant physician told Mr. Anderson that he should be transferred to Community Hospital where they had the facilities to care for him. Mr. Anderson asked that his wife be notified and that they try not to "scare her to death." Transfer was made promptly. Because the hospital had been called, emergency-room personnel were expecting Mr. Anderson. At the time of his arrival, he had some, but not marked, chest pain. He was sweating profusely and his skin was cold to touch. His skin was ashen gray in color. His blood pressure had fallen to 100/80. Before he was transferred to a hospital bed for care, an electrocardiogram was made. This showed that Mr. Anderson had had a posterior myocardial infarct.

As emphasized previously, myocardial infarction usually is associated with coronary atherosclerosis. The sequence of events leading

[61] R. E. Beamish and V. Marie Storrie: "Impending Myocardial Infarction," *Heart Bull.,* **10**:41 (May–June) 1961.

[62] Milton Plotz: "Treatment in Acute Myocardial Infarction," *Heart Bull.,* **7**:58 (May–June) 1958.

to the obstruction of the coronary arteries are discussed on pages 400–401. After a coronary artery is obstructed by a thrombus, cells in the myocardium die. Depending on the size and location of the occluded vessel, the area of necrosis may extend to, and include, the endocardium and pericardium. Another consequence of arterial obstruction is an uneven distribution of blood to the myocardium. According to Beck,[63] this disturbance in the distribution of blood results in electrical changes; the electrical changes are responsible for the heart attack.

After an acute insult such as a myocardial infarction, the heart may continue to contract, but its efficiency as a pump is diminished. Sometimes sympathetic reflexes, initiated automatically, compensate for much of the failure, with the result that signs and symptoms of heart failure are minimal. The sequence of events is usually as follows: As the output of the heart falls, the pressure of the blood in the aorta and carotid artery falls. Pressor receptors are stimulated with the result that the sympathetic nervous system is activated. This increases the force of myocardial contraction and constricts peripheral blood vessels.[64] Constriction of the peripheral blood vessels, most particularly the veins, in turn, improves venous return by diminishing the quantity of blood held in them.

When cardiac output is low, renal function may be diminished. The quantity of fluid excreted by the kidney becomes lessened and the blood volume becomes enlarged. This mechanism may, within limits, further compensate for the decrease in cardiac output. Again, within limits, an increase in blood delivered to the heart is followed by more forceful contraction. This is often true of the failing, as well as of the normal, heart.

When the myocardial infarction is large or the mechanisms for adapting the diameter of the blood vessels are defective, then cardiac shock develops. As stated earlier, at the onset of symptoms, Mr. Anderson presented evidence of shock, and by the time of his admission to Community Hospital, he was in profound shock. If Mr. Anderson was to survive, the competency of his circulation had to be restored as soon as possible. Otherwise, tissue hypoxia, including hypoxia of the myocardium, with progressive deterioration of cell function occurs. Restoration of the circulation to the tissues, therefore, has a high priority in the management of any patient who has recently experienced a myocardial infarction. The improvement of the circulation is essential to the recovery of the heart and to the prevention of injury to other tissues.

[63] Claude S. Beck: "Coronary Artery Disease," *Heart Bull.*, 7:22 (Mar.–Apr.) 1958.
[64] Guyton, *op. cit.*, p. 373.

Treatment of Myocardial Infarction

To protect Mr. Anderson's heart from any unnecessary demands, Mr. Anderson's physician prescribed strict bed rest for him for 48 hours. This meant that Mr. Anderson was to do nothing for himself. He was to be washed, turned, and fed. His food intake was limited to fruit juices. Intake of water, including the intravenous solution, was not to exceed 1,500 ml. The only voluntary activity that he was permitted was to turn on his light or to ask his nurse for assistance. Insofar as was possible, his external environment was to be regulated so he was protected from all psychological, social, and physical stimuli. Visitors were restricted to the members of his immediate family. They were encouraged to sit quietly in his room or to sit on the sun porch.

As frequently occurs following a serious myocardial infarction, Mr. Anderson had pulmonary edema and was dyspneic. The head of his bed was elevated, to lessen the dyspnea and therefore to promote rest. Morphine sulfate, 15 mg (¼ grain), was prescribed to relieve pain.

Despite the relief of his pain and despite bed rest, Mr. Anderson's blood pressure did not rise to a safe level. Therefore a vasopressor (blood pressure-raising) drug was prescribed. A variety of preparations are available. One of the most potent of these drugs is norepinephrine (Levarterenol or Levophed). It causes constriction of all blood vessels, except the coronaries, which it dilates.[65] It also increases the force of cardiac contraction and stroke volume, as well as cardiac irritability. It diminishes renal blood flow. It must be administered intravenously, as it causes a slough when it infiltrates the tissues. It is rapidly destroyed and must therefore be administered continuously. Because of the problems involved in keeping the needle patent and to lessen the possibility of tissue infiltration, an Intracath may be introduced into the vein or a cutdown may be performed. Because of the potency of norepinephrine, continuous observation is required.

There are a number of other preparations of vasopressor agents with similar, but not identical, effects. In general they are less potent than norepinephrine. Some of them have more sustained effects. Some do not injure the tissues with which they come in contact and can be administered by intramuscular or subcutaneous injection. Some do not increase the irritability of the heart muscle. Before supervising the administration of a vasopressor drug to any patient, the nurse should acquaint herself with the facts about the prescribed drug. The drug pre-

[65] Clarence M. Agress: "Heart Shock in Myocardial Infarction," *Heart Bull.*, 11:27 (Mar.–Apr.) 1962.

scribed by the physician will depend on the condition of the patient and the physician's experience with and preference for a particular preparation.

Metaraminol (Aramine), 200 mg per liter of 5 per cent glucose in water, was prescribed for Mr. Anderson. In nonhypertensive patients, the critical level for the systolic blood pressure is 100 mm of mercury. In the hypertensive patient, it is somewhat higher. Following the administration of metaraminal, Mr. Anderson's blood pressure rose as expected.

Any patient who is receiving a potent vasopressor agent should be continuously attended by a competent nurse. The nurse has two general responsibilities: to lessen the demands made on the patient to respond to his environment and to observe the effects of the treatment—both therapeutic and toxic. Within the limits prescribed by the physician, she modifies the therapeutic regime. Vasopressor agents may fail to raise the blood pressure, or they may elevate it too much. Although the blood pressure rises, there may not be a comparable increase in tissue nutrition. In the absence of the latter they may be of no benefit to the patient. When they are administered in intravenous fluids, the rate of flow of the solution should be under constant surveillance. Rapid increases or decreases in the rate of the vasopressor can result in a rebound reaction causing the blood pressure to fluctuate between high and low systolic readings. When the rate of flow is too slow, blood will clot in the needle or cannula. When it is too rapid, toxic doses of the drug may be delivered. In addition, the already feeble heart may be overburdened and the capacity of blood vessels to deliver blood restricted.

Even when the blood pressure is restored to physiological levels, the patient may still be in shock. The most sensitive index of shock is urine output. It should be at least 30 ml per hour.[66] In the mid-afternoon, Mr. Anderson voided 500 ml of urine. This, along with the stability of his systolic blood pressure at 120 mm of mercury, indicated that the shock had been relieved. His condition, however, continued to be critical.

A fourth measure prescribed for Mr. Anderson was the administration of oxygen by tent. The presence of pulmonary edema was the most important indication for oxygen as congestion of the lung decreases its efficiency in oxygenating the blood. Attention to maintaining the concentration of oxygen in the tent at a therapeutic level was imperative. (See Chapter 8.) As sometimes happens, the administration of oxygen to Mr. Anderson was accompanied by some re-

lief of pain. In addition to providing Mr. Anderson with a high concentration of oxygen, the tent made it possible to control the environmental temperature. Because the day was hot and humid, temperature control was of considerable benefit to him.

At no time should the fact that the patient is an individual human being be lost from sight. Despite the need for prompt and effective treatment, there is no place for hurry in the presence of the patient. The implications of the pain can be expected to provoke anxiety in the patient. The patient should not be permitted to suffer. If the prescription left by the physician for relief of pain is ineffective, he should be notified. Shifting from an independent, active state to a dependent, inactive one is a source of further anxiety and feeling of frustration. The very fact that strict bed rest is prescribed and every effort is made to enforce it tends to reinforce the patient's belief that he is seriously ill.

Mr. Anderson had been an active man. He found it frustrating to allow his nurse to feed him like a baby. The nurse tried to indicate that she recognized how he felt. After a day or so, arrangements were made for his wife to assist him with his evening meal. This also gave Mrs. Anderson a tangible way she could be of assistance to her husband.

At least a responsible member of the family should know that the patient is critically ill. Mrs. Anderson was so informed by the physician. Though he tried not to be too pessimistic, he did indicate the uncertainty of the outcome. Relatives of patients frequently require support and sympathetic understanding during this period.

For the first 24 to 48 hours, nursing care and medical therapy are both planned to eliminate, insofar as is possible, any demands on the patient to adapt to his environment. Care is also directed toward relieving shock and restoring the adequacy of circulation to his tissues. These objectives take precedence over all others, and unless they are accomplished, the patient will not recover. The length of time that the patient is kept on strict bed rest depends on many factors. For example, the patient who has been in definite shock is likely to be maintained on strict bed rest longer than the one who has not. Some physicians are more conservative than others.

After approximately two days, the regime of the patient who has recovered from the shock phase of the illness changes. Rest continues to be important, but bed rest is no longer essential provided certain precautions are observed and rest is achieved. Medical authorities directly and by implication emphasize the importance of competent nursing to the achievement of

[66] Agress, *ibid.*, p. 28.

basal rest.[67] When a patient is allowed out of bed, he should be assisted in getting out of bed to the chair by two people. The chair should be placed beside the bed. One person should stand on each side of the patient and assist him to a sitting position with his feet hanging over the edge of the bed. He should then be helped to a standing position, turned, and supported as he sits in the chair. He should not be allowed to walk until walking is prescribed by his physician. After he sits, his position should be checked to determine whether or not the chair is supporting him. If he is short, a footstool of the proper height should be placed under his feet. A chair of the proper depth should be selected, or if one is not available, a cushion should be placed behind his back so he is supported. Pressure against the calves of the legs is to be avoided. Chair rest carries with it one hazard; that is, the patient, his family, and even hospital personnel may assume that because he is up in a chair, he is no longer sick. Nothing could be further from the truth.

After two or three days the patient is usually allowed to use a bedside commode. He should be instructed not to strain or bear down during defecation (the Valsalva maneuver). To facilitate defecation, the physician may prescribe the patient's favorite laxative, provided it does not cause griping, or one of the stool softeners. The patient is soon allowed to feed himself and to

[67] Norman Brachfeld and John S. La Due: "Congestive Heart Failure, Coronary Insufficiency and Myocardial Infarction," *Pathologic Physiology*, 4th ed., William A. Sodeman., ed. (Philadelphia: W. B. Saunders Company, 1967), p. 483.

comb his hair. Shaving himself may be delayed for a time. During this period the patient should be protected from unnecessary and preventable stress—physical as well as emotional.

Usually the pain that marks the onset of myocardial infarction disappears after a variable period of time. It does not usually last, however, more than 24 to 48 hours. Sometimes the acute pain disappears and is replaced by a dull ache that persists for a few hours to a day or so. Signs and symptoms that relate to tissue necrosis include leukocytosis, fever, and an elevated sedimentation rate. As the membrane around the myocardial cells becomes more permeable than normal or the cells disintegrate cellular enzymes, SGOT and LDH, are released into the blood with the result that their level is elevated.

Complications of Myocardial Infarction

In addition to the changes in the electrocardiogram, the intensity of the signs and symptoms presented by the patient is of value to the physician in predicting extent of injury to the heart. When any of them continue for longer than the expected period of time, this may indicate a new insult to the heart or the development of a complication. The expected changes, as well as the findings as they occurred in Mr. Anderson, are summarized in Table 10-1.

From the history, clinical course, and laboratory findings, the physician concluded that Mr. Anderson had experienced a major myocardial infarct.

As myocardial cells degenerate, substances released in the area stimulate fibrosis, and a scar is formed. This scar is essentially the same as

TABLE 10-1

Sign or Symptom	Period When It Is Likely To Be Abnormal	Usual Finding	Mr. Anderson
Pain	Variable to 48 hr	Steady Unremitting	18 hr
Leukocytosis	Begins a few hours after onset of pain; usually returns to normal after the acute stress is over—1–2 days	12,000–18,000	18,150 the evening of the first day
Sedimentation rate	Rate of elevation slower than leukocytes; lasts 3–4 weeks		42 mm per hour fifth day
Serum glutamic oxalacetic transaminase (SGOT) (8–40 units)	Usually begins to rise in 6–12 hr and reaches a peak within 24–48 hr; subsides to normal in 3–4 days	50–600	146 units first day
Lactic dehydrogenase (LDH) (200–680 units)	Usually begins to rise in 36 hr and reaches a peak in 3–4 days; subsides to normal in 11–12 days	2–8 times normal	400 units second day

one formed in any part of the body. It serves as a patch to bridge the area of necrosis. Like scar tissue in other parts of the body, it does not perform the function of parenchymal tissue. Cardiac reserve is, therefore, decreased to the extent that muscle cells are lost. During the period of necrosis and until the scar is fully mature, the area of necrosis is weak. It is, therefore, liable to rupture or to form an aneurysm. During systole the weakened area in the wall of a ventricle may give way rather than resist distention with the result that the heart does not empty completely. Furthermore, when the myocardial reserve is sufficiently reduced by the loss of cells, the heart will no longer be able to adapt the circulation to the needs of the organism. Consequently, congestive heart failure may develop. Throughout the period of recovery, disturbances in the rate and rhythm of the heart continue to be a possibility.

One of the most serious problems during the convalescence of the patient is the possibility of intravascular clotting or thrombosis. Most, if not all, patients have more than one atheromatous plaque in their coronary arteries. Atheromatous plaques in arteries in other sites such as the brain or extremities may also serve as foci for the formation of blood clots. When necrosis extends to and includes the endocardium, the area is roughened and serves as a possible site for the formation of a mural thrombus. Whether or not there is an increase in the tendency of the blood to clot before the formation of the initial thrombus has been neither proved nor disproved. After a myocardial infarction, the possibility of intravascular clotting is increased. The tendency to thrombosis is intensified by the inactivity of the patient.

The implications of the diagnosis and the nature of the required treatment may also result in psychological complications. As emphasized earlier, the highest incidence of coronary heart disease is among men, and they are usually men who are in the most productive years of their lives. They usually have families dependent on them for support. Moreover, among the implications of myocardial infarction are sudden death, the possibility of a life of invalidism, or at least major adjustments in life. These are all sources of psychological stress. Bed rest and inactivity are also accompanied by physiological and metabolic changes that are part of the total effect. Finally, the patient cannot help but be affected by the reaction of his family, friends, and business associates.

What aspect of any illness is of paramount significance varies with each individual patient. Few, if any, escape some feeling of depression. Even the patient who makes a great show of taking his situation lightly experiences some degree of depression. The patient may be making or appear to be making good recovery and be exceptionally cheerful and yet be depressed. One patient typifies this point. He was boisterous and appeared to be carefree. About ten days after his admission, he was unusually quiet as the nurse bathed him. Finally he looked up at her and said, "I beat it [death] this time, didn't I? It was a close call, wasn't it?" His usual behavior was a front to cover his true feelings.

As discussed in the preceding pages, the most frequent threats to Mr. Anderson's life during the first 24 to 48 hours included ventricular fibrillation and arrest, pulmonary edema, extension of infarction, and shock. Other ventricular arrhythmias are also of serious import. The length of the period of acute illness varies. In a few hours a patient may be feeling well and be trying to assure himself and members of his family that nothing really happened or it was just an attack of indigestion. In some patients pulmonary edema and/or shock continues for several days or until the patient dies. Nursing care during this period is directed toward preventing any increase in the shock or pulmonary edema and carrying out therapeutic measures.

As the heart muscle degenerates, rupture of the heart is a possibility. The danger is greatest from the ninth to fourteenth day. According to Harrison,[68] the danger is greatest in patients over 70 and the rupture is particularly common in older women. When the heart ruptures, blood escapes into the pericardial sac and prevents the heart from filling. Death occurs suddenly. To lessen the possibility of rupture of the heart, Mr. Anderson should be instructed to avoid straining and sudden movements. He should be assisted out of bed and with activities likely to increase venous return.

Two types of measures were utilized to prevent the formation of thromboses and the possibility of embolism. Mr. Anderson's physician ordered an anticoagulant agent, and stasis of blood in the extremities was minimized. Physicians vary in their opinion as to when or if an anticoagulant should be started and the preparation to be used. For coumarin compounds or phenindione to be used with safety, facilities need to be available to accurately check the patient's prothrombin time. When the patient continues on anticoagulant drug therapy over an extended period of time, he must continue to have his prothrombin time checked at regular intervals. The patient must understand and

[68] William H. Resnik and T. R. Harrison: "Ischemic Heart Disease," *Principles of Internal Medicine*, 5th ed., T. R. Harrison *et al.*, eds. (New York: The Blakiston Division, McGraw-Hill Book Company, Inc., 1966), p. 837.

accept the importance of regular testing. Both inconvenience and expense are involved. Adequate medical supervision is also important. Before anticoagulant therapy is started, the patient's prothrombin time is determined. Shortly after Mr. Anderson was admitted, blood was drawn for the determination of his prothrombin time.

The specific anticoagulant preparation selected by the physician depends on the rapidity with which action is desired as well as other factors. Heparin acts immediately by depressing the conversion of fibrinogen to fibrin and prevents the agglutination of blood platelets. Neither heparin nor other anticoagulants dissolve already formed blood clots. The formation of new clots is prevented. Heparin is administered intravenously or subcutaneously with a small quantity of procaine, and the anticoagulant effect is determined by the clotting time.

Derivatives of coumarin or phenindione are generally prescribed for long-term anticoagulant effects. Because they depress the formation of prothrombin, their action is delayed and their effect persists over a longer period of time than that of heparin. The dosage for each patient has to be adjusted in relation to the effect of the drug on his prothrombin time.

According to Olwin,[69] there are several factors that may influence the prothrombin level including alcohol, the nutritional state, drugs, and liver function. Specifically some tranquilizers and caffeine increase the resistance to prothrombin depressants, whereas aspirin may cause a decrease in the prothrombin level. Patients with poor liver function and/or poor nutritional states seem to be more sensitive to anticoagulants; conversely, patients with diets high in green leafy vegetables have an increased resistance to anticoagulants.

The objective of the therapy is to prolong the prothrombin time enough to decrease its tendency to clot and at the same time protect the patient from the danger of spontaneous hemorrhage or hemorrhage resulting from minor injuries. Similar to other bodily functions, there are limits within which the clotting of the blood can safely be extended. Mr. Anderson's preanticoagulant therapy prothrombin time was 15 seconds. The objective was to raise it to between 25 and 35 seconds. Prothrombin time within this range decreases the tendency to intravascular clotting without exposing the patient to unnecessary danger of hemorrhage.

The drug prescribed for Mr. Anderson was warfarin (Coumadin). It was administered by mouth. Daily prothrombin times were per-

[69] John H. Olwin and J. L. Koppel: "Anticoagulant Therapy," *Amer. J. Nurs.,* 64:110 (May) 1964.

formed. On the third day his prothrombin time was 66 seconds. The next day it was up to 75 seconds, and the fifth day 145 seconds. On each of these days the control was 15 seconds. On the fifth day the physician prescribed vitamin K, a precursor of prothrombin. The next day Mr. Anderson's prothrombin time had returned to 33 seconds or around 20 per cent. The possibility of hemorrhage was decreased to a corresponding degree.

What are the nursing responsibilities in the treatment of myocardial infarction?

The nurse has a number of responsibilities in the care of the patient on anticoagulant therapy. Until the dosage has been established, daily prothrombin times must be taken and recorded. When the prescribed drug is administered daily, the nurse should check the prothrombin time before administering it. Also the dose should be given late enough in the day so that the patient has voided and the specimen has been checked for any evidence of blood because bleeding occurs first in the kidney. Other signs of bleeding would be petechiae, bleeding from the gastrointestinal tract, subarachnoid hemorrhage, or bleeding from small injuries such as excessive bleeding from injection sites. Vitamin K should be readily available so it can be given promptly should it be required. When Mr. Anderson's prothrombin time was 145 seconds, the small injury caused by the venipuncture resulted in bleeding from the site. Pressure over the area was continued for ten minutes before the bleeding stopped. Should bleeding take place, the physician should be notified. With proper checking of the prothrombin time and adjustment in the dosage of the anticoagulant drug, the danger to the patient is minimized. Without adequate supervision, the patient may be exposed to serious harm. Supervision must be continued as long as anticoagulant therapy is continued. The nurse has a responsibility to ascertain whether or not the patient understands what procedure he should follow, and why. The patient should also understand why he should not alter the prescribed dosage. Also, the patient should be provided with an identification card stating that he is on an anticoagulant and what to do in case of an emergency.

The following instance illustrates the possible consequences of inadequate care of a patient under continued anticoagulant therapy. The patient, a 30-year-old woman, had mitral stenosis following rheumatic fever. After experiencing a cerebral vascular accident caused by an embolus originating from a thrombus in her left atrium, she was placed on anticoagulant therapy. She took the drug faithfully, but her prothrombin time was not determined for several months. One afternoon at work she commenced to bleed from a number of mucous surfaces. For a time her life was in danger. Treatment with vitamin K reduced the prothrombin time to safe limits, and she recovered. By the time treatment was instituted, however, she had lost considerable blood and had bled into her pleural and peritoneal cavities.

Nursing measures to prevent venous stasis are emphasized in Chapter 17. Because of their importance, they will be summarized, however. As soon as emergency or lifesaving procedures have been carried out, attention should be given to the improvement of venous circulation from the lower extremities. Some physicians prescribe elastic bandages from toe to groin to support the walls of the veins. Passive exercises of the legs should be instituted as soon as feasible unless interdicted by the physician. These have previously been described. Getting the patient out of bed and into the chair also aids in improving venous flow from the legs. The importance of the prevention of pressure against the popliteal space or against the calf of the leg has also been indicated. This should not be neglected.

Congestive heart failure may be a complication of a myocardial infarction. The care of a patient with congestive heart failure has been described previously.

A disabling disorder, the shoulder-hand syndrome, develops occasionally. It is characterized by pain and tenderness in the shoulder. It is followed by pain, redness, and tenderness in the hand. Occasionally, the small muscles in the hand atrophy. According to Harrison,[70] the condition occurs in 5 to 10 per cent of patients and may develop within a year following a myocardial infarction.

Hiccoughs, when they occur, indicate a poor prognosis. Why this is true is not known. Continued hiccoughs in the otherwise healthy person are fatiguing. Perhaps fatigue is a factor in the unfavorable prognosis.

The diet prescribed for Mr. Anderson was low in salt, controlled in fat, and restricted to 1,800 calories. Salt was restricted to lessen the tendency to edema formation and because there may be a relationship between salt intake and hypertension. Fat was to be restricted in amount and type. Instead of the usual 40 to 45 per cent of the diet in the form of fat, the total was not to exceed 35 per cent. A larger proportion than is ingested by the average American was to be in the form of vegetable oils. Vegetable oils contain a higher percentage of unsaturated fatty acids than animal fats. The purpose of decreasing the intake of fat is to lower the level of lipids in the blood. Although there is no

[70] *Op. cit.,* p. 837.

definite proof that altering the kind and quantity of fat ingested decreases the incidence of coronary artery disease, a number of studies suggest that it may. Although Mr. Anderson was not overweight, calories were limited to decrease the likelihood of a gain in weight.

An essential part of the care of a patient is to prepare him to return to as full activity as the condition of his heart allows. Many patients can return to full or nearly full activity. The trend toward emphasizing what the patient can or will be able to do helps some patients move from attention on what they have lost to what they have and are able to do. Mr. Anderson had been performing a type of work that required a modest expenditure of energy. His work was also performed at a steady, but moderate, rate. Neither his safety nor the safety of others would be endangered were he to return to his job. His physician advised him to take a ten-minute rest period every two hours. Because he has an understanding employer, he thinks that this can be arranged. He has hospitalization insurance. This lessens his worry about expenses. His family is grown and his wife is employed. Financial worries are at a minimum. He hopes that he will be able to work until he is 65, when he will be eligible for full social security benefits.

Not all patients have as favorable a situation as Mr. Anderson. Some, such as Mr. Strongboy, have many problems. He is only 35 years of age. He has been divorced and has no one dependent on him. Neither does he have any one on whom he can depend. Though he has worked since he was 14 years of age, he has gone from one job to another and he has not established seniority in his work. Neither does he have savings or income insurance. His doctor has told him that he should think of doing some type of work other than truck driving. He lacks either the education or the experience required for most sedentary jobs. He expressed little interest when the subject of training for a suitable type of work was introduced. At one point he suggested the possibility of a job as dispatcher in the office of the firm where he was employed. Though referral to a sheltered workshop for cardiac patients was suggested to him, he was not interested. On discharge from the hospital, he planned to go to a hotel for men where rates were low. Because of all the factors involved, Mr. Strongboy's future did not appear to be very promising. He had neither the background nor the interest to profit from retraining.

Summary

In the preceding pages the ways in which the heart may fail have been discussed along with the implications of each of these to the needs of the patient for nursing. The causes of heart failure are summarized by Wiggers as:[71] (1) failure of the pacemakers, including the main pacemaker—the sinoatrial node, (2) too many pacemakers, (3) a breakdown in the system for the conduction of impulses over the heart muscle, (4) loss of the power of contraction, (5) obstruction of the coronary arteries, and (6) defective heart valves—they may either leak or be narrowed—stenosed. In an individual patient more than one factor is frequently involved. Whether or not a specific disorder of cardiac functioning leads to the failure of the heart as a pump depends on (1) the extent to which the condition deprives the myocardium of adequate nutrition, (2) the degree to which the heart must utilize its reserve to maintain the circulation, (3) the capacity of myocardial lead cells to initiate contraction under emergency conditions, and (4) the degree to which disorders disrupt the normal rate and rhythm of the heart.

The responsibilities of the nurse as they relate to disease of the heart include

1. Participating in programs of prevention of conditions that predispose to disease of the heart.
2. Acting as a case finder in detecting individuals who have heart disease.
3. Participating in programs of education of the public and employers so that those who have or have had heart disease and who want to be employed and are able to be, are employed.
4. Providing competent nursing of the person sick with heart disease, including his fullest rehabilitation.
5. Supporting programs of research into the cause and treatment of heart disease.

This chapter has not included a discussion of congenital malformations of the heart. Usually congenital malformations are manifested in childhood. In general they affect the circulation by some defect in the one-way circuit or by an obstruction to the flow of blood. Either one or both of these place an added burden on the myocardium and, depending on the nature and location of the lesion, result in a mixing of arterial and venous lood. Because an adequate circulation of the blood is essential not only to survival, but to normal growth and development, serious congenital defects of the heart and great vessels are usually accompanied by failure of the child to grow and to mature normally. Furthermore, defective structures appear to be more prone to infection by microorganisms than do normal ones. Persons with con-

genital heart malformations are, therefore, prone to bacterial endocarditis.

Blood Vessels

As indicated in the introduction to this chapter, the blood vessels together with the heart form a closed circuit through which blood is circulated. The heart, aided by skeletal muscles, furnishes the power by which the blood is propelled through the system. Ways in which the heart may fail and the effects of failure have been discussed in some detail. Some of the causes and consequences of failure of blood vessel function have also been presented. Further, some reference is made to some aspect of circulation in most chapters. Emphasis in this area is justified because many nursing activities are directed toward preserving the circulation or protecting the individual or some part of him from a defect in his circulation. With the steady increase in the number of aged in the population, the proportion of persons with disorders in circulation is also increasing.

Stress has been on the importance of the continuous movement of blood through the circuit. Nothing would be accomplished by this movement, however, were it not for the capillaries where exchange takes place between the interstitial fluid and the blood. In a very real sense, the capillaries are the site where the ultimate function of the circulatory system is accomplished.

Structure and Function of Blood Vessels

The structure of the blood vessels varies with their location in the circuit and with their function. With the exception of the capillaries, blood vessels are composed of three layers, or coats. The outer layer, or tunica adventitia, is largely areolar connective tissue. The middle layer, or tunica media, contains varying proportions of elastic and muscular tissue. The inner, or tunica intima, is also composed of three layers: a layer of elastic tissue lying next to the media, a thin layer of connective tissue, and finally a layer of endothelial cells. Differences in structure are significant not only to their function, but to the pathophysiology accompanying disease. The walls of the large arteries, such as the aorta and the pulmonary artery, are thick and contain a large amount of elastic tissue, but relatively little muscle. In medium-sized and small arteries conditions are reversed. As arteries decrease in size, the amount of elastic tissue also decreases and their walls contain relatively more muscle. The arterioles are largely muscle.

The highly elastic structure of the aorta en-

[71] *Op. cit.*, p. 87.

ables it to distend as the blood is ejected into it during systole. As a consequence, the aorta is capable of storing about half the blood it receives from the heart during systole. During systole the elastic tissue shortens as the blood flows out into the circuit. With the decrease in the volume of blood in the aorta, the potential (stored) energy built up as the elastic tissue in its wall is stretched is released as kinetic (moving) energy. This energy aids the forward movement of the blood. The familiar example of the rubber band can be used to illustrate the above changes. An elastic band is stretched. As it is stretched, potential energy accumulates. When the band is released, it returns to its prestretched form and at the same time releases kinetic energy. The kinetic energy may be used to move a part in a model airplane or for some other purpose. When it is released by the wall of a blood vessel, it propels the blood in the vessel forward.

The elasticity of the aorta is a factor in the continuous flow of blood through the arteries, and it helps to protect the smaller vessels from the full force of systolic contraction of the heart. Were the aorta a rigid tube, the blood pressure would be higher at the end of systole and lower during diastole. This is essentially what happens when the aorta becomes sclerosed. With aging, there is a loss of elastic tissue, and the wall of the aorta becomes increasingly rigid. As the wall of the aorta increases in rigidity, the systolic blood pressure rises. The diastolic blood pressure does not always fall, although it may. Sometimes the aorta increases in size as it becomes sclerosed. The increase in capacity tends to compensate for the loss of elasticity. Atherosclerosis, characterized by a loss of elastic tissue, especially in the intima of the aorta, starts at a relatively early age. Evidence of this can be seen at the age of 20 or thereabouts. Changes in the media of other arteries also take place with aging. They lead to tortuosity and stiffening of the vessel wall. Arteriosclerosis is not the same disorder as atherosclerosis, which was discussed previously.

ARTERIES

The structure of the artery is also a factor in the limitation of bleeding after tissue continuity is disrupted. When an artery is cut, elastic tissue shortens and retracts the artery a little beneath its sheath. At the same time the muscle contracts somewhat and narrows the opening in the artery. "Self-sealing" is completed by the formation of a blood clot in the end of the artery.

Arterioles, in contrast to large arteries, are largely muscle. They are therefore capable of adapting the diameter of their lumen to the volume of blood in the body and to the localized needs of tissues. Changes in the walls of muscular arteries affect not only the diameter of their lumen, but the hemodynamics of the circulation. The outflow from the arterioles affects not only the volume and velocity of blood flowing through the capillaries but the pressure of the blood in the larger arteries. Whereas the measure of the force with which the blood is ejected into the arteries is the systolic blood pressure, the measure of the degree of constriction of arterioles (peripheral resistance) is the level of the diastolic blood pressure. Some other factors in the regulation of the arterial blood pressure as well as theories to explain essential hypertension will be presented subsequently.

As indicated previously, the function of the circulatory system is accomplished in the capillaries. Other parts serve to propel and convey blood to and from the capillaries where the exchange takes place between the blood and the interstitial fluid surrounding cells. Capillaries are composed of a single layer of endothelial cells that are continuous with the lining cells of the arteries and veins. The capillaries and the arterioles together form the microcirculation. Some capillaries are thoroughfare channels, while others are true capillaries. The thoroughfare channels enable the body to shift blood around a part. The factors involved in the exchange between the blood in the capillaries and the interstitial fluid are discussed in Chapter 9. According to Zweifach,[72] the distance from a capillary to a cell is never greater than 0.005 in. The total length of capillaries is 60,000 miles, or an average of 400 miles per pound of body weight. The potential capacity of the capillaries is large enough to hold all the blood in the body. In health the arterioles and precapillary sphincters regulate the flow of blood through the capillaries so they are not all open at one time. When tissue is observed under the microscope, capillary channels can be seen to open and close at different times. When tissues are active, the number of functioning capillaries is greater than when they are at rest. This is another way in which the body is able to adapt function to its needs. In peripheral circulatory failure, the ability to regulate the number of functioning capillaries is lost with the result that the potential capacity of the vascular system exceeds the blood volume. The volume of blood returned to the heart drops and as a consequence the cardiac output drops. Blood pressure falls and the affected person is in shock. Unless the disturbance is corrected promptly, life ceases.

[72] Benjamin W. Zweifach: "The Microcirculation of the Blood," *Sci. Amer.,* **200:**54 (Jan.) 1959.

VEINS

The veins, like the arteries, are composed of three layers. The walls of the veins tend to be thinner than those of the arteries and the media is not as well developed. They contain less muscle and elastic tissue than the media of the arteries. Because of the thinness of their walls, veins have a tendency to collapse when they are cut. They are also easily collapsed by pressure. Because the relatively thick walls of arteries resist collapse, blood continues to enter tissues in which veins have been obstructed by pressure. This leads to swelling that, if it is allowed to continue, will eventually limit the inflow of blood. Some veins, especially those in which the blood is moved against gravity, are provided with valves. These valves are important to keep the blood moving forward in the vascular circuit. When the valves in the veins are congenitally defective or are destroyed by disease, stasis of blood in the affected vein results.

In comparison with that in the arteries, the pressure of blood in the veins is low. To a great extent, the pressure of blood in the peripheral veins is determined by the pressure in the right atrium, and the pressure in the right atrium is largely determined by the efficiency of the heart as a pump. Total blood volume affects the amount of blood available to return to the heart. Within limits the veins are capable of adapting to a decrease in blood volume by constricting. The veins have a large potential capacity for blood, and this is also a factor in shock.

The return of blood from the lower extremities is facilitated by the contraction of skeletal muscles. They are sometimes referred to as a venous pump. Prolonged motionless standing or sitting with pressure against the popliteal space results in a rise in venous pressure in the legs and feet. Fainting may occur in susceptible individuals following as little as ten minutes of motionless standing. Continued sitting such as on long bus or automobile trips predisposes to edema of the feet and legs. There have been some instances reported in the literature, of elderly persons developing convulsions as a result of shifts in the distribution of body fluids during extended bus or automobile travel. Preventive measures include getting out of the car or bus at hourly or two-hour intervals and walking about. Exercises such as flexing and extending the foot at the ankle, and setting the quadriceps muscles while sitting, are also beneficial. Many older persons would be well advised to break extended journeys by spending the night in a hotel or motel.

As are other service facilities, blood vessels are subject to regulation. Through regulation the over-all needs of the body are met, priority is given to areas with high metabolic requirements, and special needs of local areas of tissue are met. The nervous system has an important role in the regulation of the diameter of arteries and veins, but there is little evidence that it directly regulates the capillaries. The capillary circulation is believed to be regulated primarily by local conditions in the tissues. Through the regulation of the caliber of arteries and veins and the force and rate of the heart, blood is delivered to and removed from the capillaries.

Many of the circumstances that obtain when sympathetic nervous system regulation is important have been previously discussed. They include the maintenance of normal blood pressure in persons who have sustained blood loss or in whom the cardiac output is low. Sympathetic reflexes prevent cerebral hypotension when shifting from the supine to the standing position. Sympathetic reflexes are also involved when blood is shifted from one area to another.

Both the sympathetic and parasympathetic nervous system participate in the regulation of the coordination of cardiac and vascular functioning. For example, an increase in the volume of blood delivered to the right atrium stimulates receptors in the vena cava and results in an increase in the heart rate. Conversely, an increase in the pressure of blood in the aorta initiates a reflex slowing the heart.

Not all the elements in the local regulation of blood flow are known. Some of the possibilities include a lack of essential nutrients and oxygen or the liberation of a substance by the ischemic tissue that is responsible for arteriolar and capillary dilatation. The hormones epinephrine and norepinephrine cause contraction of all blood vessels except the coronary arteries. Acetylcholine causes muscle cells to relax. In the process of metabolism, chemicals are formed that, when they come in contact with the precapillary sphincter, cause it to relax. In the local regulation of the blood supply, the processes are self-correcting. When the condition initiating the response is corrected, conditions tend to return to the prestimulus state. For example, blood vessels dilate in an area in response to exercise of the muscles. As a result of the increased blood flow, ischemia is corrected and products that directly dilate the blood vessels are removed. With the elimination of conditions initiating dilatation, the blood vessels automatically constrict.

Tissues are also protected from the effects of arterial obstruction by the collateral circulation, that is, the circulation around and connecting smaller branches of the main circulation. The collateral circulation offers the greatest protection when an obstruction develops slowly. New capillaries can develop in the tissues and larger vessels can be recanalized, but the body requires from one to six months to increase the vascularity of tissues. If the loss of blood supply is not so great that the basal needs of the tissues cannot be met and if the tissues are protected from increased demands, the affected part (arm, leg, or heart) can sometimes be saved until an adequate circulation is established.

Diseases of the Blood Vessels

Not unlike other organs, blood vessels are subject to abnormalities of structure and function. Diseases of blood vessels, including blood vessels of the heart, kidney, and brain, stand first on the list as causes of mortality. Equally important, if not more, they cause a high incidence of morbidity. Some localized defects occurring in blood vessels, such as a single aneurysm of an artery supplying the brain or an aneurysm of the aorta, threaten disaster to the whole individual. Disorders characterized by structural changes are said to be organic, while those in which there is a disturbance in function in the absence of a structural change are said to be functional. Functional disorders may in time lead to structural changes in the walls of affected blood vessels. When a disease of the blood vessel results in obstruction of its lumen, it is known as an occlusive vascular disease.

Areas in the walls of arteries and veins may be weakened by congenital defects, injury, or disease. Such vessels are subject to dilatation and thinning of the wall. Abnormal dilatations of arteries are known as aneurysms; those of veins, as varicosities. Although both types of disorders impede the flow of blood, and pressure against the wall of the affected vessel increases the degree of dilatation, there are significant differences between the two disorders.

ANEURYSM

An aneurysm is a saclike dilatation occurring in the wall of a blood vessel and is caused by a weakness in its structure. Common sites of arterial aneurysms include the circle of Willis and the aorta. Those in the circle of Willis are caused by congenital defects in the walls of the arteries. Aortic aneurysms may be caused by syphilis, arteriosclerosis, or trauma. In syphilis, the spirochete invades the media and weakens the wall of the artery. Whatever its cause or site, the wall of an aneurysm is weak and, therefore, predisposed to rupture. To prevent rupture, the patient should be instructed to avoid all activities that result in an increase in blood pressure, such as straining during defecation, coughing, lifting heavy objects, or having strenuous activity. When an aneurysm is believed to be very thin-walled, strict bed rest may be prescribed for the patient.

The signs and symptoms accompanying an aneurysm will, of course, be affected by its location. An aneurysm in the ascending aorta predisposes to congestive heart failure as well as to the formation of thrombi in the vessels. Rupture of an aortic aneurysm is a cause of sudden death. Rupture of an aneurysm in an artery forming the circle of Willis (they are frequently multiple) releases blood into the cerebrospinal fluid. Meningeal signs such as stiff neck occur as well as evidence of increased intracranial pressure. The outcome varies. Some patients die suddenly. Others recover, but have other aneurysms rupture at later times.

Various surgical methods have been developed to reinforce or replace the weakened wall of the aorta or other arteries in which an aneurysm has developed. In the preoperative preparation of the patient the major objective is to prevent any increase, particularly sudden increase, in pressure against the wall of the weakened vessel. Previous discussion on achieving rest is pertinent here. In the postoperative care, prevention of strain on the operated area and prevention of clotting of blood in the operated or other vessels are major objectives.

Principles basic to the achievement of both these objectives have been discussed earlier. Certain aspects of care will depend on the route of approach to the aneurysm. For example, was it through the chest or abdominal wall? It is most important that each person be considered as an individual. Repair of an aneurysm is a major procedure and, if located in the circle of Willis or aorta, is attended by the possibility that the patient will not survive the operation. To the extent to which the patient understands or imagines the degree of risk to which he is exposed, the nature of the disorder and the therapy are sources of anxiety.

VARICOSITIES

Dilated veins or varicosities, particularly those located in the esophagus, may also rupture and cause serious, and not infrequently fatal, hemorrhage. Intracutaneous varicosities in the skin of the lower extremities may also rupture and bleed. Bleeding is limited because the vessels are small and the tissue offers counterpressure against the wall of the bleeding vessel. The epithelium over the area is thin. Trauma caused by bumping may break the skin and result in profuse bleeding. Discoloration of the skin may be a cause of emotional distress, however. The anatomy of the intracutaneous vessels may, when they are dilated, be responsible for further distress. The veins draining the intracutaneous tissue are characterized by a central vein with numerous spiderlike feeder veins. Increased pressure within these veins leading to their dilatation results in a spiderlike lesion that understandably enough is called a spider angioma. They are unsightly, but relatively harmless.

Common sites where varicosities occur are the greater and lesser saphenous veins draining the lower extremities. As they dilate, pressure of blood against their walls increases causing further dilatation. The veins not only increase in diameter, but they elongate and become tortuous. Veins lying in the subcutaneous tissue are visible and unsightly. A patient may have one type of varicosity or both. According to Cooper,[73] uncomplicated varicose veins actually cause few symptoms and are rarely incapacitating. The usual symptoms are a feeling of heaviness and fullness in the legs and a stinging sensation along the course of the veins after the person has been standing for some time. There may be mild edema in the region of the ankle and mild stasis dermatitis. Ulceration of the skin is almost entirely limited to the person who has a combination of varicosities and deep venous insufficiency.[74] In the uncomplicated form, varicosities are largely hereditary, but they may also follow thrombophlebitis in which the inflammatory process destroys the valves in the veins. Varicosities occur more frequently in women than in men. They become worse during menstrual periods and with each succeeding pregnancy. Rapid weight gain and occupations requiring prolonged motionless standing are associated with enlargement of varicosities.

According to Cooper,[75] the usual reason for treating uncomplicated varicosities is cosmetic. The treatment of intracutaneous varicosities is unsatisfactory. The most satisfactory treatment of large tortuous veins is by stripping. Injection and ligation are accompanied by a high percentage of recurrence. In patients who have deep vein insufficiency, stripping the veins does not return the patient completely to normal. The legs may look better, but the patient should still wear elastic stockings and elevate the legs regularly. The new type of elastic stocking is relatively expensive but not unattractive.

Blood flow in the veins and the competency of the valves in preventing the backflow of blood into the subcutaneous veins or in veins connecting superficial and deep veins can be determined. To test the competency of the deep

veins to carry blood, the physician occludes the superficial veins with a tourniquet at the level of the knee or thigh. The patient then walks. The normal pumping action of the muscles against the walls of the veins should cause the varices to empty. If they do not, this indicates that the valves in a large perforating vein are incompetent.

Competency of the subcutaneous veins is determined by first draining veins of the leg by elevating it and then applying a tourniquet. The leg is then lowered. If the veins fill slowly, this indicates that the valves from the perforating veins are competent. If they fill rapidly, they are incompetent. If, after the tourniquet is removed, the veins fill rapidly, the valves in the saphenous veins are incompetent. A physician performs these tests, but the nurse should be able to assist the patient and physician with the tests and be prepared to answer the patient's questions.

ARTERIOVENOUS FISTULAE

As a result of defective development or trauma, direct connections between arteries and veins may exist or be formed. A common effect of the abnormal opening is that arterial blood is circulated directly to the affected vein.[76] The effects depend somewhat on the location of the fistula and the age of the individual at the time it is formed. For example, John Sparrow, aged 30, developed a fistula between his aorta and inferior vena cava as a result of a gunshot wound in the abdomen. For a time he was reasonably well. As a consequence of a chronic overloading of his heart by recirculated blood, his heart eventually failed as a pump. Such an abnormal connection between a distal artery and vein would not have as serious an effect.

PERIPHERAL VASCULAR DISEASE

Disease of blood vessels in the periphery, especially those supplying the extremities, is known as peripheral vascular disease. These diseases may be either functional or organic. Any disorder in the function of blood vessels implies some disturbance in the capacity to deliver blood to the tissues or to remove it. So-called functional disturbances of arteries may be limited to certain structures, or they may be generalized. An example of the first is Raynaud's disease and of the second hypertension. In Raynaud's disease the blood vessels of the hands and/or feet respond to cold or emotion by vasospasm. The degree of spasm may be

---

[73] F. W. Cooper: "Varicose Veins," *Heart Bull.,* 9:57 (May–June) 1960.

[74] *Ibid.,* p. 57.

[75] *Ibid.,* p. 58.

[76] In keeping with the well-known fact, fluids move from areas of high pressure to those of low pressure.

so great that no blood enters the affected areas during the height of the attack. Hypertension is a very important disease and will be discussed later.

The most common cause of peripheral arterial disease is atherosclerosis. The pathogenesis of this disease is the same in all arteries and it has been fully discussed previously. When the disease involves vessels supplying the extremities, manifestations caused by an inadequate blood supply can be observed. One further point is of some significance in nursing. Diseased as well as normal arteries (arterioles) respond to conditions in the environment. Therefore, the patient who has atherosclerosis of arteries supplying the extremities responds to cold by constriction and to warmth by vasodilatation. Other factors such as food, smoking, emotional states, and exercise may also influence the degree of arterial constriction or dilatation. Furthermore, though some disorders affect either arteries or veins, others affect both.

The signs and symptoms associated with disturbances in circulation to the peripheral tissues have been listed by Allen, Barker, and Hines.[77] They include (1) pain; (2) color changes of the skin or nails; (3) ulceration or gangrene, scleroderma, and impairment of the growth of the nails; (4) size of the extremities altered by either an increase or decrease; (5) abnormality of temperature of the extremities—either abnormally cold or abnormally warm; and (6) enlarged or abnormal pulsations of veins.

There are some other significant signs and symptoms as well, such as color changes and eczema of the skin that accompany chronic venous stasis, impaired arterial pulsation, and unusual changes with elevation or dependency of the extremity. Because of abnormalities in the flow of blood in aneurysms or in arteriovenous fistulae, murmurs may be heard. A sound that can be felt as a vibration is called a thrill. In peripheral vascular disease most of the signs and symptoms result from vasodilatation or some type of disorder decreasing the diameter of the blood vessels such as vasospasm. Both cause an alteration in the volume of blood delivered to the tissues and a failure in the capacity to adapt blood supply to tissue needs.

The objective that takes first priority in the nursing of the patient whose tissues have an insufficient supply of blood is (1) to protect these tissues from injury. Other objectives include (2) to prevent and relieve symptoms; (3) to participate in the program of education

[77] Edgar V. Allen, Nelson W. Barker, and Edgar A. Hines: *Peripheral Vascular Diseases*, 3rd ed. (Philadelphia: W. B. Saunders Company, 1962), p. 6.

for the patient, so that he learns how, and is motivated, to prevent injury to affected tissues; and (4) to carry out the part of the therapeutic regime that is expected to promote the development of the collateral circulation.

RAYNAUD'S SYNDROME

Measures to protect the affected tissues depend in part on the nature of the disorder. For example, Ann Blue has Raynaud's syndrome. Despite the discomfort associated with an attack, Raynaud's disease is almost always a harmless disorder. Miss Blue seems to have a mild form of the disease, and at this time there is no evidence that it is progressive. She has no difficulty unless her hands are exposed to cold, and attacks can be prevented by protecting her hands from the cold. By wearing warm mittens during cold weather and avoiding becoming chilled, she keeps from having difficulty. Gangrene is unusual in Raynaud's syndrome, though superficial ulcers and scleroderma do sometimes occur. From what is known about Miss Blue, there is little reason to suppose that she will develop either complication.

OCCLUSIVE VASCULAR DISEASE

Unlike Raynaud's disease, occlusive arterial disease is generally of serious import. Mr. Marker illustrates some of the problems associated with the disease. At the moment he is sitting on the edge of his bed with his left leg hanging over the edge. His right leg was amputated two years ago. There is an ulcer on his right index finger, the result of a cigarette burn. Since burning himself, he has stopped smoking. He had continued to smoke, despite the explanation given to Mr. Marker by his physician that cigarette smoking was a possible factor in causation and undoubtedly aggravated his condition. He is now faced with the possibility of having to have his left leg amputated. He is not an old man; he is only 29 years of age.

Mr. Marker has a form of occlusive peripheral vascular disease that in the past was, and still is, identified by some physicians as Buerger's disease or thromboangiitis obliterans. Some physicians doubt that Buerger's disease is a distinct clinical entity; they believe it to be peripheral atherosclerosis occurring in young men. One distinction made between peripheral atherosclerosis and thromboangiitis obliterans is the age at which it occurs. Thromboangiitis usually develops before the age of 45 to 50 years and atherosclerosis after 45 years of age. Many of the pathological features of thromboangiitis obliterans are similar, if not identical to, those of peripheral atherosclerosis. The age of the patient does influence the manner in which he responds to his illness, and many of the problems that he faces. In arterial occlusion, the manifestations are due to tissue ischemia.[78] In meeting needs of Mr. Marker for nursing, two points are of greatest significance. One is that the need of the tissues of his extremities is greater than the capacity of his body to supply blood. The other relates to the fact that he is presently suffering pain.

Several factors may enter into the causation of his pain. In ulceration and gangrene, pain is common; pain may be a forerunner of ulceration and is called the pretropic pain of ischemia. It is constant and severe. It interferes with the ability to sleep. The pain is less severe when the affected extremity is dependent. Thus Mr. Marker secures some relief by having his foot over the edge of the bed. Heat, if not too great and if it does not elevate the metabolic rate to a greater extent than it does the blood supply, may help to relieve the pain. Pain is aggravated by continuous elevation of the extremity and by cold.

A second possible cause of pain in occlusive arterial disease is ischemic neuritis. The pain may be burning, throbbing, shooting, or tearing. It may be severe and extensive. It may fluctuate in severity, the patient having paroxysms when the pain is worse than it is at other times. Acute inflammation of the arteries and veins may cause a mild pain or a dull ache. It is usually manifested on pressure as tenderness.

For some time previous to his admission to the hospital Mr. Marker had had pain in the calf of his leg after he walked for a block or so. He had noted that the distance he could walk in comfort had become progressively less and that the pain was cramplike in character. It was relieved by rest. Pain associated with exercise is believed to be caused by insufficient supply of blood—ischemia—to the contracting muscle.

OCCLUSIVE DISORDERS

Another cause of pain in peripheral vascular disorders is sudden arterial occlusion. Occlusion may be due to either a thrombus or an embolism that causes complete acute obstruction. Pain occurs at rest and is sudden and severe. The cause of the pain has not been completely explained. It may be caused in part, or intensified, by spasm of associated collateral vessels. Surprisingly, in some instances pain is slight or even absent in patients with major arterial embolism. A possible explanation is that the peripheral nerves are rendered functionless by

acute ischemia. The affected extremity is also pale and cold, further indicating severe ischemia. There is usually a sharp line of demarcation between the ischemic and normal tissue. Within a short time after onset, there is a loss of sensory as well as of motor function. The patient notes that he is unable to move his fingers or toes. The skin becomes insensitive to pain and touch. The extremity should, therefore, be protected from pressure. It is easily injured by heat, both because a rise in the temperature of tissues increases their metabolic needs and because the mechanism for cooling the tissue is defective or lacking. Pulses in the arteries distal to the site of obstruction are absent or weak when tested by palpation or by oscillometry. Unless the circulation is re-established promptly, the extremity will become gangrenous and require amputation. Accurate observation and prompt reporting are imperative. The part should be in a dependent position. When a lower extremity is involved, this is accomplished by elevating the head of the bed on blocks. Cold may be applied to the affected extremity to reduce the rate of metabolism. Measures such as sympathetic block may be performed to dilate the collateral blood vessels. The tendency of thrombi to propagate, that is, continue to grow, is combated by the use of anticoagulants. Heparin is frequently chosen because of its immediate effects and limited length of action.

How are disorders of blood vessels diagnosed and treated?

When the clot is large, it is usually surgically removed. Thrombectomy or embolectomy must be performed as soon as possible and while the tissues are still viable (living). According to Julian and Dye,[79] an embolectomy should be performed within eight hours of the onset of symptoms. Postoperatively attention should be given to the prevention of stasis of blood in the operated extremity. An anticoagulant is also prescribed to lessen the danger of thrombosis in the operated vessels and in other blood vessels as well.

Several elements contribute to the pain associated with occlusive arterial disease. For a patient such as Mr. Marker pain becomes the focus of his attention. That this should be true is not surprising, since his pain was severe and unrelenting and was more severe at night. Constant pain combined with a loss of sleep is damaging to the morale. Even when Mr. Marker secured some relief from his pain, he

[78] Eugene A. Stead, Jr.: Vascular Disease of the Extremities," *Principles of Internal Medicine*, 5th ed., T. R. Harrison *et al.*, eds. (New York: The Blakiston Division, McGraw-Hill Book Company, Inc., 1966), p. 720.

[79] Ormand C. Julian and William S. Dye: "Peripheral Vascular Surgery," *Surgery, Principles and Practice*, 3rd ed. Carl A. Moyer *et al.*, eds. (Philadelphia: J. B. Lippincott Company, 1965), p. 1250.

was depressed by the thought, "How can a man without legs possibly support himself, let alone his family?" When whiskey and aspirin did not give Mr. Marker relief, his physician prescribed meperidine hydrochloride (Demerol). According to Allen,[80] when pain at rest is severe, a narcotic may be used. Generally, however, narcotics are used with great caution and in the smallest possible dosages because of the possibility of addiction. The nurse has essentially the same responsibilities that she has any time she administers a narcotic. Does the patient have pain? What is its nature? Where is it located? How does the patient describe it? Does the pain require a narcotic or can it be relieved by some other measure? Is the pain relieved after the drug is administered? How long does its effect last? Is there anything that the nurse can do to increase the effectiveness of the analgesic narcotic?

In addition to pain, Mr. Marker also had other signs and symptoms indicating ischemia. His feet were cold to touch. There were marked changes in color on change in position. His feet were dusky red on dependency and pale on elevation. The nails on his toes were unusually thick and brittle for a man as young as Mr. Marker.

PREVENT INJURY TO TISSUES

The problem of preventing the breakdown of tissue until Mr. Marker is able to develop a collateral circulation is urgent. Even the slightest trauma or the mildest irritating chemical may be sufficient to upset the balance between the supply of food and the needs of the tissues. Viability of the tissue is protected by decreasing the local metabolic needs of the tissue and by increasing the blood flow to the ischemic part. Careful nursing is essential to the accomplishment of both objectives.

When Mr. Marker was admitted to the hospital, his physician prescribed bed rest in a constant-temperature room. A cradle was placed over his foot to prevent the bed covering from causing pressure. To minimize the danger of traumatizing his toes or foot, a cradle the width of the bed was selected. The bed linen was inspected to be certain that there were no patches or seams. Because Mr. Marker moved about freely and frequently, there was little danger of pressure from a part remaining in one position. In less active patients, attention should be given to regular changes in the position of the extremity and to the use of devices to distribute the pressure evenly.

Heat in the form of hot-water bottles or heating pads should not be used. No chemical, lo-

tion, or other agent, unless specifically prescribed by the physician, should be applied to the skin. Before cutting the patient's nails, the nurse should acquaint herself with the policy of the hospital. In some hospitals a physician's prescription is required before the toenails are cut. In others nails are cut by a chiropodist. Before the nails are cut, the feet should be soaked in warm, not hot, soapy water for ten minutes to soften the nails. Before the foot is placed in water for bathing, the temperature of the water should be checked with the hand. The water should be warm, not hot or cold. A temperature between 29.4 and 35°C (85° and 95°F) is suggested as acceptable. The nails should be cut straight across and not too close to the flesh. Should any injury, no matter how slight, be inflicted, it should immediately be brought to the attention of the physician. Because Mr. Marker's foot was dry and scaly, lanolin was applied. Care was taken when drying his foot to pat gently with a soft towel, rather than to rub. Attention was paid to drying between the toes. Skin that is continuously moist softens and becomes macerated and is thereby predisposed to infection. Lamb's wool was placed between the toes to absorb moisture. For patients whose feet tend to be moist, exposure to air is recommended.

Not only is the nurse responsible for trying to identify and remove possible sources of injury to the patient's feet, but the cooperation and assistance of the patient are essential. Furthermore, even when the treatment of the hospitalized patient is successful, a regime similar to that followed in the hospital is essential if the tissues in the extremities are to be maintained in a reasonably healthy condition. The patient must know how to care for his extremities, especially his feet, and understand why this care is important. He must also be helped to understand that although doctors and nurses will do their best to assist him, the main responsibility in the control of the disorder is his. The patient should therefore be given written as well as verbal instructions and demonstrations of the care of the feet. He should have an opportunity to practice the essential procedures under supervision. These instructions are appropriate for all patients who have peripheral occlusive vascular disease, including those who also have diabetes mellitus.

The prevention of ulceration and gangrene is easier than the cure. Almost all ulceration and gangrene of ischemic extremities can be charged to chemical, mechanical, or thermal injury, or to local bacterial infection of tissues. Injury need not be severe. Often minor injuries, especially when neglected, lead to ulceration and gangrene. The injury does not have to disrupt

80 *Op. cit.,* p. 334.

the skin. From the experience of the writer, an elderly man comes to mind who developed gangrene of his foot after he had kicked a cow in an effort to get her to move a leg. Later in the evening he noted soreness and redness in the great toe of the same foot. A week later he was admitted to the hospital. The toe was gangrenous.

Points to be emphasized in the care of the feet include

1. Cleanliness
   a. Wash no less frequently than every other day in warm, soapy water.
   b. Dry thoroughly between the toes with a soft cloth. Use a patting or mopping action.
   c. Take care not to bruise the feet or break the skin.
   d. Powder the feet if they have a tendency to perspire.
   e. Lubricate the feet with an ointment consisting of 50 parts lanolin and 50 parts petroleum jelly if they are dry.
2. Shoes
   a. Never go barefoot. Always wear shoes when out of bed.
   b. Wear well-built shoes of soft leather.
   c. Wear shoes with a broad toe and a sensible heel. They should give the feet adequate support.
   d. Never wear new shoes more than one-half day at a time.
   e. Never wear shoes with exposed nails, defects in the lining, or any other roughened surfaces that will come in contact with the feet. Have defective shoes repaired before wearing.
3. Hose
   a. Wear seamless hose without holes, darns, or patches.
   b. Wear clean stockings daily. (Cotton stockings are preferred because they can be boiled when washed.)
   c. Be sure to buy hose sufficiently long. Too short stockings are as harmful as too short shoes.
   d. Lamb's wool should be worn between the toes provided that it does not create pressure among the toes predisposing to tissue breakdown.
4. Toenails
   a. If you go to a chiropodist, tell him that you have a reduction in blood flow to your feet.
   b. Before cutting toenails, soak feet in warm, soapy water.
   c. Cut the toenails straight across and not too short, i.e., not too close to the flesh.
   d. Place cotton wicks under the corners of the great toenails if there is a tendency to ingrown toenails.
5. Corns and calluses
   a. Do not cut corns and calluses.
   b. Do not use medicated corn plasters.
   c. Have corns and calluses taken care of by a doctor or a chiropodist who understands your condition.
6. Cold and heat
   a. In cold weather, wear adequate foot covering to protect the feet from excessive cold. Wear loose, thick, warm socks. Do not stay out in the cold for long periods of time. Cold contracts your blood vessels and lessens the supply of blood to your feet.
   b. Do not place hot-water bottles, heating pads, or other heating devices near to or on the feet or legs. Do not use any form of heat without the advice of your physician.
   c. Do not place the feet in an oven, on a heating stove, or on a radiator.
   d. If your feet are cold, warm them by wearing woolen bed socks or wrapping them in a warm blanket.
   e. Remember that your feet are sensitive to both heat and cold and that both should be avoided!
7. Rest and elevation of the feet
   a. Sit down and elevate your feet on a footstool at least once every two hours. (Many industrial concerns allow rest periods, usually 15 minutes, for their employees. This time could be used for elevating your feet on a footstool or a chair. This is most important for the older diabetic patient who has arteriosclerosis.)
   b. Do not cross your knees when you sit.
8. Injury—any injury, however slight, may become ulcerous or gangrenous if treatment is delayed.
   a. Take care not to injure your feet. Avoid crowded places.
   b. A pillow may be used to prevent pressure on the feet by bed covering.
   c. Do not delay in consulting your physician should any redness, blistering, swelling, or pain develop.
   d. When tissue is cut or bruised, the part should be covered with a clean bandage and kept moist with a solution of equal parts of boric and alcohol solution.
   e. Do not use strong antiseptics such as iodine, Lysol, carbolic acid, and bichloride of mercury. No medicine should be placed on your feet, unless prescribed by your physician.
   f. Avoid sunburn and bathing in cold water

or at beaches where there is a possibility of injuring the feet.

9. Athlete's foot

A deficient supply of blood to the feet predisposes to athlete's foot. It starts out with burning and itching between the toes. You should report these symptoms to your physician so that treatment can be started immediately.

Too much emphasis cannot be placed on the importance of the care of the feet of the patient who has occlusive vascular disease. Attention should be centered not only on the measures outlined above, but on identification of conditions in the environment that predispose to injury. Any condition that increases metabolism in tissues with an inadequate blood supply may thereby upset the balance between supply and demand and result in ulceration and gangrene.

When a break in the skin occurs or an ulcer is present, the area should be protected from infection and the patient should be kept at bed rest. No weight bearing should be permitted. As repeatedly emphasized, when the blood supply decreases, resistance to infection also diminishes. With the development of infection, tissue demands are increased. If the continuity of the skin is disrupted, the area should be covered with a clean, sterile dressing. Because adhesive tape is irritating to the skin of some people, some other method of anchoring the dressing in place is advisable. If a bandage is used, care should be taken to apply it evenly without pressure at any point. Physicians differ in their opinions about the value of locally applied antibiotics. An antibiotic active against the infecting microorganism is usually administered systemically.

INCREASE BLOOD FLOW

The second objective in therapy of occlusive peripheral vascular disease is to improve the blood flow. Measures used to increase blood flow include heat, abstinence from tobacco, position, and sympathectomy. Heat is usually applied in the form of a light cradle over the extremities. Mr. Marker was placed in a warm room in which the temperature was maintained at 26.7°C (80°F). At this temperature there is generalized vasodilatation. The humidity was controlled so that 26.7°C (80°F) was not uncomfortable. By maintenance of a warm environmental temperature, the stimulus to vasoconstriction was eliminated. The cradle placed over Mr. Marker's leg was also a heat cradle in which the temperature was thermostatically controlled at 31.1°C (88°F). When this type of cradle is not available and a light bulb is used as a source of heat, no more than a 25-watt

bulb should be used and a thermometer hung in the cradle to check the temperature. The thermometer should be placed where there is little likelihood of the patient bumping it. In any type of cradle, the source of heat should be shielded in order to prevent the patient from inadvertently coming in contact with it. The temperature inside the cradle should not exceed 32.2°C (90°F). The objective is to induce maximum vasodilatation without stimulating metabolism. Should the warm environmental temperature increase the patient's pain, as it sometimes does, the heat should be discontinued and the physician notified. Under these circumstances, the rise in the temperature of the tissue increases its metabolism without a comparable increase in the supply of blood, because a sufficient degree of vasodilatation does not occur.

For many years cigarette smoking has been known to cause vasoconstriction. An interesting observation has been made that when persons who are accustomed to smoking just go through the motions of smoking, their peripheral blood vessels constrict. Any influence causing even temporary vasoconstriction may have an adverse effect on already ischemic tissues. The possibility also exists that in some individuals, the blood vessels are allergic to tobacco. Occasionally a man who stops smoking after an episode characterized by ischemia of peripheral tissues then resumes smoking only to have an exacerbation of the previously quiescent disease. Whether or not tobacco directly enters into the etiology of occlusive peripheral vascular disease, it intensifies its harmful effects by causing vasoconstriction.

People vary in the difficulty that they have in breaking the habit of smoking. Some do it relatively easily; others find it difficult or are unwilling to try. For a person to be successful, he must really want to stop smoking and feel that the discomforts experienced are worth tolerating. The nurse can be helpful to the patient by letting him know that she recognizes how he feels. Some physicians handle the problem of the patient who finds breaking the habit very difficult by suggesting to the patient that he limit himself to one cigarette after each meal and possibly one at bedtime. Others refuse to treat the patient unless he ceases to smoke. In the latter instance, the nurse may find that a patient smokes but tries to conceal his actions. She is then faced with several problems. Her sympathies may be with the patient, but she is committed to carry out the medical regime. The patient has a right to decide to follow or not to follow instructions, provided he is in condition to make a rational judgment. Does the patient fully understand what is at stake? If the patient is confined to bed, surreptitious smoking increases the danger of fire. When a nurse is confronted with this problem, she should try to convey to the patient her appreciation of the difficulty he is experiencing. When appropriate she should attempt to reinforce the physician's explanation of why smoking is contraindicated. She should also bring the problem to the attention of his physician, not because the patient has been bad or disobedient, but because the physician needs to know just as he needs to know of any failure of the patient to respond to therapy.

Position can also be used to improve blood flow. By hanging his foot over the edge of his bed, Mr. Marker secured some relief of his pain. Gravity causes blood, as well as other fluids, to run downhill. A comparable effect might have been obtained for Mr. Marker by elevating the head of his bed on 6-in. blocks.

An electrically operated oscillating (Sanders) bed is used in some hospitals to alternately fill and drain the vessels of the lower extremities. Its use is more or less limited to patients who have ischemia with pain at rest, that is, the pain associated with ischemic neuropathy, and with minor noninfected ulcers or gangrenous lesions. This bed is designed on the same principle as a seesaw. The springs are attached at the center to a fulcrum, so that when one end of the bed is elevated the other is depressed. The rate at which the bed oscillates can be adjusted. According to Horwitz,[81] the maximum increase in blood flow to the toes can be achieved by holding the foot of the bed in the down position for five minutes with the feet at a 20-degree angle from the horizontal. The bed should then be elevated to at least a 5-degree angle above the horizontal for a few seconds to drain the veins. The length of the cycle and the extent to which the bed is lowered and raised in relation to the horizontal are prescribed by the physician. The length of the cycle in a given situation may be modified by individual physicians and the needs of patients. Barker[82] states that the bed should be adjusted so that pallor occurs at the end of the up cycle and the color returns while the feet are in the down, or dependent, position. The patient should have an explanation of why the bed is used and what it is expected to accomplish. Some patients require time to adjust to the motion and to having their heads dependent part of the time. Symptoms such as dizziness, headache, and nausea are believed in many instances to be largely of psychic

origin; nevertheless they cause the patient considerable discomfort. Patients should be assured that these effects are not uncommon and that they usually disappear as the patient becomes adjusted to the bed. A little time spent with the patient, particularly when he is on the bed for the first time, is usually very helpful. A new and frightening experience can be made easier by having an experienced person whom he trusts nearby.

A third method of using position to improve blood flow to the extremities is the Buerger or Buerger-Allen exercises. In these exercises gravity is used to alternately fill and empty the blood vessels. The legs are alternately elevated and lowered with a period of rest between cycles. According to Horwitz,[83] the time that the legs are in the down position should exceed the time they are in the up position by at least 3:1. Some physicians prefer to use the color of the legs as the criterion for determining the length of time in each position. Under these circumstances the legs are kept in the down position until they are red and in the up position until they are blanched or pale. The patient then rests in a horizontal position for a few moments before again placing his legs in the down position. To take the down position, the patient can dangle or hang his legs over the edge of the bed. A well-padded chair or an over-the-bed table may be placed in the bed to support the legs when they are in the up position. Whatever is used as a support must be well padded, and the patient should be cautioned not to bump a foot against it even then. When the patient goes home, he is usually instructed to carry on the exercises. He can use a method similar to the one he used in the hospital or he can support his legs on the end of a sofa or on the wall. The greater the degree of elevation of the legs, the shorter should be the duration of the up position.

Drugs are also utilized to improve the flow of blood to the extremities by lessening vasospasm and thereby improving the collateral circulation. Vasodilator drugs are effective to the degree to which vasospasm is present. The patient who has little or no vasospasm cannot be expected to get much benefit from them. Prolonged action is also required. Short-acting vasodilators, such as nitroglycerine, are not very helpful. One of the most effective in inducing relaxation of the peripheral vessels is ethyl alcohol, but its use is limited by the tendency of patients to develop addiction to alcohol. Some patients object to its use on moral grounds. When some form of ethyl alcohol is prescribed, the nurse should observe the patient for indica-

[81] Orville Horwitz: "Peripheral Vascular Disease," *Long-Term Illness* (Philadelphia: W. B. Saunders Company, 1959), p. 160.

[82] Nelson W. Barker: "Chronic Occlusive Diseases of the Peripheral Arteries," *Heart Bull.,* 8:78 (July–Aug.) 1959.

[83] *Op. cit.,* p. 160.

tions of developing addiction. When request is made for alcohol with increasing frequency, this should be brought to the attention of the physician. The vasodilatory effects of alcohol last about four hours. Sometimes the patient solves the problem of supply by having his favorite brand brought in by a visitor. This is a problem that is seldom easy to handle. The patient secures relief from the alcohol. The fact that he is adding another to his already serious problems may not seem very important to him at the time. Because of the very real possibility of the patient becoming an alcoholic, some physicians rarely prescribe alcohol.

Many other drugs have been tried to improve blood flow by decreasing vasospasm. These include papaverine. Its most frequent use has been to relieve vasospasm that accompanies embolism. Unlike most of the alkaloids of opium, it is not habit-forming. Some patients are benefited by aminophylline (theophylline ethylenediamine) orally, 0.1 to 0.3 g three times per day. Among the newer drugs are a number that lessen or abolish the responsiveness of the alpha receptors to epinephrine or norepinephrine. These drugs are known as *adrenergic blocking agents.* They combine with the effector substance in the cells. The cell is then unable to respond to the chemical mediator released on stimulation of the sympathetic nervous system. The result of the action of adrenergic blocking agents on blood vessels is dilatation.[84] Among a number of drugs available, one example is tolazoline (Priscoline).[85]

When treatment is unsuccessful in preventing gangrene, then amputation becomes necessary. Fortunately, this is required much less frequently than in the past. Most patients view amputation of even a finger or a toe as a mutilating operation. They face the procedure with reluctance and are likely to suffer from a grief reaction afterwards. This is no less true in the patient who has an amputation as a result of gangrene than in the one who loses a part in an accident.

In addition to the occlusion of arteries by a disease process such as atherosclerosis, arteries may be occluded by bodies or emboli floating free in the blood stream. Although fat and air may be responsible, a blood clot or thrombus is the most frequent occurrence. The usual sites for the formation of thrombi are the heart and the large veins, usually the deep veins, in the leg. In the heart the two most frequent causes are atrial fibrillation and myocardial infarction

[84] Ruth D. Musser and John O'Neill: *Pharmacology and Therapeutics,* 4th ed. (New York: The Macmillan Company, 1969), p. 275.
[85] Trade name.

accompanied by mural thrombosis. In atrial fibrillation, blood tends to stand in the atrial appendages. Thrombosis of the deep veins of the leg is associated with prolonged bed rest, childbirth, and systemic infections, and may occur following operation. A portion of the blood clot is dislodged and is carried by the blood until it reaches an artery through which it cannot pass, with the result that it occludes or obstructs the artery. The effect is frequently intensified by widespread vasospasm. The spasm of the arteries may be so great that no blood circulates to the tissues in the affected area. Thus an organic factor, a blood clot, may induce a functional response, vasospasm, that is as injurious or even more so than the clot by itself.

When the blood clot originates in the venous system, it travels to the heart and from there to the pulmonary artery. When the embolus is large or the combination of the embolus and vasospasm prevents blood from entering the lung, death occurs suddenly. When blood flow is maintained to most of the lung, the area deprived of its blood supply undergoes necrosis with the development of a pulmonary infarction. Symptoms are the result of the infarct.

DIAGNOSTIC TESTS

Diagnostic tests used to study the status of blood vessels are of two general types. In one type, the effects of various procedures on function are determined. In the other, measures are used to determine the location and extent of structural change. A variety of methods are used to determine the functional status of the vascular system. Essentially all tests of function involve exposing the individual or a part of his body to a physiological stimulus and then observing his response directly or by means of an instrument.

A rough test of the capacity of an artery or group of arteries to meet the demands of tissues for nutrients and oxygen is whether or not pain and tenderness in the muscle are associated with activity. This may be determined by asking the person how far he can walk before he has pain. It can be determined more exactly by having the person step up and down on a stair step at a predetermined rate. The result is known as the claudication time.

A second method used to determine the adequacy of blood flow is to test the ability of the artery to maintain blood flow against gravity. In a man with pain at rest, such as Mr. Marker, this test provides the physician with valuable information about the degree of failure of his arterial circulation. If pallor develops when the extremity is elevated, this indicates that there is a marked degree of arterial insufficiency. When the extremity is placed in a horizontal or dependent position, a slow rate of filling further indicates arterial insufficiency. Some physicians regard this test as among the most useful in estimating the degree of arterial insufficiency.

In peripheral occlusive vascular disease the physician may wish to determine the response of the blood vessels to physiological stimuli and the degree to which vasospasm is responsible for the signs and symptoms. To determine the degree of vasospasm some method is used to remove the effect of the sympathetic nervous system. Methods include exposing the patient to a warm environment or blocking the sympathetic ganglia or the peripheral nerve supply of the area. The effect of drugs such as alcohol or nicotine (smoking) may also be studied. The changes in blood flow may be determined by measuring the skin temperature, or by the use of instruments such as an oscillometer or a plethysmograph. The oscillometer is a manometer attached to the cuff; it is used to measure the blood pressure. It is employed in a peripheral occlusive vascular disease to determine the point of pressure at which circulation through the deep vessels to the thigh or calf ceases. Essentially the same test may be performed by pressing superficial arteries with the fingers and estimating the amount of pressure required to obliterate the pulse. Neither test provides exact information. The oscillometer is most useful in demonstrating differences between the circulation to the two extremities. The plethysmograph is a more sensitive instrument than the oscillometer. It measures the actual amount of blood entering the tissue.

Skin temperature is determined by a thermometer or thermocouple held in place in contact with the skin. Except when the temperature of the skin on one extremity differs markedly from that of another, the results may not be very valuable. Conditions such as exposure to cold or heat, exercise, the ingestion of food, and the emotional state of the person all influence skin temperature. In an attempt to minimize these factors the test is performed in a warm room with the patient at rest. Other conditions prescribed by the physician should be carefully met. The patient should be apprised of the procedure to be followed and the reasons for what is done.

In addition to determination of the degree to which spasm is present in blood vessels, the assessment of the patient may include the degree to which local or generalized vasospasm can be induced by exposure to cold. The test is usually performed by having the patient plunge his hand and forearm into a container of ice water. Depending on whether the local

or general effects are of interest, the hands are checked for pallor and the other color changes characteristic of Raynaud's syndrome, or the blood pressure is taken. The latter is known as the cold pressor test. Persons who have a greater than average rise in blood pressure are known as hyperreactors.

The location and extent of lesions in blood vessels may be studied by angiography or arteriography. The specific method used in the performance of each test depends on the location of the artery under study. In all these studies a radiopaque substance is injected into the artery. Following this the area is x-rayed. Specific directions for the preparation and aftercare of the patient are given by the patient's physician or the physician performing the procedure.

All diagnostic tests are part of the total evaluation of the effect that a particular disease condition has on the patient. The nurse who cares for the patient has the continuing responsibility to assist in the preparation of the patient for what lies ahead, to assist with or to perform certain diagnostic procedures, and to provide aftercare for the patient. Sometimes a specific regime is required. Often, however, the care required relates more to the outcome of the test than it does to the test itself. When a period of time must elapse between the time the test is performed and the outcome is known, the patient and his family are likely to experience anxiety. Not all patients are relieved by a negative report. Was the test performed properly? What causes his symptoms? When the outcome is unfavorable, the patient is sometimes faced with an uncertain future. The nurse must be prepared to give the patient and his family emotional support and help him (them) learn to carry out the medical regime required.

Many problems of the patient who has an occlusive vascular disease are similar to those experienced by patients with other chronic diseases. Prevention of or delay in the progress of peripheral vascular disease often requires that the patient be willing to modify habits of eating, exercise, and smoking. Treatment and the prevention of serious complications make these measures imperative. Besides, the patient must learn and practice the measures required to protect affected tissues. As in other chronic illnesses, much of the responsibility for continued therapy depends on the patient and his family. Unless they are willing and prepared to carry out the prescribed therapeutic regime, it is likely to fail. The nurse has a responsibility to assist the patient to learn to assume the day-by-day management of his disease and its complications.

Finally, as in other types of illness, the therapeutic regime may fail to effect improvement. Instead of improving, the condition of the patient worsens. The patient still has needs, and something can be done to improve his comfort and well-being. Goals in nursing should be adapted to the needs and status of the patient.

Without the continuous movement of blood throughout the vascular circuit, life ceases. Some of the causes and effects of failure of the heart as a pump (source of power) and of occlusion of the vascular system have previously been delineated and related to the nursing needs of patients. Another crucial factor in circulatory function is the maintenance, within limits, of the pressure of the blood within the blood vessels. The effects of hypotension, or low blood pressure, have been discussed in other relationships and will not be further examined. In the following discussion some of the causes and effects of excessive blood pressure will be considered.

Blood Pressure

As indicated in previous discussion of homeostatic mechanisms, the capacity to regulate the level of the blood pressure within physiological limits is essential to survival. Despite differences in the pressure of the blood in all parts of the vascular system, there is a normal range of pressure for each part. Arterial pressure is greater than venous pressure, but both have a normal range. In the following discussion, unless otherwise specified, references are to arterial blood pressure. As with other homeostatic mechanisms, the blood pressure is not regulated at an exact level, but fluctuates within limits. It varies among individuals as well as in the same person under different conditions. The level of the blood pressure is altered by changes in position, exercise, rest, emotional status, and age. It is slightly higher when the individual is in the sitting or upright position than when he is in the recumbent position. It is higher during exercise than at rest. It often drops during sleep. Emotional states, discomfort, a distended bladder, pain—all have an effect on the blood pressure, particularly on the level of the systolic pressure. Fear, anxiety, and apprehension may influence the level of the blood pressure. In some individuals, they may cause a marked rise.

Age is a significant factor in the level of the arterial blood pressure as it rises gradually from birth to maturity. In many persons it continues to rise throughout the life-span. In the healthy newborn infant the arterial blood pressure is approximately 55 mm of mercury systolic and 40 mm of mercury diastolic. Blood pressure rises rapidly during the first few days of life,

and by the tenth day the systolic pressure is around 78 mm of mercury. Blood pressure then rises gradually until maturity. The average healthy young adult has a blood pressure of about 120 systolic and 80 diastolic. The normal range, however, extends from 90 to 140 mm of mercury systolic and 60 to 90 mm of mercury diastolic. Moia [86] states that a blood pressure of 150 mm of mercury systolic and 90 mm of mercury diastolic is widely accepted as the upper limit of normal. Goldblatt [87] sets 140/90 as the upper limit of normal for persons at the age of 40. Despite more or less general agreement as to the physiological range for arterial blood pressure, there is no exact level below or above which the arterial blood pressure is normal or abnormal. People vary greatly in the capacity of their blood vessels to tolerate pressures above established "normal" limits. The age of the individual at which the elevation occurs is also of some significance. For example, a blood pressure of 160/100 is more significant in a girl of 15 than in a woman of 60.

Another factor making the problem of determining the upper limit of "normal" difficult is that, in many persons, the arterial blood pressure tends to continue to rise over the entire life-span. This is particularly true of the systolic pressure. A blood pressure of 140/90 or higher is found in 40 per cent of individuals between the ages of 45 and 49 and in 60 per cent of those between 60 and 64 years of age. Goldblatt [88] states that in the United States, at least 50 per cent of persons who are over 50 years of age have hypertension, and in at least 25 per cent of all persons above 50 years of age, it plays some part in their deaths. Statistical studies indicate that even a small elevation in blood pressure shortens life expectancy.[89] These statistics have predictive value when applied to a group, but are of less value in anticipating the effect of elevation of the blood pressure in a specific individual. Some persons live to an advanced age despite a considerable elevation in arterial blood pressure. For example, Mrs. Timmins lived to age 88. For some time before her death, her blood pressure was 180/110, and it had been elevated for many years. Despite a marked degree of hypertension and the lack of specific therapy, she had always been well and active. In fact, she appeared to be in better health than many of her younger neigh-

[86] Blas Moia: "The Range of Normal Blood Pressure," *Cardiology,* Vol. 4, Aldo A. Luisado, ed. (New York: The Blakiston Division, McGraw-Hill Book Company, Inc., 1959), §12, p. 15.

[87] Harry Goldblatt: "Mechanism of Hypertension," *ibid.,* §12, p. 30.

[88] *Ibid.*

[89] Metropolitan Life Insurance Company: *Statist. Bull.,* **41**:6 (Aug.) 1960.

bors. For some reason her blood vessels were able to tolerate the increase in pressure without suffering a serious degree of vascular injury. One of the medical problems receiving attention is the finding of some method that will enable the physician to predict which patients with hypertension are most likely to develop progressive vascular disease.

The lower limit of normal is as difficult to define as the upper. Unlike the person whose blood pressure is at or above the upper limit of normal, the one whose blood pressure is below the norm, but who is otherwise healthy, has a better than average life expectancy. A systolic blood pressure of 90 to 100, in the absence of evidence of disease, is not usually regarded as evidence of pathology. In a sick patient a fall in the arterial blood pressure should always be questioned. The level at which blood pressure becomes abnormally low depends on the usual blood pressure. For example, Mrs. Timmins' blood pressure at rest was 190/110. A sudden fall to 120/70, though within the normal range for a healthy person, probably would indicate hypotension. Another patient's blood pressure is usually about 120/70. A blood pressure of 90/50 indicates some degree of hypotension. In the patient who has untreated adrenal insufficiency, blood pressure is usually low. A systolic blood pressure of 90 to 100 is not unusual. Unless the patient is under some kind of stress, emergency treatment is not usually required to elevate the blood pressure. In the patient who has adrenal insufficiency, even what appears to be a minor drop in the blood pressure should be considered as cause for concern and brought to the attention of the physician. In general, a marked or continuing fall in the level of the blood pressure should be regarded as abnormal and measures should be instituted to stabilize or elevate it. Patients who are being treated with hypotensive agents may be an exception. They should, however, be observed for the effects of their therapy. As a general rule, even in these patients, treatment is regulated in order to prevent sudden and marked lowering of the blood pressure. Since the pressure of the blood in the blood vessels is one of the factors in maintaining tissue nutrition, a sharp fall may result in relative ischemia of the tissues. Among the factors to be considered in evaluating the significance of one blood pressure reading are knowledge of the level compatible with the maintenance of a sufficient degree of hydrostatic pressure to maintain tissue nutrition, the height of pressure that arteries are likely to tolerate, and the usual blood pressure of the patient.

As with other homeostatic mechanisms, the maintenance of blood pressure within limits re-

quires a number of structures that are regulated not only individually but also in relation to each other. These components of the vascular system that affect the level of the blood pressure include (1) the viscosity of the blood, (2) the total volume of the blood, (3) the rebound of the elastic material in the arterial wall during ventricular diastole, (4) the total peripheral resistance, and (5) the force with which the heart pumps blood into the arteries. Blood pressure remains stable as long as alterations in one or more factors are effectively opposed by changes in others. For example, a reduction in cardiac output will not result in a fall in the blood pressure if at the same time peripheral resistance is increased. The reverse is also true. When the cardiac output rises, the arterial blood pressure remains stable provided peripheral resistance diminishes; cardiac output also rises in the absence of a compensatory decrease in peripheral resistance. A reduction in peripheral resistance will likewise be accompanied by a fall in blood pressure unless there is a compensatory rise in cardiac output. Among the factors affecting arterial blood pressure, changes in peripheral resistance have the most profound effect. Relatively great changes in blood volume, blood viscosity, or arterial elasticity are required before the level of the blood pressure is altered appreciably.

How is arterial blood pressure regulated?

Although there may be other mechanisms regulating the level of the arterial blood pressure, Guyton [90] lists three: (1) the autonomic nervous system, (2) the kidney, and (3) the endocrine glands. The capillary fluid shift mechanism should be added as it regulates the blood pressure by altering the blood volume.

CAPILLARY FLUID SHIFT

Each of the factors in the maintenance of blood pressure will be examined briefly. The capillary fluid shift mechanism effectively regulates the arterial blood pressure by altering the blood volume. When the arterial blood volume rises, hydrostatic pressure within the capillaries is elevated and fluid is rapidly transferred into the interstitial space. As the blood volume diminishes, the interstitial fluid volume is enlarged, and blood pressure is prevented from rising excessively. Under some circumstances, such as in the seriously burned patient, loss of fluid into the interstitial space in noninjured as well as burned areas may be sufficient to cause hypotension. The reverse process may also take place. With a decrease in the volume of blood,

[90] *Op. cit.,* p. 355.

the pressure of blood in the capillaries falls. Fluid then moves from the interstitial space into the capillary and the blood volume is restored. As blood volume increases, arterial blood pressure is elevated. This mechanism is very important in the protection of the individual against the effects of rapid changes in the blood volume. It may also be a source of danger. A marked increase in blood volume, particularly when combined with an inadequate renal reserve, predisposes to pulmonary edema that can be severe enough to cause death. (See Chapters 9 and 11.) A rapid increase in blood volume also places a burden on the heart and predisposes to high-output failure. Within limits the capillary fluid shift mechanism protects the blood volume and the blood pressure by rapidly removing or adding fluid to the blood.

PERIPHERAL RESISTANCE

Before discussion of the roles played by the sympathetic nervous system and the kidney in the regulation of the blood pressure, the nature of and factors in peripheral resistance will be presented.

Peripheral resistance can be simply defined as the force opposing the movement of blood. The most important factors in peripheral resistance are the arterioles and the small arteries because they have highly muscular walls and small lumens. Even small changes in the diameter of these vessels have a marked effect on peripheral arterial resistance. Guyton[91] states that by reducing the diameter of an arteriole by one half, its resistance is increased as much as 16 times, while a fourfold decrease in arteriolar diameter can increase resistance as much as 256 times. As the lumen of the arteriole diminishes in size, a larger proportion of the blood passing through it comes in contact with the arteriolar wall, which offers resistance to the movement of the blood. As arteriolar resistance or arterial peripheral resistance rises, the diastolic blood pressure is elevated. Usually, but not invariably, the systolic blood pressure also rises with the result that the pulse pressure remains within normal limits.

Although most of the peripheral resistance is due to the opposition offered by small arteries and arterioles to the flow of blood, all blood vessels offer some degree of resistance. A loss of tone in any part of the peripheral vascular bed predisposes to a drop of the blood pressure. From information gained through the use of monitoring equipment, one of the earliest changes in shock is an increase in venous pressure resulting from a loss of muscle tone in the

veins. Peripheral resistance involves two different factors, the mechanisms regulating the tone of the vascular musculature and the responsiveness of the arterial musculature to stimulation. As long as the degree of stimulation and the responsiveness of the blood vessels are within physiological limits, peripheral resistance as reflected by the blood pressure should also be within its normal range. Uncompensated abnormalities in either aspects of peripheral resistance, that is, over- or underregulation of hypo- or hyperresponsiveness of the vascular musculature, can be presumed to result in abnormal alterations in the level of the blood pressure.

The mechanisms regulating peripheral resistance include the sympathetic nervous system and humoral substances which affect vascular tone. Some of the humoral agents are secreted by the endocrine glands, some are formed by the ischemic kidney, and others are formed and act locally. Although a humoral vasodilator with widespread action has been postulated, its presence has not been proved. Certain products of metabolism, such as carbon dioxide, as well as substances released by injured cells, dilate capillaries. These substances are of particular importance in regulating blood flow to the needs of localized tissue areas. As a consequence of a variety of regulatory mechanisms, large organisms with well-developed circulatory systems are capable of adapting peripheral resistance, and as a result blood flow, so that the needs of its cells are met. Under conditions of rest and moderate activity, tissues regulate their own blood supply in accordance with their needs. Under emergency situations or when activity is greatly increased, blood flow can be modified in relation to the needs of the entire individual or to those of a particular or of a specialized tissue.

SYMPATHETIC NERVOUS SYSTEM

The nervous system, principally the sympathetic nervous system, regulates the smooth muscle in blood vessels, causing either vasoconstriction or vasodilatation. As a result of activation of the sympathetic nervous system, there may be generalized vasoconstriction of blood vessels, or those in certain regions of the body may be constricted or dilated. Apparently depending on the degree and type of stimulation, activation of the sympathetic nervous system may result in vasoconstriction or vasodilatation. Although the effect may be general, it may also enable the body to shift blood from one region to another. As an illustration, constriction of the renal arteries limits blood flow through the kidney. Because approximately

[91] *Ibid.*, p. 255.

1,200 ml of blood flows through the kidneys each minute, a reduction to 200 ml will make available 1,000 ml to circulate to more immediately vital organs such as the brain and heart.[92] Because the nervous system acts rapidly, it enables the individual to react quickly and as a whole to changes in the environment and to protect the function of vital organs. Although adjustments in the blood pressure are made rapidly by the nervous system, they are not sustained for a long period of time.

Regulation of the caliber of blood vessels by the nervous system involves higher as well as lower centers.[93] Centers for the regulation of the diameter of blood vessels are located in the cerebral cortex, the hypothalamus, and the medulla. These centers not only regulate the sending of messages to blood vessels in the periphery, usually by way of the sympathetic nervous system, but they also have an inhibitory effect on each other. Impulses arriving in these centers have their origins in receptors located in various parts of the body. Some are located within the vascular system and others are outside it. Among those situated within the vascular system are receptors in the arch of the aorta and in the carotid sinus; they are stimulated by increases in the pressure of the blood. Although they are called baro- or mechanoreceptors, they are actually stimulated by stretching or dilatation of the aorta or carotid sinus. Receptors located outside the vascular system that may initiate impulses resulting in a change in the caliber of blood vessels include those of sight, sound, hearing, heat, cold, touch, and pain. Biochemical changes, such as changes in the pH of body fluids, may stimulate vasomotor centers in the nervous system resulting in changes in the caliber of blood vessels. Because man reacts to symbols or the meaning events have for him, these too may act as stimuli and result in alterations in peripheral resistance and therefore in the level of blood pressure.

With a few exceptions, such as the coronary arteries, the sympathetic nervous system regulates both vasoconstriction and vasodilatation. Vasoconstriction results from an increase in sympathetic activity. Vasodilatation in many regions of the body results from a lessening of sympathetic tone. In some organs such as the coronary arteries and the skeletal muscles, the sympathetic nervous system actively dilates

blood vessels. This is its only effect on the coronary arteries.

Although the regulation of caliber of blood vessels by the nervous system facilitates adaptation to the environment, the lateral sympathetic ganglia can be removed and the individual will survive. His capacity to respond to stresses, such as changing his position from the recumbent to the upright, and to hemorrhage is, of course, reduced. Because increase in the activity of the sympathetic nervous system increases peripheral resistance, it may be a factor in hypertension. Some authorities suggest that although the capacity to constrict blood vessels quickly once facilitated survival, in a protected society such as ours, it may be a handicap.

In regulating peripheral resistance, the action of the sympathetic nervous system is supported by hormones secreted by the adrenal medulla, norepinephrine and epinephrine. Norepinephrine exerts a vasoconstrictor effect, and epinephrine increases the force of cardiac contraction. Both hormones lead to an elevation in blood pressure through their actions on the heart and blood vessels. These hormones probably have little effect on the blood pressure during ordinary activity, but augment the effect of the sympathetic nervous system during stress.

ROLE OF THE KIDNEY IN REGULATION OF BLOOD PRESSURE

A number of factors have contributed to the belief that the kidney has one or more roles in the regulation of the blood pressure. Exactly what its role(s) is (are) has not been proved. Such questions as whether the kidney regulates blood flow through itself are a subject of great interest and of great controversy. The fact that there is some relationship between decreased blood flow through the kidney and the level of arterial blood pressure has been established clinically and experimentally. The classical experiment of Goldblatt demonstrates that obstruction to the flow of blood through the kidney is followed by an elevation in the arterial blood pressure. In the preparation of a Goldblatt kidney, clamps are applied to the renal arteries to limit blood flow to the kidney. After a few weeks the systemic blood pressure rises above the preclamp level, and the blood pressure in the arteries distal to the clamp, that is, within the kidney, also rises. Diseases in which there is a diminished flow of blood through the kidney such as acute glomerulonephritis and chronic pyelonephritis are accompanied by hypertension.

A number of hypotheses have been suggested to explain the apparent role of the kidney in the

[92] Robert F. Pitts: *Physiology of the Kidney and Body Fluids*, 2nd ed. (Chicago: Year Book Medical Publishers, Inc., 1968), p. 151.

[93] Donald E. Gregg, revised by Jay D. Coffman: "Regulation of Pressure and Flow in the Systemic and Pulmonary Circulations," *The Physiological Basis of Medical Practice*, 8th ed., ed. by C. Best and N. Taylor (Baltimore: The Williams & Wilkins Company, 1966), pp. 746–49.

arterial blood pressure. Currently there is evidence that the kidney may affect blood pressure in two different ways: (1) Under certain circumstances the kidney releases an enzyme that reacts with a component in the plasma to form a pressor substance, (2) the healthy kidneys either destroy a pressor substance found in the blood or they release a depressor factor.[94]

Of the two possible roles of the kidney in the regulation of the blood pressure, most is known about the first. Almost 100 years ago it was learned that a substance extracted from the kidney had a pressor or blood pressure-elevating effect. Because of its origin, the material was named renin. Renin has been purified. It is released by a hypoxic kidney into the blood, where it interacts with a serum protein, an aplha-2-globulin that is formed in the liver to form a weak pressor substance called angiotensin I. Angiotensin I is converted by an enzyme found in the blood plasma to angiotensin II, a highly active pressor material. Angiotensin is destroyed by an enzyme, angiotensinase, which is present in the blood plasma and in many organs including the kidney, intestine, and liver. There is considerable doubt among scientists as to whether the renin-angiotensin system functions in the regulation of blood flow through the kidney in health. Its action may well be limited to situations in which blood supply to the kidney is threatened. Whether or not this system plays a role in the development of human hypertension is also a subject of controversy.

ROLE OF HORMONES IN REGULATING BLOOD PRESSURE

Upon stimulation of the vasoconstrictor fibers of the sympathetic nervous system, epinephrine and norepinephrine are secreted. Basically these hormones have the same effect as direct sympathetic stimulation of the cardiovascular system.

The other major hormone to affect the blood pressure is aldosterone. It controls both the extracellular fluid volume and sodium chloride content. Aldosterone acts on the renal tubules by decreasing the amount of sodium chloride excreted in the urine. In turn there is osmosis of water from the renal tubules into the extracellular fluid. As the extracellular fluid volume increases, so does the blood volume, causing the blood pressure to rise. It is apparent that aldosterone plays a major role in the regulation of the blood pressure. As the arterial blood pressure falls, an increased amount of aldosterone is secreted, causing the sequence of events as described previously to take place.

[94] Pitts, *op. cit.,* p. 155.

Hypertension

A so-called normal blood pressure results when the various components within the vascular system are functioning within limits and the regulatory mechanisms are capable of effecting appropriate adjustments among them. That the body is not always able to make appropriate adjustments is attested to by the frequency with which blood pressure falls below or exceeds the levels required to maintain blood supply to the tissues. When the level of the blood pressure exceeds physiological limits, the condition is referred to as hypertension or arterial hypertension. Depending on which component is elevated, it is called systolic or diastolic hypertension. When both the systolic and diastolic blood pressures are elevated, it is called systolic-diastolic hypertension. An abnormal elevation in the arterial blood pressure, or hypertension, is a finding associated with an abnormality of function and sometimes of structure, but it is not a disease per se any more than pain or fever is. Some authorities distinguish between hypertension and hypertensive disease. They employ the words *hypertension* to denote the elevation of the blood pressure in the absence of demonstrable changes in the vascular system and *hypertensive disease* to indicate the presence of vascular disease.

Abnormal elevations in the blood pressure may be of known or unknown origin. In about 10 per cent of persons with hypertension, the elevation of the blood pressure is secondary to some known disorder. In approximately 90 per cent the cause is not known and the disorder is classified as essential hypertension.

Among the disorders known to cause hypertension are

1. Systolic hypertension
   a. Increased stroke volume of the heart
      (1) Anemia
      (2) Thyrotoxicosis
   b. Aortic rigidity (atherosclerosis the most common cause)
2. Diastolic and systolic hypertension
   a. Disorders of the central nervous system
      (1) Diseases of the brain stem and spinal cord (poliomyelitis and tabes dorsalis)
      (2) Increased intracranial pressure
         (a) Neoplasms
         (b) Inflammatory lesions
   b. Disorders of adrenal and chromaffin tissues
      (1) Pheochromocytoma
      (2) Cushing's syndrome
      (3) Primary aldosteronism
   c. Disorders of the kidney (usually in those

disorders in which the blood supply is impaired or there is injury to the parenchyma)

    (1) Acute and chronic glomerulonephritis

    (2) Pyelonephritis

    (3) Disorders impairing the blood supply to the kidney

        (a) Acute renal ischemia

        (b) Lesions obstructing the renal artery (embolic, thrombotic, etc.)

    (4) Urinary-tract obstruction

  d. Toxemia of pregnancy (not discussed)

  e. Coarctation of the aorta

In anemia and thyrotoxicosis the abnormal elevation in the systolic blood pressure is caused by an increase in cardiac output. In either disorder, blood pressure can be restored to normal by correcting the underlying disorder.

Systolic hypertension caused by aortic rigidity is a very common finding among older individuals. By itself it does not usually seriously affect the life of the individual. The elevation in the blood pressure is permanent.

Disorders in the nervous system that impinge on the blood supply of the brain, particularly when they develop rapidly, are usually accompanied by an increase in blood pressure. As the blood pressure rises, there is often a decrease in the pulse rate. The rise in the blood pressure results from the initiation of mechanisms for the maintenance of cerebral blood flow. As such they are protective. A rise in blood pressure in a patient with a lesion likely to threaten the blood supply of the brain, such as an acute inflammatory process, a head injury, or a neoplasm, should always be regarded as indicating the possibility of cerebral ischemia. (See Chapter 15, Part B.)

Hypertension may be caused by disorders involving either the medulla or the cortex of the adrenal gland. Hypertension associated with hypersecretion of the adrenal medulla is usually caused by a tumor of the medulla or chromaffin tissue known as a pheochromocytoma. The pheochromocytoma secretes both epinephrine and norepinephrine. Epinephrine affects the blood pressure primarily by increasing the force of cardiac contraction, and norepinephine, by increasing peripheral resistance by its vasoconstrictor effect. In addition to hypertension, there are usually other manifestations indicating excessive secretion of epinephrine, including palpitation, nausea and vomiting, sweating, anxiety, dyspnea, pounding headache, paresthesia, vertigo, and glycosuria. One patient observed by the author had periodic attacks of anxiety so severe that she was diagnosed as being in an acute anxiety state. Pheochromocytoma causes

one of the curable types of hypertension, because it can be excised surgically. Although the blood pressure may be elevated continuously, periodic attacks of hypertension are common. The diagnosis of pheochromocytoma can frequently be established by the patient's response to phentolamine hydrochloride (Regitine), an adrenergic blocking agent. Following the administration of phentolamine hydrochloride, the blood pressure should drop appreciably, because the drug prevents the effector substance in the arteriole from responding to norepinephrine. In hypertension from causes other than pheochromocytoma, lowering of the blood pressure to a significant degree does not occur.

Both Cushing's syndrome and primary aldosteronism are disorders of the adrenal cortex. Cushing's syndrome results from a neoplasm or hyperplasia of the adrenal cortex. Aldosteronism results from a neoplasm. One possible factor in hypertension in these disorders is that excessive quantities of the adrenocortical hormones, most particularly the mineralocorticoids, desoxycorticosterone, and aldosterone, enhance arteriolar responsiveness. Not only does hypertension occur in disorders accompanied by hypersecretion by the adrenal cortex, but it may be precipitated by desoxycorticosterone administered in the treatment of disease. When desoxycorticosterone was first introduced in the treatment of Addison's disease (chronic adrenal insufficiency), several patients died from complications induced by the effects of rapidly developing hypertension. Persons who have adrenal insufficiency characteristically have low blood pressures.

Not all the relationships of the adrenal steroids to vascular reactivity are known. They act conditionally; that is, their effects depend on the presence of the sodium ion. The reactivity of smooth muscle is affected by the balance of ions within the cells as well as in the extracellular fluid. The adrenocortical hormones affect this balance among ions. Correction of the cause of excessive secretion of adrenocortical hormones is often followed by a restoration of the level of the blood pressure to normal.

In the discussion of the possible role of the kidney in the regulation of arterial blood pressure, the point was made that hypertension is common in any disorder in which the blood supply to the kidney is impaired. It is also found in disorders wherein the parenchyma is diseased. In some instances in which only one kidney is diseased and it is removed surgically, the blood pressure returns to normal. When both kidneys are diseased, hypertension continues.

Finally, a known and curable cause of hypertension is coarctation of the aorta. In this disorder, at some point along the aorta a constricting band reduces the size of its lumen. In some instances, the channel may be so small that a broom straw may scarcely be able to pass through the occluded portion. These patients are hypertensive in the blood vessels above the site of constriction. They are usually hypotensive in those below the constriction. When the site of narrowing can be removed surgically, the blood pressure returns to physiological limits after the obstruction is removed.

ESSENTIAL HYPERTENSION

By far the most frequent type of diastolic and systolic hypertension in the United States is essential hypertension, that is, hypertension of unknown cause. About 90 per cent of persons with hypertension have this type. About 5 per cent of the *population* have essential or primary hypertension. Despite an elevation of the diastolic and usually, though not invariably, the systolic blood pressure, the specific cause for this is not known. The constriction of the arterioles and small arteries is believed to be about equally distributed throughout the body. Schroeder [95] states that three hypotheses have been suggested to account for this vasoconstriction. They are

1. Sympathetic vasoconstrictor nerves are hyperactive.
2. There is a vasoconstrictor substance in the blood which acts directly on smooth muscle.
3. The smooth muscle becomes "sensitized" to normally acting sympathetic nerves or to constrictor substances.

Whether the cause of hypertension is primary or secondary to a specific disease, a rise in the blood pressure causes vascular damage in proportion to the degree of elevation.[96] Although it is generally true that the higher the blood pressure, the greater the damage to blood vessels, the susceptibility of different individuals to the effects of hypertension varies greatly. Some people tolerate markedly elevated blood pressures for a long time without much evidence of vascular damage. Why this is true is not known. As indicated in the discussion of coronary artery disease, hypertension accelerates the rate at which atherosclerosis and arteriolar sclerosis develop.

The serious consequences of hypertension

arise from its effects on the heart, the kidney, and the brain. As the peripheral arterioles narrow, peripheral resistance rises. The heart muscle undergoes work hypertrophy, and for a period of time at least, blood flow to the tissues is maintained within physiological limits. Eventually, for reasons already explained, the heart muscle may fail as a pump. Congestive heart failure eventually occurs in about 25 per cent of persons with hypertension. Myocardial infarction also occurs at an earlier age in hypertensive than in normotensive persons.

That the kidney is involved in essential hypertension is demonstrated by scars found in the kidneys of some persons dying as a consequence of one of the complications of hypertension. In the most rapidly progressive and serious phase of hypertension, changes in the structure of the kidney are invariably found.

Involvement of the blood vessels supplying the brain results in hypertensive headache, hypertensive encephalopathy, and cerebral thrombosis or hemorrhage. Not all persons with hypertension develop any of the cerebral complications. The reason for the headache is not known. It is usually in the occipital region and awakens the patient in the morning and disappears as the day progresses. Caffeine often gives relief.

Cerebral blood flow and metabolism in the tissues of the brains of most patients who are hypertensive are normal. Hypertensive persons are, however, predisposed to the earlier development of cerebrovascular changes than persons whose blood pressures are within normal limits. The result of cerebral hemorrhage caused by rupture of a cerebral artery, or by the occlusion of an artery supplying the brain by a thrombus, is known as a stroke or cerebrovascular accident. The manifestations experienced by the patient will depend on the location and extent to which the brain is deprived of its blood supply. Hemiplegia is a common sequela though it is not inevitable.

The blood vessels in the retina of the eye are also affected. Because they can be observed directly by ophthalmoscopic examination, information about the degree of vasoconstriction and the structural alterations in the arterioles and other vessels can be obtained by direct observation. Papilledema or swelling of the optic disc can also be observed when retinoscopy (the examination of the retina of the eye through an ophthalmoscope) is to be performed by the physician; the patient should be informed that it is a painless procedure. A drop of a cycloplegic is usually placed in each eye to paralyze the iris and the ciliary muscle. The pupils dilate and do not react to light. After the pupils are dilated, the patient will usually experience some

---

95 Henry A. Schroeder: "Biochemical Aspects of Hypertension," *Cardiology,* Vol. 4, Aldo A. Luisado, ed. (New York: The Blakiston Division, McGraw-Hill Book Company, Inc., 1959), §12, p. 20.

96 John H. Moyer: "Blood Pressure Regulation in the Treatment of Hypertension," *Amer. Cardiol.,* 9:821 (June) 1962.

blurring of near vision such as when attempting to read. With short-acting cycloplegics blurring is present for only a short period of time. With long-acting ones, such as atropine, the effect may last for a day or more. In patients with glaucoma, a disorder characterized by elevated intraocular pressure, cycloplegics are not used, because dilatation of the pupil is accompanied by a decrease in the degree of the angle of Schlemm. Drainage of fluid from the globe is thereby decreased and the intraocular pressure is raised. With the elevation in the intraocular pressure, blood flow to the tissues of the eye is diminished and damage to the eye increases. In susceptible patients, the injury may be sufficient to cause blindness. In preparation for a retinoscopic examination the room should be darkened. During the examination the patient who is able to cooperate will be asked to look at a fixed point and not to move his eye. As implied above, retinoscopy is a widely used procedure to determine the condition of the retina and its blood vessels as well as of the optic disc. In addition to information about conditions within the eyeball itself, deductions can be made about the state of the blood vessels throughout the body as well as pressure conditions within the cranial cavity.

For the sake of emphasis, we shall repeat some of the essential points about the nature and effects of essential hypertension. Although a specific cause cannot be identified in essential hypertension, the elevation in the blood pressure is believed to be due to an imbalance between sympathomimetic activity and the responsiveness of small arteries and arterioles to stimulation. With greater vasoconstriction, peripheral resistance is increased and with it the diastolic blood pressure. Some authorities suggest that the initiating event in essential hypertension is an increase in cardiac output. In response to the increase in cardiac output, small arteries and arterioles constrict to protect the capillaries from excessive pressure. Eventually arteriolar constriction becomes the prominent feature. There is also the possibility that arteriolar constriction precedes other changes. In the past some authorities believed that the elevation of the blood pressure followed rather than preceded vascular damage. Presently, however, vascular injury is more generally believed to follow the elevation of the blood pressure. In accordance with this hypothesis, arteriolar hypertrophy is the result of more or less continued contraction of arteriolar musculature. Whatever the sequence of events, arteriolar sclerosis and atherosclerosis develop at an earlier age in hypertensive than in nonhypertensive persons.

Until vascular damage occurs, other than for the elevation in the blood pressure there are often no other manifestations of the disturbance. As a result many persons are discovered to be hypertensive at the time they are examined for insurance policies or for some other purpose. Other cases are not discovered until some vascular catastrophe occurs. Although the organs most frequently involved in the complications of hypertension are the heart, the kidney, and the brain, hypertension is nevertheless a generalized disturbance in which there is excessive constriction of the small arteries and arterioles throughout the body. These changes can be directly observed in the retina of the eye. After complications have occurred, many of the needs of the patient for nursing will be determined by the nature of the complications.

As implied by the previous discussion, hypertension predisposes to vascular damage and with it serious complications involving the heart, kidney, and brain. Despite the frequency with which these conditions are associated, hypertension does not invariably injure blood vessels. There is also a difference among individuals in the length of time their blood vessels will tolerate hypertension before evidence of vascular injury occurs. As stated previously, some physicians classify patients whose blood pressures are elevated, but who do not have evidence of vascular injury, as hypertensives and those with vascular injury as having hypertensive disease. Therefore hypertension may be classified according to the phase or stage of the disease. These various phases include prehypertension, labile, benign, and malignant hypertension. Not all persons go through all phases or progress from one to another.

In the person who is in the prehypertensive phase, the arterial blood pressure is within the normal range most of the time. His blood pressure may be at the upper end of the normal range, however. He differs from nonhypertensive individuals, because he hyperreacts to vasoconstricting stimuli by manifesting a greater and more sustained rise in his blood pressure than do normotensive persons. Studies of the effect of the cold pressor test on schoolchildren indicate that although all children have some rise in blood pressure during the test, some hyperreact to the test by elevating their blood pressures to higher than expected levels. The cold pressor test is performed by determining the resting blood pressure; then the person being tested plunges his arm into a container of ice water. Because cold initiates impulses resulting in increased peripheral vasoconstriction, blood pressure rises. A rise in the diastolic blood pressure has predictive value in terms of later development of essential hypertension. According to Hines,[97] a rise in the level of the diastolic pressure during the cold pressor test predicts the development of sustained hypertension in more than 50 per cent of individuals.

Recently reported studies of the effect of emotional stress on blood pressure indicate that in some persons elevations in the blood pressure are sustained for a longer period of time than they are in others. Not all persons whose blood vessels hyperreact do, however, develop hypertension. If methods could be developed to identify those persons who are likely to become hypertensive, that is, who are truly prehypertensive, perhaps preventive measures could be instituted to delay the onset and progress of the disease.

Some persons have what is known as labile hypertension at the time they come to medical attention. The word *labile* is derived from the Latin word *labilis,* meaning "likely to slip." When used as an adjective to describe a disease or state, labile means unstable. Therefore labile hypertension is unstable; that is, the blood pressure is subject to fluctuation. During periods of stress, the blood pressure may be markedly elevated; when the individual is at rest or relaxed, it may be at or near normal levels. It is not at all unusual for a patient to be admitted to the hospital with a diastolic blood pressure of 110 or more and a systolic blood pressure of 180 or more and after a period of rest to find that his blood pressure has fallen to normal, or nearly normal, levels. These individuals have labile hypertension. Labile hypertension is an important finding inasmuch as it is frequently followed by permanent hypertension. According to Moia,[98] permanent hypertension develops three to five times more frequently in an individual with labile hypertension than in one whose blood vessels do not overrespond. Persons who are in this phase of hypertension may in some instances be able to delay the development of hypertensive disease by appropriate changes in their habits of living.

When patients are admitted to the hospital for the treatment of hypertension, they are usually in the benign or malignant phase of the disease. Formerly benign and malignant hypertension were believed to be two different diseases. Currently malignant hypertension is usually regarded as an accelerated form of hypertension. In the terminal stage of benign hypertension, it may become malignant.

When the terms *benign* and *malignant* are used as adjectives to describe the character of a disease, their true meaning should be remembered. The word benign means kindly. A benign person is kindly. Used to describe the character of a disease, it means that it is relatively harmless. It does not mean that under some circumstances it will not cause harm, however. Benign diseases, including benign hypertension, usually progress slowly. Benign hypertension is defined by Goldblatt[99] as "persistently elevated blood pressure of unknown origin not accompanied by significant renal excretory functional disturbance." In contrast to benign disease, malignant disease endangers the life of the individual, often within a relatively short period of time. At one time a patient with malignant hypertension did not usually survive for more than a year. Because of the availability and use of drugs that are effective in lowering the blood pressure, prognosis in malignant hypertension has improved. The definition of malignant hypertension that follows indicates why the prognosis is guarded.

Malignant hypertension, as defined by the Medical Advisory Board of the Council for High Blood Pressure of the American Heart Association, is as follows: "A clinical phase, rarely occurring de novo, more often appearing after a primary or secondary hypertension, characterized by diastolic hypertension and by accelerated and progressive renal damage, usually (but not necessarily) accompanied by papilledema, often by retinal hemorrhage and 'exudate' and giving rise to death from uremia, unless the course is terminated along the way by complicating brain or heart damage."

As in other chronic disorders involving a failure in a homeostatic mechanism, hypertension probably results from the interaction of a number of factors. Hypertension develops when a combination of necessary and sufficient conditions is present. One factor appearing to predispose to essential hypertension is heredity. The incidence of hypertension is higher among offspring of hypertensive parents or grandparents than among those whose parents or grandparents are normotensive. In persons who are predisposed to hypertension by heredity, elevations in the diastolic and systolic blood pressures can be induced by chilling, frustration, anger, and anxiety. According to Merrill,[100] even the anticipation of a pleasant event may be accompanied by a rise in arterial blood pressure. Although exactly how heredity predisposes

[97] Edgar A. Hines: "The Significance of Vascular Hyperreaction as Measured by the Cold-Pressor Test," *Amer. Heart J.,* **19**:412 (April) 1940.

[98] *Op. cit,* §12, p. 17.

[99] *Op. cit.,* §12, p. 31.

[100] John P. Merrill: "Hypertensive Vascular Disease," *Principles of Internal Medicine,* 5th ed. (edited by T. R. Harrison *et al.*) (New York: The Blakiston Division, McGraw-Hill Book Company, Inc., 1966), p. 706.

to hypertension has not been settled, one hypothesis is that it determines the responsiveness of the smooth muscle in the small arteries and arterioles to sympathomimetic agents.

Among other factors seeming to predispose to hypertension, or to aggravate it, are obesity and type of gender, race, body build, and personality. Hypertension is somewhat more common among women than men, but women tolerate it better. Women who are hypertensive are likely to be obese, but men do not differ in weight and stature from the ordinary population. Essential hypertension has a higher incidence and develops at an earlier age among Negroes living in the United States and in Panama than it does in Caucasians and Indians. Negroes also have a higher incidence of the disease in the accelerated or malignant form. Authorities have somewhat different views on the relationship of personality to the development of essential hypertension. Merrill [101] states that the majority of patients with hypertension have disorders of personality which may be made worse by environmental or emotional stress. Fluctuations in blood pressure of these patients can be correlated with changes in the emotional state in the individual.

Cardon [102] agrees that efforts to describe a personality pattern exclusively and always present in patients with hypertension have not been successful. He lists a number of characteristics that have been observed by different investigators. They are "(1) neurotic traits, (2) excessive dependency needs, (3) poorly handled feelings of hostility, (4) difficulties in inter-personal relationships, (5) excessive rigidity, and (6) easily injured or afraid of injuring others." Other writers describe the hypertensive person as being excessively anxious. All the above characteristics may be observed in normotensive persons. Furthermore, not all hypertensive persons manifest these traits. Another observation that may prove to be of some significance is that persons whose hypertension is associated with a specific cause show the same behavior as those with essential hypertension. Moreover, emotional tension, which is common among these persons, is relieved by surgical or chemical treatment that is effective in restoring them to a normotensive state. The behavior of hypertensive individuals may in some instances be caused by the disease, rather than be the cause of it.

The possibility that the kidney is responsible for hypertension has been extensively debated for many years. Evidence cited in support of the kidney's role includes the fact that the incidence of hypertension is higher among women than among men. Because the incidence of pyelonephritis is also higher among women, a possible relationship is suggested. Diseases of the kidney, particularly those in which the blood supply is impaired or the parenchyma is diseased, are accompanied by hypertension. The ischemic kidney is known to produce a pressor substance or a precursor to a pressor agent. Against the hypothesis is the fact that although some persons with hypertension do have kidney disease, by no means do all.

SUMMARY

At the present time the specific factors in the etiology of essential hypertension are not known. The factors contributing to the disorder appear to be caused by an imbalance between sympathomimetic activity and vascular responsiveness.[103] There is disagreement among authorities, however, about the degree to which each of these factors is responsible. Although there are specific disorders in which hypertension is associated with increased sympathomimetic activity or with increased vascular responsiveness, in most persons with hypertension the specific cause of the hypertension cannot be identified. Whatever its role in the genesis of hypertension, an increase in sympathomimetic activity aggravates pre-existing hypertension. This fact has many implications for nursing.

As a consequence of constriction of small arteries and arterioles, peripheral resistance is increased; the diastolic pressure is increased. Essential hypertension induces pathology by increasing the work of the myocardium and accelerating the rate at which atherosclerosis develops. Despite its generally deleterious effects, some individuals are able to tolerate hypertension for many years.

Although knowledge of specific causation is lacking, much can be done to slow the progress of hypertension and to prevent the development of its complications. The fact that an individual's blood pressure is or is not within the normal range is easily determined. The procedure has become so common and is so generally accepted that at least one mail-order catalogue offers: "Sphygmomanometer takes your blood pressure. No fuss, no bother, no office visits when you want a reading. Directions are also given for its use and the cost—only $19.95." A blood pressure determination is a part of almost all screening as well as diagnostic examinations.

[101] Ibid., p. 711.

[102] Philippe V. Cardon: "Psychic Factors in Essential Hypertension," Cardiology, Vol. 4, Aldo A. Luisado, ed. (New York: The Blakiston Division, McGraw-Hill Book Company, Inc., 1959), §12, p. 9.

[103] John H. Moyer: "Etiology of Hypertension," Amer. J. Cardiol., 9:651–52 (May) 1962.

How is hypertension treated?

When the blood pressure is found to be elevated, the physician tries to establish the etiology. When a specific condition that can be cured is found associated with hypertension the blood pressure can usually be expected to return to normal levels after treatment of the disorder. In patients who have incurable disorders or essential hypertension, the same degree of specificity in treatment is not available. In general, controlling and delaying the progress of the disorder—not curing it—are the principal objectives. Merrill [104] emphasizes the importance of remembering that a patient, not just an elevated blood pressure, is being treated.

There is as much disagreement among physicians as to who should be treated for hypertension and how they should be treated as there is about which factor or factors is/are responsible for its development. Different physicians hold opposing views and all shades of opinion in between. Most physicians agree that the patient in the accelerated phase of the disease should be treated. Because the patient in the accelerated phase has a high diastolic pressure and rapidly progressing lesions in the retina and kidney, he should be treated with any measure that is successful in lowering blood pressure. Methods used in the therapy of hypertension include supportive or intensive psychotherapy, diet, drugs, surgery, and modifications in the mode of life. The principal objective of all these forms of therapy is to lower the blood pressure by lessening vasoconstriction. After the blood pressure is lowered, a regime is established in an effort to maintain it within normal or near-normal limits. This objective is based on growing evidence that elevation of the blood pressure has a damaging effect on blood vessels.

Among all the types of therapy, psychotherapy is sometimes used. For most patients psychotherapy is in the form of constructive physician- and/or nurse-patient relationship. In some instances patients do undergo intensive psychotherapy. According to Merrill,[105] the results are at least as good as those of other forms of treatment. Knowledge is not yet available about whether treated patients continue to remain normotensive. After intensive psychotherapy is initiated the patient must continue treatment as long as indicated, since there is the possibility that the hypertension will be exaggerated for a time after therapy is initiated. For the patient to benefit, he must continue under treatment through this period and until the therapy is completed.

Supportive psychotherapy is administered by the patient's own physician and by others in his environment. Writers describing the characteristics of the manner of the physician use words such as quiet and calm manner, confidence, patience, and enthusiasm to indicate a helpful approach to the patient. These characteristics would seem to be no less important to the nurse.

As in other chronic disorders, one of the important objectives of therapy is to help the patient learn to cope with his disease. This objective may be stated as, "to assist the patient in the identification of situations in his life causing him to constrict his blood vessels and to then help him to learn to handle these situations so that they do not result in vasoconstriction." The attitudes of the patient toward his life, work, home, religion, members of his family, the neighbors, his co-workers, and other persons all affect the level of his blood pressure. Each patient may be expected to react to different aspects of life differently; a factor that is a cause of stress in one individual may not be so in another. What the hypertensive patient should be helped to do is to identify those things that cause him to constrict his blood vessels and then try to modify his reaction or change the situation. Sometimes this is relatively easy. For example, Martha Brown, whose blood pressure was 190/120, found that as she approached a red traffic light, she became tense and angry. She acted as if the red light were a personal affront. By starting ten minutes earlier than usual in the morning and making a conscious effort to relax her muscles when a light turned red as she approached, she was able to remove this one stimulus to vasoconstriction. Other problems required other approaches. For example, her desk at work was near that of a woman who irritated her excessively. One solution was to resign; or she could request to move into another office. Because neither of these choices was practical, Miss Brown decided, insofar as she could, to ignore the woman's remarks and to try to find the reason for her own excessive reactions to her. Another cause of stress to Miss Brown was the fact that because her invalid mother lived with her, she felt she could not take a vacation. Miss Brown recognized that, despite her protestations to the contrary, she resented not being able to take a vacation. As a result she decided to talk to her married sister about the possibility of the sister caring for their mother while Miss Brown spent two weeks at a vacation resort and of relieving her one weekend each month. With regular relief from the responsibility for her mother, her resentment diminished and her day-to-day relationship with her mother improved. The level of her blood pressure also fell. The nurse and the physician, by their manner and interest,

104 *Op. cit.*, p. 711.
105 *Ibid.*

helped Miss Brown to identify the circumstances in her life contributing to her hypertension. They were also able to suggest possible alternatives available to her. They encouraged her to continue to try to modify her behavior and approach to the troublesome aspects of her life. They could not, however, alter the circumstances in Miss Brown's environment; only Miss Brown could do that. They could and did provide her with support when she needed it.

In addition to the problems the patient brings with him at the time the diagnosis is established, the fact of hypertension is often fear-provoking. Recently the author was with Mrs. Willow when her physician told her that her blood pressure was normal. After the physician left, Mrs. Willow turned and said, "In that case, I do not have to worry about a stroke and becoming paralyzed." Mrs. Willow's son responded in a similar manner when his mother told him her blood pressure was normal. The possibility of a stroke is not an uncommon fear among hypertensive persons. A stroke and paralysis are, of course, not inevitable. They can also occur in the absence of hypertension. Should the patient express this fear to the nurse, she should try to convey to the patient her acceptance of his feeling. She should also bring to the attention of the physician the fact that the patient is afraid that he will have a stroke and be paralyzed.

When a hypertensive patient is hospitalized for diagnosis and treatment, the nurse should try to control the physical and psychosocial environment of the patient so that the stressful situations are kept to a minimum. According to Janis [106] most patients find distressing procedures easier to bear if they do not have to know about them too far in advance. Then they should be told only the necessary details. Relating all the possible sources of stress is, obviously, impossible. Two having particular pertinence are the exact level of the blood pressure and inappropriate remarks made in the presence of the patient.

In many hospitals and physicians' offices only the physician tells the patient what the level of his blood pressure is. Patients react differently to this practice. Some patients accept the statement that the nurse is not permitted to tell them. Other patients are distressed by the refusal of the nurse to provide them with the desired information. In this event, the nurse should relay the desires of the patient to the physician. She should also try to convey to the patient her understanding of his feelings, but in this matter she must defer to the wishes of his physician. There are several reasons for the desire of the physician to control the informa-

[106] Irving L. Janis: *Psychological Stress* (New York: John Wiley & Sons, Inc. 1958), pp. 386–87.

tion given to the patient. A single blood pressure reading apart from others is not highly significant. There is also some virtue in all the information about the patient and his progress coming from one source. Most patients know or soon learn what the hospital policies are in respect to their care. Sometimes they ask the nurse for information she cannot give them, to test her. They may be reassured by the suggestion of the nurse to ask their physicians. Because people are individuals, the nurse should try to evaluate the effect of withholding information from the patient. When it appears to lead to an increase in anxiety, this should be discussed with the physician.

Patients may also be subjected to unnecessary stress by hearing thoughtless or tactless remarks or by hearing "their case" discussed, as if they were not present. Physicians state in their writings that patients need stability, reassurance, and confidence; yet the advantages and disadvantages of various hypotheses about cause and treatment may be discussed in detail in the presence of the patient. When this happens, the nurse has a responsibility to remind the physician or physicians, tactfully to be sure, but firmly, of the presence of the patient. Nurses should also exercise care in what they say in the presence of the patient.

The patient with hypertension is affected by the same general causes of stress as other patients in the hospital environment. Noise, confusion, lack of knowledge of what to expect, discourtesy, visitors, unfamiliar routines, lack of routine, uncertainty about diagnosis, lack of confidence in persons providing care, concern about family—all are among the many possible sources of distress to the patient. Although causes of unnecessary stress should be identified and eliminated for all patients, this is particularly important for the patient who is hypertensive.

For most persons with essential hypertension, control is a lifetime endeavor. In a broad sense, hypertension can be compared to diabetes mellitus and other chronic disorders. Much can be done to delay its progress and prevent complications, but few persons are cured. Control involves developing a way of life that lessens the tendency to constrict blood vessels. Moderation should be the watchword. Excesses of all types should be avoided. This includes excesses of eating, smoking, and working. For the patient who is free of complications, exercises such as walking, swimming, calisthenics, golf, bicycleriding, and fishing are generally recommended. The form of exercise selected should be based on the desires of the patient. Exercise should be a pleasure, not a punishment. Moreover, it should be undertaken in the spirit of attaining relaxation and not for the purpose of excelling. Once impairment of cardiovascular function is evidenced, physical exercise should be carefully regulated. During periods when the blood pressure rises to critical levels, bed rest may be prescribed for a week or two.[107]

In addition to exercise, persons with essential hypertension require regular periods of rest and relaxation. In the early stages of the disease, the person should plan to spend eight hours in bed and, if possible, to relax after each meal. He must be aware of nervous tension and practice consciously relaxing his muscles. One suggestion sometimes made to a patient who is learning to relax is to consciously tense the muscles of a part of his body such as an arm and hand. After it is forcefully contracted, he then consciously lets it become limp. Telling most patients that they must relax frequently is of little value. They need specific help and encouragement in learning how to relax. The physician may also prescribe a mild sedative such as phenobarbital or one of the newer tranquilizing drugs to make relaxation easier.

For persons with a mild and nonprogressive type of hypertension, supportive psychotherapy with attention to the mode of living of the patients may be all that is required in therapy. Patients with more severe types, however, require other forms of therapy. Among these is diet. All hypertensive persons should limit their caloric intake to the quantity required to maintain normal weight and strength. Excess calories should be avoided as well as other excesses. Weight reduction should be carried out in all patients who are overweight. In any program of weight reduction an important goal is for the patient to develop habits of eating compatible with the desired weight.

In addition to the restriction of calories to the quantity required to maintain normal weight and strength, sodium intake may also be restricted. This is based on the observation that salt plus the adrenal mineralocorticoids can result in hypertension. In early hypertension, salt intake is not usually greatly restricted. Particularly in the later stages it may be. In the rice-fruit diet of Kempner[108] the sodium content may be as low as 150 mg per day. This diet consists of rice, raw and canned fruits and juices that may be sweetened with substances such as honey and syrups. No salt may be added to this diet. For the rice diet to be successful, it must be continued for four to six

weeks. Because of its monotonous character, some patients refuse to continue it for the required time, although others do. Physicians also vary in their enthusiasm for this diet. Many state that most patients will not continue it for any length of time. Some also emphasize its inadequacies, one of which is for protein; it contains only 15 to 30 g of protein per day. Although vitamin deficiencies can be prevented by the daily administration of vitamin pills and capsules, the pills are usually a source of sodium. In the selection of the degree of salt restriction most physicians try to follow the dictum of Griffith,[109] who is of the opinion that diet should be a source of pleasure and not another source of stress. Emphasis should be on what to eat rather than on what not to eat. Flavoring agents that do not contain salts of sodium may be used as desired. The patient requires the same general instructions as any patient on a sodium-restricted diet.

Patients whose sodium intake is limited over a long period of time, especially when restriction is combined with sodium-depleting diuretics, are in danger of excessive salt depletion. Although evidence of sodium deficiency may occur at any time, it is most likely to be precipitated by conditions accompanied by increased secretion of sweat. For example, with the advent of hot weather the patient develops one or more of the following manifestations: marked weakness, nausea, vomiting, and collapse. The physician should be notified promptly. Therapy is to correct the sodium deficiency by increasing salt intake.

Drug Therapy

Drugs having hypotensive effects have been available for some time. There are a variety of new, potent hypotensive drugs that can be used alone or in combination to lower the blood pressure to any desired level. Besides lowering the resting blood pressure, an effective drug should lower the blood pressure during exercise and, ideally, during stress situations. The drug should not have undesirable side effects nor should it interfere with the intellectual or physical working capacity of the patient when it is administered in therapeutic doses. In some patients it is not possible to lower the blood pressure to a sufficient degree and at the same time avoid all side effects. When the blood pressure must be lowered, the patient may, therefore, have to tolerate the side effects of the drug, if he is to be adequately treated.

One of the most important groups of drugs used in the treatment of hypertension is the

[107] Charles K. Friedberg: *Diseases of the Heart,* 3rd ed. (Philadelphia: W. B. Saunders Company, 1966), p. 1493.
[108] Fairfax T. Proudfit and Corinne H. Robinson: *Proudfit and Robinson's Normal and Therapeutic Nutrition,* 13th ed. (New York: The Macmillan Company, 1967), p. 640.

[109] George C. Griffith: "The General Approach to the Treatment of Patients with Diastolic Hypertension," *Amer. J. Cardiol.,* 9:824 (June) 1962.

saluretics (sodium-excreting diuretics). Either mercurial diuretics or thiazide preparations may be prescribed for this purpose. At present, the trend is to use the thiazide preparations first and to reserve the mercurials for patients in whom the thiazide preparations are no longer effective. In addition to increasing the elimination of sodium, thiazide diuretics are antihypertensive. This action is probably independent of their saluretic effect. The thiazides also potentiate the action of the antihypertensive drugs with the result that they can be prescribed in lower dosages and their side effects can be minimized. Therefore, the thiazide diuretics are often prescribed with a hypotensive drug. One possible side effect of some of the newer diuretics such as the thiazides is that in some people they cause *photosensitivity reactions.* Persons who are taking one of these preparations should observe areas of skin exposed to the sun for reddening or other symptoms indicating skin irritation. Should sensitivity of the skin to sunlight develop, the physician should be notified. The local lesions may be treated with topical medications. Usually the offending medication is discontinued and another drug substituted. The skin should be protected from the rays of the sun and sensitized persons should be warned not to use sun or ultraviolet lamps.[110]

Chemicals classified as hypotensive agents act by a number of mechanisms. Some, such as Alpha-methyldopa (Aldomet), interfere with the synthesis of catecholamines (epinephrine and norepinephrine). Others, such as reserpine, guanethidine, and bretylium, are catecholamine depleters. Still others, such as guanethidine and bretylium, are also sympatholytic agents. Although used extensively in the past, the ganglionic blocking agents are no longer used to any extent. Sedatives such as phenobarbital or one of the tranquilizing agents may also be prescribed for their relaxing effect and to diminish the degree to which the individual responds to stress.

Table 10-2 gives some information about drugs currently being prescribed for their hypotensive effects.

For some hypotensive drugs therapeutic and toxic dosages overlap. Most of them are highly potent drugs and cause undesirable side effects that may make their use difficult in a particular patient. The patient, therefore, requires careful observation. For example, rauwolfia compounds sometimes cause mental depression. Any patient who is receiving one of these preparations should be carefully observed for evidence of depression. Because it may not occur immediately, but may be delayed for as long as a year, observation over an extended period of time is required.

Some drugs, such as the sympatholytic and ganglionic blocking agents as well as the decarboxylase inhibitors, cause postural hypotension. Patients who complain of dizziness or feel faint when they assume the upright position should be taught to rise slowly, in order to prevent syncope (fainting). Until it is known whether or not the patient manifests this side effect, he should be assisted out of bed. If the patient develops postural hypotention, the physician should be acquainted with this fact.

Diarrhea is a troublesome side effect of some of the sympatholytic agents. The problem is less severe with guanethidine than with bretylium tosylate.

During the initial phase of treatment, the decarboxylase inhibitors cause drowsiness in about one third of patients. Patients receiving alpha-methyldopa (dihydroxyphenylalaline) or another similar preparation should be warned not to drive cars during the time when drowsiness is present. Fortunately, this effect usually disappears after a period of time. Patients may also develop a mild depression and psychiatric complaints such as a feeling of unreality. When these side effects develop, they should be reported to the physician. Usually they are not severe enough to be handicapping to the patient.

To lessen the possibility of side effects, a number of drugs may be given in combination. In the hospital, the problem faced by the patient is "swallowing all those pills." When the patient receives a large number of pills, attention should be given to the possibility of distributing them more frequently, but in smaller numbers at one time. When he is at home, he is responsible for selecting, counting, and evaluating their effects. At times he may feel like a walking pharmacy without a pharmacist. In a report of a study of elderly patients taking drugs at home, Schwartz [111] enumerates some of the problems they encounter as well as some procedures found to be helpful. Among the types of errors made by patients were the following: "(1) a medicine was taken by the patient, but not ordered by the physician; (2) a medicine was ordered by the physician, but not taken by the patient; or (3) a medicine ordered by the physician was taken but in incorrect doses or at the wrong time (when time was a significant factor) or with a total lack of understanding of its purpose." Schwartz,[112] in discussing the role of the nurse in helping the newly discharged or ambulatory patient, states that the nurse must

---

[110] Morton Fuchs: "The Pharmacology and Clinical Use of Diuretics in the Treatment of Hypertension," *Amer. J. Cardiol.,* 9:827 (June) 1962.

[111] Doris Schwartz: "Medication Errors Made by Aged Patients," *Amer. J. Nurs.,* **62**:51 (Aug.) 1962.

[112] *Ibid.,* pp. 52–53.

TABLE 10-2

Hypotensive Drugs

Type of Action	Forms	Action and Results of Action	Side Effects and Undesirable Aspects
Catecholamine depleters	Reserpine (rauwolfia) Guanethidine Bretylium tosylate	They deplete the store of catecholamines in the brain, myocardium, and vessel walls.	Mental depression should be carefully watched for. May occur months or even a year after drug therapy is initiated.
	See below for further information about the latter two drugs	Lower peripheral resistance. Exact mode of action not known.	
Sympatholytic agents	Bretylium tosylate		Absorption unpredictable. Many patients develop tolerance. No parasympathetic depression, but diarrhea common presumably because of lack of sympathetic damping effect on the parasympathetics.
	Guanethidine. Used in combination with saluretics. Preferred to bretylium. Effective in small dosage. Effects prolonged.	Supposedly blocks the postganglionic transmission of norepinephrine to the vascular receptors. The drug interferes with the release of the chemical mediators at the myoneural junction. As indicated above, also depletes the store of peripheral catecholamines. Little or no tolerance developed.	Postural hypotension. Worse in the morning and improves in the day. A few patients develop diarrhea. See above.
Decarboxylase inhibitors	Alpha-methyldopa (Aldomet *). Used in combination with the saluretics.	Diminish the in vivo production of catecholamines (norepinephrine) through competitive inhibition with the decarboxylase, an enzyme catalyzing the conversion of dopa to dopamine. Not known whether its hypotensive effect is due to its interference with the synthesis of norepinephrine.	Not always effective and it is not always possible to predict whether it will be effective

Some patients develop a tolerance to it

Postural hypotension in some patients

Drowsiness in initial phases of treatment

May be depression and psychiatric complaints such as feelings of unreality

Some physicians consider it to be superior to other antihypertensive agents |

* Trade name.

understand the regimen prescribed by the physician. She must also determine the extent to which the patient understands his part in his therapy as well as how he proposes to carry it out. She suggests that nurses ask themselves the following questions: "What evidence do I have that my patients understand any better or act any differently? How can I find out what they think and do? How can I help them to remember? Would medication calendars or other visual aids be useful? Are there unexplored ways of reminding patients?" What Schwartz is asking is, how effective is our instruction of patients? Do we really know? How can it be made more effective? As long as we accept what we do without question, we cannot know whether it is effective or not, nor will better approaches be developed.

Depending on the seriousness of the patient's illness and other factors, treatment may or may not require that he be hospitalized. Eventually, however, he will have to assume the major responsibility for the management of his disease. Unless the patient is hospitalized, he and his family must carry out the therapeutic regime. He must make periodic visits to his physician so that his progress can be checked and the regime modified as required by his condition. The assumption of responsibility by the patient at home can often be facilitated by one or more visits by a public health or visiting nurse. Even when the patient is given detailed instructions while he is in the hospital or in the office of the physician, he is likely to have some problems at home. The visiting nurse can help him to resolve his difficulties and to increase his confidence in his own competence. Family members also require preparation and assistance in learning what to do and in acquiring the necessary knowledge and skill.

To illustrate some of the problems encountered by the patient after discharge, let us consider Mrs. Pine, who has been in the hospital for the treatment of rapidly progressive essential hypertension. She is a 59-year-old widow whose income is barely sufficient to meet her essential needs. Although her chronological age is less than that of the patients studied by Schwartz, what reason is there to believe that she will find coping with a complicated medical regimen easy? Because hypertension is accompanied by injury to the vascular system, Mrs. Pine may be older than her age in years. Also in common with many other persons, she is frightened by the diagnosis "high blood pressure." Added to the manifestations indicating a high degree of anxiety before her diagnosis was established is the anxiety engendered by the implications of hypertension and a relatively expensive and complicated regimen. Although both her physician and nurse reviewed her therapeutic regimen with her and she had some practice in taking her own blood pressure, what assurance did either of them have that she would be able to follow the following medical regime?

1. Phenobarbital, 30 mg three times daily. One tablet to be taken at 8 A.M., 1 P.M., and 10 P.M.
2. Reserpine, 0.5 mg daily. Because this is supplied in 0.25-mg tablets, she was to take two tablets.
3. Hydrochlorothiazide, U.S.P. (Esidrix [113]), 25 mg after breakfast and 25 mg after lunch each day.
4. Multivitamin capsules, two daily.
5. Digitoxin, 0.1 mg daily.
6. A low-sodium diet. No salt was to be added to her food during preparation, and foods in which salt was used in their processing were to be eliminated.
7. She was to spend ten hours in bed each night.
8. She was to take her own blood pressure each morning and to notify her physician should her blood pressure fall below 150/70.

Before Mrs. Pine left the hospital, all the details of her regimen were carefully presented to her. With the exception of having taken her own blood pressure twice, she had had no practice in selecting the drugs to be taken or in planning her menu. When she obtained the drugs at the pharmacy, she was shocked at their cost. She was bewildered by their number. She wondered whether they were really necessary and how she would manage to keep track of all of them. After she arrived home, she was visited by Mrs. Always, who knew the exact remedy to control high blood pressure. Mrs. Always was so convincing that Mrs. Pine was sorely tempted to try her prescription: dried spinach powder dissolved in sea water and the elimination of tomatoes from her diet. Fortunately, Miss Visiting Nurse arrived the next day and went over her plans with her. Between them they worked out a plan for the medicine schedule that made the treatment program somewhat less burdensome. Meal plans were made. Mrs. Pine took her own blood pressure and then Miss V. N. checked it for accuracy. Mrs. Pine also had an opportunity to ask Miss V. N. about the effectiveness of spinach powder in the treatment of high blood pressure. As Miss V. N. left she promised to return the next day to see how Mrs. Pine was progressing.

[113] Trade name.

In patients in whom the preceding methods of treatment are unsuccessful, sympathectomy may be done. Because the drugs that are now available are highly effective, sympathectomy is seldom performed. The procedure involves either the resection of preganglionic vasoconstrictor fibers or the removal of some or all of the sympathetic ganglia. In general the less extensive operations are performed in preference to the more extensive procedures. The surgeon tries to remove enough of the sympathetic nervous system to lower the blood pressure effectively without severe postural hypotention resulting. Care of the patient after sympathectomy relates to the fact of surgery and the possibility of postural hypotension.

Complications

The complication of hypertension that is unique to the disorder is hypertensive encephalopathy. Encephalopathy is not limited to hypertension of any specific etiology, because it is very frequent in patients with acute renal disease, such as acute glomerulonephritis. It also occurs in toxemia of pregnancy (a serious complication in pregnancy) and in rapidly progressive malignant hypertension. Signs and symptoms include rapidly rising blood pressure; visual disturbances progressing to blindness; papilledema; vomiting; coma; stertorous breathing; psychosis; and convulsions. Because the damage to the brain is not permanent, the patient may recover from hypertensive encephalopathy, provided that he does not die in acute heart failure. Many of the patients with this condition are children or young adults. In caring for patients who are predisposed to hypertensive encephalopathy, the nurse should check the blood pressure of the patient not only regularly as prescribed by the physician, but at any time the condition of the patient appears to be worsening. Should the blood pressure be found to be rising, the physician should be notified and treatment initiated immediately. Unless the nurse is alert and acts promptly, the patient may die needlessly, because there are chemical means available to lower the blood pressure.

In children and some young adults, vasospasm may be lessened by the intramuscular injection of a 50 per cent solution of magnesium sulfate; 0.2 mg is administered per kilogram of body weight. It may be repeated every four hours to keep the blood pressure within a reasonable level. Later, when the most critical period is past, up to 30 ml of a 50 per cent solution may be administered orally two to three times per day. The child should be observed for increasing somnolence and respiratory difficulties. Some physicians prescribe large dosages of protoveratrine A and B or reserpine (Serpasil [114]).

SUMMARY

Hypertension is a commonly occurring condition affecting a high percentage of persons over 40 years of age. Its frequency increases with age. Although systolic hypertension occurs, the most serious type is associated with an elevation of the diastolic blood pressure. Diastolic hypertension may be of specific or nonspecific cause. The latter is known as essential, or primary, hypertension. Despite differences in causation, there are many similarities among hypertensive persons. The mechanism or mechanisms initiating and perpetuating diastolic hypertension appear to be related to some imbalance between sympathomimetic activity and vascular responsiveness. Authorities disagree about the significance of each factor in causation. They also disagree about the harmful effects of the elevation of the blood pressure on vascular integrity. Although hypertension does not kill directly, complications involving the heart, brain, retina, and kidney cripple and kill a large number of persons prematurely.

Therapy is directed toward helping the person adjust his life and habits of living so that he protects his blood vessels from overconstriction. Moderation in all aspects of life is recommended for persons suffering any degree of hypertension. For those persons with moderate and severe hypertension, therapy with drugs and diet is added to lessen directly or indirectly the degree of vasoconstriction.

Hypertension is similar to other chronic diseases because continued control is necessary. The burden of the therapeutic regime is eventually borne by the patient and his family. The nurse has a responsibility to help the patient consider his alternatives and to provide him with needed support and instruction.

As in other disorders requiring some degree of modification in the life of the individual, not all persons respond as physicians and nurses would like them to do. Some persons become so anxious that their entire attention is centered on their illness and themselves. There are others who have no wish to alter their way of living in order to gain a few more months or years of life. Steinbeck [115] describes both types of adjustment to illness. In his statement that he prefers quality to quantity, Steinbeck makes his feelings about modifying his life quite clear. It is also clear that he has a rationale for making

[114] Trade name.

[115] John Steinbeck: *Travels with Charley* (New York: Bantam Books, Inc., 1963), pp. 19–20.

his choice. When the patient selects a course contrary to that prescribed by the physician, the nurse may feel that she or the physician has been inadequate or failed in some respect. Neither is necessarily true. The patient does have a right to choose among the possible alternatives and to have his choice respected.

Although not all the answers to the problems created by essential hypertension have been found, there is optimism that in time they will be. Furthermore nothing slows progress more than blind acceptance of the status quo.

PULMONARY HYPERTENSION

In the preceding section hypertension occurring in systemic arteries has been considered. Hypertension, however, occurs not only in the systemic arteries, but in the pulmonary arteries as well. Because of differences in the characters of the pulmonary and systemic arterial beds, the causes and consequences of pulmonary hypertension differ from those of systemic hypertension. The term applied to pulmonary hypertension is pulmonary heart disease or cor pulmonale—cor meaning heart and pulmonale, lung. Spain [116] prefers the term "pulmonary hypertensive heart disease." He defines chronic cor pulmonale as "that form of hypertrophy of the right side of the heart (with or without congestive failure) that develops secondary to diseases of the lung, pulmonary blood vessels, chest cage or primary pulmonary hypertension." Some authorities also include in this classification pulmonary hypertension that is secondary to mitral stenosis and certain forms of congenital heart disease.

According to Resnik and Branscomb,[117] pulmonary hypertension resulting from disease of the lungs is one of the most frequent causes of congestive heart failure in the United States, and it has an even higher incidence in Great Britain. Its frequency appears to be related to the incidence of long-standing chronic bronchitis associated with emphysema. With an increase in the occurrence of these two conditions, the incidence of cor pulmonale is also expected to rise.

The causes and effects of pulmonary hypertension differ from those of systemic hypertension. Whereas blood is circulated through the systemic arteries under a relatively high blood

pressure, the pulmonary circulation is a relatively low-pressure system. Three factors are responsible for the low pressure: (1) the walls of the pulmonary arteries contain relatively little muscle, (2) they are highly distensible, and (3) there is a large reserve of vessels. Were it to be fully dilated, the pulmonary vascular bed would be capable of holding the entire blood volume. Mechanical and other functional factors are therefore more important in controlling pressure in the pulmonary arterial system than in the systemic circulation. Either increased blood flow or resistance to blood flow may result in pulmonary hypertension. Both factors may be contributing. The effects of these two factors on pulmonary blood pressure are explained by the following physical principle: When blood or other fluid flows through a cylindrical tube in layers (laminar flow), the volume of fluid passing per unit of time is directly proportional to the differences in pressure at the two ends of the tube and is inversely proportional to the resistance to flow factors hindering flow. In terms of this principle, pulmonary hypertension may result from any condition in which more blood is ejected by the right ventricle into the pulmonary vascular bed than is removed from it by the left ventricle, or from disorders increasing resistance to the flow of blood through the pulmonary vascular bed.

In addition to other effects of right heart failure, the problems created by pulmonary hypertension result primarily from the effect of an increase of blood and fluid in the lung on the capacity to oxygenate the blood and to remove carbon dioxide. The increase in bronchial secretions associated with pulmonary congestion interferes with oxygenation of the blood and removal of carbon dioxide. The outcome of a patient with pulmonary hypertension depends on the factors in causation as well as the degree of loss of cardiac reserve.

The nursing care problems that have been discussed previously relate to the needs of a patient as an individual or human being, (1) who has congestive heart failure, (2) who has anoxia (hypoxia), (3) who has hypercapnia (problem eliminating carbon dioxide), or (4) who has increased bronchial secretions.

SUMMARY

Cor pulmonale (right ventricle hypertrophy and congestive heart failure) is rising in incidence, and it is expected to continue to rise. It is associated with disorders in functions of the heart and lungs that increase blood flow or resistance to circulation through the pulmonary circulation. The effects differ from those of systemic hypertension because the pulmonary circulation is a low-pressure system. In addition

[116] David M. Spain: "Pathology of Chronic Cor Pulmonale," *Cardiology,* Vol. 4, Aldo A. Luisado, ed. (New York: The Blakiston Division, McGraw-Hill Book Company, Inc., 1959), §13, p. 23.

[117] William H. Resnik and Ben V. Branscomb: "Circulatory Disorders of the Lung," *Principles of Internal Medicine,* 5th ed., T. R. Harrison *et al.,* eds. (New York: The Blakiston Division, McGraw-Hill Book Company, Inc., 1966), p. 928.

to the systemic effects of failure of the right ventricle as a pump, congestion of blood in the pulmonary circulation predisposes to hypoxia and hypercapnia, which are worsened by the fact that the bronchiolar tree responds by increasing secretions. This is a very fine example of how function of one system affects that of another. Prevention depends on the elimination of conditions predisposing to disorders such as emphysema.

Finally, for the function of the circulatory system to be achieved without acceleration of the rate at which the blood vessels deteriorate, the pressure of the blood must be maintained within certain limits. Blood pressure results from a variety of factors regulated so that pressure in the system is maintained within limits and the needs of cells are met, not only during rest, but in activity. Systemic and pulmonary hypertension differ in causes and effects, but both are significant causes of disease, disability, and death.

Blood

A third element in transportation is the blood. Whereas the heart and blood vessels provide the power and the channels through which blood circulates, as well as the site of exchange between the blood and the interstitial fluids, blood is the vehicle by which materials are distributed. In addition to its significance in the transportation of substances between the cells and the external environment, the blood has a number of other functions. Blood flow is so regulated that homeostasis of body fluids is maintained. The blood participates in the maintenance of its volume and composition by regulating the functioning of organs such as the bone marrow, endocrine glands, liver, and spleen. A self-sealing mechanism protects against the loss of blood after the disruption of the wall of a blood vessel. The blood also plays a significant role in the defense system of the body. Many functions of the blood and results of their failure are discussed in detail in other chapters. Other than for a brief or summarizing review, most of the content presented in the succeeding pages will relate to the erythrocytes and thrombocytes.

Although the functions of the heart, blood vessels, and blood are interdependent, they are often classified as two different systems. The heart and blood vessels comprise the circulatory system, and the blood is part of the hematopoietic system. The hematopoietic system includes not only the circulating blood, but the red bone marrow, the lymph nodes, the spleen, and the reticuloendothelial cells, which are scattered throughout the body. One of the important sites in which reticuloendothelial cells are found is the liver. With the obvious exception of the circulating blood, the structures listed above are sites where blood cells are formed or destroyed or both. Some, such as the spleen, serve as reservoirs for the storage of blood. The liver not only forms red blood cells in the embryo, but it stores some of the materials required for the formation and maturation of blood cells. It synthesizes blood proteins, which are essential components of blood plasma and are necessary to maintain an effective osmotic pressure of the blood.

The Components of Blood

The blood is a highly complex fluid in which the blood cells are suspended. The fluid or plasma comprises about 54 per cent of the total blood volume and the cells about 46 per cent, but these figures are subject to some variation. In women the percentage of cells is somewhat lower than in men, the average being about 42 per cent. The proportion of cells to the total volume of blood is determined by centrifuging whole blood. The cells settle to the bottom of the tube, and the length of the column of cells or fluid can be measured. The result is reported as a whole number, such as 42 or 48. The number indicates the percentage of the blood that is cells and is called a hematocrit. For example, Mr. Bok's hematocrit is 47. This means that his blood cells comprise 47 per cent of his total blood volume. The other 53 per cent is plasma. Following blood loss, blood volume may be maintained by an increase in the blood plasma, and the hematocrit may fall below the lower limits of normal. After the loss of water from the body, such as following severe burns or excessive diaphoresis (sweating), the hematocrit rises. The proportion of cells to blood plasma is increased.

PLASMA

The plasma and its constituents are examined in detail in Chapter 9, and the present discussion of them will therefore be limited. The plasma is an essential part of the blood. Its high water content (it is over 90 per cent water) enables the plasma to dissolve and carry in solution a large variety of organic and inorganic substances between the cells and the external environment. It also contains the blood proteins—albumin, globulin, and fibrinogen—as well as internal secretions, antibodies, and a variety of enzymes. Water in the plasma and other body fluids participates in the regulation of body temperature.

CELLS

The cells in the blood are of three types: the erythrocytes, or red corpuscles; the leukocytes, or white blood corpuscles; and the thrombocytes, or blood platelets. The leukocytes are part of the system of defense of the body. They are discussed in Chapter 6.

The number of each of the various types of cells in the blood is determined by a balance between the production and destruction of cells. Because the number of cells per unit of blood is regulated automatically, and the cells are maintained within well-defined limits, this is another example of a homeostatic mechanism. As with other homeostatic mechanisms, the equilibrium between blood cell production and destruction may be unbalanced resulting in a loss of homeostasis. The effects will, of course, depend on the type of cell involved and in some instances on the cause of the failure. Because of the liquid nature of the blood, cells and plasma may be lost more rapidly than they can be replaced. When the loss of blood is rapid, circulation is threatened by the loss of blood volume as well as by the loss of cells.

Not all changes in the level of blood cells indicate a failure in homeostasis. In fact, a failure to alter the number of cells would point to such a failure. For example, the number of leukocytes rises above normal levels in response to certain threats to the organism. This is true in acute appendicitis or in an acute infection caused by one of the pyogenic cocci. The total number of leukocytes is expected to be elevated. The polymorphonuclear leukocytes, particularly the neutrophils, are responsible for the rise. Inasmuch as the increase in cells represents an appropriate response to a stimulus—threat of injury to cells—it is homeostatic. This conclusion is further supported by the fact that the cells involved are defensive in nature and their number returns to normal levels once the threatening agent is removed. Although the number of cells is increased and many of the cells are not fully mature, they are in a normal stage of development. The cells are released into the circulation before they are fully mature. The number of erythrocytes may also be increased above the so-called normal range in response to a chronic deficiency of oxygen such as in congenital heart disease or at high altitudes. A failure of the organism to increase the number of blood cells in response to an appropriate stimulus is indicative of a failure in a homeostatic mechanism.

In blood dyscrasias, that is, in disorders of the blood, the number and/or character of one or more of the blood cells is abnormal. Moreover, the alteration in the number cannot be explained as a normal response to a threat to the organism. For example, in leukemia both the number and character of white blood cells are abnormal. Except in late stages of the disease, the number is usually markedly increased and the cells are both abnormal and immature. In sickle cell anemia, the erythrocytes contain an abnormal hemoglobin and are abnormal in shape, that is, they are sickle-shaped. Under certain conditions they undergo increased destruction with the result that their number falls to below normal levels. Cells may be poorly or abnormally constructed, so they are too fragile or too resistant to destruction. In familial hemolytic anemia, erythrocytes are abnormally fragile. They are therefore subject to increased destruction. In hemophilia the victim may bleed to death because his thrombocytes are abnormally resistant.

What types of failure of function of the blood occur?

The disorders in function resulting from the blood dyscrasias include the following:

1. Failure to maintain the constancy of the fluid environment of cells. (See Chapter 9.)
2. Failure to transport substances required by the cells for metabolism or to remove the products of metabolism.
3. Failure to combat successfully the agents of infection. (See Chapter 5.)
4. Failure of the self-sealing mechanism.

Possible etiological factors in blood dyscrasias include genetic abnormalities, neoplasia of the bone marrow, deficiency of materials required to form the various constituents of the blood, failure of the bone marrow, infection, blood loss—acute or chronic—and allergic responses of the bone marrow. As with other tissues, the causes of some abnormalities have not been explained. The effects associated with each disturbance are related to the function of the particular component involved and the rapidity with which the condition develops.

The needs of the patient with a disorder involving the blood will be affected by the nature and effects of the disturbance as well as its possible outcome. The person with the disorder is no less important than is his disease.

ERYTHROCYTES

With the preceding discussion as a background, the role of erythrocytes in the body economy as well as the causes and effects of abnormalities will be explored. The erythrocyte is a biconcave disc with an average diameter of about 7.2 μ and a thickness of about 2.2 μ at its thickest part and of 1 μ or less in its center. It is sometimes described as a bag that is capable of great change in shape as it passes through capillaries. Although the erythrocyte lacks a nucleus, it carries out metabolic functions. For this reason, Ley [118] states that it is a living, but specialized, cell.

The average number of erythrocytes in a healthy man is approximately 5 million cells per cubic millimeter of blood with a range of ± 600,000. In women the figure is slightly lower, with the average being about 4.5 million. The range in women is also slightly narrower than in men, being about ± 500,000. Hemoglobin content also varies with sex and from individual to individual. The average for men is about 16 g per 100 ml of blood. For women, it is about 14 g.

The erythrocyte has several important functions. First, it transports hemoglobin and, by means of it, conveys oxygen from the lung to the tissues. Second, the erythrocyte contains large quantities of carbonic acid. As a consequence the transport of carbon dioxide from the tissues to the lung is facilitated. A third function of the erythrocyte is the buffering effect of the hemoglobin and the electrolytes contained in the cell. According to Guyton,[119] the erythrocyte is responsible for about 70 per cent of the buffering action of whole blood.

The sites in which erythrocytes are formed change from embryonic to adult life. In the first weeks of fetal life erythrocytes are formed in the primitive yolk sac. Later the liver serves as the principal site for their formation, though they are also formed in the spleen and lymph nodes. As the fetus matures, the site of formation of erythrocytes shifts to the bone marrow, and by the time of birth, it is the main site of erythrocyte production. The bone marrow continues to be the site of formation throughout the remainder of the life-span. Until the time of adolescence, the bone marrow in the shaft of long bones functions in erythrocyte production. After about the age of 20, it becomes quite fatty and produces no more erythrocytes, and red cell production takes place primarily in the flat bones such as the vertebrae, skull, sternum, and ribs. Because the productive bone marrow gradually lessens in amount throughout the life-span, a mild anemia is not infrequent in the aged. In emergency situations in which large numbers of red cells are required, bone marrow that has stopped producing cells may become productive.

In the formation of erythrocytes, two factors are of significance; the cell itself and the hemoglobin in the cell. Many complex processes are involved in the formation of both. Many substances must be available and a number of enzymes are required to catalyze the reactions involved in the formation and maturation of the cell and its hemoglobin. In the process of development the cell goes through a number of stages. The reticulum cell in the bone marrow forms a primordial cell known as a hemocytoblast. This cell is nucleated and it does not contain hemoglobin. In the next stage, the synthesis of hemoglobin is begun. As the cell develops, the nucleus shrinks in size, and the quantity of hemoglobin increases. The cell, at the stage in which the nucleus disappears and a full complement of hemoglobin is present, is known as a normoblast. Most cells contain no nuclear material at the time they enter the circulating blood. They are fully mature erythrocytes. A few cells containing fine strands of basophilic material do find their way into the blood, however. They are known as reticulocytes. Normally, they comprise about 2 per cent of the total circulating erythrocytes. Following hemorrhage or the treatment of anemia they may account for 10 per cent or more of the total number of erythrocytes. Because they are less mature forms of erythrocytes, the presence of an increased proportion of reticulocytes to mature erythrocytes following treatment of anemia is taken as an indication of a rise in red cell production or erythropoiesis.

ANEMIAS

Failure of the bone marrow to produce erythrocytes in adequate numbers results in anemia. This failure may be caused by a congenital defect in which the bone marrow fails to develop or may be the result of injury to the hematopoietic (blood-forming) tissues at some time following birth. In either instance, hematopoietic tissues may be absent or insufficient in quantity. Red bone marrow is either entirely or partly replaced by fatty or yellow marrow. In the absence of any evidence of hematopoietic activity, the bone marrow is said to be aplastic. Bone marrow showing less than normal activity is hypoplastic. In the absence of red cell-producing tissue, all types of blood corpuscles, erythrocytes, granulocytes, and thrombocytes will be decreased in number. The patient will have not only anemia, but granulocytopenia and thrombopenia as well. The consequences will depend on the cause of the condition. In a patient in whom there is an acute depression of the bone marrow, survival may depend on whether or not he can be protected from infection and hemorrhage until his bone marrow recovers from injury.

[118] Revised by Dorothy C. H. Ley: "The Red Cells or Erythrocytes," *The Physiological Basis of Medical Practice*, 8th ed., ed. by C. Best and N. Taylor (Baltimore: The Williams & Wilkins Company, 1966), p. 480.

[119] *Op. cit.*, p. 111.

Aplasia and Hypoplasia

There are many possible causes of aplasia or hypoplasia of the bone marrow. Bone marrow may fail as a terminal event in leukemia or as a result of metastasis of malignant neoplasms from other parts of the body. The bone marrow is highly sensitive to a variety of chemical and physical agents. Wintrobe [120] divides these agents into two groups: (1) those that inevitably cause aplasia or hypoplasia of the bone marrow if they are given in sufficient dosage and (2) those that cause bone marrow injury in some persons and not in others and are therefore thought to be caused by an idiosyncrasy. Among the agents falling in the first category are those utilized in the therapy of malignant neoplasms. They include all forms of ionizing radiation, nitrogen and sulfur mustards, triethylenemelamine (TEM), urethan, and the antimetabolites such as folic acid compounds. Aromatic fat solvents such as benzene (benzol) are used in many industries and are toxic to the bone marrow. Unless adequate precautions are taken to protect those using these agents, sufficient quantities may be inhaled to cause hypoplasia or aplasia of the bone marrow.

Among agents in the second group is a large group of chemicals including a number of drugs. Aplasia or hypoplasia of the bone marrow occurs occasionally in individuals after exposure to one of a number of drugs or other chemical agents such as insecticides. Among the drugs most frequently associated with aplastic or hypoplastic bone marrow are the arsenicals used in the treatment of syphilis, the antithyroid drugs, antihistamines, trinitrotoluene, and preparations of gold. Insecticides have also been implicated. Before prescribing a drug reported to be associated with the development of hypoplasia or aplasia of bone marrow, it is imperative that the physician weigh the possibility of danger to the patient against the possible good. Moreover, the greater the possibility of injury, the greater the need for accurate observation and follow-up of the patient. The nurse has a further obligation to participate in public education to prevent needless use of or overexposure to drugs or insecticides. Children, as well as other members of the family, should be protected from the careless handling and use of drugs.

In addition to healthy hemopoietic cells in the bone marrow, blood production depends on an adequate supply of materials needed for the formation, maturation, and release of cells. In general these do not differ from those required by other cells. They include amino acids to form the stroma of the red cell as well as the globin portion of the hemoglobin. Besides the usual requirements for materials in cell formation, iron is an essential part of the hemoglobin molecule.

Hemoglobin is formed, therefore, only to the extent that iron is available. In the presence of iron deficiency, each erythrocyte receives less than a full quantity of hemoglobin and is smaller than normal, or microcytic. Because the hemoglobin is usually decreased out of proportion to the number of erythrocytes, the color index is less than normal and the cells are pale in color. The term *hypochromic,* which means having too little color, is used to describe this characteristic of the blood. In anemias caused by iron deficiency the blood is characterized by a greater decrease in hemoglobin than in erythrocytes; small or microcytic cells; low color index; and hypochromia.

Sources of iron include organ and lean meats, egg yolk, and shellfish. Certain fruits and vegetables are good sources provided that they are eaten fairly frequently. The fruits include apricots, peaches, prunes, grapes, and raisins. Among vegetable sources of iron are green leafy vegetables, whole-grain cereals, enriched cereals, and dark molasses.[121]

Absorption of iron from the gastrointestinal tract is regulated, and once iron is absorbed, there is no mechanism for its elimination. Somewhat over one half of the iron in the body is in the hemoglobin. About 10 per cent is in the form of myoglobin. The remainder is stored in the liver, kidneys, spleen, and bone marrow.[122] Iron deficiency may result from an inadequate intake or absorption or from the loss of blood, particularly chronic blood loss. In the United States, deficiency caused by inadequate intake of iron may be less common than it once was. Enrichment of cereals and flours with iron is primarily responsible.

Attention to infant nutrition and the early addition of iron-containing foods have lessened the incidence of iron-deficiency anemias in young children. In the past and in the present among children reared in families with limited incomes, anemia was and is frequently found in the child of 1 year or 18 months of age. Ronny Little illustrates how a limited diet leads to anemia. Ronny, a slender, pale child of 18 months, was admitted to the hospital acutely ill from a respiratory infection. On examination he was found to be anemic. Investigation of his diet showed that except for orange juice,

[120] M. M. Wintrobe: "Agranulocytosis and the Pancytopenias," *Principles of Internal Medicine,* 5th ed., T. R. Harrison, ed. (New York: The Blakiston Division, McGraw-Hill Book Company, Inc., 1966), p. 644.

[121] Robinson, *op. cit.,* 13th ed., pp. 121–22, 765–807, 808–10, 811–16.
[122] *Ibid.,* pp. 119–121.

his food intake was limited to milk and a limited amount of a refined cereal. Because the iron content of milk is low, Ronny's intake of iron was insufficient to meet his needs. To prevent iron deficiency, mothers are advised to introduce egg yolk and other iron-containing foods into the dietary of the infant at an early age. One of the problems in the nursing of Ronny was to enlarge his food intake to include egg yolk, liver, and meat and to help his mother understand why these foods were important. Mrs. Little also needed some assistance in selecting an adequate diet and in budgeting a limited income to cover essential needs.

At the beginning of the century, iron-deficiency anemias caused by an inadequate intake of iron were common in the United States. Today they are more likely to be associated with chronic blood loss. One common factor predisposing to loss of blood is ulcerative lesions—whether benign or malignant—of the gastrointestinal tract. Even when the quantity lost at one time is small, a blood loss continued over time leads to development of anemia. In disorders involving the gastrointestinal tract, food intake is likely to be limited by a poor appetite or nausea. Vomiting and/or diarrhea may further aggravate the problem by removing ingested food from the alimentary canal before absorption can take place. Another source of anemia caused by blood loss is the female reproductive tract. Lesions involving the lining of the uterus and cervix and excessive menstruation are common factors. In areas where hookworm disease is endemic and going barefoot is practiced, anemia caused by blood loss also occurs. In the iron-deficiency anemias, the erythrocytes are of smaller than normal size. The number of red cells may be at normal or near-normal levels. However, the number may be less than average. The cells are of small size, or microcytic, as a result of insufficient iron to form hemoglobin and the anemia is called a microcytic anemia. In iron-deficiency anemias therapy is directed toward two objectives, to determine the cause and to correct the deficiency of iron. In the accomplishment of the latter objective, the simplest and least expensive salts of iron, such as ferrous sulfate, are said to be as effective as more complicated and expensive preparations. Some patients develop diarrhea when iron therapy is initiated. Should diarrhea occur, the drug should be temporarily discontinued and then restarted in small dosage. As the patient develops tolerance for iron, the dosage can be increased. Because iron is incompletely absorbed from the gastrointestinal tract, much of it is excreted in the stool and the stool is black in color. The patient should be told to expect this so that he will not be frightened. Persons whose food intake has been poor in iron should also be encouraged to increase the intake of iron-containing foods in their diets. This is not always easy to accomplish. Habit, limited income, misconceptions about the effects of certain foods, and lack of energy associated with ill health often interfere with any appreciable change in the diet. In the elderly, loneliness and eating alone add to the problem of securing an adequate intake of food.

Other minerals such as copper and cobalt have been demonstrated to be essential in hematopoiesis in experimental animals. Cobalt is a component of vitamin B_{12}. Because the required quantity of these substances is small, the possibility of a deficiency in man is remote.

A third factor or group of factors in the production of blood is the B vitamins. Many years ago Castle postulated that some substance in the diet is essential to the maturation of erythrocytes. He called it the extrinsic factor. Later the extrinsic factor was identified as vitamin B_{12} (or cyanocobalamin). Vitamin B_{12} is required for the growth of all cells in the body. A deficiency is accompanied by the depression of growth in all the cells in the body. Because erythrocyte-forming tissues grow and proliferate rapidly, the production of red cells is markedly inhibited. A lack of vitamin B_{12} has two effects on red cell production. The rate of production is slowed, and the cells that are formed are abnormal. The cells are larger than normal and they are also abnormal in construction. The cell membrane is poorly formed and very fragile with the result that the cell is more easily destroyed than healthy cells. One characteristic of anemias associated with marked deficiency of vitamin B_{12} is a lemon yellow color of the skin caused by increased destruction of erythrocytes. The stroma of the red cell is also thought to be abnormal. Mature red cells are not only larger than normal, that is, they are macrocytic, but they vary in size and shape. The presence of large numbers of deformed red cells is indicated by the term *poikilocytosis*. The term *anisocytosis* refers to the marked variations in size. In conditions in which vitamin B_{12} is deficient, mature red cells are generally larger than normal (macrocytic), a large proportion of them are deformed (poikilocytic), and they vary in size (anisocytic). Their cell membranes are unusually fragile with the result that the cell is destroyed sooner than a normal erythrocyte. Because the erythrocytes are poorly formed in vitamin B_{12} deficiency, vitamin B_{12} is said to be a maturation factor. Without it, the red cells are incapable of maturing normally.

Despite defects in the maturation of red blood cells in vitamin B_{12} deficiency, the formation of hemoglobin is normal and the red cells contain a full complement of hemoglobin. One hundred ml of erythrocytes (not whole blood) contain 34 g of hemoglobin. Because the cells are macrocytic, the proportion of hemoglobin to whole blood is reduced less than is the number of erythrocytes. The color index is therefore greater than one and the cells appear to be more highly colored than ordinary erythrocytes.

Unlike iron-deficiency anemias, most anemias resulting from a lack of vitamin B_{12} do not result from an inadequate intake, but from failure of absorption. Failure of absorption can be demonstrated by the Schilling or a similar test. This test is based on the discovery that the cobalt in vitamin B_{12} can be labeled, by making it radioactive. The radioactive vitamin B_{12} is administered by mouth and the urine is then collected and tested for radioactivity. Normal individuals excrete from 11 to 26 per cent of the dose within 24 hours. Excretion in patients with anemias caused by failure to absorb vitamin B_{12} is much reduced. There may, in fact, be no excretion of radioactive material.

Pernicious Anemia

An ample supply of B_{12} is provided by a small intake of animal proteins. Absorption is dependent on a mucoprotein or some substance bound to the mucoproteins in the mucus secreted by the stomach. This factor was named the intrinsic factor by Castle. It combines with vitamin B_{12} and makes it more soluble, thus facilitating its absorption. In the absence of the intrinsic factor, the absorption of vitamin B_{12} is poor. The most common cause of lack of the intrinsic factor is atrophy of the gastric mucosa. It is most frequently associated with pernicious anemia. Until the underlying defect of pernicious anemia was discovered, it led to a disabling illness and death, which accounts for the word *pernicious*. Despite the inability to cure this form of anemia, it can now be controlled by regular injections of vitamin B_{12}. Although there are individual differences, anemia and other effects of deficiency can be prevented in most persons by monthly intramuscular injections of vitamin B_{12}. Vitamin B_{12} is stored in the liver and released as needed for the maturation of erythrocytes. As stated earlier, it is also required by other cells and its deficiency in the young leads to poor growth. One of the most serious consequences of its deficiency is the development of degenerative changes in the nervous system.

The discovery of the therapy of pernicious anemia is one of the classics of American medical science. In 1925 Whipple reported a study made for the purpose of finding a method for creating a constant anemia in dogs. In 1926

Minot and Murphy introduced the treatment of pernicious anemia with liver. For the liver to be effective, the patient was required to ingest at least a pound and a half of raw or lightly seared liver each day. Some patients found this treatment almost as distasteful as the effects of the disease. Efforts were made to disguise the taste by mixing ground, raw liver with grape or orange juice. Methods were soon found to dry the liver without destroying the anti-pernicious-anemia factor, as it was called. The role of the stomach in the pathogenesis of pernicious anemia was reported by Castle in 1929.[123] He observed that the lining of the stomach of patients with pernicious anemia was atropic. Subsequently, a preparation of pig stomach was prepared to be taken orally. Not too much time elapsed until an extract was made from liver tissue that could be injected intramuscularly. Because it was made from beef liver, it contained foreign proteins to which some patients became hypersensitive. Unless crude liver extract was injected deep into the muscle, it was also likely to cause a foreign-body reaction, with the formation of an abscess. In 1948, vitamin B_{12} was isolated in pure form and identified as a chemical entity. It has now supplanted liver extracts in the treatment of pernicious anemia. It prevents not only the macrocytic anemia characteristic of pernicious anemia, but the degenerative changes in the nervous system as well.

Once the diagnosis of pernicious anemia is established in a patient, the manifestations of the disease can be corrected and controlled for the rest of his life by regular intramuscular injections of vitamin B_{12}. In the beginning, vitamin B_{12} may be administered at weekly or biweekly intervals. Later the interval can be lengthened to monthly or even bimonthly. The need for the patient to continue these injections for the rest of his life cannot be emphasized too strongly. In the present state of knowledge, no methods for the primary prevention of pernicious anemia are available. Methods for the prevention of the harmful effects are, however, highly successful. It is one of the best examples of a chronic disorder that cannot be cured, but can be well controlled. The patient should be encouraged to continue treatment and medical supervision for the rest of his life. Whether or not patients with macrocytic anemias associated with other disorders such as cirrhosis of the liver will have to continue to take vitamin B_{12} for the remainder of their lives depends on the nature of the condition predisposing to it.

Mrs. Oaks is an excellent example of the pa-

[123] W. B. Castle: "Development of Knowledge Concerning the Gastric Intrinsic Factor and Its Relation to Pernicious Anemia," *New Eng. J. Med.,* **249**:603 (Oct. 8) 1953.

tient who has had a long history of pernicious anemia. She is now 89 years of age. Despite her present state of ill health, this stems not from the presence of pernicious anemia for more than 40 years, but from other disorders. She became aware of symptoms of pernicious anemia at about 50 years of age. Manifestations of pernicious anemia are uncommon before 30 years of age. Mrs. Oaks has many of the characteristics of persons developing this disease; she is blue-eyed and has a light skin. Although she is now white-haired, in her youth she was a golden blonde. When asked, she states that she grayed early. Early graying of the hair is also frequently observed. Pernicious anemia is more common in blue-eyed blondes who are of Scandinavian descent or from the British Isles or other northern European countries. It is less common in dark-skinned individuals, though it does occur. Mrs. Oaks is of German descent. Her father died from the effects of pernicious anemia. A family history of this disease is not at all unusual. As in other persons with pernicious anemia, the mucosa of Mrs. Oaks' stomach is atrophied with the result that it does not secrete the intrinsic factor. Neither does it secrete hydrochloric acid. The finding of a macrocytic anemia in a patient with persistent achlorhydria, even after the injection of histamine, is highly suggestive of pernicious anemia. Despite the association of achlorhydria with pernicious anemia, it is not responsible for the anemia, nor does it cause the degenerative changes in the nervous system. Many patients, and Mrs. Oaks is one of them, have indigestion that is corrected by the regular replacement of hydrochloric acid with meals. It has no effect on any other manifestation of the disease, however. With the atrophy of the lining of the stomach, secretion of mucus and hydrochloric acid both fail.

At the onset of illness Mrs. Oaks presented the usual manifestations of pernicious anemia. She complained of weakness and a sore tongue that was beefy red in appearance. She had some numbness and tingling of her fingers. On examination of her blood, macrocytic anemia with both anisocytosis and poikilocytosis was found. Her red cell count was 2 million cells per cubic millimeter of blood. Her hemoglobin was about 9 g per 100 ml of blood. Other characteristic changes in the blood in pernicious anemia, that were not determined at the time the diagnosis was made for Mrs. Oaks, are granulocytopenia with relative lymphocytosis, and thrombocytopenia. The thrombocyte count usually is down to 60,000 to 70,000 cells. About two days following the intramuscular injection of crude liver extract, her reticulocytes had risen sharply. About 15 per cent of the total number of erythrocytes were reticulocytes. Later the percentage of reticulocytes fell as the number of mature erythrocytes increased. Shortly after vitamin B_{12} was demonstrated to be effective in the treatment of pernicious anemia, it was substituted for liver extract in her treatment.

Accompanying the response of Mrs. Oaks' bone marrow to treatment was improvement in her general state of health. Soreness of her tongue was relieved. Because Mrs. Oaks was not acutely ill, she was treated in the office of her physician. Patients with degenerative changes in the nervous system and those who are too ill to be treated at home are usually hospitalized. Particular attention should be paid to position and body alignment of those who are weak or who have changes in the nervous system. Extremities should be put through the normal range of motion exercises and the patient should be encouraged to move his arms and legs. Patients who are unable to turn or who do not should be placed on a regular turning schedule. An extreme and unusual example is one patient who was admitted to the hospital recently with multiple decubiti associated with neglected pernicious anemia. These sores were thought to be caused by the effect of prolonged deficiency of vitamin B_{12} on somatic cells. Because pernicious anemia is also accompanied by sensory deficits, this was probably a contributing factor.

With the exception of changes in the nervous system, most of the manifestations associated with pernicious anemia respond quickly to therapy with vitamin B_{12}. Mrs. Oaks was fortunate inasmuch as no permanent changes had taken place in her nervous system. Although therapy with vitamin B_{12} can be expected to prevent further progress of the disease and may even result in some improvement in symptoms arising from lesions in the nervous system, it will not reverse the changes that have already taken place. The patient should be encouraged to eat a diet planned to maintain a good nutritional status. In the absence of neurological changes no special foods are required. Neither is iron required unless there is evidence of iron deficiency.

Macrocytic anemias may result from a deficiency in the intake of vitamin B_{12} or from failure in its absorption. In the United States where meat is generally available, deficient intake is uncommon. Failure of absorption is much more frequent. There are, of course, other causes of failure of absorption of vitamin B_{12} than pernicious anemia. They include total gastrectomy, in which the source of the intrinsic factor is removed; sprue, in which the absorbing membrane in the small intestine is defective; removal of the small intestine, followed by impaired absorption; and strictures or anastomoses, resulting in a diversion of the contents of the alimentary canal around the absorbing surface of the intestine. The anemia in these conditions is similar to that of pernicious anemia. Achlorhydria and neurological changes are not, however, characteristic features in these conditions.

Certain infestations and therapy with certain drugs are associated with macrocytic anemia. For example, persons who are hosts to the fish tapeworm develop a macrocytic anemia. It is believed that the tapeworm competes with the host for vitamin B_{12}, but it is not known exactly how the interference is accomplished. The tapeworm may merely utilize the vitamin or it may interfere with some step in the process of its utilization. The anemia results not because the intake of vitamin B_{12} is below normal requirements, but because it becomes unavailable to the host. Fish tapeworm infestations occur most commonly among persons who eat raw fish. One of the possible toxic effects of drugs such as diphenylhydantoin sodium, U.S.P. (Dilantin Sodium), primidone, barbital derivatives, methotrexate (amethopterin), and 6-mercaptopurine is macrocytic anemia. With the latter two drugs and probably with the others, the effect is caused by a deficiency of folic acid.

An adequate intake of all of the B vitamins is undoubtedly essential to hematopoiesis. These chemicals participate in a wide variety of metabolic reactions in cells either as direct regulators or as coenzymes.

Another substance which has a hematopoietic effect is folic acid. In many patients with pernicious anemia, blood cell formation is stimulated by the administration of folic acid. It does not, however, prevent the development of lesions in the nervous system. Wintrobe [124] states that the functions of vitamin B_{12} and folic acid are interrelated. A deficiency of one or both is likely to lead to a number of abnormalities.

A serious lack in any one regulatory substance can be associated with a depression in the production of erythrocytes. Moreover, the problem of deficiency in one required element is often accompanied by a deficiency in others. For example, a diet deficient in vitamin B_{12} would almost certainly be lacking in protein and very possibly in iron. Other regulators are also necessary to the formation and maturation of erythrocytes. Anemia develops in hypothyroidism or myxedema. It may also be associated with chronic adrenal insufficiency and disorders associated with deficiencies of function of the anterior hypophysis.

All the factors in the regulation of erythrocyte formation have not been identified, but certain observations have been made. It is known that the production of red cells is stimulated by a general lack of oxygen or by the loss of blood. It is not known how hypoxia acts to stimulate erythropoiesis. One hypothesis is that hypoxia directly stimulates the bone marrow. Guyton [125] states, however, that anoxia of the bone marrow does not directly increase red cell production. Erythropoietin is formed almost as soon as the person is exposed to an atmosphere low in oxygen. Conversely when the person is exposed to an atmosphere high in oxygen, erythropoietin production ceases or falls to a very low level for a period of 24 to 36 hours. The main action of erythropoietin is to increase the rate at which stem cells are converted to hematocytoblasts. To a lesser extent it increases the rate of all phases of red cell production, including the maturation and release of red cells. In contrast, with an excess of red cells, the formation of the erythropoietin and the production of erythrocytes are depressed.

No specific mechanism is known for the destruction of erythrocytes. Healthy erythrocytes live an average of about 120 days. As the cell ages, its surrounding membrane thins and becomes more and more easily ruptured. Cell destruction may, therefore, merely be the result of the inability of the fragile membrane of the aged cell to withstand the pressure exerted against it as the erythrocyte passes through a capillary. Erythrocytes undergo a certain amount of deformity as they pass through capillaries, and this distortion in shape could place a strain on areas of the cell membrane. According to Guyton, [126] much of the destruction of red cells takes place in the spleen, where the erythrocytes pass through the pulp of the spleen to the venous sinusoids by diapedesis. The walls of erythrocytes undergoing this process need to be strong to survive. The assumption that the aging of the membrane of the red cell predisposes it to mechanical injury is supported by the observation that poorly constructed cells with fragile membranes have a shorter life-span than do normal erythrocytes.

Once the wall of the erythrocyte is disrupted, hemoglobin is released. The shell of the former erythrocyte is called a ghost cell, and it is probably quickly removed from the blood by reticuloendothelial cells. The amino acids and lipids are utilized for energy or are reused in the building of new cells including erythrocytes.

The hemoglobin is also phagocytized by re-

---

[124] M. M. Wintrobe: "Macrocytic Anemias: Pernicious Anemia and Other Megaloblastic Anemias," *Principles of Internal Medicine*, 5th ed., T. R. Harrison *et al.*, eds. (New York: The Blakiston Division, McGraw-Hill Book Company, Inc., 1966), p. 619.

[125] *Op. cit.*, p. 114.
[126] *Ibid.*, p. 119.

ticuloendothelial cells into globin and heme. The heme is the iron-containing fraction. It is further split into iron and a pigment, biliverdin. The iron enters the iron pool of the body from whence it may be drawn to form myoglobin in the muscle or hemoglobin in new erythrocytes or stored until it is needed in the liver. The biliverdin is reduced to bilirubin, which is gradually released into the blood. Bilirubin is insoluble in water, but it combines with the blood proteins and it is transported in this form to the liver. The liver separates bilirubin from the blood protein and combines about 80 per cent of it with glucuronide. Bilirubin glucuronide is highly soluble in water. The liver cells secrete it along with the other forms of bilirubin into the bile. Bilirubin is responsible for the greenish yellow color of bile. After the bile reaches the small intestine, some of the bilirubin is converted by bacterial action to urobilinogen, some of which is excreted in the stool.

Most of the urobilinogen is reabsorbed into the portal circulation and excreted in the bile. A small amount escapes into the circulation and is excreted in the urine. An increase in the level of bilirubin in the blood may be caused by obstruction in the bile ducts or by increased blood destruction. Usually the elevation is greater in the presence of obstructive lesions than in increased red-cell destruction, though there are occasional exceptions. There are also other differences. (See Chapter 12.)

As long as blood production keeps up to the demand for red cells and the rate of red cell destruction or loss does not exceed cell production, the number of red cells found in the blood remains stable. When, however, production fails to keep pace with the destruction or loss of erythrocytes, anemia develops. In the preceding discussion, some of the causes of failure of the production of erythrocytes were presented. In those conditions anemia developed because the production of red cells failed to keep pace with the normal rate of cell destruction. Anemia may also be the result of any disorder in which the rate of cell destruction or the hemolysis of cells is excessive. These anemias are classified as the hemolytic anemias. The common feature of the hemolytic anemias is an excessive rate of hemolysis of erythrocytes. The etiological agents vary widely. Depending on the nature of the cause, hemolysis may take place in the circulating blood or in the reticuloendothelial system. These disorders also differ widely in symptomatology, severity, and course. In some, the rate of onset may be rapid and the manifestations severe. In others, the onset is slow and the manifestations are mild or absent. A determining factor is whether hemolysis occurs in the circulating blood or in the reticulo-endothelial system. In all instances in which erythrocytes are hemolyzed at an abnormal rate, some degree of jaundice occurs. It may be barely perceptible or it may be of marked degree. It may develop slowly or rapidly, but jaundice is present to some degree. In chronic hemolytic anemias the liver and spleen are frequently enlarged and complications such as cholelithiasis and leg ulcers may develop.

When the onset of hemolysis is rapid and a large number of red cells are hemolyzed as occurs following the transfusion of incompatible blood, the patient may have a severe shaking chill followed by a high fever, headache, and pain in the back, abdomen, and extremities. The abdominal pain may be so severe that abdominal rigidity results. When the hemolysis is great enough, shock may develop. As in shock from other causes, oliguria and anuria may follow. The urine that is voided is dark in color.

Hemolytic Anemias

A very large number of etiological agents have been implicated in the hemolytic anemias. Wintrobe [127] classifies them as causes arising outside the erythrocyte, or extracorpuscular causes, and those associated with defects in the structure or construction of erythrocytes, or intracorpuscular defects. Among the extracorpuscular (outside-the-cell) causes are the acute hemolytic anemias caused by immune body reactions. Common examples include the transfusion of incompatible blood and hemolytic disease of the newborn caused by the Rh factor. Excessive hemolysis of red cells is secondary to a number of diseases, particularly those involving structures forming part of the reticuloendothelial system. Some examples include Hodgkin's disease, chronic lymphocytic leukemia, metastatic carcinomatosis, and liver disease. A variety of infectious agents are also responsible for increased hemolysis of erythrocytes. Although not common in the United States, malaria on a world-wide basis is probably the most frequent reason for anemia caused by increased hemolysis of red cells.[128]

[127] M. M. Wintrobe: "Hemolytic Anemias," *Principles of Internal Medicine,* 5th ed., T. R. Harrison *et al.,* eds. (New York: The Blakiston Division, McGraw-Hill Book Company, Inc., 1966), p. 630.

[128] Malaria is a protozoan disease in which the parasites reproduce asexually in the erythrocytes. After they undergo several divisions, they fill the cell and it ruptures, releasing parasites to invade more erythrocytes. At the time the parasites are released by the hemolysis of the erythrocytes, the patient experiences a severe shaking chill, followed by a high fever, malaise, headache, and muscle pain. The spleen is frequently enlarged. As in other disorders associated with hemolysis of erythrocytes, jaundice occurs. The attack is terminated by a drenching perspiration. There are some differences in the manifestations, in their severity, and in the frequency of attacks, depending on the species of *plasmodium* infecting the individual.

A wide variety of chemicals may also be associated with increased blood destruction. The effect of some such as acetophenetidin (phenacetin), methyl chloride, acetanilid, benzene, and lead depends on the size of the dose to which the individual is exposed. Others such as the sulfonamides, quinine and quinidine, amphetamine sulfate, U.S.P. (Benzedrine), phenantoin (Mesantoin), and vitamin K substitutes depend on hypersensitivity to the chemical agent. It may be noted that some of these chemicals may also cause hypoplasia or aplasia of the bone marrow.

Physical agents such as severe thermal burns are also associated with increased hemolysis of erythrocytes. This is one of the factors predisposing to anemia in the severely burned patient.

Besides exposure to a variety of physical and chemical agents, defects in the construction of red cells or in the type of hemoglobin also predispose to an increased rate of blood destruction. A number of these disorders are hereditary. Among them are hereditary spherocytosis (familial or congenital hemolytic jaundice, hereditary leptocytosis also known as thalassemia or Mediterranean anemia) and sickle cell anemia.

To summarize, anemia results when blood production fails to keep up with red-cell destruction. The balance between the factors may be upset by a failure in blood production, by the demands for erythrocytes exceeding the capacity of the bone marrow to produce them, or by an increase in the rate of destruction of erythrocytes over the functional capacity of the bone marrow. Anemia is also caused by the loss of blood. When the loss of blood is rapid, the most acute problems are created by a loss of blood volume.

Anemias have a great number of causes. They may be primary, that is, arise from some disturbance in the functioning of the hematopoietic tissues, or they may be secondary to disturbances in other parts of the body. There are few chronically ill patients who, because of the effects of their diseases on blood production or destruction or both, as well as on food intake, escape some degree of anemia. It is not unusual for the chronically ill patient with a marked degree of anemia to feel much improved after his anemia is corrected. The characteristic feature of all anemias is a reduction in the normal number of erythrocytes or in the total quantity of hemoglobin or both. Anemias arising from various etiological factors differ from one another in some respects. In the hemolytic anemias, the products of increased blood destruction are responsible for some of their major manifestations. One aspect common to all anemias is that the oxygen-carrying power of the blood is diminished. In slowly developing anemias, the major manifestations are usually caused by the decreased oxygen-carrying power of the blood. The severity of the symptoms experienced by the patient depends in part on the rapidity with which the anemia develops and the degree to which the erythrocyte count and hemoglobin fall below normal. The latter will determine the degree to which the oxygen-carrying power of the blood is reduced. Severity also depends on the effectiveness of the adaptive mechanisms of the patient. The status of the circulatory system is a significant factor in adaptation to anemia.

When the loss of blood is slow, a patient may have a marked decrease in oxygen-carrying power and yet have few symptoms. Allen Maple illustrates this point very well. Allen, a 14-year-old boy, was admitted to the hospital for the purpose of determining why he was subject to fainting spells. Neither his mother nor his teachers had noted any other change in his behavior. To everyone's amazement, his hemoglobin was found to be 2.5 g per 100 ml of blood. Apparently his cells had adapted quite successfully to a very slow loss of blood. Needless to say, Allen was somewhat less active than a healthy boy.

The functions of the organs of most systems of the body are affected by the decreased oxygen-carrying power of the blood. In some individuals, anemia is associated with pallor of the skin. Despite the widespread belief that pallor indicates anemia, it is not a very reliable sign. Many factors affect the color of the skin, such as the thickness of the epidermis, the quantity and color of the skin pigment, and the number of blood vessels in the skin, as well as the nature and quantity of hemoglobin carried in the blood. Some persons have naturally sallow complexions and are not anemic. Certain diseases are accompanied by a pallor, though anemia is absent. Pallor of certain parts of the body such as the finger- and toenails or of the mucous membranes does indicate anemia.

Inasmuch as the respiratory system, the circulatory system, and the blood function together to deliver oxygen to the cells, many of the effects on respiratory and circulatory systems have been previously described as symptoms of circulatory distress. In moderate degrees of anemia, they are initiated by exertion or by excitement. When anemia is severe, they may even occur at rest. Among the signs and symptoms referable to the respiratory system are dyspnea and rapid breathing. Both are adaptive inasmuch as dyspnea discourages exertion, and the increase in the rate of breathing, if not excessive, increases ventilation.

The most frequent cardiac manifestation is palpitation, or awareness of the heart pounding.

The heart also adjusts to anemia by increasing its rate and stroke volume. Arterial pulsation and pulse pressure increase. Sometimes the capillaries in the fingertips can be seen to be pulsating. Under some circumstances the patient may have angina or present evidence of developing congestive heart failure. Cardiac failure occurs when adaptation is inadequate or fails.

Any person reporting symptoms of circulatory distress should be encouraged by the nurse to seek medical attention. Relief of these and other symptoms depends on the identification and correction of the cause. In patients with marked symptoms, the nursing requirements of the patient are similar to those of the patient in congestive heart failure. As the anemia is relieved, symptoms lessen and the patient is able to assume more responsibility for his own care.

The neuromuscular system is also affected in anemia. Among the signs and symptoms referable to this system are headache, dizziness or vertigo, fainting, sensitivity to cold, tinnitus (ringing in the ears), muscular weakness, easy fatigability, and irritability. Paresthesias, or abnormal sensations, are common. The headache may be very severe. The patient who is dizzy or faint should be protected from falling. These symptoms may be less troublesome if he learns to change position slowly. The patient requires a warm room, extra blankets and clothing, and protection from drafts. Although the patient should also be protected from overexertion, he should not be allowed to be in one position for endless periods of time. If he is unable to move himself, he should be moved and turned, and his extremities should be put through the normal range of motion exercises. As the patient improves, he can be expected to be more energetic.

In anemia, a number of signs and symptoms indicative of disturbances in the function of the alimentary canal are frequent. Most patients have a loss of appetite. They may need to be encouraged to eat and may require some assistance. Nausea, vomiting, flatulence, abdominal discomfort, and diarrhea or constipation may also occur. When one or more of these are present, they may also discourage the patient from eating. In pernicious anemia, glossitis with a sore tongue is a common event. In aplastic anemia, leukemia, and agranulocytosis, necrotic lesions develop in the mouth and pharynx. In these latter conditions gums tend to bleed either spontaneously or on slight trauma. These patients not only have problems in eating, but also their mouths are difficult to keep clean and relatively free from crusts.

For the patient with a painful tongue or who has sores in his mouth, the diet should be low in roughage and bland. To spare the patient unnecessary discomfort and to encourage eating, hot, spicy, or highly acid foods should be avoided. If a toothbrush is used to cleanse the teeth, it should be soft and brushing should be gentle. Application of toothpaste with large cotton balls or well-moistened pieces of cotton is less likely than a toothbrush to traumatize fragile tissues and thus cause bleeding. In some patients the cleansing of the mouth should be limited to the use of a mouthwash. Solutions such as 1 per cent hydrogen peroxide or sodium perborate, Dobell's solution, or flavored mouthwashes may be tried. The mucous membranes can be kept moist by rinsing the mouth with milk of magnesia. It forms a coat over the mucosa, which can be removed later by rinsing the mouth with water. Carbonated beverages may be used to break up the crusts collecting in the mouth without causing bleeding. Potentially toxic agents should not be used unless they are prescribed by a physician and the patient should be able to cooperate. In patients in whom the lips have a tendency to crack, liquid petrolatum or some other substance should be applied to keep the skin soft. Whenever mouth care is given, an outstanding feature should be great gentleness.

In severe anemia, menstrual disturbances in the female and loss of libido in the male are not infrequent. The most frequent menstrual disturbance is amenorrhea, although menorrhagia, excessive menstruation, also occurs.

Among the other signs and symptoms frequently associated with severe anemia are increased metabolic rate, a slight degree of fever, and enlargement of the spleen.

In long-standing anemia, changes take place in the skin and its appendages. The skin loses its elasticity and tone, the hair thins, and, in iron-deficiency anemias, the nails lose their luster, become brittle, and break easily. They may also become concave instead of being convex. Bruised spots, ecchymoses, and purpura may also be observed in the skin.

From this review of the effects of anemia on the various systems of the body, it should be clear that anemia has widespread effects. Some, such as those in the respiratory and circulatory systems, represent adjustments to lessen the effects of the lowered oxygen-carrying capacity of the blood. Others, such as those arising in the gastrointestinal and nervous systems, warn the individual that something is wrong, but do not add to his capacity to adapt. Some, such as loss of appetite, may, when continued, aggravate the pre-existing disorder.

How is anemia diagnosed and treated?

The first step in the treatment of anemia is the identification of its presence and the nature

of the cause. The appearance and general behavior of the patient provide clues leading the
physician to suspect the presence of anemia.
With experience and careful examination of the
patient, he may be able to estimate with some
accuracy the degree of anemia. Pallor of the
palms of the hands, the nail beds, and the
mucosa is present when the anemia is fairly
severe. The physician also examines the patient
for evidence of circulatory and respiratory adjustments to the anemia as well as for the previously listed effects on other systems of the body.
Examination of the blood establishes the presence or absence of anemia. Other evidence may
be required to establish its cause.

Besides counting the total number of each
type of cell, the blood may be examined in one
or more of the following ways:

BLOOD CELLS

Erythrocytes. Total count per cubic millimeter
of blood; percentage of mature cells; percentage of immature cells and stage of immaturity; presence of abnormal cells; size; variations in size as well as in the shape of cells;
fragility test (osmotic and mechanical).

Leukocytes. Total count per cubic millimeter
of blood; differential white count (percentage
of various types of leukocytes); presence and
percentage of immature cells and degree of
immaturity; presence and description of abnormal leukocytes.

Thrombocytes. Number.

Hemoglobin. Grams per 100 ml of blood (may
be reported in percentage of normal value
such as 100 per cent, 50 per cent).

Hematocrit. Volume of packed red cells in proportion to volume of plasma—in some institutions this is used in preference to hemoglobin determination because the result is
likely to be more dependable.

Icterus index. Determination of the bilirubin
content of the blood.

Sedimentation rate of erythrocytes. Rate at
which the red cells settle out of whole blood.
The height in millimeters of the column of
plasma that is formed at the top of a tube of
blood in one hour. Range 1 to 3 mm per
hour.

Schilling test. Vitamin B_{12} absorption.

Bone marrow. State of activity, percentage
composition, morphology.

Urine. Urobilinogen and bilirubin content; evidence of blood in the urine.

Stool. Bilirubin, urobilinogen content; occult
(hidden) or obvious blood in the stool.

Gastric juice. Presence or absence of free
hydrochloric acid, including response to histamine.

Isotope studies. Red cell survival (^{51}Cr), iron
turnover (^{59}Fe).

Bleeding and clotting times.

Capillary fragility test (Rumpel-Leede).

As a result of the examination of the blood
and the bone marrow the physician learns
(1) the degree of the anemia, (2) something
about its cause, (3) the extent to which blood
production is normal or abnormal, and (4) the
degree to which blood destruction is increased.

Obviously not every patient is subjected to
all the above examinations. Moreover, in individual instances other tests may be utilized in
the process of making the diagnosis. Most of
these tests do not require special or elaborate
preparation of the patient. The patient may
need some help in understanding why blood
must be removed for the purposes of examination. Even when the patient accepts, on an intellectual level, that blood is required, he may not
accept it on an emotional level. He expresses
this lack of acceptance in a number of ways.
He repeatedly asks questions, such as, "Is it
really necessary to take all that blood?" "Doesn't
the physician know that I am already short of
blood?" "How can I get well when they take my
blood each morning?" He calls the laboratory
technicians, nurses, or doctors who take the
blood "blood suckers." Among healthy people
the loss of a few milliliters of blood can be
frightening or believed to be dangerous. Understanding how the patient feels about the removal of blood for examination should help the
nurse to be supportive to him. Because the
anemic patient is frequently hyperirritable, the
taking of blood may be associated with expressions of this irritability. As the patient responds
to treatment, he will be better able to tolerate
frustration and discomfort.

Therapy in anemia must be directed to the
cause and pathogenesis of the disorder in each
patient. In anemias caused by blood loss, the
condition causing the loss of blood must, if
possible, be corrected. In acute blood loss, the
first consideration is the maintenance and restoration of the blood volume. When there is a
great loss of blood with a marked decrease in its
oxygen-carrying power, the cellular elements
must also be replaced. In serious hemorrhage,
replacement of blood cells, although not life
saving, may facilitate the recovery of the
patient.

In chronic blood loss such as occurs in hookworm disease or other disorders accompanied
by prolonged loss of small amounts of blood,
volume is not a problem. The loss of iron from
the body is. Therapy is therefore directed
toward identifying and eliminating the cause

and restoring the level of iron in the body to normal. Iron is administered as ferrous sulfate or as whole blood. Attention is also paid to the state of nutrition of the patient.

There are few disorders in which knowledge of the underlying disorder is more important to the therapy than in the treatment of the anemias. In iron-deficiency anemia, the patient responds to an increased intake of iron, but does not benefit from an increased intake of vitamin B_{12} unless it also is lacking. The same is true of patients who have a vitamin B_{12} deficiency. In some instances, such as in the patient with sickle cell anemia or thalassemia, an increase in the intake of iron, particularly in the form of red cells, may actually be harmful, because the body has no mechanism by which it can eliminate iron once it is absorbed into the body. Probably the greatest harm to the largest number of people comes from the waste of money spent on "shotgun" preparations prepared to cure all blood deficiencies. Many of them are expensive and, with the possible exception of one constituent, useless. In the absence of a disease of the blood or a condition causing the loss of blood, money spent for a nutritious diet is a good anemia preventative.

The patient who suffers from a deficiency of vitamin B_{12}, either from lack of absorption or from an actual dietary deficiency, requires this substance in his treatment.

Although not effective in all anemias characterized by periods of increased blood destruction, in some types removal of the spleen may prevent episodes of massive hemolysis of blood. In certain anemias, such as sickle cell anemia, there is no specific therapy and no way to prevent the progress of the disorder.

POLYCYTHEMIA

As in other homeostatic conditions, homeostasis may fail because too few cells and/or too little hemoglobin are produced or erythrocytes are formed in excess. The latter condition is known as polycythemia. The term itself means a large or excessive number of blood cells. In some instances polycythemia results from a physiological stimulus, that is, generalized hypoxia. In a few persons, there is no ready explanation for the disorder. This form is called polycythemia vera.

DISORDERS OF THE SELF-SEALING MECHANISM

A second function of the blood that may be disordered is the self-sealing mechanism. As the term implies, this mechanism defends the body against the loss of blood. Three elements enter into the self-sealing mechanism. They are (1) the surrounding tissues (extravascular), (2) the blood vessels (vascular), and (3) the coagulation of the blood (intravascular). Were it not for the self-sealing mechanism, even minor tears in a blood vessel would permit enough blood to escape to cause death. In every individual, small blood vessels are disrupted many times a day. When the self-sealing mechanism is effective, little or no loss of blood occurs. When for some reason it is defective, blood loss may threaten or take the life of the individual. Defects in the self-sealing mechanism may be acquired or hereditary. Walter Thomas is an example of an individual with one of the hereditary disorders of the self-sealing mechanism. He lacks one of the factors necessary to the clotting of the blood, the antihemophilic factor. As a result of this hereditary defect, minor trauma or other injuries induce severe bleeding. Despite his youth (he is only 15 years of age), he has been hospitalized 29 times for episodes of bleeding. His weight-bearing joints are ankylosed (rigid) from bleeding into the joint capsule. Were it not for excellent medical and nursing care, Walter would not have been able to survive. An older brother died from hemorrhage at the age of two.

The characteristic tissues in which the ruptured blood vessels are located have a significant influence on the extent of bleeding. Firm or nondistensible tissue tends to limit bleeding because the addition of blood quickly raises the tissue hydrostatic pressure. With the elevation of the pressure in the tissue, blood flow is impeded. In contrast, when bleeding occurs in distensible tissues or from an area where the blood escapes from the body, hydrostatic pressure may be slow to rise or not rise at all. Consequently, bleeding into an area involving a break in the skin, mucosa, or serous membrane is likely to be more profuse than bleeding into a solid tissue, because the flow of blood is unopposed by tissue hydrostatic pressure. To illustrate, some months ago while closing a car door, Mary Silver slipped and her thumb was caught between the door and the frame of the car. Many blood vessels were ruptured and the soft tissues appeared bruised. The actual quantity of blood lost into the injured area was minimal because the nail is nondistensible and the skin of the thumb is firm. The hydrostatic pressure rose rapidly in the bruised area and bleeding was stopped promptly.[129]

The use of tissue hydrostatic pressure in con-

---

[129] Needless to say, the pain was exquisitely severe. Loss of the nail can usually be prevented if the nail is pierced with a red-hot pin and the blood is allowed to escape.

trolling bleeding is illustrated by the following instance. A young man was admitted to the emergency service of a well-known hospital. He was bleeding profusely from a gash in his right thigh made by a sharp razor. As far as the physician could determine, large nerves and muscles had escaped injury. The intern who was assigned to care for the wound was busily trying to ligate all the severed blood vessels when an experienced nurse came into the room, evaluated the situation, then leaned over his shoulder and said in a low tone of voice, "Sew it up, and it will stop itself." What she was saying was that if the wound is closed, pressure within the tissues will soon exceed the hydrostatic pressure of the blood and bleeding will stop.

In contrast, in the absence of increasing hydrostatic pressure, disruption of a blood vessel may lead to copious and at times fatal bleeding. Examples such as a ruptured esophageal varix and a bleeding peptic ulcer have been discussed previously.

To recapitulate, one factor in the self-sealing mechanism is the character of the tissues into which bleeding takes place. In tissues relatively resistant to distention, a small amount of bleeding may quickly elevate the intratissue pressure above the hydrostatic pressure of the blood. Blood flow is thereby impeded and other factors in the self-sealing mechanism can come into play and plug the rent in the blood vessels. Where bleeding is into distensible tissue or cavities and the blood escapes from the body, bleeding is likely to be more profuse because the opposing hydrostatic pressure is not developed rapidly or does not develop at all.

Another factor in the self-sealing mechanism is the blood vessel. Following disruption the cut end of the blood vessel constricts. An interesting point about this is that the more the tissue is traumatized, the greater the degree of constriction. Thus instances have been known in which amputation of an extremity by crushing was associated with little bleeding. Vasoconstriction is least with the type of injury in which the blood vessel is subject to minimum trauma. Three factors contribute to vasoconstriction, the spasm of the muscle in the wall of the blood vessel, reflex nervous stimulation, and the release of serotonin by the injured tissues. One other factor enters into the decrease in the diameter of the cut end of the vessel; as the clot retracts, it pulls the blood vessel together. This will be discussed in more detail.

The third factor in the self-sealing mechanism is the clotting of the blood. Healthy blood is capable of clotting in response to a break in the wall of a blood vessel and surrounding tissue. If, however, blood is to accomplish its function

as a transporting medium, it must be in a fluid state. Two general elements protect the blood against clotting. One is the structure of the blood vessel and the nature of blood flow; the other is the presence in the blood of anticoagulant chemicals.

Healthy blood vessels have a smooth endothelial lining that lessens trauma to blood cells as they pass through. A second source of protection is a layer of negatively charged protein absorbed on the lining surface of the intima. It repels the negatively charged platelets and thereby prevents them from sticking.

Furthermore, the flow of blood in the blood vessels is laminar, that is, in layers. The fluid elements are on the outside and the cellular elements are in the inner core. This enables blood cells in larger vessels to slip along with little or no contact with the lining. When blood flow is slow because of lack of exercise of the extremities or obstruction of a vessel, cellular elements tend to settle to the wall of the vessel. The possibility of intravascular clotting is therefore increased. Patients confined to bed can be protected from venous stasis by exercising the extremities and avoiding pressure at points where blood flow is likely to be impeded. The blood contains two types of substances, the anticoagulants and the procoagulants. The function of the anticoagulants is to keep the blood in its circulating or fluid state. Among the substances postulated are those with antithromboplastin and antithrombin activity. A chemical known to act as an anticoagulant is heparin. Heparin is believed to be secreted by basophilic mast cells located around capillaries throughout the body. These cells are most abundant in the liver and lungs.[130] Heparin is thought to act by preventing the conversion of prothrombin to thrombin. It may also destroy thrombin. Healthy blood is capable of clotting in response to a break in the wall of a blood vessel. The proclotting factors are normally kept in check by anticoagulant factors in the blood. This is necessary if the blood is to carry out its defensive and transporting functions.

Important as the fluid state of the blood is to its functions, its capacity to clot is an essential defense against the loss of blood. Normal blood contains a number of substances capable of acting together to cause the blood to clot. Some of these substances are normally held in check and do not act unless they are activated by some other substance. Once blood clotting is initiated, however, the process tends to keep itself going. Blood clotting acts as a positive feedback system; that is, it is a process that is self-perpetuating or creates more of the same.

[130] Guyton, *op. cit.*, p. 169.

This is different from many homeostatic mechanisms in which a change in one direction is counteracted by a change in the opposite direction.

Among disorders in which the positive feedback effect in blood clotting can be seen are thrombophlebitis and phlebothrombosis. In these disorders, a blood clot is formed on the wall of a vein. When such a vein is opened, the clot is frequently seen to be in all stages of development from the well-organized clot adherent to the wall of the vessel to the amorphous newly forming clot in its tail. The stimulus to clot formation is usually some type of injury to the wall of the blood vessel. Occasionally, however, the clots are formed in the blood vessels in the absence of apparent damage. This situation is maladaptive.

Knowledge of the final stages of blood clotting is fairly complete, but less is known about the initial stages. A deficiency or absence in any one of the essential factors results in defective coagulation of the blood. Traditionally four factors have been identified as being necessary. They are thromboplastin, prothrombin, calcium, and fibrinogen. Wintrobe [131] lists 12 different factors. In some instances three or more substances are included under one of these factors. All of these, and possibly others, are believed to play a role in blood coagulation. Although a deficiency of calcium was once believed to be a cause of failure of the blood to clot, this is no longer thought to be true. Calcium must be present in the ionized form, but the quantity required is small. Because calcium is also required to regulate the irritability of nerve tissue, a significant fall in the level of calcium causes disturbances in neuromuscular functioning before it affects blood coagulability. Before the quantity of calcium could drop enough to affect the clotting of the blood, death would have occurred from respiratory failure.

BLOOD CLOTTING

The first step in the clotting of the blood is the activation of thromboplastin that is released by the injured tissues or platelets. Pure platelet thromboplastin cannot by itself initiate blood clotting. Three plasma cofactors are especially important in the activation of platelet thromboplastin. A deficiency of any one of them will prevent the clotting as a consequence of a lack of degeneration of platelets. The three factors include (1) antihemophilic factor, (2) plasma thromboplastin component, and (3) plasma thromboplastin antecedent. Walter Thomas,

[131] M. M. Wintrobe: "Bleeding," *Principles of Internal Medicine*, 5th ed., T. R. Harrison *et al.*, eds. (New York: The Blakiston Division, McGraw-Hill Book Company, Inc., 1966), p. 165.

who was described previously, had difficulty in the coagulation of his blood because he had a hereditary lack of the antihemophilia factor.

The presence of ionized calcium is believed to be essential for the activation of thromboplastin as well as for the conversion of prothrombin to thrombin. As stated previously, sufficient ionized calcium is always available for this reaction to occur. The same cannnot be said for prothrombin. One of the precursors of prothrombin is vitamin K. In diseases in which bile fails to reach the small intestine, vitamin K is not absorbed. As a fat-soluble substance, its absorption depends on the presence of bile. Formerly, patients with obstructive jaundice often continued to bleed for hours from minor breaks in the skin, such as those caused by the introduction of an intravenous needle into a vein. Needless to say, in these patients surgical procedure was fraught with great danger. Vitamin K can now be administered by intramuscular injection. Within about four hours, provided that the patient has sufficient liver tissue, enough prothrombin will be synthesized to make a surgical procedure safe. Occasionally a baby is born who experiences serious bleeding because the store of vitamin K in his liver is inadequate. Like the patient with obstructive jaundice, he bleeds because he lacks a sufficient quantity of prothrombin.

Because prothrombin is manufactured by the liver, in disease involving the parenchyma of the liver, prothrombin levels may be low. The production of prothrombin may also be depressed by certain anticoagulant preparations of coumarin. These substances are employed in disorders in which there is a tendency for the blood to clot in the blood vessels. Although the danger of spontaneous hemorrhage is less with some of the newer anticoagulant preparations, it is always a possibility. Any bleeding should be brought to the attention of the physician immediately, and the patient receiving an anticoagulant on an outpatient basis should be under regular medical care. The patient may bleed spontaneously from the gastrointestinal or genitourinary tract or into serous cavities. Areas of purplish discoloration of the skin or mucous membrane may indicate bleeding into these tissues. When these areas occur in the skin, they are called ecchymoses. The term *purpura* is also used to describe spontaneous bleeding into the skin and mucous membrane. For reasons not completely understood, large doses of salicylates also decrease the prothrombin content of the blood plasma.

In the third step in the process of blood clotting, thrombin catalyzes the conversion of fibrinogen, a blood protein synthesized in the liver, to fibrin. In the process the fibrinogen molecule is split and the resulting fragments are polymerized [132] and form a threadlike structure. The fibrin strands run in all directions and form a mesh that catches plasma, blood platelets, erythrocytes, and leukocytes. As the fibrin strands contract, they squeeze out fluid or serum, and the size of the clot is reduced. This process is called clot retraction. Large numbers of platelets are required for the formation and satisfactory retraction of the clot. Because the fibrin threads are sticky, they adhere to the wall of the damaged blood vessel. As they shorten they pull the blood vessel wall together, thus diminishing its diameter and acting as a plug or cork.

Sometimes in surgical procedures involving the surface of a mucous membrane, a large, loose clot forms over the surface. It acts as a curtain with the vessels behind it continuing to bleed. For bleeding to be controlled, the sheltering clot must be prevented from forming, or, if it does, it must be removed so that the blood clots in the end of the exposed blood vessels. Common sites of hemorrhage of this type are the pharynx following tonsillectomy and the urinary bladder after prostate surgery. Following the latter type of surgery, the physician often prescribes bladder irrigations frequently enough to prevent the formation of blood clots. If one or more clots form, they can also be removed by irrigation. Unless the bladder irrigations are performed thoroughly, the patient may lose an unnecessary quantity of blood.

Although primary fibrinogenemia or fibrinogenopenia can cause bleeding, this is a rare event. As a rule, a low level of fibrinogen in the blood is associated with diminished quantities of other procoagulation factors such as prothrombin and the blood platelets and is secondary to a serious injury or illness. Massive and spontaneous hemorrhage may occur. The events leading to spontaneous bleeding are complex and are not well understood. One hypothesis suggested to explain the changes is that the elements required for clotting are used more rapidly than they can be replaced by the body. In other words, demand exceeds supply. This is followed by an increase in the destruction of fibrin, or fibrinolysis. The presence of this condition is heralded by large ecchymoses in the skin and spontaneous bleeding from mucous membranes. Wintrobe [133] lists five different types of pathological disorders in which fibrinolysis is observed. They are (1) following severe traumatic injuries or burns, (2) following surgical procedures such as those involving the

[132] The joining of like molecules so that the resulting compound is a multiple of each unit.
[133] Wintrobe, *op. cit.*, p. 172.

lung, (3) obstetrical complications such as abruptio placentae, (4) neoplastic disease, and (5) a variety of disorders such as leukemia, polycythemia vera, and cirrhosis of the liver.

The bleeding resulting from acquired fibrinolysis is often massive. The nurse should observe the patient for indications of an increased tendency to bleed, such as ecchymosis in the skin. Bleeding from any area should be brought to the attention of the physician immediately. The life of the patient depends on the prompt administration of fresh whole blood and fibrinogen.

SUMMARY

The self-sealing mechanism consists of the tissue of the body, the blood vessels, and the blood-clotting mechanism. The importance and effectiveness of any one of these elements in health depends on the nature, location, and extent of injury to blood vessels. Through the efficient operation of the self-sealing mechanism, breaks in blood vessels are repaired before appreciable amounts of blood escape from them. For the blood to perform its function as a vehicle in the transportation of materials throughout the body, however, its fluid state must be preserved. The blood-clotting process must be held in check so that blood does not clot in the blood vessels, thereby obstructing the flow of blood to or from the tissues. Whether or not blood clots depends on the balance between the anticlotting and the proclotting factors.

The process of blood clotting is very complex. Despite significant advances in knowledge of the process, it still is not completely understood. Certain substances such as thromboplastin must be present and activated to initiate blood clotting. Thromboplastin is released by injured tissues and thrombocytes. Platelet thromboplastin further requires a number of plasma factors for its release and activation. A lack in any one of these factors is accompanied by an increase in the tendency to bleed. The platelets release serotonin, a vasoconstrictor substance, and they are required in large numbers to fill in the spaces in the fibrin network of the clot. Any considerable decrease in the platelet count is a potential source of bleeding. Abnormalities in the structure of the platelets increase the difficulty with which they disintegrate and thereby increase the tendency to bleeding.

Activated thromboplastin acts on prothrombin to produce thrombin. For the liver to synthesize prothrombin, vitamin K must be available in adequate quantities. Prothrombin deficiency accompanies diseases of the liver in which large numbers of parenchymal cells are destroyed or in which there is failure to absorb vitamin K from the gastrointestinal tract. As a fat-soluble substance, vitamin K requires bile for its absorption. Any disorder preventing bile from reaching the gastrointestinal tract will therefore result in inadequate absorption of vitamin K and a deficiency in prothrombin. A not uncommon cause of insufficient prothrombin is iatrogenic; that is, it results from treatment. Therapy with anticoagulants such as preparations of coumarin is most likely to be responsible.

Fibrinogen, also synthesized by the liver, is acted on to form fibrin. Strands of fibrin form the structural framework for the clot. Being sticky, fibrin adheres to the lining of the blood vessel and catches the constituents of the blood in its mesh to fill in the spaces. As the fibrin contracts, the wall to which it adheres follows and diameter of the vessel diminishes. Contraction, or retraction, of the clot, as it is called, makes a strong, firm clot.

The principal anticoagulant agents used in therapy interfere with blood clotting by preventing the formation of prothrombin or by inhibiting a step in the clotting process.

In the therapy of disorders characterized by bleeding, the most frequently used agent is fresh whole blood. It is employed because it provides not only for the replacement of blood volume and blood cells, but for the replacement or addition of the substances required in blood clotting. There are a number of hemostatic agents, that is, substances causing the blood to clot rapidly, used to accelerate coagulation of the blood. These include thrombin and purified fibrinogen. Gel foams containing procoagulant substances are sometimes applied to bleeding surfaces to hasten coagulation.

Nursing the patient with a disorder characterized by a tendency to bleed can challenge the most competent nurse. As emphasized previously, the loss of even small quantities of blood provokes fear in almost everyone. A large hemorrhage with a sudden onset may frighten the nurse as well. Some of the disorders characterized by a tendency to spontaneous hemorrhage, such as leukemia, have a poor prognosis. Patient, family, and nurse live day by day in the presence of death. Especially when the sick person is a child or a young adult, family members may suffer from a variety of negative emotional states including grief, disappointment, depression, panic, and guilt. Their demands on the nurse and physician for emotional support may be greater than those of the patient. Parents and families can be referred to local branches of the Leukemia Foundation for help and emotional support. This does not mean that the nurse is thereby relieved of all further responsibility in this area. What it means is that she

shares it with others. In working with the patient with a poor prognosis, the situation for both the patient and his family can often be improved by concentrating attention on what can be done rather than on the hopelessness of the situation. Attention to the comfort of the patient when he is ill, acceptance of his behavior as part of his illness, as well as gentleness and kindness, may not lengthen his life, but they should ease his suffering. The trend toward care of the patient at home, when this is feasible, often makes individualized care easier to attain.

Team conferences, in which nurses, doctors, social workers, occupational and physical therapists, and dietitians meet to discuss the problems involved and possible solutions to them, can do much to improve the quality of care of a patient. When appropriate, the patient and/or a member of his family may also be invited to participate. If this is done, they should be treated as a contributing member of the group. These conferences can also be used to provide support to the various members of the team. A planning conference in which goals and problems are identified, difficulties recognized, and plans made to utilize available resources often helps the personnel to gain a positive perspective in a difficult situation.

For persons such as Walter Thomas, medical and nursing care may save the life of the patient for extended periods of time. However, progressive disability is more difficult to prevent. This leads to a variety of social, economic, psychological, and educational problems. At the last admission of Walter to the hospital, he was bedfast and had been for some time. After the age of nine, he no longer attended school. Although he was assigned a visiting teacher, his progress was slow. His one interest was to be a "ham" radio operator. Because this seemed possible, his nurse encouraged him in his ambition. After discussing possible activities with him and his physician, the help of the occupational therapist was enlisted. Walter illustrates some of the problems involved in the life of an individual who has a severe bleeding tendency from early life. Economic problems were not as great as they are in many instances, since his father had a high income.

In addition to emotional support, another goal in the nursing of the patient with a tendency toward bleeding is to prevent incidents predisposing to tissue trauma. Care of the mouth is discussed previously in this chapter. Bleeding from the nose, or epistaxis, is a common problem. Crusting of the mucosa of the nose predisposes to and follows episodes of bleeding. The crusting may be lessened by inserting a wick of cotton soaked with mineral oil.

Only one nostril should be treated, and all excess of oil should be removed from the wick before it is inserted to prevent the possibility of its aspiration.

Another problem arises when subcutaneous or intramuscular injections are administered. To minimize the danger of bleeding, a sharp needle of as small diameter as is compatible with the solution to be injected should be selected. The selection of the sites to be used for injection should be discussed with the physician. When repeated injections are required, the sites should be rotated according to a plan and recorded each time. Steady pressure over the injection site for a period of 3 to 5 minutes lessens the likelihood of bleeding into the tissue and the formation of a hematoma.

Patients who are ambulatory should be instructed to avoid bumping themselves against furniture or other hard objects. Care should be taken to perform nursing procedures with extra gentleness. The patient should be protected from sources of infection, not only to protect him from unnecessary discomfort, but because infection increases his tendency to bleed.

Despite every effort to prevent hemorrhage, bleeding does occur, and the nurse should be alert to evidences of it. Petechiae, small capillary hemorrhages, occurring about the ankle or in the antecubital space after a blood pressure determination is made may be the first warning that bleeding is threatened. Purpura and ecchymosis of the skin should be watched for. Bleeding or serous drainage from the nose, gums, or vagina or the vomiting or expectoration of blood should be noted and the quantity of blood loss estimated. The first evidence of bleeding may be as bright red blood in the stool or in the form of tarry stools. Bright red blood in the urine is easily recognized, but lesser amounts causing urine to be smoky may be missed.

To summarize briefly, the maintenance of the conditions required for the healthy functioning of cells depends on a system to supply the needed substances and to remove the products of cell activity. In large multicellular organisms such as man, conduits deliver and remove materials from the capillaries where exchange takes place between the blood and the interstitial fluid. A variety of mechanisms are required to regulate the diameter of the blood vessels and the pressure of the blood within the system. A source of power is necessary to keep the fluid circulating through the system. Through regulation, blood supply to vital organs is maintained and the localized needs of tissues are met. Because the transporting medium is in a fluid state, it must be kept fluid and at the same time be capable of being converted into a solid state when blood vessels are disrupted. In health, tissues are protected from a failure of supply by the capacity to adapt function to needs and by a reserve that can be called on. In disease, cell function or even survival is threatened by failure of supply and/or removal of cell products. Care is directed toward reducing the requirements of affected tissues and/or improving the functioning of diseased organs.

REFERENCES

BOOKS

Allen, Edgar, Barker, Nelson, and Hines, Edgar: *Peripheral Vascular Diseases,* 3rd ed. (Philadelphia: W. B. Saunders Company, 1962).

Baker, Wiley F. (ed.): *Surgical Treatment of Peripheral Vascular Disease* (New York: McGraw-Hill Book Company, Inc., 1962).

Friedberg, Charles K.: *Diseases of the Heart,* Vol. 1 and Vol. 2, 3rd ed. (Philadelphia: W. B. Saunders Company, 1966).

Hoebler, Sibley W.: *Hypertensive Disease: Diagnosis and Treatment* (New York: A Hoeber-Harper Book, 1963).

Hurst, J. Willis, and Logue, R. Bruce (eds.): *The Heart—Arteries and Veins* (New York: McGraw-Hill Book Company, Inc., 1966).

Luisada, Aldo A. (ed.): *Cardiology: An Encyclopedia of the Cardiovascular System.* Vol. 1. *Normal Heart and Vessels.* Vol. 2. *Methods.* Vol. 3. *Clinical Cardiology.* Vol. 4. *Clinical Cardiology-Therapy.* Vol. 5. *Related Specialty Fields* (New York: McGraw-Hill Book Company, Inc., 1961).

Meltzer, Lawrence E., Pinneo, Rose, and Kitchell, J. Roderick: *Intensive Coronary Care—A Manual for Nurses* (New York: The Charles Press, 1965).

Modell, Walter, *et al.: Handbook of Cardiology for Nurses,* 5th ed. (New York: Springer-Verlag, 1966).

Nite, Gladys, and Willis, Frank N.: *The Coronary Patient* (New York: The Macmillan Company, 1964).

Pitorak, Elizabeth F., *et al.: Nurses' Guide to Cardiac Surgery and Nursing Care* (New York: McGraw-Hill Book Company, Inc., 1969).

Powers, Maryann, and Storlie, Frances: *The Cardiac Surgical Patient* (New York: The Macmillan Company, 1969).

Whitby, Sir Lionel E. H., and Britton, C. T. C.: *Disorders of the Blood,* 9th ed. (New York: Grune & Stratton, Inc., 1963).

White, Paul D., and Donovan, Helen: *Hearts:*

Their Long Follow-up (Philadelphia: W. B. Saunders Company, 1967).

Wintrobe, Maxwell M.: *Clinical Hematology,* 6th ed. (Philadelphia: Lea & Febiger, 1967).

P E R I O D I C A L S

Blood Dyscrasias

Gurski, Barbara M.: "Rationale of Nursing Care for Patients with Blood Dyscrasias," *Nurs. Clin. N. Amer.,* 1:23–30 (Mar.) 1966.

King, Harold E., and Cooper, Talbert: "Thrombocytopenia," *Postgrad. Med.,* 31:532–38 (June) 1962.

Kupfer, Henry G.: "Etiology, Symptoms, and Therapy of Anemias," *Clin. Med.,* 71:807–20 (May) 1964.

"Symposium: Hematologic Disorders," *Med. Clin. N. Amer.,* 40:entire issue (July) 1956.

Wintrobe, Maxwell M.: "Blood Dyscrasias," *Amer. J. Nurs.,* 60:496–500 (Apr.) 1960.

Zucker, Marjorie B.: "Blood Platelets," *Sci. Amer.,* 204:58–64 (Feb.) 1961.

Cardiac Arrhythmias

Hurst, J. Willis, and Myerburg, Robert J.: "Cardiac Arrhythmias: Evolving Concepts. I.," *Mod. Conc. Cardiovasc. Dis.,* 37:73–78 (Jan.) 1968.

Hurst, J. Willis, and Myerburg, Robert J.: "Cardiac Arrhythmias: Evolving Concepts. II.," *Mod. Conc. Cardiovasc. Dis.,* 37:79–84 (Feb.) 1968.

Starke, Rodman D., Chamberlain, Francis L., and Jahn, Lois: "Cardiac Arrhythmias—Diagnosis and Clinical Treatment," *Cardiovasc. Nurs.,* 1:15–18 (Fall) 1965.

Unger, Paul N.: "Electrical Conversion of Cardiac Arrhythmias," *Amer. J. Nurs.,* 66:1962–65 (Sept.) 1966.

Cardiac Surgery

Coleman, Doris: "Surgical Alleviation of Coronary Artery Disease," *Amer. J. Nurs.,* 68:763–66 (Apr.) 1968.

Effler, Donald B.: "Surgery for Coronary Disease," *Sci. Amer.,* 219:36–43 (Oct.) 1968.

Fernandez, Peggy L.: "The Insertion of Cardiac Implants and the Nursing Care Problems Involved," *Nurs. Clin. N. Amer.,* 2:559–69 (Sept.) 1967.

James, Edwinia E.: "The Nursing Care of the Open Heart Patient," *Nurs. Clin. N. Amer.,* 2:543–58 (Sept.) 1967.

Kennedy, Mary Jane: "Coping with Emotional Stress in the Patient Awaiting Heart Surgery," *Nurs. Clin. N. Amer.,* 1:3–13 (Mar.) 1966.

Maclean, Donna M., and Fowler, Elizabeth A.: "Heart Transplant—Early Postoperative Care," *Amer. J. Nurs.,* 68:2124–27 (Oct.) 1968.

Pitorak, Elizabeth Ford: "Open-Ended Care for the Open Heart Patient," *Amer. J. Nurs.,* 67:1452–57 (July) 1967.

Powers, Maryann E., and Storlie, Frances: "The Apprehensive Patient," *Amer. J. Nurs.,* 67:58–63 (Jan.) 1967.

Cerebrovascular Disease

Brocklehurst, J. C.: "Cerebrovascular Disease," *Nurs. Times,* 63:880–82 (July 7) 1967.

Large, Helen, *et al.:* "In the First Stroke Intensive Care Unit," *Amer. J. Nurs.,* 69:76–80 (Jan.) 1969.

Newman, Louis B.: "Physical Medicine and Rehabilitation for Stroke Patients," *J. Amer. Geriatrics Soc.,* 15:111–28 (Feb.) 1967.

Wilcoxson, Harriett L.: "Cerebrovascular Accident: The Role of the Public Health Nurse," *Nurs. Clin. N. Amer.,* 1:63–72 (Mar.) 1966.

Circulation

Bing, Richard J. (ed.): "Heart Disease—Selected Aspects of Pathophysiology, Evaluation and Treatment," *Med. Clin. N. Amer.,* 46:entire issue (Nov.) 1962.

Bing, Richard J., Danforth, William H., and Ballard, Fred B.: "Physiology of the Myocardium," *JAMA,* 172:438–44 (Jan. 30) 1960.

Gilbo, Dona: "Nursing Assessment of Circulatory Function," *Nurs. Clin. N. Amer.,* 3:53–63 (Mar.) 1968.

Johnson, Bonnie Jean: "The Hazards of Immobility: Effects on Cardiovascular Function," *Amer. J. Nurs.,* 67:781–82 (Apr.) 1967.

Kottke, Frederic J., and Blanchard, Russell S.: "Bedrest Begets Bedrest," *Nurs. Forum,* 3:56–72 (No. 3) 1964.

Levine, Samuel A.: "Chair Rest Versus Bed Rest," *Hosp. Med.,* 2:2–5 (Jan.) 1966.

Sasahara, Arthur A., and Foster, Vivienne L.: "Pulmonary Embolism: Recognition and Treatment," *Amer. J. Nurs.,* 67:1634–41 (Aug.) 1967.

Spain, David M.: "Atherosclerosis," *Sci. Amer.,* 215:48–56 (Aug.) 1966.

Wood, J. Edwin: "The Venous System," *Sci. Amer.,* 218:86–96 (Jan.) 1968.

Coronary Artery Disease

Crawley, Mildred: "Care of the Patient with Myocardial Infarction," *Amer. J. Nurs.,* 61:68–70 (Feb.) 1961.

Cross, Joseph: "Back to Work After Myocardial Infarction," *Amer. J. Nurs.,* 62:58–61 (Feb.) 1962.

Dawber, Thomas R.: "The Risk of Coronary Heart Disease," *Heart Bull.,* 18:43–46 (May–June) 1969.

Day, Hughes W.: "The Coronary Care Unit," *Heart Bull.,* 18:41–42 (May–June) 1969.

"Diet and Risk Factors of Coronary Heart Disease," *Nutr. Rev.,* 25:203–205 (July) 1967.

Frank, Charles W., *et al.:* "Physical Inactivity as a Lethal Factor in Myocardial Infarction Among Men," *Circulation,* 34:1022–33 (Dec.) 1966.

Friedman, Meyer, and Rosenman, Ray H.: "Emotions in Cardiovascular Disease," *Heart Bull.,* 13:21–23 (Mar.–Apr.) 1964.

George, Joyce: "Monitoring the Myocardial Infarction Patient," *Nurs. Clin. N. Amer.,* 1:549–57 (Dec.) 1966.

Griep, Arthur H., and DePaul, Sister: "Angina Pectoris," *Amer. J. Nurs.,* 65:72–75 (June) 1965.

Katz, Louis N.: "Physical Fitness and Coronary Heart Disease," *Circulation*, 35:405–14 (Feb.) 1967.

Kurtz, Chester M.: "The Management of the Patient with Acute Myocardial Infarction," *Med. Clin. N. Amer.*, 46:317–29 (Mar.) 1962.

Mordkoff, Arnold M., and Parsons, Oscar A.: "The Coronary Personality: A Critique," *Psychosom. Med.*, 29:1–14 (Jan.–Feb.) 1967.

Seltzer, Carl C.: "An Evaluation of the Effect of Smoking on Coronary Heart Disease," *JAMA*, 203:127–33 (Jan. 15) 1968.

Shillingford, John, and Thomas, Michael: "Hemodynamic Effects of Acute Myocardial Infarction in Man," *Progr. Cardiovasc. Dis.*, 9:571–93 (May) 1967.

"The Patient with Myocardial Infarction," *Special Supplement, Amer. J. Nurs.*, 64:C1–C32 (Nov.) 1964.

Diagnostic Tests

Coodley, Eugene L.: "Significance of Serum Enzymes," *Amer. J. Nurs.*, 68:301–304 (Feb.) 1968.

Eastridge, Charles E., and Hughes, Felix A.: "Central Venous Pressure Monitoring," *Amer. J. Surg.*, 114:648–52 (Nov.) 1967.

Kelly, Ann E., and Gensini, Goffredo G.: "Coronary Arteriography," *Amer. J. Nurs.*, 62:86–90 (Feb.) 1962.

Mignault, J. De L.: "Cardiac Catheterization," *Canad. Nurs.*, 60:240–42 (Mar.) 1964.

Scher, Allen M.: "The Electrocardiogram," *Sci. Amer.*, 205:132–41 (Nov.) 1961.

Failure of the Heart

Bristow, J. David, and Metcalfe, James: "Physical Signs in Congestive Heart Failure," *Progr. Cardiovasc. Dis.*, 10:236–45 (Nov.) 1967.

Gauder, Peter J., Blaisdell, F. William, and Vonmorpurgo, Doris: "Cardiac Resuscitation: From Theory to Practice," *Postgrad. Med.*, 30:228–32 (Mar.) 1963.

Hanchett, Effie S., and Johnson, Ruth A.: "Early Signs of Congestive Heart Failure," *Amer. J. Nurs.*, 68:1456–61 (July) 1968.

Heap, Beth: "Sodium Restricted Diets," *Amer. J. Nurs.*, 60:206–209 (Feb.) 1960.

Larson, Elaine L.: "The Patient with Acute Pulmonary Edema," *Amer. J. Nurs.*, 68:1019–21 (May) 1968.

Smith, Barbara C.: "Congestive Heart Failure," *Amer. J. Nurs.*, 69:278–82 (Feb.) 1969.

Steinberg, Joel S., and Hurst, J. Willis: "The New Role of the Nurse in Cardiac Arrest," *Nurs. Clin. N. Amer.*, 2:245–54 (June) 1967.

Vieira, Zairo E. G., and Collins, Vincent J.: "Emergency Cardiorespiratory Resuscitation," *Postgrad. Med.*, 41:418–27 (Apr.) 1967.

Hypertension

Callow, Allan D.: "A Surgeon Talks About Hypertension," *Amer. J. Nurs.*, 64:74–78 (Dec.) 1964.

Dustan, Harriet P.: "Diet and Diuretics in the Treatment of Hypertensive Cardiovascular Disease," *JAMA*, 172:2052–56 (Apr. 30) 1960.

Osmundson, Philip J.: "Preoperative and Postoperative Management of Patients with Hypertension," *Med. Clin. N. Amer.*, 46:963–64 (July) 1962.

Page, Irvine H.: "The Changing Outlook for the Hypertensive Patient," *Ann. Intern. Med.*, 57:96–109 (July) 1962.

Page, Irvine H. (ed.): "Hypertension and Its Treatment," *Med. Clin. N. Amer.*, 45:entire issue (Mar.) 1961.

Thomas, John, and Holiday, Ernestine: "Detecting Secondary Hypertension," *Amer. J. Nurs.*, 64:94–96 (Feb.) 1964.

Medications

Chou, Te-Chuan: "Early Recognition and Management of Digitalis Intoxication," *Heart Bull.*, 15:24–26 (Mar.–Apr.) 1966.

Frohman, I. Phillips: "Digitalis and Its Derivatives," *Amer. J. Nurs.*, 57:172–75 (Feb.) 1957.

Olwin, John H., and Koppel, J. L.: "Anticoagulant Therapy," *Amer. J. Nurs.*, 64:107–10 (May) 1964.

Schneider, William J., and Boyce, Barbara A.: "Complications of Diuretic Therapy," *Amer. J. Nurs.*, 68:1903–1907 (Sept.) 1968.

Seal, Anna L.: "The Nurse's Responsibility in Anticoagulant Therapy," *Nurs. Clin. N. Amer.*, 1:325–31 (June) 1966.

Pacemakers

Heller, Anne F.: "Nursing the Patient with an Artificial Pacemaker," *Amer. J. Nurs.*, 64:87–92 (Apr.) 1964.

Merkel, Rebecca, and Sovie, Margaret D.: "Electrocution Hazards with Transvenous Pacemaker Electrodes," *Amer. J. Nurs.*, 68:2560–63 (Dec.) 1968.

Moore, Sister Mary Consilium: "Nursing Care of a Patient with an Implanted Artificial Pacemaker," *Cardiovasc. Nurs.*, 2:19–22 (Winter) 1966.

Peripheral Vascular Diseases

Ajemian, Sylvia: "Bypass Grafting for Femoral Artery Occlusion," *Amer. J. Nurs.*, 67:565–68 (Mar.) 1967.

Breslau, Roger C.: "Intensive Care Following Vascular Surgery," *Amer. J. Nurs.*, 68:1670–76 (Aug.) 1968.

Elizabeth, Sister Mary: "Occlusion of the Peripheral Arteries," *Amer. J. Nurs.*, 67:562–64 (Mar.) 1967.

Fulcher, Audrey J.: "The Nurse and the Patient with Peripheral Vascular Disease," *Nurs. Clin. N. Amer.*, 1:47–55 (Mar.) 1966.

Lofgren, Karl A.: "Treatment of Varicose Veins," *Mod. Treatm.*, 2:1121–40 (Nov.) 1965.

McKusick, Victor A., *et al.*: "Buerger's Disease: A Distinct Clinical and Pathologic Entity," *JAMA*, 181:5–12 (July 7) 1962.

Roth, Grace M.: "The Effects of Smoking on Normal Persons and Patients with Peripheral Vascular Disease," *Heart Bull.,* 14:117–19 (Nov.–Dec.) 1965.

Wood, J. Edwin, III: "The Veins: Clinical Implications of Physiological Findings," *Heart Bull.,* 14:41–44 (May–June) 1965.

Rehabilitation

"Symposium on Rehabilitation in Cardiovascular Disease," *Amer. J. Cardiol.,* 7:315–85 (Mar.) 1961.

Rheumatic Heart Disease

Freimer, Earl H., and McCarty, Maclyn: "Rheumatic Fever," *Sci. Amer.,* 213:66–74 (Dec.) 1965.

WHO Expert Committee: "The Prevention of Rheumatic Fever," *WHO Chron.,* 21:27–32 (Jan.) 1967.

11

Nursing the Patient in Shock

We begin with some general considerations. The forces which give meaning to our perceptions of biology are so ramified and interrelated that the boundaries by which we isolate biological entities (cell, organ, organism, species, etc.) are boundaries of our patience, not boundaries on the relations. The more exacting we become, the more smeared these boundaries get. This is one of the most salient features of the biological world.[1]

Overview

SHOCK illustrates more clearly than most disorders the intimate relationship of all parts of the body at all levels of organization. Shock may be initiated by any serious external or internal disorder or agent that impairs the ability to provide cells with required nutrients or interferes with their ability to utilize them. In a way, shock can be the result of a failure of any of the functions discussed in previous chapters. Thus this chapter serves to emphasize and to integrate some of the content presented earlier.

During each war, including the Vietnam conflict, advances have been made in understanding and controlling the effects of serious injuries, including those resulting in shock. Unfortunately, as in many other severe disease states, the identification and control of one phase of the problem uncover a later and more difficult derangement. For example, abnormalities of the circulation and the body responses to them are now understood and can usually be corrected. The dangers of renal failure have also been identified and the patient can be pro-

tected from hyperkalemia and other metabolic fluid and electrolyte problems by dialysis until the kidney recovers adequate function. Many patients who previously would have died of the cardiovascular and/or renal disorders now survive only to die later of pulmonary failure or of certain cellular metabolic derangements.[2]

What are the responsibilities of the nurse in the care of the patient who is in shock, or likely to go into shock?

Under such circumstances, the nurse has three general responsibilities: (1) making and reporting observations on the state of the patient, (2) regulating the environment in relation to the needs of the patient, and (3) carrying out treatments as prescribed by the physician, such as those directed toward correcting circulatory and respiratory disturbances. To fulfill her responsibilities the nurse should understand

---

[1] John M. Myers: "On Limitations of Theories of Biology," *Perspec. Biol. Med.,* **10**:238 (Winter) 1967.

[2] Because of the inadequacy of knowledge of the pathogenesis and treatment of pulmonary failure, a conference was conducted by The Committee on Trauma, Division of Medical Sciences, National Academy of Sciences—National Research Council in Washington, D.C., on "Pulmonary Effects of Nonthoracic Trauma." The Proceedings of this Conference are published in the *Journal of Trauma,* **8**:625–946 (Sept.) 1968.

the current concepts of the prevention, causes, nature, effects, and treatment of shock.[3] Although some aspects of shock are fairly well understood, there is still much to be learned. Unfortunately, most of the initial knowledge on the subject was derived from experimental work done on dogs. Now authorities are finding that many of the changes occurring in dogs and people are not the same. In human beings, shock caused by hemorrhage has been most intensively studied and is best understood.

Because the term *shock* has been applied to a wide variety of clinical syndromes, it has been difficult to find a generally agreed upon definition. The term *shock* was first used by a French writer to convey the idea of a violent impression, jolt, commotion, or blow. In 1895, Warren[4] called shock "a momentary pause in the act of death."

Thal and Wilson[5] have defined shock as "a state of continuing impairment of tissue perfusion, resulting initially in cellular hypoxia and finally in asphyxia. The clinical picture reflects the homeostatic adjustments made by the body in response to inadequate blood flow. Regardless of etiology, shock begins with a fall in capillary blood flow below the levels needed to maintain cellular function. Although advanced shock is associated with failure of several organ systems, the initiating hemodynamic events may be used to form the basis of a simple classification." Although most authors stress the role of tissue perfusion, Wilson[6] emphasizes that shock is related to or caused by inadequate cellular metabolism that is not always caused by poor tissue perfusion but may also be caused by other factors, such as the direct cellular effects of endotoxin.

Jacobson[7] defines shock as "an acute circulatory insufficiency characterized by a cardiac output inadequate to provide normal perfusion for major organs." Among the hemodynamic effects are (1) generalized resistance to blood flow, (2) pooling or loss of blood, (3) arterial hypotension, and (4) inability of the heart to overcome peripheral resistance.

Because cellular survival depends on a constant supply of oxygen and nutrients, as well as the removal of products of metabolism, the eventual effects of shock are on cellular metabolism.

The Cardiovascular System and Shock Mechanisms

As a basis for understanding the pathophysiology of shock and the measures used in treatment, some understanding of the elements involved in tissue perfusion and cell metabolism is essential. The circulatory system is a closed circuit consisting of a pump (the heart), the blood, and a system of tubes or pipes carrying blood to and from the heart and the microcirculation. The components of the tubular system are (1) resistance vessels (arterioles), (2) exchange sites (capillaries), (3) shunts (vessels carrying blood directly from arterioles to venules), and (4) capacitance vessels (veins). Circulation is so regulated that the needs of all tissues are met.

Page[8] summarizes some of the tasks involved in distributing blood to the tissues in the following:

The body faces the difficult problem of distributing blood to tissues, each making its own special demands. Blood must be withdrawn from areas not in need of it. For example, the spleen and liver can act as reservoirs from which blood can be safely withdrawn during severe demand. The brain has a special controlling system to insure its supply in preference to less vital areas. To accomplish this constant redistribution of blood requires an elaborate system of sensing devices as well as the means. The complexity of this self-regulating system is almost unbelievable. Not only must it function efficiently, but it must continue to function if some of the control mechanisms are lost. The circulation does not depend on just one vital mechanism.

The Heart as a Pump

The heart applies force to the blood delivered to it by the veins, pushes it through the lungs and then drives it into the arteries. Cardiac output depends on three interrelated elements: the amount of blood the heart receives from the veins, the strength of its contraction, and its rate. The force of contraction or energy expended by the heart muscle is proportional to the diastolic fiber length (Starling's law of the heart). The quantity of blood remaining in the heart at the end of systole does not increase appreciably nor does it accumulate in the veins. (For a more complete description of cardiac function, see Chapter 10.)

[3] This discussion is not intended to meet all the needs of nurses working in shock research units or in intensive care units equipped with the latest monitoring and supportive devices. The references contain additional information. Because of the intense interest in this field, new papers will probably be published while this material is being printed.

[4] J. C. Warren: *Surgical Pathology and Therapeutics* (Philadelphia: W. B. Saunders Company, 1895), p. 279.

[5] Alan P. Thal and Robert F. Wilson: "Shock," *Curr. Probl. Surg.,* p. 8 (Sept.) 1965.

[6] Robert F. Wilson: Personal communication.

[7] Eugene D. Jacobson: "A Physiological Approach to Shock," *New Eng. J. Med.,* 278:834 (Apr. 11) 1968.

[8] Irvine H. Page: "The Mosaic Theory of Arterial Hypertension—Its Interpretation," *Perspect. Biol. Med.,* 10:327 (Spring) 1967.

Peripheral Resistance

Essentially, peripheral resistance is determined by the diameter of the blood vessels, particularly the arterioles. When there is no resistance to the flow of blood, the diastolic blood pressure falls to zero. To account for the ability to alter resistance, two types of receptors have been postulated, alpha and beta.[9] Alpha receptors in the arterioles respond to stimulation by catecholamines (epinephrine and norepinephrine from the sympathoadrenal system) and sympathomimetic agents by constriction. As the diameter of the arterioles diminishes, the resistance to the flow of blood increases. To overcome this resistance, the heart beats more forcefully, causing the arterial blood pressure to rise. As the blood pressure rises, stretch receptors in the aorta and carotid sinuses are stimulated. They initiate reflexes that can reduce cardiac output and cause the arterioles to dilate. Stimulation of beta receptors results in

arteriolar dilatation (especially in skeletal muscles), decreased venous pooling, and an increase in the rate and force of the heartbeat. Through appropriate alterations in peripheral resistance, blood flow to a tissue or an organ can thus be increased or decreased according to the needs of that tissue relative to the rest of the body.

The Capillary Unit

The capillaries are the site of exchange of essential nutrients and cellular wastes between the blood and the tissues. The capillary unit, often called the microcirculation, consists of microscopic arterioles, metarterioles, precapillaries, true capillaries, collecting and distal venules, and small veins.[10] (See Figure 11-1.)

The movement of fluid between the capillary bed and the interstitial fluid space is regulated by the filtration pressure within the capillary and the colloid osmotic pressure in the plasma.

[9] Raymond P. Ahlquist: "A Study of Adrenotropic Receptors," *Amer. J. Physiol.*, **153**:596 (June) 1948.

[10] B. W. Zweifach: "The Microcirculation of the Blood," *Scien. Amer.*, **200**:54 (Jan.) 1959.

FIGURE 11-1. Basic scheme of microcirculation. (After an original drawing by Leola Hogan.)

Filtration pressure increases when the arterioles or precapillary sphincters relax and the venules or postcapillary sphincters constrict; this increased filtration pressure tends to drive fluid from the capillaries into the interstitial space. These vessels appear to be regulated not only by the factors affecting larger vessels, but also by locally produced chemical agents such as tissue metabolites, proteolytic by-products, enzymes, and polypeptides.

In health as well as in shock, blood can be shunted through thoroughfare channels without nourishing or removing materials from the tissues. This mechanism enables the body to shift blood rapidly to the most active and vital cells and organs. Although this ability to shift blood, especially to the heart and brain, may be of temporary advantage, if long-continued it can lead to damage of other important organs such as the kidney, liver, and gastrointestinal tract.

Capacitance Blood Vessels

The capacitance vessels, especially the larger veins, normally hold about 50 to 70 per cent of the blood volume. When veins constrict, the capacity of the vascular system may be greatly reduced. The veins are important in the return of blood to the right atrium. Depending on their degree of constriction they can rapidly return blood to the heart for distribution to the tissues or serve as a reservoir for blood. Unlike the arteries the pressure within the veins is low. Factors affecting venous pressure are discussed subsequently.

Classification of Shock

In general, classifications of shock are based on either etiology or clinical manifestations.[11] Based on the initiating conditions, shock can be classified as hypovolemic (caused by loss of fluid or blood), cardiogenic (caused by inadequate pumping by the heart), septic or endotoxic (caused by infection), or miscellaneous types.[12] With a slight difference in emphasis, Wilson[13] classifies shock according to the hemodynamic derangement: (1) hypovolemia, (2) cardiac insufficiency, and (3) inadequate vascular tone.

[11] For a summary of different classifications by a number of different investigators, see Joseph H. Pollock: *A Survey of Surgical Shock* (Springfield, Ill.: Charles C Thomas, Publisher, 1966), pp. 5–6.

[12] Thal and Wilson, *op. cit.,* p. 8.

[13] John N. Wilson: "Rational Approach to Management of Clinical Shock," *Arch. Surg. (Chicago),* **91**:92 (July) 1965.

Shock Caused by Failure of the Heart as a Pump

Shock caused by the failure of the heart as a pump is characterized by an extremely low cardiac output. Some of the more common causes include myocardial infarction and arrhythmias in which the heart rate is excessively rapid, slow, or irregular. In these disorders, adequate tissue perfusion cannot be maintained because too little blood is forced into the arteries. Cardiogenic shock may also be caused by any disorder interfering with ventricular filling or emptying. Cardiac tamponade caused by excessive fluid or blood in the pericardial sac prevents blood from entering and filling the ventricles. A massive pulmonary embolism obstructs the flow of blood from the right ventricle. Unless the basic disorder is corrected, cardiogenic shock is self-perpetuating and the heart fails to perfuse not only other organs but also its own coronary vessels.

Shock Caused by a Decrease in Venous Return

Failure of or a significant reduction in venous return to the heart results whenever the intravascular volume of blood fails to adequately fill the vascular capacity. This is usually caused by excessive loss of fluid or blood or decreased vasomotor tone. Although hemorrhage is the classic example of hypovolemic shock, there are a variety of other causes. These include loss of gastrointestinal fluid from excessive vomiting or diarrhea, from excessive sweating, and through burned surfaces. An uncommon cause of hypovolemic shock is failure to replace the fluid loss from excessive urination. As an example of the latter, Mr. Compo experienced extreme diuresis following the removal of a benign brain tumor from the region of the pituitary gland. Edema and possible damage to the posterior hypophysis resulted in failure to release the antidiuretic hormone. Water lost in his urine was not replaced and as a result his blood volume fell to a point where his circulation could not be maintained. Mr. Compo went into profound shock from which he failed to recover. His life might have been saved had fluid replacement and the administration of ADH followed the observation that his urine output was greatly in excess of his fluid intake.

When the rate of fluid loss is slow, blood volume can be reduced by as much as 10 to 20 per cent without noticeable effects on tissue perfusion. Greater reductions, however, may result in sudden severe cardiovascular insufficiency. As blood volume diminishes, the quantity of blood returned to the heart and cardiac output are also reduced, although usually not by a proportionate amount.

Besides low blood volume, any condition leading to pooling of blood in the capillary or venous circulation can lessen venous return to the heart. Loss of venous tone leads to venous pooling. Loss of arteriolar tone with continued venous constriction leads to capillary pooling. In the latter condition, capillary hydrostatic pressure rises, fluid escapes into the interstitial space, and the blood volume falls. In addition, stasis of blood in the capillary bed favors intravascular clotting that may further interfere with blood flow in the capillaries and venous return.

Septic Shock

According to Weil and Shubin [14] bacterial shock is the third most frequent cause of shock at the Los Angeles County Hospital. Its incidence approaches that associated with myocardial infarction, which is exceeded only by hypovolemic or fluid-loss shock. The exact mechanisms involved in septic shock are not completely clear. Much of the knowledge of septic shock has been gained from animal experiments and the findings do not necessarily apply to human beings. It is called septic because it results from the action of toxic substances produced directly or indirectly by bacteria on blood vessels and other cells. Although these changes are most commonly caused by endotoxin from gram-negative organisms, exotoxin from gram-positive bacteria may occasionally play a role.

Dying or damaged cells may release certain substances such as histamine and proteolytic enzymes that may interfere with the normal cardiovascular activity. Histamine, for example, appears to interfere with the normal reactivity of blood vessels. Vasoactive substances, such as bradykinin, a very potent vasodilator, may be released from alpha-2-globulin fraction of the blood by the proteolytic enzymes.

There is a wide spectrum of cardiovascular findings in septic shock. When sepsis occurs without any complicating problems such as hypovolemia or cardiac insufficiency and does not involve the lungs, the patient is often warm and his blood vessels appear to be dilated. The cardiac output is normal or increased and the total peripheral resistance is either normal or reduced. It is not clear at this time how much of

this decreased resistance and hypotension is caused by arteriovenous shunting. There is evidence suggesting that although total blood flow or cardiac output may be adequate, the cells involved directly or indirectly by the septic process may have impaired aerobic and anaerobic metabolism.

If hypovolemia, cardiac insufficiency, or widespread advanced pneumonia is present, the patient tends to have a higher total peripheral resistance and he may be cold and clammy, as typically seen after blood loss or myocardial infarction.

The Role of the Nervous System in Shock

Because the nervous system regulates the contraction and relaxation of the muscles in the blood vessels, shock may result from the effect on it of injury or drugs. It should be remembered, however, that shock from head trauma is quite rare. Increased intracranial pressure characteristically increases blood pressure until shortly before death. Shock caused by the vasodilator action of the nervous system is classified as neurogenic shock and is usually transitory. The nervous system itself does not have to be directly injured. Fainting, or syncope, may be considered a form of neurogenic shock. Spinal anesthesia, as a consequence of its depressing effect on the nerve supply to the anesthetized area, may also be considered a cause of neurogenic shock.

Summary

As indicated previously, shock may be the result of a large number of unrelated disorders, only a few of which have been mentioned. Whatever the initiating factor, much of the injury in shock results from the damage done to cells by failure to supply the proper amounts of oxygen, glucose, and other substances and failure to adequately remove the products of metabolism.

Homeostatic Responses to Shock

When the body is injured it responds by a complex set of interrelated mechanisms that tend to minimize the effects of the injury and to restore normal functioning. "Nowhere is the capacity for self-preservation better demonstrated than in 'Shock'." [15] Physiological responses are of three general types: (1) cardiovascular, (2) water conservation and expansion of blood volume, and (3) respiratory. All serve directly or indirectly to maintain tissue perfu-

[14] Max Harry Weil and Herbert Shubin: *Diagnosis and Treatment of Shock* (Baltimore: The Williams & Wilkins Company, 1967), p. 10.

[15] Thal and Wilson, *op. cit.,* p. 9.

sion, most particularly to the high-priority structures, the heart and brain. Within limits these responses facilitate survival. As do other body responses, when they are inadequate or excessive, they intensify or worsen the degree of shock.

Cardiovascular Responses

Of the cardiovascular responses in shock, the body is more effective in maintaining arterial blood pressure than in correcting other derangements. When the cardiac output falls, stretch receptors in the aorta and carotid sinuses initiate impulses that stimulate vasomotor centers in the medulla. The vasomotor centers, in turn, respond by activating impulses via the sympathetic nervous system and releasing from the adrenal medulla epinephrine and norepinephrine, which act to increase the rate and force of cardiac contraction.

A second mechanism for increasing vasoconstriction is initiated by the kidney. As blood flow to the kidney falls, the juxtaglomerular apparatus releases renin, which activates angiotensin, a powerful vasoconstrictor. Despite a considerable decrease in blood volume or cardiac output, arterial blood pressure may be maintained within physiological limits by the following mechanisms. Arteriolar constriction raises peripheral resistance. Cardiac output is elevated by an increased force of cardiac contraction and an increased heart rate. The effective circulating blood volume is increased by contraction of the capacitance veins. Although veins do not respond as forcefully as arteries, venous constriction is a critical factor in the return of blood to the right atrium.

How may the degree of cardiovascular response be determined?

Arterial pressure can be measured with the familiar blood pressure cuff attached to a mercury or aneroid manometer. A more accurate but less convenient method consists of introducing a catheter into the radial or brachial artery and attaching it to an electronic pressure transducer. Not only can the levels of the systolic and diastolic pressures be determined, but certain deductions can be made from the pulse pressure, which is equal to the difference between the systolic and diastolic pressures. These deductions include an estimation of the (1) strength of the heartbeat, (2) degree of peripheral resistance, (3) amount and viscosity of blood in the arteries, (4) elasticity of arterial walls, (5) distensibility of the heart, and (6) force of venous return to the heart.

Although arterial pressure can be measured relatively easily, one cannot rely on it to reflect the severity of shock. In fact a patient's arterial blood pressure may be within physiological limits and yet his tissues may be poorly supplied with blood. The reason for this inadequacy of perfusion is that most arterioles respond to stimulation by the sympathoadrenal system by undergoing powerful constriction. This response reduces the vascular capacity and brings it into an appropriate relationship with the blood volume. It is useful inasmuch as the coronary and cerebral vessels are relatively less responsive to the sympathoadrenal system than other blood vessels and they continue to be supplied with blood. It can be detrimental, however, if it is severe and persistent, because constriction of the vessels in the extremities, heart, kidneys, and other organs deprives them of an adequate blood supply.

VENOUS PRESSURE

Whereas the arterial blood pressure is a reflection of the state of constriction of the arterioles and the force with which the heart drives blood into the arteries, venous pressure is what remains of that force after the blood passes through the capillaries. Actually, venous pressure is affected by right atrial pressure. With an increase in right atrial pressure, peripheral venous pressure must also rise if blood is to return to the heart. Pressure in peripheral veins also is affected by the distance and relationship of the vein to the right atrium. Hydrostatic pressure is caused by the weight exerted by a fluid against the wall of a tube. The higher the column of fluid, the greater is the pressure against the wall of the tube. When an individual is standing absolutely still, venous pressure is greater in the lower extremities than it is at the right atrium. Although peripheral venous pressure has been measured for many years, it is now known that it does not consistently reflect atrial pressure.

CENTRAL VENOUS PRESSURE

The pressure of blood in the right atrium, or central venous pressure (CVP), is normally from 0 to 5 cm of water. A CVP of 15 to 20 cm usually indicates that the blood is being returned to the right heart more rapidly than the heart can pump it into the arterial circulation. By continuous monitoring of the central venous pressure, the physician can estimate how the circulating blood volume compares to the pumping action of the heart at any given time. The trend of the response is often more important than the specific level.[16] When a small amount

[16] John N. Wilson *et al.:* "Central Venous Pressure in Optimal Blood Volume Maintenance," *Arch. Surg.* (Chicago), **85:**568 (Oct.) 1962.

of fluid is administered rapidly and the CVP rises abruptly, this response often indicates that the heart is overloaded. Thal and Wilson [17] state that the competence of the myocardium in the patient whose CVP is no greater than 10 cm of water can be measured by administering 500 ml of water in 20 minutes. If the CVP rises rapidly, the myocardium is probably loaded to capacity and the fluid intake should be discontinued immediately. If fluids continue to be given, pulmonary edema may result. If, on the other hand, fluids are infused and the arterial pressure increases but the venous pressure does not rise, the patient is probably at least relatively hypovolemic in relation to the competency of the heart.

RESPONSES INCREASING BLOOD VOLUME

In addition to reflexes acting to reduce the capacity of the vascular system, other changes occur that tend to restore the blood volume. As the arterioles constrict, less blood enters the capillaries, thus reducing intracapillary pressure. The quantity of fluid leaving the capillary and entering it from the interstitial space is determined by the balance between (1) the filtration pressure, which the precapillary sphincters (arterioles) and postcapillary sphincters (venules) regulate, and (2) the colloid osmotic pressure of the blood, which is proportional to the concentration of the plasma proteins. Constriction of arterioles and relaxation of venules tend to cause the net filtration pressure to fall below the colloid osmotic pressure of the plasma and result in a tendency of fluid to move from the interstitial space into the capillaries. (See Chapter 9.)

The kidney helps to protect the blood volume. Increased secretion of hormones, especially the antidiuretic hormone and aldosterone, promotes the reabsorption of water and sodium by the kidney, thereby aiding in their conservation.[18]

Thirst is commonly experienced by the person in shock and is a valuable sign that should not be ignored. Usually, however, the gastrointestinal tracts of patients in shock will not tolerate oral liquids.

Respiratory Responses

The respiratory system responds primarily to changes in the pH, pCO_2, and pO_2 of the arterial blood.[19] The receptors most sensitive to

pH and pCO_2 are found in or near the respiratory center in the brain, and the main receptors for detecting changes in pO_2 are found in the aortic and carotid bodies. Increased CO_2 tension or decreased oxygen tension as well as a fall in pH act to stimulate breathing. Hyperpnea tends to compensate for metabolic acidosis occurring as a result of hypoxia by lowering the carbon dioxide tension and thus producing a relative respiratory alkalosis. One of the serious effects of prolonged hypoxia is a metabolic acidosis caused by the accumulation of lactic acid and a corresponding reduction in bicarbonate concentration. Initially the body is able to compensate for the increased hydrogen ion production by increasing the rate and depth of respiration, which in turn reduces the pCO_2 and carbonic acid. As a result of hyperventilation, the ratio of bicarbonate to carbonic acid is returned toward the normal 20:1. Because the extent of hyperventilation is usually an excellent sign of the degree of hypoxia, it is extremely important to observe not only the rate and depth of respiration but also any changes that occur.

Summary of Homeostatic Adjustments in Shock

The body responds to life-threatening situations by initiating reflexes tending to maintain, restore, and/or improve the perfusion of body tissues. Because survival depends on maintenance of function of the heart and brain, the initial response to a diminished cardiac output or fall in arterial blood pressure is to redistribute the circulating blood to maintain adequate blood flow in these organs. By arteriolar and venous constriction, the capacity of the vascular system is reduced, thereby increasing the relative blood volume. Blood volume is also increased by movement of water from the interstitial and cellular spaces into the capillaries. The excretion of salt and water by the kidney is reduced because of the influence of aldosterone and the antidiuretic hormone. The respiratory system attempts to reduce the effects of metabolic acidosis by increased ventilation, thereby producing a compensatory respiratory alkalosis.

Effects of Shock on Specific Organs

Any patient with a serious injury or illness is in danger of developing shock. Shock occurs in all degrees from mild to so-called refractory or irreversible shock. Impending or mild degrees may be compensated for readily by the body's intrinsic homeostatic mechanisms. Depending on circumstances, however, it may

---

[17] *Op. cit.*, p. 36.
[18] See Chapters 9 and 15, Part A, for the factors influencing the secretion of these hormones.
[19] The p in pCO_2 and pO_2 stands for pressure of the gas carbon dioxide or oxygen, respectively.

progress to a partially compensated and reversible stage and finally to irreversible shock. The term *irreversible* means that the changes in the cells have progressed to the point where present methods of treatment are incapable of reversing the pathophysiological changes. Sometimes shock develops slowly, and at other times it develops with great rapidity. Unless the patient is rapidly and adequately treated, he may go into irreversible shock and die. By means of modern methods of treatment, survival is occasionally possible in some patients who appear to be in irreversible shock.

The Heart and Blood Vessels

If shock continues and is severe enough all tissues eventually suffer. The various parts of the circulatory system deteriorate and a vicious circle may develop. To illustrate, the force of contraction of the myocardium depends on the adequacy of its blood supply. In any condition with a decreased cardiac output, arterial blood pressure falls, leading to decreased systemic blood flow and decreased nutrition of all tissues, including those of the heart. As the nutrition of the heart muscle is further impaired, the force of cardiac contraction becomes increasingly ineffective. With marked tissue ischemia, toxins are believed to be released from the cells. They intensify the condition by (1) increasing capillary permeability, (2) predisposing to intravascular clotting, and (3) depressing the myocardial and vascular responses to catecholamines.

As systemic blood flow diminishes, stasis of blood develops and the tendency of the blood to clot is increased. Thrombosis within capillaries contributes to the progression of shock, and further reduces blood flow. Thus a vicious circle may be initiated with each factor intensifying the severity of the preceding one. Unless the cycle is reversed, death ensues.

With decreased blood volume because of hemorrhage, a similar cycle is initiated. Because of an inadequate blood volume, venous return to the heart is diminished. There is corresponding decrease in cardiac output and a series of events leading to myocardial and tissue ischemia.

The Kidney

In shock, there is decreased renal perfusion because of constriction of the afferent and efferent arterioles and shunting of the blood away from the glomeruli. This results in reduced renal function and urine volume. The formation of renin by the kidney in response to inadequate blood flow has been described previously. Because of the decrease in blood flow, glomerular filtration diminishes and the kidney loses its ability to regulate electrolyte and acid-base balance. Unfortunately the renal vasoconstriction may continue long after the blood pressure has been restored to normal levels. If the shock progresses, severe oliguria and tubular necrosis may develop. With appropriate therapy and prevention of overloading with fluid, the patient may survive until the kidney repairs itself sufficiently so that normal function returns. This repair takes about 10 to 14 days.

Recognition of impending renal failure even before oliguria appears is essential to the proper treatment of the patient. Among the changes in the urine indicating that the patient is in non-oliguric renal failure are (1) reduced specific gravity and osmolality of the urine, (2) reduced creatinine clearance, and (3) a rise in sodium urine concentration relative to the amount in the serum. Examination of the blood may reveal a progressive rise in urea nitrogen, creatinine, and potassium that will be especially rapid if there is associated tissue damage or infection.

The Intestinal Mucosa

The combination of decreased cardiac output and vasoconstriction also limits blood flow to the intestine. As a result of inadequate perfusion, the capillary endothelium in the intestinal mucosa is damaged, and edema, hemorrhage, and congestion of the intestinal wall may occur. The most serious effect of these changes is the reduced effectiveness of the intestinal mucosa as a barrier between the bacteria and toxins in the intestinal lumen and the blood stream.[20]

The Reticuloendothelial System

All structures and systems deprived of their blood supply tend to function poorly. In shock, the function of the reticuloendothelial system is depressed. As a consequence, the ability of the body to detoxify harmful agents may be greatly reduced.

The Lungs

Not only may the lungs suffer direct structural and functional changes in shock, but their function may also be impaired because of pulmonary edema secondary to heart failure. The reason for these changes are not well understood. Moreover, unlike the heart and kidney, there is as yet no good, practical way to main-

[20] Jacobson, *op. cit.,* p. 836.

tain life while lung function is being restored. Some of the possible causes of lung damage include left heart failure, circulating toxins such as histamine and bradykinin, and constriction of the small pulmonary veins. As a result of experiments with dogs, Veith [21] believes that humoral agents are primarily responsible.

Recently, much attention has been directed toward surfactant, a lipoprotein whose main property is the ability to reduce surface tension within the alveoli. If surfactant is destroyed or produced in inadequate quantities, as may occur with shock, anoxia, and trauma, surface tension rises in the alveoli and atelectasis results.

Simeone [22] and others have wondered whether trauma alone can destroy the integrity of the alveolocapillary membrane and promote the development of congestive atelectasis. Can hypoxia such as that associated with atelectasis affect the integrity of this layer and promote further and more intense atelectasis? Do certain aspects of therapy aggravate these problems?

STRUCTURAL CHANGES IN THE LUNG

Among the structural changes in the lungs in shock are a loss of elasticity, pulmonary congestion, edema, alveolar hemorrhage, and atelectasis. A condition that may develop in patients with various types of trauma, thoracic or nonthoracic injury has been called "wet lung." As a consequence of the changes in the capillaries and congestion in the lung, the transfer of oxygen into the blood and removal of carbon dioxide are impaired. In other words, hypoxia is made worse and carbon dioxide accumulates with resultant or increased metabolic acidosis and respiratory acidosis. In the early stage of shock, if the patient's lungs are clear and he hyperventilates spontaneously, he may develop respiratory alkalosis caused in part by an increased elimination of carbon dioxide. Hyperventilation is often the first sign of sepsis, shock, or pulmonary emboli. Endotoxin can stimulate the respiratory center even before there is other evidence of sepsis.

Martin [23] reports that in 100 patients who underwent autopsy following death from shock and/or trauma, the lungs were more frequently

involved than any other organ. The lesions included pulmonary edema, congestion, bronchopneumonia, pleural effusions, and pulmonary emboli.

Cell Damage

As discussed in Chapter 12, cellular functions and survival depend on the release of energy from the glucose molecule. Energy is released in the mitochondria by a series of minute steps. The first steps that involve the conversion of glucose to pyruvic acid can take place under anaerobic conditions. Each glucose molecule forms two molecules of pyruvic acid, hydrogen, and a small amount of a high-energy phosphate molecule, adenosine triphosphate (ATP). For the steps in glucose metabolism to continue beyond this point, oxygen is required. Under normal circumstances, pyruvic acid is converted to acetic acid and then to acetyl CoA, which enters the Krebs cycle. In the Krebs cycle, the acetyl CoA is broken down into CO_2 and H. The hydrogen is taken up in the electron transport system, and if adequate oxygen is present, the hydrogen and oxygen combine to form water. The completion of this reaction releases a great deal of energy in the form of ATP. If adequate oxygen is not available, the Krebs cycle stops and the pyruvic acid is converted into lactic acid. If oxygen becomes available again, the lactic acid can be converted into pyruvic acid that can then enter the Krebs cycle. As lactic acid accumulates, it causes metabolic acidosis, which can have a further detrimental effect on cell activity.

The Krebs cycle requires oxygen; in the absence of oxygen or the presence of some condition interfering with the cell's using oxygen, the Krebs cycle is seriously impaired. Insufficient ATP is formed to provide energy to maintain vital functions. The permeability of the cell membrane increases with potassium leaving the cell and sodium and water entering. Other functions necessary to life such as the synthesis of protein and enzymes also fail.

Because of a lack of oxygen and the development of acidosis the membranes or borders around the lysosomes, tiny particles within the cell, may be damaged. When the lysosomal membrane breaks down, powerful hydrolytic enzymes that may play a role in intracellular digestion are released. These enzymes can damage or destroy the cell and surrounding tissues. It may be that lysosome-related injury continues even after hypoxia and acidosis are corrected. This may be one reason that a patient may continue to deteriorate despite correction of the hemodynamic aspects of shock. The injured or

[21] Frank J. Veith et al.: "Pulmonary Microcirculatory Response to Shock, Transfusion, and Pump-oxygenator Procedures: A Unified Mechanism Underlying Pulmonary Damage," *Surgery*, **64**:95–109 (July) 1968.

[22] F. A. Simeone: "Pulmonary Complications of Nonthoracic Wounds: A Historical Perspective," *J. Trauma*, 8:640 (Sept.) 1968.

[23] Arthur M. Martin et al.: "Pathologic Anatomy of the Lungs Following Shock and Trauma," *J. Trauma*, 8:687–99 (Sept.) 1968.

anoxic cell may also liberate histamine or similar substances that can interfere with cardiovascular response to catecholamine-like drugs.

These enzymes, especially those with proteolytic activity, may also cause the release of certain very powerful vasoactive substances, kinins, from the alpha-2-globulin fraction of the blood. These proteolytic enzymes, or proteases, convert the inactive precursors, kininogens, into the very active and very powerful kinins. The best known of these kinins is bradykinin, which is the most potent vasodilator known to man.

What are the signs and symptoms of shock?

One of the most significant contributions the nurse makes to the care of ill patients is observing them for evidence indicating whether they are or are not progressing satisfactorily. All patients who experience traumatic injury, extensive surgery, myocardial infarction, pancreatitis, or other serious illness should be observed for any indications that shock is developing. This observation should be continued until such time as it is *known* that the patient is in a stable state. It is possible for a patient to be treated for shock and to appear to be making a satisfactory recovery only to go later into an even more severe stage of shock. The importance of informed observation cannot be overemphasized because shock must be treated early and vigorously if the patient is to survive.

Because shock involves the entire individual, signs and symptoms reflect changes in function of organs as they respond to altered blood volume, myocardial contraction, and/or vascular tone. Early signs and symptoms result from the activation of the sympathoadrenal system, which may correct or compensate for hypovolemia or other hemodynamic derangements. Early signs and symptoms serve as warning signals that something is wrong. These signs and symptoms usually reflect (1) the response of the sympathoadrenal system; (2) diminished perfusion of blood to the nervous system, heart, kidney, skin, lungs, gastrointestinal tract, and other organs; (3) the primary injury or illness.

NERVOUS SYSTEM

Many of the signs and symptoms relating to the nervous system are caused by activation of the sympathoadrenal system. The resultant hyperventilation, anxiety, agitation, apprehension, and restlessness may precede the development of other signs of shock. When they occur, the possibility that the patient is in early shock should be considered, and their presence should be promptly reported to the physician. Not infrequently, restlessness is interpreted as indicating that the patient is in pain when in fact he is suffering from hypoxia, which can produce a very similar picture. Eventually, as blood flow to the brain fails, the patient becomes more confused and finally he may become comatose.

ARTERIAL AND VENOUS TONE

Blood pressure depends on the interrelationship of blood volume, the force of myocardial contraction, and the degree of arterial and venous constriction. Arterial blood pressure tends to rise if there is an increase in cardiac output, blood volume, or vasoconstriction. The reverse is also true; that is, the arterial blood pressure tends to fall if there is a drop in cardiac output, blood volume, or if vasodilatation occurs. The pulse pressure should be noted. As cardiac output decreases, there is generally a corresponding fall in pulse pressure and increased difficulty in breathing.

The state of constriction of the peripheral blood vessels is also reflected by the skin. With peripheral vasoconstriction, the skin is cool and moist. With peripheral stasis it is mottled or cyanotic. The mucous membranes tend to be pale and dry. Nail beds are cyanotic and, when pressed, refill slowly. Although neck and peripheral veins may be distended in cardiac failure, in other forms of shock they are likely to be collapsed. Although these changes are characteristic of most types of shock, in many patients with sepsis there is a normal or increased cardiac output and the skin is warm, dry, and pink.

CARDIAC FUNCTION

The quality of the pulse and its fullness, rate, and rhythm should be noted. A thready pulse is often noted and usually indicates a low cardiac output.

KIDNEY FUNCTION

When the arterial blood pressure or cardiac output is low, blood is shunted away from the kidney, resulting in a decreased glomerular filtration rate of the fluid. Sodium and water reabsorption in the tubules increases, and urine output falls. Measurement of the output of urine is of great importance. A urine output of 25 ml or more per hour is usually a satisfactory minimum. To accurately and continuously measure urine output an indwelling catheter is inserted. Efforts should be made to improve the hemodynamic status of the patient to maintain adequate urine flow. To a certain extent, the kidney is the "window of the viscera." That is, if there is adequate urine (without the use of a diuretic), one can generally assume that the kidney is adequately perfused. If the kidney is adequately perfused, one can usually assume that the other organs are also well perfused. If the urine volume is low and the specific gravity is high, it can usually be assumed that the patient is hypovolemic, has impaired cardiac output, and/or reduced perfusion of the kidney.

Summary

All seriously ill and injured patients require regular and careful observation. In the patient in shock, pulse rate, arterial blood pressure, and central venous pressure may need to be checked every 15 minutes or continuously. At the time these measurements are made, the general condition of the patient should also be noted. Slowing of the pulse, widening of the pulse pressure, and an increase in urine output are usually indices that the patient is improving. ECG monitoring with a cardioscope is also indicated in most critically ill patients.

TESTS TO ESTIMATE DEGREE OF CELLULAR HYPOXIA

To estimate the degree of cellular hypoxia and the extent to which respiratory mechanisms are effective in compensating for metabolic derangements, arterial pH, blood lactic acid, pCO_2, and standard blood bicarbonate levels may be determined. Venous carbon dioxide content and the carbon dioxide–combining power give only an approximate estimate of the degree of metabolic acidosis. A more accurate estimate of the degree of hypoxia is the arterial lactate. This test is, however, generally limited to research laboratories. Other tests such as the blood hematocrit, cardiac output, and blood volume can also be employed. The hematocrit is easily performed and is useful in determining the need for red cells or the extent of hemoconcentration in disorders such as burns.

Even in the absence of highly sophisticated methods of determining such factors as cardiac output, degree of vasoconstriction, and blood lactic acid, a knowledgeable nurse can detect evidence that shock is developing or becoming progressively worse. The sophisticated tests often confirm what has been discerned by clinical observation.

Treatment of Shock

The fundamental objective in shock is to maintain and/or restore cellular metabolism.

To achieve this objective, the cells must be provided with adequate amounts of oxygen and glucose and be able to utilize them. The prevention and treatment of shock therefore require attention to the following: (1) identification and correction of the cause of the shock; (2) adequate respiratory function; (3) adequate circulatory function, blood volume, cardiac pumping action, and vascular tone; and (4) correction of any condition that impairs cellular metabolism.

Maintenance of Respiratory Function

Wilson [24] states that the importance of deficient ventilation and oxygenation in the etiology of shock cannot be overemphasized. An adequate supply of oxygen and the removal of carbon dioxide are essential to biochemical homeostasis. (See Chapter 8 for causes of failure of ventilation.) The first step in treatment of shock is to be certain that the airway is open and functioning. In severe respiratory failure, the patient may need ventilatory support from a respirator. An endotracheal tube may be inserted or a tracheostomy performed and a cuffed tracheostomy tube inserted (see Chapter 8). Because high concentrations of oxygen are known to damage the lung, the physician prescribes the lowest concentration that will maintain a pO_2 of 60 mm of mercury or higher.

Maintenance of Adequate Blood Volume

Despite a loss of as much as 25 to 35 per cent in the blood volume, if it is not too rapid there may be only a moderate drop in blood pressure. With a loss of 50 per cent or more, the shock is very severe or lethal. When a patient is hypotensive as a result of hypovolemia, his blood pressure may rise rapidly when as little as 500 to 700 ml of fluid are administered.

Fluid Replacement

When enough fluid is lost to seriously affect venous return, then sufficient fluid must be introduced to produce an adequate cardiac output. The best gauge for measuring the adequacy of fluid replacement is the response of the central venous pressure to the administered fluid. In general, if a patient is hypovolemic, he will have a low central venous pressure, but more important, his central venous pressure rises slowly or not at all as fluid and/or blood is given to the patient. The reverse is true of pa-

[24] John N. Wilson: "The Management of Acute Circulatory Failure," *Surg. Clin. N. Amer.*, **43**:469–95 (Apr.) 1963.

tients where the cardiovascular system is already handling as much fluid as it can. A less accurate index of blood volume is the degree of filling of the neck veins. When fluid is added rapidly and the central venous pressure rises, the neck veins, which are normally collapsed, distend. This response usually indicates that the heart is handling about as much fluid as it can. More fluid may precipitate heart failure. When the central venous pressure fails to rise and the veins remain collapsed, hypovolemia still exists and fluid may continue to be administered.

Even when the fluid deficit appears to be corrected, the patient requires continued observation until such time as it is certain that he is in a stable state. The survival of the patient depends on the consistency and accuracy of the observations that are made. As stressed throughout, appropriate actions must be taken if the observations are to benefit the patient.

The kind and amount of fluid used in the treatment of shock depend on the nature and quantity of fluid lost, the urgency of the situation, and the type of fluid available. In general, fluids used in replacement are of three types: blood and plasma, plasma expanders, and electrolyte solutions. In emergency situations, electrolyte solutions such as Ringer's lactate or saline with bicarbonate may be used to expand blood volume, because only a fraction of the erythrocytes is required to carry oxygen.

BLOOD

A rapid loss of as many as 500 ml of blood can usually occur without significant evidence of hypovolemia. In some individuals as many as 1,000 ml may be lost with only mild signs. When more than 1 liter of blood is lost there are usually clinical signs and hemodynamic changes. If bleeding has stopped, fluids that expand the plasma volume will often be adequate to restore homeostasis. When bleeding continues, blood must be used in replacement. Because of the dangers inherent in blood transfusion,[25] it should not be used if another fluid can satisfactorily increase blood volume and maintain adequate oxygen-carrying capacity. Bank blood always presents the danger of hemolysis from mismatched blood and/or serum hepatitis.

PLASMA EXPANDERS

In disorders such as acute pancreatitis, burns, and peritonitis in which the loss of plasma is excessive, fluids containing molecules large enough to be retained in the blood vessels are essential. Plasma, dextran of high or low molecular weight, or electrolyte solutions containing albumin may be used. Dextran of high molecular weight, 72,000 or more, is useful because it tends to remain in the blood. It has a disadvantage, however, because it induces cell aggregation, an already undesirable tendency in slow-moving blood in shock.

Low molecular dextran (40,000) is less effective as a direct plasma expander than the high molecular form. It acts mainly to prevent or hinder cell aggregation and to lessen the viscosity of the blood. As a result, it may improve the circulation of blood and prevent sludging of the red cells.

Before dextran is administered, blood should be taken for blood grouping and cross matching. Dextran should be administered slowly and the patient should have his central venous pressure continuously monitored.[26]

ELECTROLYTE SOLUTIONS

Electrolyte solutions such as Ringer's lactate or saline buffered with bicarbonate are useful in expanding the extracellular fluid volume. Wilson [27] states that electrolyte solutions have the advantage of reducing viscosity and preventing sludging and aggregation of erythrocytes. He favors the use of albumin in either isotonic saline or Ringer's lactate solution. Bicarbonate is also useful in correcting metabolic acidosis. Solutions containing sodium are often contraindicated in cardiac disorders.

Support of the Heart

Some estimate of the condition of the heart can be made by monitoring the ECG and noting the character of the pulse.

Any arrhythmia should be converted because it tends to reduce cardiac efficiency. Quinidine and procaine amide may be used to treat various arrhythmias but it should be remembered that they also tend to reduce myocardial contractility. Digitalis is often very useful in shock because it improves the strength of the failing heart and may reduce the heart rate to more normal values. Isoproterenol (Isuprel) is a sympathomimetic amine that acts primarily on the beta receptors. It increases the strength and rate of cardiac contraction and lowers peripheral vascular resistance, especially in certain muscles.

[25] The mortality rate associated with blood transfusion is comparable to that of appendicitis.

[26] James T. Gladish, Alon P. Winnie, and Vincent J. Collins: "Shock: Recognition and Treatment," *Postgrad. Med.,* **42**:49 (July) 1967.

[27] *Op. cit.,* p. 487.

Regulation of the Size of the Vascular Chamber

Until recently, emphasis has been on maintaining the level of the arterial pressure within so-called normal limits, the belief being that arterial blood pressure is a good index of tissue perfusion. With additional knowledge, however, it is now known that other factors are of equal or even greater importance. In the treatment of shock, the physician must try to evaluate the state of each part of the circulatory system. When in the opinion of the physician the degree of vasoconstriction is insufficient to maintain blood flow, especially to the heart and brain, he may prescribe any one of a number of vasopressor agents. Perhaps the most frequently used are metaraminol (Aramine) and norepinephrine (Levophed). Maintenance of adequate arterial pressure is especially important in older patients in whom blood flow through narrowed coronary or cerebral vessels may be pressure-dependent.[28] Both of these drugs can be administered by intravenous infusion and metaraminol can also be injected intramuscularly. However, absorption from the intramuscular site is not reliable enough to be useful in shock.

Norepinephrine is a very powerful vasoconstrictor and care must be taken to prevent it from infiltrating the tissues. If this drug does get outside a vein, it can cause the tissue to slough. It should be injected into large and central veins. The arterial blood pressure of the patient receiving norepinephrine should be under constant surveillance in order to detect undesirable rises in the blood pressure. Moreover, as the patient changes position, the rate of flow may be altered and the patient receive more or less drug than necessary to produce the desired effect.

Although these drugs may initially be beneficial by maintaining perfusion of the heart or brain, if their use is prolonged they can cause death or irreversible damage in the tissues supplied by the severely constricted vessels. Further, heart failure may be precipitated by a sudden and/or excessive rise in the arterial blood pressure. Therefore vasopressor therapy is used for as short a time as possible. Although vasoconstriction helps to maintain blood flow to the heart and brain in early shock, if prolonged it can result in irreversible injury to the tissues of other organs such as the kidney, lungs, liver, and gastrointestinal tract. If this vasoconstriction is severe and persistent despite

[28] See Louis S. Goodman and Alfred Gilman: *The Pharmacological Basis of Therapeutics,* 3rd ed. (New York: The Macmillan Company, 1965), for a complete discussion of these and other vasoconstrictor drugs.

the infusing of adequate amounts of fluid or blood, a vasodilating drug may be of value. When vasodilators are used it must be remembered that there is dilatation not only of arterioles but also of the capacitance veins. One to three liters of additional fluid or blood may be needed to fill the additional vascular capacity created by the vasodilator drug.

Among the vasodilator drugs that are being studied are phenoxybenzamine (Dibenzyline), phentolamine (Regitine), and chlorpromazine. According to Thal and Wilson [29] phenoxybenzamine is the most powerful. It blocks the alpha adrenergic receptors in the walls of the blood vessels. Thus the blood vessels do not respond to the naturally produced norepinephrine and peripheral resistance is reduced. It also reduces the response of small blood vessels to agents such as serotonin and histamine. Because phenoxybenzamine does not alter the response of the heart to the catecholamines (epinephrine and norepinephrine), the relative effectiveness of the heart is increased. Although the arterial blood pressure may be lower than normal, tissue perfusion is usually improved. Young patients can usually tolerate vasodilation and low blood pressure quite well, but older patients with sclerotic vessels may not be able to tolerate this hypotension. Under these circumstances a cardiogenic drug used in combination with the vasodilator may be able to maintain or raise the blood pressure by increasing the cardiac output.

Patients who receive vasodilator drugs must be continuously observed for evidence of improvement or of failure of the circulation. Particularly in the patient in hypovolemic shock, a rapid expansion of the vascular capacity without adequate volume to fill the space may lead to a precipitous drop in blood pressure. To protect the patient, central venous pressure must be continuously monitored and the blood volume increased as the vascular chamber enlarges. Because there is some evidence that phenoxybenzamine can cause cardiac damage, it is given slowly.

MAINTENANCE OF RENAL FUNCTION

Measures used to increase blood volume and cardiac output should benefit the kidney as well as other tissues. Correction of metabolic acidosis (discussed subsequently) is essential, because severe metabolic acidosis is injurious to the kidney and other organs. Mannitol, an osmotic diuretic, is a 6-carbon atom sugar. It is filtered in the urine and is neither reabsorbed

[29] *Op. cit.,* p. 43.

nor metabolized. It has two uses. By promoting diuresis it helps to prevent the accumulation of hemolyzed cells and other debris in the renal tubules. This action is of most benefit when hypotension is temporary. It is also useful in identifying the patient who has suffered renal damage in shock. The patient whose urine output does not improve after an adequate fluid load of 25 g of mannitol given in 100 to 500 ml of glucose in a 10- to 30-minute period can usually be assumed to have renal damage.[30]

Specific Therapeutic Techniques

ADRENAL STEROIDS

Among other drugs used in the treatment of shock are the adrenal steroids. Enthusiasm for their use waxes and wanes. Weissman and Thomas [31] demonstrated that steroids stabilize the lysosomal membrane and prevent intracellular release of enzymes. They also increase blood volume by increasing sodium retention. Adrenal steroids appear to be of most benefit in patients in septic shock caused by gram-negative organisms.

HYPOTHERMIA

Besides measures planned to improve cellular metabolism, reducing the metabolic requirements of cells also should increase the patient's chances for survival. With a 10°C reduction of the body temperature, the needs of cells can usually be reduced by about 50 per cent. In actual practice, the beneficial effects of hypothermia are offset to some extent by the slowing of the heart that accompanies it. In addition, there is an increased possibility of ventricular fibrillation, blood viscosity is increased, and tissue perfusion is impaired. In the patient with a high fever, hypothermia may be helpful in reducing the temperature to a level slightly below normal.

ANTIBIOTICS

In almost any type of shock, especially that caused by sepsis, antibiotics are an important adjunct to treatment. As stated earlier, the most frequent cause of septic shock is the gram-negative organisms. Despite the desirability of determining the sensitivity of the causative organisms to antibiotics, there usually is not time.

The antibiotic most likely to be selected is the one that, according to the most recent laboratory test, is most likely to attack the offending organism.

Summary

After the patient is in shock, continued observation is required to determine the effectiveness of the corrective measures that have been instituted. It is well to remember that shock is a dynamic, not a static, process. The condition of the patient in shock is usually either improving or deteriorating. Therefore, careful observation accompanied by the prompt reporting of signs and symptoms indicating impending or worsening shock is imperative. Regardless of whether or not the physician has requested that a given patient be observed for evidence of shock, the nurse should nevertheless assume this responsibility with all patients who (1) undergo major surgery or are seriously injured by physical trauma or burning, (2) bleed from a hollow organ or continue to hemorrhage, or (3) have an acute myocardial infarction. This list is suggestive rather than exhaustive. The significant question that the nurse should ask herself is: "Does this patient have a disorder or treatment that is likely to result in failure to perfuse the tissues?" If the answer is yes, the patient should be investigated for signs and symptoms indicating impending or fully developed shock. When they occur, they should be brought to the attention of the physician immediately.

Nursing the Patient in Shock

Signs and symptoms have been previously discussed in relation to the pathophysiology of shock. Careful and systematic observation is essential to the survival of the patient. Although monitoring devices have been made that can collect certain types of information more accurately and reliably than can man, they cannot and do not replace the knowledgeable nurse and physician. For example, machines can monitor the temperature, pulse, respiration, ECG, EEG, and arterial and venous pressures. They cannot, however, note pink fluid on a dressing, the flaring of nasal alae, or the onset of pain or abdominal distention.[32]

If they are to be useful, monitoring devices must be properly attached to the patient and in good working order. The significance of whatever information is collected must be inter-

---

[30] *Op. cit.*, p. 47.
[31] C. Weissman and L. Thomas: "Studies of Lysosomes: I. Effects of Endotoxin Tolerance, Entotoxin Tolerance, and Cortisone on Release of Acid Hydrolases from a Granular Fraction of Rabbit Liver." *J. Exp. Med.*, 116:433 (Oct.) 1962.

[32] James V. Maloney, Jr.: "The Trouble with Patient Monitoring," *Ann. Surg.*, 168:605–14 (Oct.) 1968.

preted and applied to the patient in an intelligent manner. The rational use of monitoring devices involves recognition of what kinds of information can best be secured by monitors and what their limitations are. Those using monitoring devices must recognize that clinical judgment cannot be replaced by a machine. As an example, Miss Golden is a highly experienced nurse who works in an intensive-care unit. One morning she noted a slight flaring of the nostrils of a patient who had a stab wound in his chest. Had she been less informed and experienced, she might have overlooked the change or discounted its significance. She immediately notified the physician.

Although some intensive-care units are equipped with machines that monitor the infusion of fluids, nurses are often responsible for noting the rate of flow and the response of the patient to the solution. Furthermore, they may be responsible for adjusting the rate of flow in terms of the response of the patient. Because a rapid rise in CVP indicates a relative hypervolemia (it may or may not be a true hypervolemia) in relation to cardiac competency, the nurse slows the rate of flow of the solution under such circumstances and calls the physician. Continued infusion may cause congestive heart failure or even pulmonary edema.

Perhaps the most unique nursing function in the care of the patient in shock is the control of the environment of the patient so that demands made on him are kept at a minimum. By so doing, the nurse can help to reduce the gap between the need and supply of oxygen and nutrients to the tissues. Quiet efficiency, competence in giving care, and promptness in attending to his needs can do much to reassure the patient that the personnel are doing what should be done.

When the patient is alert and anxious, the nurse should be particularly careful to be unexcited and optimistic so that the patient's anxiety does not increase. One patient reported that the most distressing part of his stay in an intensive-care unit was hearing physicians and nurses talk about him as if he were absent. Furthermore, he was not informed about the purpose of the monitoring equipment or his progress. Attention should be given to maintaining a quiet and calm atmosphere. Visitors should be limited to members of the immediate family. The effect of family members should be evaluated and the length of their visits adjusted to their effect on the patient.

The effects of the flashing lights and the beeps of monitoring and other equipment should also be evaluated. When machines have a disquieting effect on the patient a screen can be placed so that the patient is less aware of them. The nurse, however, must always be able to see the patient and the monitoring equipment.

Attention should be given to the room temperature. At one time a warm room and warm blankets were used. It is now known that warming the patient increases his metabolic rate 7 per cent for each degree of body temperature. If the patient sweats it also increases the loss of body fluids. Currently, a comfortable room temperature is advocated. In a study made on rats, Redding and Mueller [33] found that contrary to belief that 20° to 24°C (68° to 75°F) were most favorable to the survival of the animals, those kept at 17° to 20°C (63° to 68°F) had the best survival rate. These authors state that the shocked animal is not poikilothermic but is unable to create sufficient energy to maintain core temperature by peripheral vasoconstriction and loss of water by evaporation.

As stated previously, one of the problems of the patient in shock is the maintenance of adequate respiration. The patient should be moved and turned regularly if at all possible. Because the lung is unevenly perfused and the dependent portions receive the most blood, turning should help to distribute blood to all parts of the lung. Movement also improves ventilation and adds to the patient's comfort. The physician may perform a tracheotomy to reduce the respiratory dead space. A respirator may be prescribed as needed to provide adequate ventilation. Depending on the circumstances, pressure-cycled respirators such as the Bird, or volume-controlled respirators such as the Engström may be necessary in the patient with very high airway resistance or low lung compliance. In cooperative patients with mild ventilatory problems, either the Bird or Bennett is all that is required.[34]

All these measures improve oxygenation of the blood and the removal of carbon dioxide. Further, they reduce the work of breathing and thus help to reduce demand in relation to supply. As a point of emphasis, none of these measures or devices achieves its purpose unless properly applied and cared for. As an example, a tracheotomy does more harm than good unless the airway is kept open, by suctioning, if necessary.

Positioning

Until the very recent past, the moment a patient was in shock, he was immediately placed

[33] Marshal Redding and C. Barber Mueller: "Effects of Ambient Temperature upon Responses to Hypovolemic Insult in the Unanesthetized, Unrestrained Albino Rat," *Surgery,* **64**:110–16 (July) 1968.
[34] Max Harry Weil and Herbert Shubin: *Diagnosis and Treatment of Shock* (Baltimore: The Williams & Wilkins Company, 1967), p. 328.

FIGURE 11-2. Modified Trendelenburg position. (After an original drawing by Leola Hogan.)

in the Trendelenburg position. It was postulated that this position facilitated venous return from the lower portion of the body and improved the circulation to the brain. Recent experimental evidence has demonstrated that this position does not improve cardiac output. At times, circulation through the brain is actually decreased.[35] The decrease in blood flow to the brain in the Trendelenburg position may be caused by the initiation of aortic and carotid sinus reflexes causing constriction of blood vessels supplying the brain.

In the position recommended by Simeone [36] the patient lies supine with his legs elevated to a 45-degree angle. The knees should be straight and the pelvis slightly higher than the thorax. The head should be supported in a comfortable position on one pillow.

SHOCK RESEARCH UNITS

As in other areas in which active research is being performed, nurses are assisting with medical research in shock. In addition, nurses should be investigating how they can contribute to the prevention of shock and how they can alter or correct the problems before the shock becomes irreversible. Nurses who are employed in shock research units face many problems. Patients brought into the unit are frequently in a moribund condition. New as well as old methods of treatment are utilized and evaluated. Doctor and nurse alike may be so occupied with only the shock or their machines that

---

[35] F. A. Simeone: "The Treatment of Shock," *Amer. J. Nurs.,* **66:**1290 (June) 1966.
[36] *Ibid.,* p. 1290.

little attention is given to the patient as an individual human being. There are at times so much equipment and so many people in the unit that the nurse has difficulty getting to the bedside of the patient. In some institutions, remote monitoring devices allow the nurse to stay away from the bedside for long periods of time. Some physicians and nurses are questioning the wisdom of this practice.

Summary

Enough is known about the hemodynamic derangements in shock that they can usually be controlled. Much still remains to be learned about the respiratory complications and the metabolic cellular derangements that may result. Much has been learned about shock through experimental work on dogs and other animals, although much of this knowledge does not apply to human beings. To understand and treat shock in man, tests and treatments must eventually be evaluated on human beings. Each time this is done the physician and the patient or a responsible member of his family must weigh the possible hazards to the patient as against the possible benefits. To learn whether a measure is truly effective, human beings may have to be used as controls. Thus one may be denied a treatment while another receives it. This may be a source of stress to the nurse, the patient or his family, and the physician. Despite the limitations of current knowledge, under the care of knowledgeable physicians and nurses working as a team, patients are now surviving injuries or illnesses that would have been uniformly lethal only a few years ago.

REFERENCES

BOOKS

Ayres, Stephen M., and Gianelli, Stanley: *Care of the Critically Ill* (New York: Appleton-Century-Crofts, 1967).

Birch, C. Allan: *Emergencies in Medical Practice*, 8th ed. (Baltimore: The Williams & Wilkins Company, 1967).

Burton, Alan C.: *Physiology and Biophysics of the Circulation* (Chicago: Year Book Medical Publishers, 1965).

Moyer, C. A., and Butcher, H. R.: *Burns, Shock, and Plasma Volume Regulation* (St. Louis: The C. V. Mosby Company, 1967).

Powers, Maryann, and Storlie, Frances: *The Cardiac Surgical Patient* (New York: The Macmillan Company, 1969).

Shoemaker, William C.: *Shock: Chemistry, Physiology and Therapy* (Springfield, Ill.: Charles C Thomas, Publisher, 1967).

The Twelfth Hahnemann Symposium: *Shock and Hypotension: Pathogenesis and Treatment*. L. C. Mills and J. H. Moyer, eds. (New York: Grune & Stratton, Inc., 1965).

Weil, Max Harry, and Shubin, Herbert: *Diagnosis and Treatment of Shock* (Baltimore: The Williams & Wilkins Company, 1967).

PERIODICALS

Berdjis, Charles C., and Vick, James A.: "Endotoxin and Traumatic Shock," *JAMA*, 204:191–94 (Apr. 15) 1968.

Bradley, Edward C., and Weil, Max Harry: "Vasopressor and Vasodilator Drugs in the Treatment of Shock," *Mod. Treat.*, 4:243–55 (Mar.) 1967.

Carruthers, R. K., and Parsons, F. M.: "The Value of Central Venous Pressure Monitoring in the Treatment of Acute Renal Dysfunction," *Brit. J. Surg.*, 54:845–49 (Oct.) 1967.

Cohn, J. N.: "Central Venous Pressure as a Guide to Volume Expansion," *Ann. Intern. Med.*, 66:1283–87 (June) 1967.

Freidberg, Charles K.: "Shock in Acute Myocardial Infarction," *Postgrad. Med.*, 42:183–86 (Sept.) 1967.

Gray, Edward B.: "Evaluation and Treatment of Shock, Respiratory Failure," *Hosp. Top.*, 47:95–98 (Mar.) 1969.

Ingle, D. J.: "Editorial: Judgments in Medicine: The Assumption of Risk," *Perspect. Biol. Med.*, 11:525–26 (Summer) 1968.

Jacobson, Eugene D.: "A Physiologic Approach to Shock," *New Eng. J. Med.*, 278:834–38 (Apr. 11) 1968.

Kellermeyer, R. W.: "Kinins—Possible Physiologic and Pathologic Roles in Man," *New Eng. J. Med.*, 279:754–59 (Oct. 3) 1968.

Leaf, A., and McCully, K.: "Acidosis and Shock in a Patient with Diabetes, Cirrhosis, and Renal Failure," *New Eng. J. Med.*, 278:1004–13 (May 2) 1968.

Leffall, L. D., Jr.: "Current Concepts in the Management of Surgical Shock," *J. Nat. Med. Ass.*, 60:401–407 (Sept.) 1968.

Mostert, J. W.: "Shock-Blood Volume vs. Central Venous Pressure," *New Eng. J. Med.*, 280:51 (Jan. 2) 1969.

"The Nurse in Research. ANA Guidelines on Ethical Values," *Amer. J. Nurs.*, 68:1504–1507 (July) 1968.

Ratnoff, Oscar D., and Ratnoff, Marian F.: "Ethical Responsibilities in Clinical Investigation," *Perspect. Biol. Med.*, 11:82–90 (Autumn) 1967.

Russell, Margaret W., and Maier, Willis P.: "The ABC's of C.V.P. Measurement," *RN*, 32:34–35 and 66–67 (Mar.) 1969.

Said, Sami: "The Lung as a Metabolic Organ," *New Eng. J. Med.*, 279:1330–34 (Dec. 12) 1968.

Schumer, William: "Localization of the Energy Pathway Block in Shock," *Surgery*, 64:55–59 (July) 1968.

Schumer, William, and Sperling, Richard: "Shock and Its Effect on the Cell," *JAMA*, 205:215–22 (July) 1968.

"Shock: Kinds, Causes and Treatment," *RN*, 31:66–67 (Jan.) 1968.

Simeone, F. A.: "The Nature of Shock," *Amer. J. Nurs.*, 66:1286–89 (June) 1966.

"Treatment of Shock Associated with Myocardial Infarction," *Med. Lett.*, 11:29–31 (Apr. 4) 1969.

Weil, Max H.: "A New Look at the Critically Ill," *Hosp. Pract.*, 2:27–37 (Jan.) 1967.

Wilson, John N., and Owens, J. Cuthbert: "Continuous Monitoring of Venous Pressure in Optimal Blood Volume Maintenance," *Surg. Forum*, 12:94–98, 1961.

12

Nursing the Patient Having a Problem with Some Aspects of Nutrition*

Spurred by hunger from his remote past, man suffered, starved, struggled for food, survived, and is there to tell the tale. But only just.[1]

Overview

FOR their survival and maintenance of functions, cells require a continuous supply of oxygen, water, and nutrients. Oxygen, of course, must be furnished moment by moment, whereas the need for food is less acute. Nutrients are stored to a varying degree within the body so that the cells may be constantly supplied. Cells are able, within limits, to sacrifice some of their sub-

stance for use as energy and to adapt energy output to energy intake. Despite some degree of protection against a lack of food intake, continued deprivation threatens survival. Moreover, unless the supply of food more than meets minimum requirements, growth, health and productivity are threatened.

The earliest written record describing the effects of hunger caused by famine could be written today in many parts of the world. The following record was found on a stone in the tomb of an Egyptian Pharaoh:

[1] Morris Sinclair: "Another Man's Hunger," *World Health*, **15**:8 (Sept.–Oct.) 1962.

---

* Revised by Corinne Robinson, Consultant in Nutrition Education and Professor of Nutrition, Emeritus. Formerly, Head, Department of Nutrition and Food, Drexel Institute of Technology, and Instructor, Normal and Therapeutic Nutrition, School of Nursing, Jefferson Medical College Hospital, Philadelphia.

Pharaoh: From my throne I grieve over this calamity. During my reign, the Nile has failed to flood for seven years. Corn is scarce and there is no other food. My people thieve and pillage their neighbors. Those who would run cannot even walk. Children weep and the young falter and totter like old people. Their legs drag or give way under them. Their spirits are broken. My council chamber is deserted, my food stores have been pillaged and emptied. It is the end of everything.[2]

An exact understanding of several terms is essential in order that the nutritional needs of people can be described. All too often the words nutrition and diet are used synonymously.

Nutrition includes all the bodily processes involved in the use of foods. Good nutrition implies that the supply of food is adequate in quantity and quality to the needs of the cells, and that the cells are able to utilize nutrients in a physiological manner.

Nutrients are those substances in foods that are required for any of the cell functions; for example, amino acids, fatty acids, carbohydrates, minerals, and vitamins are nutrients.

Diet is the regimen of food required to support nutrition. A good or nutritious diet is one providing all the nutrients to sustain good nutrition. Whether such a regimen results in good nutrition depends on many other factors. The food must be eaten, digested, absorbed, transported, and finally utilized by the cells.

Nutritional status is the condition of health of the individual as influenced by the utilization of the nutrients. It can be determined only by correlating the information from a careful medical and dietary history, a thorough physical examination, appropriate biochemical tests on blood and excretions, and x-ray examinations. The methodology for such studies has been described.[3]

Nutrition and Health

Health, well-being, strength, and the ability to resist and recover from disease are all influenced for good or ill by the nutritional state. Not only is nutrition a significant factor in the capacity to survive, but adequate nutrition is also essential for productive and zestful living. Health is threatened by either an excess or a deficiency of food. As with other homeostatic mechanisms, within limits the individual is able to adapt to variation in supply. Although the nature of the effects differ, either a deficiency

or an excess in supply of food may impair structure and function.

Diseases such as certain types of anemia, scurvy, kwashiorkor, pellagra, beriberi, and goiter result from the lack of specific nutrients. Resistance to others, such as tuberculosis and pneumonia, is diminished among the undernourished. The mortality rate of children of ages one to five who do not get proper food may be as much as 15 times that of children who do.[4] Malnutrition remains as one of the major health problems of the world, and is by no means unknown even in the United States and Europe.

Nutritional therapy is a primary consideration for deficiency diseases and for errors of metabolism such as diabetes mellitus, phenylketonuria, hyperinsulinism, and others. It must be carefully adjusted to the body's ability to metabolize nutrients and to eliminate wastes; for example, protein-restricted, potassium-restricted, and sodium-restricted diets for renal failure. Nutritional therapy is supportive in the care of all patients.

In addition to problems of supply of food per se, selection of food is also a factor. The American public is constantly exposed to unjustified claims about foods and diets, as well as vitamin and mineral supplements. All communications media present information in the form of scientific or pseudoscientific articles or reports of research and in advertisements. The accuracy and validity of some of these are open to question and others are actually misleading or false. For example, a newspaper quoted two "nutrition experts." The first is purported to have said that the average person who eats a variety of foods is supplied with all the nutrients that he needs. He does not require extra vitamin or mineral supplements, and money spent for unnecessary food supplements is wasted. The second was cited as saying that few, if any, diets contain an adequate quantity of vitamins and minerals. To be well nourished, supplementation is necessary. What is the average lay person to believe? What, if any, function does the nurse have in interpreting present-day knowledge to the public?

What is the role of the nurse in meeting the need of the patient for food?

In general, the physician prescribes a diet designed to meet the individual requirements of the patient for food. The dietary prescription is based on knowledge of the nutritional state of the individual as well as the modifications imposed by the nature of his illness. To illustrate, Mrs. Smith, aged 65, has a diagnosis of diabetes

---

[2] *World Health,* **16**:30 (Mar.) 1963.
[3] *Manual for Nutrition Surveys,* 2nd ed. (Bethesda, Md.: Interdepartmental Committee on Nutrition for National Defense, National Institutes of Health, 1963).

[4] *World Health,* **16**:5 (Mar.) 1963.

mellitus and obesity. The dietary prescription written by her physician is based on the following knowledge of Mrs. Smith. She is a 65-year-old woman who leads a sedentary life. She is 25 lb overweight and has diabetes mellitus. A loss of excess weight will probably be accompanied by a lessening in the severity of her diabetes mellitus. The physician prescribes a low-calorie diet approximately meeting her basal needs. The prescription allows an adequate quantity of protein, minerals, and vitamins. By reducing the calories, the carbohydrate and fat are correspondingly restricted. Thereby the physician hopes to lessen the quantity of insulin required by Mrs. Smith. The low-calorie diet will result in gradual loss of weight and some reduction in the severity of her diabetes.

In many hospitals, dietitians translate the dietary prescription into food. They plan the menus and supervise the preparation of food. Like the physician, they depend to a considerable extent on the nursing staff to relay problems encountered by the patient that interfere with his ability to eat or to enjoy his food. Dietitians also counsel the patient who will continue to modify his food intake after he leaves the hospital. In public health agencies dietitians may act as consultants to nurses, as well as instructors to patients and their families.

The responsibilities of the nurse in meeting the nutritional needs of patients are many and varied. The extent of these responsibilities differs somewhat in different hospitals and health agencies. In the small community hospitals nurses frequently perform many of the functions of dietitians. No matter how highly organized the food service is, however, the nurse has a significant contribution to make in meeting the nutritional needs of patients. Her objectives are to help the patient to understand why food is essential to his health, and to help him accept and follow the diet as prescribed by his physician. To achieve these objectives, the nurse has the following responsibilities: (1) to obtain the diet prescription, if one has not been provided; (2) to plan with food service so that the patient receives food suited to his needs and, inasmuch as is possible, his desires; (3) to prepare the environment of the patient so that it is conducive to eating; (4) to prepare the patient so that he is in a comfortable position and in condition to eat; (5) to prepare the patient for what to expect, if his diet is different from his usual food pattern and to explain the reasons for modification in his diet; (6) to observe and report the appetite and food preferences of each patient; (7) to observe and report the adequacy of the food intake of the patient; (8) to observe his attitude toward food; (9) to feed or supervise the feeding of patients who are unable to feed themselves; (10) to give appropriate emotional support to those who must be fed or must learn to feed themselves or whose food habits require modification; (11) to give appropriate assistance to those who need some help; (12) to instruct the patient and his family and to answer his questions about his diet [5]; (13) to assist in the collection of data about the food pattern of the patient, his likes and dislikes, and the methods of and facilities available to him for food preparation or for the securing of food after he leaves the hospital; (14) to identify those patients who will require some assistance in obtaining or preparing a suitable diet after dismissal from the hospital; (15) to communicate with the patient, his family, the physician, and the dietitian in such a way that the needs of the patient are met and the lines of communication are kept open; (16) to assist the patient and/or members of his family in meal planning, budgeting, buying, and preparing a nutritious diet [5]; (17) to provide assistance to patients and/or members of the family in the home to: (a) make required adjustments at home after he is discharged from the hospital; (b) provide assistance to the patient who requires a therapeutic diet, but does not require hospitalization; (c) assist the patient to modify his usual food pattern so that his basic and special needs are met [5]; and (18) to feed the patient by an abnormal route and to aid the patient and/or members of his family in learning how to perform the necessary procedures.

Information Required by the Nurse

The maintenance of the nutrition of cells involves the same general processes and structures as do other homeostatic conditions. Food must be available in adequate quantity and quality and of the type accepted as being suitable to eat. Food requires a special service facility, the digestive system, to receive and to transfer nutrients from the external to the internal environment. Because many of the nutrients contained in food are not in an absorbable form at the time they are eaten, foods must undergo digestion, which consists of a series of physical and chemical changes by which nutrients are prepared for absorption. The residue remaining after digestion and absorption is then ejected from the alimentary canal.

Like oxygen, nutrients must be transported to the cells where they are utilized. The various nutrients provide cells with materials required for energy, for building or replacement of cell structure, and for the regulation of cellular processes. Excesses of supply are stored for

[5] These functions may be referred to others.

future use or are excreted. Cells are, within limits, capable of adapting to differences in supply. Like other physiological needs, the need for food must be met before higher needs can be manifested. Ill health can result from an imbalance between food intake and cell requirements. The causes for this imbalance are many and varied. There are few, if any, illnesses of any length or severity in which nutrition is not of significance.

An understanding of the nutritive processes of the body is not sufficient for effective nutritional care. Of paramount importance is knowledge of the factors affecting the food supply and of physiological, psychological, cultural, and socioeconomic influences on food acceptance. To reach people of all socioeconomic classes with nutrition information and to motivate them to alter the quantity and quality of foods consumed requires application of principles of education and use of all media of communication and techniques of teaching.

Food Supply, Nutritional Status, and Food Habits

What are some of the factors in the supply of food?

FOOD SCARCITY

Despite a plethora of food in a few areas of the world, such as in the United States, a lack of sufficient food to meet minimum nutritional requirements is one of the most critical public health problems in the world. In many countries, the vast majority of the population is adapted to a chronic state of undernutrition. In fact, the effects of nutritional deficiency may be accepted as a normal condition. For example, in the Andean Altiplano, where goiter caused by a deficiency in iodine has been present for generations, dolls are made with the characteristic neck deformity of goiter, indicating that it is accepted as usual or normal.

Insufficient food is not a new problem, nor is it one subject to easy solution. For thousands of years man in most parts of the world has led a hand-to-mouth existence. Most, if not all, of his energy is expended in obtaining just enough food to sustain life. Food supply, and with it survival, are continuously threatened by drought, floods, windstorms, and pestilence. Lack of facilities for preserving and transporting food may result in relative abundance during the warm months of the year and scarcity during the cold winter months. In other areas, hunger is always present. Food supplies are limited to plants and animals indigenous or native to the region. As is true in the United States, not all plants and animals suitable for food are utilized.

AGRICULTURE AND FOOD SUPPLY

In the early history of mankind and among some present-day primitive societies, the principal methods for obtaining food were hunting and fishing or gathering berries, nuts, and roots. One of the most significant steps in the progress of man occurred when he began to cultivate plants and animals as sources of food. The cultivation of plants and animals is known as agriculture. Not until agriculture became a reality did the prevention of periodic or continuous hunger become a real possibility. In addition to increasing the supply of food, the development of agriculture has other far-reaching effects. Successful cultivation of sources of food made it necessary for man to give up being a nomad and to settle in one place. Once man was able to produce more than enough food to feed himself and the members of his immediate family, some members of the group were released for other activities. Thus specialization was born. In addition to the food producers or farmers, other men became butchers, bakers, carpenters, and teachers. As the food supply became relatively secure, man had time and energy to think of ways by which his external environment might be changed or improved. Without the development of agriculture, the industrialized societies of today would be impossible.

FOOD PRESERVATION

Despite the importance of the development of the tools and techniques essential to modern agriculture, food supply also depends on suitable means for its preservation and distribution. Without suitable means of preserving food, it is likely to deteriorate in quality or actually spoil before it reaches the consumer, who may live far from where food is produced. Food preservation also makes it possible to save perishable foods for use throughout the year. Modern methods of food preservation combined with efficient and economical methods of transportation make possible the distribution of food far from its site of production. The accomplishment of all these requires highly trained and skilled manpower. Thus, in Big City one Sunday in January, the menu consisted of fresh chicken from Alabama, lettuce from Arizona, potatoes from Idaho, peas from Minnesota, and ice cream and butter from Wisconsin.

FOOD DISTRIBUTION

Although remarkable progress has been made in developing methods of food production, preservation, and transportation, too little available food remains a problem in much of the world. Sinclair [6] states that, according to one estimate, one third of the population eats three quarters of the food of the world. This means that about two thirds of the people subsist on one quarter of the available food. Many factors contribute to the unequal availability of food. In some parts of the world food supplies are limited by either a lack of, or a failure to exploit, natural resources. An increase in food supplies in these areas depends on the modernization of agricultural methods, the introduction of suitable methods of food preservation, and the development of transportation facilities. The introduction of suitable methods of home preservation of foods by drying, smoking, and pickling, and in some instances by home canning, may do much to bring about immediate improvement in the supply of food.

Nutritional Status

Malnutrition is worldwide in scope and differs only in the degree of severity among people living in the affluent and poor nations. Hidden hunger, detected by laboratory studies, comes to the surface as starvation and the classic deficiency diseases when inadequate intake of foods is severe and prolonged, and when filth and disease are the way of life. Infections producing only transient illness in the well-nourished are likely to lead to death or, at best, to prolonged convalescence in the poorly nourished.

What is the evidence for malnutrition in the United States?

The plight of millions of Americans has been brought to the attention of the American public by such slogans as "War on Poverty" and, more recently, "War on Hunger." A national nutrition survey is now in progress under the auspices of the Department of Health, Education, and Welfare, and directed by Arnold E. Schaefer and Ogden C. Johnson.[7] This survey will eventually assess the nutritional health of lower-income America. It is a broad-scale study of food consumption, general health, and environmental factors, and includes clinical, biochemical, dietary, dental, and socioeconomic studies. Each person in the survey gives about 200 bits of information.

The preliminary results of the study based on the findings in a few states were presented to

the Select Committee on Nutrition and Human Needs of the United States Senate in January 1969. One half of all families so far studied had incomes under $3,000, and half of these families had four or more members. About 80 per cent of all families in the survey had less than $5,000 annual cash income. Negroes accounted for 55 per cent and Spanish-Americans for 25 per cent of the total sample. More than half of the persons are in especially vulnerable groups, children under 16 years of age accounting for 44 per cent and adults over 60 years for 13 per cent.

Every kind of malnutrition observed by the investigators in other studies in Asia, Africa, and Central America has been seen in the United States. Clinical signs become evident only after nutrition has been inadequate for a prolonged time. But in this survey 4 to 5 per cent of preschool children had clinical evidence of vitamin D deficiency, protein-calorie malnutrition, and retarded growth. Rickets was found in 18 cases and severe malnutrition (kwashiorkor and marasmus) in 7 cases. Enlarged thyroid glands were found in 5 per cent of all people and gum lesions attributable to lack of ascorbic acid in 4 per cent of all people.

Decayed, filled, or missing teeth were reported in 96 per cent of all persons examined. For each 100 persons examined, 90 had need of fillings or extractions, 45 had some degree of periodontal disease, 20 of them severe, and 18 had difficulty or pain in biting or chewing. The role of nutrition in dental health is important but not the only factor to be considered, as the authors point out.

Laboratory studies gave further confirmation of the clinical findings of malnutrition and also revealed hidden hunger. Blood levels of hemoglobin, total protein, serum albumin, vitamin A, and ascorbic acid, and urinary excretions of thiamine and riboflavin, were low in 9 to 19 per cent of all persons examined. The results were similar to those in the developing countries. Of special concern was the finding that one third of children under 6 years of age had hemoglobin levels classed as anemia; also, one third of the children had low serum levels of vitamin A. The laboratory studies are a sensing device whereby high-risk individuals are identified. When such individuals remain long on an inadequate diet, any additional stress imposed by work or illness will reduce the physical and mental performance. Poor nutrition is now known to place a limitation upon mental development in the very young—an impairment that cannot be corrected by later improvement in diet.

Dietary analyses, although incomplete at the present time, have shown that many people con-

---

[6] *Op. cit.*, p. 8.
[7] Arnold E. Schaefer and Ogden C. Johnson: "Are We Well Fed? The Search for an Answer," *Nutr. Today,* 4:2–11 (Spring) 1969.

sume diets that provide less than 50 per cent of the calories, iron, vitamin A, and vitamin C considered adequate. The iron intake is low for 60 per cent of young children, and vitamin A intake is low in 40 per cent of adolescents and older individuals. The preliminary data suggest good correlation between the dietary information and the laboratory studies. The problem of malnutrition is one of multiple deficiencies of protein, minerals, vitamins, and calories.

The authors of this report have speculated that the causes for widespread malnutrition in a country so abundantly supplied with food are (1) too little money to spend for food, so that the poor man cannot afford to make mistakes in buying; (2) not knowing what foods to buy; and (3) laxity in the fortification programs that would improve nutrition—enrichment of breads and cereals, vitamin D fortification of whole milk, vitamin A and D fortification of nonfat dry milk, and iodization of salt.

WORLD NUTRITION PROBLEMS

Insufficient calories and protein, both in quantity and in quality, are the most important lacks in the diets of people in most of the world. Chronic starvation is the lot of millions. According to one estimate, anywhere from 300 to 500 million people suffer from calorie deficiency and one third to one half of the world's population from protein deficiency.[8] India, Pakistan, China, and Indonesia account for two thirds of the people who are undernourished but Latin America and Africa also have a serious incidence of undernutrition. Preschool children and mothers are especially vulnerable to the effects of malnutrition, the mortality rate being especially high among infants and young children in the most seriously affected countries. Lack of a sanitary food supply and pure water, poor disposal of sewage, and filth among the undernourished result in a high morbidity and mortality rate, even from infections not ordinarily serious. Malaria, a major world health problem, increases the nutritional requirements of the people it infects, rapidly debilitates the already undernourished, and keeps millions from producing the food that is desperately needed.

Surveys conducted principally by the Interdepartmental Committee on Nutrition and National Defense in many developing countries have shown calorie undernutrition, protein malnutrition, anemia, and vitamin A and riboflavin deficiencies to be highly prevalent. Also, rickets, scurvy, pellagra, and beriberi occur with great frequency.[9]

PROGRAMS FOR NUTRITIONAL IMPROVEMENT

The solution of nutritional problems obviously must be tailored to the conditions existing among people of a given country. Within the United States the efforts to improve the level of income assume major importance inasmuch as food is abundantly available to all who have the money to purchase it. Closely related is the need to improve the general education of low-income people so that their ability to earn a better income is improved. More specifically, nutrition education must become an integral and important part of the curriculum for every child in the elementary and secondary schools of our nation so that he can learn in early life to make wise food choices. Particular attention to the education of mothers and mothers-to-be can be expected to yield good results. Because of the rapid changes in the food products available in today's market, people need continuing information on the products that they buy—their nutritive contributions, comparative costs, methods of preparation, and so on.

The nutritional problems in the poor countries of the world almost seem to defy solution. These countries produce too little food for their populations and they do not have the money to purchase the food they need. The United States has continued to play a significant role in helping to combat malnutrition through the Food for Peace program. The Departments of Agriculture and State, including the Agency of International Development (AID), implement this program by providing shipments of food surpluses under arrangements with governments of receiving countries or with United Nations organizations. In addition the United States, through voluntary and governmental agencies, has conducted surveys of nutritional status and provided technical assistance in agriculture, food processing and marketing, and education.

Several groups in the United Nations are directly concerned with global problems of nutrition, namely, the Food and Agriculture Organization (FAO), World Health Organization (WHO), United Nations Children's Fund (UNICEF), and United Nations Educational, Scientific, and Cultural Organization (UNESCO). Through these organizations the efforts include the provision of food supplies, technical assistance, family planning for control of population growth, and general and home

[8] David Simpson: "The Dimensions of World Poverty," *Sci. Amer.*, 219:33 (Nov.) 1968.

[9] James M. Hundley: "Malnutrition—A Global Problem," *Fed. Proc.*, 18:76 (Dec.) 1959.

economics education. The technical assistance is provided for program planning by governments; the development of improved agricultural techniques; the reclamation of land; the improvement of strains of plants and animals; pest control; improved facilities for storage, preservation and distribution of food; the fortification of foods; the development of protein-rich foods; the improvement of sanitation and housing; and the development of programs in education for the lay public and the health worker. Such a brief listing of programs can scarcely convey the urgency of the problem or the exciting potential in these areas.

Factors Influencing Food Acceptance

Food acceptance is determined by the physiologic response of the senses, biochemical changes taking place in the body, and the many meanings that food holds for the individual. In the following pages some of the physiological, biochemical, psychological, social, economic, and educational factors affecting the acceptance of food will be discussed. References have been included at the end of this chapter for those who would like to explore one or more of these aspects in greater detail.

What are some of the factors influencing food acceptance?

Appetite, hunger, satiety, and *anorexia* are terms used to indicate some aspects of desire for food. *Appetite* and *hunger* are sometimes used synonymously but they are not the same physiological state.

Hunger is the most basic drive for food. There is an awareness of the need to ingest food that is accompanied by increased salivation and food-searching behavior. It is associated with unpleasant or even painful contractions of an empty stomach or intestine. As hunger increases, it occupies more and more of the attention of the individual. For example, Mr. Francis arrived at his hotel late last night. He had not stopped for dinner because he expected to eat after arriving at his destination. The dining room was closed, as were all the nearby restaurants. After retiring, Mr. Francis tried to sleep, but he could not. He finally arose and drove 20 miles to find an all-night restaurant where he ate a large meal. Despite the consumption of a high-calorie meal, Mr. Francis continued to experience hunger pangs for an hour or so after eating.

The extent to which the physiological changes characteristic of hunger are initiated by biochemical changes in the body is not completely understood. Hunger, however, is one of the frequent manifestations in certain hormonal imbalances such as in hyperthyroidism, as well as in both hyper- and hypoinsulinism. In the preceding example the individual did not experience a desire for any particular food; the need was for food. In certain disorders, the individual is aware of a craving for a special food. For example, in adrenal insufficiency, the patient is often aware of an increased consumption of sodium chloride.

Appetite implies a psychic desire for food and is a pleasant sensation. Unlike hunger, it may persist after sufficient food has been ingested to appease hunger. It is conditioned by previous experiences and habit as well as by the sight, smell, and taste of food. For example, Mr. Francis arrives home in the evening. As he enters the house, he smells the aroma of his favorite stew. His mouth waters as he anticipates eating his dinner, although he has eaten a big lunch and is not particularly hungry.

Appetite and hunger also appear to be affected by the hormonal responses to a severe injury or to a major surgical procedure. During the adrenergic and glucocorticoid responses to injury, appetite and hunger are suppressed and anorexia is the rule. In fact, the sight or smell of food may induce nausea and other unpleasant sensations. During the glucocorticoid withdrawal phase, appetite begins to return. During convalescence, appetite may, unless curbed in time, be so great as to lead to an excessive gain in weight.

Satiety is defined as a state of satisfaction or lack of desire for food following its ingestion. Unless an unusually large quantity of food is ingested, it is a pleasant state. For example, after eating a big dish of stew, Mr. Francis leaned back from the table, relaxed and comfortable. *Anorexia* is descriptive of an abnormal state, because it implies an absence of hunger under circumstances in which it should be expected. At lunchtime John, aged 14, refuses to eat, saying, "I'm not hungry." Because he has not eaten since breakfast, and then only lightly, his mother asks him, "Are you ill?" John has anorexia. He is not hungry under circumstances in which he should be expected to be. When his mother investigates further, she finds that he has a fever and a rash.

THE SENSES AND FOOD ACCEPTANCE

The sensations of taste and smell also affect appetite and the acceptability of food. Everyone has experienced the lack of enjoyment of food which accompanies a common cold. Inasmuch as taste and smell enable the individual to identify poisonous substances, these senses are protective. Because both senses are subject to conditioning, they are not completely reliable guides to the selection of foods that are safe. Familiar foods prepared in accustomed ways taste and smell "good." Unaccustomed foods, most particularly those with strong odors, are rejected because they taste and smell "bad." Thus Limburger cheese is a delicacy to one person and spoiled cheese to another.

TASTE

Because taste buds disappear gradually throughout life, taste becomes less acute as the individual grows older. Because children have more taste buds, they may well have different taste sensations from those of adults. Although conditioning is probably a factor, greater sensitivity to taste may account for the tendency of young children to reject strongly flavored foods. With advancing years the preference for sweet foods tends to lessen and tart, fruity flavors are preferred. As in many other aspects of life, the ability to taste varies among individuals as well as in the same individual from time to time.

Most sick people have some defect in their ability to taste food, with the result that they complain of its being tasteless or flat. Although illness is responsible for the inability to taste food, something can be done to improve the acceptability of food to the patient. Because a clean, moist mouth minimizes the loss of taste, the patient should be provided with the opportunity to brush his teeth or have them brushed before food is offered, and the mouth should also be cleansed after meals to remove food particles. The nurse can also relate the tastelessness of the food to the illness. Loss of taste is usually temporary and taste will return as the patient recovers. When the consumption of food is important to the recovery of the patient, he should be encouraged to eat. Eating is a way whereby he can help himself to recover. Recognition by the nurse that eating is difficult when food is without taste may also strengthen the efforts of the patient.

SMELL

Although few people distinguish between the sensations of taste and smell, much of what is loosely called taste results from the odor of food. Odors may also be responsible for unpleasant sensations associated with food. Most persons are aware that when they have a cold, food seems "flat" or tasteless. In healthy persons, the fragrance of baking bread or broiling steak arouses pleasant sensations. To the sick person, these same odors may be highly unpleasant. Odor is often accepted as an indication of the safety of a food; for example, meat smells fresh or spoiled. A procedure now being

advocated is to smell all canned food before tasting it. If it has a peculiar smell, canned food should be discarded without tasting. Appetite may be depressed by disagreeable odors and stimulated by pleasant ones. Patients with foul-smelling wounds may find eating difficult. Keeping dressings clean and minimizing the odor may do much to promote appetite.

TEXTURE

Smooth, creamy foods are preferred to lumpy or grainy foods. Cooked vegetables that are tender yet slightly crisp are likely to be more acceptable than those that are soft, mushy, water soaked, or stringy. Generally speaking, young children like soft, smooth foods. Many older people also prefer soft foods because they may have poorly fitting dentures or find biting and chewing to be painful. Diets that are varied in texture are more likely to be nutritionally adequate than those that are restricted to soft foods. Moreover, chewing of foods helps to improve dental hygiene.

TEMPERATURE

The temperature at which food is served also influences its acceptability. Despite provisions made in hospitals to ensure the correct temperature of the food served, foods do not always arrive at the bedside of the patient at either the proper temperature or consistency. For example, hot foots such as coffee, soups, and entrees are all too frequently tepid by the time they reach the patient. Cold foods, such as gelatin salads and ice cream, may melt before they are served to the patient and are therefore unacceptable. When a tray must be delayed, hot food should be kept hot or heated and cold food should be refrigerated during the delay. Attention to the condition of the food at the time it is presented to the patient not only increases the likelihood of its being eaten, but affords an opportunity to reinforce the feeling of the patient that what happens to him is important to those responsible for his care.

How does the body maintain homeostasis with respect to food intake?

HORMONAL REGULATION OF FOOD INTAKE

Hunger, in addition to unpleasant gastric contractions, is accompanied by feelings of weakness, emptiness, and sometimes headache and nausea. That a low blood glucose level is related to the gastric contractions has been known for many years. Such hunger contractions were intensified when insulin was given. On the other hand, glucagon, another hormone produced by the pancreas, has the effect of inhibiting gastric contractions. Glucagon exerts its action by releasing glycogen from the liver, thereby increasing the blood glucose level. (See Carbohydrate Metabolism.)

The gastric responses to hunger are correlated with metabolic and neurologic factors in the brain. These are complex mechanisms that are not fully understood. Satiety and feeding or appetite centers have been identified in the hypothalamus. In an experimental animal, if the nuclei in the central area (satiety centers) of the hypothalamus are destroyed, it continues to eat and becomes extremely obese.[10] If the lateral nuclei (feeding or appetite centers) are destroyed, the animal refuses to eat and will eventually starve to death unless it is force-fed.

By ingenious experiments, Mayer has shown that the food intake of the animals is closely correlated with the rate of glucose utilization. The satiety centers have a high affinity for glucose and are extremely sensitive to the availability of glucose in the blood. When the satiety centers take up glucose this is translated into an electrical impulse to other centers of the central nervous system and in turn translated into sensations of hunger or satiety. The satiety centers act as a brake to control the feeding center.

In other experiments on animals, Mayer has shown that glucagon will no longer inhibit gastric contractions if the ventromedial area of the hypothalamus is destroyed. The satiety center is believed to be highly responsive to the effects of this hormone and serves as the control center for gastric contractions.

PSYCHOLOGICAL AND SOCIAL FACTORS

Despite the significance of biochemical and physiological factors in influencing the acceptability of food, psychological factors are probably even more important. Although knowledge of the psychological and social factors in eating is incomplete, there is an increasing literature emphasizing that eating is motivated not by logic but by feelings. Mead[11] summarizes the psychological, social, and cultural aspects of food as follows: "In most societies, food is the focus of emotional associations, a channel for interpersonal relations, for the communication of love or discrimination or disapproval; it usually has a symbolic reference." Galdston[12] emphasizes the importance of psychological factors by saying: "Few functions in life are more freighted with emotions, prejudices,

taboos, and prestige symbols than is eating." He further states that a person does not eat for health, but because he is hungry, jealous, or frustrated.

The hypothesis that likes and dislikes are more important factors in the selection of food than health is supported by a study reported by Shapiro et al.[13] Food selection was studied in families from different income groups. All families had sufficient income to purchase an adequate diet. Little difference was found in the food selected by families of the various economic levels. In all groups, likes and dislikes far outweighed health as a consideration in food selection.

Both physiological and psychological factors influence the acceptance or rejection of food. For example, a healthy person who has been exercising out of doors is likely to be hungry at mealtime. This same person may develop anorexia on being frightened or angry. Neither is he likely to feel like eating or to be hungry if he is in the acute phase of an illness or in pain. When at all possible, painful procedures should be performed between meals and not just before or during meals. One reason for encouraging activity in the chronically undernourished is to increase appetite and hunger.

Not only do many factors influence what man eats, but his behavior is affected by whether he is hungry or well fed. He may be irritable, withdrawn, or restless when hungry, and happy and relaxed when he is well fed. Shakespeare relates the behavior of men to food when he has Caesar say, "Let me have men about me who are fat; sleek-headed men and such as sleep o' nights. Yon Cassius has a lean and hungry look; he thinks too much; such men are dangerous."

If the nurse is to be really effective in helping people to meet their nutritional needs, she must know not only what people should and do eat but what food and eating mean to them, as well as what some of the possible consequences of suggested changes may be. Clear distinctions between the cultural, social, and psychological aspects of food and eating are not easy to make. Some of these will be discussed and illustrated in the discussion that follows.

CULTURAL INFLUENCES

Among many potentially nutritious plants and animals available as food, only a few are used by any group of people. An explanation offered to account for this failure to use all suitable and nonpoisonous plants and animals

[10] Jean Mayer: "Obesity, Causes and Treatment," *Amer. J. Nurs.*, **59**:1732 (Dec.) 1959.

[11] Margaret Mead: *Cultural Patterns and Technical Change* (UNESCO, 1953), p. 213.

[12] Iago Galdston: "Nutrition from the Psychiatric Viewpoint," *J. Amer. Diet. Ass.*, **28**:40 (May) 1952.

[13] Leona R. Shapiro, Ruth L. Huenemann, and Mary C. Hampton: "Dietary Survey for Planning a Local Nutrition Program," *Pub. Health Rep.*, **77**:257–66 (Mar.) 1962.

as food is that the definition of food is of cultural origin. Some plants and animals are designated as being fit for human consumption without regard for their nutritional value. In some cultures, there are religious prohibitions against certain foods. In Moslem countries pork is forbidden. Hindus do not eat beef. Even in the absence of religious proscription, nutritious foods may be rejected. To most Americans, horse meat is not fit for human consumption. In America sweet corn is a treat; in France it is considered fit only for animals. In the southeastern United States grits are served with every meal. In the North they are seldom, if ever, eaten. Children learn very early which plants and animals are not acceptable to eat. Not quite five-year-old Mary supported this by commenting during a conversation about the use of horse meat as food, "I like horses, but not to eat."

Something can be learned about the food habits of different groups by visiting supermarkets in various areas in a city or the country. For example, beef or pork is preferred to lamb in Iowa, with the result that lamb is seldom available in a market. In a community in which Jewish people are concentrated, kosher corned beef and bagels are easily obtained. In non-Jewish communities, these foods are frequently unknown. In Minneapolis during the Christmas season, lutefisk is found in every grocery store. In one section of Detroit, signs on store windows advertise mustard greens and possums. In northern Michigan, pasties—beef, potatoes, and onions enclosed in pastry and baked—remind one of the Welsh miners who brought their food habits with them when they migrated to America. To any one person, depending on conditioning, some of the preceding foods are delicacies, others are unknown, and still others are rejected as being unfit to be used as food, although all are nutritious and wholesome.

FAMILY INFLUENCES

Within the framework of a culture, the family translates and modifies the cultural attitudes toward food and eating for its members. In the family, food is an important and continuing aspect of the mother-child relationship. From the beginning, the mother not only provides or makes available nutrients for the child, but, by the manner in which she feeds him, shows her love and affection.

In the family, mealtime provides more than food. In a modern industrial society, the evening meal may be the only time when the entire family regularly meets together as a group. This coming together of the family contributes to morale and a sense of unity among the members. Experiences of the day can be shared, plans made, and events reviewed. For a little while each day, every person can feel a part of a group in which he is accepted and respected. In some families, eating food is looked on as a pleasure, and much time and effort are spent in its preparation. Foods may be prepared to please one or more of the family members. Mother communicates her love and affection by preparing the foods they enjoy. Significant events are celebrated with food, and individual members are made to feel important by being served a dish that they particularly enjoy.

In other families, eating may be merely a necessary activity; food is prepared and eaten and the dishes are washed promptly. Little or no sociability accompanies eating; for members of the family, eating is necessary to sustain life but has few other tangible values. In still others, mealtime is utilized to discipline the children and settle the problems of the day. Instead of a relaxed atmosphere, meals are accompanied by strife and tension.

Whatever the attitude of the adults in the families, children develop values associated with food and eating. They learn what is and is not fit to eat and how it should be prepared. From their parents they learn not only what foods are good for them, but what foods are not good to eat. They learn to enjoy, tolerate, or reject food and eating.

In addition to defining the types of plants and animals suitable for use as food, the superstitions and beliefs adhered to by the family also designate those to be eaten during illness and how they are to be prepared. The old saying, "Feed a fever and starve a cold," is well known. Milk may be eliminated from the dietary of the sick because it is believed to be constipating, or, in the treatment of diarrhea, it may be boiled to make it constipating. Tea and toast are frequently believed to be suitable foods for sick people. Other foods such as rich desserts and cucumbers are designated as unsuitable.

FOOD AND THE EMOTIONS

The individual eats to satisfy a psychological as well as a physiological hunger. He may eat or refuse to eat to gain some measure of control over others. Mary Ellen feels comforted by eating when she feels depressed, lonely, or sad. She knows that she eats too much and is too fat, and she envies her slender classmates, but she continues to seek solace in food. She also knows that she gets more attention from her mother when she is fat than when she is thin. Despite the negative character of the remarks made by her mother and the fact that they increase her depression, Mary Ellen has her mother's attention.

REWARD VALUE OF FOOD

Some of the psychological implications of food stem from the value placed on certain foods as rewards. In the American culture, desserts such as cake, pie, ice cream, cookies, and candies have a reward value. They are served at the end of the meal after "wholesome" foods such as meat, bread, potatoes, and vegetables have been eaten. Whether or not desserts are included with the meal depends on specific conditions. They may be withheld if the individual fails to eat the foods that are "good for him" or as a punishment for some transgression. They are also used as a treat or as a reward for good behavior. They play a significant role in special events such as birthday parties, teas, and weddings. Although using specific foods as rewards may accomplish a desired result at the time, this practice may also be responsible for engendering negative attitudes toward food.

Increasing recognition is being given to the knowledge that certain foods have a reward value in the planning of modified diets. For example, ice cream is included in the diabetic diet. The food industry has recognized the psychological value of candy and other reward foods and makes them available as diabetic candy and cookies. Education is needed to acquaint parents and teachers with the undesirable effects of using food as a threat or reward. The reward-and-punishment aspect of food should also be taken into account in planning to meet the food requirements of any patient. In the past, this aspect has often been neglected.

The basis for the use of food as a reward or punishment is to control the behavior of another. Thus a parent seeks to control his child by rewarding him with food or withholding it. The child or other individual, however, can gain some measure of control in the situation by rewarding him with food or withholding it. win the approval of his mother and other members of the family. By refusing to eat, he may be able to arouse the concern and attention of his mother and gain some measure of control over her.

SYMBOLIC VALUE OF FOOD

A study of the symbolic reference of different foods in various cultures could easily take a lifetime. Only a few examples will, however, be cited. At the Seder feast which is celebrated at the beginning of the Passover, food is used to symbolize certain events in Jewish history. Three matzo crackers, or pieces of unleavened bread, are placed in a linen napkin on the table to represent the unity of Israel and to recall the departure from Egypt, which was so rapid that there was no time to take leaven. A roasted egg symbolizes life and its continuity, and bitter herbs symbolize the bitterness of slavery in the land of bondage.

In the Christian religions the egg is the symbol of the rebirth of the spiritual life of man through the death and resurrection of Christ. Eggs are colored and, in some cultures, highly intricate designs convert the egg into a thing of beauty.

Outside the realm of religion, certain foods are symbolic of certain events, status, wealth, or hospitality. Although turkey is available in the United States throughout the year, it remains the symbol of Thanksgiving. In terms of status, hamburger may be eaten by family members, but except for a cookout, it is not served to guests, as it is equated with a limited income.

Evidence of a high or low food intake can also be a status symbol. In some groups, plump children and a wife of ample proportions are accepted as evidence that "mama" is a good cook and "papa" is a good provider. In contrast, to be employed as a high fashion model, a young woman is required to restrict her food intake sufficiently to maintain a lean look.

CONDITIONING AND FOOD SELECTION

Although the culture into which the individual is born defines what is fit to eat and how and under what circumstances foods are to be eaten, conditioning or habit influences what he will eat throughout his lifetime. Although some foods are accepted more readily than others and some infants accept new foods more easily than others, babies learn to eat the foods offered to them. Food habits are established quite early in life. Most individuals prefer foods to which they became accustomed as young children, and they may be quite resistant to changing their food habits. Some may even prefer ill health or starvation to eating unaccustomed or unfamiliar foods or known foods prepared in unfamiliar ways. One of the difficult adjustments that international students in the United States frequently have to make is the adjustment to American food. Nor is the problem of adjusting to strange food limited to persons from other lands, because some Americans insist on familiar foods when they visit other countries. For example, to attract American tourists, signs on restaurants in Quebec advertise hamburgers, hot dogs, and steaks. In Santiago, Chile, a waitress, eagerly approached the writer with "Ham and eggs for breakfast?" The usual Chilean breakfast consisted of a hard roll and coffee with milk. Americans working in Chile had taken their food habits with them and Chilean hotels had adapted to their demands.

Although the foods eaten by an individual

are usually those to which he is conditioned early in life, most individuals eat more food if there is a variety of foods from which to select and a variety in methods of preparation. Variety is as important to the sick as to the healthy. The effects of the repeated serving of one food to hospitalized patients were well illustrated when a general hospital was given several hundred bushels of apples. Storage space was limited and the apples were served several times a week. Because most patients remained in the hospital only a short time, no problem was anticipated. However, a near rebellion occurred among patients undergoing rehabilitation following poliomyelitis. After several weeks, the monotony of almost daily servings of apples in some form resulted in these patients organizing a mass protest. Particular attention should be given to planning for variety for the patient who is chronically ill or who is faced with numerous adjustments and frustrations.

CHANGING FOOD HABITS

Probably the most frequent reason for a change in food habits is illness. Travelers to parts of the world where food differs from that to which they are accustomed are likely to have to make some alterations in their pattern of eating. In the past, health workers acted on the premise that if the person was properly instructed about what he should eat, and if he had enough money to buy food, he would eat a nutritious diet. Although knowledge is of significance, by itself it is not sufficient.

After food habits are established they are very difficult to change, and they cannot be changed overnight. Immigrants change their language before they change their pattern of eating. During a period of famine in the rice-eating part of India, wheat was sent to relieve starvation, but the population preferred death by starvation to eating wheat. Not only was wheat a strange food, but the familiar methods of food preparation were suited to rice and not to wheat. Before the people could be expected to use wheat as food, they would have to accept it as being suitable to eat and learn new methods of food preparation. At best, changing food habits is a slow process. It took more than 200 years to establish the potato as a food in Europe. It had been introduced during the sixteenth century by Spanish explorers but was not accepted as a food. In the eighteenth century, Count Rumford gave the potato prestige by planting it in the royal gardens and feeding it to the soldiers. Guards were stationed about the garden, but they were instructed to look the other way when the potatoes were stolen. Acceptance was furthered by feeding the po-

tatoes to the soldiers so that they developed a taste for them. In our present state of knowledge and with the variety of communications media available, it should be possible to change eating habits more rapidly. Nevertheless, food habits, once developed, continue to be difficult to alter.

PRINCIPLES BASIC TO CHANGE

Several general principles should be observed by those who desire to assist others to change their food habits. The first is to study existing beliefs, values, and practices before attempting to make a change. The reason for food practices should also be identified if possible. For example, in the United States frequent causes of inadequate diets are lack of money, poor money management, lack of interest in food, insufficient knowledge, food fads, and misguided dieting. As in other parts of the world, food intake is sometimes limited by misconceptions about food or by values ascribed to it. Beliefs about certain foods may bear little relation to their actual characteristics. For example, Mrs. Thomas never serves milk with acid foods because she believes that acids curdle milk. The following illustration, which was observed in a primitive culture, shows the relation of beliefs to practices. Despite the continued efforts of health workers and an adequate supply of eggs, the women refused to eat eggs. Eggs were not taboo because the men and children ate eggs. It was finally learned that the women believed that eggs made them aggressive and therefore were undesirable. Attention was given to changing this belief, and as the belief was changed, eggs were eaten by the women.

In the United States, values motivating people to eat or not to eat include staying slim, looking well, and keeping up with the neighbors. Studies indicate that the majority of people do not eat to be healthy per se. Motivation is through feelings, not logic. Unless the feelings of people about food are understood, information may fall on sterile soil. To date, relatively little attention has been paid by health workers to the factors motivating eating and to the utilization in practice of what is known.

Another general principle that must be observed if change is to be effected is to avoid direct or implied criticism of what is done or believed. The principal effect of criticism is to arouse stubborn resistance to change. An instance is related in which a public health nurse who was trying to encourage a group of mothers to feed their babies milk instead of beans was unsuccessful. Finally she suggested that the babies be given the water in which the beans were cooked. Later, when visiting the mothers, she found that they were feeding milk to their babies. When the nurse expressed surprise, one of the mothers said, "You accepted our way. We do your way."

One of the problems that nurses and other health workers have is that they expect the recipients of their services to accept their direction and advice without question. Moreover, they themselves may not follow the advice they give to others. Furthermore, nurses may not recognize that patients have at least two alternatives—to reject or to accept advice. The point of view of patients may be quite different from that of nurses trying to be helpful. Unless these differences in points of view are clarified by the nurse she may never know why the patient fails to "cooperate." After the point of view of the patient has been identified, his alternatives can also be clarified.

At least a minimum amount of money must be available to purchase the food required for an optimum nutritional state. Persons whose incomes fall below the minimum are likely to have difficulty securing enough food of good quality and variety.

Any plan made to assist a person to change his food habits should also include an exploration of the wants of the individual that are competing for his income. For example, a young woman with a baby had just enough money to buy a small can of peaches or a box of oatmeal. After much thought and indecision, she bought the peaches. Other individuals may want items other than food. When a person has an increase in salary, he may be faced with a number of alternatives. Should the new money be spent on nonfat dry milk, candy, carbonated beverages, cigarettes, liquor, or a television set? Objectively, the answer seems clear. To the individual who makes the choice, other answers may well take priority.

NUTRITION AND THE ADOLESCENT

Nutritional problems of the adolescent have received considerable attention. Numerous studies of the diet of teen-aged girls indicate that their intake of nutrients is deficient in some respects. The diet of boys is less likely to be inadequate. Some authorities believe that the large quantity of food ingested by teen-aged boys may be a factor in the earlier development of coronary artery disease in men than in women. Like the adult, the adolescent has little interest in nutrition and diet as such.

A number of characteristic features of adolescence influence how and what he eats. The adolescent wants respect and understanding as an individual. He wants those who work with him to believe in him and in his potential for becoming a mature adult. He wants to be liked and to do what his peers do.

Because adolescence occurs at different ages in different individuals, they differ in rate of growth, size, and general appearance. The adolescent is concerned about the changes he is undergoing and his relationships with members of the opposite sex and with his peers. He worries about pimples and being attractive. Girls are terrified lest they become fat. They skip breakfast, try fad diets, and take other shortcuts to a slender figure. The adolescent is in a period in which he has an exaggerated concern about himself. He wants others to be interested in him and to make their interest known. He requires respect. At the same time, adolescence is a period when the individual is developing an independent life. He may be torn between his wish to remain a child and his desire to be an adult. During adolescence he is developing his own ideas and making plans for his future. Physiologically, adolescence is a period of rapid growth. Especially in boys, food is required to build muscles. Girls are preparing themselves for pregnancy and lactation. Boys and girls require the proper quantity and quality of food for growth and development into healthy adults, as well as for their current activities.

NUTRITIONAL PROBLEMS IN LATER YEARS

Another period of life when nutritional problems may be exaggerated is in late maturity. An individual brings to his 60 years or more the food habits of a lifetime. Appetite may, however, be impaired by gradually diminishing activity, loss of the sense of taste, and loss of teeth. Ability to masticate food may be lessened by failure to replace teeth or by poorly fitting dentures. For some old people, money may be a real or perceived problem. Persons living on pensions, welfare, or social security may have barely enough to take care of their needs. Others have sufficient funds, but fear their money will be exhausted before they die. The cost of illness or other emergencies may strain the budget to the point where the amount left for food is inadequate. Pride or lack of knowledge of the means available to supplement the income may be responsible. Sometimes the food money is spent for food for a dog or cat. To a lonely, aged man or woman, a pet may have more value than an adequate or nearly adequate diet. To feed her dog, Mrs. Frisk eats meat only twice a week. She speaks with pride when she says that Skippy has a nice, juicy hamburger every day. A deficient food intake may result from a lack of incentive or energy to secure or prepare food. People who live alone, such as the elderly or the chronically ill, are especially prone to neglect their food intake. In some cities, *Meals on Wheels* have been developed to make meals available to the homebound at a reasonable cost.[14]

Poverty among the elderly is not limited to money. With the passage of time, the elderly man or woman often becomes increasingly isolated. As relatives and friends die or move away, the opportunity to share meals with others diminishes. With the decrease in or loss of the social aspect of eating, incentive for eating diminishes. The positive effects on the appetite of eating with others can be observed when company comes for dinner or the elderly person is invited out to eat. Mrs. Marshall illustrates this point very well. She lives alone in a small apartment. When she prepares her own meals and eats alone, she, in her own words, "eats like a bird." On Sundays, when she is invited to the home of her granddaughter, she eats about as well as the other members of the family. Her explanation is, "The food tastes better." The combination of well-prepared food, friendly conversation, and the example of others eating with pleasure has a favorable effect on Mrs. Marshall's appetite.

In some hospitals, particularly those for the chronically ill, group dining rooms are provided in order to create a social atmosphere at mealtime. For patients who are confined to their rooms, attention to the environment before food is served may help to improve the appetite. The presence of a family member or a good friend at mealtime, or a flower on the tray, may aid in creating a more homelike atmosphere, thereby encouraging eating. When failure of a patient to eat is a problem, attention to the social aspects of eating sometimes contributes to the solution.

Summary

Survival, growth, productivity, and health all depend on a continuous supply of food. In some areas of the world the amount of food available is insufficient to support the population at much more than a survival level. The reasons for the inadequate food supply include poor soil or unfavorable climate and lack of transportation or food preservation facilities. As the result of experiences during and following World War II, there has been growing appreciation of the fact that a supply of food is only one aspect of eating. Eating is a voluntary act. Before a plant or animal is utilized as food, it must be accepted as being fit or suitable to eat. This acceptance involves a variety of psychological and social factors having little or nothing to do with the nutritional value of a substance. A man as well as a hen may starve

[14] M. D. Keller and C. E. Smith: "Meals on Wheels: 1960," *Geriatrics*, **16**:237–47 (May) 1961.

to death while sitting beside a sack of wheat. There are few events in the life of the individual where food does not play a part. Often the improvement of the nutrition of an individual or of a nation depends on a change in food habits. Though knowledge of how to effect change is limited, a few guides to action have been suggested. They include the following: (1) Take time to discover the what and why of the pattern of the group. (2) Do not criticize, because criticism only arouses stubborn resistance. (3) Remember that changing food habits is a slow process. (4) Motivation for eating is more psychological and social than it is intellectual. (5) Although knowledge of what constitutes good nutrition is usually insufficient to effect change, it is one factor in change.

As stated earlier, nutrition plays a role in the etiology of or recovery from almost all diseases. It may be important throughout the course of an illness. The biochemical, physiological, and psychological changes taking place during illness frequently affect the desire for food. Not uncommonly the sick person is faced with a change—temporary or permanent—in his pattern of eating. Sometimes the problem is easily solved, as it was for Mrs. Brown who was wondering how she could ever adjust to a diabetic diet. She thought that she would be denied greens, corn bread, and ice cream. The greens presented no problem. Within limits, neither did the corn bread nor the ice cream.

When significant changes are required, the patient may appear to accept the change but may actually continue his usual food pattern. Mrs. Smith, also a diabetic, was such a person. At one time she was under the supervision of a physician who believed in strict control of the diet. Later she was cared for by a physician who believed a diabetic person could and should eat the same food as a nondiabetic. When asked by a nurse about how confusing the change must have been, she said, "Not at all. I've followed about the same regimen all the time. Both physicians were so enthusiastic that I couldn't bear to disappoint them."

Some patients react with what appears to be unreasonable resistance to change. If the professional staff reacts with hostility or indifference, the resistance of the patient is likely to increase. If the cause of the reaction of the patient can be determined, then the patient may be more willing to modify his behavior. Not infrequently the reasons for the rejection of the diet plan are reasonable, not only to the patient but, when the trouble is taken to identify them, to the nurse. What appears to be irrational behavior to the observer may be rational to the behaver. Often the diet plan can be altered in such a way as to make it more acceptable to the individual. Success is dependent, at least in part, on learning what the change means to the individual and working with him in making an acceptable plan.

The Service Facility

Because nutrients are usually ingested in a complex state, foods must be subjected to a series of physical and chemical changes whereby they are converted to a state in which they can be absorbed. Large multicellular organisms such as man have specialized structures that receive, temporarily store, and convert by chemical and mechanical means crude materials to utilizable forms, whereupon they are transferred from the external to the internal environment. The remaining residue is temporarily stored, water is absorbed and eventually the residue is ejected at regular intervals.

Before discussion of individual organs, some of the common features of the digestive system and the effects of disturbances in function on the body economy as well as on the general nutritional state will be presented. The alimentary canal and the accessory organs of digestion function as a unit. Under nervous and hormonal control, the activity of each organ of the digestive system is coordinated and integrated so that food is in the right place at the right time for digestion and absorption to be accomplished.

The Alimentary Canal

The alimentary canal is a hollow muscular tube passing through the center of the body and extending from the mouth to the anus. As in other structures in contact with the external environment, there are structural and functional defenses against injurious agents. In health, the mucosa is protected against the digestive action of gastric and other juices. The two primary functions of the alimentary canal are the digestion and the absorption of nutrients. Despite the importance of the regular evacuation of the residue remaining after digestion is completed, in health the alimentary canal plays only a secondary role in the elimination of substances from the internal environment.

UPPER ALIMENTARY CANAL

Functionally, the alimentary canal can be divided into three general regions: upper, middle, and lower. The upper alimentary canal includes the esophagus, stomach, upper duodenum, liver, and pancreas. As do other regions, the upper alimentary canal conveys food from upper to lower parts. Its other principal functions are (1) the secretion of digestive juices, (2) the breaking up and mixing of food particles with these juices, (3) storage, and (4) the beginning of chemical digestion. The importance to life and health of the various structures comprising the upper alimentary canal varies. Persons with strictures of the esophagus can and do live for many years. Removal of the stomach is compatible with life but is frequently associated with some loss of health.

MIDDLE ALIMENTARY CANAL

The middle alimentary canal extends from the duodenal papilla to the mid-transverse colon. From the viewpoint of function, it is the most important region of the alimentary canal, for it is here that digestion is completed and absorption takes place. In our present state of knowledge, adequate nutrition cannot be maintained without the absorbing surface of the mid-alimentary canal. The available surface for absorption in a healthy person is greater than is required, and although the small intestine cannot be removed in its entirety, some of it can be removed without threatening the nutritional status of the individual. Many nutrients can be supplied parenterally, but only by exceptional procedures can calories and amino acids be infused in sufficient quantities to meet tissue requirements. The middle portion of the alimentary canal is therefore a vital organ.

LOWER ALIMENTARY CANAL

The lower portion of the alimentary canal extends from the mid-portion of the transverse colon to the anus. Its primary function is to store refuse until it can be conveniently evacuated. The lower alimentary canal is not necessary to either life or health. An artificial opening in any portion from the lower ileum downward can be made to function satisfactorily in the elimination of wastes. Because the ascending and transverse portions of the colon absorb water from the fluid content of the alimentary canal, the lower the opening, the less physiological adjustments have to be made. For example, the drainage from an ileostomy is watery, but the feces in the sigmoid colon are semisolid. Following an ileostomy, the lower ileum adapts by increasing water absorption, but the process of adaptation takes time and the patient needs to be protected from the loss of water and electrolytes. The skin around the ileostomy requires protection from the fluid feces. Following a sigmoidostomy, the feces may be fluid or semifluid for a few days, primarily as a result of hypermotility, but within a short time the feces assume their normal semisolid consistency.

BLOOD SUPPLY

Most of the regions of the alimentary canal have a rich blood and lymphatic supply. The exceptions include a portion of the esophagus and of the colon. The parts richly supplied with blood have the advantage of healing rapidly after surgery or accidental injury. The abundant blood supply also makes hemorrhage a greater possibility when blood vessels are ruptured. Venous drainage from the alimentary canal is through the portal system which supplies the liver. In diseases of the liver in which there is obstruction of the portal venous system, varicosities of the esophageal and hemorrhoidal veins occur. Rupture of esophageal varices is attended by massive hemorrhage.

What mechanisms are provided for the regulation of gastrointestinal function?

The function of the alimentary canal is regulated by the nervous and hormonal systems in relation to the needs of the entire organism. The alimentary canal is exceedingly sensitive to conditions in the body as a whole. The various organs of the alimentary canal are also regulated in relation to each other. Food in one organ acts as a stimulus to alert the next organ to prepare for it or to delay the rate at which the preceding organ empties. For example, a factor in the rate at which the stomach empties into the duodenum is the degree of fullness of the small intestine. When the intestine is distended, inhibitory messages are sent to the stomach in the form of an inhibitory hormone, enterogastrone, secreted by the intestinal musosa.

HORMONAL REGULATION

Two groups of hormones participate in the regulation of the alimentary canal. The first consists of the hormones participating in the regulation of activities throughout the body. The second group is classified as local hormones because they are secreted by some part of the alimentary canal and alter action by stimulating or inhibiting another part. Examples of hormones of the first group are the adrenal glucocorticoids. They probably reduce the resistance of the mucosa to the digesting action of gastric juice. In some individuals, the administration of the adrenal glucocorticoids predisposes to peptic ulcer formation. A history of peptic ulcer is therefore a relative contraindication to the employment of adrenal glucocorticoids in treatment. When they are prescribed, the patient should be observed for symptoms associated with ulcer formation. Antacids may be prescribed as a preventive measure.

NERVOUS REGULATION

The alimentary canal is richly supplied with nerves from the autonomic nervous system and from an intramural (within the wall) nerve plexus. This plexus extends all the way from the esophagus to the anus. It consists of two layers of neurons. The outer layer lies between the longitudinal and circular muscles of the digestive tube and is known as the myenteric (or Auerbach's) plexus. The inner layer of neurons lies in the submucosa and is known as the submucous (or Meissner's) plexus. These plexuses, often referred to collectively as the myenteric plexus, regulate many of the local actions of the digestive tube. The plexuses increase the muscle tone, the intensity and rate of rhythmical contraction, and the speed with which excitatory waves spread along the gastrointestinal wall.

The alimentary canal receives nerves from both the parasympathetic and sympathetic divisions of the autonomic nervous system. Centers in the central nervous system act through the parasympathetic and sympathetic nervous systems to increase or decrease the activity of the gastrointestinal tract. In general, these two divisions of the autonomic nervous system have opposing actions. The parasympathetic nervous system increases activity of the alimentary canal, and the sympathetic nervous system has, with three exceptions, inhibitory effects. Stimulation by the sympathetic nervous system increases the activity of the ileocecal and internal anal sphincters and the smooth muscle of the muscularis mucosae throughout the alimentary tract. The action of the entire digestive tube can be blocked by intense stimulation of the sympathetic nervous system because the wall of the gut is inhibited and two major sphincters are contracted. Inhibition of the alimentary tract is to be expected during the period immediately following severe trauma or major surgery, or during the acute phase of serious illnesses such as pneumonia. (See Chapter 6 for further discussion.) Excitement, anxiety, and fear can also stimulate the sympathetic nervous system so that it greatly diminishes the activity of the digestive tube. Attention given to minimizing the anxiety of the sick person may therefore contribute to diminishing the degree to which the alimentary canal is inactivated.

In contrast to the sympathetic nervous system, the parasympathetic nervous system increases the activity of the alimentary canal, including the secretion of digestive juices. Cannon describes the functions of the parasympathetic nervous system as being concerned with nutrition. The gut is supplied from both the cranial and sacral divisions of the parasympathetic nervous system. With the exception of some parasympathetic fibers in the mouth and pharynx, the entire cranial supply is through the vagus nerve. Whereas the loss of the sympathetic nerve supply to the gut has little or no effect on function, interruption of the parasympathetic almost always has. For example, vagotomy, a surgical procedure in which a branch of the vagus nerve is severed, is sometimes used in the treatment of intractable peptic ulcer. It is followed by reduction in muscle tone and decrease of peristaltic activity in all the following regions: the distal portion of the esophagus, the stomach, and the proximal portion of the intestine. There is also a decrease in secretions in the stomach. Severing of the sacral parasympathetic nervous system is followed by diminished tone of the descending colon, the sigmoid, and the rectum with the result that defecation is seriously impaired.

CHARACTERISTICS OF MOVEMENT

The rate at which the contents are moved diminishes progressively from the mouth to the anus. Motion is accomplished by smooth muscle arranged in longitudinal and circular layers. The muscle fibers lie so close together that contraction initiated at one point tends to spread to adjacent areas. The muscles of the alimentary canal exhibit the two types of contraction characteristic of smooth muscle in any part of the body—tonus contraction and rhythmical contraction. Tonus contraction determines the degree of pressure in any organ and the resistance to movement by the sphincters. Rhythmical contraction, or peristalsis, moves the contents toward the anus. Excessive tonic contractions of a segment or of a sphincter may interfere with the forward movement of the contents of the digestive tube. They may also be a source of pain.

PERISTALSIS

Peristalsis mixes the contents of the alimentary canal and propels them forward. Peristalsis is characterized by contraction of the muscle behind the bolus and simultaneous relaxation of the muscle ahead of it. Any increase or decrease in the activity of smooth muscle disturbs in some manner the capacity of the alimentary canal to receive, retain, digest, or absorb food.

Both the tone and the rhythmical contractions of the alimentary tract are regulated by the nervous system. As a consequence of the action of the nervous system, the rhythmical contractions of the alimentary canal can be increased or decreased in intensity or rate. In addition, peristalsis (the major propulsive movements of the gastrointestinal tract) is coordinated and the secretion of digestive juices is regulated so that each ferment is provided at the time and place it is needed.

SPHINCTERS

Each major segment of the alimentary canal is separated from other segments by sphincter muscles. Sphincters control the rate at which the contents of the gastrointestinal tract are moved from one organ to another, and they prevent backflow. The sphincters at the inlet and at the outlet of the stomach also regulate the size of particles allowed to move forward. Food is retained in the stomach until particles are finely divided and converted into a fluid state and acidified. The resulting mixture is known as chyme.

INTEGRITY OF THE ALIMENTARY CANAL

Another anatomical characteristic of the alimentary canal, of importance in understanding possible effects of disease, is that the lumen of the gut lies outside the body proper. The entire lumen from the mouth to the anus is surrounded by the body, but it is not part of it. (See Figure 12-1.) The wall surrounding the lumen of the alimentary canal either is impermeable to its contents or is permeable only to water, alcohol, small molecules, and ions. In fact, many molecules and ions require a transport or carrier system to move across semipermeable membranes in appreciable quantities.[15] Any break in the integrity of the wall therefore carries with it the possibility of the escape of the contents of the alimentary canal into the internal environment. Superficial disruption of the mucous membrane is not usually serious. If, however, the break penetrates all the layers and extends through the entire wall, the contents of the organ escape into a body cavity.

DEFENSES OF THE ALIMENTARY CANAL

ROLE OF THE SENSES

As with other structural facilities serving as points of exchange between the internal and external environment, some system of defense or protection against the ingestion of harmful substances is required. The senses of sight, taste, and smell all function in protection. Foods are accepted or rejected on the basis of general appearance, odor, taste, and feel. Meat may be accepted when it is bright in color or rejected when it is dull red or black. If the meat smells

---

[15] Fat solvent liquids such as carbon tetrachloride are readily absorbed.

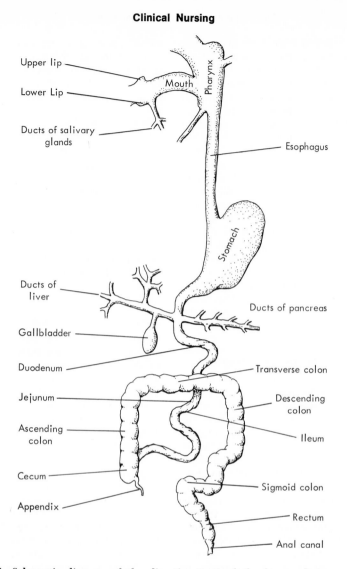

Upper lip
Mouth
Pharynx
Lower Lip
Ducts of salivary glands
Esophagus
Stomach
Ducts of liver
Ducts of pancreas
Gallbladder
Duodenum
Transverse colon
Jejunum
Descending colon
Ascending colon
Ileum
Cecum
Sigmoid colon
Appendix
Rectum
Anal canal

FIGURE 12-1. Schematic diagram of the digestive tract of the human being and accessory organs. (Adapted with permission of The Macmillan Company from *Anatomy and Physiology*, 14th ed., Fig. 41, p. 54, by Diana Clifford Kimber, Carolyn E. Gray, Caroline E. Stackpole, and Lutie C. Leavell. Copyright © The Macmillan Company, 1961.)

fresh, it is more likely to be eaten than if it has a peculiar odor or is putrid. The same is true of taste. Inasmuch as these senses enable the individual to correctly evaluate the safety of a food, they are protective. Because they are subject to conditioning and are not very accurate, wholesome food may be rejected and harmful foods accepted. When there is any doubt about the safety of food, it should be rejected.

THE MUCOUS MEMBRANE

The mucous membrane which extends from the mouth to the anus acts as a barrier to the entrance of excessively large molecules and of some microorganisms into the body proper. As in other areas of the body, the mucous membrane must be unbroken or intact. Glands in the mucous membrane secrete mucus which tends to coat the mucous membrane lining the alimentary canal and to lessen the extent of direct contact with its contents. The mucous membrane is thereby protected from mechanical injury by fibrous foods and from the digesting action of enzymes contained in the digestive juices. As in the respiratory tract, the mucous glands in the membrane lining the alimentary canal respond to irritation by increased secretion. After a harsh laxative has been taken or hard feces are defecated, mucus can sometimes be seen in or around the stool. In a disorder known as mucus colitis, hyperactivity of the colon may be sufficient to be accompanied by the discharge of large quantities of mucus. Sometimes the sheets of mucus are in the form of a cast of the bowel. In disorders in which there is a disruption of the mucous membrane lining of the large intestine, such as in chronic ulcerative colitis, mucus secretion is also increased over the normal. Any break in the integrity of the mucous membrane predisposes to the entrance of microorganisms and/or other foreign particles into the internal environment.

A third barrier to the entrance of microorganisms into the internal environment is the character of its secretions. The acid gastric juice is of particular importance. Under conditions of health, few microorganisms are found in the gastric secretions.

ANOREXIA, NAUSEA, VOMITING

Three closely related mechanisms serve to protect the individual against the ingestion of harmful material or remove it from the gastrointestinal tract after it has been ingested. They are anorexia, nausea, or vomiting. The person suffering from anorexia says, "I have no appetite," or "I don't feel like eating," or "Nothing tastes good." He may dawdle with his food or force himself to try to eat. Whereas anorexia is characterized by loss of appetite, nausea is an unpleasant or disagreeable sensation characterized by a revulsion for food. When food is offered to the nauseated patient, he says, "Take it away," or "I can't stand the sight or smell of it," or "It makes me feel sick even to think of it." He looks and feels miserable. Usually the nauseated person cannot force himself to eat. As a rule, he has other symptoms caused by imbalance in the autonomic nervous system, such as increased salivation and secretion of mucus, sweating, and tachycardia. Evidence of increased activity of the vagus nerve may result in bradycardia and hypotension. In nausea, the tone and activity of the stomach and small intestine are probably diminished.

Although nausea and vomiting are frequently associated, they may appear independently of each other. Because of the close relationship of nausea to vomiting, factors in its cause and treatment will be discussed with vomiting. Vomiting is defined as the sudden forceful ejection of the contents of the stomach, duodenum, and proximal jejunum through the mouth. It is frequently, but not invariably, preceded by nausea. A projectile type of vomiting, occurring without warning nausea, accompanies rapidly increasing intracranial pressure, such as follows head injuries.

VOMITING REFLEX

Although all vomiting results from reflex activity, the point at which the reflex is initiated varies. The basic pattern for the vomiting reflex is similar to that of any reflex. It involves a receptor connected by way of nerve fibers and cells to an effector. As in other reflexes, a group of nerve cells located within the brain, the vomiting center, regulates and coordinates the act of vomiting. Sensory receptors capable of initiating the vomiting reflex are located outside as well as within the wall of the alimentary canal. Within the alimentary canal, receptors are located in the fauces and pharynx, the stomach, and the intestine. The most acutely sensitive area is the first portion of the duodenum. Outside the alimentary canal, sensory receptors for vomiting are located in the uterus, kidneys, heart, and semicircular canals. Receptors may be stimulated by excessively irritating substances or by overdistention of an organ supplied with sensory receptors. The degree of excitability of the receptors is an element in the intensity of stimulation required to trigger the vomiting reflex. The more irritable the receptor, the easier it is to stimulate it.

Even a cursory glance at the variety of sites containing sensory receptors for vomiting and the types of conditions likely to stimulate them suggests that vomiting is a frequent event in disease. Moreover, it occurs not only in disorders involving the gastrointestinal system, but in those of the heart, kidney, uterus, and semicircular canals. Inflammatory conditions of the alimentary canal, such as acute appendicitis and gastroenteritis, frequently cause vomiting. The vomiting associated with motion sickness results from the effects of motion on the semicircular canals in sensitive persons. Motion sickness is caused by any form of transportation in the air, on water, or on land. As in many other situations, fear and anxiety increase the tendency to motion sickness.

Because the fauces and pharynx are areas where the vomiting reflex may be triggered, care should be taken during mouth hygiene to avoid initiating the vomiting reflex by mechanical stimulation of these areas. Particular attention should be paid to this in patients who have been vomiting. Mechanical stimulation of the pharynx or fauces during the passage of a nasogastric tube or the introduction of a nasopharyngeal catheter initiates the gag reflex in many people. Procedures such as asking the patient to breathe deeply or to swallow are often beneficial as they distract the attention of the patient and help him to relax. Moreover, the voluntary initiation of swallowing suppresses the vomiting reflex.

Easy access to receptors initiating the vomiting reflex can be life saving in some instances. After a toxic substance has been ingested, vomiting can sometimes be induced by stimulating the fauces with a finger or a blunt instrument. This is a commonly used technique for self-induction of vomiting. Emotionally disturbed persons sometimes induce vomiting by this method. Should a person be observed to be inducing the vomiting reflex, this fact should be recorded and brought to the attention of the physician.

Receptors in the stomach can be stimulated by drinking water containing an irritating substance or by the rapid distention of the stomach. A common, though not always effective, method is to drink a glass of tepid water to which a teaspoonful of dry mustard has been added. Mustard has the undesired effect of increasing any previous irritation. Distention of the stomach is accomplished by drinking ordinary tap water or starch water as rapidly as possible, and will always induce vomiting when ingested in sufficient quantities. Water has the advantage of diluting the contents of the stomach and it facilitates the removal of toxic substances.

Vomiting may also be initiated by impulses at the vomiting center by way of the cerebral cortex. Unpleasant sights, sounds, odors, tastes, and thoughts, as well as sensations such as severe pain, can initiate the vomiting reflex. In some persons, the sight of blood induces vomiting. It is not unusual for a person arriving at the scene of an accident where blood has been spilled to complain of nausea or actually to vomit. Fetid odors or the odor of vomitus can have a similar effect.

A third general site where vomiting may be initiated is the chemoreceptor zone, located in the medulla, but outside the vomiting center. At one time it was thought that circulating toxic agents caused vomiting by acting on the vomiting center. Emetic drugs such as apomorphine, toxic dosages of digitalis, and the "toxins" of acute infectious disease, as well as the retention of products normally excreted by the kidneys, are believed to induce vomiting by stimulating the chemoreceptor center. Vomiting is a problem in disorders accompanied by disturbances in metabolism such as pernicious vomiting in pregnancy, diabetic acidosis, and addisonian and hyperthyroid crises. As indicated earlier, vomiting also occurs in patients with traumatic head injuries, with infections involving the brain and meninges, and with increasing intracranial pressure.

In Figure 12-2, the location of common receptors which, when stimulated, initiate the vomiting reflex can be seen. Impulses are carried from these receptors to the vomiting center by way of peripheral, cranial, and autonomic sensory fibers. The vomiting center is located in the lateral reticular formation of the medulla oblongata. It is one of a number of visceral centers such as the vasomotor, the defecation, the respiratory, and the salivation centers. These are all centers regulating the autonomic nervous system. During vomiting, there is additional evidence of autonomic activity such as increased salivation, sweating, and bradycardia.

The Act of Vomiting

From the vomiting center, impulses travel over efferent fibers of the vagus and phrenic nerves as well as those supplying the abdominal muscles. The act of vomiting usually begins with nausea, increased salivation, the secretion of large amounts of mucus, and what, for want of a better name, are called disagreeable sensations. During the period of nausea, the contents of the jejunum and the duodenum are emptied into the pyloric end of the stomach by strong sustained contraction of the small intestine. The pyloric sphincter and the pyloric end of the stomach contract and force the material into the body and fundus of the stomach, thus filling them. Vomiting is caused by the diaphragm and abdominal muscles contracting against the walls of the dilated stomach and forcing the contents through the open cardiac sphincter into the esophagus. Vomiting cannot occur unless the cardiac sphincter relaxes. The hypopharyngeal sphincter also relaxes. The glottis is closed and is kept closed after inspiration, which takes place just as vomiting begins. Contrary to an old belief, the principal force in evacuating the stomach during vomiting is not reverse peristalsis of the stomach and esophagus, but contraction of the diaphragm and abdominal muscles. The unconscious patient, whether from general anesthesia or from some other cause, may aspirate vomitus because of failure to close the glottis during vomiting. Unconscious patients who are vomiting or are likely to vomit should be placed in a position favoring drainage from the tracheobronchial tree.

Possible Effects of Vomiting

From the preceding discussion it is apparent that vomiting is a commonly occurring condition. The vomiting reflex can be initiated by a wide variety of intrinsic and extrinsic factors. Frequently more than one element is involved in a patient who is vomiting or who continues to vomit. The prevention and treatment of vomiting depend on its cause and how long it continues. Although vomiting removes irritating materials from the gastrointestinal tract, it also removes water and electrolytes and interferes with the ingestion of food. In a well-nourished person who vomits for a brief period of time,

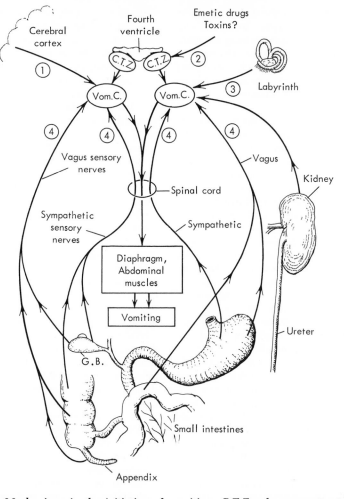

FIGURE 12-2. Mechanisms in the initiation of vomiting. *C.T.Z.*, chemoreceptor trigger zone; *Vom. C.*, vomiting center; *G.B.*, gallbladder; *1*, cerebral stimulation of vomiting center; *2*, drug stimulation of chemoreceptor trigger zone; *3*, labyrinthine (motion, etc.) stimulation of vomiting center; *4*, visceral afferent stimulation of vomiting center. (Adapted with permission of The Macmillan Company from *Modern Pharmacology and Therapeutics*, 4th ed., 1969, Fig. 27-1, p. 491, by Ruth D. Musser and John J. O'Neill.)

the latter effects are of little moment. Some emotionally disturbed persons who vomit do not lose weight because they actually vomit very little food. In the patient who is debilitated or who continues to vomit not for a few hours but for days, vomiting may result in dehydration, metabolic alkalosis, and serious loss of weight. It may also contribute to the problem of maintaining or improving the nutritional state of the individual. In patients who have had surgery, vomiting may place strain on the site of the incision by increasing pressure within the abdominal, ocular, and cranial cavities. Vomiting after surgery on the eye predisposes to intra-ocular bleeding. If vomiting occurs in a patient who has undergone surgery on the eyes, it

should be brought to the attention of the physician immediately. Orders for antiemetic drugs should be carried out faithfully.

Treatment of Vomiting

Treatment of the patient who is vomiting is based on its cause and effects. If vomiting is associated with acute appendicitis or diabetic acidosis, the obvious treatment is to remove the inflamed appendix or restore glucose metabolism, and to correct the disturbances in water and electrolyte balance. When treatment is directed toward the control of vomiting, procedures are selected which relieve vomiting by (1) removing irritating substances from the stomach, (2) relieving or preventing distention of the stomach, (3) diminishing the sensitivity of the chemotherapeutic trigger zone, (4) discontinuing the administration of drugs stimulating the chemoreceptor trigger zone, (5) correcting metabolic disorders in which circulating "toxins" activate the chemoreceptor trigger zone, and (6) correcting imbalances and deficits in water and electrolytes.

As stated earlier, irritating materials may be removed from the stomach by drinking water and vomiting or by suction through a nasogastric tube. When the stomach is distended because of failure to empty, nasogastric suction is usually prescribed. The advantages of this method of emptying the stomach are that distention can be prevented, and repeated and prolonged vomiting can be controlled.

A number of antiemetic drugs act by raising the threshold of the chemoreceptor trigger zone to stimulation. The first drug found to be effective was chlorpromazine. Other drugs include diphenhydrinate (Dramamine [16]), other phenothiazines, trimethobenzamide (Tigan [16]), and the barbiturates. These drugs are useful, not only in the treatment of vomiting, but in its prevention in motion sickness.

Physical and chemical agents used in the treatment of disease may induce vomiting. Therapy with x-ray or radioactive isotopes, particularly when applied to the upper abdomen, frequently causes some degree of nausea and vomiting. Usually treatment with radioactive substances is continued, despite the presence of vomiting. Some drugs such as digitalis cause nausea and vomiting when toxic dosages have been reached. When it has been established that vomiting is due to the toxic effects of a drug, it may be discontinued temporarily or permanently or its dosage reduced. Other drugs such as morphine and meperidine (Demerol [17]) induce vomiting in susceptible persons. When nausea and vomiting regularly follow the administration of a drug and diminish in severity as time elapses after it is given, idiosyncrasy to the drug should be suspected. The discontinuance of the drug is usually all that is required to correct the nausea and vomiting.

Nursing the Patient

In addition to the treatment prescribed by the physician, the nurse can do much to lessen the discomfort of the patient who is vomiting. There are few more disagreeable or unpleasant symptoms than nausea and vomiting. For many persons, the presence of a kindly and solicitous person makes vomiting more bearable. The nurse, or other person, herself may experience nausea as she assists the patient, with the result

[16] Trade name.
[17] Trade name.

that she finds it difficult to stay with him. The nurse can suppress the vomiting reflex by swallowing and by concentrating on what she can and should do to assist the patient. Should simple measures be ineffective, the nurse should discuss her problem with her instructor, supervisor, or physician.

During vomiting, nursing care of the patient should be based on two objectives: (1) to prevent the aspiration of vomitus and (2) to increase the comfort of the patient. To lessen the possibility of aspiration during emesis, if at all possible the patient should be turned to one side and the head should be flexed at the neck. Factors predisposing to nausea and vomiting in susceptible patients should be identified and controlled. Insofar as possible, pain should be prevented or kept under control. The room should be well ventilated. Strong odors—dressings, emesis, perfumes—should be eliminated from the environment. The emesis basin should be emptied and washed immediately after use. Because there is a psychic element in vomiting, the suggestion is usually made to keep the basin within easy reach, but out of sight. If, however, the patient is more relaxed when the basin is where he can see it, this factor should be taken into consideration. After vomiting, the patient should have an opportunity to rinse out his mouth. Soiled bed linen should be changed. Because moving predisposes to an attack of nausea and vomiting, necessary changes in position should be made slowly. Sometimes the vomiting reflex can be suppressed by deep-breathing and by initiation of the swallowing reflex. If the condition of the patient allows, carbonated beverages such as ginger ale, or soda may be tolerated when other fluids are not. Either cold or hot fluids are generally better tolerated than tepid ones. A combination of measures is sometimes necessary to control vomiting. The patient should be encouraged in the belief that something can be and is being done to control the vomiting.

The following case illustrates the value of simple measures in the control of vomiting triggered by anesthesia and prolonged by metabolic and emotional factors. Alexandra Berry, who was attending college far from home, fell and fractured the radius of her left arm. The fracture site was placed in a splint immediately, but several hours elapsed before Miss Berry was admitted to the hospital and the fracture reduced under Pentothal Sodium [18] anesthesia. As soon as Miss Berry regained consciousness, she was discharged to the college dormitory. For the next 24 hours, she continued to vomit. Since psychic factors were undoubtedly impor-

[18] Trade name for thiopental sodium.

tant, the dormitory nurse cleared the room of anxious friends. She also removed the bucket being used as an emesis basin. She obtained a large bottle of chilled ginger ale and encouraged Alexandra to sip it slowly. Each time Alexandra retched, the nurse encouraged her to swallow and breathe deeply. After an hour or so, Alexandra was able to rest comfortably without vomiting. The nurse bathed Alexandra, changed her bed, aired the room, and suggested firmly that the measures that she had instituted would cure her. They did.

Although vomiting was probably induced by the effect of the anesthetic on the chemoreceptor trigger zone, psychic factors were undoubtedly important in its continuance. Miss Berry had a frightening experience, she was far from the comforting presence of her family, and she was treated by a strange physician. Furthermore, with the loss of fluid and failure to ingest food, some degree of electrolyte imbalance presumably increased the activity of the chemoreceptor trigger zone. Factors contributing to the control of vomiting included deep-breathing, swallowing, and the drinking of ginger ale. The ginger ale provided fluid required to correct dehydration, and it provided a ready supply of glucose. With the correction of glucose starvation, the rate of mobilization of fat is depressed and the degree of metabolic acidosis is lessened. The probability also exists that Miss Berry responded in a positive way to the presence of an individual who was in control of the situation and who appeared to be convinced that the vomiting could and would disappear. Of course, not all patients are as easily helped as was Alexandra. The specific measures utilized in the therapy of vomiting depend on its cause and its effects.

Among the pertinent observations are the nature of the onset and the circumstances surrounding vomiting. Has the patient been apparently well and then become suddenly ill or has he been unwell for a period of time? How long has the patient been vomiting? Is vomiting preceded by nausea? What other signs and symptoms does the patient have? When does the patient vomit in relation to food intake or to the ingestion or injection of drugs? The emesis should be observed for amount, odor, general appearance, and presence of blood. Fresh blood is bright red, while flecks of partly digested blood give the vomitus a coffee ground appearance. In addition to the making of pertinent observations, they should be accurately recorded. Whether or not they are immediately drawn to the attention of the physician will depend on the extent to which prompt action is required. When in doubt, the nurse should notify the physician.

OTHER DEFENSE MECHANISMS

Like vomiting, diarrhea results in the removal of irritating substances from the alimentary canal. It is, however, almost always associated with a disease process or with an emotional disturbance. It will be discussed with disorders of motility.

Despite the effectiveness of primary defense mechanisms in preventing harmful agents from getting beyond the first lines of defense, they sometimes do. The internal environment is protected from general dissemination of injurious agents from the alimentary canal by lymph nodes and phagocytes. They function in protection just as they do in other parts of the body. The internal environment is further protected from the general dissemination of microorganisms and some potentially toxic agents by the liver. Bacteria in the blood circulating through the liver are destroyed by reticuloendothelial or Kupffer cells. Chemicals of extrinsic or intrinsic origin are detoxified or inactivated in the liver. To illustrate, the liver is the chief site of degradation of most barbiturates. Barbital and phenobarbital are exceptions, because they are mainly excreted by the kidney. Barbiturates excreted by the kidney have a more prolonged effect than those that are inactivated by the liver. Because persons who have severe liver damage are dependent on the kidney for the excretion of barbiturates, they are likely to experience toxicity when receiving barbiturates other than phenobarbital or barbital. Steroid hormones such as estrogen are degraded by the liver.

As in other structures in the body, tissues of the alimentary canal are capable of responding to injury by inflammation and by the formation of scar tissue. Inasmuch as these responses help to limit the extent of injury and to restore the continuity of tissue, they are beneficial. Scar tissue located near or at the orifice of an organ or duct or encircling a part can cause obstruction as it contracts with maturity.

To recapitulate, in a structural facility where materials are transferred from the external into the internal environment, provisions for the protection of the internal environment from harmful agents are required. The internal environment is protected from the ingestion, absorption, and dissemination of potentially injurious substances by a variety of structures and mechanisms. The senses of sight, taste, smell, and touch serve to warn the individual of the possible unsuitability of food or water for ingestion. Because they are not very accurate and are subject to conditioning, wholesome substances are sometimes rejected and harmful ones ingested. A continuous sheet of mucous membrane extending from the mouth to the

Clinical Nursing

anus acts as a mechanical barrier to the transfer of substances from the external to the internal environment. Mucus, secreted by the glands of the mucous membrane, provides a protective layer of material between the contents of the alimentary canal and the mucosa. Vomiting and diarrhea provide means for the removal of irritating materials. Semipermeability of the gastrointestinal mucosa as well as specific transfer mechanisms determines the size and type of materials absorbed into the internal environment. All of the above are only partly effective in preventing the absorption of injurious substances. The individual is protected from absorbed substances by phagocytic cells in the blood, lymph nodes, and liver. In addition to phagocytizing bacteria and other foreign substances, the liver decreases the activity of a variety of chemicals by altering their structures.

The mucous membrane lining the alimentary canal also requires protection from mechanical, chemical, and living agents, and from the digesting action of enzymes. It is really quite remarkable that the protective mechanisms are successful in preventing self-digestion as the protein-digesting enzymes of the alimentary canal do digest living tissue. The capacity of protein-digesting enzymes to act on living tissue can be observed when unprotected tissue is exposed to intestinal and pancreatic secretions or when the balance between the mechanisms protecting the lining of the alimentary canal from the proteolytic actions of digesting secretion is upset, as in peptic ulcer.

What determines the effects of disease or injury of the alimentary canal?

Any disorder interfering with the capacity to ingest, digest, or absorb one or more nutrients will interfere with the nutritional status of the affected individual. Other effects will depend on the nature of the disorder and the organ or organs affected. As repeatedly emphasized, the gastrointestinal tract is sensitive to the general condition or status of the body as a whole. Disorders in other parts of the body are frequently accompanied by one or more disturbances in the gastrointestinal function.

The structures forming the gastrointestinal system are subject to the same types of disorders as other portions of the body. Disturbances in gastrointestinal functioning may result from messages sent by the mental apparatus, from direct injury to cells, or from a response to injury or threat of injury. Because the system is a muscular structure, under control of the autonomic nervous system, disorders of motility and secretion are frequent.

As is true of all cells, blood supply is necessary to survival. The rich blood supply of the mucosa, the relationship of the veins draining the alimentary canal and the portal circulation to the liver, and the fact that any bleeding into the lumen of the gut is not opposed by a rapid rise in tissue fluid pressure mean that life-threatening hemorrhages are a frequent problem.[19] Massive bleeding into the lumen of the alimentary canal usually initiates the vomiting or defecation reflex, and blood is evacuated in vomitus or from the rectum. Bleeding into the lumen of the alimentary canal is not always massive. Small quantities may be lost at one time or continue to be lost over an extended period of time causing a microcytic anemia.

Blood supply to a portion of the alimentary canal may be cut off by arterial or venous thrombosis, by twisting of the small intestine, or by incarceration of a viscus or the mesentery by a ring through which one or more body structures normally pass. For example, the mesentery of the intestine may slip through the inguinal or femoral ring. Neither the mesentery nor the intestine normally passes through either of these rings, and protrusion into one of them is known as an inguinal or femoral hernia.[20] Should the contents be trapped, the venous return is impeded and swelling occurs. Unless the incarcerated tissue or organ is removed from the hernial sac, the intertissue pressure will be raised sufficiently to prevent blood from entering the area, and tissue necrosis will occur.[21]

Epithelial and other types of cells in the mucosa of glands along the alimentary canal can and do undergo neoplastic change. Neoplasms can be either benign or malignant. For some unexplained reason, neoplasms rarely are found in the small intestine. Neoplasms in the alimentary canal cause harmful effects by obstructing the lumen of the gut and thereby preventing the normal passage of food. Pedunculated neoplasms may twist on their pedicles and cause symptoms associated with the necrosis. In the small intestine they may act as a focus predisposing to the twisting or volvulus of the intestine. The neoplasm may undergo necrosis and predispose to bleeding from ulcerations formed at its surface. Specific effects of any neoplasm will depend on its nature and location

[19] In solid tissues, bleeding raises the intertissue pressure, which opposes further bleeding.

[20] A hernia is the protrusion of the contents of a body cavity through a defect in the wall of the cavity. When the protrusion occurs near the surface of the body, it can be felt as a bulge.

[21] When herniated tissue can be returned to its proper cavity, the hernia is said to be reducible. When it cannot be removed, it is irreducible or incarcerated, and when the venous return is obstructed and swelling takes place, it is said to be strangulated.

in the alimentary canal. Neoplasms are discussed in detail in Chapter 14.

The lining mucosa is exposed to a variety of mechanical, chemical, and living agents of extrinsic origin, as well as to the digestive juices. Cells may be sensitive to ordinary harmless substances; that is, they are or become allergic. Depending on the nature of the etiology and the extent of the injury, the mucosa may be acutely or chronically inflamed, infected, or ulcerated. If there is sufficient tissue destruction, scar tissue may be formed in the process of healing. Depending on its location and extent, the scar tissue, as it matures and contracts, can reduce the size of the lumen of the gut or block a duct opening into it.

To illustrate the above, Mr. Brave has a peptic ulcer in the proximal portion of his duodenum. Ulceration is due to an imbalance between the capacity of the mucous membrane lining his duodenum to resist digestion and the action of the digestive ferments. In the healing of the ulcer, scar tissue was formed, and as it matured, it contracted. Because the area of ulceration was small and not close to the opening of the ampulla of Vater,[22] healing took place without causing obstruction.

The wall forming the alimentary canal acts as a barrier protecting the internal from the external environment. In health, the internal environment is protected not only from unusable or partly digested nutrients, but from the entrance of digestive enzymes and large numbers of microorganisms. When, as a result of surgery, trauma, or disease, the wall of the alimentary canal is penetrated, its contents escape into the surrounding cavity.

ESOPHAGEAL PERFORATION

When the esophagus is perforated, secretions and food can enter the trachea or mediastinum depending on the level of the lesion. Either is serious. The effects of food and fluids entering the trachea have been discussed in Chapter 8. In the mediastinum, the esophagus is near the heart, aorta, lungs, vagus nerves, thoracic duct, vertebral column, and diaphragm. Food escaping into the mediastinum carries bacteria with it. Either food or bacteria can be responsible for abscess formation. Because of its location and poor blood supply, lesions of the esophagus are difficult to treat. For example, Mrs. Bird swallowed a large fish bone. It became lodged in and perforated her esophagus, resulting in secretions and microorganisms gaining access to the mediastinum. A mediastinal abscess was

[22] The duct formed by the union of the common bile duct from the liver and the duct of Wirsung from the pancreas.

formed as a result. Because of the possibility of perforating the wall of the esophagus, a person should neither manipulate nor allow anyone except a physician to attempt to remove an object caught in his esophagus. Should a chicken or fish bone or other object become lodged in the esophagus, no time should be lost in seeking assistance from a physician. No other person should be allowed to try to remove it.

PERITONEAL PERFORATION

Penetration of structures below the diaphragm allows the contents of the stomach or intestine to escape into the peritoneal cavity. Depending on the site of perforation, digestive juices and bacteria gain access to the peritoneal cavity. Certain anatomical features increase the hazard to the patient. They include (1) the large continuous surface of the peritoneum; (2) the aid given to the distribution of the contents entering the peritoneal space by respiratory, abdominal, and intestinal movements; and (3) the inhibition of phagocytosis and the enhancement of bacterial growth provided by the intestinal contents.

Despite its liabilities, the peritoneum is well adapted to defending itself provided that contamination is not too great or prolonged. As in other areas, the basic defense mechanism is inflammation. A second defense mechanism is the ability to form fibrous adhesions. They cause the mesentery and omentum to adhere together, aiding in the localization of the infection.

When leakage is small, the body may be able to wall off the area and prevent the dissemination of the contents of the alimentary canal throughout the peritoneal cavity. At the time Mr. Brave had a recurrence of his ulcer, it penetrated through the wall of the duodenum and into the peritoneum. He did not have generalized peritonitis, however, because his body was able to wall off the area. Mary Alice Todd had acute appendicitis with the formation of an appendiceal abscess. The inflammatory process around the diseased appendix was sufficient to wall off the leakage from it and to prevent generalized peritonitis.

When, however, a viscus is suddenly perforated and a large quantity of stomach or intestinal content enters or continues to gain entrance to the peritoneal cavity, the protective and reparative powers of the peritoneum may be overcome, resulting in generalized peritonitis. Even with a fairly large opening, the peritoneum is able to defend itself against most bacteria for a few hours. Thereafter, its defensive capacity fails rapidly. Prompt closure of an opening between the digestive tube and the peritoneal cavity is therefore of the greatest importance.

PERITONITIS

Peritonitis is frequently secondary to perforation of the alimentary tract, or leakage from the liver, biliary tract, or pancreas. Disease or injury of the alimentary tract, in which perforation of viscus occurs, includes stab and gunshot wounds in the abdomen, perforated peptic ulcers, ruptured appendices or diverticuli, postoperative leakage, and strangulating obstruction of the intestine. One of the hazards in cholelithiasis (gallstones) is that a stone can act as a ball valve, allowing bile to enter the gallbladder, but not to escape. As the wall of the gallbladder distends, its blood supply lessens and predisposes the wall to necrosis and gangrene. With necrosis of its wall, bile escapes into the peritoneal cavity and causes peritonitis.

The manifestations of peritonitis are caused by (1) the responses of the peritoneum, (2) the systemic responses to injury, and (3) sepsis. In generalized peritonitis, from 4 to 12 liters of inflammatory exudate may be formed. Because of its large "weeping" surface, the situation of the patient is similar to that of one who has been burned.

When contents of the alimentary canal escape into the peritoneal cavity, the patient usually experiences abdominal pain. This pain is usually severe and may be either generalized or localized. The patient also presents signs and symptoms of increased sympathoadrenal activity: pallor, sweating, an anxious expression, and rapid pulse and respiration. He will eventually have signs and symptoms of sepsis; fever and rapid pulse and respirations. The alimentary tract responds first by vomiting. Eventually gastrointestinal activity is depressed, absorption ceases, and the abdomen becomes distended. The abdominal wall is tender and rigid, and splinting of the diaphragm results in shallow, grunting respirations. Leukocytosis indicates a general response to the injury. Patients who fail to develop leukocytosis generally have a poor prognosis.

NURSING CARE

The responsibilities of the nurse differ somewhat with the potential causes of peritonitis. Individuals who have an acute gastrointestinal disorder or what is commonly referred to as "stomach flu" should avoid ingesting food or fluid during the attack. They should *not* take either a laxative or an enema. When a patient who has a peptic ulcer experiences sudden, severe pain, his physician should be notified immediately. Time should not be wasted on the hypothesis that, given time, the pain will disappear. No fluid, food, or drugs should be administered orally. When there is any doubt about the cause of abdominal pain, or when pain continues for more than a few hours, a physician should be consulted.

Should the pain be caused by perforation of the alimentary tract and the physician decide that the opening is to be closed surgically, the operation is usually performed as soon as possible. The care of the patient following closure is similar to that of any patient having abdominal surgery. Whether or not surgical closure is effected, the prevention of gastrointestinal distention is important. To prevent distention, a long tube is introduced by way of the nose, pharynx, esophagus, and stomach into the small intestine. Suction is applied to establish and maintain decompression. Because the patient is unable to take fluids and foods orally, fluids must be administered parenterally to maintain and correct fluid and electrolyte balance and to provide calories and amino acids. Whole blood may be administered to restore blood proteins. Antibiotics and sulfonamides are usually prescribed to combat bacterial infection.

Pain should be prevented, without unduly depressing the patient. Small doses of morphine or one of the morphine substitutes may be used for this purpose. Morphine has the particular advantage of splinting the intestine.

Care directed toward making and keeping the patient comfortable is very important. Because the patient with peritonitis is very ill, he should be allowed to be sick. His needs should be anticipated and the responsibility for his care assumed by his attendants. He should be placed in a comfortable position. Some physicians recommend that the head of the bed be elevated and the patient placed in a semi-Fowler's position. He should be moved and turned regularly to prevent respiratory and circulatory complications. He should have a quiet, nonstimulating environment. Talking should be limited to that required for his care. Personal care, such as mouth hygiene and bathing, should be performed by the nurse. The patient should be protected from unnecessary exertion. As the patient recovers, his activity should be increased.

From the preceding general background discussion, it should be clear that no serious disorder in the structure or function of any part of the digestive system is without its effects on the functioning of the entire system or on the body as a whole. It is easier, however, and the presentation is likely to be clearer, if the function or functions of each organ and the effects of alterations in function are presented separately. Discussions will be related primarily to the effects of disturbances in functions of the various organs and the implications of these to nursing. Specific diseases are outlined at the end of this chapter in Table 12-1.

ASSISTING WITH DIAGNOSIS

Although the making of the medical diagnosis is a primary function of the physician, the nurse assists in a number of ways. One of the most valuable contributions a nurse can make is accurately to observe, report, and record her observations. The nurse uses her senses of hearing, touch, sight, and smell to gain information about the patient and the effects of his disease and therapy. One of the significant aspects of observation is an alertness to changes in the behavior of the patient and to any conditions in his environment that appear to be related. For example, Mrs. Smathers vomits in 15 to 20 minutes each time she receives morphine sulfate. Mrs. Cletus, who has had a gastric resection, suffers an attack of severe pain during each of her husband's infrequent visits. After Mr. Brave returned to his room following a gastric resection, he vomited bright red blood. Each of the preceding has implications for the diagnosis and treatment of the respective individuals. Mrs. Smathers probably has an intolerance to morphine, and another drug should be substituted for it. Unless the nurse makes the connection between the time the drug is administered and the time vomiting occurs, Mrs. Smathers may continue to be made uncomfortable. Unless the observation is made about the time Mrs. Cletus' pain occurs, the emotional factors in her illness may be missed. Finally, unless the nurse knows how much blood Mr. Brave has vomited and knows whether it is within the amount to be expected, the survival of the patient may be threatened.

In addition to collecting information through observation of the patient, the nurse assists in diagnosis by preparing the patient for examination, by performing certain parts of some diagnostic tests, and by collecting secretions or excretions from the alimentary canal. Examinations for disease of the alimentary canal are of three different types. The canal or some part of it is directly or indirectly visualized, the contents are collected for examination, or determinations are made of the effects of the disorder on the nutritional status of the individual.

The details for the preparation of patients for different diagnostic tests vary from one institution or physician to another. A few generalizations will, however, be made that should be helpful. The different types of tests will be defined or described and the conditions necessary to their performance suggested.

The direct observation of the lining mucosa of an organ is known as endoscopy. The term for a particular endoscopic examination is formed by joining the combining form for the organ with the suffix *scope:* thus, esophagoscope, laryngoscope, gastroscope, or proctoscope. Direct visualization of the mucosa is limited to the organs that are accessible from the natural orifices, the mouth and the anus. An exception is a peritoneoscopic examination. A small incision is made in the abdominal wall to gain entrance into the peritoneal cavity. In addition to providing a means for the examination of the appearance of the mucosa or peritoneum, tissue and secretions can be removed for purposes of examination.

X-ray is utilized in fluoroscopy and in making shadow photographs of all organs of the alimentary canal from the esophagus to the anus. In both procedures a contrast medium is introduced into the organ to be studied. In fluoroscopy the progress or movement of the contrast medium through the canal can be followed. As the roentgen rays pass through the body, they are projected onto a fluorescent screen. X-rays are shadow photographs that provide a permanent record.

Secretions from the upper and mid-portions of the alimentary canal can be removed for examination. Secretions are examined for the concentration of normal constituents and for substances not normally present in the secretion. The capacity of the glands of the stomach to respond to food or other secretory agents can be determined. Both secretions and excretions are examined for blood, pus, and microorganisms. Feces are also examined for parasites and ova.

What factors must be considered in examining a patient for nutritional disorders?

STUDIES ON NUTRITIONAL STATUS

Examination for the effect of disease on the nutritional status of the individual includes weighing the patient, measuring skin-fold thickness, and observing for signs of rapid loss of weight and dehydration. Changes in the skin, fissuring of the lips, a sore mouth, bleeding gums, and changes in the color of the tongue may also be indicative of nutritional problems. Determinations on the blood levels of specific nutrients or their metabolites and on urinary excretions of metabolites indicate abnormalities in metabolism that result from dietary inadequacy or from interference with nutrition caused by some pathological state. For example, the hemoglobin level, erythrocyte count, and hematocrit provide evidence for or against iron-deficiency anemia. But in a seriously dehydrated patient the levels might appear normal; thus the laboratory determinations would be misleading if the physical examination did not make note of the state of dehydration. Low total protein and serum albumin levels give evidence of protein deficiency that has, in most instances, persisted over a long period of time inasmuch as general tissue depletion has taken place before the blood levels were lowered. Urinary excretions may indicate tissue depletion of some vitamins, or may indicate inability to complete certain metabolic sequences.

PREPARATION OF THE ALIMENTARY CANAL FOR EXAMINATION

The preparation of the patient for examination of the alimentary canal depends on the nature of the test to be performed. In general, food and fluid are withheld in preparation for examinations of the upper and middle alimentary canal and previous to roentgen examination of the large bowel. Food or fluids in the stomach or intestine interfere with the performance of the examination by getting in the way of the instrument or by occupying space. In studies made on gastric juice, the physician is interested in determining the concentration of hydrochloric acid before and sometimes after the acid-secreting glands are stimulated. Therefore, gastric juice is tested for acid while the patient is in the fasting state. The patient may then be given a test meal consisting of dry toast or arrowroot cookies and weak tea or water, and the test repeated. Secretion of gastric juice can be further increased by the ingestion of ethyl alcohol or the subcutaneous injection of histamine. Because histamine dilates arterioles and capillaries, susceptible patients may experience a marked drop in blood pressure. It is well for the patient who is to receive histamine to be in bed. If the fall in blood pressure is marked, it may be necessary to place the patient in a supine position. Other effects of histamine include intense headache, shortness of breath, vomiting, and diarrhea. Gastric analysis no longer occupies the position of importance that it once did in the diagnosis of disease of the stomach and intestine.

In endoscopic examinations of the upper alimentary canal, food and fluid should be withheld, because the swallowing reflex is depressed when the pharynx is anesthetized before the tube is passed. Should the patient vomit, he is in danger of aspirating food or fluid into the airway. Care of the patient during and following endoscopic examination of the esophagus is similar to that following bronchoscopic examination.

In preparation of the large intestine for examination by x-ray or endoscopy the bowel is emptied. One or more enemas with or without a drastic cathartic such as castor oil are used. When enemas "until clear" are prescribed they should be conscientiously performed, as either feces or gas interferes with the filling of the bowel with the contrast medium and thereby distorts the resulting shadow.

Following roentgen examination of the gastrointestinal tract, particularly after colon x-rays, the barium sulfate introduced into the bowel as a contrast medium should be evacuated. The patient may be instructed to take, or be given, an enema to wash out the barium remaining at the end of the procedure. Unless it is removed, it may form a hard mass in the bowel because the water is absorbed.

SUMMARY

During the period when the patient is undergoing diagnosis, the nurse makes a number of valuable contributions. Through conscientious and informed observations, she collects information about the patient and his reactions to his disease, to diagnostic procedures, and to therapy. She helps to prepare the patient both physically and psychologically for the different diagnostic procedures. She cares for the patient during and after the examinations are performed. One point that bears emphasis is that many of the methods utilized in the examination of the alimentary canal are unpleasant. They require that meals be withheld and the contents of the canal be removed by catharsis, enema, and stomach tube. In the performance of some examinations a tube may be introduced into the mouth or the anus. Although the patient knows that the various procedures are necessary, he still feels miserable. In all probability he is anxious about the outcome of the various examinations. He may, with or without reason, fear that he has cancer. Insofar as is possible, the patient should be protected from preventable sources of distress. He should be prepared for what to expect and what he can do to help himself. Attention to his personal hygiene and to serving his meals promptly after a test is completed may not seem to be crucial to the onlooker, but can do much to remove controllable sources of irritation.

The Mouth

FUNCTIONS

The normal entrance to the alimentary canal is the mouth, which also serves as a second entrance and exit for air. The function of the mouth in nutrition is to prepare food for digestion and swallowing. The taste and aroma of food stimulate the flow of saliva and initiate the reflexes that increase secretion in the stomach. In persons who are unable to taste or smell food, not only is the enjoyment of food diminished, but there may be some impairment in digestion. Food is broken into small particles in the mouth, mixed with saliva, and converted to a semisolid state. Saliva contains an enzyme, ptyalin, that initiates the digestion of starch.

Enzymes act only on the surfaces of particles. Therefore, if enzymes are to be effective, large particles must be broken up into smaller ones so that the surface area exposed to the action of enzymes is increased. Reduction in the size of food particles also facilitates swallowing. The changes in the food are almost entirely physical, but they are indispensable to digestion. When, for any reason, an individual is unable to chew food, it must be liquefied before it is introduced into the alimentary canal. Either liquid or semiliquid foods such as milk, cream, oils, eggs, and fruit and vegetable juices or solid foods may be liquefield in a blender.

INABILITY TO MASTICATE

Lack of teeth is the most common cause of failure to chew food adequately, but teeth that are painful and carious (decayed) also interfere with chewing. Painful lesions of the gums, tongue, or buccal mucosa interfere with the chewing and mixing of food. Inability to open or close the jaws will obviously make chewing difficult, if not impossible. As the result of rheumatoid arthritis, Mr. Gerald has an ankylosis (stiffness or fixation) of the mandibular joints. He can separate his teeth only about 2 cm, which makes it difficult to introduce food into his mouth and for him to grind it. He is given soft and liquid foods. Mr. Elmer fractured his mandible in an automobile accident and his jaw has been wired. All food and fluids have to be introduced into his mouth through a tube.

Patients who cannot properly masticate their food should be served food in a liquid or semisolid form. The nurse has a responsibility for determining whether or not the patient needs to have some or all of his food altered in order to eat it. For example, some people with poor natural teeth or dentures can eat most foods but cannot eat meat unless it is tenderized or ground.

In addition to the grinding surface provided by the teeth, the act of chewing requires the power or energy to open the jaws and to close them with force on the food. Power is provided by the muscles of mastication. In disorders such as myasthenia gravis [23]—great muscle weakness

[23] Myasthenia gravis is a disorder in which there is a defect in transmission of impulses at the myoneural junction. The patient experiences weakness. For some reason, many patients with this disorder have difficulty in breathing and swallowing before other muscle function is seriously impaired.

—the patient may quickly tire if he is required to masticate an ordinary diet. To conserve his energy and maintain his food intake, his food may have to be ground or be soft in character.

MOUTH CARE

Because the teeth are essential to proper mastication of food, their care is important. According to some dentists, the baby should be taught to brush his teeth when his first tooth appears. Regular dental care, as well as good nutrition, is important in the care of teeth. The salivary glands are the site of the common infectious disease mumps. Debilitated patients, in whom oral intake is restricted, are susceptible to an infection called surgical parotitis, a serious complication. Its prevention is based on an adequate fluid intake, cleanliness of the mouth, and stimulation of the flow of saliva. An adequate intake of fluid makes an important contribution to keeping the mouth clean and moist. In sick and debilitated patients this requires time, planning, and attention of nursing personnel, and should not be left to chance. Mouth care, including the brushing of the teeth, should be performed at least every four hours. Stimulation of the flow of saliva is essential. Measures such as chewing gum and sucking on lemon or orange slices or lemon sour balls are all useful in encouraging salivation. After the introduction of antibiotics, the incidence of surgical parotitis decreased, but it is again increasing.

SWALLOWING

After food has been masticated, it passes from the mouth, by way of the pharynx and esophagus, to the stomach by the act of swallowing. Swallowing takes place in three stages. The first, or oral, phase is voluntary. The second, or pharyngeal, stage and the third, or esophageal, stage are involuntary. In the act of swallowing, food passes through the pharynx, which also serves as a passageway for air; therefore food must be transferred without entering either the nares or the glottis. Furthermore, particles too big to pass easily through the esophagus must be prevented from entering the pharynx.

ORAL STAGE

The first stage of swallowing is initiated after the food has been masticated and mixed with sufficient saliva to form a soft mass. It is then squeezed and rolled toward the posterior portion of the mouth by the pressure of the tongue moving upward and backward toward the palate. The tongue forces the bolus of food into the pharynx. At any time before the bolus reaches the pharynx, the act of swallowing can be stopped.

PHARYNGEAL STAGE

As the food is pushed back, sensory receptors located in and around the pharynx are stimulated. Impulses are carried to the swallowing center located in the brain stem. Messages are sent from the brain to the pharyngeal area and a number of automatic actions are initiated. These begin with the closure of the posterior nares by the upward movement of the soft palate. This action prevents food from entering the nares. One of the characteristics of disorders wherein the soft palate is paralyzed or defective is the escape of food or fluid into the nose. In the patient who has a lesion in the nervous system, including the peripheral nerves, the escape of fluid or food through the nares should be regarded as prima facie evidence of paralysis of the soft palate. Food and fluid should be discontinued until the patient has been examined by his physician, because the patient is in danger of inhaling food or fluids.

Even more important than preventing food from entering the nares is protecting the airway below the glottis from the introduction of food. The swallowing, or deglutition, center in the brain acts to inhibit respiration as well as to facilitate the passage of food through the pharynx and into the esophagus. The glottis is closed by the approximation of the vocal cords, and the epiglottis moves backward to shield the superior opening into the larynx. The larynx is raised and moved out of the way and the esophagus is opened. All of this happens very quickly, and the bolus of food is moved rapidly through the pharynx into the esophagus. The pharyngeal stage of swallowing takes only about two seconds. Failure to closely approximate the vocal cords during swallowing always results in the introduction of food or fluid into the trachea. (See Chapter 8.) When food or fluids enter the larynx and trachea, a paroxysm of coughing or choking is initiated. Particularly in patients who have lesions in the nervous system, choking should be regarded as an indication that food and fluids should be discontinued until the patient has been examined by his physician.

ESOPHAGEAL STAGE

The third stage of swallowing takes place in the esophagus. After the bolus of food enters the esophagus, it is conveyed by peristalsis to the stomach. If the primary peristaltic wave, which begins when food enters the pharynx and continues over the length of the esophagus, is insufficient, secondary waves are initiated at the sites where the esophagus is distended.

Under normal conditions, the average length of time it takes food to pass through the esophagus is about five seconds.

FAILURE OF SWALLOWING REFLEX

Although the most immediate and serious danger attending failure of the swallowing reflex is aspiration of food or fluid into the airway, other problems are also created. One troublesome problem is the handling or disposal of saliva and other secretions in the mouth and upper respiratory tract. About 1200 ml of saliva is secreted per day, or about 100 ml each waking hour. When swallowing fails, saliva must be removed from the mouth by suction or by expectoration. Drooling is not only unpleasant and unesthetic, but saliva is injurious to the skin around the mouth, because a continuous state of wetness predisposes to maceration of the skin. When drooling cannot be prevented, the skin should be protected by the application of some water-repelling agent, such as aluminum paste or zinc oxide.

TUBE FEEDING

Another problem created by the inability to swallow is the maintenance of the fluid intake and the nutritional status of the patient. Although fluids can be administered by intravenous infusion, at the present time nutrients are not available on a practical basis for the maintenance of nutrition. If the individual is unable to swallow, but a tube can be passed through the esophagus, a nasogastric tube may be introduced into the stomach. Food or fluids may be introduced into the tube at regular intervals or continuously. The latter method requires some means of keeping the food cold to prevent the multiplication of bacteria that cause food poisoning. When a tube cannot be passed through the esophagus, a tube may be placed directly into the stomach by way of an incision in the abdominal wall and stomach (gastrostomy) or jejunum (jejunostomy). Following either a gastrostomy or a jejunostomy, food and fluid are introduced by the tube into the stomach or the jejunum.

For food to be introduced through a tube, it must be in a liquid state. Tube feedings prepared from the foods of a normal diet are preferred to formula feedings because they are generally more appealing to the patient, and they are less likely to produce diarrhea. Any foods that make up a nutritionally adequate normal diet may be blended with liquid in a high-speed blender and strained several times to remove fiber that is likely to clog the tube. For convenience, infant foods including strained meats, vegetables, fruits, and fruit juices, as well as milk, eggs, and cereals, are used because they are low in fiber. The frequency whereby eggs are contaminated with Salmonella makes it advisable to cook the eggs with milk in the form of a soft, thin custard.

Some patients prechew food before placing it in the tube. Though the spitting of food into a funnel after it is chewed may appear unesthetic or even revolting to the onlooker, one should make an effort to concentrate on the benefit the patient receives from this practice. The patient should be protected from onlookers and embarrassment by adequate screening. Unless the patient plans to chew his food before it is placed in the tube, it should be liquefied. When the patient is physically able and emotionally ready to feed himself, he should be taught to perform the procedure. The nurse should be certain that the food served to the patient has been properly liquefied. For weeks Mr. Good, who had developed an esophageal fistula following a laryngectomy and radical neck resection, was repeatedly served lumpy wheat cereal for breakfast. The lumps were large enough to obstruct the feeding tube and they could have been removed easily by straining the cereal. Because of the nature of his surgery, Mr. Good was not able to chew the cereal before introducing it into the tube. Quite understandably Mr. Good interpreted the lumps to mean that the hospital personnel were persecuting him.

DYSPHAGIA, PAIN, AND HEARTBURN

Difficulty in swallowing is known as dysphagia. Its effects depend on its cause and the degree to which the passageway is obstructed. The person with dysphagia may be unable to swallow either food or fluids, or he may be able to swallow foods of one consistency, for example solids, and not be able to swallow those of another, possibly liquids. The patient may also have periods of dysphagia with little or no difficulty in between them. Accurate descriptions of the type and timing of the difficulty in swallowing experienced by the patient are very important in establishing the cause of dysphagia. When an individual is unable to swallow any food or fluid, evidences of dehydration and starvation appear very quickly.

The following anatomical and physiological features of the pharynx, as related to swallowing, and the esophagus influence the nature of the disorders to which the esophagus is prone. (1) The act of swallowing is regulated by the nervous system. (2) The pharynx and esophagus constitute a tube connecting the mouth and stomach. The tube can become obstructed by scars or neoplasms, and it can be perforated by foreign bodies. (3) The tube, being lined with mucous membranes, is subject to the growth of benign or malignant neoplasms. (4) The esophagus passes through the mediastinum; any neoplasms or abscesses of the mediastinal structures may obstruct the esophagus. Perforation of the esophagus allows the esophageal contents to leak into the mediastinum, a most serious event, as it is bounded by the pleurae and pericardium. (5) The esophagus is drained by the azygos veins, which serve as an alternate route when the portal vein is obstructed. They are poorly supported by connective and epithelial tissue. In cirrhosis of the liver the blood flow through the portal vein is impeded and seeks alternate routes; one route is the azygos veins. With elevation in venous pressure, the veins dilate, developing varices. As the walls become thin, they are increasingly susceptible to rupture and bleeding. Unlike the situation in solid tissues, the bleeding is not opposed by rising interstitial fluid pressure. Blood is vomited and also evacuated in the feces. (6) The esophagus is incompletely protected by the cardiac sphincter from the effects of gastric juice. Features (1) to (4) may make swallowing difficult because of functional or mechanical obstruction.

Dysphagia may be of reflex origin or caused by an obstruction in the pharynx or esophagus. Reflex disturbances are usually responsible for interference with the second stage of swallowing, while obstructing lesions are more likely to be responsible for dysphagia in the third stage.

The factors in dysphagia caused by a disturbance in reflex activity are similar to those that cause disorders in reflexes in any part of the body. Dysphagia can conceivably arise from disordered function in any part of the reflex arc —receptors, centers in the central nervous system, or effector nerves or cells.

The swallowing centers in the brain can be stimulated or inhibited, with the result that swallowing or the coordination of the various activities involved in swallowing fails. Inhibition of or failure to transmit impulses over some part of the reflex arc may also be responsible for failure in swallowing.

FUNCTIONAL DYSPHAGIA

As do other centers regulating bodily functions, the swallowing center receives messages from the higher centers in the brain, including the cerebral cortex. Dysphagia may therefore be a manifestation of emotional disturbance. Frequently the patient says that he cannot swallow because he has a lump in his throat that he believes is caused by a neoplasm. Despite a thorough examination of the esophagus and the information that his esophagus is healthy, the patient states that he knows there is a tumor even though it cannot be seen.

Although it is sometimes difficult to demonstrate, the interference with swallowing may be a spasm at some point of the esophagus. Mrs. Clifford is a good example of a patient who is starving because she believes that she has an invisible tumor. She is a lonely widow whose husband died after a long and trying illness. Her children are married and live at a distance. For Mrs. Clifford, life holds little promise. She suffers from marked dysphagia. As far as can be demonstrated by fluoroscopy, esophagoscopy, and studies of cells taken from the mucosa, her esophagus is free from any evidence of neoplasia or other structural disease. Despite evidence to the contrary, Mrs. Clifford believes that she has cancer. When she tries to swallow, she says, there is a lump in her throat that prevents swallowing.

Mrs. Clifford's food intake is limited almost entirely to small quantities of milk. She has lost so much weight that her skin hangs loosely. As is characteristic in starvation, she lacks energy. The preparation of adequate meals requires more effort than she can muster. Although Mrs. Clifford's illness was precipitated by the loss of her husband, she is now physically ill from a lack of food. Unless her food intake is increased in quantity and quality very soon, irreversible changes will take place in her cells and she will die from the direct effects of starvation. Attention must therefore be given to improving the nutritional status of Mrs. Clifford, if she is to survive. There are no easy answers to the problem of bringing about an increase in food intake in patients such as Mrs. Clifford. In the instance of Mrs. Clifford, a close relative spent some weeks with her. The relative planned the meals around what Mrs. Clifford could and would eat. Progress in the beginning was slow, but as Mrs. Clifford made an effort to eat, she gained strength and her general outlook improved. More food did not cure her basic problems, but it did contribute to her capacity to cope with them. The maintenance of food intake is of no less importance in the patient whose dysphagia is caused by an emotional problem than it is in the patient who has an organic lesion.

LESIONS IN THE CRANIAL CAVITY

In addition to dysphagia caused by disturbances in function, lesions within the cranial cavity interfere with the function of the swallowing centers in the brain stem. Lesions are of two general types: those that lessen the blood supply to the area and those that result in inflammation. Inflammation, by causing swelling also diminishes the blood supply. The blood supply to the swallowing center may be lessened by an obstruction of a blood vessel by a thrombus or an embolus. Intracranial pressure may be raised by neoplasms, particularly those obstructing the free flow of cerebrospinal fluid, and by edema of the brain resulting from the response of the brain tissue to injury. Infections such as bulbar poliomyelitis are accompanied by difficulty in swallowing. Usually the difficulty with swallowing is manifested as a failure to coordinate swallowing with breathing, so that the patient is in danger of aspirating saliva and secretions from the nasal and pharyngeal cavities, as well as food and fluids. Disturbances in the regulation of swallowing can originate from injury to peripheral nerves supplying the muscles involved in swallowing. Finally, failure of transmission of nerve impulses from a nerve to a muscle will cause dysphagia.

Because the patient cannot manage his own secretions, they must be removed by gravity and suctioning. Oral fluids, food, and drugs must be withheld until the patient is able to swallow. The objective is to protect the patient from aspiration of foreign material into his airway. The patient with myasthenia can swallow normally until he becomes fatigued; therefore, measures should be taken to limit fatigue.

OBSTRUCTIVE LESIONS

In the esophagus itself, dysphagia can be caused by a variety of disorders that obstruct the lumen and block the passage of food and/or fluid. Among the causes of obstruction of the esophagus are neoplasms, malignant and benign, inflammatory strictures, congenital defect, hiatus hernia,[24] foreign bodies, achalasia, and extrinsic pressure. The most frequent causes of mechanical obstruction of the esophagus are neoplasms and strictures caused by the formation of scar tissue. All obstructing lesions have a common effect. They interfere with the ability of the individual to ingest enough food to meet his nutritional needs. Patients with one of the above disorders are often in poor nutritional condition when admitted to the hospital. As a matter of fact, they are all too often in a state of near starvation. They are usually treated surgically after the diagnosis is made and the gross nutritional, water, and electrolyte deficiencies and anemia are corrected. Because the route of approach to the esophagus is through the thorax, attention must be paid to re-establishing and maintaining the expansion of the lungs during the immediate postoperative period.

OBSERVATION OF PATIENTS

Careful and accurate observation of the patient who is dysphagic is important. What, if

---

[24] A hiatus is a gap or opening in the diaphragm. In hiatus hernia, contents of the abdominal cavity escape through the hiatus into the thoracic cavity. A lay term for hiatus hernia is "upside-down stomach."

anything, is the patient able to swallow? Are there any circumstances that affect the ability of the patient to swallow? If the patient regurgitates, what are the characteristics of the emesis? For example, does the regurgitated material contain digested or undigested food particles? Does it contain blood? Does the patient complain of pain or other sensations before, during, or after swallowing? When are the symptoms intensified or relieved? The patient may be aware of the point where food is delayed as it passes through the esophagus. When the patient complains of pain or discomfort, where is it located and what is its general character?

PAIN

Other symptoms associated with alterations in the function or structure of the esophagus include pain and heartburn. Painful sensations accompany the ingestion of irritating substances such as dilute hydrochloric acid. Regurgitation of the acid chyme from the stomach into the esophagus also causes pain and may cause ulceration. Spasm or distention of the esophagus, particularly when associated with ulceration of the esophagus, is a cause of pain. When the pain-evoking stimulus is continuously present, the pain is burning in character. When the stimulus is applied intermittently, it is likely to be griping and intense.

HEARTBURN

Heartburn, or pyrosis, is a condition experienced by most persons at some time in their lives. Despite its name, heartburn has no relation to the heart or to its function. It is characterized by a burning sensation over the precordium or beneath the sternum and is accompanied by the regurgitation into the esophagus or mouth of the acid gastric juice. Heartburn is one of the discomforts of pregnancy. In persons with hiatus hernia or cardioesophageal hernia, foods such as cake, sweet rolls, and orange juice induce heartburn. The mechanism for this disorder is not known, though the associated sensations may be due to the lowering of the pH in the esophagus by the regurgitation of the contents from the stomach.

The Stomach and Proximal Duodenum

Because the stomach and the adjacent portion of the duodenum perform common function and are the site of several serious diseases, they will be discussed as a unit. The diseases are peptic ulcer, gastric carcinoma, and hypertrophic pyloric stenosis. Inflammation of the stomach, or gastritis, is not uncommon. Knowledge of the physiology of the stomach and duodenum is essential to understanding the disorders of this region. (See Table 12-2 at the end of this chapter.)

STRUCTURE AND FUNCTIONS

The lower end of the esophagus is guarded by the cardiac sphincter, which prevents the reflux of acid chyme from the stomach into the esophagus. The esophageal mucosa is not protected against the digesting action of gastric juice, and repeated reflux of the acid gastric juice predisposes the esophagus to acid ulceration. The pyloric sphincter regulates the movement of gastric contents into the duodenum.

The functions of the stomach to be discussed are those relating to the preparation of food for absorption. The secretion of the intrinsic factor that facilitates the absorption of vitamin B_{12} is no less important in nutrition; however, because vitamin B_{12} is essential to the maturation of red blood cells, its functions are discussed in Chapter 10.

The stomach is divided into three parts: the fundus; the corpus, or body; and the antrum. The antrum is frequently, though incorrectly, called the pyloric or prepyloric region. Because the wall of the stomach has relatively little tone and the mucous and submucous coats form folds, or rugae, as the stomach empties, the size of the stomach is determined by the quantity of its contents. As food enters the stomach, it forms concentric rings with the most recently ingested food, which lies nearest to the cardiac sphincter; food that has been in the stomach longest is nearest the pyloric sphincter.

During the time food remains in the stomach, it is mixed with the gastric secretions until a semifluid mixture called chyme is formed. When the stomach is empty and the pyloric sphincter relaxed, liquids may not remain in the stomach, but may pass immediately from the esophagus to the duodenum. When, however, a mixed diet is ingested, food remains in the stomach for varying periods of time and is slowly emptied into the duodenum. The rate of emptying depends on two factors: the fluidity of the gastric chyme, and the receptivity of the duodenum to receiving more chyme. The fluidity of the gastric chyme is determined by the type of food ingested, the completeness of mastication, the length of time food has been in the stomach, and the intensity of peristaltic waves. A meal of foods rich in fat remains in the stomach longer than a meal rich in carbohydrate but low in fat. Relatively large particles of food must be reduced in size before they can be emptied into the duodenum. The more intense peristaltic waves are, the less time chyme is likely to remain in the stomach.

PROTECTION OF DUODENUM FROM
OVERLOADING

The duodenum is protected from overloading by regulation of its receptivity, which is determined by the quantity of chyme already present in the upper intestine, the acidity of the chyme, and the type of food in the chyme. As the duodenum fills, receptors initiate impulses which depress gastric peristalsis and at the same time increase contraction of the pyloric sphincter. A high concentration of fats in the chyme also diminishes gastric secretion. As fat or fatty acids enter the duodenum, glands in the mucosa secrete a hormone called enterogastrone which is carried by way of the blood to the musculature of the stomach. Enterogastrone has an inhibitory effect not only on gastric muscle but also on secretion of the gastric glands. In the presence of powerful inhibitors of the activity of the stomach, such as fat, peristalsis may be reversed and intestinal secretions regurgitated into the stomach. In general, products of protein digestion, acid, and nonspecific irritants in the duodenum act reflexly to diminish gastric activity and secretion. The effect of fats and fatty acids is mainly through the hormone enterogastrone. The coordinated functioning of the stomach and duodenum enables the stomach to be a storehouse for food and to prepare it for digestion. The duodenum is protected from overdistention and is provided with a more or less continuous stream of chyme. The importance of the regulation of the rate at which chyme enters the intestine is illustrated by the dumping syndrome.

THE DUMPING SYNDROME

After gastroenterostomy or gastrectomy, the individual is no longer able to regulate the rate at which chyme enters the intestine, with the result that the intestine is dilated by a large volume of concentrated material. The resulting manifestations are known as the dumping syndrome because the contents of the stomach are rapidly "dumped" into the jejunum. Shortly after a meal, particularly one containing large amounts of carbohydrate, the patient experiences weakness, profuse perspiration, nausea, dizziness, flushing, epigastric fullness, and palpitation. His symptoms may be so severe that he is forced to lie down.

Stemmer et al.[25] state that after gastrectomy as many as 70 to 80 per cent of patients have the dumping syndrome. For most patients, symptoms are mild and disappear within a month or so, but it remains a significant prob-

lem for 5 to 10 per cent. A few are so incapacitated that they cannot work.

None of the theories proposed explain the mechanisms of the dumping syndrome in a completely satisfactory way. The effects are generally described as being caused by the rapid distention of the jejunum with a hypertonic fluid. Because of the sudden distention, peristalsis is increased and sympathetic reflexes are initiated. The hypertonic fluid attracts water and electrolytes, thereby lowering blood volume and potassium.

Two to three hours after eating, hypoglycemia may occur. The sequence of hypoglycemia is as follows: The rapid entry of a large amount of carbohydrate into the circulation causes a marked, but transient, hyperglycemia. Insulin is secreted in excess of the quantity required to restore the level of glucose in the blood to physiological limits, resulting in hypoglycemia.

A high-protein, high-fat, low-carbohydrate diet given in small, frequent feedings helps to control the symptoms. Meat, fish, poultry, eggs, cheese, and fats are liberally used. Complex carbohydrates such as those in cereals, breads, and vegetables are gradually added, but sugars and sweetened foods are rigorously avoided. Liquids are taken between, but not with, meals. Some patients lie down after eating, whereas others eat in a reclining or semireclining position. Sedatives or antispasmodic drugs may be prescribed.

Although the manifestations accompanying the dumping syndrome are frightening and unpleasant, they usually disappear with time. The patient should therefore be reassured that the disorder is not dangerous and that in time he will recover. In the words of Barborka,[26] "Reassurance seems the best treatment and time the best cure." For the American who judges the success of therapy by the immediacy of results, the waiting period may well be a trying one.

GASTRIC SECRETION

Secretion into the stomach and duodenum is important in both health and disease. In the stomach and small intestine, foods undergo chemical and physical changes in preparation for absorption. Chemical reactions are catalyzed by enzymes capable of digesting not only food but also living cells. One of the factors in the activity of each enzyme is the pH of the fluid in which it works. Pepsin, an enzyme secreted into the stomach, is most active in an acid medium. In the absence of hydrochloric

[25] Edward A. Stemmer et al.: "A Physiologic Approach to the Surgical Treatment of the Dumping Syndrome," JAMA, 199:909–13 (Mar. 20) 1967.

[26] Clifford J. Barborka: "The Stomach," in Christopher's Textbook of Surgery, 7th ed. (Philadelphia) 1960), W. B. Saunders Company, p. 661.

acid, pepsin is inactive. Chemical digestion in the stomach therefore depends on the presence of both hydrochloric acid and pepsin. Direct contact with the cells lining the stomach is prevented by the secretion of mucin. Other factors, such as the blood supply to the mucosa, are also important to the defense of the gastroduodenal mucosa. Any condition upsetting the balance between digestion and protection predisposes to ulceration.

The secretion of hydrochloric acid in the stomach involves the neurogenic, chemical, and mechanical mechanisms, as well as systemically and locally acting hormones. As a result of the interaction of the various regulators, a balance between stimulation and inhibition is maintained. Digestion is accomplished, and at the same time the mucosa is protected.

Hydrochloric acid is secreted by the parietal cells in the corpus of the stomach. Three phases, cephalic, antral, and intestinal, are involved. The cephalic phase of secretion is under nervous control. Stimulation of the vagus nerve increases the production of hydrochloric acid, while stimulation of the sympathetics, either by their direct effect on the acid-secreting glands in the stomach or by inhibition of the action of the vagi, lessens it. Usual stimuli initiating the cephalic phase of gastric secretion include the sight, smell, and taste of food. Even thoughts of good food, such as a thick steak or luscious lemon pie, may be sufficient to initiate the cephalic phase of gastric secretion. Impulses from distance receptors, such as the retina of the eye, travel to the cerebral cortex, where they are relayed to the hypothalamus. From the hypothalamus, secretory impulses are relayed to the glands in the stomach by way of the vagi. The cephalic phase of gastric secretion can be prevented by the sectioning of the vagus nerves. The procedure is known as vagotomy.

The second phase in gastric secretion is the antral phase. Whereas the cephalic phase prepares the stomach for food, the antral phase regulates the amount of acid secreted after food enters the stomach. The antrum does not secrete hydrochloric acid, but it secretes a hormone, gastrin, that stimulates the acid-secreting glands in the corpus of the stomach. When the acidity of the chyme is high, gastrin secretion lessens. When partial gastrectomy is performed in the therapy of peptic ulcers, the antrum is often removed, not because it secretes hydrochloric acid, but because it regulates the production of hydrochloric acid. Marginal ulcers [27] are more frequent in patients in whom the antrum has not been removed.

The third phase in the secretion of hydrochloric acid is the intestinal phase. A hormone similar to, but not as powerful as, gastrin is believed to be secreted by the intestinal mucosa, but it has not been identified. The basis for this hypothesis is that gastric juice continues to be secreted when the stomach is empty. As indicated earlier, a high concentration of fat in the chyme entering the duodenum stimulates the production of enterogastrone which decreases both gastric secretion and motility. Thus secretion into the stomach is regulated by nervous and hormonal factors. In health, secretion in the stomach illustrates one of the characteristics of a homeostatic mechanism; that is, a change in one direction is counteracted by increasing activity of processes acting in the opposite direction.

The mucosa lining the stomach is protected from digestion by a covering sheet of mucus. Mucous glands are located in the mucous membrane throughout the stomach. The mucosa of the duodenum is protected by alkaline mucus secreted by Brunner's glands. Secretion of mucus is constant, though the volume can be increased by the ingestion of irritating agents. Any failure to secrete mucus in adequate quantities reduces the protection of the underlying mucosa and increases its susceptibility to digestion.

In health, the mucosa of the stomach and adjacent duodenum is protected from digestion by the gastric juice, but other parts of the alimentary canal, such as the esophagus, lower duodenum, jejunum, and ileum, do not have the same degree of resistance. However, because bile and pancreatic juices are alkaline in reaction, they neutralize the acid chyme with the result that the lower duodenum, jejunum, and ileum are protected from injury.

ULCERATION

When the mucosa of organs lacking protection is exposed to acid chyme over a period of time, ulceration is likely. In the past, benign ulcers in areas exposed to acid-pepsin have been categorized as peptic ulcers. All ulcers in the gut have similarities. They can be shallow or deep, hypertrophied or proliferating, benign or malignant. They differ in fundamental respects such as etiology, natural history, prognosis, and treatment.[28] (See Table 12-2 at the end of the chapter for details.)

What are the causes of ulceration?

More exactly, ulceration results from an imbalance between the digesting action of gastric juice and the capacity of the gastric and duodenal mucosa to resist digestion. In effect, the

[27] Ulcers formed at the site of junction or anastomoses of the stomach and jejunum.

[28] John C. Krukal: "Gastric Ulcer: An Appraisal," *Surgery,* 63:1024–36 (June) 1968.

digesting action of the gastric juice may be increased, or the resistance of the mucosa lining the stomach and duodenum decreased, or both. Continuous or intermittent hypersecretion of hydrochloric acid is believed to be responsible for the increase in the digesting action of the gastric juice. Hypersecretion can be the result of (1) overstimulation of the secretory mechanisms, (2) failure of the mechanisms inhibiting secretion, or (3) failure of the mechanisms for neutralizing hydrochloric acid. Failure to regenerate epithelium at a rapid rate, failure to secrete an adequate quantity of mucus, and a poor blood supply can all reduce resistance of the mucosa. Although ulcers in the duodenum are always benign, ulcers in the stomach can be either benign or malignant. Malignant neoplasms in the stomach may eventually ulcerate. Although peptic ulcers are usually chronic, they may also be acute.

Acute ulcers are of two types: Cushing's and Curling's. The acute ulcer of Cushing is found in disorders of the nervous system, particularly in disorders involving the anterior hypothalamus. It sometimes occurs in bulbar poliomyelitis.

Curling's ulcer was first described by Curling, who noted the formation of ulcer of the stomach and duodenum in patients who had been burned. More recently, the formation of acute gastric and duodenal ulcers has been reported in patients who have experienced various types of trauma. Because some degree of stress is involved, one explanation for the formation of Curling's ulcer is that it results from the effect of the adrenocortical hormones on the secretion of gastric juice. They may also decrease the thickness of the protective layer of mucus.

Patients who are predisposed by disease or injury to acute ulcer formation should be observed for symptoms and signs indicating ulcer development. Any type of pain or discomfort in the upper abdomen should be brought to the attention of the physician. Onset may be ushered in with hemorrhage or perforation. Either is an emergency and should be treated as such; that is, the physician should be notified immediately. Fluids and food should be withheld until the physician indicates that they can be safely given. The patient should be kept quiet and as comfortable as his situation permits.

DUODENAL ULCER

To summarize some of the aspects of duodenal ulcer, including methods of treatment, Mrs. Carrie Maple, a 43-year-old charwoman, will be presented. Five years previous to her present admission to the hospital, Mrs. Maple had undergone a subtotal thyroidectomy for the treatment of hyperthyroidism. Shortly thereafter, she experienced pain in the epigastric region about one and one-half to two hours after eating. X-ray examination of her stomach and duodenum revealed an ulcer in her duodenum. She was treated by diet and an aluminum hydroxide antacid. She responded well and treatment was discontinued after three months. Mrs. Maple continued to be well until two days prior to her admission to the hospital, when she noted that her stools were tarry. The following day she had lower abdominal pain radiating to her upper abdomen and several loose, tarry stools.

At the time of her admission she was feeling weak and dizzy. Her hemoglobin was 7.8 g per 100 ml of blood and her erythrocyte count was 2,370,000 cells per cubic millimeter of blood. Both the hemoglobin level and the erythrocyte count were reduced to approximately half of normal, indicating serious blood loss. Although her hematocrit was 28 per cent (the normal is about 48 per cent), her blood pressure was 142/88, indicating that the blood volume had been maintained despite the loss of blood. See Chapters 10, 11, and 17. She required 2,000 ml of blood to raise her hemoglobin to 13.4 g.

In many respects, the history presented by Mrs. Maple is characteristic of the patient with duodenal ulcer.

As stated previously, duodenal ulcer occurs where there is an imbalance between the digesting action of gastric juice and the capacity of the mucosa in the stomach and duodenum to resist digestion. Exactly why ulceration occurs is not known. Authorities agree that certain factors are predisposing. One is that too much acid secretion must have a role in ulcer formation. Not all patients, however, can be shown to have hyperchlorhydria, as there is some overlapping between the level of secretion in patients with ulcer and the upper limits of normal secretion. No information was available about acid secretion by Mrs. Maple's stomach. She had been in another hospital at the time of her first illness and was in no condition at this time to have her gastric acidity evaluated. It can be assumed that she did have either absolute or relative hyperchlorhydria, because there is general consensus among authorities that supports the maxim: no acid, no ulcer.

In duodenal ulcer, secretion of hydrochloric acid is increased as are the number of parietal cells. Some investigators have found an increase in the secretion of gastrin. A number of other hypotheses have been suggested and found wanting. Why any of these conditions occur is not known. What is known is that ulcers heal and remain controlled providing that acid secretion can be neutralized or reduced by one third to one half by medical or surgical means.

Despite disagreement about the mechanisms involved, direct observation of the stomach indicates that it responds to different stimuli by hypersecretion and engorgement. The first to report this effect was Beaumont. He made direct observations on the lining of the stomach of Alexis St. Martin who had a gastric fistula. The later work of Wolf and Wolff [29] further supported and extended the concept that the stomach responds to many forms of stimuli by secretion. Prolonged emotional disturbance associated with anxiety, guilt, resentment, anger, or hostility has been demonstrated to evoke vascular engorgement accompanied by increased secretion and motility of the stomach.

The possibility that duodenal ulcer may have a genetic basis stems from the observation that it occurs more frequently among persons of blood group O than among other groups. It is also associated with the nonsecretion by the stomach of ABH substances. Both of these are hereditary traits which are inherited independently of each other, but their effect is additive. The person who belongs to blood group O and who secretes the ABH substances is less likely to develop duodenal ulcer than the person who inherits both traits. Although these observations have been made, proof is lacking that there is an hereditary factor predisposing to duodenal ulcer. Mrs. Maple had type A blood and was Rh-positive. No determination was made of the secretion of ABH substances in her gastric juice or saliva. As far as she knew, no one in her family had ever had an ulcer or bleeding into the alimentary canal. There was no evidence suggesting that heredity directly contributed to her development of a duodenal ulcer.

It will be remembered that the onset of ulcer symptoms in Mrs. Maple followed thyroidectomy to correct hyperthyroidism. As with peptic ulcer, the onset of hyperthyroidism may be coincident with a period of emotional stress. As a shy, retiring person, Mrs. Maple did not conform to the stereotype of the "ulcer personality" of the hard-driving, anxious-to-succeed, "wants what he wants when he wants it" person. She gave some evidence of being depressed, because she was found crying on several occasions. She may have felt angry but turned her anger against herself.

In the previous discussion of the factors in the development of duodenal ulcer, the roles

[29] Stewart Wolf and H. G. Wolff: *Human Gastric Function*, 2nd ed. (New York: Oxford University Press, 1947).

of the nervous and endocrine systems were presented. The effect of stress on the capacity of the stomach to resist digestion and on the secretion and motility of the stomach is mediated by the nervous and the hormonal systems. In terms of the above, duodenal ulcer is a localized manifestation of a constitutional disease.

A number of elements including genetic predisposition, emotional stress, sex, and age, as well as other factors, combine to upset the balance between resistance to digestion and the digesting action of acid-pepsin. As in other chronic diseases, duodenal ulcer is probably caused by the interaction of multiple factors.

Mrs. Maple's ulcer illustrated an almost textbook picture of the behavior and manifestations of duodenal ulcer. Five years prior to her present attack, she had had pain and nausea, appearing one and one-half to two hours after eating. The pain responded to treatment with hourly feedings on the hour alternated with hourly doses of an aluminum hydroxide antacid taken on the half hour. As a result of this schedule, she ingested either food or medication each half-hour. *Pain, food, relief* is the most common manifestation.

Pain is the most frequent symptom associated with peptic ulcer. The two main hypotheses advanced for it are that (1) hydrochloric acid irritates the exposed sensory nerve endings in the edges and base of the ulcer, and (2) pain results from increased motility or spasm of the muscle at the ulcer site. The second view is favored because pain occurs in the absence of an increase of hydrochloric acid.

Although Mrs. Maple did not remember the exact nature or location of the pain associated with her first ulcer, the pain of uncomplicated ulcer is almost always located in the epigastrium and is limited to a small localized area. When an ulcer is located on the posterior wall of the duodenum, the pain sometimes is referred to the back. Pain is steady, and it may be described as gnawing, or it may be dull, aching, or burning.

Three characteristic features of the pain, its chronicity, periodicity, and relationship to the ingestion of food, are considered to be pathognomonic of the disease. Although not true of Mrs. Maple, patients not infrequently have periodic attacks of pain for five or six years before seeking medical attention, and ulcers may have been present for as many as 40 or 50 years. Recurrences are common, even among patients who continue under medical supervision, and are often triggered by a situation associated with an increase in stress. Sources of stress may include a traumatic injury or a frustrating situation at the office.

During her first attack, the pain experienced by Mrs. Maple demonstrated the characteristic relationship to the ingestion of food inasmuch as it occurred from one and one-half to two hours after meals. Most patients have pain from one to three hours after eating and secure relief by the ingestion of food or antacids.

At the time of Mrs. Maple's current admission to the hospital, she had one of the complications associated with peptic ulcer—hemorrhage. At the time of her admission, the priority objective in her care was to stop the bleeding and to restore the elements lost as a result of hemorrhage. (See Chapters 9, 10, 11, and 17 for details.)

The most common complication of the ulcer is intractability, or the failure to heal with treatment. Jim Snow was a 19-year-old pre-medical student who had an intractable duodenal ulcer. Despite intensive medical therapy, his ulcer did not heal and so about four fifths of his stomach was removed. A few months later, he returned to his physician with a marginal ulcer. Possibly Jim was born 15 years too soon, inasmuch as neither vagotomy nor anticholinergic drugs were available to him. He does illustrate, however, the persistence of ulcer formation in some individuals.

The dangers and problems of the two other relatively frequent complications, penetration of the duodenal wall (perforation) and obstruction of the pylorus, have been discussed previously. Obstruction may be caused by edema, inflammation, muscle spasm, or the contraction of scar tissue. Unless there are frequent recurrences of the ulcer with the formation of scar tissue in healing, obstruction is likely to be temporary.

THERAPY OF DUODENAL ULCER

As knowledge of the natural history of duodenal ulcer has increased, two problems have become evident. The disease has a tendency to undergo spontaneous remission as well as spontaneous recurrence. Further symptoms tend to be relieved long before the ulcer heals.

Based on the observation that duodenal ulceration does not occur in the absence of hydrochloric acid, medical and/or surgical treatment is instituted to reduce its secretion or to neutralize it. Four types of measures are employed—diet, antacids, antisecretory compounds, and attention to psychic or emotional factors. Surgical therapy may also be utilized to bring about a similar effect. Gastric resection with the removal of the part of the stomach containing the parietal cells or vagotomy, or the two in combination, may also be performed to decrease gastric secretion. Mrs. Maple was successfully treated by medical means.

Diet

Diet and antacids are usually prescribed in relation to each other in order to secure and maintain the continuous neutralization of the gastric juice. Physicians vary in the emphasis they place on the traditional bland diet. Some physicians prescribe half-hourly feedings of milk and antacid during the phase of acute ulcer activity. Mrs. Maple was allowed clear liquids and milk for the first two days of her hospitalization. She was given 3 oz of milk every two hours and 1 oz of Maalox [30]—a creamy white, colloidal suspension of magnesium and aluminum hydroxides. By the third day of her hospitalization there was no longer any evidence that Mrs. Maple was bleeding, and the physician prescribed a bland diet with six feedings for her. The bland diet is a transitional diet between milk feedings and an ordinary house diet.

The underlying principles for dietary management in duodenal ulcer are these: (1) A nutritionally adequate diet, often with emphasis on protein, iron, and ascorbic acid, is essential so that the nutrients required for rapid healing of the ulcer are readily available. Many patients, in fact, have some degree of undernutrition because they have consumed inadequate and restricted diets, either prescribed or self-imposed. (2) Regularity of meals requires particular emphasis inasmuch as many patients have eaten hastily at irregular intervals or have skipped meals. Five or six small meals including a light meal at bedtime are recommended. Frequent meals dilute the stomach contents and have some effect on the neutralization of acid. Some protein food, for example, whole or skim milk, should be included in each of the feedings. Although protein foods stimulate acid secretion, they also have a buffering effect that more than balances the acid production. (3) Food selection should be based on individual tolerances. Physicians now question the need to restrict the menu choices to refined cereals and breads, ground meats, and puréed fruits and vegetables; such foods, over a long period of time, are unappetizing and poorly accepted.[31] Schneider *et al.*[32] have shown that, except for pepper, chili powder, cloves, mustard, and nutmeg, spices and herbs do not alter the appearance of the gastric mucosa or retard the speed of healing of ulcers. Intolerance to strongly flavored vegetables and to fibrous foods is so

[30] Trade name.
[31] Louis Weinstein *et al.:* "Diet as Related to Gastrointestinal Function," *JAMA,* 176:935 (June 17) 1961.
[32] M. A. Schneider *et al.:* "The Effect of Spice Ingestion upon the Stomach," *Amer. J. Gastroent.,* **26**:722 (Dec.) 1956.

variable from one individual to the next that it is impractical to set up arbitrary restrictions.[33] He who has discomfort when he eats cabbage will, of course, avoid it; but he who has no intolerance to it should not be denied the eating of it.

Some clinicians have also questioned the advisability of prolonged use of milk-cream feedings inasmuch as the high saturated fat content of these regimens may predispose to atherosclerosis and coronary thrombosis. In addition to the three principles described above, the diet is sometimes modified to restrict saturated fats to a minimum and to emphasize polyunsaturated fatty acids. Thus skim milk is used; only lean meats, fish, and poultry are included; and vegetable oils and special margarines are substituted for butter and hydrogenated fats. See also "Lipid Metabolism," p. 561.

Antacids

Antacids are effective in preventing as well as in relieving ulcer pain. Although soluble antacids such as sodium bicarbonate and calcium carbonate neutralize acid most effectively, they cause systematic alkalosis in some patients. As a consequence, nonabsorbable antacids such as aluminum hydroxide gel or magnesium trisilicate are prescribed. Aluminum gels have a tendency to be constipating and magnesium salts to cause diarrhea. Therefore, magnesium and aluminum oxides are frequently combined.

Nothing should be ingested that stimulates the secretion of acid without neutralizing it or that directly irritates the gastric mucosa. For example, alcohol is a potent stimulator of gastric secretion, but it does not neutralize the acid after it is secreted. Neither should the patient be given, or take, a drug that directly irritates the gastric mucosa, such as the salicylates. They appear to exert a direct irritating effect without increasing acid secretion. The most frequently used form of this drug is acetylsalicylic acid, or aspirin. The daily or very frequent ingestion of aspirin appears to predispose to hemorrhage from the stomach. Mrs. Maple was given codeine, 32 mg, when she complained of headache. A patient with a diagnosis of peptic ulcer should be instructed *not* to take either aspirin or drugs containing it or other salicylates without a specific prescription from a physician who knows that he has an ulcer.

Because there is evidence that smoking increases the secretion of acid by the stomach, physicians generally discourage their patients from smoking. In fact, some physicians feel so strongly about smoking that they refuse to treat patients who do not cooperate. (See Chapters 10 and 14 for a discussion of some of the aspects of discontinuing smoking.)

Anticholinergics

Because hydrochloric acid is one of the essential factors in ulcer formation, an ideal drug would appear to be one that depresses its secretion. Such a drug would, in effect, produce a chemical vagotomy. There are a number of drugs available that do block the action of acetylcholine on smooth-muscle and gland cells. Because stimulation of the vagus nerve results in the release of acetylcholine and increases gastric secretion and motility, the effect of the anticholinergics or cholinergic-blocking agents is to decrease secretion and motility. Among the most widely used anticholinergics or cholinergic-blocking agents are the alkaloids of belladonna. Authorities differ as to the effectiveness of the alkaloids of belladonna in decreasing gastric secretion and motility in human beings. They do decrease both in experimental animals.

Among the synthetic anticholinergic agents are methantheline bromide (Banthine Bromide [34]) and propantheline bromide (Pro-Banthine Bromide [34]). Methantheline has been largely replaced by propantheline, which is said to be more effective in reducing gastric secretion and motility and to have fewer toxic effects. Readers who wish a more detailed description of these drugs should refer to a textbook on pharmacology.

Psychic Factors

One of the most important aspects in the care of the patient with a peptic ulcer is attention to the psychic factors in his illness. As indicated previously, gastric secretion, motility, and blood supply to the gastric mucosa are all responsive to a wide variety of stimuli in the environment. Some patients respond positively, that is, by healing their ulcers, when they are removed from a stressful environment. For example, Mr. George fits the stereotype of the patient with a peptic ulcer. He was a tense, hard-driving executive. He smoked cigarettes excessively, and, although he never became intoxicated, he consumed several cocktails in the course of most days. He often took work home at night, and his weekends were spent playing golf with business associates. When his ulcer symptoms finally became so severe that he could no longer ignore them, he consulted a physician and the diagnosis of peptic ulcer was confirmed. Mr. George and his physician decided that, instead of being admitted to a hospital, he should take a long-planned hunting trip with his wife. Plans were made for the trip. Mr. George agreed to eliminate smoking and the drinking of alcoholic beverages. He also took a bottle of an aluminum hydroxide antacid with him. Most of all, he planned to relax and enjoy himself. Within a few days of his arrival at the hunting lodge his symptoms had disappeared. At the time of his return to his physician one month later, his ulcer was found to be healed and he was free from symptoms.

For some patients, hospitalization is therapeutic because it provides a setting in which the patient can be dependent without feeling guilty about wanting to be dependent. A hospital is a place where he can be looked after. He can feel comfortable in allowing others to assume responsibility for his care. For this patient, the healing of his ulcer is favored by an atmosphere in which he is allowed and encouraged to be dependent. He not only wants, but needs, to have his needs anticipated and met. He wants and needs to be freed from responsibility for a time. If he is a patient who is undemanding, his need for dependence may be overlooked. Mrs. Maple, who was shy and quiet, was such a patient. One statement that she made to the nurse indicated that she had the desire to be dependent. She said, "I'm so glad to have a nurse who does things for me. At home, Joe always makes me decide how the money is to be spent and when to discipline the children. I wish that he would take more responsibility."

At the other extreme is the patient who is unable to allow others to assume responsibility for his care and overtly overreacts at the slightest frustration. For example, Mr. Johns watches a clock to be sure that he gets his medication at the exact time it is scheduled. As the hour approaches, his muscles become tense and he becomes more and more angry. Should the nurse be two minutes late, he becomes highly distraught. The nurse knows that she cannot possibly distribute medications to 30 patients at the same time and that a reasonable interval before or after the hour is acceptable. Because the patient attacks an approved practice and the nurse herself feels attacked, she too may feel angry. If she can recognize that the behavior of the patient is his usual way of reacting in frustrating situations and that she just happens to be the person who is present, then she may be able to avoid personalizing his remarks and to remain objective. She will be better able to develop a plan to increase the confidence of the patient that he will, in fact, receive the care he requires. Instead of respond-

ing with anger, she may try to administer Mr. Johns' medication at the scheduled hour. When the medication is one that can be safely left at the bedside of the patient, this possibility may be discussed with the physician and, with his approval, the drug may be left with the patient. Patients in some hospitals are encouraged to assume responsibility for their own medications. After the nurse has established a trusting relationship with the patient, problems such as the above tend to be less acute.

Because of the importance of psychic stimuli in promoting gastric secretion and motility, drugs are also prescribed to decrease the responsiveness of the individual. The physician prescribed phenobarbital, secobarbital (Seconal [35]), and prochlorperazine (Compazine [35]) for Mrs. Maple. Phenobarbital, 30 mg, was administered every four hours during the daytime. Because of its relatively prolonged sedative action, phenobarbital maintained Mrs. Maple in a continuous state of relaxation. Secobarbital 0.1 g, a relatively short-acting barbiturate, was prescribed for the hour of sleep, should Mrs. Maple require it for restful sleep. After the first evening, Mrs. Maple did not require it. Mrs. Maple, as well as other patients who are receiving relatively large doses of barbiturates, should be observed for indications of excessive depression of the nervous system. Furthermore, the patient who sleeps most of the time should be moved and turned regularly as well as be offered fluids. Sedative drugs should be given only if there is a specific indication for them.

In place of, or in combination with, phenobarbital, any one of a number of tranquilizing agents may be prescribed for the patient. The desired effect is to lessen the response of the individual to stimuli. These drugs modify the cephalic phase of gastric secretion; that is, they lessen secretion in response to sight, smell, or taste of food. Because of a decrease in the cephalic phase, the gastric phase of secretion may also be less intense.

The indications for and the effects of surgical therapy in the treatment of peptic ulcer have been discussed previously. Should bleeding recur or her ulcer fail to heal, surgery may be considered in the treatment of Mrs. Maple.

To summarize briefly, at the time of the admission of Mrs. Maple to the hospital, she was suffering from the effects of blood loss. Because an adequate volume of blood is essential to maintaining tissue nutrition, the restoration of the lost blood was the objective receiving priority. As soon as bleeding stopped and the blood

[35] Trade name.

that had been lost was replaced, attention was then directed toward treating her ulcer. Because an ulcer is a local manifestation of a constitutional disease, attention to Mrs. Maple as a person was as important as treating her ulcer. The fundamental objective of care was to reduce the effect of acid-pepsin in gastric juice on the lining of the duodenum. Since the stomach responds to a wide variety of stimuli by increased secretion and motility, treatment was planned to decrease Mrs. Maple's responsiveness to environmental stimuli as well as to neutralize gastric acidity.

Because peptic ulcer is a chronic disease characterized by periodic recurrences, Mrs. Maple should know that the ulcer may be reactivated at a later time. She should be advised to see her physician immediately should she develop pain or nausea. Delay not only increases the difficulty in healing the ulcer, but predisposes to complications. Inasmuch as she is able, Mrs. Maple should try to avoid situations that are upsetting to her. Possibly, Mr. Maple could be encouraged to assume more responsibility for family matters. Before approaching this problem with either Mr. or Mrs. Maple, the nurse should discuss the problem with the physician, who may decide to refer Mr. and Mrs. Maple to social service or to some other agency, such as the Family Service Society. As in other chronic illnesses, one of the important factors in the control of peptic ulcers is the strengths and resources of the patient and his family.

The Middle Alimentary Canal

STRUCTURE AND FUNCTION

The middle portion of the alimentary canal extends from the duodenal papilla to the mid-transverse colon. It consists, therefore, of the lower duodenum, the jejunum, the ileum, the cecum, the ascending colon, and the first portion of the transverse colon. This portion of the digestive tube functions, as do other parts of the alimentary canal, to move its contents analward (toward the anus). Its specific functions are to dilute, digest, and absorb nutrients. Because the mid-portion of the alimentary canal is where nutrients are transported from the external to the internal environment, the most critical function of the alimentary canal as a service facility is accomplished here. With the exception of water, absorption of nutrients is largely completed before the intestinal contents reach the ileocecal valve. In terms of survival, the mid-alimentary tract is the most important region of the alimentary canal. Although a portion can

be sacrificed, enough of the ileum must remain for the absorption of nutrients. Large quantities of fluid enter the jejunum from the duodenum and stomach, and secretions are added by the jejunum.

The ileocecal valve regulates the movement of material into the cecum and normally prevents the reflux of the contents of the colon into the small intestine. Acute obstruction of the colon distal to the ileocecal valve induces reverse peristalsis and relaxation of the valve. Reverse peristalsis may be sufficiently active to carry fecal material to the stomach, after which it is vomited. The emesis that results has a fecal odor. Needless to say, observation of the odor of vomitus is important.

Disturbances in the motility, secretion, or absorption in the midportion of the alimentary canal impair nutrition and hydration by decreasing the length of time that nutrients and water remain in the intestine or by interfering with their absorption. The middle part of the alimentary canal is subject to many of the same types of disorders as other parts of the gut. It can be obstructed by neoplasms, twisting (volvulus), scar tissue, incarceration in a hernial ring, or motor failure. Its blood supply can be cut off by twisting, by incarceration, or by thrombosis of the mesenteric artery. Inflammation occurs as the result of the effects of unknown and microbial agents. As in other areas, diverticula occur. Digestion and absorption may be impaired because of failure of delivery of digestive enzymes and bile salts. Fistulae may allow intestinal contents to escape before they can be digested and absorbed. Important disorders are summarized in Table 12-2 at the end of this chapter.

MALABSORPTION

The effects of ischemia of tissues and of perforation of the intestine have previously been considered. In malabsorption there is a failure to digest or to absorb one or more nutrients. The effects depend on the cause and degree of failure, the suddenness of onset, and which nutrients are not absorbed. For example, in the absence of pancreatic enzymes, fat is not digested. It is evacuated in the stool, which is large, bulky, and foul-smelling. The patient usually loses weight because fat is an important source of calories. The absence of bile salts interferes with the digestion of fats and the absorption of fats and fat-soluble vitamins. Inability to absorb vitamin K means that prothrombin will not be adequately formed and the tendency to bleed is increased. Briefly, as a consequence of failure to digest and absorb food, (1) nonabsorbed food appears in the stool; (2) secondary deficiencies caused by failure of absorption of nutrients develop; and (3) symptoms relating to gastrointestinal function such as diarrhea, anorexia, and nausea occur.[36]

The Lower Alimentary Canal

FUNCTIONS AND DISEASE

The lower portion of the alimentary canal extends from the mid-portion of the transverse colon to and including the anal sphincters. Because the portion distal to the ileocecal valve forms the large intestine and many of the disorders involving these structures are similar or involve the whole area, the entire large intestine will be discussed here.

Although the surgical removal of the entire large intestine is possible, it is attended by considerable risk. A part of all of the large intestine can be bypassed by anastomosing two sections or by bringing a portion of it through the abdominal wall. Complete or partial resection or bypassing of the large intestine, with or without the formation of an artificial anus after the individual has adjusted to the change, is compatible with a full and active life. Although the large intestine completes the absorption of water and stores and evacuates the residue left from the digestion of food, these functions can be accomplished by the remaining portion or by the distal end of the ileum.

The large intestine is the site of a number of important diseases. They include cancer, chronic ulcerative colitis, diverticulitis, and hemorrhoids. Abscesses and fissures in the region of the external anal region are not uncommon. The above disorders are summarized in Table 12-2.

Two common effects of disease or disturbances on the function of the large intestine include diarrhea and constipation. Lesions, such as benign and malignant neoplasms or strictures formed in the process of healing, that narrow the lumen of the intestine will in time prevent the passage of the contents through the large intestine, that is, block or obstruct it.

DIARRHEA AND CONSTIPATION

Diarrhea and constipation are terms used to indicate alterations in the normal pattern of defecation. Because of the wide range in bowel habits among healthy individuals, these terms are difficult to define precisely. For the purpose of this discussion, diarrhea is defined as the

[36] For a list of disorders characterized by malabsorption, see Thomas R. Hendrix and Theodore M. Bayless: "Malabsorption," *The Principles and Practice of Medicine,* 17th ed. A. McGehee Harvey *et al.* eds. (New York: Appleton-Century-Crofts, 1968), p. 983.

passage of several unformed stools as a result of the rapid movement of the fecal contents through the large intestine. By way of contrast, constipation is associated with delay in the passage of feces. Because the feces remain in the intestine for an unduly long period of time, water is absorbed and they are hard and dry. Defecation may be accompanied by discomfort. Both diarrhea and constipation are relatively common, and either can be caused by a disturbance in the regulatory mechanisms controlling the functioning of the large bowel or by mechanical interference with the progress of its contents. Inflammatory disorders of the large intestine are more likely to cause diarrhea than constipation. Hyperactivity of the stomach and small intestine predisposes to diarrhea for reasons to be explained subsequently.

Acute disturbances in the function of the digestive system are second only to acute respiratory disease as a cause of morbidity. Any acute disorder increasing the activity of one part of the alimentary canal is likely to affect the function of other parts. An affected individual is likely to experience both vomiting and diarrhea. Like vomiting, diarrhea is one of the defense mechanisms utilized by the gastrointestinal tract to rid itself of harmful agents. In diarrhea, the intestine is hyperactive.

The intestine, like other areas in the alimentary canal, is under control of the autonomic nervous system. Although defecation is largely a reflex action, it is subject to some voluntary control. Unless the contractions of the bowel are very powerful, defecation can be delayed for a time. The defecation reflex is similar to other reflexes in the body. Receptor cells in the rectum, which is normally empty, are stimulated by material entering the rectum. Impulses are carried to the defecation centers in the hypothalamus, where they are relayed to the intestinal muscles. Interconnections between the hypothalamus and the cerebral cortex make it possible for messages that modify the activity of the defecation center to be sent from the cerebral cortex to the hypothalamus. Feces are normally stored in the sigmoid and adjacent portions of the colon. The fecal content is moved to the storage areas and to the rectum by the same type of peristaltic action found in other parts of the alimentary canal.

A mass type of movement, known as the gastrocolic reflex, also occurs. It usually follows a meal or the ingestion of a glass or two of cold water or fruit juice on arising in the morning. The cold fluid moves rapidly through the stomach and into the duodenum and acts as a stimulus to activate the gastrocolic reflex. The entire small intestine is excited and the wave of contraction passes rapidly along the colon with the result that feces enter the rectum. Whether or not the anal sphincters are relaxed at this time will depend on the propulsive power of intestinal contractions and the cooperation of the individual with the reflex. For this treatment to be successful, the person should pay attention to the call to defecate. If he successfully inhibits defecation, future efforts to defecate will be increasingly unsuccessful.

As defined earlier, diarrhea is a condition in which a number of unformed stools are defecated. From the preceding description of the defecation reflex, it is evident that diarrhea can result from any condition in which peristalsis becomes hyperactive. As in other reflex activity, stimuli may act on receptors in the lining of the alimentary canal or be of central origin. Simply, diarrhea can be caused by irritation of the lining of the intestine resulting in hyperactivity of the intestine or it may be of nervous origin. See Table 12-1 for causes.

Two examples of diarrhea of neurogenic origin follow. One is Joan Book, who usually has diarrhea just preceding an examination. She calls her condition "nervous diarrhea." Jean Servus is the second example. When Jean consulted her physician because she had had repeated attacks of diarrhea over the past few months, no evidence of an organic lesion was found to account for her difficulty. After some discussion, Jean remembered that her episodes of diarrhea began following a violent quarrel with her father. The problem had not been resolved and she felt that her father was continuing to harass her. Each time Jean and her father had an argument, Jean had an episode of diarrhea. After she understood the relationship of her feelings to diarrhea, it became less troublesome.

Although diarrhea of neurogenic origin is not uncommon, the usual cause is some agent irritating the intestinal mucosa. Irritants can be of endogenous or exogenous origin. Microorganisms are among the more frequent causative agents of acute diarrhea. In the United States infection is most frequently caused by a virus, a Salmonella or the *Endamoeba histolytica*. The nature of each of these is summarized at the end of this chapter. Diarrhea, as well as nausea and vomiting, is frequently associated with the onset of acute diseases of the gastrointestinal tract.

Whenever a person experiences repeated attacks of diarrhea, he should be examined by his physician because they may be associated with a serious disorder that may respond if treated early. Furthermore, when diarrhea continues, important nutrients and fluids are lost from the body. In severe diarrhea there is probably always some impairment in absorption. In disorders in which absorption is markedly reduced, large quantities of fat and protein may be lost. For example, in sprue, failure to absorb fat and protein results in large, bulky, foamy feces with a foul odor. Maintenance of even a minimal nutritional status may be difficult.

In obstructive lesions of the large intestine, diarrhea alternates with constipation. As the lumen of the bowel is reduced in size, liquid feces are moved past the site of the obstruction and evacuated. During periods when the feces accumulate behind the obstruction, constipation occurs. The most serious cause of this type of diarrhea is cancer. Fecal impactions can, however, be responsible for the same combination of symptoms. Diarrhea is a manifestation in a number of generalized disorders, such as hyperthyroidism, lymphosarcoma, and tuberculosis. It, too, can be of allergic origin. Radiation therapy of pelvic and abdominal organs predisposes to diarrhea.

From the preceding, the logical conclusion is that diarrhea occurs frequently and is associated with a variety of disorders. The effects of diarrhea depend on its cause and severity as well as how long it persists and the age and state of health of the individual who has it. Age is a significant factor, because diarrhea in a young infant can soon cause a serious depletion of electrolytes, water, and nutrients. Unless the disorder is promptly corrected, the life of the child can be threatened. A bout of diarrhea in a youth or adult is likely to cause some feeling of unfitness, but need not be a source of alarm unless it is very severe or continues for more than a few hours.

Although few persons escape or fail to recover from an occasional episode of diarrhea, excessive or prolonged diarrhea leads to the loss of water and nutrients from the body and predisposes to malnutrition. Undernutrition may be worsened by the fact that anorexia, nausea, and vomiting discourage the intake of food. When cramping accompanies diarrhea, the individual may be afraid to eat. Loss of nutrients may be exaggerated when diarrhea is caused by failure to digest or absorb food, or when there is a large outpouring of mucus into the alimentary canal. Erosion of blood vessels accompanied by bleeding is a frequent observation in patients whose diarrhea is due to an ulcerating lesion or lesions. In chronic or severe diarrhea, nutrition is always affected to some extent by failure to ingest food and by losses of nutrients, mucus, and blood.

What are the nurse's responsibilities in caring for the patient with diarrhea?

The physician will try to determine the nature of the cause of the diarrhea and what effect, if

TABLE 12-1

Causes of Diarrhea

Psychogenic and/or Neurogenic Innervation

1. Vagal (generalized hypermotility of entire alimentary tract)
   a. Stomach
   b. Small intestine   Treatment: surgical   a. Vagotomy
   c. Ascending colon   b. Gastrectomy
   d. Transverse colon
2. Sacral (diarrhea alternates with constipation; irritable colon, mucous colitis)
   a. Descending colon

Classification of Diarrhea

1. Inflammatory
   a. Regional enteritis: distal portion of small intestine
   b. Ulcerative colitis: distal portion of descending colon
2. Irritative
   a. Mechanical: small intestine, transverse and descending colon
      (1) Fecal impaction
      (2) Foreign body
      (3) Neoplasm
      (4) Intussusception
      (5) Extraluminal compression
      (6) Angulation
   b. Chemical: descending colon
      (1) Poisons
      (2) Cathartics
   c. Bacterial: small intestine, descending colon
      (1) Salmonellae
      (2) Shigellae
      (3) Staphylococci
      (4) Streptococci
      (5) *B. coli*
      (6) Clostridia *et al.*
   d. Parasitic: descending colon
      (1) Amebiasis
      (2) Trichinosis
      (3) Ascariasis
3. Malabsorption: small intestine
   a. Tropical sprue
   b. Symptomatic sprue
   c. Celiac disease (adult celiac disease)
   d. Nontropical sprue
   e. Whipple's disease
4. Osmotic: small intestine and descending colon
   a. Saline cathartics
5. Endocrine
   a. Thyroid
      (1) Hyperthyroidism
   b. Adrenals
      (1) Adrenocortical insufficiency
   c. Liver
      (1) Secreting carcinoid tumors (serotonin)
6. Dietary: descending colon
   a. Food intolerance
   b. Vitamin deficiencies
7. Allergic: descending colon
   a. Drug sensitivity
   b. Food sensitivity

---

any, it has had on the nutritional status of the individual. The medical plan of therapy will then be dependent on the cause of diarrhea and the general status of the individual. The nurse contributes to diagnosis through observations of the patient and by assisting with medical examinations. The nurse usually participates in the therapy by administering medications and other forms of treatment. In addition, the nurse carries the responsibility for the comfort of the patient and for improving his nutritional status. When the patient is known to harbor or is suspected to harbor agents that are transmissible to others, the nurse has the responsibility for planning and enforcing suitable procedures to protect herself and others.

Observations

One important way in which information is collected is by observation of the feces. Pertinent observations include color, odor, consistency—formed, liquid, frothy—number and frequency, and the presence of foreign matter such as blood, mucus, pus, and worms. What symptoms accompany defecation; that is, does the patient have cramping, urgency, pain, or tenesmus on defecation? Tenesmus is the term for the sharp, unpleasant contractions in the lower-left quadrant associated with straining during defecation. Following defecation, the patient feels only partly relieved. The nurse is more helpful when she describes the sensations as they are related by the patient in his own words than when she names them. Does he have abdominal or other pain? Where is it located? Under what conditions are the symptoms of the patient worsened? Improved? For example, is defecation initiated by eating or activity? Is the patient relieved following defecation, or does he feel as if he had only partly evacuated his bowels? Observations of vital signs are of particular significance when diarrhea is associated with infection or hemorrhage. The nursing of the patient who suffers from a disorder accompanied by chronic diarrhea taxes the patience and ingenuity of any nurse.

To illustrate the problems of the patient with chronic diarrhea, Mrs. Reddy is presented. Mrs. John Reddy, who is 24 years of age, has a diagnosis of chronic ulcerative colitis. A year ago, shortly after her marriage to a promising young businessman, she suffered an attack of diarrhea with pus, blood, and fibrin in the stool. At the time of her admission to Special Hospital, she looked and felt sick. She presented evidence of a poor nutritional state because she had lost 20 lb in weight, her hemoglobin was reduced to 6 g, and her blood proteins were 5.2 g per 100 ml. Each day she passed from 10 to 20 rectal discharges of blood, mucus, and pus. With each defecation, she experienced intestinal cramping and straining. Despite frequent defecations, she was not relieved by defecation. The area around the anus was inflamed and sore. When she tried to eat, cramping was intensified. She was aware of the disagreeable odor of her stools. Because of the urgency associated with defecation, Mrs. Reddy was not always able to get on the bedpan in time, and the bed was soiled. Because she was chronically ill and many aspects of her illness were unpleasant, if not repugnant, to others, Mrs. Reddy worried about her marriage and the reaction of her husband to her illness. Quite understandably, she was anxious and depressed.

The Nursing Care Plan

In making a nursing care plan for Mrs. Reddy, her nurse established two objectives. The *first* was to increase her comfort and the *second* to try to improve her nutritional status. To accomplish the first objective, the nurse planned to wash, dry, and powder the anal region after each defecation. To protect the bed from soiling, an absorbent pad of the type used in disposable diapers was placed under Mrs. Reddy's buttocks. It was changed each time it was soiled. The bedpan was washed after every use. To help minimize odor, the room was aired after each defecation. Because the outside temperature was cold, a screen was placed in front of the window and an extra blanket was spread over Mrs. Reddy to prevent chilling. After each defecation, Mrs. Reddy was provided with an opportunity to wash her hands. For the first few days, the nurse gave care to Mrs. Reddy; that is, she allowed her to be sick and dependent. She made few demands on her, accepting her as a very sick woman whose behavior could be explained by her illness and who needed a high quality of nursing care.

The objectives of medical therapy are (1) to improve the general well-being of the patient, (2) to induce a remission of the disease, and (3) to eliminate histological evidence of the disease. For the first three days Mrs. Reddy was in the hospital, fluids containing multivitamins were administered by intravenous infusion and she was given 1,000 ml of whole blood. To decrease intestinal peristalsis, her physician prescribed tincture of opium (Laudanum), 0.6 ml (10 minims), every four hours during the daytime. If required, a fifth dose could be administered during the night. For two weeks, she was given 50 ml of water containing 20 mg of prednisolone rectally, each evening. In addition, each day prednisolone 0.60 mg was given orally. Because of her improved condition, a soft, high-protein diet was prescribed to be started on her fourth day in the hospital. Before Mrs. Reddy's food arrived, she was prepared for the meal by having an opportunity to brush her teeth and wash her face and hands and was assisted to a comfortable position. The room was aired and a clean bedpan was conveniently placed, but covered. Mrs. Reddy had been encouraged to choose what she wanted for breakfast. She asked for a white wheat cereal and toast. The suggestion was made that she eat slowly and drink only a minimum of fluid during her meal. Fluids were encouraged between meals. Iced fluids are generally avoided because they tend to stimulate peristalsis. When Mrs. Reddy complained of a cramping sensation, the suggestion was made that she contract her buttocks and pull them together and try to contract the anus. By practicing this maneuver, she was sometimes able to prevent defecation.

As her nutritional and general status improved, Mrs. Reddy widened her selection of foods. To occupy her time and attention, and to promote relaxation, her physician prescribed occupational therapy. The occupational therapist suggested she make pot holders on a "Weave It" frame. By using different colored strands, she could design varying patterns. The motions are repetitive and relaxing. The product is useful and can be sold or given to relatives and friends. To encourage relaxation, her nurse planned regular rest periods for her. She tried to control conditions in her external environment, so that Mrs. Reddy was protected from unnecessary stimulation or irritation. Because any kind of stress, including infection, aggravates the disorder, people with colds were banned from her environment.

In addition to medical therapy, surgical procedures are sometimes indicated. To provide rest and allow the diseased portion of the bowel to heal, an ileostomy may be performed. Because there is a tendency for islands of healthy tissue that are surrounded by areas of disease and cicatrization (scarring) to undergo polyp formation and malignant degeneration, resection of the diseased bowel may be required.

Whatever form of therapy is instituted, the patient with chronic ulcerative colitis is sick. Minimizing the disagreeable effects of the disease includes the control of odors, protection of the skin, and control of conditions in the environment tending to stimulate peristalsis. Because of the nature of the disease, nutrition is a problem. One of the major problems in nursing the patient is to improve his intake of food. Unless his food intake is improved, recovery is doubtful.

CONSTIPATION

In constipation, in contrast to diarrhea, evacuation of feces is delayed, and when they are finally evacuated, feces are frequently hard and dry. Because of the great variability among people, constipation is difficult to define exactly. Many people, though by no means all, defecate once daily. Probably the most frequent cause of constipation is neglect to respond to the normal defecation reflex. Because of failure to respond, the reflex itself becomes less powerful and constipation results. Constipation can also be the result of a disease process or of agents used in the treatment of disease. Constipation occurs in degenerative diseases of the central nervous system, in severe psychoses, and with the use of drugs such as the ganglionic blocking agents and morphine.

The treatment of simple constipation is primarily education. A regular and convenient time should be selected for defecation. For most people, the defecation reflex is most active after meals, particularly after breakfast. In a family of six or eight with only one bathroom, obviously it will not be available to all members of the family immediately after breakfast. The time selected should be one when the individual can be comfortably relaxed. The individual should be encouraged to "obey" the urge to defecate when it does occur. A diet containing a reasonable amount of bulk and regular exercise, especially before breakfast, are other useful measures in the prevention and treatment of constipation.

For the elderly patient who is poorly motivated or who has a disease that makes change difficult or impossible, the correction of constipation by changing habits of living may not be possible or practical. Measures such as bulky laxatives and oil-retention or other types of enemas may be the most reasonable solutions to the problem. In elderly patients and in those who have neurological disorders affecting bowel function, observation of the regularity of defecation as well as the size and consistency of feces is important to the prevention and early detection of fecal impactions. Sick and debilitated individuals, especially if elderly, and persons with lesions in the nervous system that interfere with the regulation of bowel function are especially predisposed to impaction. Size of the stool is significant because the patient may pass a small amount of feces while retaining and accumulating feces in the lower bowel. Water is absorbed from the fecal material remaining in the bowel, increasing the difficulty with which it is evacuated. In patients who are predisposed to fecal impactions, measures such as bulk-producing cathartics and oil-retention enemas may be successful in the prevention of their formation. After an impaction is formed, it usually has to be broken up manually and removed. Impactions should not occur if the patient is observed and appropriate actions are taken when there is evidence that feces are being retained. Prevention is to be preferred to cure.

CAUSES AND EFFECTS OF OBSTRUCTION

Any disorder interfering with the forward movement of the contents of the alimentary canal is called an obstruction. As indicated previously, an obstruction in the esophagus interferes with the ability to ingest food. An obstruction of the outlet of the stomach delays or prevents chyme from entering the duodenum. Either the small or large intestine may be the site of an obstruction. For the most part, the discussion of obstruction that follows will be related to blocking of the intestine, large or small. Whatever the nature of obstruction or its site or location, however, it interferes with the accomplishment of the function of the alimentary canal. Three primary types of disturbances predispose to obstruction. They are mechanical blocking of the lumen, reduced or absent peristalsis, and impaired circulation caused by the occlusion of the blood supply. Mechanical blocking may have its origin in abnormalities within the wall of the alimentary canal or outside it. Neoplasms, unreduced volvulus, and incarcerated hernias are a few of many causes of mechanical obstruction.

Neurogenic Obstruction

Absent peristalsis is usually caused by some disturbance in the function of the autonomic nervous system associated with surgical or other trauma. As a result of reflex inhibition of the gastrointestinal tract, the stomach may be acutely dilated by retained secretions and swallowed air. Complete cessation of motor activity of the small intestine produces a functional obstruction and is referred to as paralytic or adynamic ileus. Impairment of the circulation may be caused by a thrombosis of the mesenteric artery, or by distention of the inactive intestine.

In both the neurogenic and the vascular types of obstruction, the lumen of the bowel is open. The effect is that of obstruction, however, because the affected parts of the bowel do not propel its contents forward. As a result of the obstruction the intestine and stomach are distended by gas and fluids. The gas is presumed to have its origin in the air that is swallowed. As the pressure within the bowel increases, absorption decreases. When the pressure within the intestine equals the diastolic blood pressure, absorption ceases. The effect of distention on the circulation of blood to the wall of the intestine is similar to that of pressure on any tissue. First the venous outflow from the tissue is impaired. This leads to a slowing of the blood flow through the tissue and the development of edema. If the condition is allowed to continue, arterial blood flow is impaired and finally ceases. Because of the failure in the flow of blood to the tissue, tissue necrosis occurs. Death of a portion of the alimentary tract may lead to perforation of the viscus and to the death of the individual.

Obstruction in the gastrointestinal tract also leads to shock. One of the factors in the development of shock is that distention of the stomach and intestine is a powerful stimulus to secretion. Secretion combined with a failure of absorption leads to the trapping of a large volume of fluid within the gastrointestinal tract and to a reduction in the blood volume. Therefore, when obstruction is allowed to progress, shock eventually develops. As the stomach and/or bowel distends, the increase in their volume has an adverse effect on respiratory and circulatory function. Increased intra-abdominal pressure reduces vital capacity by interfering with the depression of the diaphragm. It also interferes with the return flow of blood from the lower extremities by direct pressure on the veins.

Decompression

Before definitive treatment can be instituted, the stomach and/or intestine must be deflated by the removal of gas and fluid. Decompression is accomplished by the introduction into the stomach or intestine of a tube to which suction is applied. The principles on which decompression therapy is based are described in Chapter 17. As the bowel is decompressed, the blood supply to the wall improves. Because of the improvement of the nutrition of the wall, functional disorders such as adynamic ileus tend to correct themselves. Structural lesions usually require some form of surgical therapy to remove or relieve the effects of obstruction. One of the important responsibilities of the nurse in the care of the patient who has a gastric or intestinal obstruction is to maintain the suctioning apparatus in good working order. Because respiratory and circulatory functions are impaired, attention must be given to nursing measures that support these functions.

HERNIATION—TYPES AND EFFECTS

The alimentary canal is subject to two general types of herniation. In the first type the mucosa prolapses through the muscle wall forming a sac or pouch known as a diverticulum. Multiple diverticula are known as diverticulosis. The two most common sites for the formation of diverticula are the colon and the esophagus. As may the appendix, the diverticula may become filled with food or feces and become inflamed or perforated. Inflammation of a diverticulum is known as diverticulitis.

In the other types of herniation, the mesentery or one or more of the organs escape through a ring through which body structures pass. Common types of hernias involving the alimentary canal include esophageal hiatus hernia and inguinal, femoral, umbilical, and postoperative ventral hernia. The name indicates the ring through which the organ prolapses. Thus in an esophageal hiatus hernia, contents of the abdominal cavity protrude through the gap in the diaphragm into the thoracic cavity. Most types of hernia predispose the patient to two dangers, obstruction of the alimentary canal and necrosis of the trapped tissues.

SUMMARY

Understanding of the effects of disease on some portion of the alimentary canal requires knowledge of the following:

1. The structure and function of each part.
2. The mechanisms regulating each part, so that it performs its function and its activity is coordinated with that of other parts of the alimentary canal.
3. The mechanisms for regulating the function of the alimentary canal so that the nutritional needs of the individual are met.

Disease may be caused by disorders in the regulation of function or to alteration in the structure of the alimentary canal. The manifestations of disease of the alimentary canal result from the effect of injuring agents (in a broad sense) on the structure and function, from failure of the canal to defend the integrity of its lining, and from interference with the intake of food and water. Furthermore, most of the wall of the alimentary canal is richly supplied with blood. Disorders in which the lining membrane is damaged predispose to bleeding. Thrombosis of arteries or veins supplying any part of the alimentary canal predisposes to tissue necrosis. Esophageal and hemorrhoidal veins have the tendency under certain circumstances to dilate and become tortuous, that is, to form varicosities. Although rupture of varices may occur in either location, those in the esophagus are more likely to be the site of serious hemorrhage. Varicosities of hemorrhoidal veins (hemorrhoids) may become thrombosed and painfully inflamed.

The Liver and Biliary Tract

In the preceding sections, the functions of the alimentary canal, as well as something about the nature of disorders in function, have been discussed. In addition to the secretions from glands in the mucosa of the alimentary canal, secretions from two glands external to but emptying into the duodenum have a significant role in digestion. These glands are the liver and pancreas.

The liver is not only the largest, but it is the most complex, organ in the body. The liver has four main systems—blood vessels, reticuloendothelial Kupffer's cells, parenchymal cells, and the biliary channels.[37] All these systems are so intimately related that any considerable or continuing pathology in one inevitably leads to disturbances in others. Injury can be the result of direct extension of a pathologic process or the response of the tissues to injury. In the adult, the vascular system of the liver stores and filters blood. Kupffer's cells—a specialized type of reticuloendothelial cells—in the lining of the venous channels of the liver play an important role in defense because they phagocytize potentially harmful agents circulating through the liver. Parenchymal cells secrete bile and play an essential role in the intermediary metabolism of most nutrients. The biliary channels store, concentrate, and conduct bile from the liver to the alimentary canal.

In the study of the liver, one is impressed with the interrelatedness of body functions and structure. For example, the most frequent cause of vascular congestion in the liver is congestive heart failure resulting from the failure of the right side of the heart as a pump. (See Chapter 10.) In right-sided heart failure, stasis of blood in the right atrium impedes the flow of blood from the inferior vena cava with the result that the blood pressure rises in the inferior vena cava. As the blood pressure rises in the inferior vena cava, pressure is transmitted to the hepatic veins and blood accumulates in the liver, causing the liver to swell and to enlarge. Because the capsule surrounding the liver offers resistance to swelling, pressure within the liver rises. As in any other tissue in which venous congestion occurs, blood supply to the tissue is impeded by failure to remove blood at about the same rate as it enters.

The liver receives 20 per cent of the cardiac output. Approximately three fourths of the blood delivered to the liver is venous blood and is carried by the portal system. The other one quarter is arterial blood conveyed by the hepatic artery. Because such a high proportion of the blood circulated to the liver is venous blood,

[37] Franz J. Ingelfinger: "The Liver," *Pathologic Physiology: Mechanisms of Disease,* 4th ed. William A. Sodeman and William A. Sodeman, Jr., eds. (Philadelphia: W. B. Saunders Company, 1967), p. 661.

oxygen supply, under the most favorable circumstances, tends to be marginal. Any disorder decreasing the blood supply through the liver, therefore, predisposes to some degree of hypoxia. In addition to causing a deficient supply of oxygen to liver cells, congestion in the liver elevates the blood pressure in the veins forming the portal system. Because fluids move in the direction of least resistance, the elevation of blood pressure within the portal system is reflected by congestion of the wall of the stomach, esophagus, and duodenum. In the esophagus, elevated venous pressure predisposes to esophageal varices. In the stomach and duodenum, elevated portal pressure predisposes to peptic ulcer.

In the liver itself, swelling interferes with parenchymal cell function and may, when severe, obstruct ducts of the biliary canal. Jaundice caused by a failure to remove bile pigments is a frequent sign in severe right-sided heart failure.

What is the function of the liver in digestion?

At this point, the function of the liver in digestion and absorption will be presented. Metabolic functions will be discussed later in this chapter. The liver functions in digestion by the secretion of bile. Because bile contains substances that are discharged into the internal environment, it is an excretion as well. From 600 to 800 ml of bile are formed each day. Drainage of all of the bile secreted each day results in the loss of fluid and requires its replacement. In addition to water, the important constituents of bile are cholesterol, bile salts, bile pigments, and lecithin. Because the biliary tract is lined with mucous membrane, bile contains some mucus.

BILE

Bile formed in the liver is conveyed by a series of channels or ducts to the duodenum. Liver cells are arranged around ducts that join together to form larger ducts and finally leave the liver as the hepatic duct. The hepatic duct branches to form the cystic duct leading to the gallbladder where bile is stored and concentrated. The duct formed by the hepatic and cystic ducts is the common bile duct. It opens, usually in common with the duct of Wirsung from the pancreas, into the duodenum. The terminal portion of the common bile duct and the duct of Wirsung are known as the ampulla of Vater. The opening into the duodenum is guarded by a muscle called the sphincter of Oddi. For the structural relationships of these organs see Figure 12-3.

STORAGE OF BILE

Between meals, bile, which is secreted more or less continuously, is stored in the gallbladder, where it is concentrated. When fat enters the intestine, a hormone, cholecystokinin, is secreted by the intestinal mucosa and carried to the gallbladder by way of the blood. It stimulates the muscle in the gallbladder to contract, thus forcing the bile out into the bile ducts. At the same time the sphincter of Oddi relaxes and bile enters the duodenum along with the pancreatic juice.

EVALUATION OF BILE DUCTS AND GALLBLADDER

The patency of the bile ducts and the capacity of the gallbladder to store and concentrate bile are evaluated by x-ray following the administration of an iodinated organic compound. The usual method for the administration of the dye is by mouth, but it may be given by intravenous injection. Dye may also be injected directly into biliary canals in patients having a T tube or at the time of surgery involving the biliary tract. After absorption of the dye into the blood, it is removed by the liver and secreted into the bile. When the substance is administered orally to a healthy person, sufficient dye will have been excreted into the biliary canals to render them opaque to x-ray in about 12 hours. The success of the examination depends on (1) normal motility and absorbing powers of the alimentary canal, (2) normal liver function, (3) patent biliary channels, (4) an empty gallbladder at the time the test is initiated, and (5) a gallbladder capable of concentrating and storing bile. To make sure that the gallbladder has been emptied before the dye is administered, the patient may be given a fatty meal the morning and noon before the tablets are administered. The evening that the dye is given, the patient has a liquid low-fat meal. Following the initial x-rays, the capacity of the gallbladder to empty can be checked by the ingestion of a fatty meal. Throughout the period of the examination, foods and fluids are limited to those indicated in the directions for the examination. Stimulation of gastric motility and foods stimulating the flow of bile into the alimentary canal are to be avoided after the dye is administered and until the first x-rays have been taken, because they will prevent the dye from being concentrated in the gallbladder.

FUNCTIONS OF BILE SALTS

Of the constituents of bile, the only ones functioning in digestion and absorption are the bile salts. Bile salts are formed by the neutralization

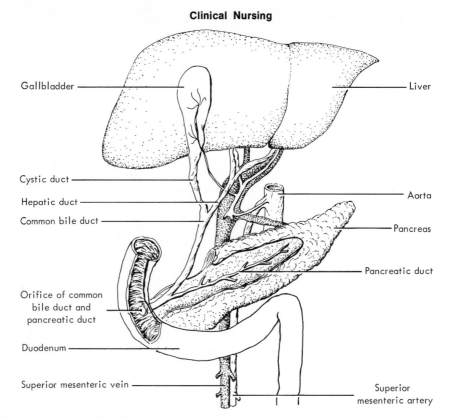

Gallbladder

Liver

Cystic duct

Hepatic duct

Aorta

Common bile duct

Pancreas

Pancreatic duct

Orifice of common
bile duct and
pancreatic duct

Duodenum

Superior mesenteric vein

Superior
mesenteric artery

FIGURE 12-3. Diagram showing relationships of the pancreatic and bile ducts and their entrance into the duodenum. Where might obstructions be located to produce jaundice? (Adapted with permission of The Macmillan Company from *Textbook of Physiology*, Fig. 100, p. 278, by Caroline E. Stackpole and Lutie C. Leavell. Copyright © The Macmillan Company, 1953.)

of cholic acid in the liver and secreted as sodium and potassium salts. Cholic acid is probably formed from cholesterol. The action of bile salts is similar to that of a detergent. They lower the surface tension of fat so that the fat globules suspended in the watery chyme can be broken up and prevented from merging again. Many small droplets offer a larger surface on which enzymes can act.

Even more important than their action in facilitating the digestion of fat, bile salts are required for the absorption of fatty acids, mono- and triglycerides, and fat-soluble vitamins. In the absorption of fats, bile salts are reabsorbed and returned to the liver to be resecreted. One of the earliest effects of injury of liver cells is a decrease in the secretion of bile salts. Obstruction of the common hepatic or the common bile duct can prevent bile salts from reaching the intestine. One of the most distressing effects observed in patients with lesions associated with obstruction of the biliary tract is pruritus. It is believed to be caused by excessive amounts of bile salts in the blood. Mr. Pine,

who was admitted with a diagnosis of cancer of the head of the pancreas obstructing the common bile duct, had deep scratches over every part of his body that he could reach. To minimize itching he was given tepid baths to which starch was added and calamine lotion was applied to his skin. Room temperature was regulated so that it did not exceed 68°F because heat increases the intensity of itching. To lessen the damage to his skin from scratching, his nails were cut short. If obstruction is incomplete, cholestyramine, an anion exchange resin, may be prescribed to prevent the reabsorption of bile salts from the intestine. It takes 4 to 6 days to be effective.

In the absence of bile salts, a large part of the ingested fat is lost in the stool in the form of soaps. The stool is pale and frothy in appearance. Fat-soluble vitamins A, D, E, and K are also lost in the stool. Because vitamins A and D are stored in sufficient quantities to last for some time, evidence of vitamin A or D deficiency does not usually occur unless the deficiency continues for months. In contrast, absence of bile salts for more than a few days leads to deficiency in vitamin K. Vitamin K acts as a catalyst in the formation of prothrombin. In its absence, whether due to a vitamin K deficiency or to the administration of one of its antagonists such as bishydroxycoumarin, the blood fails to clot in the usual period of time. Before the discovery of vitamin K, the surgical treatment of the patient with a common bile duct obstruction was difficult because of the tendency of the patient to bleed. Even small breaks in a blood vessel resulted in bleeding that was difficult to control.

Because bile is alkaline in reaction—its pH is between 8.0 and 8.6—it helps to neutralize the acid chyme entering the duodenum. Under some circumstances bile is regurgitated into the stomach, where it has a similar effect. Enzymes in pancreatic and intestinal juice require a pH of about 7 for optimum function.

CHOLESTEROL

In addition to the secretion of bile salts, bile contains substances that are excreted from the body, such as cholesterol and bilirubin. Cholesterol is synthesized in the body and ingested in food. The liver is the chief organ in which cholesterol is synthesized but it is formed in lesser quantities in other tissues, such as the adrenal cortex and skin. Cholesterol is readily absorbed from the intestine. Although the level of cholesterol in the blood can be lowered by decreasing the quantity ingested in the diet, synthesis by the liver and other tissues prevents it from being eliminated from the blood. Cholesterol continues to appear in the bile despite its elimination from the diet. The quantity of cholesterol in the bile is not affected by its contration in the blood. (See also "Lipid Metabolism," p. 561.)

From what are gallstones formed and what factors contribute to their formation?

Although cholesterol is nearly insoluble in water, it is kept in solution in the bile by bile salts, fatty acids, and lecithin. In some persons, cholesterol and/or bilirubin and calcium carbonate precipitate and form stones (cholelithiasis). Although one constituent may predominate, even so-called pure stones contain varying proportions of other constituents. For example, a "pure" cholesterol stone is about 98 per cent cholesterol, the other 2 per cent being pigment and calcium carbonate. Cholesterol, mixed, and pigment stones are relatively common in man. Calcium carbonate stones are uncommon in man but are common in cattle. About 50 per cent of gallstones contain sufficient calcium carbonate to be opaque to x-ray. Stones with

little or no calcium can be detected by x-ray only with the use of contrast media. Cholesterol stones are cream-colored, but pigment stones are dark in color.

Etiology

Cholelithiasis is presumed to result from some condition upsetting the balance between the factors keeping cholesterol, bile pigments, and calcium carbonate in solution and those favoring precipitation. Three factors are believed to favor precipitation: (1) obstruction, (2) stasis, and (3) inflammation. The mechanisms initiating precipitation and the growth of gallstones are unknown.[38]

The incidence of cholelithiasis is higher among women than men. At the time of death, 30 per cent of women and 15 per cent of men have gallstones.[39] Approximately 500,000 persons are hospitalized each year with gallbladder disease.[40] Women who have had several children appear to be more susceptible to cholelithiasis than nonparous women. The incidence of cholelithiasis is high among persons having hemolytic jaundice, a condition in which red blood cells are destroyed at an excessive rate. Obesity and diabetes mellitus appear to predispose to gallstones, as do infections of the gallbladder, one notable example being typhoid fever.

The number of stones found in the gallbladder of any one person varies from 1 to more than 200. They vary in shape and size. Single stones are likely to be smooth and round or oval in shape, while multiple stones are likely to be small and faceted and variable in size and shape.

Signs and Symptoms

Highly variable signs and symptoms accompany cholelithiasis. About half of the patients have no signs or symptoms referable to the biliary tract but have so-called silent cholelithiasis. In those who have stones containing sufficient calcium carbonate, their presence may be demonstrated by an x-ray over the area. Stones may be identified during abdominal surgery or after death during postmortem examination. Signs and symptoms vary from belching and bloating to periodic attacks of biliary colic. Biliary colic is characterized by attacks of pain in

[38] Donald M. Small: "Gallstones," *New Eng. J. Med.,* 279:588, 1968.

[39] Franz J. Ingelfinger: "Diseases of the Gall Bladder and Bile Ducts," *Principles of Internal Medicine,* 5th ed., Tinsley R. Harrison *et al.,* eds. (New York: The Blakiston Division, McGraw-Hill Book Company, Inc., 1966), p. 1088.

[40] "Gallbladder Disease Hospitalizes 500,000 a Year," *Statist. Bull. Metrop. Life Insur. Co.,* 46:9–11 (Nov.) 1965.

the right upper abdomen accompanied by nausea, vomiting, and difficulty in taking a deep breath. The attacks are believed to be caused by muscle spasm initiated by a stone passing through the common duct. Attacks may be precipitated by a fatty meal, but they may also occur during the night when the stomach is presumably empty.

Mrs. Helmer is illustrative of the patient who is assumed to be predisposed to cholelithiasis. She is 40 years of age, about 20 lb overweight, and has four daughters. Although gallstones do develop at any age, they are uncommon before the age of 30. Mrs. Helmer was among the 50 per cent of the persons who have cholelithiasis with symptoms. About two o'clock one night, she awakened with excruciating pain in her right upper abdomen. It extended through to the region just under the central side of the right scapula. Her pain was so severe that she arose and walked the floor, bending forward with her arms folded firmly across her chest. Although the room was cool, beads of perspiration stood out on her forehead. She complained of nausea, and her breathing was shallow. Because of the severity of her pain, Mr. Helmer called the family physician, who came and gave Mrs. Helmer 15 mg (gr ¼) of morphine sulfate and suggested that she come into his office as soon as possible for diagnostic tests and probably surgery. In the meantime, Mrs. Helmer was told to avoid greasy, fatty, or fried foods and those having strong odor when cooked such as cabbage, turnips, and kale.

The pain was relieved by the morphine and Mrs. Helmer went to sleep. When she awakened in the morning, she had some residual soreness in the affected area, but she felt much better. Although some patients have frequent attacks, Mrs. Helmer continued to feel well for several months. She found that if she avoided fatty foods and cabbage, she was free from symptoms. Being comfortable, busy, and human, she did not make an appointment to see her physician.

Possible Complications

Because Mrs. Helmer's gallbladder contained many small stones—over one hundred were found in her gallbladder at the time of cholecystectomy—she might have had biliary colic at any time. By delaying treatment Mrs. Helmer was exposing herself to the danger of several serious complications. They include acute and chronic cholecystitis, choledocholithiasis, cholangitis, fistula from the biliary tract to surrounding organs, biliary cirrhosis, carcinoma of the gallbladder, and gallstone ileus. She did develop choledocholithiasis—a stone was lodged in the common duct, causing obstruction. On examination in the laboratory her gallbladder was found to be acutely inflamed.

About a year after the attack described above Mrs. Helmer experienced several acute bouts of pain. None was as severe as the first and she could usually relate an attack to a dietary indiscretion. Her final attack was not quite as severe as the first, but instead of disappearing, her symptoms persisted. She could no longer avoid facing the fact that she was ill and she sought admission to the hospital for diagnosis and treatment. At the time of admission, she had pain in the right upper quadrant, nausea and vomiting, a temperature of 38.3°C (101°F), and leukocytosis. She looked and felt sick. Although chills may precede a rise in temperature, she had none. Careful inspection of the sclera of her eyes revealed some icterus. The level of bilirubin in her blood was 2 mg per 100 ml of blood plasma. The normal range is 0.1 to 1.2 mg per 100 ml. Even in the absence of stones in the common duct a transient icterus can occur. Jaundice is probably caused by edema, spasm, or inflammation of ducts draining the liver.

Although the history and clinical picture pointed toward choledocholithiasis, a few days were required before Mrs. Helmer was ready for surgery. In addition to the diagnostic procedures cited above, she had an x-ray of the abdomen. No preparation was required for it. Her urine was examined for, and, as expected, contained, bilirubin. Urine containing bilirubin is dark in color and forms large bubbles when shaken. Feces were pale or clay-colored.

Treatment and Nursing Care

Because Mrs. Helmer had fever and had been vomiting, she was somewhat dehydrated. She was given fluids containing glucose in physiological saline solution to correct the loss of water, chlorides, and calories. Because her biliary tract was obstructed and she had not been eating for several days, she was given multivitamins plus vitamin K in the intravenous infusion each day. Nursing of Mrs. Helmer during the period of diagnosis and preparation for surgery was directed toward providing comfort and emotional support and preventing complications as well as carrying out the aspects of diagnosis and treatment usually delegated to the nurse. Mrs. Helmer was a very sick woman who was fighting for survival and she behaved as sick people are likely to do. She regressed to a childlike state. Her tone of voice was whining. She complained repeatedly about how miserable she felt when she had to wait for care even briefly. She was petulant and irritable. She required and was provided with the same kind of care that any acutely ill person needs. She was given mouth care, was bathed, and had her back rubbed. The external environment was regulated to her for quiet and comfort. Because she was a member of a large family and had many friends, she required protection from too many visitors and from those who stayed too long. To prevent respiratory and circulatory complications, she was moved and turned and her extremities were passively exercised. Instructions were limited to preparing her for what was to be done at the time and to answering her questions. The nurse assumed full responsibility for the nursing care of Mrs. Helmer. The nurse anticipated her needs and she limited the demands made on Mrs. Helmer for adapting to her environment, including other people.

Although any change in the condition of a patient should be noted and recorded, observations of particular significance in the instance of Mrs. Helmer include increasing jaundice, color of stools and urine, and abdominal pain.

FAILURE OF THE LIVER

ETIOLOGY

In adidition to disorders involving the vascular system of the liver and the biliary canals, the liver parenchyma may fail. Because of the large reserve of liver parenchyma, evidence of failure of the metabolic and excretory functions is a relatively late manifestation in liver disease. Approximately 80 per cent of the liver can be destroyed before signs of liver failure appear. The liver is further protected by the great regenerative power of its cells. For example, in acute infectious hepatitis, areas of necrosis regenerate leaving no evidence of previous disease.

As stated previously, the most frequent cause of vascular congestion is failure of the right side of the heart as a pump. Parenchymatous cells can be injured by a wide variety of agents. Hepatotoxic agents range from the poisonous mushroom, *Amanita phalloides,* to a host of man-made chemicals.[41] Among the latter are chlorinated hydrocarbons used as solvents and chloroform, a general anesthetic; inorganic phosphorus, arsenic, and drugs such as sulfonamides, antithyroid agents, and tetracycline. Although about 30 per cent of patients with cirrhosis of the liver are alcoholics, cirrhosis was once thought to be caused primarily by the resulting malnutrition because it is well known that alcoholics eat poorly. However, fatty livers also occur in well-nourished alcoholics. Moreover, alcohol increases the susceptibility of the

liver to other toxic agents. The livers of some individuals also appear to be sensitive to agents not harmful to most persons.

Liver function, as well as the fact that the portal blood passes through the liver before entering the systemic circulation, exposes the liver to higher concentrations of pathogenic agents than other tissues. Some chemicals are concentrated 10- to 100-fold by the liver.[42] In addition to parenchymal injury from hepatotoxic agents, parenchymal damage can also result from disease or obstruction of the biliary tract.

According to Ingelfinger,[43] the effects of the various etiological agents on parenchymous cells of the liver are similar. Three principal factors probably account for similar morphological effects of different etiological agents. With the exception of hypoxia and certain specific poisons such as carbon tetrachloride and carbon trichloride (chloroform), etiological agents are poorly defined. In some patients a number of factors may be interacting to cause injury. Second, the number of ways in which liver cells can respond to injury is limited. Third, by the time the effects of disease of the liver are manifested, the defensive reactions of the liver tend to obscure the original injury.

To illustrate, Mrs. Clarence, aged 42, had a diagnosis of advanced portal cirrhosis of the liver. For the last ten years she had consumed increasing quantities of alcohol. For three or four months preceding her admission to the hospital, she had been drinking heavily and eating very little food. The only food that she ingested consistently was an 8-oz glass of orange juice on arising. Biopsy of her liver demonstrated necrosis of the parenchyma of her liver and extensive fibrosis. What factor or factors were responsible for the injury of Mrs. Clarence's liver? Was it caused by the alcohol or poisons contained in it or was it caused by lack of important nutrients such as protein and the B vitamins? Probably all these factors played a part.

LIVER FUNCTION TESTS

A great variety of tests have been used to determine abnormalities in the physiology and anatomy of the liver. Understanding of the nature and effects of liver disease has been greatly increased by a number of developments: (1) liver biopsy, (2) electron microscopy, (3) improved biochemical techniques, (4) knowledge of the role of intracellular and serum enzymes, (5) ability to study circulatory patterns, and (6) radioisotope scans.

Commonly prescribed tests with their pur-

---

[41] Hyman J. Zimmerman: "The Spectrum of Hepatotoxicity," *Perspect. Biol. Med.,* **12**:135–39 (Autumn) 1968.

[42] *Ibid.,* p. 140.

[43] Sodeman and Sodeman, *op. cit.,* p. 661.

poses and hazards are summarized. Directions for the performance of each test are not included because they vary in detail from one institution to another. The most important hazards to the patient are included, however, because some tests are accompanied by serious risks. Even when an untoward reaction is likely to occur only once in 1,000 patients, every patient should be treated as if he were that one.

BILIRUBIN—DIAGNOSTIC SIGNIFICANCE

Bilirubin, already referred to in the discussion of cholelithiasis, is a product of the degradation of heme, the pigmented portion of hemoglobin. It is discussed in greater detail in Chapter 10.

The level and type of bilirubin or its products found in the blood, feces, or urine have several uses in diagnosis. As products of the breakdown of hemoglobin, they can be used as a measure of the rate of blood destruction. As excretion products, they can be used as a measure of liver function or of the patency of the biliary tract. In some instances, the site of failure may be indicated by the form in which the substance occurs. For example, bilirubin levels in the blood rise (1) when the rate of blood destruction is excessive and the rate of formation is more rapid than the liver can excrete, (2) when certain types of injury to liver cells prevent its excretion, and (3) when the flow of bile from the liver to the intestine is blocked. With elevated bilirubin levels the skin, mucous membranes, and sclera of the eyes become a greenish yellow or jaundiced. The degree of jaundice is affected by the extent to which the bilirubin is elevated.

As it passes through the liver, the bilirubin molecule is conjugated with glucuronic acid to form bilirubin glucuronide, a water-soluble compound. Unconjugated bilirubin is not soluble in water. The van den Bergh reaction is based on the differences in the solubility of the free and conjugated forms. In the test, a color reagent is added to the blood. In obstructive jaundice an immediate change in color, known as the *direct* reaction, takes place; the concentration of bilirubin glucuronide is high. In hemolytic jaundice no color change occurs until the solubility of bilirubin is increased by adding alcohol; this is known as the *indirect* reaction and indicates a high level of unconjugated bilirubin. In inflammatory disorders such as hepatitis, the reaction may be intermediate.

Urine and stool examinations also help to distinguish between obstructive and hemolytic jaundice. In obstructive jaundice, bilirubin glucuronide is excreted in the urine. In hemolytic jaundice the urinary bilirubin is negative. In obstructive jaundice bilirubin does not enter the duodenum and the stool is clay-colored. In hemolytic jaundice bilirubin is secreted into the intestine and the color of the stool is normal.

BROMSULPHALEIN EXCRETION

The ability of the liver to remove a substance from the circulation and to excrete it can be measured by injecting a dye and measuring the rate at which it disappears from the blood. The Bromsulphalein (BSP) excretion test is the most widely used. In normal persons, 10 to 15 per cent of the dye is removed per minute. Less than 5 per cent of the dye should remain in the blood at the end of 45 min following injection. The greater the retention of Bromsulphalein, the greater is the liver injury. An occasional patient is hypersensitive to Bromsulphalein. This test should never be performed without appropriate preparation for this possibility.

TURBIDITY-FLOCCULATION TESTS

Two tests, or variations of them, are widely used to determine whether active parenchymal disease exists. These are the cephalin-cholesterol flocculation test and the thymol turbidity test. Blood serum is treated with the appropriate reagent and allowed to stand for a period of time. In the absence of disease no turbidity or flocculation takes place. In the presence of parenchymal disease a marked turbidity or flocculation, depending on the test used, appears. The flocculation is shown by most patients with acute viral hepatitis and is often positive before bilirubin levels are elevated and before jaundice appears. A negative test does not exclude hepatitis, however, inasmuch as up to one fifth of patients may give negative results. A high proportion of patients with cirrhosis shows a positive test, as do those with inflammation of the biliary tract. On the other hand, patients wtih biliary obstruction of short duration show normal values.

SERUM ENZYMES

Elevation of the level of two types of enzymes is useful in the diagnosis of liver or biliary tract disease. The tests are based on the principle that enzymes are released into the circulation following injury to a tissue. The tests are not specific for liver or biliary tract disease, and are useful only in association with other findings.

Transaminase enzymes—serum glutamic oxaloacetic transaminase (SGOT) and serum glutamic pyruvic transaminase (SGPT)—are found in high concentrations in the liver, heart, and skeletal muscle cells. When there are over 500 units of either enzyme in the blood, the patient is presumed to have liver damage, other conditions having been ruled out.

Serum alkaline phosphatase, another enzyme, is synthesized by the liver, bone, intestines, kidney, and placenta. The level of this enzyme is often elevated in conditions in which new bone is formed and in biliary tract obstruction.

LIVER SCANNING

A liver scan is based on the same general principle as the scan of any organ. The organ takes up and concentrates a chemical that can be made radioactive or labeled with a radioactive substance. In the case of the liver, ^{131}I-labeled rose bengal, or albumin labeled with ^{131}I may be used. From the liver scan, the size, shape, and location of the liver can be determined as well as the location of abnormal tissue.

What are some of the gastrointestinal manifestations of disease of the liver?

The signs and symptoms accompanying diseases of the liver depend on a number of factors such as the acuteness or chronicity of the disorder, the extent to which liver function is impaired, and the nature of the response of the liver to injury. Unless cirrhosis of the liver develops, the patient is not likely to develop ascites. Serious disease of the liver affects to a greater or lesser degree the functioning of all parts of the body.

As might well be expected, disorders of gastrointestinal function frequently accompany liver disease. Many of the gastrointestinal manifestations are caused by disorders in motility and are nonspecific, inasmuch as they are commonly seen in illness. They include anorexia, nausea, vomiting, flatulence, diarrhea, constipation, and cramping.

Anorexia is frequently observed in patients with a diagnosis of liver disease. This is of special significance in the nursing of the patient because one of the keystones in the therapy is a nutritious diet. To be of value, food must be eaten. When a patient is severely anorexic, he will usually require considerable attention and support to overcome his disinclination to eat. For example, Mr. Clarence, who has acute infectious hepatitis, is anorexic to the point that the thought of food causes a feeling of revulsion. His doctor has explained to him that anorexia is a cardinal manifestation in acute hepatitis, but that he will recover more rapidly if he can force himself to eat. Sometimes in the early stages intravenous glucose may be given until appetite returns to some extent.[44] Gradually, simple foods are added with emphasis on

[44] Charles S. Davidson: "Nutritional Aspects of Liver Diseases in Man," *Modern Nutrition in Health and Disease,* 4th ed., Michael G. Wohl and Robert S. Goodhart, eds. (Philadelphia: Lea & Febiger, 1968), p. 741.

those of high nutritional value. The patient should be expected to be a "fussy" or "finicky" eater, even if he eats everything when he is well. He should know why eating is important and he should be given whatever encouragement and assistance he requires. His food preferences should be taken into account in the selection of his meals.

Large meals may only serve to increase the anorexia and nausea. It is better to serve three small meals and to use interval feedings of a liquid formula. A variety of milk beverages reinforced with protein can be offered; they may be taken slowly over a period of time and may be well tolerated. If adequate nourishment cannot be given by mouth, tube feeding may be necessary as the main source of nutrition or as a supplement to the small meals eaten.

If the patient becomes exhausted before he has completed eating, he should be fed. Sometimes the relationship of the family or friends is such that he will eat when they feed him. The tray should be checked at the end of the meal, and the quantity of food not eaten should be recorded. If the patient will accept a substitute at a later time, this should be provided. One of the important functions of the nurse is to keep the lines of communication open between the patient, dietitian, and physician.

In disorders of the liver and biliary tract, digestion of food proceeds normally unless bile is prevented from reaching the alimentary canal. When bile does not reach the duodenum, the usual cause is biliary tract obstruction.

Changes in gastrointestinal function can also be caused by organic changes associated with liver disease. In portal cirrhosis, the alimentary canal may be congested as a consequence of portal hypertension.

CHANGES IN BLOOD CONSTITUENTS

Disease of the liver is accompanied by changes in a number of blood constituents resulting from the response of the organism to infectious agents or to cellular necrosis. In infectious hepatitis, neutrophils are frequently decreased and monocytes increased, probably caused by a response of mesenchymal tissues to the infectious agent and not by the involvement of the liver per se.

BLOOD PROTEINS

The liver synthesizes the blood proteins, including the serum albumin, which is especially important in maintaining the osmotic pressure; the fibrinogen, which is essential for blood clotting; and the globulins, which are involved in the immune processes. In serious liver disease the serum albumin level may be less than half the normal value. One effect of this decrease is the tendency of the tissues to hold fluid. By contrast the serum globulin level is increased, and the total serum protein (albumin + globulin) level may appear to be normal. The ratio of albumin to globulin is often less than 1:1, as compared with a normal ratio of 2:1 or 2.5:1.

ANEMIA

Many patients with disease of the liver have anemia, the type depending on the factors contributing to its incidence. Mrs. Helmer, for example, whose biliary tract was obstructed, developed hypoprothrombinemia from failure to absorb vitamin K. She had a microcytic hypochromic anemia; that is, her red cells were small in size and pale in color. Patients with repeated bleeding from esophageal varices may also have a microcytic anemia. Mrs. Clarence had a macrocytic anemia. Her red cells, though decreased in number, were larger than normal size. Normocytic and macrocytic anemias are common in the patient wtih cirrhosis of the liver. This type of anemia may be the result of increased blood destruction, or folacin deficiency, or some unknown factor.

HEMORRHAGIC TENDENCY

An increased tendency to bleed is a frequent finding in patients with disease of the liver. Failure to absorb vitamin K is a common cause. It is also thought that the liver, in some instances, is unable to utilize vitamin K to form prothrombin. Some patients who have a tendency to bleed have normal prothrombin levels; increased permeability of the capillaries or the lack of some other clotting factors may be at fault. Patients with disorders of the liver or biliary tract should be carefully observed for any evidence of hemorrhage. When bleeding occurs, the physician should be apprised of this fact.

SPIDER TELANGIECTASES

A phenomenon associated with cirrhosis of the liver is spider telangiectases. These are small, dilated blood vessels resembling a spider in form. They may be observed in the skin in various parts of the body.

THERAPY

Diet and rest are the basic considerations in the therapy of patients with disease of the liver. At least 1 g of protein per kilogram of body weight should be included; somewhat more liberal intake (90 to 120 g) is beneficial to many patients. The protein should be of good quality so that a complete assortment of amino acids is continuously available for maximum regeneration of liver tissue and for replacement of tissue and blood proteins. Sufficient calories from carbohydrates and fats should be provided so that protein can be used for tissue synthesis rather than for energy. The improvement in the level of serum albumin is sometimes exceedingly slow. Yet a nutritionally adequate diet improves the general sense of well-being, restores protein tissues of the body, and may reduce the tendency to edema.

The choice of food depends on the patient's preferences, provided that they are in accord with a nutritionally adequate diet. The restrictions in fat and the omission of spicy foods or strongly flavored vegetables are no longer considered to be necessary. Obviously, intolerance of particular foods should be respected, just as discretion should be used in menu planning. For example, many fried foods, very fatty meats, and rich pastries could produce discomfort, but butter, margarine, cream, ice cream, salad dressing, or an occasional piece of pastry might be enjoyed.

When anemia is present, the type and cause must be determined before satisfactory therapy can be instituted. Supplementary iron salts are prescribed for iron-deficiency anemia because the diet will seldom furnish more than 15 mg of iron per day; this is far too low to be of therapeutic value. Folic acid is often prescribed for macrocytic anemia, especially in alcoholic hepatitis.[45]

In addition to a nutritious diet, the other form of treatment used in the therapy of patients with disease of the liver is rest. Currently the subject of the extent to which rest should be prescribed is highly controversial. Some, but not all, physicians advocate complete bed rest until the serum bilirubin is reduced to 3 mg or less per 100 ml. Bed rest is thought to shorten the length of illness. Everything should be done to promote relaxation of the patient. All activities that can be done by someone else should be performed for the patient, and the physical, emotional, and social climate should be regulated so that rest is encouraged.

Although the physician prescribes the therapeutic regime for the patient with a disease of the liver, much of the responsibility for carrying it out is borne by the nurse. Whether the food served to the patient is eaten frequently depends on the patience and the persistence of a nurse who appreciates the importance of a nutritious diet to the recovery of the patient. Whether the patient is provided with an environment in

[45] Carroll M. Leevy: "Clinical Diagnosis, Evaluation and Treatment of Liver Disease in Alcoholics," *Fed. Proc.*, 26:1479 (Sept.–Oct.) 1967.

which rest is possible also depends on a nurse who understands the importance of rest to recovery and who acts in accordance with her understanding.

EDEMA

As the severity of disease of the liver increases, the patient retains sodium and water. Retained water may be distributed over the body as generalized edema or be concentrated to some extent in body cavities, particularly in the abdominal cavity as ascites and in the pleural cavity as hydrothorax. A number of mechanisms are usually implicated in the development of edema in liver disease. Not all are involved in every patient. Some authorities state that failure to inactivate aldosterone leads to increased retention of sodium and water by the kidney; others state that this failure is doubtful.

Another factor predisposing to edema formation is a decrease in the synthesis of albumin, which is the most important blood protein in the maintenance of the colloid osmotic pressure of the blood. A significant fall in the concentration of serum albumin, therefore, decreases the water-holding power of the blood.

In the liver itself, two changes may occur that increase the likelihood of the development of ascites. In cirrhosis of the liver, contraction of the liver by scar tissue leads to portal hypertension and to an elevation of the hydrostatic pressure of the blood in the portal capillaries. With increased capillary permeability, albumin and fluid escape into tissues and serous cavities and increase the water-holding power of the tissue and serous fluids.

Treatment of Edema

The treatment of edema in the patient with disease of the liver is similar to that for patients with healthy livers but who are edematous because of cardiovascular or renal disorders. To be sure, the edema associated with liver disease sometimes responds slowly to conservative measures and often reforms rapidly.

Restriction of sodium and an adequate to liberal intake of protein are important aspects of diet therapy in edema. Sodium restriction must usually be severe, ranging from no more than 200 to 500 mg daily. Not only must all foods be prepared without salt or other sodium compounds, but the amounts of meat, fish, poultry, eggs, and milk are carefully controlled because these foods are naturally high in sodium. Low-sodium milk is often substituted for regular milk. The sodium-restricted diet is probably one of the most difficult regimens for patients to accept, but by ingenuity in the use

of spices and herbs, much can be done to improve the flavor of foods. The patient needs to know why it is important for him to omit salt and any foods that contain other sodium compounds. In addition, medications that contain sodium should be avoided.

An occasional patient receiving a severely restricted sodium diet may show signs of sodium depletion, including abdominal pain, muscle cramping, weakness, lethargy, confusion, and convulsions.[46] This is especially true in patients who have cirrhosis and chronic renal disease. When any of these signs are detected, the physician should be notified.

The importance of protein for albumin synthesis has been pointed out in a preceding discussion. At a 500-mg sodium level of restriction, it is possible to include about 70 g of protein using regular milk and unsalted meats; when the sodium restriction is lower, low-sodium milk must be used to ensure an adequate intake of protein.

Paracentesis

When ascites or hydrothorax becomes so great that either interferes with the function of the alimentary canal or with breathing, fluid may be withdrawn from the peritoneal or thoracic cavity. Removal of fluid from either cavity involves intrusion in the internal environment, and both procedures should therefore be performed under sterile conditions. The general precautions to be taken when the pleural cavity is entered are discussed in Chapter 8.

Paracentesis is usually performed in the room of the patient or in the treatment room. The nurse has two general responsibilities. One is to prepare the patient and to support and comfort him during the procedure and the other is to assist the physician. The latter is also a service to the patient, inasmuch as assistance given by the nurse to the physician facilitates the care provided for the patient. The patient should be so prepared that he knows what to expect. Emphasis should be placed on the fact that as the result of the removal of fluid, he will be able to breathe more easily, move about more freely, and eat better. To prevent puncturing of the bladder during the procedure, the urinary bladder should be emptied by the patient or by catheterization before the procedure is attempted. If the paracentesis is performed on the patient in bed, he should be brought to the side of the bed and supported in a sitting position. If he is able, he may sit in a chair or with his feet over the edge of the bed. In whatever position he is placed, his back should be adequately

---

[46] Davidson, *op. cit.,* p. 750.

supported. The skin should be shaved if necessary and thoroughly cleansed.

To lessen the danger of puncturing the colon, the cannula is introduced at the mid-line and below the umbilicus. After the cannula has been introduced into the peritoneal cavity, tubing is attached to it and the ascitic fluid is drained into a pail or a bottle. Although either is a satisfactory receptacle, the physician may wish to collect the fluid under sterile conditions for purposes of examination or for infusing it into the patient.

After the procedure is completed, the skin at the site of puncture may require a stitch or two to close the incision. A small dressing may be all that is required. When it becomes wet, it should be replaced. The clothing of the patient and bedding should also be checked at the same time and changed as often as necessary. When ascites develops rapidly and the patient requires repeated paracenteses, the problem of keeping him dry may be considerable.

During the performance of paracentesis, fluid is withdrawn slowly to prevent syncope resulting from a too rapid reduction in intra-abdominal pressure. At the completion of the procedure a scultetus binder may be applied until the patient has adjusted to the decrease in intra-abdominal pressure.

Throughout the procedure the patient should be apprised of what is expected of him, of what is being done, and of his general progress. For example, when the nurse cleanses the skin, she should tell the patient what she is doing. When a solution that evaporates rapidly is placed on the skin, the patient should be prepared for the fact that it will be cold. As the physician injects the anesthetic into skin, or introduces the cannula into the peritoneal cavity, the patient should be informed of what is happening. After the peritoneal cavity has been entered and the fluid has started to flow, the patient should be informed. Whether the patient is undergoing paracentesis for the first or the hundredth time, he should be included as a participating member of the team. Attention should be given to the physical status of the patient. His pulse, respiration, and color should be noted and any undue change reported to the physician.

SIGNS OF SERIOUS LIVER DISEASE

In patients with serious disease of the liver, changes in the mental status, from mild confusion, disorientation, and irrational behavior to stupor and deep coma may appear. Hyperventilation and flapping tremor may also occur. In hyperventilation the depth of respiration is increased, but not the rate. In fact, the rate of respiration may be slower than normal. Not all patients with severe liver disease develop coma, nor do those who become comatose necessarily present the milder signs before developing coma.[47]

Although the reasons for the development of mental changes have not been completely identified, two mechanisms appear to be involved. They are the accumulation of metabolites, probably of a nitrogenous nature, in the internal environment of cells and an abnormal sensitivity of cerebral cells to changes in their fluid environment. Among the nitrogenous substances, ammonia and ammonia-bearing compounds are implicated. Hepatic coma can be precipitated in susceptible patients by orally administered ammonia compounds as well as by certain bacterial metabolites containing methionine. In the healthy liver, substances absorbed from the intestine, such as ammonia, are detoxified before they reach the general circulation. Ammonia is converted to urea. In severe liver disease, the liver cells are assumed to be unable to convert ammonia and other potentially harmful nitrogenous materials to harmless ones. Another possibility is that blood containing these substances does not pass through the liver before it enters the general circulation. Blood flow may be detoured around the liver by naturally occurring or surgical shunts.

Coma can be precipitated in susceptible patients by agents increasing the load of nitrogenous substances or by sodium-excreting diuretics. Thus a high-protein diet predisposes to coma because of the increased production of ammonia by the deaminization of the amino acids. When there is impending coma, a protein-free diet or a very low-protein diet (20 to 30 g) is usually prescribed. The calorie intake should be maintained as high as practical by fruit juices reinforced with glucose in order to minimize tissue breakdown. The catabolism of tissues is a source of ammonia through the breakdown of the constituent amino acids. Even 500 to 600 calories per day can be quite effective in keeping tissue breakdown to a minimum.

Ammonium drugs such as ammonium chloride increase the load of nitrogenous substances to be excreted. Carbonic anhydrase inhibitors such as acetazolamide (Diamox[48]) also increase the possibility of coma by increasing the excretion of the sodium ion. Because these agents are also of value in the therapy of the patient with liver disease, the physician may prescribe one or more for a given patient. The nurse should be alert to and promptly report

[47] In stupor, the patient can be, but is not easily, aroused. In coma he cannot be aroused.

[48] Trade name.

any changes in the patient's mental alertness and status. Nursing of the comatose patient is discussed in Chapter 19, Part C.

Metabolism and Some Related Nutritional Problems

Cellular Functions

The quality of nutrition depends not only on the kinds and amounts of food supplied to the body and its preparation by the digestive tract for absorption but also on the capacity of the organism to carry out its physiological and biochemical functions. *Intermediary metabolism* is used to describe all the changes taking place within cells of the internal environment, including the building-up, breaking-down, and functional activities. It is often thought of as those activities beginning at the point when digestion has been completed. The intestinal wall, thought of as part of the external environment, is involved in the active transport of materials and in the synthesis of many compounds, and these activities are properly included in intermediary metabolism. Thus one cannot draw a sharp line of demarcation.

ANABOLISM

The synthesis of larger molecules from smaller ones is known as *anabolism;* for example, the production of the various structural components of the cell itself or the synthesis of compounds secreted by the cells such as enzymes, hormones, and others. Cellular proteins are synthesized from amino acids, fats from fatty acids or glucose, and so on. The anabolic activities are energy-saving.

CATABOLISM

On the other hand, *catabolism* is the breaking up of large molecules to smaller ones. Thus glucose, fatty acids, glycerol, and amino acids are oxidized to yield the energy required for the synthetic and functional activities of the cell. The breakdown of energy-containing compounds yields lower energy compounds or carbon dioxide and water, and, in the case of amino acids, urea.

METABOLIC BALANCE

Anabolic and catabolic activities take place continuously throughout life and are equal in the healthy adult who has no net change in body size. When new tissues are being added to the body, the anabolic activities exceed the catabolic activities, as in the growth of children, during pregnancy, and in the period of recovery from illness or injury. Catabolic processes exceed anabolic processes during weight loss whether planned or occasioned by starvation, serious illness, or trauma from injury.

FUNCTIONAL ACTIVITIES

Among the functional activities of the cells are contraction of the muscles, the transmission of nerve impulses, the secretion of glands, the selective absorption from the intestine, and the excretion of waste products by the kidneys and other organs. Homeostasis is maintained by continuous regulation of the transport of materials across the cell membranes and of the extracellular fluid environment of the cells. For example, the sodium ion is continuously entering the cell, yet in health it does not accumulate in it. Energy is required to prevent the sodium ion concentration in the cell from approaching the concentration of the extracellular fluid.

Energy, glucose, fatty acid, amino acid, and calcium metabolism represent just a few examples of the many aspects of intermediary metabolism. Space as well as the complexity of each of these aspects of metabolism permits only the briefest summary in this text. Many textbooks of biochemistry are available for the student who desires further details of a specific aspect of metabolism.

Some General Aspects of Metabolic Processes

OXIDATION REDUCTION

The chemical reactions within the cell that release energy are primarily oxidative. According to the electron theory, oxidation is a process whereby one or more electrons are given up. As a result, electrons are lost, valence raised, oxygen added, or hydrogen removed. The compound that causes oxidation is always reduced. Therefore, oxidation always involves reduction, the basic change in the latter being a gain in electrons; that is, the valence is lowered, oxygen is lost, or hydrogen is added. Thus to have oxidation reduction, a substance donating electrons and another accepting electrons must be present.

How does the body maintain a constant supply of materials for metabolic activities?

THE METABOLIC POOL

The body maintains a supply of nutrients instantly available for the regulation of its activities and the maintenance of homeostasis. This is often referred to as the *metabolic pool,* which is an intimate combination of the nutrients available through absorption from the intestinal tract plus those that are constantly released by the catabolic and secretory activities of the cell. The metabolic pool must not be thought of as having a specific body location; it is rather that instant availability of essential nutrients at any given site to carry out any given activity. For example, the metabolic pool of amino acids would include those from the intestinal tract, those released by the breakdown of cellular proteins, and those derived from cellular synthesis. From this assortment, cells could withdraw the exact kinds and amounts of amino acids required for the synthesis of any given protein.

NUTRITIONAL NEEDS OF CELLS

Cellular function depends on an adequate supply of (1) energy-producing materials, chiefly glucose, fatty acids, glycerol, and amino acids; (2) tissue-building materials including a complete assortment of about 20 amino acids, some fatty acids, carbohydrates, and mineral elements such as calcium, phosphorus, sodium, potassium, magnesium, and many others; and (3) materials for the synthesis of a myriad of regulatory substances such as enzymes and hormones. Many of these regulatory substances are of a protein nature and therefore require varying assortments of amino acids. Some incorporate specific carbohydrates or lipids, or both. Trace elements such as iron, manganese, fluorine, iodine, molybdenum, selenium, zinc, copper, and others are essential as are also the fat-soluble and water-soluble vitamins. In all, more than 50 nutrients are required for cellular function.

ENZYMES AS CATALYSTS

Oxidation-reduction reactions depend on innumerable enzymes, each of which acts on a specific chemical bond. Each enzyme either donates or receives electrons. The maintenance of metabolic activities depends on the capacity of the cell to synthesize enzymes and to synthesize or recover chemicals needed to keep the process going. For example, pyruvic acid ($CH_3COCOOH$) is subjected to oxidative decarboxylation and reacts with coenzyme A to form acetyl coenzyme A. The acetyl coenzyme A is combined with oxaloacetic acid to form citric acid. For the cycle to continue, oxaloacetic acid must be either recovered or synthesized. See Figure 12-4.

The activity of the enzymes is related to the concentration of materials on which they act, the pH of the environment, and the temperature. The use of hypothermia in certain surgical procedures is based on the fact that the rate of metabolism in cells is reduced by lowering of body temperature. As body temperature is lowered, enzyme activity is reduced and the rate of metabolism is diminished.

ENZYME COFACTORS

Many enzymes require coenzymes or cofactors for their activity. These usually are compounds of low molecular weight that may be tightly bound as a prosthetic group to the protein part of the enzyme molecule or they may be loosely attached to the protein. Most vitamins function as coenzymes in enzyme systems that control cellular activity. For example, thiamine pyrophosphate, a coenzyme known as cocarboxylase, is the prosthetic group for the enzyme carboxylase. This enzyme is essential for the removal of the carboxyl group from pyruvic acid, an intermediate product in the metabolism of glucose (see Figure 12-5). When thiamine is lacking in the diet, insufficient carboxylase is available for decarboxylation to proceed, and pyruvic acid accumulates in the blood. The interference with carbohydrate metabolism at this point is serious, and, if uncorrected, leads to the classic deficiency disease, beriberi.

Riboflavin, niacin, pantothenic acid, biotin, vitamin B_{12}, folacin, and vitamin B_6 are also constituents of coenzymes and therefore are intimately associated with energy and amino acid metabolism. Ascorbic acid and vitamins E and K probably have coenzyme functions, but these are not clearly understood at the present time. The role of vitamins in enzyme activity helps to explain the correlation of dietary requirements of them with the caloric and protein needs of the individual. A deficiency of any of the coenzymes interferes with the metabolic machinery so that succeeding steps in anabolism or catabolism cannot take place. Hence the resulting symptoms are those of multiple deficiencies rather than of specific failure of one metabolic step.

Mineral elements are also important cofactors for enzyme activity. They include magnesium, iron, copper, molybdenum, zinc, manganese, and others.

ENZYME INHIBITORS

The action of enzymes may be inhibited by the action of heavy metals and by certain drugs. One way that mercury is believed to produce toxicity is by inhibiting enzyme reactions. Chemicals such as cyanide are highly toxic because they inhibit enzyme systems catalyzing oxidation-reduction reactions. Death occurs in a matter of minutes following the ingestion or inhalation of cyanide.

The actions of many drugs depend on their ability to depress enzymatic activity. Barbiturates may depress the nervous system by depressing specific enzymes. Acetazolamide (Diamox) induces diuresis by interfering with the ability of the enzyme carbonic anhydrase to catalyze the reaction enabling the kidney to

FIGURE 12-4. Glycolysis—the conversion of glucose to pyruvic acid and lactic acid. (Adapted with permission of CIMA from *The Ciba Collection of Medical Illustrations*, Plate V, by Frank H. Netter, M.D. Copyright © CIBA.)

FIGURE 12-5.—Protein metabolism. (Adapted with permission of CIBA from *The Ciba Collection of Medical Illustrations*, Plate IV, by Frank H. Netter, M.D. Copyright © CIBA.)

reabsorb the sodium ion. As a result, the kidney excretes an increased volume of sodium ion in the urine. Sulfonamides are effective in the control of certain bacteria because they depress the enzyme system, enabling them to synthesize folic acid from para-aminobenzoic acid.

INBORN ERRORS OF METABOLISM

Disorders of metabolism result from the inability of the cell to synthesize a specific enzyme. The capacity to synthesize enzymes depends on the genetic inheritance of the individual. A single gene is involved in a single metabolic reaction. A defective gene may be inherited as a mendelian recessive or dominant. When inherited as a recessive trait, the defect is evident only in individuals inheriting the same trait from both parents. In the absence of the necessary enzyme, a metabolic process is stopped at the point where the missing enzyme acts.

Numerous enzyme-deficiency diseases are now recognized, including such widely known conditions as phenylketonuria, galactose disease, maple syrup urine disease, and leucine-induced hypoglycemia. The metabolic errors produce marked changes in the infant shortly after birth, mental retardation being particularly severe. In some of the diseases it is possible to prevent the severe abnormalities by the early institution of a diet that is carefully regulated to limit or omit the nutrient that cannot be adequately metabolized.

In phenylketonuria, the enzyme that is essential for the conversion of phenylalanine to tyrosine is missing. As a consequence the central nervous system fails to develop and severe mental retardation results. The early detection of the abnormality means that a low-phenylalanine diet can be initiated, thereby making possible essentially normal development of the infant. Galactose disease, resulting from the inability to convert galactose to glucose, likewise leads to severe mental retardation and other abnormalities. It is amenable to treatment, the omission of all sources of milk being essential. Some success has been achieved with the use of very expensive synthetic formulas restricted in isoleucine, leucine, and valine in the treatment of maple syrup urine disease. No treatment has currently been developed for a number of metabolic errors.

How is the rate of energy metabolism controlled?

HORMONAL CONTROLS

The rate at which enzymes catalyze chemical reactions is subject to control by hormones, or "chemical messengers." More than 20 hormones have been isolated and studied. They include those produced by the ductless glands, such as the thyroid, parathyroid, pancreas, adrenal, and pituitary. Some of their effects will be detailed in the sections that follow.

SOURCES OF ENERGY

The carbohydrates, fats, and proteins of the diet are the ultimate sources of all energy for the body. In typical diets of the United States, carbohydrates furnish about 45 to 55 per cent,

fats about 40 to 45 per cent, and proteins about 15 per cent of the calories. In the underdeveloped countries of the world carbohydrate is responsible for as much as three fourths of the total energy value of the diet.

The body itself is provided with energy reserves that are utilized throughout each day and that can maintain the organism for a surprising length of time when no food is ingested. Glycogen constitutes a relatively small, readily available reserve, but, at best, it can supply the energy needs for only part of one day. Adipose tissue, on the other hand, furnishes a substantial and continuous reserve of energy that can, in emergency, be relied on for days or even weeks. When starvation continues, some cellular substance is also sacrificed to supply calories. Because of the loss of fat and other tissue substance, weight declines. The loss of weight decreases the quantity of tissue requiring support; and because of a loss of strength, less energy is utilized for nonsurvival purposes. The body's own substance is thereby used more slowly and life can be further prolonged.

ENERGY TRANSFER

The central mechanism in bringing about the transfer of energy is in the reversible system of adenosine triphosphate (ATP) and adenosine diphosphate (ADP). When glucose, for example, is converted to glycogen, energy is required to bring about the reaction. The energy is furnished by splitting off a high-energy phosphate group from ATP. The remaining compound, having one less phosphate group, is ADP. When glucose is oxidized to carbon dioxide and water, some of the energy set free in the reaction is used to rebuild ATP from ADP. In this way the body maintains a constant source of high-energy bonds.

This system operates in a wide range of anabolic activities including the synthesis of acetylcholine for the transmission of the nerve impulse, sugar phosphates, proteins from amino acids, urea by the liver, and ammonia by the kidney. ATP also provides the energy for the absorption of sugars from the intestine and the reabsorption of glucose by the kidney.

Muscle cells also synthesize creatine phosphate, another high-energy phosphate compound. This is an available store of energy for the contraction of the muscle fiber.

COMMON DENOMINATOR

Three major stages characterize the degradation of carbohydrates, fats, and amino acids to furnish energy for cellular activities. In the first, glucose, fatty acids, and amino acids are converted through a series of independent steps

FIGURE 12-6. Oxidative breakdown (the Krebs cycle). (Adapted with permission of CIBA from *The Ciba Collection of Medical Illustrations*, Plate VI, by Frank H. Netter, M.D. Copyright © CIBA.)

and catalyzed by individual enzymes, to molecules serving as "common denominators" for all. These are pyruvic acid, acetyl coenzyme A, and alpha-ketoglutaric acid. Little energy is released in this stage. These common molecules then enter the last two stages to be converted to energy, carbon dioxide, and water.

THE CITRIC ACID CYCLE

The second stage in the release of energy is known as the citric acid, tricarboxylic acid, or Krebs cycle. The first molecule in the ring to be metabolized is citric acid. The molecules in the cycle are three-carbon groupings, and

Krebs first described the reactions. The routes by which carbohydrates, fats, and proteins reach the cycle, as well as the changes taking place within the cycle, are shown in Figures 12-4, 12-5, and 12-6. The reactions are cyclic because the series of compounds involved are utilized and regenerated so that the chain can start over again whenever another molecule of pyruvic acid or acetyl coenzyme A is available for oxidation.

RESPIRATORY CYCLE

The third stage is known as the respiratory cycle. It consists of the removal of carbon dioxide from the body via respiration and the combination of hydrogen atoms with oxygen available through respiration into water. Each of the steps in the transfer of hydrogen to oxygen requires specific enzyme activity.

ENERGY REQUIREMENT

Food energy is required to maintain the resting metabolism, the body temperature, the voluntary activity, and the synthesis of new tissues. The recommended allowance for the 22-year-old male engaged in light activity and weighing 70 kg (154 lb) is 2,800 calories, and for the 22-year-old female weighing 58 kg (128 lb) it is 2,000 calories.[49] By age 65 these allowances for men and women who have maintained their same weights and levels of activity have been reduced to 2,400 and 1,700 calories, respectively. The 10- to 12-year-old boy weighing 35 kg (77 lb) needs 2,500 calories, and the girl of the same weight and age needs about 2,250 calories. These allowances take into account such factors as body size, age, activity, climate, and growth needs.

BODY SIZE

In general, the large individual has a greater energy requirement than the small one. An obese adult, however, because of less lean body mass and less activity, may not have a greater energy requirement than the person of normal size. Small animals have a higher metabolic rate than larger ones with the result that they require more food per unit of mass. A bird or mouse requires more food per gram of body weight than an elephant. An infant with his relatively large surface area and high rate of metabolism requires more calories per kilogram of body weight than does the adult.

LEAN BODY TISSUE

Males generally require more calories than do females, because of greater body size and greater proportions of lean body tissue. Beginning with early adulthood (about 22 years), a steady decline in caloric need takes place. This is explained in part by the reduction in lean body mass and hence in basal metabolic rate and in part by a gradual diminution in voluntary activity. Nevertheless, there is no decrease in the number of calories required by an older person to perform any given activity. Mrs. Bird requires as many calories to walk a mile as does her 16-year-old grandson who weighs the same as she does.

ACTIVITY

Voluntary activity is an important factor in determining the energy requirement but it is somewhat difficult to make a precise estimate for the various levels of work and play. The recommended allowances have been set up for people whose activity may be described as "light." For many inactive persons in the United States these allowances could result in weight gain. The individual who is engaged in heavy labor might require up to 1,500 calories in excess of the stated allowances.[50]

CLIMATE

Extremes of climate will affect the need for energy, but for most people in the United States the heating of buildings in winter and their cooling in summer together with adjustments in the clothing worn tend to equalize the calorie requirements throughout the seasons. Exposure to severe cold weather increases the calorie expenditure to maintain the body temperature, and shivering rapidly increases the energy expenditure. The wearing of heavy cold-weather clothing and footwear further adds to the energy need. Surprisingly, physically active people living in tropical areas have a higher calorie requirement than those in temperate climates at the same level of activity because of the energy needed to dissipate additional heat from the body.

GROWTH

Rapid growth greatly increases the calorie requirement. Infants, for example, require 100 to 120 calories per kilogram to support their growth, their considerable activity, and their proportionately large surface area. By comparison, the calorie allowance for a 13-year-old boy is about 63 calories per kilogram and for his 45-year-old father is only 37 calories per kilogram.

The development of the fetus and the maternal tissues during pregnancy represents a considerable need for energy as well as for all

[49] *Recommended Dietary Allowances,* 7th rev. ed. (Washington, D.C.: 1968), Pub. No. 1694. Food and Nutrition Board, National Academy of Sciences, National Research Council.

[50] *Op. cit.,* p. 6.

nutrients, most especially during the last trimester. Many women decrease their activity during this period so that the addition of about 200 calories usually suffices. During lactation each 100 ml of milk secreted entails an expenditure of 120 calories; thus a daily secretion of 850 ml of milk would increase the need by 1,000 calories.

Obesity

Although the incidence of obesity is high among Americans, obesity is neither confined to Americans nor a new problem. It is found among the wealthy, sedentary individuals in all parts of the world. Art objects uncovered in the ruins of ancient civilizations attest to its antiquity. The Venus of Willendorf is a limestone statuette named for the Austrian village in which it was discovered, and the figure is indistinguishable from the present-day fat woman. The Venus of Willendorf, however, is the figure of a Stone Age woman and antedates the development of agriculture by 10,000 years. The group in which the Venus of Willendorf lived were hunters. They probably gorged themselves when food was plentiful, as after a successful hunt, and fasted or starved when food was scarce. In fact, the fatty deposits stood them in good stead during the periods of scarcity.

Considering so many factors affecting energy balance, one must marvel at the homeostatic mechanisms by which most people are able to maintain desirable weight throughout life. Yet, a substantial proportion of the population, perhaps 10 per cent of all school children, and 20 to 25 per cent of all adults, experiences overweight and obesity to some degree. Food in the United States is so plentiful and attractive in its many forms that overeating can easily become a habit. Many people lead sedentary lives at work and in leisure so that they can ill afford the calorie-rich foods so widely available for meals and snacks. Too many people lack knowledge concerning calorie and nutrient values of foods and often do not realize that even small intakes beyond daily energy needs lead, in time, to gross obesity. This growing public health problem requires a careful study of the many reasons obesity may occur and of ways by which it may be prevented or treated. How is the determination of obesity made?

DEFINITION OF OBESITY

Obesity is an excessive accumulation of fatty or adipose tissue. On the average, adipose tissue contains about 72 per cent fat and 23 per cent water. Protein and mineral elements account for the remainder of the tissue, including the structural components of the cells, blood vessels, and nerves.[51] Thus adipose tissue differs markedly from lean tissue, which contains somewhat over 70 per cent water. Contrary to earlier beliefs adipose tissue is not inert but participates actively in energy metabolism by synthesizing triglycerides from fatty acids or glucose and by releasing free fatty acids to the circulation. (See "Lipid Metabolism," p. 561.)

Height-weight tables have long been used to determine the degree of overweight and obesity. Because it is generally agreed that it is undesirable to gain weight throughout life, weight considered to be normal for height and body frame at age 22 years is accepted as desirable throughout life. A weight increase of 10 per cent over the desirable level is usually defined as overweight, and an excess of 20 per cent or more is designated as obesity. Those individuals who are grossly obese are detected visually, but for people who are moderately overweight the height-weight tables do not provide an accurate guide for body fatness. Jim Johnson is a college athlete who weighs 20 lbs more than tables indicate he should. He has a well-developed musculature and no evidence of thick folds of fatty subcutaneous tissue; he is not obese. Sally Brown is within 5 lb of her desirable weight but leads a very inactive life. She has moderately thick folds of fatty tissue around the abdomen. She is slightly obese, although the tables do not so indicate.

The normal fat content of the body increases steadily from infancy, girls becoming fatter than boys by the early school years. The percentage of body fat increases throughout life as lean tissue decreases, even though weight remains stationary. The occasional exceptions are those individuals who remain vigorously active throughout life. At all ages women have a higher percentage of body fat than do males. By methods used in the research laboratory, body fat content in excess of 20 per cent for adolescent males and 25 per cent for adolescent females is classed as obesity. In adults, obesity is considered to be present if the fat content exceeds 20 per cent in males and 30 per cent in females.[52] The thickness of subcutaneous tissue is a more reliable indicator of the degree of fatness than are height-weight tables. Clinicians often make a rough estimation by simply pinching up a fold of skin. By using calipers,

[51] Edward Staunton West et al.: Textbook of Biochemistry, 4th ed. (New York: The Macmillan Company, 1966), p. 416.

[52] Ruth Huenemann et al.: "Adolescent Food Practices Associated with Obesity," Fed. Proc., 25:4–10 (Jan.–Feb.) 1966.

the exact thickness of the tissue may be determined at selected points such as the triceps and subscapular skinfolds and compared with normal standards for fatness.

What are the effects of obesity on health?

HAZARDS OF OBESITY

Obesity is of concern primarily because it has an adverse effect on health and life expectancy. Adipose tissue places a double burden on the individual. Excess tissue has to be carried as a weight on the individual. Mrs. Albert carries a 55-lb weight with her everywhere she goes, upstairs and down as well as on a level. Obese tissue also has to be supported with nutrients. Each pound of adipose tissue contains 0.7 mile or more of capillaries through which blood circulates.

Diabetes mellitus in adults is highly associated with obesity. It is now believed that obesity is not a cause of diabetes but that it is an early manifestation of the metabolic defect that in later life leads to the typical symptoms of diabetes. Gout and diseases of the liver and gallbladder are also found more frequently in the obese. With a positive energy balance, fatty components in the blood rise and predispose the individual to atherosclerosis and coronary disease. Those individuals who have arthritis or osteoporosis find that the burden of fat to be carried around is an additional handicap.

Although a moderate degree of overweight (10 to 20 per cent) is not always regarded as harmful, statistics indicate that the mortality rate goes up as the weight rises above the desirable level. According to the findings of the Build and Blood Pressure Study made in 1959 by the Society of Actuaries [53] on men aged from 51 to 69 years, the mortality rate for those who were 10 per cent or more overweight for height and age was one fifth higher than for those insured at standard risks. Among men who were 20 per cent or more overweight, mortality was one third higher. The mortality rate rises with increasing weight. The adverse effects of obesity were greater in the 40-to-69 age group than in the 15-to-39 group. Disorders of the cardiovascular and renal systems accounted for a high percentage of the excess mortality among the overweight men.

CAUSES OF OBESITY

In the final analysis obesity is caused by an energy intake in excess of the body's expenditure of energy. There are, however, many causes for this imbalance.

[53] *Statist. Bull. Metrop. Life Ins. Co.,* **41**:6–9 (Feb.) 1960.

OVEREATING

Excessive ingestion of food has been the most frequently cited cause of obesity. Overeating may be related to the cultural pattern or may be an expression of some psychologic disorder. Great importance is attached to food in social situations, the food industries entice the consumer with attractive advertising for calorie-rich foods, and snacks have become a way of life in America. The dietary patterns of some families predominate in calorie-rich foods. Unfortunately, overemphasis on excessive eating as a cause of obesity has led many health workers to adopt an unjustified moralistic stand against the individual.

PSYCHOLOGICAL FACTORS IN OVEREATING

Because the nervous system participates in the regulation of eating, overeating frequently has a psychological basis. In some persons overeating accomplishes two psychological purposes or gains. The first is a primary gain. Food is used to substitute for gratification in life situations. Eating relieves unpleasant feelings —loneliness, frustration, guilt, depression, insecurity, or anxiety. As an example, everyone is acquainted with someone who eats when bored or who makes additional trips to the refrigerator when preparing for an important examination.

Secondary psychological gains involve the use of eating not for its direct effect on relieving unpleasant feelings, but to bring about desired changes in interpersonal relationships. It may be used offensively to control or gain attention of others. For example, a youngster overeats because by so doing he pleases his mother. Overeating may be a defensive maneuver utilized by the individual to protect himself from contact with others. For example, Dorothy, aged 15, is 50 lb overweight. She is a shy, anxious girl who fears rejection by her peers. She uses her obesity as a reason for avoiding others. In effect, a thick layer of fat serves to insulate her from people in her environment.

INACTIVITY

One of the most neglected factors in the incidence of obesity is relative inactivity rather than excessive eating of food. In the American culture, machines have largely replaced human beings in the performance of manual labor. In fact, the machine has greatly reduced physical activity in all aspects of the life of man. The farmer not only uses a tractor to cultivate his fields, but both he and his city cousin use a machine to mow their lawns. When a man plays golf, he rides a motorized cart because it speeds his game and is easier. When he needs something from the corner store, he rides in a car. Even children ride to school or to the park. Elevators make it unnecessary to walk from one floor to another. The home is equipped with labor-saving devices from vacuum cleaners to electric beaters and dishwashers. Many recreational activities are for the spectator rather than the participant. Because machines have reduced the need for physical exercise, control of caloric intake combined with regular exercise is necessary for control of weight.

People of middle age and older continue to eat about as much throughout their lives as they did in their youth. Mrs. Simon, age 45, is a good example. Despite lessening activity, she eats about as much as she did when her children were young and she was very active. She has gained 10 lb over the last 8 to 10 years and complains of her thickening waist. Her weight gain is probably caused by failure to adjust her food intake to her diminishing energy requirements.

Insufficient activity has been established as a primary cause of obesity in many boys and girls. During the winter months obese girls gained excessive amounts of weight. They ate less than nonobese girls but spent much less time in occupations requiring exercise. Even during exercise periods obese girls were observed to stand around more and to exercise less than normal-weight girls.[54]

ENDOCRINE IMBALANCE

Aberrations of the hormonal control of energy metabolism are responsible for only a small percentage of obese individuals. Hypothyroidism is the best known of these. The lessened secretion of thyroxine reduces the basal metabolic rate, sometimes as much as 30 to 40 per cent, so that the required number of calories to maintain the resting metabolism is reduced. These individuals are likely to be inactive, thereby further decreasing the energy expenditure. Consequently, obesity is likely unless the calorie intake is maintained at levels considerably below the expected normal.

Adrenocortical hyperfunction may lead to a condition known as Cushing's syndrome or moonface obesity. A lesion of the pituitary results in Fröhlich's syndrome, a type of obesity occasionally seen in children. These obesities are characterized by abnormal fat deposits in certain regions of the body.

HEREDITY

Mr. Johns says, "I'm fat. My father and mother were fat, as were their mothers and fathers." Perhaps heredity is used too often by people as an explanation of their obesity. Frequently the explanation for obesity in several members of a family lies in a cultural pattern dictating the hearty eating of many rich foods. This is not always the case, however. Mayer has found that 80 per cent of children are obese if both their parents are obese, 40 to 50 per cent of the children are obese if one parent is obese, and only 10 per cent of children are obese if neither parent is obese.[55] He states that there are "constitutional and genetic factors operating in the predisposition to obesity."[56]

The endomorphic (soft, round) individual must continuously control his diet and increase his activity to control his weight, whereas the ectomorphic (lean, wiry) individual is able to follow the dictates of his appetite without fear of growing fat. Inasmuch as these body types are inherited, the tendency to obesity may likewise be said to have a genetic origin. The point most worthy of emphasis is that early recognition of body types in children could result in the initiation of effective measures relating to food intake and activity so that obesity could be prevented in these highly prone individuals.

METABOLIC OBESITY

An error in fat and carbohydrate metabolism has not been conclusively demonstrated as a cause of obesity in man, although studies on experimental animals suggest the possibility of such genetic defects. Certain strains of obese mice have been developed that demonstrate a number of metabolic abnormalities.[57] These mice were much less active and had a lower oxygen consumption. Hyperglycemia, glycosuria, and high blood cholesterol levels were present. The mice were resistant to insulin, but the pancreas produced more insulin than normally. Lipogenesis was increased, but the amount of endogenous fat burned was less than normal.

Biochemical abnormalities have also been observed in some obese adolescents and adults.[58,59]

[54] Jean Mayer: "Physical Activity and Anthropometric Measurements of Obese Adolescents," *Fed. Proc.*, **25**:11–14 (Jan.–Feb.) 1966.

[55] Jean Mayer: "Obesity: Causes and Treatment," *Amer. J. Nurs.*, **59**:1732 (Dec.) 1959.

[56] Jean Mayer, *op. cit.*

[57] Jean Mayer: "An Experimentalist's Approach to the Problem of Obesity," *J. Amer. Diet. Ass.*, **31**:230–35 (Mar.) 1955.

[58] Felix P. Heald: "Natural History and Physiological Basis of Adolescent Obesity," *Fed. Proc.*, **25**:1–3 (Jan.–Feb.) 1966.

[59] Marshall Goldberg and Edgar S. Gordon: "Energy Metabolism in Human Obesity," *JAMA*, **189**:616–23 (Aug. 24) 1964.

The insulin levels were significantly elevated and a glucose infusion resulted in a still greater production of insulin. However, these individuals were resistant to insulin as demonstrated by hyperglycemia and the lessened ability to mobilize free fatty acids from adipose tissue. Whether these abnormalities are related to the cause of the obesity or are the result of the excess weight has not been ascertained.

Meal spacing in animals has also resulted in variations in the rate of fat deposition. Rats are natural nibblers, eating 20 to 30 times per day. When they are force-fed only twice per day with the same quantity and quality of food, they exhibit a number of changes. Among these is an increase in body fat.[60] The American who eats a small breakfast and lunch and a large dinner might, in fact, be placing undue stress on the mechanisms of fat metabolism and the deposition of fat could be favored.

PREVENTION OF OBESITY

About 80 per cent of obese children remain obese in later years. Because chronic obesity is especially resistant to treatment, particular emphasis should be given to its prevention in childhood and adolescence. Infant-feeding practices may need to be modified so that the mother does not force the last bit of formula or other food; the fat baby is not necessarily the healthiest baby. Preschool children need to have sufficient diversion by various activities so that they do not become unduly preoccupied with eating. Throughout the school years the child and adolescent should have opportunity to learn about the nutrient and calorie values of food, to know something of food selection for daily meals, and to understand the role of food in weight control. In some instances attention must be given to cultural patterns that encourage excessive food intake through emphasis on calorie-rich foods with great values being attached to eating. The programs of physical education should aim toward physical fitness throughout life by encouraging activities that can be continued into the later years.

Adults in their 20's and 30's need to be aware of the ease with which they may gain 5 or 10 lb in a year, and that these gains are often the results of small daily excesses of food or of gradual decreases in daily activity. Watching one's weight, engaging in physical activity, and taking prompt steps to correct small gains will eliminate the problems of later obesity.

[60] Clarence Cohn: "Meal-Eating, Nibbling, and Body Metabolism," *J. Amer. Diet. Ass.,* 38:433–36 (May) 1961.

TREATMENT OF OBESITY

The treatment of obesity would appear to be a relatively simple matter, namely, to reduce the energy intake below that of the body's expenditure. Yet, in actual practice, obesity is difficult to treat, and the failures are many. Those who have become obese in middle age are most likely to succeed, whereas those who have been obese since childhood or adolescence are seldom successful.

The satisfactory treatment of obesity should meet the following aims: (1) weight loss to a level desirable for the individual, (2) the maintenance of good nutrition throughout the period of weight loss, and (3) lifetime modification of food habits so that the desirable weight is maintained. A newspaper columnist, in writing of his experience with a reduction diet, stated that he was waiting for the day when he had attained the desired loss of weight. On that day he planned to eat all the rich foods he desired so greatly. Apparently his aim was to lose weight and not to maintain a desirable weight.

To achieve the desired goals, professional guidance is essential throughout. A thorough evaluation of each individual must be made by the therapist to determine the causes of the obesity, the factors that may be useful in bringing about motivation, and whether any psychological factors would contradict the imposition of a weight-losing regimen.

Unless the obese individual has developed for himself sound reasons for weight loss and is determined to follow a prescribed regimen, any efforts by the therapist are doomed to failure. Among the more common reasons are pride in personal appearance, improved health status, avoidance of jibes of family, friends, and business associates, and desire to improve health or to avoid one of the chronic disorders associated with obesity. Sometimes the obese person finds that, to obtain a particular job, he must lose weight. The nurse can sometimes assist the patient in expressing why he wishes to reduce and to support his efforts to continue.

As an example, Mrs. Albert, aged 35, was 55 lb overweight. Her mother had diabetes mellitus, and Mrs. Albert's glucose tolerance curve was indicative of stress diabetes. On this basis, the physician recommended that she lose her excess weight over the next year. To encourage her, her husband offered to buy her a new wardrobe when she reached the desired weight. Both Mr. Albert and the physician frequently complimented her on her improved appearance.

One must be certain that the advantages of weight loss are not counterbalanced by the severe depression that is experienced by some who use overeating as a defense against their feelings. Psychiatrists consider obesity in these individuals to be the lesser of two problems.[61]

CALORIE LEVEL OF THE DIET

The caloric intake generally prescribed permits a weight loss of 1 to 2 lb per week. Because the loss of 1 lb of adipose tissue is equal to roughly 3,500 calories, it is apparent that the loss of 1 lb per week would necessitate reducing the daily diet by 500 calories below the maintenance level. Thus the man who ordinarily needs 2,800 calories per day would lose 2 lb in a week if he reduced his intake to 1,800 calories per day. The 65-year-old woman who needs 1,700 calories per day would lose 1 lb in a week if her diet furnished 1,200 calories per day.

Extremely low-calorie diets (300 to 900 calories) are sometimes prescribed because the rapid weight loss that results gives encouragement to the patient. Nutritionally, such diets are inadequate in minerals and vitamins and they may also provide less protein than is desirable. Diets containing less than 1,000 calories are seldom warranted except for bed patients in a hospital. Not infrequently such diets lead to weakness, dizziness, and, for those with coronary insufficiency, to an increase in anginal attacks. In older persons, too rapid loss of weight may lead to loose, flabby skin, scrawny necks, and sunken cheeks, thus attracting adverse comments from relatives and friends.

Starvation regimens varying from two weeks to several months have been used by Duncan,[62] Drenick,[63] and others for the grossly obese. The patient is given no food except noncaloric beverages and vitamin-mineral supplements. Weight loss is rapid, thereby encouraging the patient. Starvation over periods of 1 to 3 months, as described by Drenick, resulted in significant losses of protein tissue and the tendency to gout in some patients.[64] When patients were placed on diets containing as few as 32 g of protein and 300 calories, nitrogen equilibrium was again established. Starvation should never be used for weight loss except in patients who are under constant medical supervision in a hospital.

[61] Robert I. Simon: "Obesity as a Depressive Equivalent," *JAMA,* **183:**208–10 (Jan. 19) 1963.
[62] Garfield G. Duncan *et al.:* "Intermittent Fasts in the Correction and Control of Intractable Obesity," *Amer. J. Med. Sci.,* **245:**515–20 (May) 1963.
[63] Ernst J. Drenick: "Weight Reduction with Low-Calorie Diets. Practical Management," *JAMA,* **202:** 118–20 (Oct. 9) 1967.
[64] Marian E. Swendseid, Dorothy B. Mulcare, and Ernst J. Drenick: "Nitrogen and Weight Losses During Starvation and Realimentation in Obesity," *J. Amer. Diet. Ass.,* **46:**276–79 (Apr.) 1965.

NUTRITIVE ADEQUACY

The nutritive requirements of the obese, except for energy from food, are the same as those of the nonobese person. Although a protein intake of 55 to 65 g is satisfactory for adults, many people find that a somewhat higher level of protein (80 or 90 g) results in a more satisfying diet. When foods are chosen from the Meal Exchange Lists,[65] including milk, vegetables, meats, and breads and cereals, the mineral and vitamin intakes are likely to be adequate for diets of 1,000 calories or more. If lower calorie levels are prescribed, mineral and vitamin supplements must be added.

FOOD VALUES

The patient must have a thorough knowledge of food values if he is expected to follow a diet and to maintain desirable weight throughout his life. The Meal Exchange Lists furnish a good starting point for becoming familiar with food values because the calorie and other nutritive values of foods within each list are similar. The initial restriction of food choices to these lists also helps to ensure adequate intakes of all nutrients. Leverton[66] has given some clues to foods low in calories by describing them as thin, watery, or dilute; bulky or with lots of fiber; and with crispness from water, not fat. By contrast, she describes foods high in calories as oily- or greasy-crisp; thick and smooth; sweet and gooey; or alcoholic.

Various methods of food preparation illustrate further how readily the calorie value may be increased. For example, one egg—raw, soft- or hard-cooked, or poached—furnishes 80 calories. But when the egg is fried in 1 tsp of fat about 45 calories have been added. When the egg is beaten with 1 tbsp of cream and cooked as an omelet with 2 tsp of butter, the calorie value has been increased to 175. Cream, butter and other fats, sugar, and flour are ingredients that rapidly increase the calorie content.

The obese individual should recognize that relatively small daily intakes of food in excess of calorie needs are additive in terms of body weight. An average daily excess of 50 calories amounts to 18,250 calories in a year, or the deposition of about 5 lb of fat. But 50 calories represent a very small amount of food: 1 tablespoon of heavy cream, or 3 level teaspoons of sugar, or ⅓ cup of whole milk, or 4 ounces of carbonated beverage, or ½ cup of orange juice, or 1½ teaspoons of butter, and so on.

[65] The American Dietetic Association, Chicago.
[66] Ruth M. Leverton: "Food Needs and Energy Use in Weight Reduction," *J. Amer. Diet. Ass.,* **49:**23–25 (July) 1966.

EXERCISE

Activity has not been sufficiently emphasized as a means of control of weight because many people have felt that too much exercise was required to lose a small amount of weight, and that exercise had the tendency to increase the appetite. An individual who learns that he must walk 36 miles to utilize the calories of 1 lb of fat tends to become discouraged. Yet, over the period of one year, a walk of 1 mile per day will result in the loss, or in the prevention of gain, of 10 lb. This may be stated in another way: Reducing the daily intake by 500 calories below the body's needs will result in a 4-lb weight loss in one month. If the activity is also increased by a daily 1-mile walk, the increased output each day of 100 to 125 calories will result in the loss of almost an additional 1 lb each month.

Moderate exercise such as walking on a daily basis is preferred to occasional vigorous exercise. Moderate exercise does not increase the appetite, but intense physical activity sometimes does. Even though 18 holes of golf may utilize 800 to 1,000 calories, the expenditure is nullified if the nineteenth hole includes considerable quantities of beverages and food. In addition to its effect on weight loss, exercise increases muscle tone and improves the physical and mental well-being. The amount of exercise recommended must be adjusted to each individual's health status; a sudden and marked change in exercise patterns is ill advised for older persons.

VARIATIONS IN WEIGHT LOSS

The actual weight loss may vary widely from that calculated. Norma Sims has conscientiously followed her 1,200-calorie diet but has lost no weight in two weeks. The nurse reassures her by telling her that it is not uncommon for tissues temporarily to hold water and that she will soon begin to lose weight if she continues to adhere to her diet. Many women experience fluid retention prior to onset of the menstrual period, and this should also be kept in mind. Of course, if there is continued failure to lose weight, the therapist will need to determine whether the prescribed calorie level was appropriate and whether the patient is, in fact, rigorously controlling portion sizes and methods of preparation.

Variations in activity from week to week will also affect the degree of weight loss. Mrs. Thomas, 60 years old, follows her prescribed diet and takes a walk every afternoon. Several weeks of cold weather and icy walks have kept her indoors, and she finds that she is not losing much weight.

PSYCHOLOGICAL SUPPORT

Losing weight is a day-to-day endeavor in which the results become apparent only with the persistent attention to diet and activity. The patient must be given confidence in his ability to control his food intake. He needs the continuing support of his family. The therapist must give "understanding, sympathetic, non-threatening, unjudging, and unchastizing therapeutic support." [67] Because the obese individual often has a sense of inferiority and guilt, the therapist must be careful not to add to this burden for this will only increase the patient's withdrawal and lead to further inactivity.

Aldrich, a psychiatrist,[68] indicates that obesity should be viewed as any other addiction. He recommends that it be studied from the point of view of impulses, controls, and consequences. Obesity is a consequence of failure to control the impulse to eat. According to this concept of obesity, the problem faced by the patient and by those who are working with him is to help him to learn to control the quantity of food he eats. Emphasis is on the patient exercising the control rather than the control being external. For example, Mrs. Leslie, who is chronically obese, sees her physician about every six weeks. For the two weeks preceding her visit to her physician she literally starves herself. After her visit, she exercises little control over what she eats. Her control is from the physician. Mrs. Leslie wishes to please him or to avoid being scolded. She blames her employer and husband for tempting her with food.

As a consequence of her behavior, Mrs. Leslie feels ashamed. "I should lose weight, I'm a sight." She also rationalizes, "How can I lose weight when you make pie and sweet rolls and leave them out where I can see them?" and "Ben won't eat broiled, roasted, or boiled meat. It has to be fried." Many obese people react in a similar manner. They need help in identifying their own responsibility in controlling their weight.

DRUGS IN WEIGHT REDUCTION

Appetite depressants, as well as agents purported to suppress the appetite, come and go. Drugs suppressing the appetite center in the brain usually cause nausea as well as anorexia. Drugs such as amphetamine phosphate and related compounds depress the appetite by inducing a sense of well-being. Because some drugs have dangerous side effects, they should

[67] Charlotte M. Young: "Some Comments on the Obesities," *J. Amer. Diet. Ass.,* **45:**134–38 (Aug.) 1964.
[68] C. Knight Aldrich: "Mechanisms and Management of Obesity," *Med. Clin. N. Amer.,* **47:**77 (Jan.) 1963.

not be taken by persons who are not under medical supervision.

Metabolic stimulants, including hormones, have been tried in weight-reduction regimens. Because the thyroid hormone stimulates metabolism, it has been used to increase weight loss. In the euthyroid individual, the ingestion of exogenous thyroid hormone decreases the secretion of the thyroid gland. When excessive dosages of thyroid are ingested, symptoms of thyroid toxicity appear.

GROUP THERAPY

Some people are better able to achieve weight loss when they ally themselves with a group such as TOPS (Take Off Pounds Sensibly) or Fattys Anonymous. In such groups individuals are able to talk over their problems with others and to compare methods for coping with them. Group meetings provide opportunity for information on dietary control, methods of food preparation, how to resist overeating, the value of exercise, and so on.

Any individual who joins a group should be advised initially by a physician that it is safe for him to undertake weight loss. Preferably, he will have had some individual counseling regarding his diet prior to joining the group. So that members of a group do not fall prey to misinformation or faddism, it is advisable that a nurse, nutritionist, or physician be available for consultation and guidance.

SUMMARY

Obesity, an excessive accumulation of fatty tissue, is a major public health problem that increases the incidence of chronic diseases and the mortality rate. Although it results from an excess of calorie intake over the energy expenditure, multiple causes are involved. Cultural dietary patterns, ignorance of food values, overeating as a compensation for emotional problems and to meet life stresses, and relative inactivity are the principal factors leading to obesity. Those who have endomorphic body types are more prone to obesity than those of ectomorphic body types. Hormonal imbalance rarely accounts for obesity, and errors of metabolism of fat or carbohydrate have not been firmly established as causes of obesity. The prevention of obesity with emphasis on nutrition education and physical activity during the school years is likely to be much more rewarding than attempts to treat obesity. Successful treatment of obesity requires the extended and sympathetic guidance of the physician, nurse, or nutritionist; the sustained motivation of the patient; adequate counseling regarding control

of the diet; and emphasis on a program of physical activity.

Undernutrition

The term *undernutrition* as used here refers to the condition in which weight loss has occurred, or is in progress, because of an inadequate supply of calories to meet body needs. It is a generalized state of deficiency in which the deficient calorie supply is accompanied by insufficient proteins, minerals, and vitamins. Manifestations of specific deficiency diseases may become evident when lack of one nutrient predominates. For example, in beriberi thiamine is the principal nutrient lack; in pellagra the primary lack is that of niacin; and in kwashiorkor protein is deficient. However, in each of these conditions the body is supplied with inadequate quantities of most, if not all, nutrients, and some signs characteristic of multiple deficiency are also present. Although particular emphasis in therapy may focus on the predominating deficiency, the diet must be nutritionally balanced to correct for the multiple nature of the deficiency.

What are the principal causes of undernutrition?

ETIOLOGICAL FACTORS

On a worldwide basis and even in the United States most of the existing undernutrition is of primary origin; that is, the dietary intake is below that required to meet normal body needs. The inadequate dietary intake is occasioned by one or more of these factors, as discussed in the beginning of this chapter: (1) insufficient food supply because of poor agricultural practices and land use; (2) inadequate facilities for food preservation, food storage, and food distribution; (3) ignorance, superstition, food taboos, and food faddism; and (4) poverty.

Infections and parasitic infestations accentuate the effects of inadequate diet. The calorie and nutrient requirements are increased because of fever and losses through the gastrointestinal tract. Infections, in turn, become more acute because of the body's lowered resistance. Hence, a vicious cycle is created. For example, measles becomes especially virulent among already malnourished children and the ensuing complications and mortality rate are much higher than among well-nourished children. The overall high morbidity and mortality of infants and young children in the developing countries is the result of a synergism among infection, parasites, and undernutrition.

Undernutrition is frequently brought about by some pathologic condition that interferes with adequate food intake, digestion, absorption, or metabolism. The nutritional problems associated with many pathologic conditions have already been discussed in this and other chapters of the text. (See Table 12-2 at the end of this chapter.) Unless careful adjustment is made in the diet, one can expect some degree of undernutrition when one or more of the following conditions exist.

Anorexia is frequently associated with organic disease as well as psychologic disturbances. In the latter, extreme emaciation sometimes results. Acute illness in the well-nourished and the temporary loss of appetite are not likely to be serious. In the chronically ill patient, or in those who are undernourished at the onset of illness, anorexia is of more serious import.

Increased nutritional requirements are imposed by fever, burns, hyperthyroidism, severe anemia, and advanced neoplastic disease. Effects of illness, such as restlessness, dyspnea, or orthopnea, intensify the need of the patient for food.

The degree to which the basal metabolic rate is elevated in the orthopneic patient is illustrated by Mrs. Thims. She had a basal metabolic rate of $+100$ per cent. Unless there is a corresponding increase in food ingested, weight loss accompanies any condition in which tissue requirements are increased. In some disorders such as congestive heart failure, retention of salt and water may mask the loss of body substance. Upon the removal of the edema fluid the patient is found to be emaciated. Sometimes the state of nutrition of the edematous patient is so poor that he does not respond to the usual measures to eliminate the edema until his nutrition is improved.

In some disorders, the total quantity of food required by the patient may be increased, not by an increase in the requirement of cells, but by excessive losses of nutrients from the body. For example, some disorders of the alimentary tract are accompanied by loss of nutrients. Patients who have large burns or draining wounds or abscesses may lose enormous quantities of nutrients. Large quantities of protein may be lost through abnormally permeable glomeruli in the kidney. In uncontrolled diabetes mellitus, weight loss results from the loss of glucose in the urine. Inasmuch as protein and fats are mobilized for energy and to form glucose, they are also lost. Whatever the cause of the loss, the extent and type of nutrient lost must be estimated and every effort made to restore the balance between supply and demand. The nurse contributes to the estimation of the extent of tissue requirements by making pertinent observations.

SIGNS AND SYMPTOMS

Undernourished infants and children gain weight slowly, remain short in stature, show delayed maturation of the skeletal structures, have a poor resistance to infection, and may be mentally retarded. The younger the child, the more severe are the effects of undernutrition. As the deficiency progresses the child is less able to digest foods, presumably because of a decreased output of digestive enzymes. The serum albumin level gradually falls and the serum globulin level rises, indicating some interference with liver function. The skin becomes dry and pigmented, and the hair pigment also changes with grayish or reddish streaking. In severe undernutrition the fluid and electrolyte imbalance may be so serious as to threaten the life of the child. The term *marasmus* describes the severe undernutrition of the infant suffering from protein and calorie lack; the term *kwashiorkor* refers to the condition in which the quality of the protein is the principal lack.

Adults who are moderately undernourished show few signs except loss of weight. As undernutrition proceeds they will do less and less work unless forced to do it. They become much more susceptible to infections and convalesce more slowly from any illness. The pregnant woman is especially vulnerable, and undernutrition increases the possibility of spontaneous abortions, stillbirths, and premature births. By repeated pregnancies, the poor condition of the mother and the fetus is further aggravated.

As undernutrition progresses in the adult, numerous changes take place in body tissues: lowered basal metabolic rate in accord with lowered cell mass and reduced cell activity; changes in hair, skin, and mucous membranes, including dry, pigmented skin, glossitis, and stomatitis; reduction in gastrointestinal enzymes, intestinal ulceration, abdominal distention, diarrhea; neurological changes such as polyneuritis; lowered serum albumin sometimes accompanied by edema; fatty liver; macrocytic or microcytic anemia; and many other changes.

TREATMENT

Correction of the undernutrition is effected through an increase in the intake of calories and protein. Easy as this may appear to be to those who have a problem with overweight, the correction of caloric and protein undernutrition may take weeks and months of effort. It often requires (1) a fundamental change in attitudes of the individual and/or his family, (2) a building up of the tolerance of the gastrointestinal tract for food, (3) more money to buy food, as well as (4) the patience, understanding, and cooperation of the various members of the health team to achieve success. The reasons for undernutrition vary from one person to another. Therefore, inasmuch as is possible, each person must be treated as an individual.

When undernutrition is extreme, little is gained by suddenly initiating a high-protein, high-calorie diet; in fact, force feeding may be dangerous. Neither the digestive tract nor the cardiovascular system is able to cope with the additional demands posed by large amounts of food. The patient's appetite, during severe undernutrition, often appears to be easily satisfied, and this appears to be, in fact, a protective mechanism. The management of patients with severe undernutrition is, therefore, complex and requires attention to fluid and electrolyte balance, control of any existing diarrhea, and gradual replacement of nutrients. Initially, small meals of nutritionally balanced foods are given. When the tolerance to small quantities of food is well established, gradual additions are made to the diet.

EXAMPLES OF UNDERNUTRITION

The following individuals illustrate some of the problems that contribute to calorie undernutrition. Some questions that might be considered here are the following: What is the presenting problem or problems in each of the four individuals? What are the possible outcomes? Suggest appropriate ways in which a nurse might contribute to the solution of each. In which of the patients presented below is the prognosis favorable, if appropriate action is taken in time?

Sharon, aged 15, had been a plump baby and child and had always eaten well. At the close of the school year she decided to lose weight so that she would be more nearly like her friends in appearance. Because her previous attempts had been unsatisfactory, she felt that her situation was desperate. With the exception of a glass of skim milk and a piece of fruit, three times per day, she refused to eat. Her parents became frantic. The less she ate, the more they scolded and the greater was Sharon's determination to stick to her diet and to lose weight rapidly.

Mrs. Ross, aged 75, lives across town from Sharon. She lives alone in a one-room apartment. Although she has a modest income, her meals consist of health bread and tea. She says other foods disagree with her and that her food intake is adequate. She supports her position by stating that printed on the wrapper covering of the bread is a statement that this bread contains all of the elements required for health. Mrs.

Ross has never been fat. She is weak and tired, but after all, as she says, she is an old woman. Her family and friends are gone. She lived during the period when family life was the most intense at any time in American history. When she was a child and until her children left home and her husband died, meals were a social event. The entire family gathered round an abundantly supplied table to eat and enjoy each other's company. Now all that is gone and Mrs. Ross has little incentive to eat.

Mary Alice, aged 17, has arthritis. She was hospitalized for rehabilitation, during which time she made considerable progress. After her return home, she soon returned to almost full-time bed rest. She says that she is too weak and tired to get out of bed. A three-day food-intake study revealed that her caloric intake was only about 800 calories. Among a number of possible factors contributing to the situation, the easiest to identify and correct is the fact that Mary Alice's mother is a poor cook.

Many of the elements that contribute to problems that arise in the chronically malnourished patient are well illustrated by Mrs. Muncie. As is often true, Mrs. Muncie's malnourished state did not arise suddenly nor was it the result of a single cause. At the time of her admission to the hospital Mrs. Muncie presented an emaciated appearance. Her skin was tightly drawn over her slight frame. She had a large infected decubitus ulcer over her sacrum. Although she had not felt well for some years, she had been able to care for a five-room flat, prepare meals for herself and her husband, and be active in church work. Her present illness had its onset about a week previous to her admission for an episode of diarrhea. Her husband had cared for her at home, because he wanted her to die in peace. A neighbor finally persuaded him to have her admitted to the hospital.

Some of the factors contributing to Mrs. Muncie's chronically malnourished state were revealed by her personal history. She was the thirteenth child born to sharecropper parents in Mississippi. She had completed about the fourth grade in school. Her diet throughout her lifetime was that which she ate as a child. She and her husband had moved to Big City 25 years ago. Insufficient income to cover expenses had been a constant problem. At the time of her admission to the hospital, her husband's wages as a janitor were only $270 a month, but he did have sufficient hospital insurance to cover Mrs. Muncie's hospital expenses. Only by the most careful management were they able to meet all of their obligations. Because her appetite was poor and her husband left early in the morning, she usually ate only two meals a day. The first consisted of either tea or coffee and toast and soup or orange juice. The second meal, which she shared with her husband, usually consisted of a vegetable, preferably greens cooked with fat pork, and cornbread or hot biscuits. Mrs. Muncie had worn dentures since she was 25 years of age. When she was between the ages of 13 and 25, her father pulled her teeth, one by one, because they were painful. When asked about her weight, she said that she had always been "skinny." Based on her dietary history, Mrs. Muncie's nutrient intake was probably always marginal. Significant factors in her background include poverty, a low educational level, loss of her teeth at an early age, and customs in food selection and preparation that tended to restrict her intake of protein and calories as well as other important nutrients.

An appropriate question at this point is, "How is it that Mrs. Muncie managed to live for more than 60 years on a diet of cooked vegetables, corn bread, and fat pork?" Adults show considerable resistance to food deprivation. In the presence of an inadequate supply of nutrients, cells adapt by decreasing their rate of metabolism. Stores of fat and protein are mobilized and utilized for energy. The only evidence that food intake is less than that required may be loss of weight or a weight that is less than normal. Although the individual is able to do heavy work, he rests at every opportunity. During the period in which the individual is able to adapt the metabolic rate of his cells to his limited food intake, his malnourished state is said to be compensated. He may survive in this state for a long period of time. When some condition develops, such as an infection, that places added stress on the individual, adaptation fails and evidence of uncompensated undernutrition appears.

Mrs. Muncie indicated that she had been underweight most of her life when she said, "I've always been skinny." Until she had a nephrectomy six years ago, she had always been reasonably well. Since that time she had been in her words "poorly." Her present illness was ushered in by an episode of diarrhea. Although she attributed this to some cabbage that she had eaten, diarrhea is frequently the first evidence that chronic undernutrition has entered the uncompensated phase. When she entered the hospital a week later, she was also found to have pyelonephritis in her remaining kidney. As stated previously, an infection is frequently the stress that upsets the unstable balance in chronic undernutrition. Soon after the onset of her illness a decubitus ulcer formed at the base of her spine. It was infected. After compensation failed, Mrs. Muncie was no longer able to protect her tissues from the effects of pressure. Resistance to infection was also impaired.

On physical examination, Mrs. Muncie presented many signs and symptoms of chronic undernutrition. Despite the fact that she was 5 ft 5 in. tall, she weighed only 88 lb. The desirable weight for a woman of small frame and 65 in. tall is from 111 to 119 lb.[69] She did not give the appearance of having lost weight recently. In older individuals, rapid losses of weight are usually accompanied by wrinkling of the skin and loose folds of skin over areas where subcutaneous fat is stored. As the skin ages, it loses its elasticity, and with the loss of elasticity, the ability to adapt the skin to the size of the underlying tissue is diminished. After 50 years of age or so, the skin of the person who loses weight rapidly is likely to be too large for him. The severely undernourished person tends to retain water. Although this is more likely to occur in children than in adults, the absence of wrinkling of Mrs. Muncie's skin may have been caused in part by water retention.

Among the other signs and symptoms of chronic undernutrition presented by Mrs. Muncie were wasting of tissues including her muscles; edema; dry, scaling skin; numbness and tingling of her toes; hyperesthesia of feet and legs; weakness and pallor; glossitis (sore tongue); diarrhea; poor wound healing; and anorexia.

Her laboratory findings, which are summarized below, were consistent with a state of chronic undernutrition.

It will be noted that her total blood proteins are within the lower limits of normal, but that the albumin-globulin ratio is reversed. This indicates that albumin is being broken down or lost from the body more rapidly than it can be replaced. Multiple factors probably account for the deficit of albumin. Lack of sufficient intake of protein to provide the amino acids required to replace albumin lost from the body, loss of albumin in the exudate from the decubitus ulcer, and possibly in the diarrheal fluid, utilization of serum albumin to provide energy, and possibly inability of the liver to synthesize albumin—all probably contribute to the reversal of the albumin-globulin ratio. This condition also occurs when large quantities of albumin are lost in the urine. Loss of albumin by this route was not a factor in the instance of Mrs. Muncie. The relatively high serum globulin level accounts for the total protein level being within the normal range, and indicates the response to the prevailing infection. Some degree of dehydration may have also contributed to maintaining the level of protein within normal limits. The blood urea nitrogen elevation may be

[69] Metropolitan Life Insurance Company, "New Weight Standards for Men and Women," *Statist. Bull.,* 40:3 (Nov.–Dec.) 1959.

Laboratory Test	Finding—Mrs. Muncie		Normal Range
Blood protein—total	6.6	g/100 ml	6.5–8.3
Serum albumin	1.82		3.5–5.5
Beta globulin	2.51		0.52–1.01
Gamma globulin	2.25		0.61–1.39
Blood urea nitrogen	35	mg/100 ml	10–20
Electrolytes			
Sodium	120	mEq/liter	125–147
Potassium	4.8	mEq/liter	3.5–5.5
Carbon dioxide	26.1	volumes per cent	50–70
Hemoglobin	8.1	g/100ml	12–16
Hematocrit	31	per cent	36–47
Urine			
Albumin		Negative	Negative

caused by some degree of dehydration. The lowering of her carbon dioxide-combining power is consistent with acidosis. It will be noted that her serum sodium is slightly decreased; this indicates some loss of cations. Acid-base balance is discussed fully in Chapter 9. Acidosis is common in starvation. As might be expected, Mrs. Muncie's hemoglobin is low. Associated with this is a low hematocrit. Anemia is a common occurrence in menstruating women who are undernourished. Although Mrs. Muncie is well past the menopause, she had been undernourished for much, if not all, of her life.

After Mrs. Muncie was admitted to the hospital, three interrelated problems required immediate attention. The first and central problem was to improve her nutritional status. The second and third were to heal the decubitus and to eliminate the infection in her kidney—the pyelonephritis. In the early part of her hospitalization, these problems required urgent attention. Others were secondary. To correct her undernutrition, a plioform nasogastric tube was introduced into her stomach. The formula was made by liquefying natural foods in a blender. It contained 1,500 calories per liter. In the beginning the formula was administered over a 24-hour period with the pump adjusted at the slowest rate of speed. In addition, she was served an 1,800-calorie diet and a multivitamin capsule that contained the recommended daily allowance of vitamins. Nutrients were not administered parenterally.

To prevent the loss of nutrients and fluid by diarrhea, she was given 1 dram of paregoric (camphorated tincture of opium) in each liter of formula. Paregoric was discontinued when the diarrhea ceased. The tolerance of the digestive tube for food is diminished in undernutrition. Therefore, the ingestion of more than the usual amounts of food is likely to aggravate or induce diarrhea. Paregoric acts by increasing the tone of the stomach and intestine and by decreasing propulsive peristalsis. The latter action is important in the control of diarrhea.

In addition to efforts to improve her nutritive state, measures were instituted to hasten the healing of her decubitus ulcer. She was placed on a Stryker frame that was turned every two hours day and night. Attention was paid to all sites of pressure in order to prevent further tissue breakdown. Warm saline compresses were applied to the decubitus twice daily for an hour, followed by exposure of the area to a heat lamp for one-half hour. When she was first admitted to the hospital she was incontinent of urine. A retention catheter was inserted. Every effort was made to keep the area clean and dry. Plastic surgery was considered, but not performed because of her poor nutritive state.

Mrs. Muncie's progress was slow. During the first three weeks of therapy she gained only 2 lb in weight but she had gained enough strength so that she was able to walk with assistance. She was encouraged to walk because ambulation improves morale and appetite as well as the normal functioning of the alimentary canal. To increase her food intake, her request for a soft diet was granted. Because she tired when eating, she was given assistance at mealtime.

Mrs. Muncie had some assets not available to all patients. She had a devoted husband. She had a strong religious faith. Her husband, who had an excellent work record, was assisted by his employer in establishing that he was 65 years of age and therefore eligible for social security. He planned to retire so that he could care for his wife at home. As soon as the decubitus ulcer was healed, Mrs. Muncie was to be discharged home under the supervision of the outpatient clinic and a visiting nurse. Efforts were made to instruct the husband and wife in selection of food that would meet at least minimum nutritional requirements. Because of their age, limited education and money, and a life-time of habits, the outlook for marked improvement was poor.

There were also other problems in the care of Mrs. Muncie. The purpose, however, of introducing her case here was to present some of the problems that cause and result from chronic undernutrition. Mrs. Muncie was not from a far-off land, but lived in a large city in the United States. The factors in her condition are those that underlie undernutrition over the world—poverty and illiteracy perhaps being the most fundamental. She did not have a so-called deficiency disease, such as arises when one nutrient is lacking in the dietary. Rather she suffered to a greater or lesser extent from a lack of all nutrients, calories, proteins, vitamins, and minerals.

Had Mrs. Muncie's state been discovered before decompensation occurred, her illness might have been prevented. This would have taken an increase in the ingestion of all nutrients. For each pound gained, an intake of 3,500 calories in excess of those utilized is required. In persons whose food habits and patterns are set, an increase in food intake is often difficult to achieve. It takes time and patience. The individual needs to understand and accept that increase in the intake of food is necessary to health and well-being and to want to improve his food habits.

Carbohydrate Metabolism

DIETARY SOURCES

Wheat is the chief cereal grain in the North American diet, but corn and rice are also widely used. Potatoes and sugars are also significant sources of carbohydrate, with other fruits and vegetables contributing much smaller amounts. In worldwide use rice leads all grains. Other rich sources of carbohydrate used in some parts of the world are millet, plantain, cassava, and a variety of legumes. No specific requirements have been established for dietary carbohydrate. Moreover, no particular level of carbohydrate is most conducive to health.

DIGESTION AND ABSORPTION

About 98 per cent of the carbohydrate in the typical American diet is hydrolyzed to the simple sugars, chiefly glucose, and lesser amounts of fructose and galactose; the remainder is indigestible fiber. The principal mechanism for absorption is by active transport, involving the phosphorylation of glucose (the addition of a molecule of phosphate available from ATP). The capillaries of the intestinal wall empty into the portal vein, which in turn carries the glucose to the liver.

How is homeostasis maintained in the metabolism of carbohydrates?

BLOOD GLUCOSE

The intermittent ingestion of carbohydrate and the constant requirement of the body for energy suggest the need for mechanisms to maintain homeostasis at all times. The blood glucose level, kept within a limited range, is the key to this control, just as the liver is the principal organ for the regulation of the blood sugar. A number of hormones complement or oppose one another in the maintenance of the blood sugar and in the metabolism of carbohydrate by the tissues. The nervous system is also involved in the control mechanism.

The sugar of the blood is glucose, just as the principal carbohydrate metabolized in the tissues is glucose. The relatively small amounts of fructose and galactose from digestion are converted to glucose by the liver. Normally, the blood sugar level ranges from 70 to 110 mg per 100 ml of blood. Immediately after a meal it rises to 130 mg per 100 ml or so, but drops relatively soon to the lower levels. The level of glucose at any given moment is the balance between the sources of glucose to the blood and the demands made on it by the tissues. A change in one direction is counteracted by the activation of mechanisms that correct the change. The result is change within limits. Only when there is a disturbance in these mechanisms does the blood sugar rise to abnormal levels (hyperglycemia), as in diabetes mellitus, or fall abnormally (hypoglycemia), as following an overdosage with insulin.

BLOOD SOURCES OF GLUCOSE

Three general sources of supply for the blood glucose are (1) the simple sugars resulting from absorption from the small intestine; (2) glycogenolysis, or the breakdown of glycogen in the liver; and (3) gluconeogenesis, or the formation of glucose from the amino acids and other substances by the liver.

Less than 1 lb of glycogen is stored in the body, about four fifths of this being in the liver. Muscle glycogen is available for glucose in the muscle cell, but it does not add to the glucose level of the blood. Glycogen reserves within the liver would be depleted within a few hours by a fasting individual in order to maintain the blood glucose. Thus the liver glycogen may be thought of as a short-term or emergency supply to meet the tissue energy needs.

When glycogen levels are depleted the blood sugar level is maintained through the breakdown of amino acids by the liver. About half of the amino acids deaminized in such a situation yield available glucose. The glycerol fraction of the fats that are broken down is also a source of glucose and accounts for about one tenth of the fat molecule.

REMOVAL OF GLUCOSE

Six ways to remove glucose from the blood are listed by West and his associates: [70] (1) by the cells for utilization as energy; (2) by the liver for storage as glycogen; (3) by conversion to fat and storage in adipose tissue; (4) for the synthesis of compounds such as lactose, mucopolysaccharides, glycolipids, and nucleic acids; (5) by glycolysis in the red blood cells; and (6) by excretion in the urine when the renal threshold has been exceeded. The renal threshold is that level of the blood glucose beyond which sugar will appear in the urine. It is somewhat variable from one individual to another, but generally it is about 160 to 180 mg per 100 ml of blood. During prolonged hyperglycemia, as in uncontrolled diabetes mellitus, the renal threshold is often above 200 mg per 100 ml. The formation of fat in the form of adipose tissue from glucose represents the body's mechanism for ensuring a long-term reserve of body fuel, as contrasted to the short-term stores available from glycogen.

HORMONAL CONTROL

The pancreas, adrenal, and pituitary glands secrete hormones that influence the blood sugar level and the metabolism of carbohydrate by the tissues. Increased blood glucose levels stimulate the secretion of insulin, the pancreatic hormone produced by the beta cells of the islands of Langerhans. Insulin increases the rate of oxidation of glucose by the tissues and the rate of glycogen and fat formation. Thus the blood sugar is lowered. Glucagon, another pancreatic hormone, probably produced by the alpha cells, increases the rate of glycogen breakdown to glucose, thereby increasing the blood sugar level.

The cortex and medulla of the adrenal gland produce a number of hormones that influence the blood sugar level. If an experimental animal is adrenalectomized, it becomes extremely sensitive to insulin, but this sensitivity is reduced when glucocorticoids are injected. Patients with Addison's disease have reduced function of the adrenal cortex and characteristically have a hypoglycemia. This is corrected when glucocorticoids are administered. The

[70] Op. cit., p. 1039.

glucocorticoids secreted by the adrenal cortex increase the production of glucose and glycogen from amino acids and decrease the use of glucose by the tissues. Because the glucocorticoids are antagonistic to insulin, their administration would increase the severity of diabetes mellitus. The accelerated breakdown of amino acids brought about by the glucocorticoids results in a greater excretion of nitrogen in the urine. In fact, undesirable breakdown of tissue protein may accompany the administration of these hormones.

Epinephrine, sometimes described as an emergency hormone, is secreted by the adrenal medulla under conditions of severe emotional stress or activity. Its effect is to bring about a rapid breakdown of liver glycogen to glucose and to increase the rate of use of muscle glycogen. In extreme emotional states, the amount of hormone secreted may be sufficiently great to produce a transient hyperglycemia.

The hormones of the pituitary affecting carbohydrate metabolism are of two types: (1) those having a direct effect, and (2) the tropic hormones having an effect on the secretion of other glands, thus indirectly affecting metabolism. Somatotropin (the growth hormone) increases the blood glucose levels by increasing gluconeogenesis, by antagonistic effects on the activity of insulin, or by the release of glucagon or other hyperglycemic factors. Adrenocorticotropic hormone (ACTH) stimulates the secretion of the adrenal cortex and thereby glucose and glycogen production by gluconeogenesis.

The thyroid hormone increases the rate of absorption of glucose from the intestine to raise the glucose level of the blood. Because the thyroid hormone regulates the rate of metabolism in the tissues, any excess or deficiency of the hormone would correspondingly affect the rate of glucose metabolism.

UTILIZATION OF CARBOHYDRATE

The chief source of energy to the body is carbohydrate. One gram of dietary carbohydrate, on the average, yields 4 calories. Brain tissues use glucose exclusively, and even after a short period of severe hypoglycemia the brain ceases to function, and irreparable damage may result.

Glucose is utilized as a source of energy according to the steps outlined in Figures 12-4 and 12-5. The glucose is phosphorylated by the addition of first one and then a second phosphate group and is broken down anaerobically (without the addition of oxygen) to lactic or pyruvic acid. Within the muscle cell the breakdown of glucose to lactic acid produces a small release of energy that permits the muscle to operate until sufficient oxygen is brought from the blood. About four fifths of the lactic acid produced in the muscle are reconverted to glycogen, and the remainder is converted to pyruvic acid. The pyruvic acid is decarboxylated by carboxylase to acetic acid, is activated by coenzyme A, and enters the citric acid cycle, as described in a preceding section of this chapter (p. 541).

Glucose is essential to prevent the excessive metabolism of fats. Whenever the breakdown of fatty acids exceeds the availability of glucose to "prime" the citric acid cycle, an accumulation of short-chain fatty acids takes place in the blood, and the condition is known as ketosis or acidosis. In the normal individual a temporary ketosis is produced by a very low-carbohydrate or low-calorie diet or by starvation. Gradually, the normal individual adjusts by increased glycogen production from amino acids. In diabetes mellitus, however, the failure to utilize glucose is accompanied by excessive breakdown of fats and their accumulation as keto acids. The effects of acidosis are discussed in Chapter 9. Occasionally, ketosis is intentionally produced in the therapy of epilepsy by using diets high in fat, somewhat restricted in protein, and reduced to less than 40 g of carbohydrates per day.

Glucose is also said to be protein-sparing. In other words, when ample glucose is available through the absorption of dietary carbohydrate or from liver stores of glycogen, amino acids need not be used to form glucose.

HYPOGLYCEMIA

Despite the effectiveness of regulatory mechanisms in keeping the level of glucose in the blood within physiological limits in most people, they sometimes fail. Depending on the nature of the failure, the level of glucose in the blood falls outside physiological limits. When the concentration of glucose in the blood falls below 70 mg per 100 ml, the condition is known as hypoglycemia.

Causes

Theoretically, hypoglycemia could result from a failure in the supply of glucose. In diseases of the liver in which its capacity to store glycogen is below physiological limits, hypoglycemia is at times a problem. Hypoglycemia may also result from failure of the mechanisms for adding glucose to the blood. As a consequence, hypoglycemia is associated with adrenal insufficiency. Probably the most frequent cause of hypoglycemia of a severe degree is overactivity of the mechanism for lowering the level of glucose in the blood, that is, an oversupply of insulin. The insulin may be of endogenous or exogenous origin. If the supply of insulin is excessive, the level of glucose in the blood falls below 70 mg per 100 ml of blood. The effects of lowering the level of glucose in the blood will depend on the suddenness and the extent to which it falls below normal limits.

Signs and Symptoms

Most of the manifestations of hypoglycemia result from failure to supply sufficient glucose to the cells of the nervous system. Glucose is the only fuel from which it can derive energy. Early symptoms and signs in hypoglycemia result from increased autonomic activity. Hunger, often marked, sweating, increased pulse rate, restlessness, irritability, and headache occur early. The patient who is experiencing hypoglycemia for the first time may say, "I feel funny," or "I feel peculiar." Changes in the usual behavior of a patient who is receiving insulin are frequently the result of hypoglycemia. For example, Steven Anderson, who had been a model patient, suddenly became very amorous. Mary Sema was found sitting upright in bed, her eyes fixed and her arms rigidly extended in front of her. Mild-mannered Mr. Boas became violent when treatment of hypoglycemia was delayed until blood could be drawn for glucose analysis. Mr. Johns was admitted to the hospital in coma. Buddy Reiman, aged 12, developed nocturnal enuresis (bed wetting). Each of the above patients was suffering from the effects of hypoglycemia. In each instance, treatment with a readily available form of glucose restored the patient to his usual mode of behavior. With the exception of Mr. Johns, glucose was administered by mouth in the form of fruit juice. Moments after an intravenous solution of glucose was begun, Mr. Johns regained consciousness and was demanding to know why he was in the hospital.

Treatment

Because of the possibility of permanent damage to the brain, patients who receive insulin in the treatment of diabetes mellitus should learn to recognize early symptoms and signs of hypoglycemia and how to treat it. Modified insulins create a problem, inasmuch as hypoglycemia may develop without causing warning signs. Persons under insulin therapy should also be taught that exercise improves the utilization of glucose and that hypoglycemia is more likely to develop when unusual amounts of exercise are taken. They should be subject to regular observation when they are hospitalized. Should they develop signs or symptoms indicating hypoglycemia, it should be treated promptly. Usually 100 ml of orange or other fruit juice provide sufficient glucose to correct the condition. Observation of patients receiving long-acting insulin who experience hypoglycemia should be continued. Because of the possibility of recurrence of hypoglycemia in persons receiving long-acting insulin, milk and crackers may be used in treatment because they provide a more sustained source of glucose than do fruit juices or sugar.

Excessive secretion of insulin associated with hyperplasia or an adenoma of islet cells may also be responsible for hypoglycemia. Adenomas are believed to be of infrequent occurrence. Cure is effected by surgical removal. Functional hypoglycemia is a common occurrence. It is usually associated with anxiety and increased nervous tension. Symptoms such as weakness, faintness, tachycardia, and headache follow a meal. The ingestion of carbohydrate alleviates the symptoms temporarily but because carbohydrates act to stimulate the secretion of insulin, a vicious circle, or positive feedback, is initiated.[71] Most patients respond well to a high-protein, high-fat, and low-carbohydrate diet. They should be instructed to avoid the ingestion of highly concentrated carbohydrates because they stimulate the secretion of insulin.

HYPERGLYCEMIA

In contrast to hypoglycemia, hyperglycemia is a condition in which the level of glucose in the blood rises above 110 to 120 mg per 100 ml of blood. It can result from the excessive ingestion of glucose, from overproduction of glucose within the organism, or from inadequacy or failure of the mechanism for the removal of glucose from the blood. More than one mechanism may be involved. The condition in which hyperglycemia follows the excessive ingestion of concentrated carbohydrates is known as alimentary glycosuria. The term *alimentary* refers to the fact that glucose is absorbed from the alimentary canal. The presence of glycosuria indicates that the renal threshold for glucose has been exceeded with the result that glucose appears in the urine. Therapy is obvious: Avoid eating excessive quantities of carbohydrate, especially in the form of sugars, at a given meal.

Overactivity of one or more of the mechanisms for the endogenous formation of glucose follows the administration of epinephrine, and this results in an elevated blood glucose. It can also be expected to rise as a part of the reaction of the individual to stressful situations. Many

patients have some elevation in blood glucose following a coronary occlusion or major surgery. Because epinephrine stimulates the liver to convert glycogen to glucose, the elevation of the blood sugar depends on glycogen being present in the liver.

Hyperglycemia of sufficient degree to cause glycosuria may also occur in persons with hyperfunctioning adrenal cortices. It is also a finding in acromegaly, a disorder associated with hyperexcretion of the growth hormone by the anterior hypophysis. In these conditions the failure in the homeostasis of glucose is thought to be the result of the overproduction of glucose by the organism. The possibility also exists that some of these hormones also antagonize the action of insulin or interfere with its secretion.

A third source of hyperglycemia derives from a failure of the mechanisms for the removal of glucose from the blood. Although the mechanism that immediately comes to mind relates to the action of insulin, failure of the liver to store glucose is also a cause of hyperglycemia. In serious liver disease, hyperglycemia after a meal, followed by a sharp drop in blood glucose to hypoglycemic levels, is a common finding.

The second souce of failure to remove glucose from the blood at a normal rate is a deficiency in the supply of insulin. Although this is generally believed to be the result of inadequate secretion, it may possibly be caused by an increase in the rate at which insulin is destroyed. Whatever the cause, hyperglycemia occurs when the supply of insulin is insufficient to remove glucose from the blood as rapidly as it is added. All degrees of failure are possible. In some individuals sufficient insulin is secreted to maintain the level of glucose within physiological limits provided the ingestion of glucose is moderate or there is no increase in the activity of mechanisms for increasing the production of glucose. In others the deficiency of insulin may be so great that only by restricting the intake of carbohydrate and the administration of exogenous insulin can the blood sugar be maintained within normal limits most of the time. The disease resulting from a failure of the mechanism to remove glucose from the blood at a normal rate is diabetes mellitus.

GLUCOSE TOLERANCE TEST

Individuals who are unable to adapt normally to a heavy load of glucose can be identified by a glucose tolerance test. The details for performance of this test differ from one physician or agency to another. In all instances the purpose of the test is to determine the adequacy of the mechanism of the patient for removing

---

[71] In a positive feedback, a change in one direction intensifies the tendency to change in the same direction.

glucose from the blood, thereby restoring homeostasis.

For 2 to 3 days preceding the test, the patient should eat a diet that provides 250 to 300 g of carbohydrate. The nurse has a responsibility to make sure that the patient understands the instructions and, when he is in the hospital, to encourage him to eat the food served to him. On the day of the test, fasting specimens of blood and urine to be used as controls are obtained before the glucose is administered. The patient is then given a weighed amount of glucose (usually 100 g for an adult) dissolved in water and flavored with citric acid or lemon juice. Blood samples and specimens of urine are obtained ½, 1, 2, and 3 hours later.

The results obtained in individuals with normal and abnormal glucose-tolerance curves differ in several respects. The individual who has a normal capacity to respond to an increased supply of glucose has a sharp, but limited, rise in the concentration of glucose in his blood plasma. The maximum elevation should not exceed 150 mg per 100 ml of blood plasma. There is a sharp rise in one-half hour, with little rise thereafter. By the second hour the concentration of glucose in the blood has returned to normal.

The individual with an inadequate capacity to remove glucose from the blood responds to overloading with glucose differently. The fasting blood sugar is higher than normal. The rise in the blood sugar following the ingestion of glucose is higher, and the return to the pretest level is delayed. This type of curve is observed in the patient in the early phases of diabetes as well as in those whose diabetes mellitus is known.

Several modifications of the glucose tolerance test have been developed. In one of these the test dose of glucose is divided into two parts. The second half is given one-half hour after the first. In the person who has a normal adaptive capacity, the level of glucose in the blood does not rise after the second dose of glucose. In the person whose adaptive capacity has been impaired, the level of glucose in the blood continues to rise. When hyperinsulinism is suspected, blood and urine samples may also be collected at 4, 5, and 6 hours after the ingestion of glucose. In patients who produce too much insulin the blood sugar drops to hypoglycemic levels.

The early detection of diabetes mellitus is often accomplished by performing two glucose tolerance tests. Eight hours and again 2 hours before the second test 50 mg of cortisone are administered orally. The cortisone intensifies the strain on the mechanisms for removing glucose from the blood. In persons with an inadequate insulin reserve, the blood glucose curve obtained during the second test resembles that found in diabetes mellitus. Persons who respond positively to this test are encouraged to follow a regime to decrease the likelihood of developing diabetes mellitus, that is, to avoid gaining weight.

For example, Mrs. Hale, aged 27, has stress or stage II diabetes mellitus. Both her parents are diabetics. When Mrs. Hale is well and eats moderately and exercises actively and regularly, her fasting blood sugar is within normal limits. When she overeats, has a cold, or is pregnant, her blood glucose tends to rise. She sees her physician regularly and eats moderately. She tries to adjust her food intake so that she maintains her ideal weight. In contrast Mrs. Hale's sister Clara's response to glucose-tolerance tests indicates that her capacity to adapt to glucose is within normal limits. Present-day knowledge is insufficient to be sure that Clara will never develop diabetes. Because the ideal weight favors health and longevity, Clara has been advised to avoid obesity and to exercise regularly. She has also been assured that she does not have diabetes.

Lipid Metabolism

Lipids include fats, oils, and many other fatlike substances. Body lipids include triglycerides or neutral fats, phospholipids, free fatty acids, cholesterol, and other substances of a fatlike nature.

NUTRITIONAL ROLE

The chief contribution made by dietary fats is to the energy needs of the body. Typical American diets supply about 35 to 45 per cent of calories from fats. In some parts of the world, especially in the Orient, the fat intake may account for only 10 to 15 per cent of the calories. When metabolized, 1 g of fat yields about 9 calories. Fats improve the flavor of many foods thereby increasing food acceptability, increase the satiety value of the diet by reason of the longer time required for digestion, and serve as carriers for the fat-soluble vitamins.

Lipids are distributed in all body cells and tissues. Most of the body fat occurs as neutral fat in the adipose tissue located beneath the skin, in the abdominal area, and surrounding the organs. Adipose tissue normally represents about 15 to 20 per cent of the body weight. It is the long-term reserve of body fuel, for we have seen that the glycogen stores would suffice for less than a day in the absence of food.

Body fats serve in the cushioning of the organs and as insulation against changes in the environmental temperature. Phospholipids and cholesterol abound in active tissues and are essential for the absorption and transport of fats. Phospholipids and glycolipids are also integral components of nervous tissue. Arachidonic acid, a polyunsaturated fatty acid, is required for growth and normal skin health in infants. This fatty acid is probably required for the transport of lipids and is involved in the permeability of the cells.

DIETARY SOURCES

About 60 per cent of dietary fat is supplied by "invisible" sources: meats, poultry, fish, dairy products (excluding butter), egg yolks, and baked foods. The remaining 40 per cent is furnished by "visible" fats including butter, margarine, lard, hydrogenated shortenings, oils, and salad dressings.

The type of fat is an important dietary consideration inasmuch as saturated fats are believed to increase the level of the blood cholesterol whereas fats predominating in polyunsaturated fatty acids appear to have a cholesterol-lowering effect. Beef, pork, lamb, whole milk, cream, cheese made from whole milk, ice cream, butter, and egg yolk are rich in saturated fatty acids; poultry and fish contain somewhat higher proportions of the polyunsaturated fatty acid, linoleic acid. Most vegetable oils including safflower, sunflower, sesame, cottonseed, corn, and soybean oils are rich sources of linoleic acid. By contrast, peanut oil is only moderately high, and coconut and olive oils are low in linoleic acid.

By hydrogenation, oils become solid fats, the level of saturated fatty acids increases, and the level of linoleic acid is reduced. Thus even a vegetable oil high in linoleic acid is no longer a good source when it is converted to margarine or a hydrogenated shortening. Special-type margarines that have been only lightly hydrogenated are now available in most markets. It is obviously an oversimplification and error to state that animal fats are saturated and vegetable fats are unsaturated.

Phospholipids and cholesterol are readily synthesized by the liver and other organs and a dietary source is not essential. High dietary intakes of cholesterol are believed to increase the blood cholesterol levels. Rich dietary sources include egg yolk, liver, brains, kidney, shellfish, and sweetbreads. Butter, cream, whole milk, ice cream, and fatty meats are moderately high. Plant foods contain no cholesterol.

DIGESTION AND ABSORPTION

A small amount of emulsified fat may be hydrolyzed in the stomach, but the chief site of fat digestion is in the small intestine. Bile reduces the surface tension and increases the emulsification of fats so that they are more readily attacked by pancreatic lipase. The products of hydrolysis include monoglycerides, free fatty acids, and glycerol. The intestinal mucosa resynthesizes new fat so that the products absorbed include triglycerides and phospholipids, free fatty acids, and glycerol.

Normally about 95 per cent of dietary fats are digested and absorbed. Fats high in saturated fatty acids are more slowly digested than those that are unsaturated, but there is little if any difference in the amounts that are eventually absorbed. Likewise, fried foods are more slowly digested although the completeness of digestion is not, as a rule, adversely affected.

The absorption of fats is facilitated in the presence of bile and phospholipids. Short-chain fatty acids and glycerol are water soluble and enter the capillaries of the intestinal wall and in turn the portal vein. The insoluble longer-chain fatty acids, triglycerides, phospholipids, cholesterol, and fat-soluble vitamins proceed into the lacteals, the lymph circulation to the thoracic duct, and then to the left subclavian vein.

BLOOD LIPIDS

Because they are insoluble in water, lipids are transported in the blood associated with more or less protein, phospholipid, and cholesterol. The complexes are broadly classed as alpha and beta lipoproteins. The alpha lipoproteins remain relatively constant throughout life, but certain classes of the beta lipoproteins increase with age.

The serum or plasma of a sample of blood taken after a meal rich in fat will be milky in appearance because of the high level of circulating lipids. After a few hours this turbidity disappears resulting from the action of clearing factors including heparin, lipoprotein lipase, and arachidonic acid.

Increased levels of certain classes of beta lipoproteins are believed to correlate with the incidence of atherosclerosis and coronary disease. The determination of total lipid, cholesterol, phospholipid, and triglyceride levels in the blood is less expensive and appears to be as useful for identifying high-risk individuals. When such determinations are ordered they should be made on blood samples drawn after an overnight fast.

What mechanisms control the anabolism and catabolism of fats?

THE LIVER AND FAT METABOLISM

The key organ in fat metabolism is the liver. It shortens or lengthens fatty acid chains; synthesizes triglycerides, cholesterol, or phospholipids and attaches them to proteins for transport to the tissues; and hydrolyzes the triglycerides brought to the liver. The normal metabolism of fats in the liver proceeds only when one or more lipotropic factors are present; these are methionine, betaine, choline, vitamin B_{12}, and inositol. When these factors are missing, fats accumulate in the liver.

The liver is the chief source of the ketone bodies—acetoacetic acid, beta-hydroxybutyric acid, and acetone. The acetoacetate molecule is not efficiently metabolized by the liver and passes to the peripheral tissues that normally oxidize ketones at the rate they are produced by the liver. During fasting the oxidation of endogenous fat is increased to compensate for the decreased energy available from glycogen. The production of ketones by the liver may exceed the ability of the tissues to use them so that a mild ketosis results, and 5 to 10 g of ketones may be excreted in the urine. This is corrected by giving carbohydrate to replenish liver glycogen. In uncontrolled diabetes mellitus, ketones are produced at a rapid rate but the peripheral tissues have a decreased capacity to oxidize them; in severe diabetes the excretion of ketones may exceed 100 g per day, and acidosis is severe. The ketosis is corrected by giving insulin to restore carbohydrate metabolism.

HORMONAL CONTROLS

The uptake of glucose from the blood by adipose tissue is facilitated by the action of insulin. Fatty acid and triglyceride synthesis is also stimulated by insulin. The release of free fatty acids from adipose tissue to the circulation is brought about by epinephrine, norepinephrine, glucagon, adrenocorticotropic hormone, growth hormone, and thyrotropic hormone.

SYNTHESIS OF FATS

Many body organs and tissues including the liver, lactating mammary glands, kidney, intestinal mucosa, arterial walls, and adipose tissue itself can synthesize fats. Adipose tissue consists chiefly of triglycerides. Contrary to widely held opinions it is a rapidly changing tissue with free fatty acids being constantly released to the circulation and new triglycerides being resynthesized. Thus adipose tissue is effective in maintaining blood lipid levels within limits.

Fats, carbohydrates, and amino acids are donors of acetate, which, activated by coenzyme A, is the key unit in the synthesis of fatty acids. Thus an energy supply in excess of body needs, whatever the source of calories, will lead to rapid synthesis of adipose tissue. The acetate unit can be condensed with another unit to form acetoacetate; in turn, another acetate unit may be added, thereby gradually lengthening the fatty acid chain.

Various tissues also possess the ability to modify the degree of saturation of fatty acids as well as the length of the fatty acid chain. Thus arachidonic acid can be synthesized from linoleic acid by adding an acetate unit and introducing two additional double bonds. On the other hand, the tissues are not able to introduce a second double bond into the oleic acid molecule to produce linoleic acid. Therefore, linoleic acid is an essential fatty acid that must be present in the diet.

Phospholipids are produced by the small intestine, liver, and kidney. Cholesterol is readily synthesized from acetate units by the liver, adrenal, kidney, and lung. Just as acetate units available from excess calorie intake lead to increases in adipose tissue, so also the synthesis of cholesterol increases when calories are in excess of body needs.

OXIDATION OF FATS

Beta oxidation, first described by Knoop, is probably the main pathway for fat oxidation. According to this theory, two carbon atoms are split off from the fatty acid chain at the time. The acid (COOH) group is combined with coenzyme A and through a series of steps the acetate unit is split off. For example, stearic acid, containing 18 carbon atoms, would eventually yield 9 acetate units. The acetate units, as we have seen, may be used to resynthesize fatty acids or cholesterol, or they may be further oxidized by combining with oxaloacetate and entering the citric acid cycle to yield energy, carbon dioxide, and water. The glycerol fraction of triglycerides follows the pathway of glucose in its oxidation. (See Figures 12-4 and 12-5.)

ABNORMALITIES OF FAT METABOLISM

Obesity, underweight, and diabetes mellitus are widely recognized abnormalities of fat metabolism discussed at other points in this text. A great deal of evidence has accumulated over the last decade to implicate the diet in the elevation of blood cholesterol and other blood lipids and in the incidence of atherosclerosis. (See also Chapter 10.) Blood cholesterol levels are increased when diets are high in saturated fats and low in polyunsaturated fats and by diets high in cholesterol. Blood triglyceride levels are increased by diets containing large amounts of sucrose. On the other hand, diets designed to maintain normal weight, very low-fat diets, and diets normal in fat content but modified to give high proportions of polyunsaturated fatty acids to saturated fatty acids bring about lowering of the blood cholesterol levels. The American Heart Association [72] now recommends that Americans reduce the risks by replacing saturated fats with polyunsaturated fats as much as possible, by eating less food that is high in cholesterol, and by counting calories to lose weight or to keep weight down. These diet changes mean that more poultry and fish are eaten and less meat, skim milk is used in place of whole milk, vegetable oils are used instead of solid fats, and eggs, organ meats, and shellfish are restricted.

Protein Metabolism

NATURE OF PROTEINS AND DIETARY SOURCES

Proteins are composed of 20 or so amino acids, each of which contains an acid (COOH) group and an amino (NH_2) group. Eight of the amino acids are classed as dietary essentials because they cannot be synthesized in the body. The remaining 12 or so amino acids are nonessential because the body can synthesize them, provided that some source of nitrogen is available. Proteins that contain all of the essential amino acids in sufficient amounts to synthesize new tissues as well as to maintain them are known as *complete*. Milk and milk products (except butter), eggs, meats, poultry, and fish are excellent sources of complete proteins.

When a protein lacks one or more of the essential amino acids, or has a deficient quantity of them, it is classed as *incomplete;* it is not able to meet the needs for synthesizing tissues. The proteins in cereal grains, legumes, nuts, fruits, and vegetables are incomplete. Nevertheless, cereal grains and legumes are important sources of protein because they are staple foods for much of the world's population; the amounts of these foods eaten usually meet the protein needs for the maintenance of the healthy adult. On the other hand, plant-food diets, for the most part, do not contain sufficient amounts of some amino acids to meet the growth needs of infants, children, or pregnant or lactating women or the replacement needs of people convalescing from severe undernutrition. Even a small quantity of complete protein foods eaten at the same meal with these less expensive

plant-food sources will yield an amino acid combination that is satisfactory for growth needs. For example, bread is a relatively inexpensive source of protein and of calories. If bread is served with milk the combination of amino acids will be satisfactory; nonfat dry milk is an inexpensive way to improve the protein quality of bread.

Most of the world's population has little complete protein available, the result being severe protein malnutrition among millions of infants and children. A number of approaches are being used in an effort to solve this problem. (1) Foods are developed that contain proteins from several plants. The mixtures are based on the principle that some plants are good sources of certain of the essential amino acids, whereas others supply a different assortment of amino acids. By combining the foods, the final product yields all the essential amino acids in satisfactory amounts; one food is said to *supplement* another. *Incaparina* is such a product developed in Central America for feeding infants and young children and consisting of corn and cottonseed meals, yeast, and sorghum. Many similar products have been developed in other countries of the world, using foods native to the countries. (2) Fish is an excellent source of protein and relatively inexpensive but has not been utilized as widely as it might be. Fresh fish farming has been introduced, especially in the rice-growing countries. The fish are grown in the rice paddies. Also, fish protein concentrate is now prepared in the United States and in some developing countries. This is a creamy white, practically flavor-free powder containing about 80 per cent protein. Its keeping qualities are good, an important consideration in countries of the world where refrigeration is practically nonexistent. It can be used to reinforce the protein content of breads and other foods. (3) Agricultural geneticists have developed strains of corn and wheat that are richer in some essential amino acids than the usual varieties of these grains. This approach holds considerable promise for improvement of the quality of the protein of the diet. (4) The lacking amino acids may be added in synthetic form to foods to improve their protein quality. Reinforcement of wheat flour with lysine, one of the essential amino acids, is now being tested in India. Some of the essential amino acids are still too expensive to make this a practicable method for improving the diets of poverty-stricken people. (5) Leaves, yeasts, fungi, and algae currently seem to be exotic and improbable sources of protein. Yet, with rapid technological developments, some or all of these potential sources probably will be widely used in the future.

---

[72] *Reduce Your Risk of Heart Attack* (New York: American Heart Association, 1966).

UTILIZATION OF PROTEIN

About 92 per cent of dietary proteins are hydrolyzed to amino acids in the small intestine and then absorbed into the capillaries of the intestinal wall. The amino acids are carried by the portal vein to the liver and then enter the general circulation. The amino acids are rapidly incorporated into the existing tissues or used for synthesizing new tissues; they may be used for the production of numerous regulatory compounds; they may be deaminized and used for energy or stored in the form of glycogen or fat.

Proteins are part of the structure of every tissue in the body and are components of all body fluids except bile and urine. Tissue proteins are in a state of dynamic equilibrium; that is, cells are constantly disintegrating and new ones are replacing them. For example, the cells of the intestinal mucosa are completely replaced every few days and those of the liver almost as rapidly. The turnover rate is somewhat slower in muscle, but the large mass of muscle tissue represents a sizable daily interchange.

Proteins have innumerable regulatory functions inasmuch as they are components of enzymes and hormones. The blood proteins include hemoglobin involved in the transport of oxygen, fibrinogen as one of the factors in blood clotting, globulins that function in the defense against disease, and serum albumin for the maintenance of the osmotic pressure of the blood and fluid balance of the tissues. The amino acids have specific functions; for example, tryptophan is a precursor of niacin and of serotonin, a vasoconstrictor; methionine has lipotropic activity in the liver and is essential for the formation of phospholipids; and glycine is involved in the detoxication of benzoic acid in the liver and the formation of bile acids, purines, and fatty acids.

Proteins are also a source of energy, each gram of protein yielding about 4 calories when oxidized in the body. Amino acids that are not used for building tissues are deaminized, that is, the amino group is split off. The remainder of the molecule is an organic acid that can enter the citric acid cycle to yield energy (see Figure 12-6) or that can be transformed into glycogen or fat. The energy needs of the body take priority over the synthesis of tissues. Therefore, if the diet does not supply sufficient calories from carbohydrates and fats, the protein of the diet as well as body glycogen, fat, and tissue protein will be used to complete the energy requirement. Under these circumstances the synthesis of tissue proteins will be curtailed. If optimum tissue building is to take place, whether in childhood or in recovery from illness, the caloric adequacy of the diet—as well as that of protein—is essential.

Most of the deamination of amino acids takes place in the liver where the amino group is used to synthesize urea, the principal nitrogen compound in the urine. The liver may also bring about the transfer of an amino group (transamination) to an organic acid, thus forming the nonessential amino acids. The kidney is able to utilize the amino group for the synthesis of ammonia that, in the form of ammonium salts, helps to conserve the sodium ion and thus aids in maintaining acid-base balance.

NITROGEN BALANCE

The level of protein metabolism can be determined by measuring the nitrogen balance. Because protein is approximately 16 per cent nitrogen, 1 g of nitrogen is equivalent to about 6.25 g of protein. In nitrogen balance studies the nitrogen content of the food consumed is compared with the nitrogen content of the excretions. Most of the nitrogen excreted is in the urine, chiefly as urea. The measurement of the nitrogen in a 24-hour collection of urine is a reliable indicator of the preceding metabolism of protein that has taken place. The daily excretion of nitrogen in the feces usually ranges from 0.5 to 1.5 g depending on the nature of the diet ingested. The fecal excretion includes the nitrogen from undigested protein and from bacterial cells and the disintegrated proteins of enzymes and cells of the intestinal mucosa.

If the nitrogen intake and excretions are equal, the individual is in *nitrogen balance,* this being the normal state for the healthy adult. If the nitrogen intake is greater than the nitrogen output, the individual is in *positive balance.* This means that anabolic processes are greater than catabolic processes, the expected situation in growth of infants and children, in the development of maternal and fetal tissues during pregnancy, in the production of milk during lactation, and in the recovery from illness, injury, or surgery. *Negative nitrogen balance* is an unfavorable sign for it means that nitrogen is being lost from the body more rapidly than it is supplied by the diet. The underlying reasons for a negative nitrogen balance are many, including (1) insufficient intake of protein in terms of quality or quantity or both, (2) insufficient calorie intake so that dietary protein and body tissues are being used to meet the energy needs, (3) defect in absorption of amino acids from the digestive tract because of enzyme deficiencies or diseases of malabsorption, (4) inability to metabolize one or more amino acids because of a genetic defect, and (5) excessive losses of protein in exudates of burns and draining wounds or in the urine because of renal damage.

The body does not store protein in the same sense that it stores fat. Nevertheless, the tissues are able to yield some protein to maintain important functions when the intake is inadequate. These *labile* reserves permit the adult to function for comparatively long periods of time with a deficient intake of protein. For young children, the consequences of protein deprivation are much more acute.

RECOMMENDED ALLOWANCE

The recommended allowance for protein for the adult is 0.9 g per kilogram of desirable body weight, or about 0.4 g per pound.[73] Because of anabolic requirements, the needs for infants and children and for pregnant and lactating women are somewhat higher per unit of body weight. The calorie needs should be essentially met from carbohydrates and fats. At least one third of the dietary protein of adults should be derived from complete protein foods; one half to two thirds of the child's protein allowance is preferably furnished by complete protein foods.

What are the effects of a lack of protein?

The effects of protein deficiency have been described in this chapter under the heading "Undernutrition" (p. 552). Because protein foods are generally good sources of the B-complex vitamins and iron, the signs of deficiency are those of multiple nutrient lacks. Loss of weight, strength, and ability to respond to infection and stress are frequent but nonspecific indicators of deficiency. Anemia is often present because of the lack of both protein and iron for the synthesis of hemoglobin. The colloid osmotic pressure of the blood is gradually reduced as the level of serum albumin falls. Fatty livers have been noted in severe protein undernutrition.

Protein deficiency occurs in many serious illnesses because of inability to ingest protein or because of excessive losses. The deficit is aggravated by the fact that there is an increase in the rate of tissue breakdown for the first few days after a severe injury or a surgical procedure. Proteins may be lost in excessive amounts into the urine, from draining wounds such as burned surfaces, and in accumulations of serous fluids such as ascites. Chronic abscesses, decubiti, or osteomyelitis may be accompanied by an excessive loss of protein. Continued bed

[73] *Recommended Daily Dietary Allowances,* 7th ed. (Washington, D.C.: Food and Nutrition Board, National Research Council, National Academy of Sciences, 1968).

rest, even in the healthy, is accompanied by loss of protein for the first three or four days— then the loss of protein tapers off and the nitrogen balance is restored. Loss of protein from the body is, therefore, one of the undesirable effects of bed rest. Loss of protein-containing fluid represents a loss not only of protein but of minerals, vitamins, water, and other substances from the body. The effects on the organism will depend in part on the suddenness with which the losses occur, the conditions that are responsible, and the length of time that they persist. Sudden large losses of fluid into serous cavities may, by reducing blood volume, lead to shock. Smaller losses over a period of time lead to malnutrition with a loss of weight, strength, and ability to respond to stress. Resistance of tissue to pressure is less in the undernourished than in the well-nourished. When decubiti form, they resist treatment unless and until protein and other nutritional deficiencies are corrected. Recovery depends on the restoration of nutritive elements.

Mineral Elements and Vitamins

Mineral elements and vitamins have numerous metabolic roles, many of which have been discussed in some detail in other chapters of this book. The discussion that follows is intended to summarize briefly some of the pertinent facts regarding these important body components. A number of texts in nutrition may be consulted by the student who desires more detailed discussion of one or more of these nutrients.

What is the scope of the regulatory functions of the minerals and vitamins?

METABOLIC ROLE

Mineral elements constitute only about 4 per cent of the body weight. Calcium alone accounts for about half of this and phosphorus for about one fourth, the bones and teeth being the chief site of the calcium-phosphate salts. Magnesium is also an important element in the bone structure, and sodium and fluorine occur in small amounts. Potassium is the chief mineral element within the cells of the soft tissues. Sulfur, a constituent of the amino acids methionine and cystine, is present in all protein tissues.

The regulatory functions of minerals are numerous, such as the maintenance of fluid and electrolyte balance, involving principally sodium, potassium, and phosphorus (see Chapter 9); the transport of materials across cell membranes—for example, phosphorus as a constituent of the phospholipids; the maintenance of nerve irritability and muscle contraction based on the precise concentrations of the sodium, potassium, magnesium, and calcium ions in the body fluids; the activity of the parathyroid and thyroid hormones, involving calcium and iodine, respectively; and the transport of blood gases by hemoglobin of which iron is an essential constituent. Trace elements, sometimes called micronutrients, are constituents of, or catalysts for, enzymes and hormones. For example, zinc is a component of insulin, iodine of thyroxine, and cobalt of vitamin B_{12}. Copper, chromium, selenium, and molybdenum were once considered to be contaminants of the diet and in the body but are now established as essential for the activation of specific enzymes.

Vitamins are organic compounds that are required in minute amounts in the diet for specific functions in the body. They differ greatly in their molecular structure, from the relatively simple ascorbic acid molecule to the exceedingly complex vitamin B_{12} molecule. Likewise, they differ in their physical and chemical properties and in their biologic functions. Generally speaking, vitamins function as coenzymes and are involved in highly specialized metabolic processes that have been described previously in this text. For example, vitamin B_{12} and folacin are required for the synthesis of red blood cells in the bone marrow (see Chapter 10); thiamine, riboflavin, and niacin are essential for the activity of many enzyme systems including those for the release of energy from carbohydrates and fats as discussed in this chapter; pantothenic acid is a component of coenzyme A that activates the acetyl group for its entrance into the citric acid cycle or for the synthesis of fatty acids and cholesterol; vitamin B_6 is essential for the metabolism of amino acids and for the conversion of linoleic acid to arachidonic acid; and so on. Ascorbic acid, or vitamin C, is essential for the formation of collagen, and thus is important in the integrity of the blood vessel walls and the connective tissues; its lack results in poor wound healing, hemorrhages, and eventually scurvy. (See Table 12-2.) The B-complex vitamins and ascorbic acid are stored in the body only to a limited extent. A moderate diet deficiency leads to gradual depletion of the tissues and within a period of a few months to such nonspecific signs as fatigue, weakness, neuritis, and poor resistance to infection. If the deficiency in the diet is great, the symptoms of classic deficiency disease will become manifest within months. For example, infants who are given a formula that is deficient in ascorbic acid and with no supplementary foods that are rich in this vitamin will show unmistakable signs of scurvy by the age of 6 to 8 months.

Vitamin A is essential for the integrity of the epithelial tissues, including the mucous membranes and in the regulation of vision in dim light. The liver stores vitamin A so that a person who has had a good intake will suffer few if any ill effects even after months of dietary lack. Yet it should be remembered that many people, especially adolescents, are consuming diets that fail to supply the recommended allowances. As a consequence nutritional surveys have shown lowered blood levels of vitamin A and associated night blindness. Severe vitamin A deficiency, as characterized by keratinization of the epithelium, xerophthalmia, and permanent blindness, is a major health problem particularly in the Far East.

Vitamin D is required for the utilization of calcium and phosphorus (see Chapter 15, Part A); its lack is responsible for rickets in young children. Vitamin E is important for its antioxidant properties, and vitamin K in the formation of prothrombin.

PROBLEMS OF DIETARY ADEQUACY

Of the 15 or so mineral elements required by the body, special attention is needed for calcium, iron, iodine, and fluorine. When the allowances for protein and for these elements are met, the needs for other mineral elements will be fully realized.

The dietary survey conducted by the United States Department of Agriculture in 1965 showed that only 70 per cent of families were consuming diets that met the recommended allowances for calcium.[74] This study indicated a lower consumption of milk and greater intake of carbonated beverages, fruit drinks, coffee, and tea. Some improvement in the milk consumption would correct the calcium lack in the diet. A nurse often finds it difficult to convince people of the need for calcium inasmuch as the effects of deficiency usually are manifest only after years of inadequate intake. Moreover, many individuals have the ability to adapt to relatively low intakes. Perhaps the best argument that can be made for adequate calcium intake throughout life is on the basis of insurance in terms of normal bone structure. Teen-aged girls often drink too little milk in the mistaken notion that it is fattening. Their actual calcium needs are high to meet the requirements for bone growth and maturation. When the demands of pregnancy are superimposed on these already high needs, the young mother-to-be is quite likely to be in negative balance. Osteoporosis, a bone disease affecting large numbers of older people, especially

[74] Sadye F. Adelson: "Changes in Diets of Households, 1955 to 1965," *J. Home Econ.,* **60**:448–55 (June) 1968.

women, has a complex etiology, but it seems clear that those who drink little milk throughout life are more susceptible than those who are milk drinkers. Sometimes the ill effects of low calcium intake become evident in the failure of bones to heal following fracture, particularly in older persons.

The most serious dietary problem with respect to the mineral elements is that of iron. Infants, young children, adolescent girls, and pregnant women are especially vulnerable to iron-deficiency anemia. To correct this problem, the recommended allowance for iron is 18 mg for girls and women and 10 mg for men.[75] A good diet based on suggested intakes from each of the four food groups will supply about 6 to 7 mg of iron per 1,000 calories. Thus the man experiences no difficulty in obtaining the recommended allowance. Not so for women! Most women require about 1,800 to 2,400 calories daily, and even good diets would therefore supply only about two thirds of the recommended iron allowance. In nutrition education, emphasis must be placed on rich sources of iron including the organ meats, especially liver, enriched and whole grain breads and cereals, some dark green leafy vegetables, meats, egg yolk, legumes, dried fruits, and molasses. The contribution made by these foods, of course, depends on the frequency with which they are consumed as well as the amounts used. Nutrition scientists are currently considering the advisability of fortification of foods with iron. A first step in this direction would be the mandatory enrichment of all cereals and flours.

Iodine deficiency is most common in the parts of the world far from the sea. During the history of the world, soil has been leached of iodine and iodine washed into the streams and thence into the seas and oceans. Soil in the great plains, such as the center of the United States, and in mountainous regions, such as the Andean Altiplano or the Swiss Alps, is deficient in iodine. In these areas evidence of iodine deficiency has been common. Conditions increasing the need for thyroxin intensify the deficiency. Pregnancy, adolescence, or infections may be associated with enlargement of the thyroid gland in iodine-deficient areas. Prevention of iodine deficiency is achieved by the use of iodized salt.

When added to water in the amount of 1 part per million of water, fluorine has been demonstrated to reduce the rate of dental caries. Excessive concentrations of fluorine cause mottling of the enamel of the teeth. Despite convincing evidence of the value of fluorides in the prevention of dental caries,

there has been organized resistance to the introduction of fluoride into drinking water. Some of the opponents claim the fluorine increases the incidence of heart disease in the areas where it is used. Objective analysis of the statistics indicates the falsity of this belief. Other persons object on the basis that fluorine is of value only to the young and that cities should not use tax funds to support a procedure that benefits only a part of the population. Still others object on religious grounds. Some even object on the ground that it violates the right of the individual to choose what he will or will not ingest. A review of the history of chlorination of water indicates a similar story.

Adelson [76] reported that only 73 per cent of American families had good diets with respect to ascorbic acid and 74 per cent of diets rated good for vitamin A. These dietary inadequacies stem primarily from failure to supply sufficient amounts of fruits and vegetables in the diet. The rules for dietary planning to ensure sufficient intake are relatively simple: (1) some dark green or deep yellow vegetable or deep yellow fruit at least every other day to supply ample carotene, the precursor of vitamin A; and (2) some citrus fruit or other good source of vitamin C such as tomato juice, raw cabbage or dark green leafy vegetable, broccoli, or cantaloupe.

Summary

In this chapter, the role of the nurse in facilitating the maintenance of nutrition in the patient has been presented. Content has been selected to emphasize the importance of nutrition to health and productivity as well as to the susceptibility to disease and the ability to recover therefrom. Emphasis has been placed on the manner in which the body uses nutrients in its processes and the manner in which these processes may be disturbed. Although stress has been placed on the biochemistry of nutrition, the importance of food in the emotional and social life of the individual has been included. Survival depends on the supply to the cells of at least a minimum level of nutrients. Growth, reproduction, and all the higher functions also depend on the nutritional state of the individual.

As with other needs, satisfaction of the need depends on adequate supplies to meet the requirements of the tissues, a facility whereby materials may be taken from the external environment and altered so that they can be transported to the internal environment, transporta-

---

[75] *Recommended Dietary Allowances, op. cit.*

[76] *Op. cit.*, p. 449.

tion from the point of entry to the cell, the capacity of the cell to utilize the nutrients, regulation of the processes so that the needs of the cells are met, and the integration of all activities so that the needs of the whole organism are met. Because some nutrients are stored, provisions for converting them into appropriate substances and storage facilities are necessary.

Facilities are also required to eliminate excesses of intake or end products of metabolism. A disruption or disturbance at any point may interfere with the capacity of the cell to carry on its processes.

Because of the importance of food, physiologically, emotionally, and socially, it provides the nurse with a natural medium through which to convey to the patient her concern for him as a person and as a human being. It is often through her efforts to meet his individual wishes and desires that the food is "transferred from the plate to his stomach." Although it may be a cliché to say "It isn't the food that is served to the patient, but what he eats that is important," it is true, nonetheless.

For short periods of time, diets inadequate in one or more nutrients may be ingested without causing serious harm. More or less permanent modifications in the diet must meet basic nutritional requirements if malnutrition is to be avoided. In general, diets are modified to (1) accommodate to a disturbance in the structure or function of the gastrointestinal tract, (2) correct the effect of an excess or deficit of essential nutrients, and (3) accommodate to a defect in the capacity to utilize one or more nutrients.

The theme of this chapter is summarized in the words of King:

Nutrition is the science of food, the nutrients and other substances therein, their action, interaction and balance in relation to health and disease, and the processes by which the organism ingests, absorbs, transports, utilizes, and excretes food substances. In addition, nutrition must be concerned with certain social, economic, cultural, and psychological implications of food and eating.[77]

[77] C. Glen King, in Ogden C. Johnson: "A Conference on Nutrition Teaching in Medical Schools," *Nutr. Rev.,* **21**:34 (Feb.) 1963.

TABLE 12-2

A Survey of Some Disorders of Nutrition and Conditions Involving the Alimentary Tract and Related Structures

Diagnostic Category	Etiological Factors	Incubation Period and Nature of Onset	Part of Gastrointestinal Tract and/or Associated Structures Involved	Severity of Illness and Course; Signs and Symptoms	Effect on Adequacy of Nutrition	Major Medical and/or Surgical Treatment
Psychogenic and/or Neurogenic						
Achalasia (cardiospasm)	Physiological obstruction. Emotional disturbances may precipitate.	Dysphagia of the kind in which there is a delay of ingested food entering the stomach.	Esophagus: tortuous, elongated, lower end fails to relax with each peristaltic wave. Esophageal dilation of varying degree except at distal end, which is undilated. Substernal pain, intermittent dysphagia, regurgitation.	Chronic condition. Progression of dysphagia inconsistent. Regurgitation in recumbent position. Nocturnal wakefulness caused by excessive cough. Pulmonary complications may occur if food is aspirated into the tracheobronchial tree. Esophageal carcinoma sometimes develops because of prolonged irritation.	Initially satisfactory; then malnutrition caused by insufficient food intake. Weight loss.	Bougienage. If not curative, hydrostatic or pneumatic forceful dilatation is done. Cardioesophagomyotomy if the above methods fail.
Irritable colon	Excessive irritants (laxatives, foods, enemas), or emotional disturbance, or both.	Distention and fullness induced by ingestion of food or liquid, to severe cramplike abdominal pain. Sudden or gradual onset lasting for hours to years depending on duration of the emotional disturbance.	Colon: often palpable and tender. Normal rectum and sigmoid on proctoscopy. Small intestine and colon irritability noted on barium enema.	Defecation or passage of flatus may afford temporary relief or initiate more cramps and tenesmus. Nausea, belching, rumbling, gurgling in abdomen, burning tongue with a brassy taste.	Usually well-nourished but occasionally varying degrees of malnutrition are seen.	Relief of anxiety about organic disease. Deeper psychotherapy if needed. Education of patient in relation to diet and fluids, in obtaining and maintaining satisfactory bowel habits.

Diverticulum (one) Diverticulosis (many) Diverticulitis (Inflammation of) (An outpouching or herniation of the mucosa through a defect in the muscularis.)	In general, weakness of the muscular wall of the alimentary canal caused by congenital defect or loss of muscle during the process of aging.	Depends on site, size, and presence or absence of inflammation.	Common sites: esophagus, duodenum, and colon. May occur anywhere along the alimentary canal. In the presence of diverticulitis, signs and symptoms of acute inflammation. Effects intensified by peritonitis or mediastinitis.	Diffuse spasm of lower third of esophagus. Hypermotility of the stomach.	Excessive flatus.	Avoidance of fecal impaction during initial therapy.
				May be symptomless, acute, chronic, or recurring. Perforation results in mediastinitis or peritonitis depending on location. Symptoms of mechanical obstruction are present. Occasionally, symptoms of the genitourinary tract are present. Fistula formation and hemorrhage may complicate course of illness.	Other physical symptoms related to psychogenesis of disease.	Rest and exercise determined on individual basis.
					Patient usually wants bowel movement daily and takes laxative or enema to achieve this.	Antispasmodics.
					Absence of organic disease.	None, a diet avoiding nuts, seeds and fibrous foods, to surgical removal and closure of the defect.
					Depends on site and effects.	
			Esophagus. Diverticula are present for years before producing symptoms and then symptoms are correlated with the size of the diverticula and the distortion of the esophageal lumen.	May be few if any symptoms or minor difficulty in swallowing. Prominent complaint is regurgitation of undigested food particles on assuming the horizontal position. Gurgling noises in the	Weight loss. Malnutrition in later stages caused by failure of food to enter the digestive tract.	Surgical treatment when symptoms occur.

TABLE 12-2 (cont.)

A Survey of Some Disorders of Nutrition and Conditions Involving the Alimentary Tract and Related Structures

Diagnostic Category	Etiological Factors	Incubation Period and Nature of Onset	Part of Gastrointestinal Tract and/or Associated Structures Involved	Severity of Illness and Course; Signs and Symptoms	Effect on Adequacy of Nutrition	Major Medical and/or Surgical Treatment
				neck, nocturnal choking and weight loss may occur. Pulmonary complications occur as a result of aspiration into the trachea.		
	See above	Two thirds of persons living to 85 years of age have them. See general comments.	Colon. See general comments.	See above.	None usually.	See Meckel's diverticulum.
Meckel's	Persistence of omphalomesenteric duct.		Large intestine. Ileum.	May parallel signs and symptoms of acute appendicitis when inflamed.	Malabsorption syndrome.	Surgical removal if necessary.
						Bed rest.
	Outpouching of serosa and mucosa at point where nutrient artery perforates muscularis layer.	Lower abdominal pain worsened by defecation.		May cause volvulus, intussusception, or strangulation.		Heat to tender abdominal area.
						Antibiotic therapy.
				Signs of peritoneal irritation.		Very soft diet during acute phase; then diet avoiding nuts, seeds, and fibrous foods.
				Muscle spasm.		
				Fever.		Oil enemas.
				Guarding.		

	Etiology	Symptoms	Pathology	Clinical Course	Complications	Treatment
Chronic non-specific ulcerative colitis	No known single cause. Relationship between emotional stress and onset and exacerbations.	Diarrhea, abdominal pain, blood, pus, fibrin in stools, or excreted as pure exudate.	Rectum and/or colon, ileum: inflammatory reaction involving mucosa and submucosa.	Anemia, weight loss, anorexia, malaise.	Malnutrition. Avitaminosis. Hypoproteinemia. Anemia.	Correction of nutrition and electrolyte loss. Vitamin and iron supplements. Discourage bacterial invasion: anti-microbial therapy. Bed rest.
Acute ulcerative colitis		Diarrhea, toxicity, fever, abdominal pain, distention, tenesmus, spasm, contraction. Constipation rather than diarrhea may be present.	Rectum and rectosigmoid: intensely red, edematous mucous membrane; tissue friable. Ileocecal valve to anus: as above. Colon: engorged, hyperactive. Covered with thick, opalescent, tenacious mucus, high in lysozyme concentration; increased friability of mucous membrane; eventual ulceration and submucosal bleeding.	Exacerbations and remissions. Little systemic sign of active inflammation. Course varies with patient. May have local reaction and involvement. May develop carcinoma (3–5% do). May have hyperimmune response.		Control diarrhea by opiates initially and later by sedation and antispasmodics. Psychological support. Parenteral feedings. Adrenocortical steroids. Surgery may be necessary. All the above apply to both forms of the disease.
Acute ulcerative proctitis			Rectum: see above. Inflammatory reaction of the rectum with the mucosa being friable and edematous.	Bloody exudate on stool with no systemic manifestation. Rectal urgency if upper rectum involved.		

573

TABLE 12-2 (cont.)

A Survey of Some Disorders of Nutrition and Conditions Involving the Alimentary Tract and Related Structures

Diagnostic Category	Etiological Factors	Incubation Period and Nature of Onset	Part of Gastrointestinal Tract and/or Associated Structures Involved	Severity of Illness and Course; Signs and Symptoms	Effect on Adequacy of Nutrition	Major Medical and/or Surgical Treatment
Peptic ulcer						
Duodenal	Unknown—imbalance between digesting action of contents of the stomach and resistance of stomach and duodenum to digestion—see discussion.	Right epigastric pain. High midline pain usually 1 to 3 hours after eating. Nocturnal pain between 2:00 A.M. and 4:00 A.M.	First portion of duodenum: progressively a crater develops in which there is coagulation necrosis at base with infiltration and accumulation of acute and chronic inflammatory cells.	Characterized by exacerbations and remissions. Exacerbations occur most frequently in autumn and spring in temperate climates. Increased muscular activity initiates pain. May perforate. Pain relieved by eating or alkali.	Protein, iron, and ascorbic acid deficiency with long dietary restriction.	Hospitalization for therapy if possible. Reduction of volume, acidity, and peptic content of gastric juices. Bland diet with 6 or more feedings; may start with milk-cream feedings, increasing diet in 3 to 4 stages.
Gastric	Unknown. May be induced by adrenal steroid therapy; adrenergic blocking drugs (tolazine hydrochloride, hydralazine, and hexamethonium). May develop in connection with practically all diseases.	Left epigastric pain. Pain usually one to several hours after eating, often not relieved or even aggravated by ingestion of food. History of six to seven years of attacks. Exacerbations occur frequently in spring and fall.	Stomach: usually in prepyloric area of lesser curvature. Crater develops and area around becomes hyperemic, edematous, and infiltrated.	Vomiting when obstruction occurs. Anemia. Constipation. Chronic disease may lead to perforation. Frequently fails to respond to medical treatment and recurs.	Anorexia and weight loss frequent. Malnutrition may occur if fear of eating is present or with prolonged vomiting.	Antacids. Parasympatholytics. Sedatives and tranquilizers. Therapy individualized because of role of stress (emotional and physical) in exacerbations. Surgery (subtotal gastrectomy) may be indicated. Bland diet. Rest in hospital.

		Pain. Hemorrhage.	Stomach-duodenum.	Nausea and vomiting.		
Curling's	Following extensive burns of the skin.					
Vascular						
Varices Esophageal	1. Increased pressure in veins of portal system—cirrhosis. 2. Thrombosis of portal and/or splenic vein (uncommon).	Hematemesis following local injury to the vessels or sudden elevation of portal pressure. Pressure is increased by straining at defecation, vomiting following a large meal or forceful exertion.	Esophagus: veins are distended and tortuous.	Chronic illness. Blood loss. Weight loss.	If etiology is cirrhosis, there is usually generalized malnutrition.	Symptomatic therapy of clinical picture presented. Possible surgery—various shunts, ligation of varices. Low-fiber diet.
Mechanical Obstruction Neoplasia—benign or malignant neoplasms may occur at any level of the alimentary canal. Occurrence in the small intestine is rare. See Chapter 14.						
Hemorrhoids (dilation of either the internal or external hemorrhoidal plexus or both).	Predisposing factors—constipation, motionless standing, pregnancy, hereditary weakness of the wall of the hemorrhoidal vein. May be found in patients with cancer in the rectum or sigmoid colon.	May be present with few symptoms, or may be highly acute, depending on the type of hemorrhoids, the degree of involvement, and complications.	Hemorrhoidal veins in anal canal.	When infected, strangulated, thrombosed, and prolapsed through the anus, symptoms may be exceedingly acute. Severe pain is common. Although bleeding is usually minimal, the loss of large quantities of blood does occur.	None unless continued or excessive loss of blood.	Surgical removal—after-care is very important. Operated area must be kept clean and strictures prevented from forming. Immediately after operation an ice bag may be placed over the dressing to lessen pain. Sitz baths are

TABLE 12-2 (cont.)

A Survey of Some Disorders of Nutrition and Conditions Involving the Alimentary Tract and Related Structures

Diagnostic Category	Etiological Factors	Incubation Period and Nature of Onset	Part of Gastrointestinal Tract and/or Associated Structures Involved	Severity of Illness and Course; Signs and Symptoms	Effect on Adequacy of Nutrition	Major Medical and/or Surgical Treatment
				Tenesmus accompanies strangulation, thromboses, and usually prolapse. Itching follows bowel activity.		started about 24 hours after surgery. Mineral oil to keep stool soft. In the treatment of acutely infected and thrombosed hemorrhoids: Sitz baths, stool softeners, keep area clean.
Choledocho-lithiasis	Calculi in common duct.	Varies from no symptoms to acute attacks of colic with an unusual degree of nausea and vomiting.	Extra- and intrahepatic biliary passages may become dilated and edematous.	Jaundice may or may not be present. If present, its severity dependent on extent of obstruction. If persistent may lead to distention of the gallbladder.		Vitamin K when jaundice present. Surgical removal of stones
Hernia (protrusion of the contents of the peritoneal cavity through a defect in the wall).	Developmental defects —trauma, aging, infection, surgery.	Depends on location. Some hernias can be seen and felt as a bulge in the affected area.	Depends on location and whether or not strangulation occurs. With gangrene of the intestine, peritonitis occurs. Locations include Inguinal (Direct or Indirect) Femoral Umbilical	May be few symptoms or signs until hernia becomes incarcerated (irreducible), and intestinal obstruction and strangulation occur. If allowed to continue, bowel becomes gangrenous and peritonitis occurs.	Depends on location.	Surgical repair, preferably before complications develop.

Ventral Postoperative incisions Hiatus or diaphragmatic hernia.					
Hiatus hernia	Gradual onset resulting in substernal or epigastric pressure precipitated by eating. Belching. Hot sensations in the back of the throat. Symptoms increase in severity when in recumbent position and are relieved when in the upright position. Sudden respiratory distress follows trauma and has rapid onset.	Stomach and esophagus. Stomach herniates into thorax, leads to esophagitis after regurgitation of gastric contents, continues for a long time. Hyperemia of gastric mucosa, caused by compression of venous drainage, renders it easily susceptible to trauma.	Chronic illness that may be quiescent or lead to development of respiratory embarrassment, cardiac irregularities. Bleeding, slow but persistent.	When acute episode of esophagitis interferes with food ingestion, there is an inadequate quality of nutrition. Anemia, microcytic type.	Avoid excessive filling of herniated pouch: diet is based on small meals, bland foods; restriction of sweets, coffee, alcohol. No food for three hours prior to retiring. Antacids. Sleep with head of bed elevated. Surgical treatment depends on the severity of symptoms.
Parasites					
Cestodes (tapeworms)	Asymptomatic.		Transient abdominal discomfort; diarrhea, hunger, anemia. Infrequently: severe cramping, vomiting, weakness, loss of weight. Usually seeks medical attention because part of parasite is passed per anus.	Malnutrition. Avitaminosis. Weight loss. Anemia. Protein and vitamin deficiency.	Anthelmintics. High-protein, high-calorie diet. Iron therapy.
	Diphyllobothrium latum. *Taenia solium.* *Taenia saginata.* *Hymenolepisnana.* Sparganosis. Echinococciasis.				
Hookworm disease	Have been known to survive 5 years in intestine. "Ground itch" or lesions on feet at point of entry.	Larvae penetrate skin, enter circulation, go to lungs, enter alveoli, ascend respiratory tree, enter pharynx, and	Severity depends on the number of worms and the nutritional status of the host and his age.	Anemia. Generalized malnutrition. Poor diet influences course unfavorably.	High-protein, high-calorie diet. Iron therapy. Anthelmintics.
	Necator americanus (New World). *Ancylostoma duodenale* (Old World).				

TABLE 12-2 (cont.)

A Survey of Some Disorders of Nutrition and Conditions Involving the Alimentary Tract and Related Structures

Diagnostic Category	Etiological Factors	Incubation Period and Nature of Onset	Part of Gastrointestinal Tract and/or Associated Structures Involved	Severity of Illness and Course; Signs and Symptoms	Effect on Adequacy of Nutrition	Major Medical and/or Surgical Treatment
			are swallowed. In intestine they mature and adults attach themselves to intestine, sucking about 0.5 ml of blood daily. Primarily in jejunum.	Epigastric pain. Abdominal tenderness. Sometimes nausea, vomiting, and diarrhea because intestine is attacked. Anemia, dyspnea, palpitation, lassitude, tachycardia, constipation may be manifested as infestation progresses.		
Ascariasis	*Ascaris lumbricoides.*	Temperature elevation 4-5 days after ingestion of eggs.	Early transient pulmonary stage followed by larval migration and intestinal infestation.	Physical and mental retardation may result from severe chronic infections. Cough and hemoptysis during pulmonary migration. Passage of worms via rectum, epigastric pain, abdominal distention, tenderness, vomiting, and constipation may occur during intestinal infestation.		Symptomatic during pulmonary stage, then use chemotherapy.

Disease	Etiology	Clinical Features	Pathology	Complications	Sequelae	Treatment
Amebiasis	*Endamoeba histolytica* as motile trophozoite and nonmotile cyst in the colon.	Chronic:: intermittent diarrhea, foul-smelling; abdominal cramping; mild fever. Acute: high fever, severe abdominal cramps, bloody diarrhea, tenesmus, diffuse abdominal tenderness.	Ileum: cyst wall disintegrates and 8 trophozoites result; these pass to colon, attack mucosa, and divide by binary fission; amebic ulceration: cecum, ascending colon, rectum, sigmoid, appendix, terminal ileum.	Vague intestinal symptoms; symptoms of appendicitis, gallbladder disease, peptic ulcer. Dysentery or diarrhea. May eventually enter circulation and infest liver. May infest lung from site in liver. May cause granuloma that encroaches on lumen.	Dehydration. Electrolyte imbalance. Weight loss.	Acute: replace fluid, electrolyte, and blood losses; bed rest; relief of pain and tenesmus; specific drug chemotherapy. Chronic: specific drug therapy. Hepatic or pulmonary: chloroquine and terramycin are given concomitantly.
Enterobiasis.	*Enterobius vermicularis.*	Perianal pruritus most troublesome at night.	Cecum and colon: adults attach themselves to mucosa. Ingested.			Communal treatment. Piperazine citrate.
Trichinosis	*Trichinella spiralis.*	Complaints vary with the severity of infestation and range from mild to severe. Diarrhea characterizes development of adults in the intestine 24 hours after ingestion.	Encysted larvae are ingested and parasites are liberated in duodenum and jejunum. There the parasites anchor themselves to mucosa and extract oxygen and liquid food. Nervous system and heart are frequently involved.	Myositis and systemic reaction when larvae migrate and infest skeletal muscle on seventh day after ingestion; may last up to 6 weeks. Edema, usually periorbital, conjunctivitis, nausea, vomiting, diarrhea, abdominal cramps, and fever within 2–7 days. Mortality rate in epidemics is 5%.	Hypoproteinemia. Dehydration.	Symptomatic therapy. Relief of pain. Maintain adequate fluid and caloric intake. Rest; if necessary, sedation. ACTH and adrenal steroids in severe cases. Anthelmintics.
Bacillary dysentery	*Shigella.*	1–6 days; median 48 hours. Colicky abdominal pain followed by profuse diarrhea, fever,	Sigmoid and rectum: acute inflammation leading to coagulation necrosis and ulceration. Mild	Passage of pus and mucus. Fever. Nausea. Vomiting. Headache. Malaise. Spontaneous recov-	Dehydration. Depletion of electrolytes.	Symptomatic. Isolation. Sulfonamides. Fluid replacement. Bland diet.

TABLE 12-2 (cont.)

A Survey of Some Disorders of Nutrition and Conditions Involving the Alimentary Tract and Related Structures

Diagnostic Category	Etiological Factors	Incubation Period and Nature of Onset	Part of Gastrointestinal Tract and/or Associated Structures Involved	Severity of Illness and Course; Signs and Symptoms	Effect on Adequacy of Nutrition	Major Medical and/or Surgical Treatment
		tenesmus, chills, nausea, vomiting, headache. Onset sudden and severe in children.	case: mucosa is strawberry red tint with diffuse inflammation and hyperemia, bleeding when traumatized.	ery in 2–7 days. 3–6 weeks in severe cases.		
Deficiencies						
Scurvy	Deficiency of ascorbic acid.	Weakness, fatigue, aching in muscles, joints, bones after 90 days of depletion. Hair follicles become prominent after 120 days of deprivation; perifollicular hemorrhage after 165 days. Peak incidence in infants at 8 months with tenderness and swelling of lower extremities.	Skeleton in children: periosteum and costal cartilages separate from bone shaft. A dense, calcified cartilaginous matrix forms in the cartilage shaft junction. Generalized hemorrhages in adults.	Aching muscles, joints, bones. Swollen, painful lower extremities. Swollen gums with hemorrhage; eventual loss of teeth. Rapid improvement with therapy.	Anemia is often an associated finding.	Ascorbic acid.
Pellagra	Niacin deficiency. Low-protein diet with tryptophan deficiency will accelerate the progress; tryptophan is pre-	Follows several months of low intake of niacin, protein, and B-complex vitamins.	Skin: erythema, vesical formation, rough and scaly. Alimentary tract: glossitis, inflammation of the esophagus,	Dermatitis, anorexia, glossitis, lassitude, stomatitis, diarrhea. Later leads to dementia. Symptoms begin to	Anorexia. Weight loss. Anemia.	Niacin. High-protein, high-calorie, soft diet. Water and electrolyte replacement. Bed rest.

Condition						
(pellagra, continued)	cursor for niacin. Contributing factors are gastrointestinal disease, liver disease, alcoholism.		ulcer formation in the colon. Nervous system: vertigo, headache, paresthesia, anesthesia, diminished tendon reflexes, coarse tremors, mental disturbances. Degeneration of peripheral nerves, nerve roots, and spinal cord tracts; atrophy of cerebral neurons.		disappear after 24 hours of therapy; almost absent after 3–4 days, except for polyneuritis.	Symptomatic therapy.
Beriberi	Thiamine deficiency. Protein, calorie, and multiple B-complex deficiencies coexist. Prevalent in Far East, especially in prisons, asylums, in infants, pregnant and lactating women, and alcoholics. Rare in United States.	Insidious onset. Fatigue, muscle weakness, pain, and atrophy in neurologic form.	Loss of reflexes. Paresthesias and anesthesias. Symptoms progress until patient is bedridden. Dry form: peripheral neuritis. Wet form: edema, muscle cramps. Cardiac form: palpitation, precordial pain, dyspnea, tachycardia, edema, increased pulse and venous pressure.	Myelin degeneration of peripheral nerves with loss of exoplasm. In alcoholics, bilateral hemorrhagic foci in the mammillary bodies, hypothalamic nuclei, and midline structures. Optic nerve damage and spinal cord lesions. Heart dilatation and occasional hypertrophy of the right ventricle.	Weight loss. Anorexia. Multiple deficiencies of B complex and iron.	Thiamine. High-protein, high-calorie diet.
Undernutrition	Calorie deficiency. Protein deficiency. Associated lack of vitamins and minerals. Endemic undernutrition results from inadequate food supply, poverty, ignorance.	Weight loss is initial sign in adults. Other signs only after months of severe deprivation or when aggravated by disease. Infants weaned to low-protein diets show rapid deterioration	Reduced production of digestive enzymes; reduced liver function. Affects growth and mental development of infants and young children.	Children: failure to gain, short stature, retarded mental development. Edema or severe dehydration. Fatty liver, low serum albumin, anemia. Changes in skin and hair pigment. Adults: course usu-		Gradual addition of nutritionally balanced meals; milk for infants.

TABLE 12-2 (cont.)

A Survey of Some Disorders of Nutrition and Conditions Involving the Alimentary Tract and Related Structures

Diagnostic Category	Etiological Factors	Incubation Period and Nature of Onset	Part of Gastrointestinal Tract and/or Associated Structures Involved	Severity of Illness and Course; Signs and Symptoms	Effect on Adequacy of Nutrition	Major Medical and/or Surgical Treatment
	Infections, gastrointestinal parasites accelerate effects. Infants, young children, pregnant and lactating women are vulnerable.	in growth, development.		ally determined by associated disease.		
Inflammatory						
Glossitis	Secondary to chronic malabsorption.®		Tongue becomes hyperemic. Small ulcers sometimes occur.		Anorexia because swallowing is painful.	Correct underlying disorder.
Stomatitis, catarrhal	Poor oral hygiene. Excessive use of tobacco or alcohol. Associated with debilitated persons. Uremia.		Mouth. Mucous membranes erythematous; increased exudate.			As above.
Aphthous ulcer	Unknown.		Vesicle develops, ruptures, and leaves ulcer.			No treatment; heals spontaneously.
Ulceromembranous	*Bacillus fusiformis.* *Borrelia vincentii.*	Painful, irregular-shaped ulcer covered with whitish gray membrane.	Oral and pharyngeal membranes, particularly gingival tissue. Inflammation and induration surround ulcerations.	Moderate fever, enlargement of submaxillary lymph nodes.	Temporarily modifies diet.	Penicillin. Dental hygienic measures to eradicate ulcerations.

582

Parotitis	Hemolytic streptococcus through ducts, blood stream, lymphatics, or extension from adjacent structures.	Acute inflammation of salivary gland; usually parotid but may be any salivary gland. Blockage of Stensen's duct by a calculus.	Enlargement of salivary glands associated with pain and swelling.	Leukocytosis; rapid pulse; trismus; pressure on gland usually produces purulent discharge from duct; fever and chills.	Temporarily modifies diet.	Antimicrobial agents. Therapeutic doses of irradiation are used if antimicrobials fail. Removal of obstruction and local heat application. Surgical drainage if conservative measures fail.
Regional enteritis	Granulomatous response of submucosa to unknown agent(s).	Duodenum: usually leads to stenosis. Upper jejunum: usually leads to stenosis. Terminal ileum: encroachment of lumen, scarring of muscle, slow spread to other areas of intestine; beefy red appearance. Usually leads to ulceration. Nonstenotic. Fistula forms.	Acute right lower quadrant pain and tenderness; disturbance in bowel motility.	Acute stage can lead to perforation and generalized peritonitis. In nonacute onset, history of intermittent chronic diarrhea, fever, weight loss, crampy pain or distention, anemia. Two thirds develop chronic enteritis. Eventual obstruction of lumen.	Impairment of absorption of amino acids, fats, fat-soluble vitamins, folic acid, iron. "Malabsorption syndrome." Undernutrition.	Surgery: end-to-side ileotransverse colostomy. Provide mental and physical rest. Chemotherapeutics and antibiotics to treat purulent complications. Corticosteroids to convert a subacute obstructing lesion into a nonstenotic one. Diet: high-calorie, high-protein (2 g per kg of ideal body weight per day), low in seasoning and cold fluids. Therapeutic vitamins. Fluid and electrolyte balance restoration.

Table 12-2 (cont.)

A Survey of Some Disorders of Nutrition and Conditions Involving the Alimentary Tract and Related Structures

Diagnostic Category	Etiological Factors	Incubation Period and Nature of Onset	Part of Gastrointestinal Tract and/or Associated Structures Involved	Severity of Illness and Course; Signs and Symptoms	Effect on Adequacy of Nutrition	Major Medical and/or Surgical Treatment
Sprue	Nontropical: adult form of celiac disease. Primary form involves defect of intestinal epithelium. Secondary form exists in wide range of malabsorption states.	Insidious onset. Diarrhea: 2–3 (or more) mushy, light-colored, foul-smelling stools associated with explosive flatus. Intermittent constipation.	Jejunum: villi become short and blunt, width of crypts of Lieberkühn increases; microvilli become sparse, blunted, and fused. Distortion of columnar cells of the epithelium. Plasma cells of the lamina propria become infiltrated. Mitochondria are enlarged and vacuolated.	Chronic disease. Severe fatigue. Moderate to severe weight loss. Nausea and vomiting and abdominal pain may occur. Nocturnal diuresis. Clinical manifestations of malnutrition. Eventually fractures of bones and tetany. Anemia.	Malnutrition results from inability of food products (properly prepared for absorption) to pass through the mucosa. Vitamin A, C, D, B$_{12}$, K deficiencies. Deficiencies in electrolytes, potassium and calcium. Hypoproteinemia. Progressively reserves of iron, folic acid, and B$_{12}$ are depleted. Malabsorption of fats and fat-soluble nutrients. Lowered serum cholesterol and phospholipids, copper, prothrombin.	Gluten-free diet (do not eat food containing wheat, barley, rye gluten). Takes about 6 months to evaluate this therapy. In presence of nutritional deficiencies, corrective therapy instituted. In presence of malnutrition, adrenocortical hormone therapy initially with diet therapy. Tetany treated with 10% calcium gluconate I.V. Electrolyte therapy: potassium chloride, 2–3 g daily. Hemorrhagic complications treated with menadione intramuscularly, 10 mg daily. Antibiotic therapy when sprue is secondary to diverticula, infection, blind loops, and intestinal strictures.

						Treatment
						Recognize secondary causes of sprue and institute therapy. Postgastrectomy: small, frequent feedings; addition of pancreatin to diet. Androgens for anabolic effect; antibiotics.
Hepatitis	Filtrable virus A (infectious hepatitis).	15–50 days. Abrupt onset with high temperature, G.I. symptoms, and nonspecific constitutional symptoms lasting a few days to 2 weeks.	Liver: cellular damage ranges from swollen or shrunken cells with disintegrating nucleus to massive central necrosis of every lobule of the liver. Kupffer cells are often swollen; edema and cellular infiltration of portal and periportal areas; biliary stasis.	Preicteric stage: fever, anorexia, fatigue predominate. Nausea, vomiting, chilly sensations, indigestion, abdominal pain, headache, pain on eye movement, and arthralgia may occur. Enlarged lymph nodes are common. Icteric stage: jaundice, increases rapidly reaching a maximum in 10–14 days; few days in which anorexia, lassitude, and nausea are striking; right upper abdominal pain. This stage may last a few days to a few weeks, depending on severity. Sudden reappearance of appetite plus sense of well-being indicates beginning of recovery period. Jaundice clears in 4–6 weeks.	Undernutrition as a result of anorexia.	Bed rest. Isolate. Blood and stools considered infectious until fever and jaundice subside. High-protein, high-calorie diet except in massive hepatic necrosis. Parenteral feedings if nausea, vomiting, or anorexia is present.
	Filtrable virus B (serum hepatitis).	60–160 days. Insidious onset with minimal symptoms and little if any fever.				

TABLE 12-2 (cont.)

A Survey of Some Disorders of Nutrition and Conditions Involving the Alimentary Tract and Related Structures

Diagnostic Category	Etiological Factors	Incubation Period and Nature of Onset	Part of Gastrointestinal Tract and/or Associated Structures Involved	Severity of Illness and Course; Signs and Symptoms	Effect on Adequacy of Nutrition	Major Medical and/or Surgical Treatment
Cholecystitis						
Acute	Biliary calculi, or the action on the wall of the gallbladder caused by a stone. Bacterial infection. Chemical irritants in the bile.	Upper abdominal pain, gradual or acute, associated with biliary colic. Fever.	Gallbladder is distended; serosa is injected; wall is tense and swollen; mucosa is congested. Frequently small amounts of fibrinopurulent exudate.	Becomes chronic but with severe upper abdominal distress. Fever and chills usually. Nausea and vomiting. Mass sometimes palpable.		Removal of calculi after subsidence of acute phase. Symptomatic therapy. Restoration of fluid and electrolyte balance. Low-fat diet. Water-soluble form of vitamins K, A, D, and E. Choledochal exploration. Cholecystectomy.
Chronic	Biliary calculi.	Distinct attacks occurring days to years apart with abrupt onset of abdominal pain, fever, intermittent mild jaundice and digestive complaints.	Chronic inflammatory gallbladder with degenerative changes.	May lead to persistent gallbladder distention as with acute, but having chronic form of jaundice.		Cholecystectomy for cholelithiasis. Medically with antispasmodics, antacids, laxatives, and sedatives. Moderately low-fat diet.
	Unknown.			Belching, bloating, and epigastric distress after meals. Variety of digestive and systemic complaints. Symptoms aggravated by ingestion of fats. Insomnia.		
Cirrhosis	Malnutrition. Alcoholism. Hepatitis.	Insidious onset, with nonspecific complaints of anorexia,	Liver enlarges and is pale initially; then fibrosis in portal	Anorexia, weight loss, eventually (1) hepatocellular fail-	Malnutrition in terms of essential nutrients although caloric	Normal to high-protein, high-calorie diet. Prohibition of

	weakness, and unusual fatigability.	areas and around central veins. Lobular structure becomes distorted with regeneration.	ure, manifested by: ascites, edema, jaundice, pleural effusion, alteration in serum electrolytes, spider nevi, palmar erythema, gynecomastia; testicular atrophy, loss of axillary and pubic hair, bleeding tendency; (2) portal hypertension manifested by splenomegaly, esophageal varices (with or without massive hemorrhage), visible venous collateral circulation over abdomen, rectal hemorrhoids; and eventually may have (3) hepatic coma; rapid fluctuation of mental and neurological signs, flapping tremor, and occasionally fetor hepaticus.	intake may be adequate or even high. Anemia.	alcohol (where it is etiological factor). Supplemental water-soluble vitamins. Regulation of salt and water balance. Prompt control of hemorrhage and replacement of blood loss. Bed rest. Antimicrobial therapy in presence of infection. Prednisone. Diuretics. Sodium-restricted diet if ascites present. Paracentesis and/or thoracentesis if needed. Surgery is sometimes used: portacaval shunt. Coma: (1) restriction of protein intake, but calories supplied from fats and carbohydrates; (2) correction of deficiencies in fluids and electrolytes; (3) neomycin; (4) administration intravenously of L-arginine monohydrochloride (25 g in 500 ml water); frequency depends on response of blood ammonia.
Pancreatitis, acute	Obstruction to outflow of pancreatic juices in common duct. Direct injury of	Destruction of parenchyma of pancreas and ductal obstruction. Varying: edema of head	Sudden moderate or severe and prolonged upper abdominal pain and vomiting.	Loss of weight although excessive amounts of food are ingested; leading to obstipation; vomit-	
				Incomplete hydrolysis of starches, fats, and proteins and hence incomplete absorption. Marked	

TABLE 12-2 (cont.)

A Survey of Some Disorders of Nutrition and Conditions Involving the Alimentary Tract and Related Structures

Diagnostic Category	Etiological Factors	Incubation Period and Nature of Onset	Part of Gastrointestinal Tract and/or Associated Structures Involved	Severity of Illness and Course; Signs and Symptoms	Effect on Adequacy of Nutrition	Major Medical and/or Surgical Treatment
	acinar tissue by toxins, ischemia, inflammation, or trauma. Cancer of ampulla of Vater. Secondary pancreatic edema. Epithelial metaplasia in duct. Alcoholism. Peptic ulcer. Trauma. An occasional complication of pregnancy and mumps.		of pancreas to patchy or diffuse necrosis of gland. Extensive fibrosis.	ing, distention, and ileus may occur. Tetany may develop. Leads to destructive process in pancreas and fibrotic contracture may cause compression of common duct, producing jaundice. Repeated attacks result in chronic pancreatitis. This, if it progresses sufficiently, may result in calcification of pancreas and diabetes mellitus and steatorrhea.	malnutrition. Avitaminosis. Hypocalcemia.	N.P.O. Aspiration of gastric contents. Anticholinergic drugs. Analgesics (opiates sparingly and in small doses). Antibiotics. Restoration of fluid and electrolyte balance.
Appendicitis	Obstruction caused by fecalith or stricture. Ulceration. Diffuse phlegmon. Infection.	Acute periumbilical or epigastric pain, followed by anorexia, nausea, and vomiting.	Appendix: inflammatory response to cause.	Anorexia, nausea, vomiting progressing, fever, high leukocyte count. Perforation of the appendix and ensuing peritonitis.	Loss of fluid and electrolytes caused by vomiting. Inadequate nutrient intake because of nausea, anorexia, and vomiting.	Surgical removal of appendix. Correction of dehydration and electrolyte imbalance. Restoration of physiological function (in absence of peritonitis).

REFERENCES

BOOKS

Brown, Charles H.: *Diagnostic Procedures in Gastroenterology* (St. Louis: The C. V. Mosby Company, 1967).

Mitchell, Helen S., *et al.: Cooper's Nutrition in Health and Disease,* 15th ed. (Philadelphia: J. B. Lippincott Company, 1968).

Robinson, Corinne H.: *Proudfit-Robinson's Normal and Therapeutic Nutrition,* 13th ed. (New York: The Macmillan Company, 1967).

Sherlock, Sheila: *Diseases of the Liver and Biliary System* (Philadelphia: F. A. Davis Company, 1968).

Wayler, Thelma J., and Klein, Rose S.: *Applied Nutrition* (New York: The Macmillan Company, 1965).

Wohl, Michael G., and Goodhart, Robert S. (eds.): *Modern Nutrition in Health and Disease,* 4th ed. (Philadelphia: Lea & Febiger, 1968).

PERIODICALS

Nutritional Care and Dietary Counseling

Dawson, Marlene J.: "New Patients Dine with the Nurse," *Amer. J. Nurs.,* 66:287–89 (Feb.) 1966.

Johnson, Doris: "Effective Diet Counseling Begins Early in Hospitalization," *Hospitals,* 41:94 (Jan. 16) 1967.

Moore, Mary Lou: "When Families Must Eat More for Less," *Nurs. Outlook,* 14:66–69 (Apr.) 1966.

Morris, Ena: "How Does a Nurse Teach Nutrition to Patients?" *Amer. J. Nurs.,* 60:67–70 (Jan.) 1960.

Piper, Geraldine M.: "Nutrition Services in Home Health Agencies," *J. Amer. Diet. Ass.,* 50:23–25 (Jan.) 1967.

Skiff, Anna W.: "Programmed Instruction and Patient Teaching," *Amer. J. Public Health,* 55:409–15 (Mar.) 1965.

Zitnik, Ruth: "First, You Take a Grapefruit," *Amer. J. Nurs.,* 68:1285–86 (June) 1968.

Food Supply, Nutritional Problems, and Nutritional Status

Council on Food and Nutrition: "Improvement of Nutritive Quality of Foods," *JAMA,* 205:868 (Sept. 16) 1968.

Expert Committee on Medical Assessment of Nutritional Status: *Tech. Rep. Ser.* No. 258 (Geneva: World Health Organization, 1963).

Goldsmith, Grace A.: "More Food for More People," *Amer. J. Public Health,* 59:694–704 (Apr.) 1969.

Mayer, Jean: "The Nutritional Status of American Negroes," *Nutr. Rev.,* 23:161–64 (June) 1965.

Schaefer, Arnold E., and Johnson, Ogden C.: "Are We Well Fed? The Search for the Answer," *Nutr. Today,* 4:2–11 (Spring) 1969.

Sebrell, William H., Jr.: "Clinical Nutrition in the United States," *Amer. J. Public Health,* 58:2035–42 (Nov.) 1968.

Wilson, Christine S., *et al.:* "A Review of Methods Used in Nutrition Surveys Conducted by the Interdepartmental Committee on Nutrition for National Defense," *Amer. J. Clin. Nutr.,* 15:29–44 (July) 1964.

Food Acceptance and Food Habits

Berkowitz, Philip, and Berkowitz, Nancy S.: "The Jewish Patient in the Hospital," *Amer. J. Nurs.,* 67:2335–37 (Nov.) 1967.

Bernard, Viola W.: "Why People Become the Victims of Medical Quackery," *Amer. J. Public Health,* 55:1142–47 (Aug.) 1965.

Cantoni, Marjorie: "Adapting Therapeutic Diets to the Eating Patterns of Italian Americans," *Amer. J. Clin. Nutr.,* 6:548–55 (Sept.–Oct.) 1958.

Hacker, Dorothy B., and Miller, Eleanor D.: "Food Patterns of the Southwest," *Amer. J. Clin. Nutr.,* 7:224–29 (Mar.–Apr.) 1959.

Halsted, James A.: "Geophagia in Man: Its Nature and Nutritional Effects," *Amer. J. Clin. Nutr.,* 21:1384–93 (Dec.) 1968.

Kaufman, Mildred: "Adapting Therapeutic Diets to Jewish Food Customs," *Amer. J. Clin. Nutr.,* 5:676–81 (Nov.–Dec.) 1957.

MacGregor, Frances C.: "Uncooperative Patients: Some Cultural Interpretations," *Amer. J. Nurs.,* 67:88–91 (Jan.) 1967.

Mayer, Jean: "Why People Get Hungry," *Nutr. Today,* 1:2–8 (June) 1966.

Rice, E. P.: "Changing Social Values in Public Health," *Amer. J. Public Health,* 58:1323 (Aug.) 1968.

Torres, Rosa Marina: "Dietary Patterns of Puerto Rican People," *Amer. J. Clin. Nutr.,* 7:349–55 (May–June) 1959.

Valassi, Kyriake V.: "Food Habits of Greek Americans," *Amer. J. Clin. Nutr.,* 11:240–48 (Sept.) 1962.

Upper Alimentary Canal—Functioning

George, J. D.: "Gastric Acidity and Motility," *Amer. J. Dig. Dis.,* 13:376–83 (Apr.) 1968.

Griffin, Ward O.: "Antral Regulatory Mechanism —An Hypothesis," *Surg. Clin. N. Amer.,* 47:1335–39 (Dec.) 1967.

Grossman, Morton I.: "Gastrointestinal Hormones," *Med. Clin. N. Amer.,* 52:1297–1303 (Nov.) 1968.

Hunt, J. N., and Knox, M. T.: "Control of Gastric Emptying," *Amer. J. Dig. Dis.,* 13:372–75 (Apr.) 1968.

Ingelfinger, Franz J. "Gastrointestinal Absorption," *Nutr. Today,* 2:2–10 (Mar.) 1967.

Joint Committee, American Dietetic Association and American Medical Association: "Diet as Related to Gastrointestinal Function," *J. Amer. Diet. Ass.,* 38:425–32 (May) 1961.

Jordan, Paul H.: "Clinical Aspects of Gastric Secretion and Gastric Analysis," *Med. Clin. N. Amer.*, **52**:1305–13 (Nov.) 1968.

Upper Alimentary Canal—Disorders
(*See also Ulcers; Surgery*)

Boyle, James D., and Goldstein, Howard: "Management of Pyloric Obstruction," *Med. Clin. N. Amer.*, **52**:1329–37 (Nov.) 1968.

Castleman, Benjamin and McNeely, Betty U.: "Long-standing Hiatus Hernia with Vomiting and Epigastric Pain," *New Eng. J. Med.*, **278**:725 (Mar. 28) 1968.

Cummins, Alvin J.: "Nausea and Vomiting," *Amer. J. Dig. Dis.*, **3**:710–21 (Oct.) 1958.

Edwards, D. A. W.: "Esophageal Pain and Motility," *Amer. J. Dig. Dis.*, **13**:340–45 (Apr.) 1968.

Flood, Charles A.: "Clinical Features in the Management of Esophageal Hiatal Hernia," *JAMA*, **172**:314–19 (Jan. 23) 1960.

Mackby, M. Judson: "Treatment of Bleeding Esophageal Varices," *JAMA*, **171**:1916–22 (Dec. 5) 1959.

Menaker, Gerald: "The Physiology and Mechanism of Acute Abdominal Pain," *Surg. Clin. N. Amer.*, **42**:241–48 (Feb.) 1962.

Rumball, John M.: "The Emergency Management of Upper Gastrointestinal Hemorrhage," *Med. Clin. N. Amer.*, **46**:531–35 (Mar.) 1962.

Upper Alimentary Canal—Gastric and Duodenal Ulcers (*See also Surgery*)

Fortran, John S. and Collyns, J. A. H.: "Antacid Pharmacology in Duodenal Ulcer," *New Eng. J. Med.*, **274**:921–27 (Apr. 28) 1966.

Hartroft, W. Stanley: "The Incidence of Coronary Artery Disease in Patients Treated with the Sippy Diet," *Amer. J. Clin. Nutr.*, **15**:205–10 (Oct.) 1964.

Kirsner, Joseph B.: "Peptic Ulcer: A Review of Recent Literature on Various Clinical Aspects," *Gastroenterology*, **54**:611–41 (Apr.), 945–75 (May) 1968.

Kukral, John C.: "Gastric Ulcer: An Appraisal," *Surgery*, **63**:1024–36 (June) 1968.

Palumbo, Louis T., and Sharpe, Wendell S.: "Active Bleeding Duodenal Ulcer," *Surg. Clin. N. Amer.*, **47**:239–54 (Feb.) 1967.

Review: "Dietary Misconceptions," *Nutr. Rev.*, **26**:18–19 (Jan.) 1968.

"Symposium: Clinical Management of Peptic Ulcer," *Amer. J. Clin. Nutr.*, **15**:191–245 (Oct.) 1964.

Upper Alimentary Canal—Surgery

Foster, Frank P.: "Peritonitis: A Plan when Treatment Fails," *Med. Clin. N. Amer.*, **50**:551–63 (Mar.) 1966.

Gilmore, Stuart I.: "Rehabilitation After Laryngectomy," *Amer. J. Nurs.*, **61**:87–89 (Jan.) 1961.

Hansen, Donald E.: "Abdominal Hernias," *Amer. J. Nurs.*, **61**:102–104 (Mar.) 1961.

Holinger, Paul H., Johnston, Kenneth C., and Mansireto, Mario D.: "Cancer of the Larynx," *Amer. J. Nurs.*, **57**:738–43 (June) 1957.

Klug, Thomas J., *et al.*: "Gastric Resection," *Amer. J. Nurs.*, **61**:73–76 (Dec.) 1961.

Machella, Thomas E.: "Mechanism of the Postgastrectomy Dumping Syndrome," *Gastroenterology*, **54**:721–22 (Apr.) 1958.

Magruder, Lucinda, *et al.*: "Gastric Resection—Nursing Care," *Amer. J. Nurs.*, **61**:76–77 (Dec.) 1961.

Stemmer, Edward A., *et al.*: "A Physiological Approach to the Surgical Treatment of the Dumping Syndrome," *JAMA*, **199**:909–13, (Mar. 20) 1967.

Willis, Mildred T., and Postlewait, R. W.: "Dietary Problems After Gastric Resection," *J. Amer. Diet. Ass.*, **40**:111–13 (Feb.) 1962.

Middle and Lower Alimentary Canal—Disorders (*See also Colitis; Enzyme Deficiency; Sprue; Surgery*)

Dobbins, William O., III: "Drug-Induced Steatorrhea," *Gastroenterology*, **54**:1193–95 (June) 1968.

Finkelstein, James D.: "Malabsorption," *Med. Clin. N. Amer.*, **52**:1339–54 (Nov.) 1968.

Gardner, Frank H.: "Nutritional Management of Chronic Diarrhea in Adults," *JAMA*, **180**:147–52 (Apr. 14) 1962.

Grey, Chester C., and Hunter, Harry L.: "Rectal Bleeding," *Surg. Clin. N. Amer.*, **38**:235–55 (Jan.) 1958.

Hefferson, E. W.: "The Irritable Colon—A Common Mimic," *Med. Clin. N. Amer.*, **47**:425–29 (Mar.) 1963.

Horner, John L.: "Natural History of Diverticulosis of the Colon," *Amer. J. Dig. Dis.*, **3**:343–50 (May) 1958.

Sleisenger, Marvin H., Jr.: "Some Implications of Current Research in Gastroenterology," *Med. Clin. N. Amer.*, **52**:1269–72 (Nov.) 1968.

Symposium: "Malabsorption and Malnutrition in the Tropics," *Amer. J. Clin. Nutr.*, **21**:939–1127, 1968.

Middle and Lower Alimentary Canal—Colitis (*See also Enzyme Deficiency*)

Jay, Arthur N.: "Colitis," *Amer. J. Nurs.*, **59**:1133–35, 1959.

McKittrick, John B., and Shotkin, Jane M.: "Ulcerative Colitis," *Amer. J. Nurs.*, **62**:60–64 (Aug.) 1962.

O'Connor, John F.: "Psychological Considerations in Ulcerative Colitis," *New York State J. Med.*, **68**:1055–65 (Apr. 15) 1968.

Rider, J. Alfred, and Moeller, Hugo C.: "Food Hypersensitivity in Ulcerative Colitis," *Amer. J. Gastroent.*, **37**:497–507 (May) 1962.

Zetzel, Louis: "Treatment of Ulcerative Colitis," *New Eng. J. Med.*, **271**:891–95 (Oct. 27) 1964.

Middle and Lower Alimentary Canal—Enzyme Deficiency

Dahlqvist, Arne, *et al.*: "Intestinal Lactase Deficiency and Lactose Intolerance in Adults," *Gastroenterology*, **54**:807–10 (Apr.) 1968.

Gryboski, Joyce D., *et al.*: "A Defect in Disaccharide Metabolism after Gastrojejunostomy," *New Eng. J. Med.*, **268**:78–80 (Jan. 10) 1963.

Ingelfinger, Franz J.: "For Want of an Enzyme," *Nutr. Today*, **3**:2–10 (Sept.) 1968.

Peternel, W. W.: "Disaccharidase Deficiency," *Med. Clin. N. Amer.*, **52**:1355–65 (Nov.) 1968.

Middle and Lower Alimentary Canal—Sprue

Harkins, Robert W., and Sarett, Herbert P.: "Medium-Chain Triglycerides," *JAMA*, **203**: 272–74 (Jan. 22) 1968.

"How to Eat Well on a Gluten-Free Diet," *Today's Health*, **43**:38 (Oct.) 1965.

Menendez-Corrada, Rodrigo: "Current Views on Tropical Sprue and a Comparison to Nontropical Sprue," *Med. Clin. N. Amer.*, **52**:1367–85 (Nov.) 1968.

Schizas, Alyette Asselin, *et al.:* "Medium-Chain Triglycerides—Use in Food Preparation," *J. Amer. Diet. Ass.*, **51**:228–32 (Sept.) 1967.

Middle and Lower Alimentary Canal—Surgery

Dericks, Virginia C.: "Rehabilitation of Patients with Ileostomy," *Amer. J. Nurs.*, **61**:48–51 (May) 1961.

Donaldson, G. A.: "Current Concepts in Therapy Management of Ileostomy and Colostomy," *New Eng. J. Med.*, **268**:827–30 (Apr. 11) 1963.

Hallburg, Jeanne C.: "The Patient with Surgery of the Colon," *Amer. J. Nurs.*, **61**:64–66 (Mar.) 1961.

Ray, John E., *et al.:* "Postoperative Problems of Ileostomy and Colostomy," *JAMA*, **174**:2118–23 (Dec. 24) 1960.

The Liver and Biliary Tract—Gallbladder

Juniper, Kerrison: "Cause of Gallstone Disease," *Mod. Treatm.*, **5**:480–92 (May) 1968.

Small, Donald M.: "Gallstones," *New Eng. J. Med.*, **279**:588–93 (Sept. 12) 1968.

"Symposium on the Treatment of Gallbladder Disease," *Mod. Treat.*, **5**:479–540 (May) 1968.

The Liver and Biliary Tract—Diseases of the Liver

Carey, James B.: "The Pruritus of Jaundice," *GP*, **37**:118–22 (Apr.) 1968.

Chalmers, Thomas C.: "The Management of Hepatic Coma. A Continuing Problem," *Med. Clin. N. Amer.*, **52**:1475–81 (Nov.) 1968.

Davidson, Charles S.: "Is Life Worth Living? It Depends upon the Liver," *New Eng. J. Med.*, **274**:894–96 (Apr. 21) 1966.

Hayter, Jean: "Impaired Liver Function and Related Nursing Care," *Amer. J. Nurs.*, **68**:2374–79 (Nov.) 1968.

Leevy, Carroll M.: "Cirrhosis in Alcoholics," *Med. Clin. N. Amer.*, **52**:1445–55 (Nov.) 1968.

Nefzger, M. Dean, and Chalmers, Thomas C.: "The Treatment of Acute Infectious Hepatitis: Ten-Year Follow-Up Study on the Effects of Diet and Rest," *Amer. J. Med.*, **35**:299–309 (Sept.) 1963.

Pearlman, D. M.: "Hepatogenic Ascites: Pathogenesis and Management," *New York J. Med.*, **68**:1837–42 (July) 1968.

Read, A. E.: "Cirrhosis of the Liver," *Brit. Med. J.*, **1**:427–30, 1968.

Rubin, Emanuel, and Lieber, Charles S.: "Malnutrition and Liver Disease—An Overemphasized Relationship," *Amer. J. Med.*, **45**:1–6 (July) 1968.

Schimmel, Elihu M.: "Diagnostic Procedures in Liver Disease," *Med. Clin. N. Amer.*, **52**:1407–16 (Nov.) 1968.

The Liver and Biliary Tract—Pancreas

Knight, William A.: "The Basis of Therapy in Pancreatic Disease," *Amer. J. Dig. Dis.*, **9**:832–35 (Nov.) 1964.

McDonough, Francis E., and Reaves, Leonard E., III: "Chronic Relapsing Pancreatitis. Recognition and Management," *Postgrad. Med.*, **40**:593–98 (Nov.) 1966.

Nardi, G. L.: "Pancreatitis," *New Eng. J. Med.*, **268**:1065–67 (May 9) 1963.

The Liver and Biliary Tract—Surgery

Ferris, Deward O., and Sterling, William A.: "Surgery of the Biliary Tract," *Surg. Clin. N. Amer.*, **47**:861–75 (Aug.) 1967.

Fisk, Jean E.: "Nursing Care of the Patient with Surgery of the Biliary Tract," *Amer. J. Nurs.*, **60**:53–55 (Jan.) 1960.

Onstad, G. R.: "Treatment of Some Problems Occurring after Cholecystectomy," *Mod. Treatm.*, **5**:528–40 (May) 1968.

Obesity

Albrink, Margaret J. (ed.): "Symposium: Endocrine Aspects of Obesity," *Amer. J. Clin. Nutr.*, **21**:1395–1485 (Dec.) 1968.

Christakis, G., *et al.:* "Effect of a Combined Nutrition Education and Physical Fitness Program on the Weight Status of Obese High School Boys," *Fed. Proc.*, **25**:15–19 (Jan.–Feb.) 1966.

Duncan, L. J. P., and Munro, J. F.: "The Present Status of Anorexiant Drugs," *Practitioner*, **200**:167–73, 1968.

Dwyer, Johanna T., Feldman, Jacob J., and Mayer, Jean: "Adolescent Dieters: Who Are They? Physical Characteristics, Attitudes, and Dietary Practices of Adolescent Girls," *Amer. J. Clin. Nutr.*, **20**:1045–56 (Oct.) 1967.

Grande, Francisco: "Energetics and Weight Reduction," *Amer. J. Clin. Nutr.*, **21**:305–14 (Feb.) 1968.

Mayer, Jean: "Obesity Control," *Amer. J. Nurs.*, **65**:112–13 (June) 1965.

Mayer, Jean: "Some Aspects of the Problem of Regulation of Food Intake and Obesity," *New Eng. J. Med.*, **274**:610–16 (Mar. 17), 662–73 (Mar. 24), 722–31 (Mar. 31), 1966.

Peckos, Penelope S., and Spargo, John A.: "For Overweight Teenage Girls," *Amer. J. Nurs.*, **64**:85–87 (May) 1964.

Undernutrition: Calorie; Protein-Calorie; Mineral

Béhar, Moises: "Progress and Delays in Combating Goiter in Latin America," *Fed. Proc.*, **27**:939–44 (May–June) 1968.

Committee on Nutrition: "The Relation between

Infantile Hypercalcemia and Vitamin D—Public Health Implications in North America," *Pediatrics,* 40:1050–61 (Dec.) 1967.

Council on Foods and Nutrition: "Iron Deficiency in the United States," *JAMA,* 203:119–24 (Jan. 8) 1968.

Cravioto, Joaquin, DeLicardie, Elsa R., and Birch, Herbert G.: "Nutrition, Growth and Neurointegrative Development. An Experimental and Ecologic Study," *Pediatrics,* 38:319–72 (Aug.) 1966.

Iskrant, Albert P.: "The Etiology of Fractured Hips in Females," *Amer. J. Public Health,* 58:485–90 (Mar.) 1968.

Lotz, Myron, *et al.:* "Evidence for a Phosphorus-Depletion Syndrome in Man," *New Eng. J. Med.,* 278:409–15 (Feb. 22) 1968.

Review: "Malnutrition, Infection, and Socio-Economic Status," *Nutr. Rev.,* 26:100–103 (Apr.) 1968.

Review: "Mental Development following Kwashiorkor," *Nutr. Rev.,* 27:46–49 (Feb.) 1969.

Scrimshaw, Nevin S., and Béhar, Moises: "Malnutrition in Underdeveloped Countries," *New Eng. J. Med.,* 272:137–44 (Jan. 21), 193–98 (Jan. 28) 1965.

Sours, J. A.: "Clinical Studies in Anorexia Nervosa Syndrome," *New York J. Med.,* 68:1363, 1968.

Metabolism—Carbohydrates, Fats, Proteins

Browe, John H., *et al.:* "Diet and Heart Disease in the Cardiovascular Health Center," *J. Amer. Diet. Ass.,* 50:376–84 (May) 1967.

Brown, W. Duane: "Present Knowledge of Protein Nutrition," *Postgrad. Med.,* 41:A109–16 (Feb.), A107–12 (Mar.), A119–26 (Apr.) 1967.

Christakis, George, *et al.:* "The Anti-Coronary Club: A Dietary Approach to the Prevention of Coronary Heart Disease—A Seven-Year Report," *Amer. J. Public Health,* 56:299–314 (Feb.) 1966.

Council on Foods and Nutrition: "The Regulation of Dietary Fat," *JAMA,* 181:411–29 (Aug. 4) 1962.

Hodges, Robert E., and Krehl, W. A.: "The Role of Carbohydrates in Lipid Metabolism," *Amer. J. Clin. Nutr.,* 17:334–46 (Nov.) 1965.

Hurley, Lucille S.: "Nutrients and Genes: Interactions in Development," *Nutr. Rev.,* 27:3–6 (Jan.) 1969.

McGandy, R. B., *et al.:* "Dietary Carbohydrate and Serum Cholesterol Levels in Man," *Amer. J. Clin. Nutr.,* 18:237–42 (Apr.) 1966.

Yudkin, John: "Sucrose and Heart Disease," *Nutr. Today,* 4:16–20 (Spring) 1969.

Metabolism—Minerals

Callender, Sheila T., and Warner, G. T.: "Iron Absorption from Bread," *Amer. J. Clin. Nutr.,* 21:1170–74 (Oct.) 1968.

Cohen, Nina L., and Briggs, George M.: "Trace Minerals in Nutrition," *Amer. J. Nurs.,* 68:807–11 (Apr.) 1968.

Crosby, William H.: "Control of Iron Absorption by Intestinal Luminal Factors," *Amer. J. Clin. Nutr.,* 21:1189–93 (Oct.) 1968.

Goulding, Peter C.: "Why Doctors Vote Yes to Fluoridation," *Today's Health,* 43:8 (Oct.) 1965.

Schade, Stanley G., Cohen, Richard J., and Conrad, Marcel E.: "Effect of Hydrochloric Acid on Iron Absorption," *New Eng. J. Med.,* 279:672–74 (Sept. 26) 1968.

Staff Report: "Iodized Salt," *Nutr. Today,* 4:22–25 (Spring) 1969.

Wacker, Warren E. C., and Parisi, Alfred F.: "Magnesium Metabolism," *New Eng. J. Med.,* 278:658–63 (Mar. 21), 712–17 (Mar. 28), 772–76 (Apr. 4), 1968.

White, Hilda S.: "Iron Nutriture of Girls and Women. A Review," *J. Amer. Diet. Ass.,* 53:563–69, 570–74 (Dec.) 1968.

13

Nursing the Patient with an Alteration in Body Temperature

The biologist who investigates the quantitative responses by which organisms self-regulate each property and component of their bodies finds reproducible responses which accurately compensate for the specific property or component suffering disturbance. The specificity applies to hundreds of properties. Apparently the responses are prepared ones and are triggered by specific detectors. The detectors communicate with effectors of varying degrees of specificity; but, in general, the possible non-specific responses appear to have been filtered away in the course of evolution so that the more specific ones remain. The problems of identifying the exact kinds of information used in the effectors are largely unsolved; but the over-all results as seen in compensatory responses can be evaluated now. Organisms compress large numbers of specific response systems into a surprisingly few organs and organelles.[1]

Overview

One of the most common methods used in medical diagnosis is the measurement of body temperature. When accurately determined, a number of inferences can be made about the state of the patient as well as the nature of his illness. As with other measurements, the value of a temperature reading depends on the accuracy of the measuring device and the care with which the determination is made.

Temperature Regulation and Variation

As are other homeostatic conditions, body temperature is regulated by a negative feedback

[1] E. F. Adolph: "How Specific Are Physiological Regulations?" *Perspect. Biol. Med.,* 3:68 (Autumn) 1959.

system or more likely a number of interrelated systems. Unlike some other homeostatic conditions, not all animals are capable of regulating their body temperatures despite environmental changes. Depending on their ability to regulate their temperatures, animals are classified as homeothermic (warm-blooded) or poikilothermic (cold-blooded). Homeothermic animals maintain their body temperatures within limits, whereas poikilothermic animals do not. Although this classification is generally useful, it is not completely accurate, because hibernating animals are homeothermic when they are active and poikilothermic during periods of hibernation. Their body temperature is subject to homeostatic control when they are active and is determined by the temperature of the environment when they are hibernating. Individuals who have low cervical cord injuries become poikilothermic.

Although man is homeothermic, the temperature of his tissues varies from one part of his body to another. According to DuBois [2] there is no one body temperature but a series of gradients. As an example, the temperature of the liver is about 100°F, whereas that of the uncovered skin is from 10° to 15°F lower. Factors such as metabolic activity and nearness to the surface of the body affect tissue temperature. Authorities agree that the temperature of the core tissues, the nervous system, and the organs in the abdominal and thoracic cavity is regulated. Whether the temperature of the peripheral tissues is regulated is not known. In Figure 13-1, thermometer readings of rectal and oral temperatures determined under different conditions are shown. It will be noted that the range is greater for rectal than for oral temperatures.

In Figure 13-2, DuBois indicates that the possible range of body temperatures is greater than that shown in Figure 13-1. In this diagram DuBois [3] shows zones of temperature regulation. It can be seen that between 34°C (93°F) and 41°C (105.8°F) temperature regulation is efficient. He notes that, except in patients who have brain lesions or heat stroke or are moribund, temperatures seldom rise above 41°C. Then he asks the question, why should the temperature not rise higher? He answers thus:

If in disease a thermoregulatory thermostat can be set quite accurately at 39° or 40°C, why not at 42°C or higher? From the physical standpoint it is no more difficult to raise body temperature from

[2] Eugene F. DuBois: *Fever and the Regulation of Body Temperature* (Springfield, Ill.: Charles C Thomas, Publisher, 1948), p. 31.
[3] *Ibid.*, p. 9.

40°C to 42°C than from 38°C to 40°C. It is hard to escape the conclusion that there is some sort of secondary temperature regulation in exercise and in disease that vigorously opposes any rise in temperature above 40.5°C. Such a mechanism would appear to be absolutely essential to life.[4]

All bodily processes are affected by temperature. Within the limits of the tissue tolerance, biochemical reactions within cells are accelerated by increasing body temperature and slowed by decreasing body temperature. With increased body temperatures, oxyhemoglobin is dissociated more rapidly than at normal temperatures, the heart rate is increased, and wound healing is accelerated. The metabolic rate is accelerated 7 per cent for 1°F of elevation.

As with other homeostatic conditions, body temperature depends on a supply of what is needed and the regulation of processes whereby the condition is maintained constant. Unlike some substances required by the body, heat is one of the products of cellular activity. The direction of exchange is generally from the internal to the external environment rather than the reverse. Although heat may be regarded as a by-product, it is necessary to the biochemical activities of the cell. Temperatures in the neighborhood of 24°C (75°F) are probably minimal for survival.

Factors Increasing Body Temperature

In Table 13-1 the factors tending to elevate and to lower body temperature are summarized. As long as these opposing forces are in a state of dynamic equilibrium a relatively constant

[4] *Ibid.*, p. 62.

FIGURE 13-1. Thermometer readings, rectal and oral, under various conditions. (Adapted with permission of Charles C Thomas, Publisher, from *Fever and the Regulation of Body Temperature*, 1948, p. 8, by E. F. DuBois.)

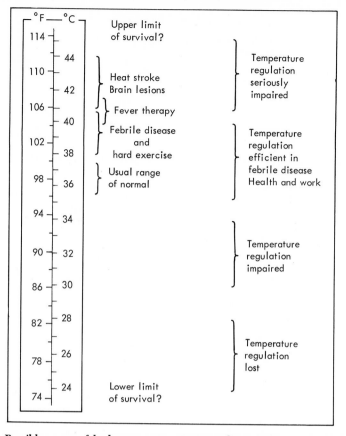

FIGURE 13-2. Possible range of body temperatures: upper limit and lower limit of survival of the human being. (Adapted with permission of Charles C Thomas, Publisher, from *Fever and the Regulation of Body Temperature*, 1948, p. 717, by E. F. DuBois.)

temperature which ranges from 35° to 39°C is maintained.

Factors tending to increase body temperature are of two types: (1) those producing heat from the metabolism of fats, carbohydrates, and proteins and (2) those preventing heat loss or introducing heat from the external environment. As examples, exercise, shivering, and the thyroid hormone increase the production of heat. Peripheral vasoconstriction, subcutaneous fat or edema, clothing, or still or moist air lessen heat loss.

Factors Lowering Body Temperature

On the other side of the balance, heat is lost by (1) radiation, (2) convection, (3) conduction, and (4) evaporation.

Radiation is defined as the transfer of heat by means of waves. These waves are like radio waves in all respects except length. Radiation differs from other means of transferring heat inasmuch as it does not need a medium to pass through space. Convection can be defined simply as the movement of heat from one site to another by currents of air or fluid. As air warms it tends to expand; it becomes less dense and therefore rises. As it rises cooler air takes its place. It in turn warms, expands, and rises and is replaced by cooler air. In conduction, heat is transferred from one molecule to adjacent ones. A good example of conduction is the transfer of heat from a metal coffee pot to its handle. The wall of the pot is heated by the hot water and the heat is transferred directly to adjacent metal in the handle. This movement of heat can be observed by holding the handle and feeling it warm. Evaporation is a process whereby water is converted to steam.

Heat loss through the skin is primarily by radiation, convection, and evaporation. Some is lost in the urine, feces and expired air. In the deeper tissues and the muscles, blood absorbs the heat produced in the tissue and transports it to the skin, where it is transferred to the external environment, thereby cooling the

TABLE 13-1

Factors Influencing Body Temperature

Tending to Elevate	Tending to Lower
Body temperature	Body temperature
Dehydration	Peripheral vasodilatation
Peripheral vasoconstriction	Warming and humidifying inspired air
Ingestion of hot foods and liquids	Exhaling warm air—panting
Increased metabolic rate (rate increased by thy-	Urine and feces
roxin and adrenal hormones)	Evaporation from the skin—sweating
Exercise	Decreased metabolic rate as with decreased thy-
Shivering—unconscious tensing of muscles	roxin during sleep
Body position—decreasing exposed surface	Body position—increasing body surface
Insulating layer of subcutaneous fat or edema	Lack of subcutaneous fat
fluid	Lack of or diminished body covering
Body covering	
Still, warm, moist air	Cool, dry, moving air
Excitement, strong emotion (mostly in children)	Alcohol increases heat loss by increasing periph-
	eral dilatation (when ingested)
Heat production as the result of the metabolism	Mechanisms for heat loss
of fat (9 calories per g), carbohydrate, and	Convection
protein (4 calories per g of each used as fuel)	Radiation
	Conduction
	Evaporation

blood. The transfer of heat from the tissue to the blood and from the blood to the tissue ilustrates one of the laws of thermodynamics; that is, energy travels from an area of greater energy to an area of lesser energy; that is, heat moves from the warmer to the cooler tissues.

Heat is not necessarily always lost to the external environment. In the extremities heat may be transferred from the arteries to the cooler blood in the veins by a countercurrent heat transfer mechanism. Heat loss may be facilitated by increasing the circulation of blood through the skin, by increasing the amount of skin exposed to the environment, and by increasing the capacity of the air surrounding the body to take on heat or moisture. Body structure also affects the rate at which heat is lost. The apron of fat, the omentum, that hangs in front of the abdominal organs protects them from the loss of heat. A layer of fat under the skin insulates the deeper tissues and reduces heat loss. As stated previously, the layer of fat under the skin of the Eskimo plus his short, stocky frame is a type of adaptation to a cold climate, as fat acts as insulating material. Conversely, obesity is a handicap in a tropical climate because the fatty subcutaneous tissue interferes with heat loss. In tropical regions of Africa, adaptation has been in the direction of a long, lean trunk.

Clothing decreases heat loss because it is a poor conductor of heat and it traps air, which is also a poor conductor. Because air is trapped in the spaces between fibers, loosely woven woolens are effective in preventing heat loss under certain conditions (when the air is still). In windy climates, close-woven or impervious materials may be more effective than heavy ones, because the body heat is trapped and prevented from dissipation by the wind. Still air limits heat loss, whereas moving air promotes heat loss by replacing the warm, moist layer or air that surrounds the body with a layer of cooler, drier air. Therefore, an electric fan increases comfort on a hot day, and the wind increases the danger of frostbite on a cold one. Chilling is, therefore, related not only to the temperature but to the movement of air. Thus a "windbreaker" coat may offer more protection from the cold on a windy day than a heavier, "warmer" coat.

The extent to which the air is saturated with moisture is also a factor in heat loss. One of the ways in which heat is transferred from the skin to the external environment is through the evaporation of the water secreted by the sweat glands in the form of perspiration. Conversion of a liquid to a vapor requires energy in the form of heat to overcome the cohesion of molecules. Water requires more heat to vaporize than any other liquid. This property is called the latent heat of vaporization, because the heat remains in the steam until it forms water and releases the heat. There is a limit to the amount of water vapor that the air can hold before it becomes saturated. This amount varies with the temperature. The lower the temperature, the lower the absolute amount of water the air will hold before it is saturated. This is demonstrated in hot weather when the humidity is relatively high. During the night and in the early morning when the temperature is low, the capacity of the air to hold moisture is reduced, and although it remains saturated, or nearly so, some of the air vapor is precipitated as dew. As the humidity falls, the grass dries slowly or quickly, depending on the degree of saturation of the air and whether or not there is a wind. For example, this morning the temperature was 63°F and the humidity was 93 per cent. At noon the temperature was 85°F and the humidity was 63 per cent. The absolute amount of moisture in the air is as great as or greater at noon than it was earlier in the day. The amount that the air is capable of holding has been increased by the increase in temperature.

Another factor in comfort is the relationship of the humidity to the temperature. This is expressed as the comfort index. As the humidity rises in relation to the temperature, comfort declines. Cooling systems are designed differently for use in hot moist and hot dry climates. In hot moist climates an essential feature of a cooling system is a device to remove moisture as well as heat. In fact, unless the temperature is extreme, comfort can be greatly increased by the removal of excessive moisture, despite little or no decrease in temperature. In hot dry climates cooling may be effected by increasing evaporation. Rather than removing moisture, it is added as air is circulated. The windows may be open to supply fresh dry air. Temperature in the room falls because of the heat used in evaporation. Persons driving through a hot dry region sometimes utilize a similar device to cool their cars. They hang wet towels in the car. Cooling is effected by evaporation. The dripping water bags hung on the fenders of cars driven through the desert are based on the same principle.

In addition to its high latent heat of vaporization, water has other properties that facilitate heat loss and therefore help to protect the tissues from overheating. They include its high specific heat and its high conductivity. Specific heat is defined as the amount of heat required to raise the temperature of 1 g of water 1°C. Water has a specific heat of 1, which is the highest of all liquids. All others have a specific heat of less than 1. Defined in terms of numbers, 1 g of water absorbs 1 calorie of heat in rising 1°C. As a consequence, body fluids are capable of absorbing relatively large amounts of heat with little change in temperature.

What factors influence the ability to regulate body temperature?

Although body temperature is regulated, the temperature of the external environment affects the ease with which this is accomplished. Heat loss may be facilitated by cooling the environment, by removing moisture or dehumidifying it, by removing clothing, by increasing air currents, and by applying fluids that are cooler than the body to the skin. Conversely, heat loss may be diminished by increasing the environmental temperature, by adding moisture or humidifying it, by covering the body, by reducing air currents, and by immersing the body in warm water.

Similar to other bodily processes, the temperature of the body is subject to nervous and hormonal control.

Despite a lack of knowledge of the number of circuits involved in the nervous control of body temperature, it behaves as if it were a closed-loop negative feedback system. Information is fed into the hypothalamus by the temperature of the blood circulating through it and/or by sensory receptors in other parts of the body. In the hypothalamus the information is interpreted and converted (transduced) into neural impulses that initiate behavior that increases or decreases rates of heat loss and heat production.[5]

Centers for the coordination and integration of those processes that result in a balance between heat produced and heat lost are located in the hypothalamus. Stimulation of the area increasing heat production results in inhibition of the area facilitating heat loss. There is some evidence indicating that there are heat-regulating centers in the spinal cord. The principal centers are, however, in the hypothalamus and nearby preoptic nuclei. A center in the anterior hypothalamus integrates the responses that prevent overheating, or hyperthermia. Stimulation of this area initiates panting, dilatation of surface blood vessels, and sweating. All these activities promote heat loss. Injury to this area results in elevation of body temperature. A center in the posterior hypothalamus integrates responses that prevent chilling, or hypothermia. Stimulation of this area results in constriction of blood vessels, shivering, and increase in muscle tone. These activities either prevent heat loss or increase heat production. Messages from the hypothalamus are conveyed to the surface of the body by the sympathetic, or thoracolumbar, division of the autonomic nervous system. It innervates both the sweat glands and the periph-

[5] H. T. Hammel: "Regulation of Internal Body Temperature," *Ann. Rev. Physiol.,* **30:**641–710 (1968).

eral blood vessels. Although the postganglionic fibers supplying the sweat glands are cholinergic, they respond to stimulation of the sympathetic nervous system. According to Hemingway and Price [6] nonshivering heat production in the cold-adapted individual is controlled or influenced by the sympathetic nervous system.

HORMONAL FACTORS

Heat production is also regulated by the hormones thyroxine and epinephrine. Thyroxine augments the rate of cellular oxidation and thereby increases the production of heat. In hyperthyroidism, body temperature is elevated a degree or so. Epinephrine, which is secreted at the sympathetic nerve endings, increases heat production by affecting the rate of metabolism. Female sex hormones have an influence on body temperature. During the proliferative phase of the menstrual cycle, body temperature is low. At the time of ovulation the temperature often falls and then rises. During the period that follows, the temperature remains up and then falls just prior to the onset of menstruation. Fluctuations in body temperature may be used as a basis for determining the so-called safe period in family planning.

AGE

Although the newborn infant has been thought to be poikilothermic at birth, this belief is now being questioned. According to Silverman and Parke, [7] heat loss in the infant exceeds his capacity to produce heat. Although he responds to cold by shivering and by increasing his metabolic rate, his losses are too great to maintain heat balance. Because he lacks subcutaneous fat and has a relatively larger body surface, the premature infant has more difficulty in maintaining a stable body temperature than the full-term infant.

In infants and children the temperature response in illness is often greater than in adults. They have a higher metabolic rate; therefore, there is more heat to eliminate. Normally they have a larger proportion of their body water in the interstitial fluid space, and their kidneys do not concentrate urine as effectively as do those of adults.

In contrast to the child and younger adult, who respond to a variety of etiologic agents by developing a fever, elderly and debilitated per-

---

[6] Allan Hemingway and William M. Price: "The Autonomic Nervous System and Regulation of Body Temperature," *Anesthesiology,* **29**:693 (July–Aug.) 1968.

[7] William A. Silverman and Priscilla C. Parke: "Keep Him Warm," *Amer. J. Nurs.,* **65**:81 (Oct.) 1965.

sons may have little or even no elevation of temperature when ill. Therefore, other evidence that the elderly person is ill should not be discounted because he does not have a fever. A failure to develop a fever under circumstances when it is usual is generally a poor prognostic sign.

Adaptation to Extremes in Temperature

Within limits man is capable of adapting to extremes in temperature. Most individuals have an excess of sweat glands, not all of which function at the same time. Persons born in tropical climates have more sweat glands functioning at one time than those who are born in temperate climates, but they do not have visible drops of sweat. Given time, a nonadapted but healthy person adapts physiologically to elevated environmental temperatures. Evidence that adaptation to heat occurs is that the first hot days of summer are more uncomfortable than later hot days. Changes taking place during adaptation to heat include increased salt conservation, probably caused by increased aldosterone secretion, and a small decrease in metabolic rate. The ability to retain salt takes longer to develop than the other changes. The pulse rate, which is increased in the beginning, returns to normal levels. Flushing of the skin because of vasodilatation decreases as adaptation develops. Edema of the hands and the feet is common until adaptation occurs and the individual may have many signs and symptoms similar to those observed during illness. Some people, especially those with a limited cardiac reserve, have a limited capacity to adapt to heat. This is evidenced by an increase in pulse rate. Also, in the adaptive process the tendency to conserve salt may aggravate previous salt and water retention and place an added strain on a limited cardiac reserve. For further discussion, see the References.

Persons who are elderly or who have a cardiac disorder should be encouraged to reduce physical activity during hot weather. This is most important at its onset. Other measures reducing the burden on the heart and the thermoregulatory systems include the wearing of lightweight clothing and use of electric fans and air conditioning. It is also important for the person to maintain his fluid intake without exceeding his excretory capacity. When sweating is profuse, it is often difficult to replace the fluid loss by voluntary drinking. When air conditioning is not available, patients who are in congestive heart failure are sometimes placed in oxygen tents in hot weather. Although the increase in oxygen supply may be beneficial, the air conditioning reduces the demands made on the circulatory system to facilitate the loss of heat. When the patient is removed from the tent, he may be called on to adapt both to a reduction in environmental oxygen and to an increase in the temperature of his surroundings. Consequently, the tent may be removed gradually. When this is done, it is well to take it off during the cooler parts of the day and to replace it when it is hot.

To summarize the physiology of temperature regulation, temperature is one of the conditions that is homeostatically controlled by the nervous, hormonal, and circulatory systems. The heat-regulating centers in the nervous system regulate body temperature primarily by increasing or decreasing the diameter of blood vessels in the skin and by shivering. The hormonal system influences heat production and salt retention, which in turn increase water retention and in this way aid in the transfer of heat from the interior of the body to the external environment. The temperature known to be regulated is that of the deeper, or core, tissues of the body. Body temperature varies with such factors as activity, emotion, environmental conditions, and the time of day. Body temperatures can be elevated by procedures interfering with heat loss, such as hot baths, hot weather, and strenuous muscular exercise. Children are likely to respond with greater swings in temperature than adults. Elderly people often respond less actively than younger persons.

One of the most common findings in disease is some disturbance in temperature regulation. Although temperatures below the lower range of normal do occur, the most common change is an elevation above the upper limits of normal. Because some people normally maintain a temperature somewhat higher than average, the upper limit of normal is difficult to define exactly. However, for persons resting quietly in bed, an oral temperature of 37.5°C (99.5°F) is usually accepted as the upper limit of normal. The condition in which the body temperature is elevated above normal in disease is called fever.

Measuring the Body Temperature

Whether or not the temperature recorded by the thermometer accurately reflects the temperature of the body depends on the care with which the procedure is performed and the accuracy of the thermometer. Even for the rectum the temperature may vary as much as 1°F.[8] Whatever site is selected, the purpose is the same, that is, to estimate as accurately as possible the temperature of the interior of the body. To do this the thermometer should be placed in an area of the body that contains large blood vessels and that is protected insofar as possible from outside influences. It should be kept in place long enough to register the true temperature. Finally, care should be taken to shake the mercury down before the thermometer is reused.

Not only do the temperatures of various parts of the body differ, but the temperatures at the same site vary from one time of the day to another. Temperature is one of the functions for which there appears to be a biological or circadian rhythm. The lowest temperature is reached sometime between 3 and 5 A.M. Then it begins to rise until it reaches its highest point between 7 and 10 P.M. When temperatures are taken once a day, the time selected should reflect the peak temperature. For most moderately well patients a temperature reading taken about 7 P.M. is most satisfactory. When a patient's temperature rises rapidly, readings may need to be made every 10 to 15 minutes in order to determine the peak temperature as well as to protect the patient should his temperature rise excessively.[9] If knowledge of the peak and trough is desired, suitable times are 7 A.M. and 7 P.M. Sims [10] further suggests that a six-hour schedule beginning at 7 A.M. provides sufficient information about the temperature of most patients.

SITES USED FOR TEMPERATURE DETERMINATION

Although the tympanic membrane and other sites have been used for experimental studies, the sites commonly used are the mouth, rectum, and axilla. Authorities differ as to the range of normal for each of these sites. Despite the assumption that the rectum most accurately reflects core body temperatures, some authorities believe that equally or more accurate temperature readings may be made in the mouth or axilla.

From the studies made by Nichols and her associates,[11] factors influencing the accuracy of temperature readings included the reliability of the thermometers and the time they were left in place. Of 52 oral thermometers tested for reliability, 35 were accurate at 95.4°F. At 105.8°F only 5 were accurate. Of 52 rectal

[8] Jere Mead and C. Lawrence Bonmarito: "Reliability of Rectal Temperatures as an Index of Internal Body Temperature," *J. Appl. Physiol.*, 2:97 (Aug.) 1949.

[9] R. S. Sims: "Temperature Recording in a Teaching Hospital," *Lancet*, 2:535–36 (Sept. 11) 1965.
[10] *Ibid.*, p. 536.
[11] Glennadee A. Nichols *et al.*: "Oral, Axillary, and Rectal Temperature Determinations and Relationships," *Nurs. Res.*, 15:308 (Fall) 1966.

thermometers tested, only 16 were accurate at 95.4°F and 3 at 105.8°F.

The time necessary to obtain an accurate reading in the different sites varied from those generally suggested. Nichols et al.[12] found that individuals required from 1 to 12 minutes to reach their maximum oral and axillary temperatures and 1 to 9 minutes to reach their maximum rectal temperature. Differences between oral and axillary temperatures varied from 0° to 4.2°F. A few subjects had higher axillary temperatures than oral temperatures. More than one half of the subjects' rectal temperatures were less than 1°F greater than their oral temperatures. The range was 0.2° to 2.8°F. As a result of their study, Nichols et al.[13] recommend the following placement times if reasonably accurate readings are to be obtained: oral, 7 minutes; axillary, 10 minutes; and rectal, 2 minutes.

Other studies challenge accepted practices. Woodman and her associates [14] studied the effects of drinking iced water and of smoking cigarettes. Smoking and iced water produced statistically significant changes in temperature.

Verhonick and Werley [15] concluded, as a result of their studies, that the ingestion of hot and cold fluids does make a difference in the degree of temperature of afebrile patients. Contrary to general opinion, cigarette smoking or chewing gum does not make a difference.

Kintzel [16] could not support the assumption that the administration of oxygen by either nasal catheter or tent had a significant effect on oral temperature readings. In fact, she suggests that by changing from oral to rectal thermometers at the time oxygen therapy is instituted a greater error may be introduced than if oral temperatures are continued. On the basis of her findings, Kintzel recommends that no change be made in the site used for temperature determination when oxygen therapy is prescribed.

What environmental temperature factors must the nurse consider in caring for the patient?

The nurse not only is responsible for the procedure but for being certain that each reading accurately reflects the temperature of the site at which the determination is made. Studies in-

[12] *Ibid.*, p. 309.

[13] *Ibid.*, p. 310.

[14] Ellen A. Woodman, Susan McConnell Parry, and Lillian Simms: "Sources of Unreliability in Oral Temperatures," *Nurs. Res.,* **16:**276–79 (Summer) 1967.

[15] Phyllis J. Verhonick and Harriet H. Werley: "Experimentation in Nursing Practice in the Army," *Nurs. Outlook,* **11:**205 (Mar.) 1963.

[16] Kay Corman Kintzel: *A Comparative Study of Oral and Rectal Temperatures in Patients Receiving Two Forms of Oxygen Therapy,* ANA Clinical Sessions (New York: Appleton-Century-Crofts, 1966), p. 102.

dicate that the time oral thermometers are left in place have been too short to give an accurate reading in many patients. The time required varies with the individual and with the site. The assumption that the rectal temperature is 1°F higher than the oral temperature and that the axillary temperature is 1°F lower than the oral temperature has been shown to be untrue. When the mouth is used, recent ingestion of hot or cold liquids affects the temperature reading.

Knowledge of temperature regulation has a bearing on meeting the needs of all patients as well as those with fevers. One general objective in the nursing of patients is to protect the patient from conditions that place strain on the adaptive capacity of the individual. Certainly temperatures outside the range of comfort increase metabolism and, as a result, the activity of all tissues and organs. Although the effect of small or moderate changes in environmental temperature may be of no consequence as far as the heat-regulating center is concerned, they may place serious strain on the heart or blood vessels. In heart disease or shock, they may well have serious consequences. Methods that can be used to protect the patient from the consequences of high environmental temperatures have already been suggested. Patients should also be protected from chilling by adequate bed covering and warm clothing. Hot-water bottles to the feet, with attention to their temperature, bed socks, bed jackets, and sweaters, help to protect patients from chilling. People, especially the elderly, who are accustomed to wearing their underwear in bed should be permitted to continue the practice when at all possible. Screens in front of open windows or doors may reduce drafts, which some patients find chilling. When bathing patients, especially during those times of the year when the environmental temperature is low, care should be taken that the bath water is warm and that the person is kept covered and the skin is thoroughly dried.

The second objective is to make, record, and report observations basic to planning the nursing care of the patient and pertinent to the diagnosis and treatment of the patient's condition. The first relates directly to the practice of nursing and the second to the role of the nurse as a co-worker of the physician. Although the physician has the responsibility for establishing the medical diagnosis and for planning the patient's therapeutic regime, the nurse can and should contribute both by observing signs and symptoms indicating deviations from health and by clearly describing her observations.

Two Abnormalities in Body Temperature

Body temperature varies widely among individuals as well as in the same individual from one time of day to another. Environmental conditions also affect body temperature. Depending on the circumstances a healthy person's temperature may range from 35.8°C (96.6°F) to 37.8°C (100°F). Particularly at the upper limits of normal, there is some overlapping between what in one person may be a normal temperature and in another hyperthermia or fever. In general, persons who are ill with a temperature of 37.4°C (99.2°F) or above may be suspected of having a low-grade fever. Similarly persons whose temperatures are below 35.8°C (96.4°F) may be hypothermic.

Fever

Fever is associated with two quite different situations. In the more common and usually less serious one, the individual behaves as if his temperature-regulating center were reset at a higher level. Body temperature continues to be regulated, but it is regulated at a level above normal. In the other type of fever, as a result of injury or disease of the hypothalamus or midbrain, temperature regulation fails and the temperature continues to rise unless external measures are employed to increase heat loss. When the condition injuring the heat-regulating center is temporary and tissues are protected from excess heat, recovery is possible. For example, in thyroid crises, or heat stroke, temperature regulation may fail. If body temperature is controlled within levels tolerated by the tissues, until such time as the thyroid hormone level falls toward normal, the patient may be saved.

Pathogenesis

Although fever has been recognized as a cardinal sign of disease since the time of Hippocrates, why it occurs or what purpose it serves is not known. A number of theories have been advanced to explain fever. The one most generally accepted is that fever results from the effects of pyrogenic (fever-producing) substances liberated by injured cells. Granulocytic leukocytes are known to contain a pyrogenic agent. Other cells may also contain them. The body responds to tissue injury with an inflammatory process. The exudate formed in inflammation has been demonstrated experimentally to contain a substance that, when injected, induces fever. If this theory is correct, then fever, whether it occurs in the patient with cancer, diphtheria, an infected wound after suffering a crushing wound, or an infarction in the heart or lungs, has a common denominator, that is, a pyrogen released by the granulocytic leuko-

cytes or other cells. The nurse should keep in mind that fever is not a disease but part of the body's response to tissue injury.

Although the value of fever is in most instances not known, in certain chronic conditions such as neurosyphilis, some gonococcal infections, and rheumatoid arthritis, fever is followed by an improvement in the patient's condition. Fever, particularly when it is high or continued for long periods of time, has a number of harmful effects.

Description of Fever Patterns

The onset of fever may be abrupt with a shaking chill, or fever may develop without the patient being aware that he has it. The course may be constant or fluctuate greatly. Fever may terminate suddenly with a drenching diaphoresis or it may decline slowly. It may last a predictable period of time or continue indefinitely. It may disappear only to return. When this occurs it may mean that the patient is developing a complication or it may reflect the nature of the disease causing the fever. As an example, malaria is characterized by attacks of chills and fever alternating with afebrile periods. The length of time between attacks of chills and fever varies from 48 to 72 hours, depending upon the species of malarial parasite.

What physiological changes are responsible for the rise in temperature in fever?

Heat production is increased in much the same way as in exercise. Heat loss, however, does not increase to the same degree. In fact, the body responds much as it does when exposed to cold. The peripheral vessels constrict and limit the circulation of blood through the skin. The person may shiver and his muscle tone increase. The muscles attached to the hair in the skin contract and elevate the hair; accompanying this are elevations of the skin commonly called goose pimples. The person feels cold and piles blankets over himself or turns the electric blanket on high even when the room is hot. When the temperature of his tissues reaches the new level, shivering stops and the patient may feel warm. Whereas during the chill he was pale, his skin becomes pink. A new equilibrium between heat production and heat loss has been set. Return of body temperature to normal levels is preceded by the regulator being reset at a lower level. The mechanisms responsible for the lowering of the body temperature are the same as those accompanying exercises; that is, sweating and vasodilatation occur.

The mechanisms responsible for the elevation of the temperature in patients who have a chill are easy to explain. The mechanisms responsible in the patient who does not have a chill are less clear. Elevation in temperature may be brought about simply by a decrease in heat loss. It is also possible that the metabolic processes are stimulated by a specific fever-producing substance. Of all the discomforts accompanying fever, chills and sweating are probably the most unpleasant.

What are the nurse's responsibilities in caring for the patient who has a chill?

When a patient has a chill or his temperature is rising rapidly, his temperature should be checked frequently enough during and after the chill to determine the height and trough of the fever. For example, during the chill the temperature may be measured every ten minutes. After the chill ceases, it may be measured every half hour until the last reading is no higher or is lower than the preceding one. Readings may then be taken every two to four hours until the patient maintains a normal temperature. Whatever the hospital routine, temperature determinations may be necessary at more frequent intervals than those prescribed by the physician. When the temperature of the patient is rising very rapidly or is at a very high level, his safety may depend on frequent determinations and on the institution of effective measures of control.

Although instances have been recorded in which patients have survived temperatures as high as 44.4°C (112°F) for a short period of time, a temperature as high as 42.2°C (108°F) for an extended period of time can be expected to do permanent damage. Furthermore, when temperatures exceed 41.0°C (105.8°F), regulatory mechanisms cannot be depended on to resist further rise. (See Figure 13-2.) Excessively high temperatures endanger the body by irreversibly inactivating essential enzyme systems and by producing permanent alterations in the structure of body proteins. Therefore, when a patient's temperature is elevated to, or approaches, 40.56°C (105°F) and continues to rise, measures are instituted to reduce it.

When the heat-regulating centers are injured, the only effective measures are those that increase heat loss by increasing the temperature gradient between the skin and the external environment. To increase the difference in temperature gradient, measures are instituted to increase the evaporation of moisture from the skin, or the patient is placed in a cold environment, so that the heat moves from his tissues to the surrounding media. Thus the patient may be sponged liberally with water or alcohol. When his skin is cool, the sponging should be accompanied by rubbing in order to encourage the circulation of blood through the skin. Another point to be remembered when giving a sponge bath is that it should be continued for as long a period of time as is necessary to lower the temperature. A quick "splash" may do more harm than good as it may only stimulate heat production. In young children temperature may be effectively lowered by cooling rectal irrigations.

For the patient whose temperature is dangerously high, placing him in a tub of iced water may be lifesaving. When hypothermia blankets are available, a patient may be placed between them. "Space suits" that may be either cooled or warmed are also available. These procedures must be prescribed by the physician. When drastic measures are taken to reduce body temperature, regular and frequent checking of the patient's temperature is essential. Since the temperature continues to fall after the decline is established, the physician should be asked to indicate the level at which the temperature-reducing procedure should be discontinued. During the chill, the patient should be covered and protected from drafts. A hot-water bottle applied to his feet and an ice cap to his head may increase his comfort.

Signs and Symptoms of Fever

The signs and symptoms accompanying fever result from (1) the increase in the metabolic rate as a result of the elevation in body temperature, (2) the response of the cardiovascular and respiratory systems, (3) the nonspecific responses of the body to injury, and (4) the nature of the causative agent.

As the metabolic rate rises in fever, utilization of calories and protein catabolism increases. Unless carbohydrate and protein intake is increased in proportion to the elevation of body temperature, weight loss occurs. Attention to the patient's food intake is of particular importance when fever lasts more than a few days. Weight loss does not need to occur, providing the patient's food intake is adequate.

Another effect of the increased metabolic rate is increased sweating. As much as 3 liters of water may be lost each day by the patient with fever. Salt is also lost. To maintain fluid balance, the patient must be given assistance to replace this fluid. The higher his temperature, the more fluid he loses and the more help he needs to ingest sufficient fluids to keep fluid intake equal to fluid loss. An inadequate fluid intake is accompanied by a low output of concentrated urine and sordes in his mouth. When his fluid intake is adequate, he does not develop sordes and he excretes at least 1000 ml of urine daily. In those patients who have drenching sweating (diaphoresis), comfort is increased by sponge baths and by replacing wet with dry clothing and linen. In patients who continue to feel chilly, such as those with influenza, bathing may increase discomfort.

The cardiovascular and respiratory responses to fever are those one expects when the metabolic rate is increased. They include an increase in the heart and respiratory rates and dilatation of the peripheral blood vessels. As a result of the vascular changes, the patient appears flushed and complains of feeling warm. In a patient with a limited cardiac reserve, the extra burden placed on the heart by the increased heart rate may precipitate heart failure.

Among the nonspecific responses to fever are nausea, vomiting, and diarrhea. The leukocyte count may be elevated above 12,000 cells or be lower than 5,000 cells per cubic millimeter of blood. There may be an increase in the sedimentation rate.

Although patients who have a fever may have few or no subjective symptoms, they may feel unpleasantly warm, have headache and malaise, muscle aching, and photophobia, and feel miserable. For the relief of headache, applying an ice cap to the head or sponging the patient's face may be helpful. Protection of the patient with photophobia from bright light is essential and may lessen the headache. The doctor may prescribe aspirin for the headache. However, some patients prefer the headache to the sweating that follows the ingestion of aspirin. Adults tolerate fever quite well unless it continues for an extended period of time.

In addition to the signs and symptoms that accompany fever, the patient is likely to have others that are related to the condition causing the fever. For example, the sputum of the patient with pneumococcal pneumonia has specific characteristics. The type of fever and the length of time it lasts are related to the fact that the pneumococcus is the causative agent. In many disorders in which fever occurs, the type of fever as well as the length of time it lasts is generally predictable.

The possibility that the cause of the fever may be an infectious agent should not be overlooked in those patients in whom there is a problem of differential diagnosis. Measures appropriate to the prevention of the spread of infection to personnel and to other patients should be instituted. These measures should take into account the avenues by which organisms leave the host, vehicles whereby they can be transported to others, and portals of entry to others. See Chapter 5.

Hypothermia

Just as the tissues can, within limits, tolerate temperatures higher than the normal range, they can tolerate temperatures that are lower. The usual response to cold is shivering and constriction of the peripheral blood vessels. Shivering is accompanied by an increase in the production of heat and by changes decreasing heat loss. When these mechanisms are adequate or the environmental temperature is not too low, they may be sufficient to maintain body temperature within normal limits. When, however, heat loss exceeds heat production, hypothermia (abnormally low body temperature) ensues. As an example, a hunting party is lost in the woods or mountains or on the prairie in freezing or near-freezing weather. The seriousness of their predicament depends not only on the temperature of the environment but on the adequacy of their clothing, whether or not it is wet or dry, and their ability to find or construct a shelter for protection from the wind. As indicated previously, water is a better conductor of heat than air. As air warms, it tends to form an insulating layer around the body; water does not. Chilling is more rapid when evaporation takes place and/or there are air currents than when clothing is dry and the air is still.

A more common incident is the elderly person who is exposed to cold after a fall either outside or indoors. If he is inebriated at the time, heat loss is increased because alcohol causes vasodilation. Should the temperature reading of any patient be 95°F, the lowest reading on a standard clinical thermometer, a low-reading thermometer should be obtained and the patient's true temperature determined. Another cause of hypothermia is depression of the nervous system by drugs such as morphine and the barbiturates. When the patient is found to be hypothermic, he is slowly rewarmed by placing him at ordinary room temperature and by covering him with light bed covering. His temperature should rise about 1° to 2°F per hour. As the patient warms, he is in danger of developing hypovolemic shock as his arterioles dilate. To prevent this complication the physician may prescribe intravenous fluids. They should be administered slowly because rapid infusion of fluids may overload the circulatory system. The skin of the hypothermic patient is susceptible to heat. Therefore, external heat is applied cautiously. The skin should be inspected regularly for reddening or other signs of overheating.

The patient's blood pressure, temperature, pulse, and possibly central venous pressure should be checked regularly. In addition to shock the hypothermic patient is susceptible to ventricular fibrillation and cardiac arrest as he warms. Electrocardiac monitoring may be used to identify early cardiac irregularities. Cardiac irregularities may be caused by metabolic acidosis, which occurs as a consequence of anaerobic metabolism. Irregularities of pulse or ECG should be promptly reported. A defibrillator and emergency drugs should be on hand to use if needed.

Artificial Induction of Hypothermia

The method employed to induce hypothermia depends on why it is used, how long it is to be maintained, and the equipment available. Hypothermia is induced by three methods: (1) *external or surface cooling*, (2) *internal or body cavity cooling*, and (3) *extracorporeal cooling*.

The fastest method of external cooling is by immersion of the trunk and extremities in a tub of iced water. Because they are easier to use, refrigerated blankets are more commonly used for surface cooling. These blankets contain coils through which a refrigerant is circulated.

Hypothermia or even freezing of body cavities such as the stomach has been used to treat diseases such as peptic ulcer. The purpose is to decrease the activity of the acid-secreting glands. In the hands of physicians skilled in the technique, it may be beneficial to some patients.

In open heart surgery, blood is cooled by circulating it through the cooling system of the pump oxygenator. The same system is used to warm the patient after the procedure is completed.

Effects of Hypothermia

As the body temperature falls, the metabolic rate also falls. The most important effect of the decreased metabolic rate is that the oxygen requirements of the tissues are likewise decreased. As an illustration, when tissue temperature is decreased to 25.5°C (78°F), oxygen consumption is reduced by approximately 50 per cent. One of the important uses of hypothermia is, therefore, in surgical procedures requiring interruption of the circulation to important structures, such as the brain. By induction of hypothermia, the length of time the circulation is stopped can be prolonged. It is used in open heart surgery and in operations on the aorta to protect the brain from the effects of hypoxia. It is also employed in the therapy of patients with serious injuries to the brain as well as in the treatment of uncontrolled hyperthyroidism.

What are some of the nurse's responsibilities in the care of the patient who undergoes hypothermia?

The responsibilities of the nurse vary with the method used and the length of time hypothermia is maintained. When hypothermia is induced by circulating the blood through a pump oxygenator, most of the responsibility is borne by the physician and the technician who runs the pump. When the blanket is used and the patient is maintained in a hypothermic state for several days, much of the responsibility is delegated to the nurse.

SHIVERING

One of the problems in hypothermia is the control of shivering. It must be controlled as the temperature will not fall unless heat loss is greater than heat gain. In the conscious patient, shivering is a source of great discomfort. The patient should be observed regularly for evidence of shivering, which starts with a quivering of the chest muscles. One of the phenothiazines, usually chlorpromazine, is prescribed, to be given before hypothermia is instituted and every two hours as needed. Other drugs such as Demerol may be prescribed to reduce discomfort.

In all phases of hypothermia—induction, maintenance, and warming—regular and accurate observation of the patient is essential. During induction and also during rewarming the temperature tends to overshoot the desired mark.

OBSERVATION

The nursing care of the patient who has had hypothermia artificially induced is similar to that in which hypothermia is accidentally induced. When induction is artificial, the temperature, blood pressure, central venous pressure, and rate and rhythm of the pulse should be monitored continuously. The blood pressure and pulse rate are expected to decrease. Especially during the warming period, ventricular fibrillation and cardiac arrest are possible. Irregularity of the pulse may herald this event. Urine output diminishes. The urine has a low specific gravity. Because hypothermia depresses the activity of tissues, bodily responses to infection may be diminished. Respiratory infections may develop in the absence of the usual signs and symptoms.

The size and shape of each pupil as well as their response to light should be noted. Because tearing is likely to be minimal, the condition of the conjunctiva should also be observed. Irrigations of the eyes and/or applications of eye patches may be necessary to keep the cornea moist and protect the eyes from injury.

DRUGS

With the depression of metabolism and of organs such as the liver and kidneys, reactions to drugs may well be abnormal. Absorption may be delayed or the mechanisms for their destruction or elimination impaired. The nurse should know the expected as well as the toxic effects of drugs given to the patient.

To illustrate, Mrs. Molly McRobin was admitted to the emergency room for treatment of a stab wound in her chest. Although she was fully conscious at the time of her admission, she soon lapsed into unconsciousness from which she never recovered. She was rushed to the operating room, where she was found to have cardiac tamponade caused by bleeding into the pericardial sac, and she experienced cardiac arrest for a period of from five to ten minutes.

Because of the injury to the temperature-regulating centers in the hypothalamus, Mrs. McRobin was unable to control her temperature and it began to rise. To prevent damage to the brain by hyperthermia and to decrease its oxygen requirements, Mrs. McRobin was placed on a hypothermia blanket. At this time Mrs. McRobin was deeply unconscious and she was dependent on the nurse to meet her physiologic needs. Observation not only of the status of the patient but of the functioning of all the different types of equipment was necessary. Although the only aspect of Mrs. McRobin's care that will be discussed is the hypothermia, she required special attention to maintenance of oxygen supply, fluid intake and output, nutrition, mouth care, protection of her skin, and attention to position and body alignment. To maintain her joints in a functional condition, her extremities were moved through a normal range of motion daily. Because respiratory insufficiency occurs during hypothermia, regular turning at two-hour intervals is necessary. A tracheostomy and respiratory assistance may be required.

Because Mrs. McRobin was unconscious, the procedure could not be explained to her. Her mother, her only visitor, was informed, however. Before Mrs. McRobin was placed on the blanket, she was bathed and her skin was covered with a thin layer of lanolin to lessen the possibility of frostbite. After she was on the blanket, she was given partial baths as needed. Cool water was used. Patting rather than rubbing motions were used in drying her.

Although the patient may be placed between two hypothermia blankets, Mrs. McRobin was placed on one. The patient may be placed directly on the blanket or it may be covered with a sheet. The latter practice is more aesthetic and may be more comfortable for the patient; when the sheet is tucked under the sides of the mattress, it may also help to keep the blanket in place. By such placement of the blanket or sheet, the rate of cooling is reduced by trapping air, which insulates the skin from the blanket.

As prescribed by Mrs. McRobin's physician, the thermostat on the blanket was set at 32.2°C (90°F). To observe her temperature, a rectal probe was introduced and connected to a battery-operated thermometer. Her temperature could be determined at any time by switching on the machine. The blanket operates automatically. Because the patient's temperature drops about 2° after cooling is discontinued, the machine should turn off before the desired temperature is attained. It should also turn on when the temperature starts to rise.

Although not a problem with Mrs. McRobin, the restless patient may move off the blanket. When this happens, either the patient or the blanket must be moved so that the patient is reclining on it.

The blanket itself requires some care. Tape rather than safety pins should be used to fasten tubing to sheets. A puncture of the blanket will allow the refrigerant fluid to escape and render the blanket useless. Hot water or strong chemicals should not be applied to the blanket as they may damage the plastic covering. The blanket can be washed with soap and tepid water or a solution of benzethonium chloride. It should not be folded when stored, but it should be rolled loosely and placed on a flat surface.

Summary

The purpose of this chapter has been to discuss some of the needs of the patient who has problems in the control of body temperature or in whom hypothermia is induced. As a basis for understanding the nature of these problems, the homeostatic mechanisms utilized by the body in maintaining temperature have been reviewed and related to the mechanisms that are involved in hyperthermia and hypothermia. Suggestions have been made as to how this content applies to the care of patients in general and to those with alterations in body temperature. Students who are interested in pursuing the study of temperature regulation in its various aspects will find references at the end of the chapter. Material has been included on studies that have been made to improve the accuracy of temperature determinations.

Despite their importance to the safety of the patient, certain problems related to temperature taking have not been discussed. They include being certain that (1) the thermometer is clean when it is inserted and that (2) the thermometer is introduced in such a manner that it does not damage body tissue.

REFERENCES

BOOKS

Adolph, E. F., *et al.: Physiology in Man in the Desert* (New York: Interscience Publishers, Inc., 1947).

PERIODICALS

Agate, J., *et al.:* "Discussion on Old People," *Practitioner,* 200:582–83 (Apr.) 1968.

Bazett, H. C., *et al.:* "II: Temperature Changes in Blood Flowing in Arteries and Veins in Man," *J. Appl. Physiol.,* 1:3–19 (July) 1948.

Beland-Marechak, N.: "Circadian Rhythms," *Canad. Nurs.,* 64:40–44 (Dec.) 1968.

Bell, Shirley: "Early Morning Temperatures," *Amer. J. Nurs.,* 69:764–66 (Apr.) 1969.

Benzinger, T. H.: "The Human Thermostat," *Sci. Amer.,* 204:134–47 (Jan.) 1961.

Bloom, Ben: "A Role for Day and Night in Evolution," *Perspect. Biol. Med.,* 10:269–71 (Winter) 1967.

Bodel, Phyllis T., Dillard, Morris, and Bondy, Philip K.: "The Mechanism of Steroid-Induced Fever," *Ann. Intern. Med.,* 69:875–79 (Nov.) 1969.

Brocklehurst, J. C.: "Various Problems in Geriatric Medicine," *Nurs. Times,* 63:1072–74 (Aug. 11) 1967.

Dubois, Franklin S.: "Rhythms, Cycles and Periods in Health and Disease," *Amer. J. Psychiat.,* 116:114–19 (Aug.) 1959.

Goldsmith, R.: "Use of Clothing Records to Demonstrate Acclimatization to Cold in Man," *J. Appl. Physiol.,* 15:776–80 (Sept.) 1960.

Hector, Winifred E., "Changes in Temperature," *Nurs. Times,* 64:353–54 (Mar. 15) 1968.

Hickey, Mary Catherine: "Hypothermia," *Amer. J. Nurs.,* 65:116–22 (Jan.) 1965.

Hoagland, Robert J., and Bishop, Raymond H., Jr.: "A Physiologic Treatment of Heat Stroke," *Amer. J. Med. Sci.,* 141:415–22 (Apr.) 1961.

Hock, Raymond J., and Covino, Benjamin G.: "Hypothermia," *Sci. Amer.,* 198:104–14 (Mar.) 1958.

Nichols, Glennadee, *et al.:* "Taking Oral Temperatures of Febrile Patients," *Nurs. Res.,* 18:448–50 (Sept.–Oct.) 1969.

Nichols, Glennadee A., and Glor, Beverly A. K.: "A Replication of Rectal Thermometer Placement Studies," *Nurs. Res.,* 17:360–61 (July–Aug.) 1968.

Nichols, Glennadee A., and Verhonick, Phyllis J.: "Time and Temperature," *Amer. J. Nurs.,* 67:2304–2306 (Nov.) 1967.

Phelps, Elbert T.: "Fever—Its Causes and Effects," *Amer. J. Nurs.,* 56:319–22 (Mar.) 1956.

Purintum, Lynn R., and Bishop, Barbara E.: "How Accurate Are Clinical Thermometers," *Amer. J. Nurs.,* 69:99–100 (Jan.) 1969.

Skinner, Earl C.: "Malignant Hyperpyrexia," *AORN,* 8:35–38 (Aug.) 1968.

Torrance, Jane T.: "Temperature Readings of Premature Infants," *Nurs. Res.,* 17:312–20 (July–Aug.) 1968.

Verhonick, Phyllis J., and Nichols, Glennadee A.: "Temperature Measurement in Nursing Practice and Research," *Canad. Nurse,* 64:41–43 (June) 1968.

Walker, Virginia H., and Selminoff, Eugene D.: "A Note on the Accuracy of the Temperature, Pulse and Respiration Procedure," *Nurs. Res.,* 14:72–76 (Winter) 1965.

Warner, C. G.: "Measurement of Thermal Environment," *Occup. Health,* 20:18–23 (Jan.–Feb.) 1968.

Williams, J. Egerton: "Treatment by Hypothermia," *Nurs. Mirror,* 126:33–40 (Feb.) 1968.

Wilson, William J.: "Heat Injury," *Amer. J. Nurs.,* 60:1124–25 (Aug.) 1960.

Wood, W. Barry, Jr.: "The Role of Endogenous Pyrogen in the Genesis of Fever," *Lancet,* 2:53–56 (July 12) 1958.

14

Nursing the Patient Having a Problem Resulting from Failure to Regulate the Proliferation and Maturation of Cells

Today about one patient in three is being saved. A few years ago the ratio was about one in four. This represents a gain in lives of about 45,000 men and women each year. Using knowledge now available, this gain can be substantially extended. Just by applying widely what we know, we could save half of the people who contract cancer:

Uterine cancer can be detected at an early and generally curable stage by using a simple, well established technique; unfortunately, relatively few women seek and obtain this examination in time.

New developments in the early detection of breast cancer hold forth the promise of similar reductions in deaths from this form of cancer.

Physical examinations using modern diagnostic techniques often lead to early recognition and successful treatment of cancer in many sites.

Lung cancer can be sharply reduced by reducing cigarette smoking.

Meanwhile medical research is opening up new pathways to diagnosis and cure.[1]

Overview

What is the role of the nurse in caring for the patient who has or fears that he has cancer?

The Pathophysiology of Neoplastic Disease

How does abnormal cell growth differ from normal cell growth?

How do benign and malignant neoplasms differ?

Factors in the Cause and Promotion of Cancer

Signs and Symptoms of Neoplastic Diseases

What are some of the psychological effects on the patient with a real or imagined diagnosis of cancer?

What are some of the possible harmful effects of withholding information about a diagnosis of cancer?

Prevention of Cancer

Therapy in Cancer

What is the objective toward which the surgical treatment of cancer is directed?

How is the patient helped to resume his normal activities?

What are the responsibilities of the nurse to the patient with widespread and progressive disease?

Overview

The President's Commission on Heart Disease, Cancer, and Stroke was established to recommend practical methods leading to the control and eventual elimination of these diseases. Not only are they leading causes of death,

[1] "A Report to the President, A National Program to Conquer Heart Disease, Cancer and Stroke," *The President's Commission on Heart Disease, Cancer, and Stroke,* 1:10–11 (Dec.) 1964.

but they may cause extended periods of disability and suffering. Since the commission's report was published in 1964, progress has been made in some areas; however, about one patient with cancer in three continues to be saved. One of the most thought-provoking statements in the quotation is that one out of every two persons could be saved were present knowledge applied. One implication is that despite the importance of knowledge of cancer, this knowledge by itself is not enough. Other kinds of knowledge and skills are also important. How can what is known be applied so that cancer is prevented, detected early, or treated adequately? This question is fundamental to the control and eradication of any disease. Until knowledge is applied, it cannot prevent or cure disease.

The purpose of this chapter, however, is to present information about neoplasia and to make some suggestions about how this information can be used in nursing practice. One point that has been emphasized throughout is that in health all body structures and functions are regulated so that the needs of individual cells and tissues as well as of the total organism are met despite changes in the environment to which the individual is exposed.

The cell, like other structures, responds to conditions in its environment. It alters its activities in relation to its food supply, to the demands made on it, and to potentially harmful agents. Depending on the quantity and nature of the injuring agent, the cell may recover, be altered in some manner, or die. The inherent characteristics of the remaining cells determine whether dead cells are replaced by like cells or by fibrous connective tissue. Certain cells can adapt to an unfavorable environment by undergoing metaplasia.

Furthermore, cells may appear to recover following injury, but at some later time, sometimes many years later, they are transformed into less differentiated cells that no longer look or behave like normal cells.

Markert [2] relates carcinogenesis to other diseases when he states that all biological processes may be deranged so that disease results. Cell growth and proliferation are no exception. Exactly what happens in the process whereby healthy cells are transformed to neoplastic cells has been very difficult to identify.

What is the role of the nurse in caring for the patient who has or fears that he has cancer?

For many reasons, the nurse has a notable contribution to make in the care of the patient who has or fears that he has cancer (a term generally understood to mean a malignant neoplasm). There are few situations in which a nurse requires more knowledge and understanding or a wider variety of skills than she does in the care of patients with a possible or positive diagnosis of cancer. The knowledge and skills of the nurse need not be limited in their application to patients with a diagnosis of cancer. One of the fears frequently expressed by patients who have other diagnoses is the fear of cancer. The patient who hesitates to

[2] Clement L. Markert: "Neoplasia: A Disease of Cell Differentiation," *Cancer Res.,* **28**:1908 (Sept.) 1968.

make his anxiety known may be encouraged to do so by a "listening and hearing" nurse. The nurse can be more helpful to patients if she accepts cancer as a disease similar to many other diseases in that it can sometimes be prevented and cured. Similar to patients with other diagnoses, the patient can be benefited by intelligent care, provided by people who care.

The services of the nurse are required and utilized in programs for the prevention and the detection of cancer, in case finding and diagnosis, and in the treatment and rehabilitation of patients. Patients with cancer are from all age and social groups. In terms of degrees of illness, they range from the healthy to those with widespread and progressive disease. The needs of the patient and his family vary from health teaching to detailed physical care and sustained emotional support.

Two developments of the last 10 to 15 years have a direct bearing on the practice of nursing. They are the use of extensive surgical procedures in the treatment of cancer and increased interest and facilities for the patients with recurrent inoperable disease. Radiotherapy or chemotherapy have particularly helped the second category of patients.

Historical Review

With the current emphasis on cancer as a cause of death, the reader may have the impression that cancer is a new disease and that it is unique to man. Nothing could be further from the truth. It is neither a new disease nor a disease of civilization per se. Evidence indicating the presence of an osteoma (a benign neoplasm) has been found in the vertebrae of a dinosaur that lived some 50 million years ago. References to neoplasms are found in the earliest medical literature. They were described by the Egyptians in 1200 B.C. Neoplasms were known to Hippocrates. The modern concept of cancer as a disturbance in cellular growth, however, is not much more than 130 years old. It probably had its origin in the work, published in 1838, of Johannes Müller, who is credited with the first description of the cellular nature of cancer. Virchow, some 20 years later, gave impetus to the idea by describing the characteristic changes in cancer cells.

Previous to the discoveries of Müller and Virchow, the relationship of cancer to certain occupations had been observed. In 1775, Sir Percivall Pott reported his observation that chimney sweeps in London had an exceptionally high incidence of cancer of the scrotum. In the sixteenth century, men working in mines in the mountains of Saxony were known to develop a progressive and fatal disease. Not until later, however, was the disease identified as cancer. The discovery that pitchblende was the causative agent did not come until still later. More than 500 chemical agents are now known to be carcinogenic.

Not only is cancer a disease of antiquity, but it is not unique to man; it occurs in both plants and animals. Cows, chickens, parakeets, horses, monkeys, dogs, and laboratory animals such as mice, rats, and rabbits develop neoplasms. Because of the contributions of these animals to the study of disease, they might be included with the dog as best friends of man. When cancer, as well as other types of neoplasms, is viewed as a phenomenon of growth, neither the fact that it is of ancient origin nor that it occurs in species other than man should be surprising. In all living creatures it has one essential characteristic: the organism is unable to control the growth and proliferation of cells.

Proliferating cells often but not always lose their ability to differentiate. They often mutate and become abnormal. The result is unrestricted growth of cells that are often poorly differentiated and without useful function. Even if they retain their original function they rarely contribute to the patient's welfare and often damage the body by flooding it with excessive amounts of their products.

Definitions

Anaplasia is the transformation of cells to a less differentiated or more primitive embryonic type, with greater capacity for multiplication but less ability to specialize.

Neoplasm. A new growth that can be accompanied by a loss as well as a gain in cells. For example, malignant neoplasms of the stomach are sometimes in the form of ulcers.

Tumor. The word *tumor* is frequently used interchangeably with neoplasm. Strictly speaking, they do not have identical meanings. A tumor is a swelling that can be caused not only by an increase in the number of cells in a tissue but by inflammation or an accumulation of blood or fluid in a localized area of tissue.

Benign neoplasm. The word, *benign* takes its origin from the latin word *benignus; bene* means "well" and *gnus*, "kind." When the word *benign* is used to describe a disease, the implication is that it is relatively harmless. A benign neoplasm is therefore one that is not of itself deadly. It may, however, cause harm by virtue of its location and by the fact that it occupies space.

Malignant neoplasm. The term *malignant* has its origin from the latin *malignans,* which means evil. Similar to the adjective *benign,*

malignant may be employed to characterize any type of disease. Malignant diseases are ones in which death is probable, unless something can be done to halt or alter their course. The separation between benign and malignant neoplasms is not always clear-cut inasmuch as many benign neoplasms, because of their location or size, can be fatal. On the other hand, some malignant neoplasms can run a relatively long course. Some of the significant differences between benign and malignant neoplasms will be discussed in greater detail where the characteristics of neoplasms are presented.[3]

Cancer is often used synonymously with malignant neoplasm. Garb[4] defines cancer as a "condition in which abnormal cells develop, multiply, and invade normal tissue, interfering with normal functions and eventually causing death unless adequate therapy is given early."

Carcinoma—Malignant. Neoplasms arising in tissues originating in the ectoderm or entoderm of the embryo are called carcinomas.

Sarcoma are malignant neoplasms (fleshy tumors) having their origin in tissues that are formed from the mesoderm, or mesenchyme.

Oncology is the study of tumors. The word is often used more broadly to include all aspects relating to tumors, including the prevention, diagnosis, and treatment of patients with tumors.

Past and Present Trends in the Incidence of Malignant Neoplasms

In the United States, as well as in other countries for which reliable statistics are available, cancer ranks second only to cardiovascular disease as a cause of death. It is known to be the second cause of death in all the countries of the modern world.[5] Besides its importance as a cause of mortality, it is one of the significant causes of morbidity. It is now the leading cause of death among women aged 30 through 54 years. Cancer causes more deaths than any other disease in children of school age.[6] Most authorities express the opinion that the incidence of cancer is probably the same all over

---

[3] The words *benign* and *malignant* are adjectives that may be used to describe the character of a wide variety of situations, conditions, diseases, and even people.

[4] Solomon Garb: "Neglected Approaches to Cancer," *Saturday Review* (June 1) 1968, p. 54.

[5] Canada, United States, Germany, Denmark, Finland, France, Norway, Netherlands, England and Wales, Scotland, Northern Ireland, Sweden, Switzerland, Australia. "The Ten Principal Causes of Death in the Modern World," *World Health*, **13**::2–3 (Jan.–Feb.) 1960.

[6] *1969 Cancer Facts* (New York: American Cancer Society, Inc.), p. 4.

the world, but the actual occurrence of the disease is difficult to verify because statistics are not reliable in many regions. Furthermore, because of lack of trained medical personnel, many persons who develop cancer may not be identified.

In some countries a smaller proportion of the people may be dying from cancer than in other countries because the average length of life is shorter. However, certain types of cancers are known to occur in some areas more commonly than others, such as liver cancer in South Africa and China, choriocarcinoma in Southeast Asia, and an unusual lymph node cancer in children, in so-called Burkitt's lymphoma, in the rain forest regions of Africa. In the United States lung cancer is the leading cause of death from cancer and cancer of the stomach is steadily declining. In Japan cancer of the stomach is the leading cause of death from cancer, but lung cancer is rising in incidence.

According to *1969 Cancer Facts and Figures*[7] approximately 320,000 Americans died from cancer in 1968, and in 1967, 314,000 died. The National Vital Statistics Division has reported that in 1966, 303,736 died. The American Cancer Society estimates that 940,000 Americans will be under treatment for cancer during 1969 and that about 615,000 persons will be diagnosed as having cancer for the first time. On the basis of a study made by Heller [8] and his associates, they predicted that by 1975 the number of new cases diagnosed each year will increase to 750,000 and that under prevailing conditions 32 newborn babies out of each 100 can be expected to develop cancer sometime during their lifetime. The American Cancer Society states [9] that one in every four Americans now living can expect to have cancer sometime during their lifetime. Cancer now causes one out of every six deaths in the United States.

FACTORS CONTRIBUTING TO INCIDENCE

The increase in the number of persons having a diagnosis of cancer is not believed to be caused by a significant rise in its actual incidence. The incidence of cancer in certain sites such as the lung and pancreas and of leukemia, has risen. In other sites, such as the stomach, the incidence is falling, and occurrence of cancer in other sites is leveling off. Similar to other chronic diseases a number of factors have contributed to the increase in the number of per-

sons diagnosed as having cancer. Some can be explained on the basis of improved diagnostic methods and facilities. The number of persons having a diagnosis of cancer is greater in areas having good medical facilities than in areas with poor facilities. The total is increased by the fact that formerly diseases such as leukemia and Hodgkin's disease were not classified as cancer, as they now are. With the lessening of the infant mortality rate and decrease in mortality from acute communicable diseases, more persons are living to be of an age when the incidence of cancer is highest. Another factor contributing to the increase in the total number of persons having cancer is the fact that the population is rising.

Although the incidence of cancer tends to rise with age, the disease occurs in all age groups from infancy to old age. As a cause of death, cancer is second only to accidents in children 1 to 14 years of age.[10] More than half the deaths from cancer occur in persons over 65 years of age.[11] The common sites in which cancer occurs differ with age. Leukemia and cancer in the brain, nervous system, and kidney are types most frequently found in children. Leukemia occurs more commonly among persons in older age groups than was once believed. Among persons in older age groups, cancer of the breast, skin, lung, gastrointestinal tract, and genital organs is most common.

Early in the century more women than men died from cancer, but the situation is now reversed. Over the years this ratio has narrowed. Since 1949 the mortality rate for males exceeded that for females. In 1969 the ratio of males to females is expected to be 55:45.[12] Two reasons are offered that partly explain the change. One is that the incidence of lung cancer has risen rapidly in men; the other is that cancer in women is generally in more accessible sites than it is in men.

Accessibility of site does not of itself guarantee a reduction in the mortality rate from cancer. The death rate from cancer of the breast remains essentially the same, despite extensive educational programs intended to facilitate early detection of neoplasms in the breast. By way of contrast, the programs for the early detection of cancer of the cervix have been accompanied by a decrease in mortality rate from this cause.

Cancer mortality is greater among nonwhites than among whites. Early in this century the reverse was true. Mortality is also higher in cities and in industrial areas than it is in rural

[7] *Cancer Facts and Figures, op. cit.*, p. 3.

[8] John R. Heller, Sidney J. Cutler, and William M. Hoenszel: "Some Observations on the Epidemiology of Cancer in the United States," *JAMA*, **159**:1628–34 (Dec.) 1955.

[9] *1969 Cancer Facts and Figures, op. cit.*, p. 3.

[10] *Cancer Statistics* (New York: American Cancer Society, Inc., 1969), p. 16.

[11] *Ibid.*, p. 4.

[12] *Ibid.*, p. 4.

and less heavily populated areas. Possibly the quantity and quality of medical care available to different groups are responsible for some of these differences.

The primary sites in which cancer leads to death have also changed in the last 30 or 35 years. As previously indicated, cancer in the lung and other parts of the respiratory system has risen markedly.[13] Furthermore, the increase in incidence in cancer of the lung is real and cannot be attributed merely to an improvement in diagnosis. Leukemia has been increasing in incidence. This increase has been greatest in children and in older people. In the United States cancer of the skin is the most common and preventable form of cancer with the highest survival rate.[14] In 90 per cent of the patients, the cause is exposure to ultraviolet rays. Prevention consists of minimizing exposure of the skin to the sun.

PATIENTS SURVIVING

Despite the emphasis on cancer as a cause of mortality, it should be remembered that a considerable number of patients are living and well many years after the diagnosis and treatment of cancer. To illustrate, acute leukemia generally is accompanied by an unfavorable prognosis; yet of 157 long-term survivors of acute leukemia, 103 are living and well and free from any evidence of the disease from 5 to 17 years after diagnosis.[15]

Commonly, patients with a diagnosis of cancer who are alive and well at the end of five years after treatment are considered cured. The figure of five-year cure is useful, however, only for the more rapidly growing cancers because some slower-growing cancers can recur or persist without any treatment for decades.

One favorable note is that the number of treated patients surviving five or more years has increased from one in five 30 years ago to one in three in 1967. Paradoxically, the death rate has risen from 125 to 153 per 100,000 population during the same time.[16]

Despite a lack of evidence indicating a decrease in the overall mortality rate from cancer, progress is being made toward the solution of

the problem of cancer. John R. Heller, as director of the National Cancer Institute, summarized in *Progress Against Cancer 1959*[17] some of the achievements of the preceding ten years. They include (1) a steady increase in basic knowledge of the nature of cancer; (2) synthesis of knowledge derived from many fields, so that the whole field of cancer research is being unified; (3) advances in knowledge of chemotherapy and virology; (4) the cytological test for cancer of the cervix; and (5) a comprehensive body of knowledge of the epidemiology of cancer.

The 1967 report[18] continues to stress the importance of expanding the basic knowledge of the nature of cancer. Cancer virology and immunology are being extensively studied. Developing sound methods of prevention, early detection, and treatment of patients in all stages of cancer are all receiving much attention. Interest in improving the care of patients with widespread and progressive disease continues. Emphasis is being placed on the fact that, like many diseases, cancer is a chronic disease for which much can be done to improve the patient's condition and prolong his useful life. Despite a not uncommon belief to the contrary, many patients live long and useful lives after the diagnosis of cancer is made.

The Pathophysiology of Neoplastic Disease

Homeostasis of Cell Proliferation and Differentiation

In the discussion of homeostasis thus far, emphasis has been on the maintenance of the conditions in the internal environment favorable to cellular activity. Homeostasis is also dependent on the ability to maintain the structure and function of tissues. The continuity of tissues and the maintenance of function require that cells lost as a result of wear and tear and of injury be replaced. Fundamental to this replacement is the capacity of cells to proliferate (multiply) and to differentiate into mature tissue. As with other homeostatic mechanisms, the usefulness of the capacity of cells to multiply depends on (1) the ability of the organism to regulate the proliferation and maturation of cells and (2) the appropriateness and adequacy of the response. The potential for growth of the different types of tissues varies. Some, such as fibrous connective tissue and reticular cells, are not only

[13] *The Health Consequences of Smoking*, 1968 Supplement to the Public Health Service Review (U.S. Department of Health, Education, and Welfare, 1968) p. 94.

[14] American Cancer Society exhibit, "Cancer of the Skin."

[15] Joseph H. Burchenal: "Long-Term Survivors in Acute Leukemia and Burkitt's Tumor," *Cancer,* **21**:596 (Apr.) 1968.

[16] A Report of the National Advisory Cancer Council: *Progress Against Cancer, 1967* (Washington D.C.: U.S. Department of Health, Education, and Welfare, 1967), p. 5.

[17] *Progress Against Cancer, 1959* (Washington, D.C.: U.S. Department of Health, Education, and Welfare, Public Health Service, National Institute of Cancer, Jan. 1960).

[18] *Op. cit.*

able to proliferate but they can differentiate into a number of types of tissue cells. Other types of tissue cells are capable of proliferation, but they can mature only into cells similar to the parent cell. The example of the ability of epithelial cells to proliferate and mature into some type of epithelial cell has been previously cited. Immature epithelial cells differentiate into the different types of epithelial tissue. In the examples just cited, tissue cells have a great potential for growth. In other types of tissues, such as nervous tissue and striated muscle, the potential for growth is exceedingly limited.

In healthy tissues, the process whereby cells multiply follows a predictable pattern known as mitosis. In mitosis the cell undergoes a complicated series of changes in which each chromosome is divided and two new, or daughter, cells are formed. In a report on the studies being made on cells by radioautography, Baserga and Kisieleski [19] state that only a small proportion of the cells of the adult animal body are capable of dividing at all. In the adult human being only about 3 per cent of the cells are able to divide for the purposes of repairing tissue. By using tritium (the radioactive isotope, ^3H), it was found that of the two daughter cells formed during cell division one remains in the tissue and divides as its parent cell does; the other daughter cell dies. Depending on the potentialities of the cell and environmental conditions, new cells may be a replica of the parent cell or may differ in some respect from it. The ways in which a daughter cell can differ at maturity from the parent cell are predictable. The daughter cells fit into the overall organization of the tissue. For example, the type of epithelial cells entering into the formation of a mucous membrane may be altered by exposure to an unfavorable environment. Following a tracheostomy, transitional cells in the mucous membrane lining the trachea undergo metaplasia and are replaced by a thick layer of squamous epithelium. The change is adaptive, as squamous cells are better able to survive chronic irritation than are transitional cells. The pattern for metaplasia is predictable and the resulting tissue organized and functional.

As with other homeostatic mechanisms, the multiplication of cells occurs in response to a need and ceases when the need is met, which indicates that the potential for growth of cells is subject to regulation. Not all the factors in the regulation of growth are understood. The growth of some tissues is influenced by both intrinsic and extrinsic factors. Among the extrinsic regulators are certain hormones; adjacent cells also appear to exert a growth-inhibiting influence on each other.

Many examples could be cited in which cell proliferation occurs in response to a need and ceases when the need is met. One such example is wound healing. Other examples include the continuous replacement of worn-out erythrocytes and leukocytes. The production of either erythrocytes or leukocytes may be greatly increased in response to appropriate stimuli. The production of erythrocytes is increased following acute hemorrhage or on exposure of the organism to a lowering of the oxygen tension in the atmosphere. Infection initiated by one of the pyogenic cocci, such as the pneumococcus or meningococcus, is accompanied by an outpouring of neutrophils. When the demand for either erythrocytes or neutrophils is very great, cells may be released from the bone marrow at an earlier stage of development than is usual. Following hemorrhage, the level of not quite mature erythrocytes—the reticulocytes—rises from the usual 2 per cent or less to 10 per cent or more. This same response can be observed in the patient who is treated for certain types of anemia. Shortly after a hemorrhage occurs, the reticulocyte count rises rapidly. The rate at which the level of mature erythrocytes rises is slower. As the normal level of erythrocytes is approached, the reticulocyte count drops to normal. This is, therefore, evidence of a mechanism operating to control the proliferation of erythrocytes. The extent to which the reticulocyte count is elevated, under conditions such as those cited, is an indication of the capacity of the bone marrow to produce blood cells.

In conditions under which the neutrophils are markedly elevated, the proportion of nonfilamented or nonsegmented leukocytes to filamented or segmented leukocytes is increased. Nonfilamented leukocytes are the not quite mature form of white blood cells. Like reticulocytes, they represent a normal stage in the development of leukocytes. When the situation calling for the increase in leukocytes is controlled, the normal level of leukocytes is restored.

The process whereby cells multiply and produce cells that are the same type and form as those found in the tissue or organ is known as hyperplasia. It occurs in response to an extracellular stimulus. With the removal of the stimulus the multiplication of cells ceases; that is, in hyperplasia the multiplication of cells is controlled. The cells are typical of the tissue from which they arise and are organized into a normal or healthy pattern, and multiple tissue elements are often involved. For example, in the healing of a wound, neutrophils, macrophages,

[19] Renato Baserga and Walter E. Kisieleski: "Autobiographies of Cells," *Sci. Amer.*, **209**:106–107 (Aug.) 1963.

fibroblasts, epithelial cells, and capillaries participate in the formation of the scar.

How does abnormal cell growth differ from normal cell growth?

The principal differences between the normal replacement of cells and abnormal growth are as follows: The proliferation of cells is homeostatic when the multiplication of cells (1) occurs in response to an appropriate stimulus, (2) is adequate to the requirements of the organism, (3) differentiates or matures into normal functioning tissue, and (4) ceases when the need of the organism is met. In contrast, the proliferation of cells is abnormal when it (1) occurs in response to an inappropriate stimulus; (2) is inadequate to, or in excess of, the needs of the organism; (3) results in immature and abnormal cells; and (4) continues growth without regard for the needs of the organism—the well-being and possibly the life of the individual are threatened. Malignant neoplasms may cause widespread toxic effects even at a time when the lesion is more or less localized.

Despite important differences between normal and neoplastic cells, difference in rate of growth is not one of them. In both normal and abnormal tissues, the rate of growth may be slow, rapid, or moderate. As examples, the bone marrow can produce erythrocytes at an extremely rapid rate. Cells in the gastrointestinal mucosa reproduce rapidly. Liver cells multiply at a fairly rapid rate. Conversely, cells of the brain, heart, and kidney do not reproduce at an appreciable rate. Neoplasms arising in the latter organs tend to grow more rapidly than the parent cells. Those occurring in epithelial cells of the skin and the gastrointestinal mucosa often grow more slowly than healthy epithelial cells.

Neoplastic cells differ from normal cells in a variety of ways. The structure and organization of cells in a neoplasm may be similar in many respects to that of healthy tissue, or they may be so different that there is little or no resemblance to normal tissue. For example, in glandular structures, goblet epithelial cells are arranged in an orderly fashion around the ducts. In some neoplasms, this pattern may be disturbed but still recognizable. In others, the pattern of organization and the character of cells are so abnormal that most, if not all, resemblance to normal tissue is lost. Some of the characteristics of neoplastic cells are the following: (1) Abnormal cells tend to be larger, with a disproportionately large nucleus, than normal cells. (2) Cells tend to vary in size and shape. (3) There is a high frequency of mitotic figures within the nucleus. (4) Although neoplastic cells have been observed to have abnormalities in the number and appearance of chromosomes, chronic myelogenous leukemia is the only disorder with a consistent chromosomal change.

SUMMARY

Although the cells in some malignant neoplasms are fairly normal in appearance and in organization, they may be so abnormal and immature that there is little or no resemblance to healthy tissues. Cells differ from healthy cells in size, shape, and staining characteristics. Whereas healthy cells are similar in size and shape, neoplastic cells may demonstrate great variability. In normal mitosis, each parent cell divides into two daughter cells, but in tissues taken from a malignant neoplasm, cells can sometimes be seen to be dividing into a number of cells, for example, three, four, or six. Neoplastic cells behave as if they were mutants with an impaired sensitivity to the organizing influence of adjacent cells. They disregard the normal regulators of growth; they often continue to multiply without limit or regard for the needs of the organism as a whole, and not infrequently at the expense of healthy cells. The extent to which neoplastic cells differ from healthy cells varies.

One of the outstanding characteristics of neoplastic cells is their ability to push between normal cells and to invade the surrounding tissue. They must have some mechanism for breaking down the gel-like substance that serves as an intercellular cement. Moreover, they have a tendency to break away from the parent growth. The free cell or cells can then be carried from the parent growth to neighboring lymph nodes or to distant sites where they set up secondary growths or metastases.

In attempting to explain the differences between normal and neoplastic cells, Warburg [20] proposed the theory that a neoplastic cell results from the adaptation of a normal cell to injury to its respiratory (enzyme) mechanism. To survive the cell adopts anaerobic rather than aerobic metabolism. The changes in the enzymes are now believed to be a secondary rather than a primary event. Moreover, a number of scientists in the United States and other countries believe that cancer develops in several stages and that different biochemical events occur at each stage. [21]

An important characteristic of neoplasms is

[20] O. Warburg, cited in S. Weinhouse: "On Respiratory Impairment in Cancer Cells," *Science,* **124:**267 (Aug. 10) 1956.
[21] *New Directions for Cancer Research,* A Report from The American Cancer Society (New York: American Cancer Society, Inc., 1967), p. 29.

that they serve no useful purpose. Some neoplasms arising in glands do produce the secretion of the gland, but this usually results in an excess of the secretion. Neoplasms arising in endocrine glands are frequently, though not always, functional. For example, neoplasms in the thyroid gland may secrete the hormones of the thyroid gland, thus causing symptoms and signs of hyperthyroidism.

Neoplasms, like other living tissues, require nutrient materials for their growth and survival. They are dependent on the host for their food supply. They grow without regard to the needs of the host and frequently at his expense. Slow-growing neoplasms may exist for extended periods of time without interfering with the nutrition of the host. Rapidly growing ones are likely to be accompanied by severe emaciation and debility of the host. Neoplasms in the alimentary canal may further interfere with nutrition by their mechanical effect. The maintenance of nutrition is one of the common problems in the care of patients with certain types of neoplasms.

Naming Neoplasms

For the most part, the system for naming neoplasms is relatively simple. The suffix *oma* is derived from the Greek and is used to denote a tumor or neoplasm. Benign neoplasms are usually classified as to site of origin. In a few instances, the term for the type of cell is used. In general, the word is formed by adding *oma* to the combining form, indicating the type of tissue. To illustrate, a benign neoplasm of fibrous tissue is a fibroma. There are some exceptions. Gliomas, which have their origin in the neuroglia, are almost always, if not always, malignant. Malignant neoplasms are also commonly classified as to site of origin. For the purpose of illustration, a brief classification of neoplasms is given in Table 14-1. For anyone wishing to examine a complete list, the *International Classification of Diseases*[22] is suggested.

When the origin of the neoplasm is uncertain, this system of naming may not be very helpful, however. For example, malignant melanoma, a tumor of pigment cells in the skin, may originate from one of two cells: melanocyte, a skin cell that actually originates from nerve tissue; or from melanophore, a pigment containing cells of the lower skin layers. In any individual tumor the exact determination of the origin is difficult and therefore leads to confus-

ing multiplicity of the names. Terms such as *melanosarcoma* and *melanocarcinoma* have been used; however, both of them probably should be abandoned for the better term, *malignant melanoma*.

When more than one tissue enters into the formation of a neoplasm, the combining forms for each type are used. For example, the so-called fibroid tumor of the uterus is actually a *leiomyofibroma,* because it contains smooth muscle and fibrous connective tissue.

Many terms are used to describe the character of the neoplasm. The term *polyp* or *polypoid* is used to indicate that a neoplasm extends from a mucous membrane into the lumen of a tube. Some polyps have a stem or stalk similar to a cherry. The stalk is called a peduncle and the polyp is said to be pedunculated. Other polyps are attached to the surface by a broad base. The term used to indicate this characteristic is *sessile*. Some neoplasms grow around the wall of tubular organs; that is, they are annular growths. Annular neoplasms tend to obstruct the tube by constricting or reducing the size of its lumen. Some neoplasms stimulate the production of large amounts of fibrous connective tissue, which causes the neoplasm to be firm or hard. A firm, hard neoplasm containing a large quantity of connective tissue is called *scirrhus*. There are many other terms used in the description of neoplasms. Satisfactory definitions can usually be found in a medical dictionary.

How do benign and malignant neoplasms differ?

Table 14-2 represents a number of important characteristics in which benign and malignant neoplasms differ.

The capsule enclosing a neoplasm is formed of fibrous connective tissue as a result of the local tissue reaction to the abnormal growth of cells. Occasionally the cells inside an encapsulated neoplasm are found to be malignant, but this is a rare occurrence. It is not known whether the connective tissue capsule has its origin in the connective tissue of the organ in which the tissue has arisen or whether it arises from the tumor itself. The capsule helps to explain why benign neoplasms are usually accompanied by a better prognosis than are malignant neoplasms. The capsule tends to confine the neoplastic cells, and the removal of an encapsulated neoplasm is not only easier but it causes less damage to healthy tissue. Because encapsulated neoplasms grow by expansion rather than by infiltration, their principal effect is pressure. Although some benign neoplasms such as ovarian cysts grow to enormous size, their growth is usually limited. Benign neoplasms do not spread to distant parts of the body, and, with rare exceptions, they do not

[22] *International Classification of Diseases* Vol. II, 8th rev. (Washington, D.C.: U.S. Department of Health, Education, and Welfare, Public Health Service, 1968) pp. 326–49.

TABLE 14-1

Type of Tissue	Type of Neoplasm	
	Benign	Malignant
Connective tissue		
1. Fibrous	Fibroma	Fibrosarcoma
2. Cartilage (chondroblast)	Chondroma	Chondrosarcoma
3. Bone (osteoblast)	Osteoma	Osteogenic sarcoma
4. Fat (lipoid tissue)	Lipoma	Liposarcoma
Muscle tissue		
1. Smooth muscle	Leiomyoma	Leiomyosarcoma
2. Striated muscle	Rhabdomyoma	Rhabdomyosarcoma
Epithelial tissue		
1. Squamous cells	Papilloma or wart	Squamous cell carcinoma
	Epidermoid cyst	
	Sebaceous cyst	
2. Basal cell	Little adenoma or sweat gland adenoma	Basal cell carcinoma
3. Pigmented layer	Mole or nevus	Malignant melanoma
4. Gland cells (adeno-)	Adenoma	Adenocarcinoma
Nervous tissue		
1. Nerve tissue	Neuroma	Neurofibrosarcoma
2. Glia		Glioma
3. Meninges	Meningioma	Malignant meningioma
4. Nerve sheath	Neurofibroma	Neurofibrosarcoma
Endothelial tissue		
1. Blood vessels	Hemangioma	Hemangiosarcoma
Lymphatic and hematopoietic tissue		Hodgkin's disease
		Leukemia
		Lymphoma
		Lymphosarcoma
Mixed tumors	Dermoid cysts	
Tumors derived from embryonic cells well differentiated	Teratoma	Malignant teratomas

TABLE 14-2

A Comparison of Selected Characteristics of Benign and Malignant Neoplasms

Characteristic	Benign	Malignant
1. Capsule	Usually	Rarely
2. Manner of growth	Expansive	Infiltrative
3. Rate of growth	Usually slow and restricted; extent limited	Compared to healthy tissue may be slow or rapid and unrestricted; varies greatly from patient to patient and with the type of lesion
4. Tendency to recur after removal	Rarely	Frequently
5. Characteristic of cells	Fairly normal	Varying degrees of abnormality; immature and abnormal in appearance and organization
6. Mitotic activity	Little	Usually great; mitosis is abnormal
7. Metastasis	Never	Usually
8. Vascularity	Slight	Moderate to marked

recur. Although some benign neoplasms eventually become malignant, this does not occur very frequently. Few, if any, persons escape having one or more benign neoplasms during their lifetime; most of them are of no significance. One interesting fact is that, according to the U.S. National Health Survey,[23] more patients are hospitalized for the treatment of benign and unspecified neoplasms than for malignant neoplasms.

Because of their manner of growth, malignant neoplasms, as the term implies, may cause death. Some malignant neoplasms, but not all, can be eradicated by present methods of treatment. Furthermore, not all malignant neoplasms behave alike. Some types may be present for many years and never cause any known ill effect. Others are so rapidly progressive that despite what appeared to be prompt diagnosis and treatment, death occurs only a few weeks after their presence becomes known. The differences in the behavior of malignant neoplasms are well illustrated by the different types of cancer occurring in the skin. Three types have been identified: basal cell carcinoma, which tends to remain localized; squamous cell carcinoma, which spreads through the lymphatics to the lymph nodes; and malignant melanoma, which has often produced systemic disease by the time it is identified. Of the three, basal cell carcinoma seldom causes death, whereas the malignant melanoma has a definite cure rate of about 40 per cent.[24]

METASTASIS

As commented on previously, malignant neoplasms tend to infiltrate or invade the surrounding tissue as they grow. They tend to disseminate throughout the body, or metastasize. The studies with tritiated thymidine [25] have also provided some information about the process of metastasis.[26] A single cell or a small group of cells separate from the parent cell and are transported by way of the lymph and blood streams to distant parts of the body. When the cells survive and lodge in a site favorable for their growth, they multiply. The new growth is not detectable, however, until it reaches a size of about 1 cm in diameter, at which time it contains about 500 million cells. The time taken to produce a detectable tumor will depend on the

length of the reproductive cycle for the neoplastic cell. If it is ten days, it will take ten months for the original cell to grow into a nodule 1 cm in diameter. If the cycle is 30 days, it will take almost three years for a detectable nodule to develop. This explains why it may take months or even years for a metastatic neoplasm to appear after a surgeon removes a primary growth.

The tendency to metastasize varies with the type of cancer and among individuals. When the surrounding tissues recognize the growth as abnormal and considerable amounts of fibrous tissue are formed, it can act as a barrier to spread. In other instances, however, the cancer cells [27] proliferate and overcome the local barriers to spread; they infiltrate or invade the surrounding tissue, and eventually, if left to itself, the malignant neoplasm can be expected to spread to the regional lymph nodes and, via the lymph or blood vessels, to distant points, where it sets up secondary or metastatic growths. Metastasis takes place as easily by way of the blood vessels as through the lymphatics. Because cancer cells have a tendency to separate from the parent growth, large numbers of malignant cells may be found in the venous blood draining a neoplasm. Moreover, the size of the neoplasm bears no relationship to the earliness with which it metastasizes. Extensive metastasis may be found in a patient with a small neoplasm and none in a patient with a large one. In some instances, the primary growth has an inhibiting effect on metastatic lesions. Following the removal of the primary growth, the rate of growth of metastasis may be accelerated.[28] The opposite is also seen; that is, with removal of the primary lesion, metastasic lesions regress.

In addition to the tendency of malignant neoplasms to metastasize, their sites of metastasis may also metastasize. Although the tendency to metastasize is inherent in all malignant neoplasms, whether or not it takes place depends on the individual and the site of origin. For reasons not understood, malignant neoplasms may spread early in one person and late in another.

SITES OF METASTASIS

Certain organs seem to be preferred sites for metastasis. The site of metastasis is primarily determined by the lymph and blood drainage

[23] U.S. Department of Health, Education, and Welfare: "Hospitalization," *Health Statistics from the National Health Survey,* Series B-7 (Washington, D.C.: U.S. Government Printing Office, 1958) p. 23.

[24] Henry M. Williams: "Malignant Melanoma," *CA,* 18:151 (May–June) 1968.

[25] Thymidine labeled with tritium, that is, radioactive hydrogen.

[26] Baserga and Kisieleski, *op. cit.,* p. 110.

[27] The term *cancer,* which is also the name of the fourth sign of the zodiac, means crab. The use of the term *cancer* to describe malignant neoplasms is based on the supposed resemblance between a crab and the manner in which the neoplasm invades the surrounding tissue.

[28] George Crile, Jr.: "The Cancer Problem," *Perspect. Biol. Med.,* 3:361 (Spring) 1960.

of the original cancer site; however, it is possible that local conditions within some organs are more favorable to cancer growth than others. Injury to the tissues appears to predispose the tissue or make it more susceptible to metastasis. Besides the lymph nodes the four most common sites of metastasis are the lung, the liver, the bone, and the brain. Cancers with venous drainage directed to one of the venae cavae tend to metastasize primarily to the lungs (various sarcomas; carcinomas of the liver, lower rectum or anus, and kidney). The venous drainage carries metastasis from the cancers of the digestive tract through the portal vein into the liver. Tumors originating closely to the intercostal or paravertebral veins tend to spread to the bones (carcinomas of the breast, prostate, thyroid, and kidney). The tumors of the lung metastasize through the arteries and therefore can spread anywhere. Because of a very high blood flow rate through the brain and lung, metastasis commonly appears there. From the preceding, the reader can note that neoplasms from some organs metastasize to a number of organs; for example, cancer of the breast can metastasize not only to the bone but also to the lung, brain, or liver. The sites of most commonly encountered metastasis are summarized in Table 14-3.

All the factors enabling a neoplasm to metastasize are not known. One factor, however, is the invasiveness of cells of the neoplasm, or their power to overcome the local barriers to spread. Another is the tendency of malignant cells to separate from the parent growth. The routes by which neoplastic cells are spread throughout the body are the same as those by which any substance can be transported from one part of the body to another. Various terms are employed to indicate the mechanism of spread. Local spread of malignant neoplasms is known as metastasis by the infiltration or invasion of surrounding tissue. When neoplastic cells penetrate and enter blood and lymphatic vessels—and they may grow along the course of the vessel—metastasis is said to take place by lymphatic or vascular permeation. When cells or groups of cells separate from the primary growth and are carried in the blood or lymph to distant points, metastasis is, logically enough, said to be by lymphatic or vascular emboli. During surgery for the removal of a malignant neoplasm, cells may be carried from the original site and be implanted in another area, including the incision. Metastasis is, therefore, by implantation. Cancer of the stomach sometimes metastasizes by sedimentation. For example, cells extending through the wall of the stomach separate from the parent growth and settle on an organ such as an ovary in the abdominal cavity where, if conditions are favorable, they set up a secondary growth.

As emphasized, a characteristic feature of malignant growth is its tendency to metastasize, or to set up secondary growths at points distant from the primary site. Some tissues appear to provide conditions that are more favorable to metastasis than others. Injury to tissue favors metastasis. The routes by which neoplasms spread are those by which materials are distributed throughout the body.

RECURRENCE

No discussion of the characteristics of malignant neoplasms would be complete without a comment about the tendency of malignant neoplasms to recur. As with other characteristics, the likelihood of recurrence varies considerably for different types of malignant neoplasms and from one person to another.

A concept introduced to explain the behavior of malignant neoplasms is that of *biological predeterminism*. By this term is meant that the course and behavior, or natural history, of a cancer is determined at the time of its inception. A slow-growing neoplasm with little power of invasion can be expected to retain these characteristics, whereas a rapidly growing and/or highly invasive neoplasm has the potential for rapid growth and invasiveness from the start.

TABLE 14-3

Sites of Metastasis

Site of Metastasis	Organs from Which Metastasis Originates								
	Breast	Colon	Kidney	Liver	Lung	Pancreas	Prostate	Stomach	Thyroid
Bone	√		√		√		√		√
Brain	√		√		√				
Liver	√	√			√	√	√	√	
Lung	√		√	√				√	

The earlier-cited example of the different types of malignant neoplasms of the skin illustrates the concept of biological predeterminism exceptionally well. (See page 616.)

VARIABILITY

A point that must be emphasized about malignant neoplasms is that, despite their general characteristics, there is great variability in their behavior in different individuals. For example, cancer cells are found in the prostate without any evidence of invasion to surrounding tissue or spread to distant parts. The fact of their presence may have been unknown to the patient or the attending physician until after death, when the prostate is examined at autopsy. Other neoplasms, such as malignant melanomas, are highly malignant from the start. Despite a small primary lesion, malignant cells may be distributed throughout the body before the primary lesion is known to be active. What appears to be the same type of lesion also behaves differently in different individuals. There is a growing appreciation that each person who has cancer is an individual and that the way in which the disease behaves in each person is also unique.

To illustrate differences in the course of malignant neoplasms in two different people, Mr. Bernard and Mr. Lester will be described. Mr. Bernard, who died last week, had always been a healthy and active man. Five weeks before his death, he complained of feeling ill. When, after a week or so, he continued to feel weak and tired, he consulted his physician who, after appropriate studies, made a diagnosis of acute leukemia. Mr. Bernard did not respond to any of the therapeutic measures and he failed rapidly.

Mr. Lester lives across town from Mr. Bernard. Eight years ago, he was found to have chronic leukemia. Unlike Mr. Bernard, he has responded well to therapy. Although he seldom feels entirely well, he has been able to continue his employment as an accountant and to support himself and his family. Recently he has not been feeling as well as he did in the past. How long he will be able to work is a matter for conjecture. Although many elements in the lives of Mr. Bernard and Mr. Lester are similar, the manifestations of leukemia have been quite different.

Factors in the Cause and Promotion of Cancer

As in most other chronic diseases, knowledge of the factors in the etiology of cancer is incomplete. Similarly, causes of cancer can be classified under the general headings of suscep-

tible host, injuring or carcinogenic agents, and the elements in the environment bringing the host and agent together. The concept of necessary and sufficient cause probably applies to some cancers. In the etiology of cancer, no single element is known to be required for its development. Whatever the factors are in its etiology, they must be of sufficient degree to initiate malignant change and to allow the abnormal growth to continue. The differences in susceptibility of various individuals to the effect of smoking cigarettes appears to illustrate the concept of sufficient causation. Not all individuals who smoke cigarettes develop bronchogenic carcinoma; a few who do not smoke do. The length and intensity of exposure are both elements, however, as the incidence of bronchogenic carcinoma rises with the length of time the individual has smoked and as the number of cigarettes smoked increases.[29] Individual susceptibility varies, but bronchogenic carcinoma develops when the injury to the cells is sufficient to overcome the protective mechanisms of the individual. In many cancers multiple factors probably interact to cause the disease.

Host Susceptibility

Among elements presumed to affect the susceptibility of the host are genetic constitution, age, hormone balance, immunity, nutritional status, and precancerous lesions. Data on the possibility that heredity is a factor in cancer are derived from several sources: the occurrence of certain types of cancer among close relatives, so-called cancer families, and the development of cancer strains of experimental animals.

GENETIC FACTORS

Accurate knowledge of the genetic factors in cancer among human beings is difficult to obtain. Persons who are predisposed to cancer may die from some other cause before the disease develops. For many reasons, information gained about disease and cause of death among family members tends to be unreliable. Persons may not know what caused the death of members of preceding generations. Some persons withhold information about family members who have had cancer because they believe it is caused by venereal disease or results from an activity that is unclean or sinful. There are undoubtedly a variety of reasons for the unreliability of data reported by persons relative to a history of cancer in the family.

Genetic factors appear to influence the devel-

[29] *The Health Consequences of Smoking, 1968 Supplement, op. cit.,* pp. 94–99.

opment of cancer either by the effect of a specific gene or as a consequence of the genetic constitution of the individual. Neoplasms for which there is known to be a familial tendency are relatively rare. They include von Recklinghausen's neurofibromatosis, osteochondroma, and pheochromocytoma. There are a few lesions that are not of themselves malignant, but they undergo malignant degeneration when they are exposed to specific conditions. As an example, xeroderma pigmentosa is hereditary, but neoplastic change is dependent on exposure of the skin to sunlight. Besides the disorders in which evidence of genetic factors is reasonably clear, there are studies indicating that a tendency to cancer of the breast is inherited. The transmission of the tendency to cancer of the breast is not consistent enough, however, to make accurate predictions possible. Although a few cancer families have been identified, the extent to which genetic factors are responsible is not known.

Heredity may predispose to cancer, not by a specific gene or genes, but by the effect of the genetic constitution of the individual. In keeping with this concept, susceptibility to or protection from cancer depends on the effects of genes on bodily processes. As one example, mutant or abnormal cells are known to be formed by persons who do not develop cancer as well as by those who do. Heredity may be a factor in the efficiency of defense mechanisms against abnormal cells. Theoretically, at least, the genetic constitution of an individual may alter the manner in which his cells respond to or metabolize potentially carcinogenic agents. In one individual the product of the metabolism of a carcinogen may be harmless and in another it may be harmful. Another possibility lies in the ease with which the cells of an individual throw off the restraints on growth. In the vast majority of persons heredity is only one of a number of factors interacting to protect the person from, or to predispose him to, neoplasia. Whether or not a given individual develops cancer depends on the net result of all these factors.

Other evidence implicating heredity as a factor in the etiology of cancer is that the neoplasia is universal in nature. Strains of experimental animals, such as mice, have been developed that demonstrate a high degree of susceptibility not only to cancer but to cancer in certain sites. Even among these animals, in some instances the tendency to the disease requires additional etiological agents to ensure its development. In studies with strains of mice inbred to develop spontaneous tumors of the breast, multiple factors are required for the mice to develop mammary cancers with any degree of consistency.

Bittner[30] found three factors to be necessary: hereditary susceptibility, the female hormones required for the growth and development of mammary tissue, and the milk factor. The milk factor is a filtrable substance that is transmitted in the milk and is generally thought to be a virus.

Certain malignant neoplasms are associated with specific abnormal chromosomes. Chronic myelogenous leukemia occurs more commonly in individuals with one chromosome 21 having one short arm. Children with mongolism usually have 47 chromosomes rather than the normal number, 46. They have an unusually high incidence of leukemia. Apparently their chromosomal abnormalities increase their susceptibility to leukemia.

Despite a growing body of knowledge about heredity as a factor in the development of cancer, exact information about how it influences its development is far from clear. For most individuals, their genetic constitution is presumed to protect them from, or to predispose them to, not only cancer but other diseases. In most instances, additional factors are involved.

HORMONES

Hormones have long been suspected of influencing susceptibility to cancer. In 1889, Schinzinger[31] suggested that hormones might be important in the development of cancer of the breast in women. In 1919, Loeb[32] demonstrated that the incidence of cancer of the breast in cancer-susceptible strains of mice could be reduced by removing their ovaries. That cancer of the breast is extremely rare in males and is the leading cause of death from cancer in the female is well known. The exact role of hormones in the induction of cancer is not clear. Knowledge is not available as to whether hormones act as inciting agents or whether they prepare the tissue so that it responds to carcinogenic agents. The hormones found to be carcinogenic in animals are those that have an influence on the growth of certain tissues. Hormones from the ovaries, testes, and adrenal cortex are necessary to the growth of some cancers. In addition to promoting growth of specific tissues, these hormones are all steroids and their chemical structure is similar to that of the carcinogenic hydrocarbons. The signifi-

[30] John J. Bittner: "The Causes and Control of Mammary Cancer in Mice," *Harvey Lect.,* **42**:224 (1946–47).

[31] James D. Hardy: *Pathophysiology in Surgery* (Baltimore: The Williams & Wilkins Company, 1958), p. 169.

[32] *Ibid.,* p. 170.

cance of these relationships is not known. That a relationship exists between certain hormones and the development of cancer is supported by animal experiments. Cancer of the breast has been induced in male mice of susceptible strains by the prolonged administration of excessive dosages of female hormones. Some cancers have been induced in animals by upsetting hormonal balance. From available knowledge, certain hormones are necessary to the growth of some cancers. Other hormones inhibit for a time the growth of some cancers. Thus a deficient supply of hormone might be a factor in the development of certain neoplasms. After a time a neoplasm whose growth is inhibited by a hormone adapts to its presence, and it is no longer restrained by it. From this and other evidence, hormones appear to be one of the multiple factors entering into the genesis of cancer.

OTHER FACTORS INFLUENCING SUSCEPTIBILITY TO CANCER

AGE

Authorities disagree as to the influence of age on susceptibility to cancer. Some interpret the fact that the incidence of cancer increases with age as evidence that age influences susceptibility, whereas others do not. According to Homburger,[33] evidence obtained from work with experimental animals is contradictory. In general these studies have indicated that younger tissues are more susceptible to carcinogenic agents than older ones. The age at which the peak incidence for cancer in various sites occurs differs. Although some of these are benign rather than malignant, some types of new growths, such as Wilms' tumors of the kidney, teratomas, neuroblastomas, neurofibromas, chondromas, hemangiomas, and nevi, are often congenital; that is, infants are born with them. Leukemia, which was once presumed to have its highest incidence in young children, actually occurs more frequently in adults than it does in children, and the rate is increasing.[34] In children, leukemia is more likely to be more acute and the course shorter than in adults. Acute lymphatic leukemia is, however, primarily a disease of childhood. Hodgkin's disease occurs most commonly in young adults.

PRECANCEROUS LESIONS

Certain lesions in the body appear to increase host susceptibility to cancer. The presence of one neoplasm increases the likelihood of developing another. The person who develops cancer

in one tissue is more likely to develop another one than is the person who has never had a cancerous lesion. Another type of lesion, the so-called precancerous lesion, may also predispose to cancer. These are lesions that at their inception are not cancerous but that tend to undergo malignant degeneration. Among the more common precancerous lesions are (1) large burn scars, particularly those resulting from third-degree burns; (2) nevi, especially moles near the juncture of the two sides of (midline) the body; (3) senile keratosis, a disease of the epidermis involving the horny layer; and (4) leukoplakia, a disorder characterized by the development of a white patch or patches on the buccal mucosa inside the cheek or on the female vulva.

On the basis of several different types of observations, there has been recurring interest in the role of immunity in cancer. Not all persons require the same degree of exposure to carcinogenic agents to develop cancer. Among those who do there is definitely a host response. Spontaneous regression occurs in 1 of 100,000 cases. Some persons have a desmoplastic, that is, fibrous tissue, reaction. Among others, the disease is manifested by rapid growth and spread. Mutant cells developing in healthy persons are rapidly destroyed. Whether or not each of the preceding represents immunity or an immune response is not clearly established.

IMMUNITY

Hamlin [35] states that human tumors have not yet proved to be antigenic. If there is host resistance, one factor is likely immunological.

Earlier Shoji and Sheffer [36] stated that some malignant neoplasms are immunologically different from others. Hodgkin's [37] disease differs from other malignant lymphomas even in their early stages.

SEX

The incidence of some sites of cancer is influenced or determined by sex. As examples, cancer of the breast is common among women but occurs rarely among men. Cancer of the stomach and lung is more common among men than among women. Not all the reasons for sex differences are known.

Carcinogens

In addition to host susceptibility, a variety of

---

[33] Freddy Homburger: *The Biologic Basis of Cancer Management* (New York: Paul B. Hoeber, Inc., 1957), p. 19.

[34] *1969 Cancer Facts and Figures, op. cit.,* p. 19.

[35] Iris M. E. Hamlin: "Possible Host Resistance in Carcinoma of the Breast: A Histological Study," *Brit. J. Cancer,* 22:383–401 (Sept.) 1968.

[36] Mamoru Shoji and Albert L. Sheffer: "Immunological Aspects of Neoplasia," *Surg. Clin. N. Amer.,* 47:785–802 (June) 1967.

[37] *Ibid.,* p. 793.

chemical, physical, and living agents are associated with neoplasia. More than 500 substances have been identified that are carcinogenic; that is, they induce malignant change in cells when applied to tissue for a sufficient period of time. No one knows how carcinogenic agents act. They may overstimulate the cell or release it from the inhibiting influence of growth regulators. Not all persons who are exposed to carcinogenic agents develop cancer. Knowledge of carcinogenic agents is important, however, for many are subject to control. The chances of developing cancer in certain sites can be lessened by reducing or eliminating contact with carcinogenic agents.

Carcinogenic chemicals include a great variety of organic and inorganic substances. Some of them contaminate the air in industrial and urban areas. Among the organic chemicals are aromatic compounds such as tar, soot, asphalt, crude paraffin oil, lubricating and fuel oils, as well as aromatic amines such as benzol and aniline dyes. Inorganic chemicals include nickel, asbestos, and arsenicals.

Physical carcinogens include heat rays, ultraviolet light, and ionizing rays and particles.

Living agents implicated as carcinogens include viruses and *Schistosoma haematobium*.

HABITS AND CUSTOMS

Because the habits and customs of a people determine to a large extent the carcinogens to which they are likely to be exposed, they are important in carcinogenesis. Some habits and customs seem strange because they are unfamiliar. All people, including Americans, have some customs and habits that result in their exposure to carcinogens. From many examples that could be cited, only a few have been selected. In England, the incidence of cancer of the scrotum, which was common among chimney sweeps in the eighteenth century, was reduced by teaching the men to bathe frequently. This form of cancer is absent among similar workers in Japan because they practice meticulous cleanliness. In Kashmir, mountaineers carry charcoal-burning stoves under their cloaks to keep themselves warm. The stoves are supported on the upper areas of the abdomen. Burns of the abdomen and chest are frequent. There is a high incidence of cancer in the burn scars. Cancer of the cheek is frequent in those who chew betel nuts. Cancer of the lip is more frequent among pipe smokers than among nonpipe smokers. More than 25 scientific studies in ten countries have demonstrated a high degree of relationship between the smoking of cigarettes and the risk of developing cancer.

CIGARETTE SMOKING

In the 1968 supplement to the 1967 Public Health Service Review, *The Health Consequences of Smoking*,[38] a total of 221 references are listed at the end of the chapter "Smoking and Cancer." Few subjects have been studied more intensively during the past two decades than the relationship of cigarette smoking and health. Based on a study made by Hammond,[39] of over 1 million men and women, a man aged 25 who smokes two packs of cigarettes per day shortens his life expectancy by 8.3 years. Even one who smokes ten or less cigarettes per day has from 2.8 to 4.6 years less life expectancy than a nonsmoker. The shortening of the life expectancy is caused by a number of detrimental effects of tobacco and not just by the higher incidence of cancer among smokers.

To emphasize the importance of cigarette smoking in carcinogenesis, however, note that the number of deaths from lung cancer rose from 18,313 in 1950 to 48,483 in 1965.[40] Since 1930, the death rate for cancer of the lung in women has increased over 400 per cent, and in the past 14 years it has increased by 50 per cent.[41] Studies made in Japan, Iceland, and other countries also demonstrate a causal relationship between cigarette smoking and lung cancer.[42]

Not only has cigarette smoking been shown to be causally related to cancer of the lung, but it is believed to be a significant factor in cancer of the larynx. A clear-cut relationship has not been established between smoking and cancer of the esophagus and the urinary bladder; there is evidence that such a relationship exists.[43]

The fact that fewer women die from lung cancer than men is explained by the following: (1) fewer women smoke than men, (2) more women who smoke are under 50 years of age than men (lung cancer in men has its highest incidence in the 65–74 age group), and (3) women's smoking habits are different. They are not as likely to smoke cigarettes down to the end where the tars and nicotine are proportionately higher. They do not inhale as deeply. They smoke more filter-tip cigarettes and low tar and nicotine cigarettes than men.[44]

Although tar and nicotine are two chemicals known to be present in cigarettes, studies indicate that tobacco smoke contains several thousand compounds. Of these, 700 to 800 have been identified.[45] Despite the evidence that cancer

[38] *Op. cit.,* pp. 106–17.
[39] *Ibid.,* p. 9.
[40] *Ibid.,* p. 94.
[41] *Ibid.,* p. 97.
[42] *Ibid.,* p. 94–6.
[43] *Ibid.,* p. 89.
[44] *Ibid.,* p. 97.
[45] *Ibid.,* p. 90.

of the lung and other organs can be prevented by the elimination of smoking, the application of this knowledge is highly complex. Some aspects of this problem include the following: (1) children, especially boys, may start smoking as early as eight or nine years of age; (2) children of parents who smoke are likely to follow their example; (3) people who smoke appear to do so for many reasons, and therefore a single approach to the problem is not likely to solve it; and (4) because the incidence of cancer caused by smoking is correlated with the length and degree of exposure, the development of cigarettes as well as of smoking habits that lesssen exposure to tar and nicotine should be encouraged. Generally less tar and nicotine are inhaled with filter-tipped cigarettes. Tobacco is being developed with a lower tar and nicotine content than that previously grown. Avoidance of inhaling cigarette smoke and discarding the cigarette after it is half smoked also reduces exposure. Rapidly burning and porous cigarette papers reduce the degree of exposure.

Despite the fact that lung cancer does occur in nonsmokers, the cigarette smoker is particularly susceptible to this disease. Were cigarette smoking eliminated, most lung cancer would also be eliminated.[46]

OTHER HABITS AND CUSTOMS

Practices by certain groups may alter the incidence of cancer. As an example, cancer of the penis has a low incidence in Jewish and Moslem men. This is believed to be related to the practice of early circumcision.

Cross and his associates [47] reported a study in which cervical smears were made on over 5,000 women who were considered to be typical of the U.S. rural population. The socioeconomic and medical standards of the group were similar. Almost half of the group were Amish, a religious group that has practiced strict endogamy and monogamy for many generations. The incidence of cancer of the cervix was lower for the Amish than for other women. The authors interpret this finding as indicating that the marital behavior of the Amish may limit the spread of an agent important in the etiology of cancer.

Cancer of the skin is more common in persons whose skin is exposed to the rays of the sun, such as farmers and sailors, than it is among indoor workers. Exposure to the rays of the sun probably accounts for the observation that cancer of the skin is more common

among persons living in the southern than in the northern part of the United States.

Those who live in cities and industrial areas of the United States have a higher incidence of cancer than those who live in rural areas. Among the factors presumed to contribute to this difference is that those who live in cities are exposed to an atmosphere contaminated by smoke and automobile exhaust gases. From these examples, the conclusion that customs and habits are a factor in cancer appears valid, for they determine to some extent the carcinogens to which the individual is exposed and the degree of exposure.

Certain occupations also increase the likelihood of exposure to chemical and physical carcinogens. A large number of chemical agents of organic and inorganic origin have been implicated as carcinogens. Included among organic chemicals that have been demonstrated to be carcinogenic in animals are the carcinogenic hydrocarbons found in tar and soot. The aromatic amines and benzol as well as many other chemicals are potentially carcinogenic. Among the inorganic chemicals with carcinogenic powers are the arsenicals, chromates, nickel, and asbestos. Many of these chemicals are either used in industrial processes or are products or by-products of these processes. Knowledge of the carcinogenic potential of chemicals is essential to the protection of workers and the members of the community. Protection involves the development of effective procedures for eliminating or minimizing contact and a program to teach workers how to use them.

A number of physical agents are known to be carcinogenic. The effect of long-continued exposure to ultraviolet light or to the rays of the sun has already been mentioned. Ionizing radiation, whether produced by x-ray or from natural or artificially produced radioactive isotopes, is of increasing significance. The increased use of ionizing radiation in hospitals, in industry, and in national defense increases the amount of and the number of opportunities for exposure. Leukemia is four times more frequent among general physicians and ten times more frequent among radiologists than it is among the members of a comparable group in the general population.[48] The incidence of leukemia is also rising and possibly some of the increase is caused by an increase in ionizing radiation in the atmosphere.

The role of physical or mechanical injury of the tissues in carcinogenesis has been a subject

[46] *Ibid.*, p. 99.

[47] Harold E. Cross, Elmer E. Kennel, and Abraham M. Lilienfeld: "Cancer of the Cervix in Amish Population," *Cancer,* **21**:102 (Jan.) 1968.

[48] Hugh Rodman Leavell and E. Gurney Clark: *Medicine for the Doctor in His Community,* 3rd ed. (New York: The Blakiston Division, McGraw-Hill Book Company, Inc., 1965), p. 271.

for debate. The possibility of a single injury being a causative factor in cancer is believed to be remote. When a neoplasm is found following an injury, the probability is that it was there at the time the injury occurred and the injury served to call the attention of the person to it. Following tissue injury, the rate of growth of a neoplasm is sometimes accelerated. This occurs frequently enough that some lay people are aware of the possibility. Some authorities discount the importance of chronic mechanical irritation as a significant etiological factor in cancer. Others regard the fact that cancer develops in old burn scars and in cells forming the walls of draining sinuses as evidence supporting chronic irritation as an etiological agent.

Living agents may also act as etiological agents. Leukoplakia is sometimes, though not always, associated with syphilis. Cancer of the liver is more common in those parts of the world where a type of flat worm, the liver fluke, is ingested in the drinking water. The fluke invades the liver, where it sets up housekeeping.

Of the possible causative agents in cancer none is of greater interest than the possible role of viruses. Interest in the virus as an etiological agent in cancer is not new, for at least 50 years ago Rous [49] demonstrated that a virus caused sarcoma of the breast in chickens. Until recently, however, there was no evidence that a virus acted as a carcinogenic agent in any species except birds and fowl. Since Bittner's discovery in 1936 that the milk factor was a necessary condition to the development of cancer of the breast in mice, a number of neoplastic diseases in animals have been shown to be of virus origin. Included among these are leukemia in mice and papillomatosis in rabbits. Warts and papillomas in man, though nonmalignant growths, are of virus origin. Until recently no virus had been found in a human malignant neoplasm; this fact had been taken as positive evidence against the virus as an initiating factor in cancer in human beings. A herpes-like virus has been detected by electron microscopy in cultures of cells with Burketts' lymphoma (a neoplasm involving the jaw that is related to leukemia).[50] A common virus located in the nose and throat of man, adenovirus 12, can cause cancer in hamsters.[51]

To date virus-like particles have been isolated from human tumor material, but no virus has been isolated that has been shown to cause cancer in man. The current view continues to reflect the statement of the Research Program of the American Cancer Society, 1963 (p. 15), "Cancer-causing viruses have been detected in chickens, frogs, mice, rats, rabbits, hamsters, deer, monkeys, even willow trees. Why not human beings?"

There is a growing body of scientific evidence indicating that a virus or viruses may be the principal cause of leukemia in human beings. Interest in the virus as a causative factor in leukemia has been stimulated by the occurrence of clusters of individuals ill with leukemia in a number of communities. One such instance occurred in Niles, Illinois, where 13 individuals were discovered concentrated in one area; this number is many times the expected incidence.[52]

Even if a virus proves to be a factor in some or all cancers, there is no evidence to suggest that cancer is contagious in the ordinary sense of the word. It is not disseminated in the same manner as measles, chickenpox, or the common cold. It is not transmitted by the blood, as healthy men have been transfused with blood from patients with leukemia without subsequently becoming ill. Mothers with leukemia have healthy babies. Neither a physician nor a nurse has ever been known to develop leukemia after caring for a patient with it.

Despite the possibility that viruses are a factor in the development of some cancers, a number of factors contribute to the difficulty in identifying their presence in tissues even when they are there. There is evidence to indicate that viruses can be present in the tissues in the absence of morphological evidence that they are there. They are apparently able to assume a latent form and to resume their virulent characteristics when conditions are favorable. In recently reported studies, cells transformed by certain cancer viruses, such as the Rous sarcoma virus, appeared to be able to transmit the genetic material of the virus from one generation of tumor cells to another without producing the virus in the infectious form. For the infectious form to appear, the tumor cells had to be subjected to special conditions.[53] The discovery that some viruses that infect animals enter into the genetic DNA is also of more than passing interest. Some viruses, such as the Rous sarcoma virus, are RNA viruses.

Summary

Two factors are involved in the development of cancer. One is a susceptible host. The other

---

[49] Dr. Peyton Rous shared the Nobel Prize in medicine and physiology in 1966 for his fundamental research in this area.

[50] *Progress Against Cancer, 1967, op. cit.,* p. 21.

[51] *New Directions in Cancer Research, op. cit.,* p. 25.

[52] *Facts About Leukemia* (New York: American Cancer Society, Inc., April 1963).

[53] "Link Viral Genes to Cancer," *Public Health Rep.,* **78:**568 (July) 1963.

is an agent or group of agents capable of injuring the cell. Except in those rare instances in which cancer appears to result from the action of a specific gene, the induction of cancer depends on the action of multiple factors. Knowledge of the epidemiology of cancer has been expanded significantly. Epidemiological studies are directed toward the identification not only of carcinogenic agents and of the characteristics of individuals who develop cancer but of the characteristics of those who do not. Present evidence points to the conclusion that cancer does not have a single cause and is not really a single disease but that it is the result of the interaction of multiple factors, some of which have their origin in the host and others in his environment.

To emphasize the natural history of cancer, its course has been compared to that of an infection. Although there are significant differences, the course of cancer has many aspects in common with infectious disease. They both involve a susceptible host, injuring agents, and conditions in the environment bringing the two together. The degree to which host susceptibility and the pathogenicity of inciting agents are significant factors in etiology differs among infectious diseases as well as neoplastic ones. In some infectious diseases, such as measles, the nature of susceptibility is largely a matter of the presence or absence of immune bodies. To date, evidence that immunity plays a significant role in cancer is not clear-cut. Because of the scientific interest in this field, answers may be found to questions about it. In infections such as tuberculosis, factors other than immunity affect susceptibility. This is probably also true in cancer. In neither tuberculosis nor malignant neoplasms are all the factors in etiology understood.

In infection, the causative agent has its origin in the external environment and is a necessary condition of disease; a microorganism is the inciting agent. In cancer, the relationship of the injuring agent to the development of the disease is not as clear and possibly not as direct as in infection. The injuring agent may have its origin in the internal environment as well as in the external environment. It may serve as an inciting or a promoting agent. An inciting agent is one that induces changes in the cell that result in cancer. A promoting agent acts to support or favor cellular growth after cancerous change has taken place.

In both infectious and neoplastic disease a period of time elapses between the moment a microorganism enters the body or a cell is injured and the development of overt disease. In infectious disease, this is known as the incubation period. During the incubation period, the organism establishes itself in a favorable tissue, multiplies, and overcomes the body defenses against its growth and spread. Disease does not occur unless the microorganism is able to proliferate to the point where it can cause some type of cellular injury either directly or by means of its products. In the development of cancer, the periods between the time the cell is injured and the overt disease develops are known as the induction and lag periods. According to Hopps,[54] the induction period is usually not less than one tenth of the life span of the individual. Two theories have been advanced to explain this observation. One is that this is the length of time required by the cell to establish a new metabolic pattern. The other is that time is required for the cancer cell to overcome the restraining influences on proliferation.

In both infectious disease and in cancer, clinical manifestations depend on the multiplication of cells—microorganisms or cancer cells —to the point where they or their products injure tissue cells. In infection, the body recognizes the microorganism as foreign or alien and mobilizes both specific and nonspecific defense mechanisms. Apparently, the body also recognizes abnormal or mutated cells and destroys them. When the body defenses are adequate, microorganisms or abnormal cells are destroyed and the individual returns to or maintains his health. In addition, in some, though not all, types of infection, the body develops a sort of recognition system that enables it to protect itself against future attacks. Cancer differs from infection in that, after the stage of overt disease is reached, the body does not appear to have an adequate system of defense against it. There have been a few authenticated instances in which cancer in a person with overt disease disappeared, but these are rare. They are, naturally, of great interest. If the reason for the regression of the cancer could be determined, this knowledge might be useful in prevention and therapy of disease in other individuals. When cancer reaches the stage of overt disease, cancer cells are more or less unresponsive to factors regulating the growth, reproduction, and differentiation of cells. Therefore, unlike an infection, the body is unable to limit the extent of injury or, by itself, to restore health.

In some types of infectious processes, the infection has its origin in a localized site. Whether or not the infection remains localized or spreads to distant points depends on the virulence and invasiveness of the microorganism and the adequacy of the defenses of the body. When the body is unable to localize the infecting microorganisms, they may infiltrate the sur-

[54] Howard C. Hopps: *Principles of Pathology*, 2nd ed. (New York: Appleton-Century-Crofts, 1964), p. 340.

rounding tissue or enter the blood and lymphatic vessels. The microorganisms entering the blood and lymphatic system may be destroyed by cells in the blood or in lymph nodes or they may be deposited in distant tissues. There they may be destroyed or conditions may favor their multiplication. When this is true, a secondary or metastatic infection is established. Cancer cells behave in a similar manner. From the available evidence, cancer usually has its origin in a single cell or group of cells. For a period of time, it remains localized at the site of origin. It may never go beyond this site and may even regress.

Cancer Research

Much of the intensive research being conducted today is for the purpose of learning more about the nature of cancer. Among the five principal goals cited in *A Cancer Source Book for Nurses* [55] two relate directly to learning more about the causation of cancer. The other three are concerned with treatment. The five goals of cancer research cited are (1) "discovery of cellular trigger mechanisms that start malignant cell growth; (2) a means of checking metastasis—the spreading of cancer; (3) chemicals effective in selectively killing, or halting division in cancer cells; (4) understanding the possible immune defense mechanisms that may work against cancer; and (5) learning if viruses are a cause of some forms of cancer in human beings." Although goals 1 and 5 appear to be more directly related to the etiology of cancer than the others, new knowledge throwing light on any aspect of the problem may result in gains in other areas. Moreover, cancer research adds to the fundamental knowledge of the cell and eventually greater understanding of the human body in health and disease.

Among the broad areas of interest in the study of the cell in health as well as in disease are included the fundamental genetic and biochemical mechanisms controlling the proliferation and maturation of cells, the mechanisms by which hormones control or regulate bodily processes, and the mechanisms by which viruses cause cancer and whether or not they are a cause of some cancers in human beings.

To review, cancer is a cellular disease. In the first stage of its development the cell interacts with an etiological agent(s). After a period of time, the cell is converted to a cancer cell. It may be destroyed or it may be able to establish itself and multiply. Depending on its characteristics, it may remain localized or overcome the barriers to spread and metastasize to the surrounding area or to distant sites. In the period when the cancer is limited to the site of origin (cancer in situ) the person is unlikely to be aware of its presence unless cells are removed and examined. As the cells increase in number, a mass may be formed. As the cells extend into the surrounding tissue, the mass may become fixed or adhere to the tissue. Depending on the location, size, and degree of spread the individual may or may not be aware of the presence of the lesion.

Signs and Symptoms of Neoplastic Diseases

The signs and symptoms accompanying cancer, as well as benign neoplasms, are caused by the local mechanical effects of the primary and metastatic growths and by the total biochemical impact of the disease. Except in neoplastic diseases that are manifested as a generalized disease from the beginning (as an example, leukemia), the early signs and symptoms are usually caused by the local mechanical effects of the primary lesion. Because of the availability of modern surgical techniques, it is usually possible to remove the primary lesion, so that it is seldom the direct cause of death. Death is usually caused by the extensive derangements of normal biochemical functions associated with the systemic or metastatic stage of the disease.[56] The effects observed in late cancer are similar to those seen in generalized sepsis—another point of similarity between infection and cancer.

Mechanical Effects

The manifestations caused by the mechanical effects of a neoplasm result from the neoplasm (1) occupying space, (2) obstructing the lumen of a tube or duct, (3) exerting pressure on overlying mucous membrane, and (4) twisting the pedicle of a polyp. The obstruction of the lumen of a tube or duct and the pressure on the overlying mucous membrane are caused by the space-occupying effect of neoplasms.

The earliness with which symptoms develop, as well as their nature, depends on the anatomical and functional characteristics of the involved organ or structures. Such factors as the size and distensibility of the space containing the neoplasm influence the period of time elapsing before the neoplasm causes signs and symptoms. The location of a lesion in a hollow or tubular organ also influences its effect. For example, a lesion near the outlet of the stomach causes symptoms earlier than one in the fundus. A neoplasm growing around a tubular organ

[55] *A Cancer Source Book for Nurses* (New York: American Cancer Society, Inc., 1963), p. 11.

[56] James D. Hardy: "Why Do Cancer Patients Die?" *Surg. Gynec. Obstet.,* **108**:368–69 (Mar.) 1959.

causes a greater degree of obstruction than one projecting into it. Each of these points is illustrated later.

Because neoplasms are formed of masses of cells, they generally occupy space and cause clinical manifestations by (1) interfering with the blood supply of tissue, (2) interfering with the function of an organ, and (3) activating compensatory or defensive mechanisms.

As stated earlier, the size and distensibility of the space or organ containing a neoplasm influence the nature as well as the earliness with which manifestations of disease occur. The examples that follow are intended to clarify the mechanical effects of neoplasms.

Mike Sunny, aged 11, has a rapidly growing neoplasm in his cerebellum. As the neoplasm increases in mass, it occupies space and presses on the tissues of the cerebellum.[57] The earliness with which local pressure is exerted is influenced by the fact that the cerebellum is surrounded by a rigid bony wall, the skull; it does not distend to accommodate the increase in the contents of the cranial cavity. Furthermore, the location of this particular neoplasm is such that it obstructs the drainage of cerebrospinal fluid from the ventricles, causing the fluid to accumulate within the ventricles and thus further raising the intracranial pressure. Because the size of the cavity containing the brain is fixed, increased resistance to the flow of blood through the brain is a consequence of an elevation in intracranial pressure.

The manifestations presented by Mike are caused by an inadequate supply of blood to the cerebellum and other parts of the brain and by the activation of mechanisms to maintain the blood supply of the brain. The signs and symptoms presented by Mike indicate disturbances in the function of the cerebellum as well as evidence of alterations in cardiorespiratory function, which tend to overcome the resistance to the flow of blood to the brain. See Chapter 15, Part B for further discussion of disturbance in the function of the cerebellum and for signs and symptoms of increased intracranial pressure.

In contrast to Mike, who had an expanding lesion within a fixed space, Mrs. Thinly had a neoplasm in a space that is highly distensible. Mrs. Thinly had a benign ovarian cyst, which, at the time it was removed, weighed more than 40 lb. It was so large that it overfilled a basin about the size of an ordinary dishpan. The day before Mrs. Thinly was admitted to the hospital

she had done the family wash and cleaned the house. For some months previous to seeking medical attention she had noticed a gradual increase in the size of her abdomen which she attributed to the fact that she had had several children and was getting old. Until the tumor reached considerable size, it had little effect on function because the abdominal wall distended to accommodate the increase in contents. As the size of the tumor increased, however, the intra-abdominal pressure rose, causing pressure against the diaphragm and decreasing the capacity of her stomach and other abdominal organs. She experienced some shortness of breath, swelling of the feet, and loss of appetite. Because of her loss of appetite she lost weight. After the tumor was removed, she weighed 85 lb, but she made a rapid and uneventful recovery. Because the neoplasm was benign, she was cured.

Mike Sunny and Mrs. Thinly have been described to illustrate how the rigidity or distensibility of the space in which a neoplasm grows influences its effects. At the time Mike Sunny's skull was opened, the neoplasm was about the size of a small orange, and it was already threatening his life by its effect on the blood supply to his brain. In contrast, because of the distensibility of the abdominal wall, Mrs. Thinly had a very large neoplasm that had little effect on the blood supply to the tissues in the abdominal cavity. Signs and symptoms observed in Mrs. Thinly were mainly caused by the interference with the functions of the respiratory and digestive systems.

OBSTRUCTION

Mr. Timothy Thomas illustrates what happens when the diameter of a tubular structure is decreased by a space-occupying mass. Mr. Thomas had a carcinoma of the prostate that, as it increased in cell mass, caused pressure on the urethra, thus increasing the resistance to the flow of urine. As shown in Table 14-4, any tubular structure may be obstructed by the

TABLE 14-4

Sites of Neoplasms May Obstruct Any Tubular Structure

1. External to structure
2. Internal, arising from lining membrane
3. Internal, arising in and encircling the wall

pressure created by a neoplasm external to it, or by a neoplasm extending from the lining membrane into the lumen of the tube, or by a

---

[57] In the cerebellum the space is less confining than that enclosing the cerebrum. Because the neoplasm is malignant, it also invades the surrounding tissue, but at this point the effect of a space-occupying mass is under discussion.

neoplasm arising in the wall and encircling it as it grows. Both benign and malignant neoplasms may obstruct by creating external pressure on a tubular structure or by extending into its lumen from the lining tissues. Neoplasms arising in the wall and encircling the lumen of a tube, such as the large intestine, are usually malignant.

In the instance of Mr. Thomas, obstruction of the urethra was caused by a neoplasm in tissue external to it. Whatever the cause of the obstruction, its primary effect is to interfere with the passage of the tube's contents. When the obstruction of a tubular structure develops slowly enough, the portion of the tube preceding the obstruction dilates, and the muscle layer in its wall hypertrophies. Muscular hypertrophy occurs as a result of the increase in resistance to the movement of the contents of the obstructed tube; it is, therefore, a compensatory mechanism. Eventually, as the degree of obstruction increases, the lumen will be blocked and the tube will cease to function as a passageway. Chronic obstruction, whatever its cause, predisposes to infection of the organ drained by the duct and, if unrelieved, to its destruction.

To return to Mr. Thomas, who has an obstruction of the urethra caused by a carcinoma of his prostate gland—as the neoplasm enlarged, it encroached on the lumen of the urethra, thus impeding the passage of urine. To overcome the effect of the increase in resistance caused by the narrowing of the urethra, the muscle in the neck of the bladder hypertrophied. As the urethra narrowed, Mr. Thomas noted that he had difficulty in starting to void and that the urinary stream was small. He also had a feeling of urgency and seldom felt that he had really emptied his bladder. As time passed and the obstruction increased, the bladder did not empty at the time of voiding. Urine accumulated and became infected. The bladder was distended by the accumulated urine. Eventually, if the obstruction is allowed to continue, the ureters and the pelvis of the kidney become distended with urine and all the structures—urethra, bladder, and kidneys—become infected. The outcome of unrelieved obstruction along the urinary tract is kidney failure.

The effects of obstruction of the alimentary canal and of the ducts emptying into it have been discussed in Chapters 12 and 17 and will not be pursued further. One effect meriting some consideration is that neoplasms in the alimentary canal usually impair nutrition before those located in other parts of the body. Patients with obstructing lesions in the upper alimentary canal not infrequently experience a rapid loss in weight and are markedly dehydrated and anemic because of impaired intake of food and fluids.

Because the effects of obstruction of ducts forming the tracheobronchial tree and the biliary tract have been discussed in Chapters 8 and 12, they will not be repeated here.

Another mechanical effect of neoplasms results from pressure created by the neoplasm on the overlying mucous membrane. Pressure on any tissue decreases its blood supply. With impairment in its nutrition the mucosa atrophies, and if the pressure is severe and unrelieved, it ulcerates. Ulceration predisposes to bleeding in benign as well as in malignant neoplasms. For example, some patients with leiomyofibromas located in the submucosa of the wall of the uterus (fibroids) are predisposed to profuse bleeding. Tumors located in the deeper layers of the wall of the uterus do not usually result in hemorrhage. To illustrate, Mrs. Beech has a leiomyofibroma located in the submucosa of the wall of the uterus. As a consequence of pressure, the blood supply to the mucosa overlying the tumor was impaired. It atrophied and eventually ulcerated. During her menstrual periods she experienced heavy bleeding, or menorrhagia. Despite the benign nature of leiomyomas, Mrs. Beech's health and possibly her life were threatened by repeated hemorrhage. Because she has multiple fibroids (leiomyomas) and she is bleeding excessively, she has been advised by her physician to have a hysterectomy.

The fourth mechanical effect of a neoplasm results from the twisting of a pedunculated polyp, benign or malignant, on its pedicle. Twisting causes severe pain and it also deprives the polyp of its blood supply. When a polyp is torn from its pedicle, massive bleeding can result.

In the preceding discussion, the manner in which neoplasms cause signs and symptoms by their mechanical effects has been presented. As space-occupying masses, they create pressure on tissues, thus impairing their blood supply; they obstruct the lumen and interfere with the function of tubular organs; and when they are pedunculated, they are likely to twist on their pedicles. All of these are local effects and may be caused by either benign or malignant neoplasms. Specific signs and symptoms depend on the location of the lesion, the degree to which function is disrupted, and the extent to which compensatory or defense mechanisms are mobilized.

Systemic Effects of Neoplasms

Benign and malignant neoplasms may also be accompanied by systemic effects. As stated earlier, neoplasms arising in glands (adenomas) may elaborate the secretion of the gland. When this occurs, symptoms of hyperfunction occur. Functioning tumors may be benign or malignant. At least in the thyroid gland, hyperfunction is more likely to be associated with a benign than with malignant neoplasms.

As indicated earlier in this chapter, malignant neoplasms differ from benign neoplasms in a number of ways. Whereas benign neoplasms are usually localized to the area where they originate, malignant neoplasms tend to invade the surrounding tissue and to be disseminated throughout the body. Some of the effects of malignant neoplasms are caused by the invasion and replacement of healthy tissue at the site of the primary growth or of metastasis. The specific effects of metastasis depend on the site affected. For example, in cancer of the lung, either primary or metastatic, the destruction of lung tissue eventually leads to asphyxia of the patient. In leukemia, the abnormal cells invade and destroy the bone marrow as well as other vital structures. As the bone marrow is invaded and destroyed, its capacity to produce erythrocytes and thrombocytes fails; this predisposes to anemia and bleeding.

A number of the manifestations accompanying malignant neoplasms are caused by their tendency to outgrow their blood supply. As in healthy cells, cells in malignant neoplasms die unless their nutritional needs are met. Death or necrosis of cells on the surface of a neoplasm predisposes to ulceration. Ulceration predisposes to infection and bleeding and is one of the important causes of pain. Ulceration with its concomitant effects can sometimes be observed in the patient with advanced and neglected cancer of the breast. Large, infected ulcerations, often with foul-smelling drainage, occur over the affected area. Signs and symptoms accompanying tissue necrosis and/or infection include fever, leukocytosis, elevation of the sedimentation rate, anorexia, and malaise. Because these symptoms and signs are nonspecific, a patient who manifests them without an obvious cause should be investigated for cancer.

In addition to infections of ulcerated lesions, the patient with metastatic cancer is predisposed to infections of the lung and urinary tract. These infections are frequently caused by obstruction of a bronchus, a ureter, or the urethra. Curing of the infection depends on relief of the obstruction and use of appropriate antibiotics. Nursing measures that can and should be instituted to prevent obstruction of the airway by secretions in the bedfast patient are discussed in detail in Chapter 8.

Bleeding not only accompanies ulceration, but it can also be the result of the erosion of one or more blood vessels. The amount of blood lost at a time may be micro- or macroscopic. Any abnormal bleeding should be investigated, as it may indicate the presence of a malignant neoplasm. Blood in the stool or urine or any unusual bleeding from the vagina should be investigated for evidence or absence of cancer. Eventually the continued loss of blood leads to anemia, with its characteristic signs and symptoms. Bleeding is not the only cause of anemia in cancer, as anemia occurs in advanced cancer in the absence of any significant loss of blood. Other factors predisposing to anemia include infection and uremia. Metastasis to the liver or bone marrow may reduce the capacity to replace blood cells. Treatment of cancer by radiotherapy or chemotherapy is usually accompanied by some degree of depression of the bone marrow, thus predisposing to anemia. With the exception of pallor, the signs and symptoms are those of circulatory distress. They are tachycardia, palpitation, dyspnea, dizziness, easy fatigability, and weakness.

Malignant neoplasms cause symptoms by utilizing nutritional elements required by normal cells. They continue to grow as long as the host remains alive. This is true even in the most emaciated patient. The rate of growth is sometimes slowed by undernutrition, but growth continues. Why malignant cells have a competitive advantage over normal cells is not known. They seem to require more of some types of amino acids and vitamins than do normal cells, but little more is known.

Malignant neoplasms located in the lung, ovaries, and breast are frequently accompanied by the effusion of serous fluid into the pleural and peritoneal cavities. The fluid can be removed by thoracentesis or abdominal paracentesis. When the fluid is formed rapidly, radioactive gold or nitrogen mustard may be introduced into the appropriate cavity to lessen the tendency to effusion; effusion is prevented in about one half of the patients so treated.

One of the most striking effects of advanced cancer is severe cachexia. In lay terms, the individual literally becomes skin and bones. The patient appears to be, and is, suffering from severe starvation. One explanation offered to account for cachexia is that the food intake of the individual is insufficient to support the neoplasm and the individual. Although an inadequate intake of food may be a contributing factor, it is probably not the sole cause of cachexia, as forced feeding is often unsuccessful in correcting it. It is probable that cachexia, as well as other manifestations of terminal cancer, is caused by derangements in the biochemical functions of the body. Whatever its cause may be, every reasonable effort should be made to encourage the patient to eat, particularly protein-containing foods.

Pain

Because pain will be discussed in some detail in Chapter 17, it will be considered here only briefly. Despite evidence that pain is neither as common nor as inevitable as generally believed, it is probably the most feared effect of cancer. The fact that people believe that cancer and pain are synonymous is unfortunate, because it contributes to the dread or fear of cancer that permeates our society. As stated in Chapter 17, the discomfort caused by pain has two sources. One is the pain sensation and the other is the meaning that the pain has for the individual. Studies of persons who are in pain-inducing situations demonstrate that the meaning that pain has for the individual frequently determines the degree of suffering experienced. The belief that pain is inevitable and frequently so severe that it is intolerable can of itself increase the severity of the pain experienced by the patient. When nurses and physicians are convinced that pain is an unavoidable aspect of cancer, it may result in a narrow or unimaginative approach to the care of the patient. The care may be such as to reinforce the fears of the patient, and other causes of discomfort may be missed or neglected. Not only does a morbid fear of pain add to the suffering of the patient who has been diagnosed as having cancer, but it may prevent persons who suspect that they have it from seeking medical attention. Persons who do not have cancer, therefore, experience unnecessary discomfort and those who do may delay until such time as metastasis has occurred. There are undoubtedly other negative aspects of the all too common belief that pain and cancer are synonymous.

When pain occurs in cancer, it is usually the result of pressure on, or the involvement of, sensory nerve endings in obstruction, ulceration, or infection. Pain can also be induced by measures employed in the treatment of cancer. For example, the patient who undergoes surgical treatment is likely to experience more or less pain. Radiotherapy, particularly when it induces an inflammatory reaction in tissues in the treated area, may be responsible for pain. Although pain may be present early in the course, it is more likely to be a late symptom. Pain in cancer of the bone is likely to be severe, for the rigidity of the bone allows for little or no expansion. Pressure on sensory nerve endings occurs early.

PREVENTION AND RELIEF OF PAIN

The prevention and relief of pain are one aspect of the care of the patient with a diagnosis of cancer. Although not all will experience pain, most patients fear that they will. Moreover, there are many other causes of discomfort besides pain that can increase the suffering of the patient or that the patient may perceive as pain. Lack of rest as well as the inevitable discomforts associated with any illness diminish the capacity of the patient to withstand pain and add to his tendency to magnify the degree of pain that he is experiencing. The nurse should be alert to, and try to relieve, whatever is causing the patient discomfort. As an example, Mr. Sands had metastatic cancer involving the ribs and sternum. Even touching his chest with a sheet caused him to cry out in pain. His nurse was able to prevent unnecessary pain by placing a large cradle over his torso as a support for the bed covering. When she moved and turned him she was gentle and moved him slowly. She supported his head and arms in a relaxed position, so that they did not pull on his thorax. Mrs. Lottie had metastatic cancer involving her cervical vertebrae. Although she had a neck brace, she found it uncomfortable. Mrs. Lottie and her nurse worked out a plan for turning her so that pain was prevented and the brace was not required. Mrs. Lottie supported her head with her hands as she turned. After she was turned, pillow supports were used to keep her head in alignment. Pain was prevented by the identification of the situations causing it and by the utilization of effective nursing measures.

In nursing the patient, gentle handling, attention to his hygienic and physiological needs, intelligent concern for his well-being, an attitude that something constructive can be done to improve his condition, and the sensible use of diversion and occupation—all when appropriately selected and utilized—can contribute to the prevention and relief of pain.

When drugs are required for the relief of pain, they must be prescribed by the physician. In selecting a drug or drugs, the physician usually considers the following points: (1) Is the pain severe? (2) Does it come in episodes or is it continuous? (3) How much anxiety does it produce and how anxious is the patient? (4) What is the patient's life expectancy? (5) What can be done about the cause of the pain? In a patient with good life expectancy, can the cause of pain be completely removed? Drug addiction can become a problem; therefore, nonaddicting drugs should be used when possible and, in some instances, patients are requested to tolerate some pain. On the other hand, when the cause of a patient's pain cannot be removed and, particularly, when the patient's life expectancy is short, withholding narcotics is cruel. For a patient who is no longer employed and who no longer is required to function as the breadwinner or family mother, the control of pain is more important than the avoidance of drug addiction, which, in a terminal cancer patient, very rarely represents a serious management problem.

The nurse has the responsibility for preparing the patient so that he is in a comfortable position and condition and for observing the effects of the drug. Although drugs are usually ordered by the clock, pain does not tell time. The nurse should, therefore, observe the length of time that the patient is relieved. Because of daytime activities, patients often require less medication during the day than at night. In some instances, small doses of a pain-relieving medication given every two hours provide more relief than do large doses given every four hours. Part of the benefit from the drug comes from the faith of the patient in its effectiveness. Nothing should be done to interfere with this by either word or deed. Occasionally a well-intentioned, though misguided, nurse decides to protect the patient from the danger of addiction by prolonging the time the patient has to wait for his medication or decides to withhold the narcotic portion of his prescription. The result of the first may well be that the patient receives little or no benefit from his medication because his pain has become intolerable. The result of the second is that the faith of the patient in the power of his medication to relieve his suffering is destroyed.

Unless the patient is presenting evidence of toxicity from the drug, the prescription left by the physician should be adhered to. Any problem related to the drug or drugs the patient is receiving should be discussed with the physician before a change is made. In the use of drugs for the control of pain in the patient with cancer, the objective is to regulate selection and use so that the patient is provided relief over the course of his illness.

Callaway [58] also emphasizes the importance of using a sympathetic approach to the patient. Mild drugs such as aspirin plus a tranquilizing agent will often give the patient the necessary relief. However, unnecessary restrictions in use of pain-relieving drugs probably contribute as

[58] Enoch Callaway: "The Misuse of Narcotics by Patients Suffering from Cancer," CA, 10:33–36 (Jan.–Feb.) 1960.

much to unnecessary suffering of cancer patients as any other single cause.

SURGICAL THERAPY OF PAIN

In addition to the use of drugs for the relief of pain, surgical procedures to correct conditions causing pain may be instituted. Ulcerated lesions may be excised, obstruction may be relieved by rerouting operations such as colostomy, or pain impulses may be prevented from reaching higher centers in the nervous systems by cutting a sensory nerve, nerve root, or tract in the spinal cord. The interruption of sensory nerve pathways is not usually performed unless all other measures fail. With the loss of their sensory nerve supply, tissues are deprived of one of their important defenses against pressure and heat. The patient should be turned and the skin inspected for redness or blanching no less often than every two hours. Protective measures should be instituted such as placing an alternating pressure mattress or flotation pad under the affected area. The bed linen should be free of crumbs and wrinkles. A cradle should be used to lessen the pressure of the bed covering on the patient.

To control the pain and odors associated with ulcerated lesions, the area may be excised surgically, or the patient may be treated with x-ray or chemotherapy. All these measures are utilized because they remove or control the tumor itself.

CONTROL OF ODORS

When the lesion remains open, the most important general measure is *cleanliness*. Odors originate from dead tissue and the effects of infection. The agent used to cleanse the lesion should be prescribed by the physician. There is usually no reason for not cleansing the area around the lesion with soap or detergent and water. Moreover, when the patient has a draining and foul-smelling wound, the nurse should take whatever initiative is required to see that it is cleansed. Dressings should be changed when soiled and replaced by clean ones. When wounds are treated by exposure to the air, the patient should be draped and screened so that he is protected from view. Ventilation of the room, with precautions to prevent chilling the patient, reduces the intensity of odors. When deodorizing agents and devices are used, they should supplement and not substitute for keeping the wound clean.

In summary, although pain is not inevitable to cancer, it does occur. Even patients who do not experience pain are almost certain to fear they will. There are few areas in which a kind, gentle, thoughtful, compassionate, and creative nurse can do more to prevent human suffering. The prescription of drugs and treatment by surgical and chemotherapeutic means are the prerogative of the physician. Whether or not the drugs are effective often depends on the quality of nursing care the patient receives. Furthermore, by attention to the hygienic, physiological, and psychosocial needs of the patient, pain and suffering from pain can be minimized.

What are some of the psychological effects on the patient with a real or imagined diagnosis of cancer?

Not by any means the least important cause of suffering in the patient who has or suspects he has cancer is its psychosocial effects. As mentioned previously, the psychological effects extend to persons who do not have cancer, inasmuch as many fear that their illness or ill health is caused by cancer. The family is also affected by a diagnosis of cancer in a family member. Their response to the diagnosis and to the individual affects the behavior of the sick person. The psychological effects are those resulting from the manner in which the individual perceives the entire cancer experience, that is, its nature and effects, and outcome, as well as the measures utilized in its diagnosis and treatment. The sociological effects of cancer stem from group attitudes toward it and its nature, effects, and treatment. Each person reading this book has attitudes about cancer and its effects and curability that were learned from the groups of which he is a part. These attitudes influence how a person feels and behaves when faced with a diagnosis of cancer in himself or in another individual. His behavior toward another individual is also influenced by the way in which the individual defines his role in the situation. The quality of care that a patient receives is affected by the attitude of all who have a relationship to him—his family, his neighbors, his nurses and doctors, and the community. As an illustration, when Mr. and Mrs. Thompkins were driving home from an appointment with her physician where Mrs. Thompkins learned that she had cancer of the breast, Mr. Thompkins asked in a tentative tone, "Don't you think that you would sleep better if I moved into the guest room?" Mr. Thompkins did not intend to be unkind; he was frightened. Despite the fact that the physician had answered his question about the possibility that cancer was infectious in the negative, he was not convinced. Besides, cancer always made him think of suffering and death.

Any person who has a diagnosis of cancer can be expected to be under severe emotional stress. For most persons in the United States, the diagnosis carries with it a threat of a prolonged and painful course, ending in death. Because of the extended course of the illness and the nature of the treatments, cancer is often an economic burden not only to the patient but also to his family.

On the discovery of a lesion or symptom that suggests cancer, most persons experience fear. With the fear, the person may have a variety of feelings—a sense of doom, anger, helplessness, shame, and disgrace. He may feel trapped or abandoned. Cameron [59] states, "in general, cancer signifies premature death, supreme physical suffering, abysmal depression, incalculable economic loss, and pathetic family disruption and dissolution." The fear and anxiety experienced by the patient are extended to his family, friends, neighbors, and community.

Nurses also have culturally derived attitudes toward cancer and what nurses ought to be able to accomplish in the care of the sick. To be successful in identifying and meeting the needs of the patient, the nurse is helped by knowing what her own feelings are. The aim of the nurse is not to avoid feeling but to manage her feelings in such a way that she can attend to those of her patients. The nurse should try to take a middle course so that she is able to identify the needs of the patient and to meet them in ways that are helpful. Neither feeling too strongly with the patient nor isolating herself from him will enable her to achieve this goal with any degree of consistency.

The person who suspects or knows he has cancer can then be expected to experience fear and its attendant feelings. How he reacts to this fear depends on the way in which he customarily behaves when he is under severe stress and the quality of support given to him by his family. If his fear is reasonable, he may be stimulated to seek medical attention and to follow through with the recommendations of his physician. In contrast, unreasonable fear leads to denial, disorganization, confusion, and panic. Denial is a very common reaction. It may be strong enough to convince a cancer patient that he is suffering from some other ailment. This conviction exists even after all the diagnostic studies have been completed and even after cancer therapies have been administered. Sometimes this denial mechanism will prevent the patient from seeking help or accepting appropriate treatment when it is offered. When denial

[59] Charles S. Cameron: "We Who Are Concerned," *Cancer News,* 8:4 (Summer) 1959.

is complete, the patient may grasp at straws, seek new treatments, and ask for constant reassurance. He asks not to know that he has cancer but to be reassured that he does not. Like many psychological reactions, the denial can also be useful, particularly to patients with cancer having a poor prognosis or terminal patients. The denial of hopelessness will frequently help the patient to remain cheerful and productive in spite of incurable cancer. A skillful physician or nurse can utilize the denial to increase the patient's comfort, whereas uncontrolled denial may force the patient to delay the diagnosis and treatment and drive him to consult "quacks" who promise cure.

Another possible source of stress is that treatment of cancer frequently involves the loss of important functions and organs. These may be important not only to the patient but to the members of his family, his friends, and the community. The lesion, because of its location or the nature of its treatment, may be the cause of psychological stress. Either benign or malignant neoplasms may cause disfigurement. Nevi or birthmarks on the exposed surface of the body may be the cause of more or less psychological stress. One small girl, Mary Lou, had a type of malignant neoplasm in which the skin on the exposed surfaces of her body was covered with wartlike growths. Life was made bearable for Mary Lou when she was given a pretty hat with a veil and encouraged to wear it. The veil served to protect her from the stares and thoughtless comments of bystanders. Because Mary Lou had a widespread and progressive disease and was not expected to live for more than a few months, one of the important objectives in her care was to make her as comfortable as possible in the time she had. Persons who have benign lesions that are disfiguring must be helped to adjust to the situation. Often a lesion can be made less conspicuous by the use of a covering type of cosmetic.

In addition to the psychological stress caused by a diagnosis of cancer, neoplasms located in certain sites may be responsible for additional stress. Neoplasms located in the head and neck not only cause obvious disfigurement, but the removal of the lesion is usually accompanied by some degree of mutilation and loss of function, including loss of the ability to swallow, to speak, or to breathe normally. After laryngectomy the patient may feel that because of his loss of speech he is something less than human. About 70 per cent of persons who have had a laryngectomy can learn esophageal speech. It takes about 12 months for the patient to reach the stage of maximum intelligibility. Some patients who cannot learn esophageal speech may be able to use an artificial larynx. It differs from the esophageal speech, which provides an internal source, by providing a sound source external to the human vocal folds.

The loss of the breast causes disfigurement and some loss of function of the muscles moving the shoulder and the arm. It also predisposes to edema of the arm on the affected side. The structural deformity can be corrected by a prosthesis. Because the breast is a symbol of femininity, the woman may feel that she is less of a woman after mastectomy. A variety of prostheses are available, from which a woman can select one best suited to her.

The removal of reproductive organs of either the male or female is usually accompanied by some feeling of loss of identity. The man who loses his testes is likely to feel that he is less a man, just as a woman who loses her uterus, breast, or ovaries feels less a woman.

The psychological problems created by a colostomy are discussed later, in the study of Mrs. Wren. The discussion of the needs of the patient who is in the terminally ill phase of the disease is included in Chapter 3.

Some of the factors causing psychological stress in the patient who has a diagnosis of cancer have been presented. Further discussion of psychosocial aspects of care are included in later sections of the chapter. For a more detailed discussion of the effects of severe psychological stress and what the nurse can do to help the patient, see Chapter 7.

Telling the Patient

A problem growing out of the fact that cancer can and often does create a high degree of psychological stress among members of the family, nurses, and physicians is the question of whether or not the patient should be told that he has cancer. In few, if any, other diseases is there any question about withholding the nature of the diagnosis. Often the cooperation of the patient in his treatment requires that the patient know what his diagnosis is. Although physicians may not inform the patient of the nature of his illness, some member of the family is informed. Practice among physicians varies. In cancer, as in other diseases, the physician carries the responsibility for informing the patient of the nature of his diagnosis and the treatment required. At one time the practice not to tell patients unless there was some reason for telling them was general, and some physicians still rarely tell a patient that he has cancer. Others always, or almost always, tell their patients and feel just as strongly that the patient should be told as do those who feel that knowledge of the nature of the diagnosis should be withheld. Many physicians try to make their decision on the basis of whether the patient wants to know and how the knowledge will affect him.

What are some of the possible harmful effects of withholding information about a diagnosis of cancer?

In the past there has been much argument about the harmful effects resulting from the patient's learning that he has cancer; not too much consideration has been given to the harmful effects of his not knowing. Making an issue over whether or not to tell the person who has cancer fosters the urge to secrecy. It also suggests that the situation of the person is hopeless and that there is something mysterious about cancer. The fact that patients know that they may not be told may cause some persons to distrust the information given them. It is not unusual to hear persons say that they are not certain whether they have or have not been told the truth about their illness. Patients who are not told that they have cancer sometimes obtain this information through questions and statements made to a nurse or doctor. When the patient is not told, this creates the necessity for treating the patient as if nothing were wrong. The patient's questions have to be answered without giving him any information. This, in turn, creates a barrier between the patient and the professional staff. He is cut off from seeking information, help, and comfort from those who, by preparation, should be able to help him. A patient may be told by a visitor or another patient that he has cancer. This can be, needless to say, an exceedingly traumatic experience. Furthermore, uncertainty usually causes more discomfort than certainty. Imagination, unless disciplined by reality, can do terrible things to an individual. According to the accounts of persons writing about their personal experience with cancer, the lives of some persons become richer and more meaningful after they know they have cancer. As emphasized by Mrs. Willis (see Chapter 3), not all persons react in this way. Not knowing that he has cancer may have an adverse effect on the course of the disease, inasmuch as the patient who does not know that he has or has had cancer may fail to keep his appointments for care and for follow-up examinations.

Against telling the patient that he has cancer is the fact that, for many people, the knowledge is very upsetting. In some people it may cause a disruptive panic and possibly lead to suicide. Actually, suicide is quite rare among patients who have cancer and its risk can be virtually eliminated by giving the patient the necessary information tactfully and sympathetically, as well as explaining to the patient all the aspects of his disease—not only the unpleasant ones but also the hopeful ones.

At the present time, two factors determine whether or not a given patient is told he has cancer. One is the feelings of the physician. The other is the distress of the patient. Unless there is an important reason for telling the patient, he is not told when he indicates that he does not want to know that he has cancer. If he never refers to cancer as a cause of his illness, or if he asks to be reassured that he does not have cancer, this is taken as an indication that he does not want to know. Conversely, when he asks the direct question, "Do I have cancer?" he is answered in the affirmative.

Frequently the intelligent patient who is not using powerful denial mechanisms probably knows that he has cancer by the time the doctor has established the diagnosis. In some of these patients, the condition is worsened by fostering denial mechanisms. They want to know whether or not they have cancer. Doctors who do inform the patient of his status try to do so in a manner that fosters his hope. Although they tell the patient the truth, they do not usually go into all the future possibilities. A friend with cancer of the breast was told by her surgeon that he had removed her entire breast because she had some abnormal cells. Over the course of the next two or three years she learned the extent of her disease. She commented later that in the beginning she did not believe that she could have tolerated knowing the full truth, but by learning it gradually, she had come to accept her situation. With time she was able to accept that she had cancer.

To summarize, whether or not, and how, the patient is told depends on the patient and his situation. The doctor and the family of the patient weigh the factors that enter into the decision. Not only the personality of the patient but also the prognosis has to be considered. The support that may be obtained from his family and even the personality of the doctor are important factors. There is not, at this time, a single answer to the needs of all patients. Decisions should be based on what will, in the long run, make it possible to meet the needs of the patient. One day the problem of telling or not telling the patient will cease to exist. Under all circumstances, every effort should be made to convey to the patient that much can and will be done to promote his welfare and the approach to a patient with an incurable cancer should be similar to the approach used in treating patients with other chronic diseases.

Phases in the Life Cycle of the Patient with Cancer

In the *Cancer Bulletin* [60] the life cycle of the cancer patient is depicted as occurring in seven phases. To these seven should be added another, the first, or preventive, phase. The phases, as listed, included (1) early diagnosis, (2) recommended treatment, (3) comprehensive treatment, (4) follow-up education for the patient, (5) regular follow-up by the physician, (6) rehabilitation, and (7) adequate terminal care. Not all patients who have a diagnosis of cancer progress through all these phases.

The discussion is organized as follows: (1) the elements in primary prevention; (2) the phase of secondary prevention, detection, and diagnosis of cancer; (3) the phase of curative and palliative treatment; (4) the nursing needs of patients; and (5) the phase of terminal illness. Because rehabilitation and instruction begin the moment the individual enters the clinic or doctor's office and continue throughout all phases of the patient's life, they will not be treated separately.

In all phases of the patient's illness, the nurse tries to convey to the patient that something can and will be done to improve his condition. This does not always mean that his life will be prolonged, but that, whatever the probable outcome, the quality of his life can be improved. The goals for each patient should take into account the phase of the patient's illness, his psychological and physiological resources, and the nature and extent of treatment. Persons who happen to have cancer are people. They have the same basic needs as do all people. Because of the manner in which cancer and its treatment are perceived, patients with cancer can be expected to be under severe stress. Each patient behaves as an individual. To meet the needs of patients, the nurse requires knowledge and competence in all nursing skills. These include skill in observing, in communicating, in providing care in such a manner that the patient feels accepted and respected, in teaching the patient and family members, in planning and organizing the patient's care, and in performing the procedures required in his physical care.

Observation is a continuous process directed toward the identification of the patient's physiological and psychological needs. From observation, data are collected that indicate improvement or deterioration of the patient's condition or the development of complications. Instruction of the patient is planned to achieve three goals: First, the patient continues to have regu-

[60] "The Cancer Program Workshop," *Cancer Bull.*, **11**:47 (May–June) 1959.

lar medical supervision for the remainder of his life. Second, within the limits of the patient's capacity, he continues as an active and productive member of his family and community; he should not be unnecessarily invalided. The third objective is an aspect of the second—if he can accept in perspective whatever limitations are imposed by his treatment, he can be helped not to allow them to become the focus of his life. The other aspects of nursing will be integrated throughout.

Prevention of Cancer

Primary Prevention

In the control of cancer, prevention is the keynote. As in other chronic diseases, prevention is of two types, primary and secondary. In primary prevention the objective is to eliminate conditions predisposing to its development. In the present state of knowledge evidence points to multiple factors interacting to cause cancer. A problem in prevention is to identify those factors that are controllable. Through the use of epidemiological studies, some of the agents in the external environment have been identified as carcinogenic. As they become known, methods can be developed to eliminate them or to protect persons from their effect. Much has been accomplished in industry to protect workers from carcinogenic chemicals. A familiar example from the health field is the precautions that are taken to protect workers from exposure to ionizing radiation. The basis for, and the nature of, these precautions have been discussed elsewhere. At times knowledge about the significance of a factor is less clear-cut, or the findings of epidemiological studies are difficult to implement. For example, the incidence of cancer of the lung is higher in urban than in rural areas. Many factors may well enter into this difference. Among these is the higher concentration of smoke discharged into the air from all sources—houses, stores, industrial plants, and automobile exhaust gases. Both smoke and exhaust gases contain carcinogenic hydrocarbons. To reduce the pollution of the air by potentially harmful substances, public education is required. The public must accept, demand, and be willing to pay for whatever is required to do this. Furthermore, permanent control of air pollution depends on continued supervision and enforcement of regulations. In the primary prevention of cancer, much has been accomplished to protect workers from the carcinogenic effects of agents used in industry. A beginning has been made in the protection of the general public from known carcinogens.

Equally difficult or possibly even more difficult to accomplish is the primary prevention involving a major change in a custom or habit. As an illustration, the Surgeon General's report stated that cigarette smoking is an etiological agent in cancer of the lung. Most of the deaths from this disease could be prevented by eliminating smoking. Yet many persons continue to smoke. Knowledge of hazards, especially when cause-effect relationships are not immediately observable, is not enough to effect changes in the habits of all people. Many other factors are involved.

A second type of primary prevention is based on the identification and removal of precancerous lesions. These have been discussed previously. One of the reasons cited for the decrease in the incidence of cancer of the cervix is that women receive better obstetrical care than in the past. By preventing injury of the cervix and providing early treatment of lesions that develop, the chances of development of cancer of the cervix are reduced.

Primary prevention of cancer is the ideal method of control. The most extensive and effective applications of the principles of primary prevention have been made in industry in the protection of workers from carcinogenic chemicals. Some cancer is prevented by treatment that eliminates the possibility of development of a precancerous lesion or by the removal of suspicious lesions. Applications of primary prevention, though significant, are limited by knowledge of the direct and indirect causes of cancer.

The nurse assists in primary prevention by (1) supporting research projects, not only those directly related to cancer, but those directed toward understanding the nature of cell growth; (2) supporting community efforts to improve environmental conditions; (3) practicing self-protection in situations in which there is a possibility of exposure to carcinogens; and (4) observing and reporting precancerous lesions in herself and others and encouraging others to do likewise.

Secondary Prevention

The secondary prevention of cancer is based on the identification of a cancer while it is still a local rather than a systemic disease. In this stage of disease, malignant change has taken place, but cancer cells have not been distributed throughout the body. In terms of the life of the patient with cancer, this is the first phase. In the past the presumption has been that if cancer could be detected, diagnosed, and treated early enough, then its harmful effects could be prevented. Emphasis has been placed on early diag-

nosis and adequate treatment. In some patients, cancer can be and is detected while it is a local disease. It can be eradicated and the patient cured. In other patients, with the present methods of diagnosis, cancer is a systemic disease by the time its manifestations are evident, and possibly from the beginning. At first sight, this is shocking. It serves to emphasize the fact that cancer is not a single disease with one cause and one method of treatment. Control depends on more knowledge than is now available. Some patients can, however, now be cured by early diagnosis and adequate treatment. Many patients can have their effective lives prolonged. In the American culture the tendency to want one complete answer that works universally appears to contribute to a person's disappointment when the problem turns out to be complex. In whatever phase the patient is when his cancer is discovered, much can be done to improve his condition. There is also the possibility that some discovery will be made that will reverse the disease process.

In the present state of knowledge, the patient's best hope of cure lies in early diagnosis followed by adequate treatment. Slaughter [61] emphasizes the difficulty in establishing a diagnosis of early cancer. One characteristic of early cancer is that it has not invaded the surrounding tissue. According to the American Cancer Society publications, about one half of the persons who have cancer could be cured if treatment were initiated early enough.

Ideally, every woman over the age of 35 and every man over the age of 45 should have a physical examination every year. According to Dr. Emerson Day [62] of the Strang Clinic, the cancer-detection examination should include the following:

History
    Family
    Environment, habits, illness
    Review of systems

Physical
    Skin and lymph nodes
    Head and neck
    Breasts
    Lungs
    Abdomen
    Genitalia
    Rectum—colon
    Extremities

Laboratory
    Hemoglobin or hematocrit
    White blood cell and differential counts

[61] Danely P. Slaughter: "What Is Early Cancer?" *Postgrad. Med.,* 27:271–73 (Mar.) 1960.
[62] Emerson Day: "What Is an Adequate Cancer Checkup?" *Postgrad. Med.,* 27:275 (Mar.) 1960.

Urinalysis
Chest x-ray
Vaginal and cervical smears
Tubeless gastric analysis
Stool guaiac

Although the doctor is responsible for making the diagnosis, the nurse should know what constitutes a thorough examination and why it is desirable. This knowledge is of value to the nurse as a person and in her practice as a professional person. In her work with patients, she requires this information in order to prepare them for what to expect and for what is expected of them. The examination is planned to elicit two types of information. One is directed toward identifying any condition that predisposes the patient to cancer and the other toward determining whether the patient has any signs, symptoms, or tissue changes pointing to the presence of cancer.

The information is utilized in two ways. The more obvious is that it is necessary to the diagnosis of the condition of the patient. The other is that, as data are collected about many patients, the data are subject to analysis and then conclusions are drawn as to their relevance. For example, the conclusion that a relationship exists between cancer of the lung and smoking is based on information obtained from the medical histories of many patients and the statistical analysis of the information.

Most physicians agree that specialized medical training is not required to do a thorough cancer examination. Any physician who is convinced that a thorough examination is important should be able to perform it satisfactorily. The first step is to obtain the family and personal history of the patient. Have other members of the family had cancer? If so, where? Did they recover or die from it? In the personal history, such data as where the person lives, whether or not in his work situation he is exposed to carcinogens, whether he smokes and what he smokes, and whether he drinks alcoholic beverages are pertinent. For women, the menstrual history as well as obstetrical data are desired.

A review of systems is made to elicit any information about previous signs or symptoms that the patient has observed. Unless this is done, the patient may not remember them or may think that observations he has made are insignificant. By the review of each system, one by one, the memory of the patient is refreshed and he is given an opportunity to relate his observations. Patients do not always understand why this is necessary. This is especially true when they seek advice for a symptom or sign in one part of the body. The nurse may help the patient by treating the patient's question cour-

teously and answering it or by referring it to the physician.

The physical examination consists of the palpation and visual inspection of organs to determine changes in color, texture, contour, and function and of listening to the heart and lungs. The physician performs the examination systematically so that no part is missed. He often begins by inspecting the skin for evidence of an increase or decrease in tissue and for changes in its appearance. Although the physician examines the entire skin surface, he pays special attention to areas exposed to the sun, to the palms and soles, to the genitalia, and to areas subject to repeated trauma, as these are the sites where cancer of the skin most commonly occurs. The skin is observed for small, scaly lesions, small ulcers or sores, lumps, senile keratoses, nevi, pigmented moles, and burn scars. Basal cell carcinoma usually makes its appearance as a small scale that later disappears and leaves a sore that increases in size. Squamous cell carcinoma may also start with a scaly lesion or a small lump or an encrusted nodule. It is frequently preceded by senile keratosis, a condition in which there are patches of horny hypertrophy of skin in the aged. They often occur on the face. Nevi, or pigmented lesions, in areas subject to chronic irritation or that have undergone a change in size or color, are ulcerated, or bleed, should be viewed with suspicion. Any person with a lesion that is suspected of being a malignant melanoma should consult or be referred to a surgeon who is experienced in treating melanomas.

The palpation of the superficial lymph nodes is an essential part of any cancer-detection examination. Enlargement of lymph nodes may point to lymphomas or leukemia or to cancer in structures drained by the lymph channels supplying the node. An increase in size in a node or group of nodes may be the first evidence of the disease.

A cancer-detection examination of the head and neck includes the inspection of the skin and the oral and nasal cavities, the visualization of the larynx, and the palpation of the oral cavity, the areas containing lymph nodes, and the thyroid gland.

One of the most publicized cancer-detection examinations is that of the breast. There has been a widespread promotional program to teach women how to examine their own breasts. Many doctors instruct their patients in the procedure. Teaching women to examine their own breasts regularly and systematically each month is based on the expectation that women will be able to detect cancer while the disease is still localized in the breast. Instructions for self-examination of the breast may be obtained from the American Cancer Society or from a local branch of the society. The woman is instructed to report immediately any findings of lumps or changes in the contour or skin of the breast or secretions from the nipple. The physician follows essentially the same pattern in examining the woman's breast that he teaches her to follow. Some patients require special types of examinations. They include those whose breasts, because of the size or because of the cystic changes, are difficult to examine as well as patients coming from cancer-prone families. The recent introduction to mammography and xerography has been shown to be helpful. Because of relatively high amount of radiation utilized for these diagnostic tests, until further advancements in these techniques are made, they should not be used routinely for examination of every woman.

The most essential tool in the detection of lung cancer is the chest x-ray. Because the lung is a common site of metastasis, the chest x-ray is useful not only in detection of primary cancer but in estimation of its prognosis. In persons who are predisposed to lung cancer by their work or personal habits, cytological examination of bronchial secretion may be performed. The presence of abnormal cells in the sputum is an indication for further examination. Physical examination of the chest is also essential. Partial obstruction of a bronchial tube by a neoplasm may cause a wheezing sound as the air passes through accumulated secretions. Furthermore, the partial obstruction may result in the incomplete expansion of a segment of the lung.

The abdomen is palpated to determine the presence of any lumps or increase in size of abdominal organs. Because the liver is a frequent site of metastasis, it receives special attention.

No examination for cancer in women is complete without a thorough investigation of the female reproductive organs. This includes (1) inspection of the external genitalia, (2) inspection of the vagina and cervix with a speculum, (3) collection and staining of cells from the vagina and cervix (Papanicolaou smear examination), and (4) bimanual palpation of the uterus and adnexa. Day [63] emphasizes the importance of the cytological examination in the detection of cancer of the cervix before it becomes invasive. In a series of 107 women examined at the Strang Clinic, approximately 90 per cent of those with cancer were found to have cancer in situ. Of these, 53 per cent were discovered in a cancer-detection examination

[63] *Ibid.,* p. 280.

and before symptoms had occurred. When cancer of the cervix is discovered in the preinvasive phase, it is almost 100 per cent curable.

In preparation for a gynecological examination, a woman should be instructed not to take a vaginal douche. Immediately preceding the examination, she should be asked to empty her urinary bladder. The bed or examining table should be screened and the patient should be draped, so that the genitalia are exposed, but the surrounding area is covered. The patient should lie on her back with her hips flat on the bed or table. When the patient is on an examining table, the hips should be brought to the edge of the table and the legs and thighs supported by stirrups. When the patient is examined in bed, the thighs should be raised so they are perpendicular with the bed. The feet should be resting with the soles flat on the bed. During the examination, the knees are moved outward.

At the beginning of the examination, the external genitalia are inspected for nevi, leukoplakia, ulcerative lesions, and other abnormalities. The vaginal mucous membrane and cervix are examined. The speculum that is used is moistened with water rather than jelly, as the jelly interferes with the cytological examination. Cells are obtained for the vaginal Papanicolaou smear by aspirating secretions from the posterior lateral fornices with a vaginal pipette. The secretions are then spread thinly on a glass slide. The slide is immediately placed in a jar containing equal parts of 95 per cent alcohol and ether. Material for the cervical smear may be obtained by swabbing the surface of the cervix with a cotton applicator and by inserting the cotton into the cervical os and gently rotating it. Another method is to scrape the cervix with a wooden tongue depressor-like device. Material may be obtained from the cervical os by a specially designed cervical scraper. The material obtained from the cervix is spread thinly on a glass slide. The slide is immediately placed in the jar containing equal parts of 95 per cent alcohol and ether or it is fixed by spraying its surface with a commercially available spray fixative. The latter method is a much more convenient way of handling the slides.

The physician also investigates the pelvic organs by means of a bimanual examination. As the prefix *bi* implies, two hands are used. One hand is placed on the abdomen, and one or more fingers of the other hand are placed in the vagina. By exerting pressure, the physician can determine changes in the size and conformation of various structures.

When areas of the cervix present a suspicious appearance, biopsy may be done to establish the diagnosis. Some physicians do a punch biopsy of the suspicious tissue. This can be performed in the outpatient clinic or in the office of the physician as well as in the hospital.

Cancer-detection examination for men should include an investigation of the male reproductive system. This examination should include the inspection and palpation of the external structures and the palpation of the internal organs. Cytological examination may be made on fluids obtained by aspiration from the testes or from a hydrocele. Prostatic fluid may be obtained by massaging the prostate. Every physical examination on an adult male should include the digital examination of the prostate per rectum. From this procedure the physician can identify changes in the size of a part or the entire gland as well as the presence of nodules. Although the enlargement of a lobe or the entire gland is often a benign condition, unless corrected it can cause serious harm by obstructing the flow of urine from the bladder.

Rectal Examination

The digital examination of the rectum serves a further purpose in that some 50 per cent of lesions in the large bowel are within reach of the examiner's finger. For this reason the physical examination of every adult should include this procedure. Because some lesions are beyond the reach of the examiner's finger and cannot be felt, the examination of the rectum and colon should include a proctosigmoidoscopy. In the proctosigmoidoscopy, a lighted tube is introduced through the anal sphincter into the rectum and sigmoid. The walls of these structures are directly visualized and abnormalities such as polyps, ulcerations, and narrowing of the lumen are noted. This is a relatively simple and safe procedure that can be performed in the office of the physician or in an outpatient clinic. Some physicians instruct the patient to take an enema the night preceding the morning of the examination. The purpose of the enema is to cleanse the bowel. The importance of cleansing the bowel to the success of the examination should be stressed. Others prefer to do the examination without any special preparation and remove any feces in the area at the time of the examination. The reason for the omission of enemas is that the solution may injure the mucosa lining the bowel and increase the activity of the intestine. The latter makes the performance of the procedure more difficult.

For the performance of the proctosigmoidoscopy, the patient must be placed in a knee-chest position. The process of assuming this position can be strenuous, and the patient may feel embarrassed. To assist the patient into the knee-chest position, he should lie face down on a table that can be adjusted to the proper position or he may be instructed to assume the proper position on the table. When the patient assumes the knee-chest position, he should turn onto his abdomen with his left arm under his chest. His hips are elevated by bringing his legs up so that he rests on his knees and shoulders. When he is in proper position, his thighs are perpendicular to the table and they form one side of a triangle. The other two sides of the triangle are formed by his back and the table. Because a proctosigmoidoscopy takes about five minutes, the patient should not be placed in position until the physician is ready. As with other procedures, unnecessary exposure of the patient should be avoided by draping and screening. Although the procedure is safe, relatively simple, and leaves no aftereffects, the introduction and movement of the tube may cause cramping. The patient should be reassured that the discomfort is to be expected and that it will cease as soon as the procedure is completed.

The laboratory examinations performed as part of a cancer-detection examination are for the purpose of uncovering clues indicating the presence of cancer in the body as well as pinpointing its location. At the present, there is no single test for the identification of early cancer. Some laboratory tests, though not specifically for cancer, should be part of every cancer-detection examination. Every examination should include a hemoglobin or hematocrit determination. An unexplained anemia is often the first symptom in cancer of the gastrointestinal and urinary tracts. A leukocyte count combined with a determination of the types of leukocytes (differential white count) may provide evidence of leukemia or lymphoma. A complete urinalysis may provide information indicating the presence of a neoplasm in the kidney or urinary tract. The finding of microscopic amounts of blood in the urine is especially significant. Occult (hidden) blood in the feces may indicate a malignant lesion somewhere along the gastrointestinal tract.

Because cancer located in the stomach is frequently, but not always, associated with a lack of secretion of hydrochloric acid (achlorhydria), gastric analysis may be performed. Secretions may be removed by a tube passed into the stomach. Because it is more acceptable to patients, a "tubeless" test may be performed. Gastric secretion is first stimulated with caffeine. The patient is then given a cation exchange resin containing the cation quininium, or azure A. When the gastric juice contains hydrochloric acid, the resin exchanges the quininium cation, or azure A, for the hydrogen ion in the gastric juice, and the released cation, or azure A, is absorbed and excreted in the urine. In the absence of hydrochloric acid, the azure A is not released and very little appears in the urine.

Implications of Suspicious Lesions

The discovery of suspicious lesions, signs, or symptoms may make further investigation necessary. The methods used are those enabling the physician to visualize the lesion directly or indirectly and to obtain tissue for microscopic examination. X-ray, endoscopic, and tissue examinations are made. These procedures have been described in other chapters and will not be repeated. The point that many of these examinations are sources of physical and psychological stress bears repeated emphasis. The patient should be prepared for what to expect and for what is expected of him. When the patient is required to prepare himself for a diagnostic procedure, he should be given written, as well as verbal, instructions.

The location of lesions and their general character may be indirectly visualized by x-ray or fluoroscopic examination. The progress of lesions may be followed by either endoscopic examination or x-ray or both. For example, a patient is found to have an ulcer in his stomach. At the time of the initial examination, it appears to be a benign lesion on both the gastroscopic and x-ray examinations. Although ulcers occurring in the stomach can be benign, they are usually viewed with suspicion. Following treatment, the patient is again examined to determine any changes in the size of the ulcer. Failure of the ulcer to diminish in size and to give other evidence of healing is presumptive evidence that the lesion is not benign.

BIOPSY

The diagnosis of cancer is confirmed by the finding of cancer cells by microscopic examination. When tissue is removed for this purpose, the entire procedure is called a biopsy. When the lesion can be reached from the surface of the body either directly or through a small incision, the procedure itself is relatively minor. Cells may be obtained in body fluids by using a needle or by introducing a punch into the tissue or by cutting out a piece. Tissue is removed from the uterus by scraping. At times a body cavity, such as the abdominal or the thoracic cavity, must be opened to obtain the necessary tissue. In the emphasis on the biopsy as the critical procedure in establishing the diagnosis of cancer, the point may be missed that it is equally useful in establishing that a patient does not have cancer. For example, only four

out of ten lumps in the breast are cancerous. Neither are all lumps in other organs malignant. When they are, treatment is initiated promptly. When they are not, the patient can be reassured that he does not have cancer.

At the time a diagnosis of cancer is made, the characteristics of the cancer and the extent of its spread are evaluated. This information is useful in estimating the prognosis of a patient. The characteristics of cancer are determined by macroscopic and microscopic examination. The macroscopic examination yields information about the size, shape, consistency, and location of the neoplasm. From looking at and feeling the growth, information is gained about whether the neoplasm (1) extends into or grows around an organ, (2) is separate from or has invaded the surrounding tissue, (3) is hard or soft, (4) is ulcerating or intact, and (5) has spread to distant points. The microscopic examination provides information about the character of the cancer cells and the degree to which they resemble or differ from healthy cells. It is also useful in determining the extent of metastasis. With few exceptions, the more cells differ from healthy cells in character and organization, the more rapidly they grow and the faster they metastasize. Pathologists have devised a way of classifying neoplasms according to the degree of differentiation and organization of cells. This is known as grading. The scale is from I to IV. Neoplasms in which the differentiation and organization of cells differ from the normal from 0 to 25 per cent are graded as I. Those that differ from 75 to 100 per cent from normal are graded IV. Grades II and III are in between. On this scale, Grade I neoplasms are slow-growing and slow to metastasize. Those of Grade IV are rapid-growing and early to metastasize.

Neoplasms in some organs are also typed according to extent of spread. The organ for which this was done the earliest was the large bowel. The extent of spread of malignant neoplasms in the large bowel is typed as A, B, and C. In a type A neoplasm, the neoplasm involves only the mucosal and muscularis coats. In type B, the neoplasm extends so that it involves, in addition to the above tissues, the serosa. A type C neoplasm not only involves the above tissues but has spread to the neighboring lymph nodes. At the time typing of neoplasms was introduced, the fact that cancer cells are shed into the venous blood was not known.

A newer method of expressing the extent of spread is to use the term *staging,* with stage I indicating that the lesion is limited to the site of origin. Stage IV indicates widespread metastasis. Because the definitions of staging for the various neoplasms differ from organ to organ, references are included at the end of this chapter for those who are interested in pursuing this subject.

The combination of grading and typing or staging provides information used by the physician to predict the prognosis of the patient. In general, poorly differentiated and disorganized cells, combined with extensive spread, indicate a poor prognosis. A slow-growing neoplasm discovered early, that is, while the disease is still localized, offers a good prognosis. The prediction of prognosis is like any other prediction; it is based on knowledge of facts as they are known today. Some patients live longer than expected. Others die sooner. New knowledge makes conditions that were untreatable now treatable.

Cancer Detection

Because the outlook of patients with neoplasms that respond to therapy depends on early diagnosis and treatment, every individual is important in a cancer-control program. Physicians disagree as to the advisability, practicality, and possibility of every person having a yearly or, as some suggest, biyearly cancer-detection examination. Some physicians suggest that efforts be concentrated on patients in high-risk groups. Women over 30 or 35 years of age and men over 40 years of age are encouraged to have yearly examinations. A family history of cancer, a past history of cancer, smoking, and employment in a hazardous occupation (involving exposure to carcinogens) are suggested as indications for a regular checkup.

Every individual has a responsibility in cancer detection. Persons who have regular physical examinations may, however, develop signs or symptoms that indicate the possibility of cancer. Many, for one reason or another, see a physician only when they are obviously ill. To help people recognize signs and symptoms that indicate the possibility of cancer, the American Cancer Society has prepared and distributed a list known as the *Seven Warning Signals*. These signs and symptoms are not positive proof that cancer is present any more than smoke in the kitchen is proof that the house is on fire—it may be or a pan may have been allowed to become dry. In either case, something needs to be done, but the seriousness of the situation varies.

Prompt action is required to prevent unnecessary damage. The seven warning signals are "(1) any sore that does not heal, (2) any lump or thickening in the breast or elsewhere, (3) unexplained bleeding or discharge, (4) persistent indigestion or difficulty in swallowing, (5) change in bowels habits, (6) any change in a wart or mole, and (7) persistent hoarseness or cough." There are a number of other warning signals. These are, however, the important ones. Prompt reporting of any of these does not necessarily ensure that the cancer is in an early stage. Prompt reporting plus regular medical examination with follow-through on advice given is the best protection available.

There has been some criticism of programs to educate the lay public to have yearly or biyearly examinations and of techniques of cancer detection. The basis for the criticism is that this may lead individuals to have an unnecessary concern about the possibility of having cancer. Those who disagree say that this happens only in persons who are predisposed to worrying about their health. If they were not concerned about cancer, they would be concerned about some other disease or problem.

Cancer detection depends on people and facilities. The term *people* encompasses everyone, not only the person who suspects or knows he has cancer but also professional personnel who understand the nature of cancer and its manifestations and have the skills that enable them to identify suspicious lesions or changes. For a lay person to participate in cancer detection he must know what to look for and where to go for help. He also needs to know that help is available if he seeks it. Professional personnel must have the conviction that cancer detection is important and that it makes a significant contribution to the well-being of people. Following the stage of cancer detection, persons with suspicious lesions go on to diagnosis.

Therapy in Cancer

With diagnosis, therapy follows. Three types of therapy are available. They are surgery, radiation, and chemotherapy. In the treatment of any patient, any one or a combination may be used. The plan of treatment is based on the condition of the individual patient; on the nature, extent, and location of the lesion; and on what can be expected from a given therapeutic agent. That is to say, therapy is individually tailored. The initiation of a plan of therapy is contingent on its acceptance by the patient. Occasionally a patient prefers to take his chances with cancer to the treatment that is suggested. This is his right and must be respected as such. In this event the plan has to be modified so that it becomes acceptable to the patient. Some patients, given time and support that recognizes their right to make their own decisions, will eventually agree to the original plan. The outcome is not always as bad as anticipated. For example, Mrs. Friend had a malignant melanoma on the sole of her left foot. At the time of diagnosis, the recommendation was made that she have a high leg amputation, but she refused to have the operation. Instead of dying within a few months, she lived for 10 or 12 years. She lived, for the most part, an active life. Sometimes children whose parents refuse amputation for the treatment of melanoma live for a number of years after the diagnosis is made. In other instances where parents allow the amputation to be done, the activity of the disease is increased and death comes soon thereafter. Although patients and parents do not always make what appears to be, at the time, a wise decision, the result is not inevitably bad. Whatever the outcome, however, they have the right to their choice. This right should be respected.

The objective of all types of therapy is to remove or destroy all the cancer cells in the body. To date, no method has been devised that is completely successful. The term *cure* is used cautiously. Although the physician may be reasonably certain that all cancer cells have been eradicated from an individual who has cancer, he cannot be positive. Terms are coined to express this caution in the use of the word *cure*. Thus patients who are alive and well at the end of five years are said to have a five-year cure. Those who are alive and well at the end of ten years have a ten-year cure. The patient who is alive and well at the end of five years is presumed to be cured, but this is not a certainty.

In patients with advanced and progressive disease, therapy has as its objective the amelioration of the condition of the patient. The same methods are used as in the curative treatment of cancer. The criterion for success is that the patient be objectively or subjectively improved. Although palliative therapy is sometimes neglected, there is much that can be done to improve the well-being and comfort of the patient for whom there is little chance of cure.

For example, Mrs. Jane Merriweather, who had a large abdominal mass, was short of breath on the slightest exertion, she was anorexic, and when she did force herself to eat, she usually became nauseated and vomited. She was losing weight and strength rapidly. She looked and felt sick and discouraged. Soon after x-ray treatment was initiated, improvement was noticeable. On palpation of her abdomen, the tumor could be felt to be smaller in size. Even Mrs. Merriweather had objective evidence that the tumor was regressing as she could again wear dresses with belts. She gained weight. Subjectively she

felt better. She was able to carry on moderate activity without becoming short of breath. She felt encouraged and stronger. Her appetite improved and she began to enjoy her meals. The basis for the use of x-ray in the treatment of Mrs. Merriweather was palliation. The x-ray did not, and was not expected to, cure. Mrs. Merriweather did have, however, several months in which she was relatively well.

Surgery in the Treatment of Cancer

According to *Primer on Cancer for Nurses*,[64] the surgical treatment of cancer goes back some 3,500 years. The Greeks and Egyptians have recorded the surgical removal of tumors. The first successful operation for cancer was performed in 1882, when Bilroth removed a cancer of the stomach. The history of the advances that contributed to the development of modern surgery is outlined in Chapter 17. Suffice it to say that as knowledge of ligatures, anesthesia, asepsis, and the physiological needs of man, as well as techniques for meeting his needs, has increased, more and more extensive surgery has been possible. As a consequence, cancer in any body cavity or any part of the body may be removed surgically. Some of the problems arising from the surgical treatment of cancer are similar to those that arise in the surgical treatment of patients for other conditions. In addition, there are problems that arise out of the fact that the diagnosis is cancer. Then, too, the surgical procedure is often, though by no means always, more extensive than it is in the treatment of noncancerous conditions.

What is the objective toward which the surgical treatment of cancer is directed?

The objective of the surgical treatment of cancer is the extirpation of the primary growth and the tissues to which it has extended. In the performance of the operation, the surgeon tries to encircle the growth without cutting into it in order to prevent its spread. Since learning that cancer cells can be found in the venous blood draining the neoplasm and the surrounding area, some surgeons tie off these veins before attempting to remove the cancer. The extent of the operation selected depends on the natural history of the cancer, the condition of the patient, and the stage of the disease. For example, a slow-growing cancer that spreads locally by invading the surrounding tissue, such as an early basal cell carcinoma, may be successfully removed by simple excision. In squamous cell carcinoma, however, the lymph chan-

[64] *Primer on Cancer for Nurses* (New York: New York Cancer Committee of the American Cancer Society, Inc., 1963).

nels and nodes are excised in addition to the primary lesion, because it spreads through the lymphatics. In treatment of malignant tumors involving an extremity, the removal of an entire limb may be necessary to permit cure of the patient.

PALLIATIVE SURGICAL THERAPY

Surgical treatment may also be undertaken as a palliative measure. Although palliative treatment is not expected to cure the patient, it is primarily performed to increase the patient's comfort or well-being, and in many instances it can prolong the patient's life.

The lesion itself may be removed, or rerouting or short-circuiting operations may be done to relieve symptoms of obstruction. The nerve supply to an area may be interrupted to relieve pain or muscle spasm. The indication for the removal of the neoplasm is that it is necrotic, infected, or bleeding. Ulcerated and infected lesions are the common cause of pain in cancer. When the lesion is at the surface of the body, the control of odors is difficult. Removal of the growth may result in relief of pain and in a general improvement of the patient. The effects of obstruction have been discussed previously.

Another type of palliative surgery is based on the observation that the growth of some tissues is dependent on certain hormones. Cancer of the breast sometimes regresses after oophorectomy. Castration in the male may be of benefit in cancer of the prostate. Adrenalectomy and hypophysectomy are also of benefit in selected patients. In these operations, the beneficial effect is presumed to result from removing a condition favorable to the growth of the neoplasm. The possibility exists that as more is learned about the factors favoring the establishment of metastatic growths these and other organs may be removed before, or at the time, the local growth is excised. If this should come to pass, then the operation would be curative.

The same principles apply to the preparation of any patient for a surgical procedure whether or not he has cancer. The patient requires emotional, physiological, and physical preparation. The patient needs to know what to expect and what is expected of him. He needs to be able to trust those responsible for his care and to know that he can count on them to meet his needs. In patients who are admitted one day and undergo a surgical procedure the following day, there is little time to develop a trusting relationship. Each step or act in the process of the admission of the patient is therefore exceedingly important. When people are under stress, they tend to magnify and personalize behavior that under happier circumstances would pass unnoticed or be dismissed as unimportant.

Patients who require special preparation because of the location of the lesion or because of the need to repair physiological deficits may be in the hospital some days before surgery is scheduled. Improvement in the patient's physiological status may be essential to his survival. The correction of anemia and protein and other nutritional deficiencies, as well as restoration of water and electrolyte balance and/or relief of obstruction, is often a required part of preoperative preparation.

Ionizing Radiation

Ionizing radiation is also utilized to eradicate cancer cells or in palliation. In either event it may be used alone or in combination with surgery or chemotherapy. It may be used prior to an operation to reduce the size of neoplasm or after a suitable period to destroy the cells that remain behind. The principle on which the treatment is based is that the tissues with larger numbers of dividing cells are more susceptible to ionizing radiation. Although all cells, regardless of whether they are dividing or not, are equally damaged by radiation, the non-dividing cells are frequently able to repair the radiation-induced damage, whereas cell division prevents such repair and often multiplies radiation injury. Many of the radiated cells will not die until they try to divide. This may occur sometimes as long as several months after radiation has been completed. Ionizing radiation may be applied to an area or may be administered as a radioactive isotope solution. The latter is used in a few instances in which the body removes the isotope from the blood and concentrates on a selected tissue or when the radioactive solution can be directly applied to tumor-affected areas. Radioactive iodine is useful in the treatment of cancer of the thyroid because the body removes the iodine from the blood and concentrates it in the gland or in the tumor originating from the thyroid. In addition the half-life of iodine is 8.1 days, which makes it suitable to practical use. Radioactive gold and radioactive phosphorus are sometimes injected into the pleural cavity to treat malignant effusions. The effects of ionizing radiation, the measures required for the protection of the patient and personnel, the nursing needs of the patient, and the therapy are discussed in Chapter 4.

Chemotherapy

Modern chemotherapy is the newest form of cancer therapy. Although some of our chemotherapy agents had been used by the ancient Egyptians and Greeks, their rational use became commonplace only in the second half of this century. With rare exceptions, the benefits of chemotherapy are only palliative. It is used primarily for treatment of disseminated, progressive, and symptomatic cancers that cannot be treated with localized measures. When effective, they can suppress all manifestations of cancer; however, unfortunately, in most instances developing drug resistance makes its use of temporary value. In some instances, chemotherapy is used in an attempt to potentiate radiation or to minimize the risk of cancer dissemination during surgery. The major usefulness of chemotherapy is in treatment of childhood tumors, leukemia, lymphoma, synovial carcinomas, and choriocarcinoma (a rare tumor originating during pregnancy). To a lesser extent, patients with other cancers can benefit from its use.

One value of chemotherapy or any other new treatment that is difficult to measure objectively is the hope that generates in the patient, his family, and those who care for him. During his illness, the patient badly needs hope and the feeling that something is being done for him. The patient is often comforted by the knowledge that he may be helping others by participating in the investigation of a drug or treatment. Even if the drug or treatment fails to meet the expectations, the psychological benefits to the patient may be considerable.

In the chemical treatment of cancer, two general classes of drugs are being used. One type (cytotoxic drugs) kills or injures cancer cells in dosages that are insufficient to kill normal cells. The other type of drugs (mainly hormones and, recently, some of the enzymes) alters the climate or environment of the cancer cell so that its growth is depressed or prevented.

To be ideal, the chemotherapeutic agent would act only on cancer cells and not on the healthy cells. At least in some forms of animal and possibly in human leukemias, this has been accomplished (the use of asparaginase in treatment of acute lymphatic leukemia). However, as more is learned about the nature of cancer, the expectation of finding a single agent that is effective in all instances seems unrealistic.

The following difficulties stand in the way of effective chemotherapeutic agents: [65] (1) Unlike microorganisms, neoplastic agents are not foreign invaders. (2) The biological characteristics, particularly in respect to cell growth and differentiation, are similar for healthy and for normal cells. (3) The patient's own defense

[65] Louis S. Goodman and Alfred Gilman: *The Pharmacological Basis of Therapeutics,* 3rd ed. (New York: The Macmillan Company, 1965), p. 1344.

mechanisms against cancer cells are much less effective than those against microorganisms. Although it has been conclusively demonstrated, at least in some instances, that the body has some mechanism to defend itself against malignant cells, these defenses are usually quite weak and not adequate to control the cancer. A great deal of research is currently being done to see how those naturally existing defense mechanisms can be enhanced.

Drugs that injure cells are of three general types. They primarily work by affecting the mechanisms involved in cell replication. The alkylating drugs and some of the new antibiotics directly damage the genetic material (deoxyribonucleic acids). This damaged material cannot be equally distributed between the daughter cells in the cell division. This, then, results in production of weakened daughter cells or even in their death. Included in this group of drugs are nitrogen mustards (chlorambucil, cyclophosphamide, melphalan, busulfan, thiotepa) and the antibiotic actinomycin-D. Like ionizing radiation, these drugs damage the DNA of all cells. The resting cells are better capable of repairing such damage, whereas the damaged dividing cells become further damaged during the cell division.

Another group of chemicals that injure cells is the antimetabolites. These chemicals simulate or compete with essential components of nucleic acids. They often inhibit the enzymes that metabolize their normal counterparts or sometimes stay incorporated in the cell substance where they can replace the normal counterparts without performing the function. Amethopterin (methotrexate, U.S.P.) has proved to be effective in the treatment of the rare cancer choriocarcinoma. It had produced complete cures of some otherwise incurable patients. It is also useful for treatment of some leukemias. Other commonly used antimetabolites are 5-fluorouracil, 6-mercaptopurine, and cytosine arabinoside.

The third group of chemicals that injure cells directly affect the mechanism of cell division. Because they alter the appearance and function of the mitotic spindle, they are commonly called spindle inhibitors. Vincristine and vinblastine are the main representatives of this class of compounds, and their main usefulness lies in treatment of childhood tumors, leukemias and lymphomas. For the complete discussion of these and other drugs used in the chemotherapy of cancer, the student should refer to a pharmacology text and to recent periodicals.

To summarize, the drugs that injure cells by chemical reaction are primarily useful in tumor palliation. All agents presently available have serious toxic effects. They depress the bone marrow and damage other rapidly dividing normal tissues. Bleeding and gastrointestinal disturbances are, therefore, not uncommon, as is hair loss and skin changes. Some of them cause severe irritation of tissues with which they come in contact. They should be administered only by a physician or a nurse thoroughly instructed in their use, and every effort should be made to prevent them from escaping into surrounding tissues. However, appropriately selected patients and careful use of these drugs can sometimes produce quite worthwhile remissions that sometimes last several years.

Because of the extreme toxicity, occasionally these drugs are used locally either by administering them directly to the tumor or to the blood vessels supplying the tumor. In that manner the systemic toxic effects of these drugs can be minimized and sometimes completely eliminated.

The main group of chemical agents used to alter the environment of cells are those hormones that affect growth of some tissues. At the present time the effect of hormones is palliative. The removal of the estrogen sources (by surgical excision or radiation destruction of the ovaries) can temporarily control some breast cancers. Similar effects can be obtained by administration of hormones. Both estrogens and androgens can be used for the treatment of breast cancer. The exact mechanism of the action is not presently understood. Similar effects can be obtained with these hormones in treatment of cancer of the prostate. Adrenocortical hormones such as cortisone can also induce remission of these tumors as well as temporary control of some forms of leukemia and lymphoma.

Because there are a number of agents that are capable of producing such tumor remissions, the fact that the patient no longer responds to one of the previously effective agents does not mean that he will not be responsive to another. Thyroid hormone has recently been shown to be effective in suppression of thyroid cancers in young individuals. For some reason it is not effective in treatment of identically appearing cancers in older patients. Progesterone sometimes helps patients with endometrial or renal cancers.

One of the new agents capable of inducing tumor remissions by affecting tumor cell environment is the enzyme asparaginase. This is an enzyme that destroys aspartic acid. This amino acid apparently is not required for growth of normal cells, but some of the cancer cells (some of the acute lymphatic leukemias, the malignant melanomas, and others) require it to survive. Complete cures of some animal tumors have been obtained with the help of this completely

nontoxic drug. Extensive evaluation of this new agent in human cancer patients is presently in progress.

Despite progress in the control of cancer, much remains to be accomplished. Not all patients who have an incurable form of the disease are diagnosed early enough to receive maximum benefit from present-day methods. New methods are required for the control of the types of cancer that do not respond to surgery, radiation, or chemotherapy. Further progress awaits greater knowledge of the factors controlling the growth of normal cells. Crile emphasizes this point in a concept that applies to all medicine when he states, "Progress comes through understanding the ways of nature rather than from trying to bend them to our will." [66]

How is the patient helped to resume his normal activities?

As the patient recovers, he is helped to resume responsibility for meeting his own needs and to prepare to return to his family and the community. Sutherland,[67] in discussing the psychological impact of cancer surgery, emphasizes the importance of considering every patient in the light of his individual problems. Each person makes his own adjustment to his kind of cancer and its treatment. Sutherland [68] also stresses that the cancer patient is under a special and severe form of stress. The psychological mechanisms of the defense that he utilizes are those he has learned to use in coping with the world. Just as patients use avoidance and denial to defend themselves against anxiety before diagnosis and treatment, they use it after surgery to protect themselves against the anxiety induced by the therapy. They also experience grief, depression, and dependency. Some patients may be so seriously depressed that they cannot recover without help. For most patients, depression is a forerunner of recovery. Instead of becoming depressed, some patients express their anger by projecting their feelings to members of the family and the nursing personnel.

In cancer and its treatment, many factors may cause psychological stress. The fact that the disease is cancer rather than some other disease is one. Stress is particularly likely to arise out of treatment when the effects of treatment are obvious or when a bodily function is altered in a way that is obvious to the individual and/ or to others. The patient often experiences shock when he realizes the extent of the opera-

[66] Crile, "The Cancer Problem," *op. cit.,* p. 380.
[67] Arthur M. Sutherland: "Psychological Impact of Cancer Surgery," *Public Health Rep.,* **67:**1143 (Nov.) 1952.
[68] *Ibid.*

tion or the nature of the change in function. He becomes concerned about how this change in appearance or function will affect his relationship with members of his family, his friends, and his co-workers. His concern extends to how this change is going to affect his ability to make a living.

In the study by Sutherland *et al.*[69] of the problems in living created by colostomy and what patients did to solve these problems, the authors emphasize that one of the most significant factors is a supportive spouse or home situation. The adjustment of the patient was in general more rapid and more satisfactory when the husband and wife relationship was favorable. In families where the relationship had been poor before the colostomy was performed, the relationship deteriorated after it. These findings point to the desirability of utilizing family members whose feelings toward the patient are positive in his rehabilitation. Nurses are not responsible for the nature of family relationships of their patients, but they can and do observe these relationships. This information can be used in planning to meet the needs of the patient. Recognition of the importance of the family to the rehabilitation of the patient should result in including them in plans made to meet the needs of the patient. Sutherland *et al.*[70] state that the family must understand the needs of the patient and why they are important to him if they are to give him adequate support. The family may require considerable interpretation. To fulfill their supportive role, family members need to have their efforts recognized and appreciated. The nurse must remember that families are people, too. There are reasons for their behavior, be it calm, kind, thoughtful, helpful, frantic, neglectful, or unkind. Whatever the behavior of relatives of the patient, they, too, should be treated with courtesy and kindness. Their attempts at being helpful should be guided and appreciated. Relatives can sometimes be of help to themselves and to the patient if they can assist with certain aspects of his care. Because nurses cannot and should not try to be all things to all people, problems with relatives of the patient should be discussed with the physician. The purpose of this discussion should be to find ways of working with the family of the patient more productively. Sometimes the physician can help by talking with one or more of the relatives. In hospitals where social workers are available, the family may be referred to them for help. Another source of help and comfort to the family is their spiritual advisor. The nurse is by no means alone in her efforts to meet the needs of the family for support.

Sutherland *et al.*[71] also reported that patients regarded a warm and supporting relationship with the nurses as important in changing their attitude and aiding in their recovery. The desire of the nurse to be helpful and her willingness to devise measures that improve the feeling of well-being of the patient are imperative. Attention to details that increase the physical comfort of the patient is sometimes neglected. Because lower needs must be met before higher needs can be manifested, the undernourished or dehydrated patient cannot be expected to feel encouraged; neither can the patient whose bed is wet with urine or feces. As an illustration, Mrs. Karlin had an ileostomy in the treatment of chronic ulcerative colitis. She wore an ileostomy bag that was glued to the skin with a type of adhesive. For the seal to be effective, both the skin and the rubber disk that attached to the skin had to be perfectly clean. Any soiling of either meant that the intestinal contents leaked under the rubber disk and out onto the skin of the abdomen, thus soiling her clothing and the bed linen. Because the contents of the ileum are liquid, enzymes contained in them come in intimate contact with the skin and cause irritation. Continuously wet or moist skin also loses its resistance to irritation. Mrs. Karlin was asked to speak to a group of nurses about the quality of care that she received. Her major criticism stemmed from the fact that, until her doctor taught her to care for the apparatus herself, she was never dry. After she assumed responsibility for her own care, she was never again wet. This patient suffered psychological stress and physical injury not because nurses were unkind or unfriendly but because a basic physical need was neglected.

To be helpful, the nurse must be able to allow the patient to become dependent without herself becoming unduly anxious. She must also be able to tolerate projection of the negative feelings of the patient and still remain accepting and kindly. This is not always easy to do, especially when the nurse has tried very hard to meet the patient's needs and wants and he still continues to be critical and dissatisfied. The behavior of the patient is, however, his way of coping with an intolerable situation. If the nurse can accept it as such, she is in a better position to be helpful to the patient. She will have less need to punish the patient or herself for his behavior. One nurse was able to help herself when she was caring for a highly critical patient by saying to herself, "There must be a reason, there must be a reason." To her surprise, when the nurse had convinced herself that the behavior of the pa-

[69] Arthur M. Sutherland *et al.*: "The Psychological Impact of Cancer and Cancer Surgery," *Cancer,* **5**:857–72 (Sept.) 1952.

[70] *Ibid.,* p. 868.

[71] Sutherland, *op. cit.,* p. 866.

tient was reasonable, her relationship with the patient improved.

Another technique that sometimes helps is a group conference in which persons responsible for the care of a patient discuss the nature of the problem presented by the patient. Knowing that others are also aware of the problem is often of help. Planning together to develop methods of coping with the patient is most essential.

Observation of the behavior of the patient is also the responsibility of the nurse. Continued disruption in his sleeping and eating patterns after the acute phase of illness or treatment is indicative of depression. Depression may also be accompanied by disturbances in cardiovascular function, which is evidenced by tachycardia and palpitation. Patients, especially women, often cry. Although some depression is to be expected, severe or prolonged depression is not.

To summarize, a warm and friendly relationship between the nurse and patient facilitates his recovery. This relationship is characterized by mutual trust. The patient knows that he and his welfare are important to the nurse and that insofar as possible she will try to meet his needs.

In the restoration of the patient to health, attention must be given to the physiological needs of the patient. If the neoplasm has been in the gastrointestinal tract or has affected its function, the patient may be both dehydrated and undernourished. Loss of weight, fatigue, and weakness may be evident. Anemia present before surgery may be a continuing problem. The ingenuity of the nursing and dietary staff is often taxed in finding ways to improve the nutritional status of the patient. In addition to trying to serve the patient foods that he can and will eat, a number of other activities may be helpful. One is to be sure that he has his dentures and that they are clean. Exercise improves not only muscle tone but also morale and the appetite. Ventilation of the room and getting the patient into a chair or into a position that facilitates eating may be of help. Eating in a community dining room may create a social atmosphere conducive to eating. Continued refusal of the patient to eat may be evidence of depression.

In addition to the psychological and physiological rehabilitation of the patient, the patient is helped to resume responsibilities for the daily activities of living and for his special requirements that result from the fact he has, or has had, cancer and from its treatment. As the patient resumes increasing responsibility for meeting his own needs, the nurse should try to communicate that (1) the shift indicates progress toward recovery, (2) she is standing by to give him assistance if he really needs it, (3) she has faith in his ability to care for himself, (4) she

will not interfere with his efforts unnecessarily, (5) she appreciates the struggle that he is making, and (6) she recognizes his successful efforts.

The nurse should try to avoid any behavior that suggests to the patient that responsibility for his care is shifted to him because the nurse is too busy or does not want to care for him. The nurse should be sure that the patient knows what is expected of him and what he should expect. She is also responsible for supervising his care so that his needs are met.

Before he is dismissed, the patient should learn to carry out required procedures. The groundwork for the instruction of the patient begins when he first contacts members of the health team with a suspicion of illness and continues throughout all phases of his care. By the time he is ready to be taught to care for his own needs he should have developed confidence in nurses and doctors. The nurses and doctors should also know what the patient wants to know, what he already knows, and something about his home and work situation, as well as his goals. The instructor should know that people learn more slowly when they are excessively anxious. The instructor should be prepared to repeat over and over, patiently and simply, the instructions to be followed. The nurse who instructs the patient should also be skilled in the performance of the procedure she is attempting to teach the patient; otherwise, the patient will distrust her and may even hold her in contempt. The patient should practice the procedure with the equipment and materials that are available to him at home, and he should learn how to care for his equipment. Enough time should be allotted for practice so that the patient has an opportunity to develop some degree of confidence in his ability to cope with the required procedures.

In communities where a visiting nurse service is available, referral of the patient to this agency should help the patient to bridge the gap between the hospital and the home. Problems that did not occur to the patient earlier may arise; minor adjustments may assume major proportions. Even patients (and their families) who seem to be well prepared for discharge frequently require some help and emotional support after discharge. In cities where home care programs are available, cooperation between the hospital and visiting nursing service often makes possible the early discharge of patients. In some instances a home care program reduces the cost of illness and facilitates the rate at which the patient recovers. When a patient is discharged from the hospital early, supervision of his care and provisions for required assistance become imperative.

In some communities, persons who have had

surgical procedures such as colostomy or laryngectomy are organized into a society for the purpose of mutual support. Members of these organizations are eager to assist persons facing surgery and to aid in their adjustment afterward. In some areas, classes are available for laryngectomized patients to learn esophageal speech. Physicians may arrange for a person who has made a successful adjustment to laryngectomy or colostomy to visit each patient who is facing a similar procedure and to continue his visits thereafter. Nurses may also make these arrangements. When they do, they should be acquainted with the wishes of the physician as well as with the nature of the adjustment made by the person called upon to help. Information about local organizations can be obtained from the local division of the American Cancer Society.

In the care of the patient with cancer, the objectives are to eradicate the disease and to assist the patient in returning to as normal a life as his condition permits. To meet his needs during detection, diagnosis, and treatment, attention should be given to (1) his needs as an individual, (2) his needs resulting from cancer and its effects, (3) his needs resulting from the method of treatment, and (4) his needs resulting from the effects of the treatment on his emotional and physiological condition.

What are the responsibilities of the nurse to the patient with widespread and progressive disease?

At the time of diagnosis or at any point thereafter, cancer may be found to be widespread and progressive. Hope for cure or even for prolonging the life of the patient is not expected; that is, death is the probable outcome. For this reason, this phase in the life of the cancer patient is called terminal. The use of the word *terminal* is unfortunate as it suggests that the patient's situation is hopeless, whereas this phase may extend over weeks, months, or years. The result has been that patients in this phase of illness have been and still are neglected. The tendency has been to give preference to those in whom cure is a possibility. Despite the improbability of cure, much can be done to improve the condition and well-being of the patient.

The basic ingredient in the care of the patient with widespread and progressive disease is the firm conviction that something can and should be done to help the patient. Emphasis is placed not on cure but on what can be done. Hope is encouraged rather than hopelessness and despair. Objectives for the patient's care include (1) to encourage and support the patient's efforts to remain independent and useful, (2) to maintain physiological function, and (3) to prevent and relieve suffering. As is often the case, some of the same procedures contribute to the accomplishment of more than one objective. To achieve these objectives the nurse requires some understanding of her own feelings toward death. Most healthy people feel uncomfortable in the presence of the dying and the dead. The words *dead* and *death* are avoided whenever possible. Instead words and phrases such as *passed away, passed on,* and *expired* are used. Until recently little has been available in the medical literature about the care of the dying. See Chapter 3 for a more detailed discussion of the care of the dying patient.

To this point, information useful in understanding the needs of patients with cancer has been stressed. In the following section the needs of Mrs. Robin, who had cancer of the breast treated by radical mastectomy, and Mrs. Alan Wren, who had cancer of the sigmoid colon treated by combined abdominal perineal resection, will be discussed.

THE PATIENT WITH BREAST CANCER

During her regular monthly examination of her breasts, Mrs. Robin found a small lump in the upper outer quadrant of her right breast. For a moment she thought that she must be mistaken, but it was there. After a sleepless night, she made an appointment with Dr. Smith, her family physician. He confirmed the fact that there was a lump and suggested that she see Dr. Surgeon for diagnosis. He reminded her that tumors in the breast are frequently harmless. Mrs. Robin asked if there was any hurry about seeing the surgeon. She had not told her husband that she had an appointment with the physician, and their daughter Margery was to graduate from high school in three weeks. Seeking to delay diagnosis and treatment is not uncommon, for the patient reasons that his or her condition cannot be serious if delay is permitted. Dr. Smith suggested that Mrs. Robin tell her husband that evening. He also stated that if she saw the surgeon within the next week and the lesion proved to be harmless, she would enjoy her daughter's graduation more than if she waited. As a result, ten days after her visit to Dr. Smith, Dr. Surgeon performed a biopsy. A frozen section of the neoplasm was made. It proved to be malignant. Dr. Surgeon then proceeded to perform a radical mastectomy.

Mrs. Robin was admitted to the hospital the afternoon previous to the morning when the biopsy was to be performed. Because the extent of the operation was to be determined by the biopsy, she was prepared for a radical mastectomy. Dr. Surgeon had explained to Mr. and Mrs. Robin that this was a possibility, and so she was not surprised. In planning Mrs. Robin's nursing care, four major elements were considered. First, Mrs. Robin is an individual human being who reacts or behaves in an individual manner; second, at the time Mrs. Robin was admitted, the nature of her illness was uncertain, but following biopsy the diagnosis was established as cancer; third, Mrs. Robin had an extensive surgical procedure; fourth, the operation was a radical mastectomy. The information required to meet the first three is presented elsewhere. The discussion that follows relates principally to meeting Mrs. Robin's requirements arising from having radical breast amputation. All elements had to be taken into account in meeting her needs for nursing.

In the postoperative period the nursing care required by Mrs. Robin was accomplished by planning to meet the following objectives: (1) to facilitate her emotional adjustment to the removal of her breast, (2) to heal her wound, and (3) to maintain the function in her right arm.

When Mrs. Robin recovered from the anesthetic she was overwhelmed by the extent of the procedure. Her entire breast had been removed along with lymph channels, axillary lymph nodes, and the pectoral muscles. Her chest and the upper part of her right arm were swathed in dressings.

In a radical mastectomy a large area of tissue is removed and many blood vessels are disrupted. This results in the formation of a large amount of fluid exudate in the wound area. Although some fluid in the wound is to be expected, large amounts delay healing, and the fluid must be removed before healing takes place. Surgeons meet this problem in different ways. One is, as was done for Mrs. Robin, to apply a large pressure dressing over the area to lessen the exudation of fluid and to prevent it from accumulating in the wound. This fluid drains from the wound into the dressings. When the dressings become saturated, they may be reinforced by the nurse. Because hemorrhage is always a possibility, the nurse must decide when the quantity of drainage is excessive. In general, the wound exudate is a straw-colored fluid that is blood-tinged. Obvious bleeding is bright red in color and should be immediately reported to the physician. Changes in vital signs, such as a fall in blood pressure and an increase in pulse rate, are also indicative of hemorrhage. When there is external evidence of bleeding, the nurse should not wait for the pulse and blood pressure to change before reporting the bleeding to the physician. A point to remember when checking dressings for blood or other fluids is that water runs downhill. Therefore, the part of the dressing next to the bed should always be checked. This same principle is also used to facilitate drainage from a wound.

A second method employed by some surgeons to remove the wound exudate is to insert catheters into the wound to which gentle suction is applied by a suction machine or a commercial device known as a Hemovac. (See Figures 14-1 and 14-2.) As wound exudate is suctioned into the Hemovac, pressures are gradually equalized. To maintain suction, the drum must be emptied of drainage and the negative pressure re-established. The inside of the Hemovac is sterile; care must be taken to maintain this sterility when the drum is emptied, as the serosanguineous exudate being suctioned from the wound provides an ideal medium for the proliferation of microorganisms.

Characteristics of drainage are easily observed through transparent walls of the drum; all pertinent facts about drainage are reported and recorded when the drum is emptied.

Because of materials used in its construction, the Hemovac cannot be resterilized. It is discarded after use for a single patient. No dressing, or only a small dressing, is applied. The catheters may be left in place for three or four days. The patient may be taught how to disconnect the suction so that he is free to walk about.

When Mrs. Robin was returned from the operating room, she was placed in bed with the head of the bed elevated to about a 15-degree angle. Her right arm was abducted at the shoulder, rotated internally with the forearm flexed at the elbow, and elevated. Some surgeons ask that the arm be abducted at the shoulder and that the forearm be flexed at the elbow with the hand above the head. Others place the arm across the chest of the patient and bandage it in that position. The latter position reduces the tension on the wound and therefore is favorable to wound healing. The first two positions are for the purpose of maintaining the function of the arm. In all three positions the arm should be supported so that unnecessary strain and discomfort are prevented. In the first two positions, elevation also supports venous return and prevents stasis of fluid or edema of the arm. The removal of the lymph nodes and channels as well as the inflammatory response in the operated area interferes with the drainage of fluid from the arm.

Whatever the position of the arm, it should be supported so that there is no unnecessary pull on the muscles. A pillow should be placed along the side of the chest and under the arm that is strapped over the chest, as well as under those parts requiring elevation. The pillows or supports should be placed so that they support

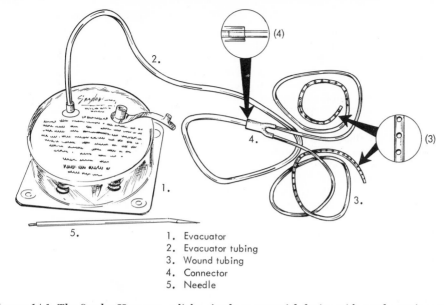

1. Evacuator
2. Evacuator tubing
3. Wound tubing
4. Connector
5. Needle

FIGURE 14-1. The Snyder Hemovac, a light, simple commercial device with gentle suction used for the removal of fluid exudate of extensive wounds. *1*, Evacuator; *2*, evacuator tubing; *3*, wound tubing; *4*, connector; *5*, needle. All wounds, clean or septic, are completely closed. Wound suction is continuously applied from the insertion of the tubes, through the wound closure, and until the tubes are removed. Drip and suction for closed circulation are started as soon as the tubes are placed and before wound closure is started. Drip and suction never cease during wound closure, during transportation of the patient from surgery, or until the permanent attachment to the mechanical pump is made for continued use. (Adapted. Courtesy of Snyder Laboratories, Division of Snyder Manufacturing Company, Inc., New Philadelphia, Ohio.)

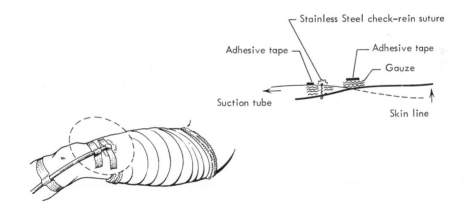

FIGURE 14-2. The Snyder Hemovac tube inserted in leg wound. Schematic of dressing: If tubes are to be in for some time as for patients with circulatory problems, the check-rein suture is used. Otherwise no suture is used. In either instance it is a great convenience to have the wound dressing completely separated from any attachment to the tubes. Manipulation, inspection, and removal of tubes can then be done without disturbing the wound dressing. Keep tubes in line with their skin exits. Do not curl them to put pressure on the skin holes or the skin will become irritated or slough. Pad lightly between skin and tube but put adhesive directly against and over the tube to anchor it firmly to the skin. Circle denotes area before gauze and tape. (Adapted. Courtesy of Snyder Laboratories, Division of Snyder Manufacturing Company, Inc., New Philadelphia, Ohio.)

the arm of the patient rather than the reverse. Because the patient can and should move about, the supports tend to become disarranged and require readjustment. The first criterion to be used in checking their placement is, because water runs downhill, that the most distal portion—in this instance the hand—should be higher than the portion proximal to it. In checking the position of Mrs. Robin's arm, her hand should be higher than her elbow and her elbow higher than her shoulder. One of the common errors in elevating the arm is to allow the elbow to be lower than the shoulder, with the result that fluid tends to accumulate at the elbow and cause swelling. The second criterion is the following: Do the muscles of the arm appear to be relaxed? Does the patient appear to be comfortable? When the patient looks uncomfortable, the arm is probably in poor position. The degree of the elevation, as well as the alignment of the arm, should be checked. When the patient is sufficiently alert she is likely to say something similar to "My, that feels good" or "That is better" when a comfortable position is finally achieved. The patient may have said that the former arrangement was comfortable. No matter how comfortable the position of the patient is at the time the pillows are arranged, she does not stay comfortable. Even if she does, one position soon becomes fatiguing. Therefore, the plan for the nursing of the patient should include provision for regular checking and changing of the patient's position.

At the same time, the hand and arm should be checked and any evidence of swelling of the hand or interference with the circulation noted. You will remember that the dressing extended over the upper part of Mrs. Robin's arm. As emphasized in Chapter 4, when swelling is allowed to continue in a part surrounded by a fixed or nondistensible wall, first the venous return and then the arterial circulation are interrupted. With a loss of the arterial blood supply, death of tissue follows.

In addition to hemorrhage and swelling of the hand and arm, pneumonia is a possible complication in the early postoperative period. This can usually be prevented by encouraging the patient to move about in bed and to deep-breathe and to cough. Mrs. Robin was encouraged and assisted to move and to cough, and she recovered without developing respiratory complications.

Mrs. Robin had some pain in her incision which was controlled by meperidine hydrochloride (Demerol) 75 mg, on request, but not oftener than every four hours. Dr. Surgeon had informed Mrs. Robin that she could have a pain-relieving medication when she needed it.

She required meperidine hydrochloride only twice.

One of the objectives following radical breast amputation is to restore the arm on the affected side to full usefulness. Two problems require control to achieve this objective. One is the prevention of limitation of motion of the arm by the scar tissue formed in healing of the wound. The other is to prevent or limit edema of the hand and arm. The restoration of the arm to full usefulness, by preventing disability caused by contractures, is accomplished by arm exercise. When exercises are to be started and what type are to be used at a given point are decisions made by the surgeon. Some surgeons start exercises early, whereas others prefer to wait until wound healing is well under way. When the quantity of tissue that has been excised is extensive, the amount of skin left to close the wound may be marginal, and additional tension on the incision may interfere with healing. In the early postoperative period Dr. Surgeon asked that Mrs. Robin's arm be put through the normal range of motion without forcing abduction. Mrs. Robin was fearful, and arm movement was painful. Dr. Surgeon reassured her that the movement of her arm would not produce harmful effects and was necessary to her recovery. The nurse reinforced Dr. Surgeon's statements. The first few times that Mrs. Robin exercised her arm, the nurse supported it and abducted and adducted it slowly and gently. She also encouraged Mrs. Robin to alternately flex and extend her elbow as well as her wrist and fingers. Because movement of the arm is painful, arm movements should be started slowly. As soon as the physician's prescription permits, the patient should be encouraged to carry on her usual activities with her arm. These include feeding herself, washing her face and hands, brushing her teeth, and combing her hair. These activities serve a double purpose. They not only exercise the arm, but they improve the morale of the patient. They are more effective than countless words in convincing the patient that the arm will in fact be restored to usefulness. The fact that the use of the arm is painful at the beginning should be recognized. The patient can be assured, however, that within a relatively short period of time pain on use will disappear and by exercising she is helping with her own recovery. As the nurse cared for Mrs. Robin, she tried to communicate to Mrs. Robin the fact that she did appreciate her discomfort but that movement of the arm was necessary if she were to recover its full use.

In preparation of Mrs. Robin for discharge from the hospital, the nurse asked that she be given the booklet *A Handbook for Your Recovery.*[72] Mrs. Robin was taught to do wall-climbing, pendulum, pulley, broom-raising, and rope-turning exercises. Dr. Surgeon told Mr. and Mrs. Robin that, as her strength returned, she should resume full activity. Household activities that involve reaching and stretching and full movements of the arm are especially helpful.

To do the wall-climbing exercise, Mrs. Robin was taught to stand with her feet about 8 in. apart and facing the wall and as close to it as possible. Both hands are placed against the wall at shoulder level. Then, using the fingers, the hands parallel to each other climb the wall until the arms are completely extended. When this exercise was started, Mrs. Robin was unable to fully extend her right arm. This is to be expected. The nurse made a small mark on the wall, so that Mrs. Robin could check her progress. In the beginning the nurse encouraged Mrs. Robin to take her time as she performed the exercise and to repeat it ten times.

In the performance of the pendulum exercise, Mrs. Robin was taught to stand with her feet 8 in. apart and to bend forward, allowing her arms to hang toward the floor. At first she allowed her arms to dangle and then she swung them back and forth. Eventually, she was able to swing them in circles.

To perform the pulley exercises, an 8-ft length of rope is placed over a door, a shower curtain rod, or a suspended pulley. The patient then alternately raises and lowers each arm. The arms are in adduction and extended.

To perform the broom-raising exercise, any horizontal bar similar in weight to a broomstick may be used. The stick or broom handle is grasped by both hands with the hands about 2 ft apart. The broom is then raised until the arms are fully extended. Then it is brought down behind the head of the patient. This exercise is somewhat harder to do than some of the others. The patient should therefore be encouraged to try it only once or twice the first few times and to gradually increase the number of times that it is performed.

The rope-turning exercise is performed by turning a rope, ribbon, or string that has been tied to a doorknob or other suitable object. The patient holds the rope in the hand on the affected side with the arm straight in front of her and places the other hand on her hip for balance. Then she moves the rope in a circle without turning her elbow or wrist. As the function of her arm improves, she will be able to form larger and larger circles.

[72] Helen B. Radlee: *A Handbook for Your Recovery* (New York: Society of Memorial Center, 1955).

In instruction of the patient, emphasis should be placed on the objective: to return the arm to its normal function. Although some patients require support and urging to return to full activity, others need to be cautioned against overuse of the arm. This is true especially in the beginning. As the patient returns to normal activity, the need for special exercises is lessened.

One of the expressed or unexpressed problems of the patient who has a radical mastectomy is the loss of the breast and the resulting disfigurement. The patient should be encouraged to discuss with her surgeon the earliest time that she can start wearing a brassiere and then to shop for the type that is suitable and comfortable for her. Mrs. Robin was very much concerned about the extent of her operation and its effect on her appearance. The surgeon and nurse both tried to reassure her that the operation was similar to what is usually done. The nurse told Mrs. Robin about the types of brassieres now available. They are sold in department stores and at specialty shops. They are made with a variety of fillers and in different sizes. Fillers contain fluid or are made of sponge rubber and other similar materials. For the patient who feels lopsided, the filler containing fluid may be preferred; the shape of the breast also changes with position. The patient should be encouraged to select a brassiere that is comfortable and fits her individual requirements.

Patients should be encouraged to resume normal activities after they return home. There is some evidence that patients tend to regress immediately after they go home and to be more dependent than they were in the hospital. If the family accepts the behavior of the patient, the increase in dependency is usually short-lived and the patient soon begins to assume more responsibility. Actually, there is some evidence that the patient who is permitted to be dependent recovers more rapidly than the one whose family is not as accepting.

Before the patient is discharged, plans should be made with her and a family member about when she will visit the doctor. If x-ray therapy is planned and the patient knows this, she may have questions, some of which the nurse may answer. Others may need to be referred to the physician. Some increase in anxiety at this time can be expected.

The patient who faces or has a radical mastectomy has a special problem. The operation itself involves removal of a large amount of tissue and disruption of many blood vessels. The nursing care has among its goals to preserve and strengthen the self-esteem of the patient as well as to contribute to the accomplishment of the medical goals to heal the wound and restore the function of the arm. The accomplishment of these goals depends on the application of knowledge of the patient, the effects of cancer, and the nature of the operation to the care of the patient.

The family may require some instruction for support. They should know what is to be expected of the patient, how they can be helpful, and that the patient may not be very active for a week or so after she returns home. The equipment required for exercise is not very complicated; her husband or son may get some satisfaction from making it. The family can be helpful to the patient by making a conscious effort to note and to comment on progress and efforts made by the patient.

In most women the breast has significance as a symbol of femininity. Some of the patients will equate the loss of the breast with the loss of their attractiveness to their husbands. This often creates major psychological problems. Many of these problems can be solved by reassurance of a thoughtful husband.

THE PATIENT WITH A COLOSTOMY

Mrs. Alan Wren—an active, vivacious, charming, fastidious, intelligent, and well-educated woman of 65—and Mr. Wren had been married for 39 years. Their position as substantial and contributing members of the community was well established. Mr. Wren's income was sufficient so that they had both a country estate and an apartment in town. Mrs. Wren was active in community affairs.

The day after her sixty-fifth birthday Mrs. Wren called her family physician to make an appointment for her annual physical examination. She had seen her physician about six months previously when she had an attack of influenza. She had always been a healthy woman who took good health for granted. She was neither overly concerned about her health nor neglectful of it.

At the time of the examination, she told Dr. Olds that she had had some discomfort in her abdomen but that she found it difficult to describe. She had had some flatulence that she considered to be embarrassing. She also had recently been constipated. On physical examination Dr. Olds found that Mrs. Wren's general state of health was good. Her weight, 125 lb, was the same as for the previous year. Her hemoglobin level was 13.8 g, which was also unchanged. Her leukocyte count at 7,500 cells per cubic millimeter was within normal limits.

The proctoscopic examination revealed a narrowing of the bowel at the junction of the rectum and sigmoid. At one point there was an ulcerated area. On x-ray of the large bowel, Mrs. Wren was found to have an encircling, or annular, lesion. As the result of these findings, Dr. Olds referred Mrs. Wren to Dr. Surgeon, who recommended and performed a one-stage combined abdominal perineal resection with a colostomy.

In Mrs. Wren, cancer was located in one of the common sites. The large intestine is among the five common sites for cancer, and the rectosigmoid is the most common site for the large intestine. According to *1969 Cancer Facts and Figures* 46,000 persons are expected to die from the effects of cancer in the colon and rectum in 1969, and 73,000 persons are expected to be diagnosed as having cancer of the colon and rectum for the first time. Almost three out of four patients might be saved by early diagnosis and proper treatment. The incidence of cancer of the rectum is higher in men than in women, whereas the reverse is true in cancer of the colon. One of the hopeful aspects of cancer of the rectum and colon is that the majority of these lesions can be discovered early by rectosigmoidoscopy when they can still be cured. If discovered early, the cure rate by surgery of these lesions is greater than the cure rate of most other tumors.

Symptoms accompanying cancer of the colon and rectum vary with the location of the lesion. Symptoms of obstruction are more commonly associated with lesions on the left than on the right side. Water is absorbed from the feces as they pass through the large intestine, and the narrowing of the lumen of the intestine offers more resistance to the semisolid feces than to liquid feces higher in the intestine. Symptoms include, as in the instance of Mrs. Wren, vague abdominal distress and a change in the bowel habit including constipation, obstipation, and diarrhea. Especially in low left-sided lesions, the shape of the stool changes and becomes smaller in diameter; ribbon-shaped stools are not uncommon. Hemorrhoids not infrequently accompany left-sided lesions. They may, in fact, be an early warning sign. Bright-red blood can be observed in the stool in left-sided, but not in right-sided, lesions. Anemia accompanies lesions located on either side. Anemia of unexplained origin may be the first indication of cancer of the cecum. Weakness and general debility occur as the cancer progresses. Mrs. Wren had not experienced any of these effects.

The treatment of cancer of the large intestine, like treatment of cancer in other parts of the body, is directed toward the eradication of all cancer cells. The same methods—surgery, ionizing, radiation, and chemotherapy—are used.

Treatment of cancer on the left side often, though not always, includes a colostomy. Cancer of the right bowel can usually be treated without a permanent colostomy; the diseased portion of the bowel is removed and the ends are anastomosed (joined).

Bowel resections with or without colostomy may be performed for conditions other than cancer. A permanent or temporary colostomy may also be constructed for the treatment of a number of noncancerous conditions. For example, a patient with colitis may have a portion of his bowel resected or a colostomy made to allow the diseased portion of the bowel to heal. Resection of the bowel may be required in the treatment of diverticulitis. Diverticula are saclike outpouchings occurring along the gastrointestinal tract, usually in the esophagus or colon. They may become inflamed as the result of food or feces accumulating in the pouch. A colostomy may also be used as a palliative measure to relieve obstruction of the colon.

The purpose of the colostomy in all instances is to provide an avenue for the discharge of intestinal contents. It may have a single opening, as in the instance of Mrs. Wren; it is then called a single-barreled colostomy. When the proximal and distal loops are brought to the surface, it is known as a double-barreled colostomy. Occasionally there is difficulty in identifying the proximal loop for irrigation; the surgeon should be asked to identify it when this is the case. When the distal loop is irrigated, the patient discharges the fluid via the rectum.

As mentioned previously, Mrs. Wren was treated by a combined abdominal perineal resection. In this operation a left hemicolectomy is performed. All of the bowel distal to the splenic end of the transverse colon is removed. In Mrs. Wren's case, the distal end of the remaining bowel was brought through the abdominal wall to form the colostomy. During the performance of this operation, Mrs. Wren had three incisions: a stab wound for the formation of the colostomy; an anterior incision for the exposure, exploration, and preparation of the area for the removal of the lesion; and, finally, a perineal incision for the completion of the removal of the tumor and the surrounding tissue. Readers who are interested in the details of the operation are referred to the References.

The surgeon had two objectives relating to the nature of the cancer and its site. His first objective was to remove all of the tumor-bearing tissue, including the lymph channels and nodes draining the area. The second was to prevent the dissemination of cancer cells in the lumen of the bowel or through the veins draining the area. Dr. Surgeon also had in mind a third objective, which he was unable to achieve, that is, to preserve, if possible, the anal sphincters.

Throughout all phases of Mrs. Wren's experience as a patient with cancer, the objectives on which her nursing care was based took into account (1) her needs as an individual human being, (2) the fact that she was diagnosed as having cancer, (3) the fact that she had had an extensive surgical procedure, and (4) her resultant colostomy.

Factors considered in meeting Mrs. Wren's needs for nursing as they relate to the first three points have been discussed previously. The discussion will be limited to the steps in the eventual adjustment of Mrs. Wren to her colostomy. It took her about a year to adjust.

Time is required to adapt to major changes in one's way of life. Although the social, psychological, financial, and health factors were favorable, she required time to adjust to the fact of the colostomy and to develop confidence that she would be able to control its behavior. During the ensuing months Mrs. Wren was to experience more or less emotional turmoil, but her adjustment began when Dr. Olds told her that, though her symptoms were vague and mild, she did have a lesion in her intestine. He suggested that he make an appointment for her to see Dr. Surgeon at her earliest convenience. Mrs. Wren's immediate reaction was a common one: to seek to delay diagnosis. Could not this appointment with Dr. Surgeon be deferred until she returned from Florida? Mr. Wren had made reservations for them to leave on Thursday. They would be gone only three months. Certainly nothing bad could happen in that time. Dr. Olds was firm, but kindly, as he urged her to delay the trip. She was quiet a moment, and then said, "You think that I have cancer, do you not?" Dr. Olds had known Mrs. Wren for a number of years and he did not evade the question. He answered her by saying, "Yes, I think so, but I think that it is an early cancer. If it is removed now, there is a good chance that it can be entirely removed. Dr. Surgeon is a competent surgeon. You will be in good hands." Mrs. Wren then said, "I never thought about it happening to me. I'd like to talk to Alan before I decide. Would it be satisfactory with you if I call you tomorrow?" Dr. Olds agreed that she should talk it over with her husband. He recognized Mrs. Wren's need to maintain some control over her situation and her reliance on her husband. Furthermore, in the difficult days ahead she would need the help, support, and understanding of her husband as well as the knowledge that she had made her own decision.

Sutherland *et al.*[73] emphasize the importance of a supportive spouse in the eventual adjustment of the patient to the colostomy. In his studies of families where rapport was poor before the operation, the relationship deteriorated afterward; in a series of patients, 4 out of 57 patients who had colostomies had to live away from home because they were unacceptable to their families. Both patients and family members studied tended to hide the fact of the colostomy from others. Of the 57 patients referred to above, 25 had not allowed even other family members to see the colostomy. Even when the patient was willing to allow family members to see the colostomy, they sometimes refused to view it. Mrs. Wren was fortunate because Mr. Wren was a kindly and dependable man who gave her understanding and support through the months that followed the diagnosis and treatment of her disorder.

To return to Mrs. Wren, who had just learned that her family physician was of the opinion that she had cancer of the colon, though she was feeling shaken, she waited until that evening after dinner to tell Mr. Wren about the outcome of her visit to Dr. Olds. After talking, they decided to visit Dr. Olds together. At this time Dr. Olds urged them not to delay treatment. They decided to follow Dr. Olds' advice, and an appointment was made with Dr. Surgeon for the following day. To give Mrs. Wren support, Mr. Wren went with her. After examining Mrs. Wren, Dr. Surgeon confirmed Dr. Olds' suspicions and explained to both Mr. and Mrs. Wren the need for prompt surgery as well as the type of procedure that would probably be required. He explained that the left half of the bowel would have to be removed and that a colostomy would have to be performed. Despite her expectation that an operation would be necessary, she felt overwhelmed and confused when Dr. Surgeon stated that she should prepare to go to the hospital without delay. Later she told members of the family that she felt that she was in a fog. She went through the necessary motions, but they were automatic. Mr. Wren was also upset but tried to hide his feelings and to comfort Mrs. Wren. He assumed the responsibility for making the arrangements for her admission to the hospital.

For the first two or three days following the operation, Mrs. Wren's needs were similar to those of other patients who have had extensive abdominal surgery. Dr. Surgeon had reassured both Mr. and Mrs. Wren that, as far as he could tell, all of the tumor had been removed. Mrs. Wren's postoperative progress was most satisfactory. On the morning of the third postoperative day, Mrs. Wren passed flatus through the colostomy. Although this indicated that normal physiological functioning of the gastrointestinal tract was returning, it also reminded Mrs. Wren that she was no longer able to control defecation. This aroused the fear that she could never again leave her home because of the danger of involuntary defecation. Her anxiety was to become more severe and to plague her for months. As Mrs. Wren recovered physically, she became more and more aware of the physiological alterations in her alimentary canal. As the function of the bowel returned, flatus and liquid feces were discharged through the colostomy stoma. When irrigations were started, Mrs. Wren found the procedure exceedingly distressing. Her discouragement and depression deepened and she was unable to eat or to sleep. Her general attitude was one of hopelessness.

Mrs. Wren's behavior was by no means unusual. Some degree of depression usually accompanies serious illness and treatment by a major surgical procedure. Furthermore, the patient who has a colostomy may suffer additional shock from seeing the colostomy for the first time, from the involuntary discharges, and from the irrigations. A more or less severe emotional reaction is to be expected, because of what a colostomy means to many individuals. Some of these meanings stem from the fact that one of the important achievements in the life of a child is the attainment of control of his sphincters. Removal of the rectum with the ensuing loss of the ability to control defecation has consequences that go beyond the physiological aspects. These consequences are largely emotional. In a few instances they may be so serious that, despite thoughtful and careful management, the life of the patient is permanently disrupted. In most instances, however, patients can be helped so that unnecessary restriction is prevented.

Two weeks postoperatively, Mrs. Wren was discharged from the hospital. She had made a good physiological recovery, but she was still depressed and fearful. Her fears were centered around her ability to control the behavior of the colostomy and to perform the irrigations. There was nothing unusual about those fears. In fact, studies made on patients having colostomies indicate that these are the common areas of concern. Because she feared spillage, she was concerned with the effect of what she ate on the activity of the bowel. Although the patient may find that certain foods, especially those that are high in roughage, such as raw cabbage and fresh fruits, or very rich foods, do stimulate peristalsis, he should be encouraged to eat a variety of foods. Foods such as cab-

[73] Sutherland *et al., op. cit.,* p. 864.

bage and rich desserts can be avoided without threatening the nutritional status of the individual. Most authorities emphasize that no special diet is required. A well-balanced diet in amounts necessary to maintain the desired weight and strength should be the objective. Mrs. Wren required support and encouragement to maintain an adequate food intake. As her physical and psychological status improved, she gradually added different foods to her diet. Eventually she found that by limiting the amount she could eat almost anything but highly seasoned foods. She rarely had diarrhea, but when she did, she selected foods that are low in residue. She used as a reference *Care of Your Colostomy*.[74]

Because she was afraid of spillage, Mrs. Wren felt that she should wear a colostomy bag. She was, however, fearful lest the bag would be noticeable and draw attention to the colostomy. Despite the reassurance of her surgeon that in time the colostomy would become regulated and that she would not require a bag, she found this difficult to believe. As is usual, in the early postoperative period Mrs. Wren had many liquid stools from her colostomy. As time passed, the number of defecations diminished and the contents became less fluid and more formed. In the early postoperative period, the bowel responds by increasing its activity and allowing less time for the absorption of water, resulting in liquid feces. As the activity of the bowel diminishes, water is absorbed and the stool becomes formed. The period in which her bowel was adapting to the artificial opening was a very trying time for Mrs. Wren, as it is for most patients. When a colostomy bag is applied soon after the colostomy starts to function, the patient is protected from spillage of intestinal contents on the wall of the abdomen, provided, of course, that it is properly applied. When absorbent dressings are used, they should be changed as soon as they are soiled. The skin around the colostomy should be washed and dried and a water-repellent powder applied. Low-lying areas such as the groin should be checked and washed as necessary. In the reapplication of dressings, the fact that water runs downhill should serve as a guide to their placement. Dressings should be fluffed to increase the surface for absorption and placed around the colostomy forming an encircling mound. They have little value when they are piled on top of the colostomy. When the bed linens are soiled, they should be changed. After the patient is clean and dry, the room should be aired.

At the time the dressing is changed, the skin

74 *Care of Your Colostomy* (New York: American Cancer Society, Inc., 1959), pp. 18–19.

around the colostomy should be checked for signs of redness or excoriation. The colostomy itself should be observed for any changes in appearance. When the patient has an anterior abdominal incision, the dressing should be protected from, and checked for evidence of, soiling. Any abnormalities should be discovered and reported to the surgeon.

An early decision that Mrs. Wren had to make was whether or not to irrigate her colostomy. Her surgeon had recommended that she irrigate it daily, but Dr. Olds had suggested to her that she might prefer to regulate the colostomy without irrigation. She decided after several weeks to irrigate. After some trial and error, she also decided to irrigate at night as this allowed time for any solution left in the intestine to be discharged. During her first few weeks at home Mrs. Wren had the help of a practical nurse, who was under the supervision of a visiting nurse who came in three times a week. In time Mrs. Wren was able to assume full responsibility for herself, including the irrigation of her colostomy, which took about an hour each evening. After about a year, Mrs. Wren had developed sufficient confidence that she and her husband took a trip around the world. She took a bottle of paregoric and the names of physicians that she could consult with should she need their services. Although she took a colostomy bag, she had graduated to wearing a piece of soft tissue lubricated with a small quantity of petroleum jelly over the colostomy. She wore an elastic girdle to hold it in place. During the entire trip, she spent only one day in her hotel room because of diarrhea. This was the only time that she needed her colostomy bag. When she returned home, she resumed her social and community activities.

Not all patients make as complete an adjustment to a colostomy as did Mrs. Wren. She was fortunate in that, as a person, she had the inner resources that made it possible for her to recover from the emotional shock created by having a colostomy. She was most fortunate in having an understanding and supporting husband as well as the financial resources to provide for her needs. Her medical and nursing care also contributed to her recovery. As a result of these and other factors, Mrs. Wren made a complete recovery.

Not all patients make as complete a recovery as Mrs. Wren. This is reflected in some degree of curtailment of their activities. Reasons given include fear of spillage, feelings of being unacceptable to others, the fear of being offensive because of odor, the fear of gas escaping, and the time required for irrigation. An occasional patient spends his entire day irrigating his colostomy. The problems confronting the patient are those illustrated by Mrs. Wren. They include (1) acceptance of the colostomy as necessary and manageable, (2) irrigations—if required, (3) what is worn over the colostomy, and (4) diet—to the end that the food intake is adequate in quantity and quality. The overall objective should be to help the individual with a colostomy to learn to manage it so that, although it is necessary to his remaining alive, it does not become the focus of his life.

Some of the factors in the patient's acceptance of the colostomy have been presented in the discussion of Mrs. Wren. To these might be added that patients regard a warm and supporting relationship with nurses as important in changing their outlook and aiding in their recovery. Moreover, an operation such as a colostomy lowers the self-esteem of the patient. Attention should be paid in the care of the patient to preventing further decrease in his self-esteem by the way in which care is given.

Patients who have a natural bowel movement at a regular time each day do not require colostomy irrigations. The patient who does not, or who, like Mrs. Wren, feels more secure if he irrigates his colostomy, is taught to irrigate it.

When irrigation is required, the patient and, if possible, a member of the family should be taught the procedure to be followed before the patient leaves the hospital. The equipment that the patient expects to use should be procured and the patient should use it when he is learning to irrigate his colostomy. Such factors as whether the patient has a bathroom that he can use and the time of day that it is available should be considered in selecting the time to irrigate the colostomy. The nurse who instructs the patient should be competent and skillful. The patient can be expected to be highly anxious, and his anxiety decreases his ability to learn. As a result, instruction may need to be repeated over and over. Learning is also easier when the person providing the instruction is understanding and supporting. A person under stress is likely to interpret the behavior of the nurse in terms of himself. If the nurse is incompetent or appears to find the performance of the procedure distasteful, her behavior is likely to increase the anxiety of the patient and impair his ability to learn.

IRRIGATION OF THE COLOSTOMY

Many hospitals have developed a procedure that they have found to be satisfactory. For hospitals lacking such a procedure, The American Cancer Society has a booklet, *Care of Your Colostomy* [75] which may prove helpful;

[75] *Ibid.,* pp. 12–14.

it outlines a procedure for colostomy irrigation adapted for use at home. This same procedure can also be followed in the hospital. The instruction of the patient should be based on the fact that the purpose of the colostomy irrigation is the same as that of an enema. The same general principles apply in both instances. There is one important difference. The anal sphincters normally prevent the fluid from returning immediately. Because there is no sphincter at the opening of the colostomy, fluid may return as rapidly as it is introduced. A guard is required to prevent the backflow of fluid while it is introduced. A guard can be made by cutting off the tip of a rubber bulb syringe (ear syringe) and making an opening in the opposite end. The catheter is then introduced through the upper part of the bulb and down through the tip of the syringe. The position assumed by the patient during colostomy irrigation usually differs from that suggested for an enema. The patient sits on the toilet or a low stool and uses the toilet or a pail to catch the return. A plastic sleeve or conduit placed over the colostomy is helpful to direct the flow of the contents of the colon into the appropriate receptacle. Before the catheter is introduced, the air should be removed and the catheter lubricated as for an enema. When there is resistance to the passage of the catheter, force should not be used as the bowel can be perforated by its forcible introduction. Rather, the clamp on the tubing should be opened and water allowed to flow into the intestine as the tube is introduced; the water opens the lumen of the bowel. Because the opening into the colostomy may narrow with the passage of time, some surgeons teach patients to dilate the colostomy by inserting a finger into its opening and gently rotating it.

The amount of solution required to effectively cleanse the bowel varies. Some patients use as little as a pint, whereas others use a quart or more. Some doctors advise patients to use warm water, whereas others suggest that 2 tsp of salt or 1 tsp of baking soda be added to a quart of water. The frequency with which different individuals require irrigation also varies. Occasionally an individual has a regular evacuation and remains clean and dry in between. Some patients irrigate daily. Others irrigate only every second or third day. Timing is something that the patient has to learn by experience. After the patient becomes adept in the performance of the procedure, the total length of time required should not be more than one half to three quarters of an hour. If he consistently takes more than an hour, he should be encouraged to discuss this problem with his physician. The patient should aim toward the development of a regular routine and schedule that he follows. The patient should be assured that after he is adjusted, the schedule does not have to be followed slavishly. Moreover, the time selected for the irrigation should take into account the needs of other members of the family as well as those of the patient. The time selected should be one that enables the patient to be comfortable and relaxed. The colon is sensitive to the feelings of the person. Feelings of pressure or tension have an adverse effect on the activity of the bowel.

The patient should be prepared for the difficulties that are encountered in the performance of the procedure. Painful cramping is caused by the too rapid introduction of fluid into the intestine or by too large a volume; the flow of water should be stopped and the height of the fluid container lowered.

Just as with an enema, the results obtained from a colostomy irrigation may be inadequate. This may be caused by constipation or by fatigue or nervous strain. When the fluid does not return after a suitable interval, it may be siphoned back. If the flow is just slow to return, massage of the abdomen may hasten its return.

Because the mucous membrane lining the colostomy is fragile, irritation may cause a small amount of bleeding; a small amount of blood staining the gauze covering the colostomy usually is indicative of irritation.

Doctors vary in their recommendations to patients about what type of covering to wear over the colostomy. Some recommend that a colostomy bag be worn. Others prefer that a small, flat dressing—gauze, paper tissue, or cloth—be worn. A small amount of petroleum jelly placed over the colostomy lessens irritation. A girdle or supporter is worn to hold the dressing in place.

With the exception of odors caused by escaping flatus, odors can be controlled by attention to scrupulous cleanliness. The skin around the colostomy should be thoroughly washed with soap and water, and any equipment used must be kept clean. Equipment includes not only the colostomy bag, if one is worn, but girdles and irrigating equipment. There are deodorizing agents that can be taken by mouth or inserted into the colostomy, but those taken by mouth often cause diarrhea.

Despite careful instruction of the patient and a member of his family before his discharge from the hospital, the patient frequently requires, or benefits from, some assistance in adjusting to his home situation. In communities where a visiting nurse service is available, referral of the patient for this service should be considered. Patients are seldom fully recovered at the time of discharge. The home situation

and family relationships may differ from those perceived by nurses and physicians who care for the patient in the hospital. For example, Mrs. Wren required continuing help and support for several months. The fact that it was available to her undoubtedly contributed to her eventual recovery. During the period of adjustment, the members of the family frequently require help in understanding the needs of the patient and their role in helping him. The visiting nurse is accustomed to working with patients and their families in the home situation. She can guide them in working out practical and acceptable solutions to problems as they arise.

In communities where there are colostomy clubs, some persons gain comfort and help from other members of the club. They learn that they are not alone, as many others have a similar problem. They have an opportunity to learn from each other and to give each other mutual support.

The successful management of a colostomy by an individual requires knowledge, skill, and confidence that it can be managed without its being an undue burden. Whether or not the patient eventually achieves success depends on the patient, his family, and the quality of professional service that he receives during the entire period of his illness and recovery. There are a few patients who are, despite excellent management, unable to adjust successfully to a colostomy, but most patients will adjust successfully with appropriate assistance. The adjustment of the patient is facilitated by all the members of the health team working with the patient and the members of his family to meet the needs of the patient at each stage of his recovery.

Cancer Quacks

No discussion of the problems created by neoplasms is complete without some consideration of why people consult cancer quacks and of the kinds of information useful in distinguishing between a quack and a bona fide physician. First, quacks are not unique to cancer. They seek out people who have a health problem that is not easily solved by available methods of treatment. Any long-term and disabling illness offers the quack an opportunity to offer sick people hope and to exploit their feelings to his own ends. Sometimes a quack treats many types of disease including arthritis, cancer, diabetes mellitus, and gout.

Possibly cancer offers a more fertile field for the quack than many other diseases because people all too often regard cancer as a mysterious and hopeless disease having a poor prognosis. Knowledge or even a suspicion that cancer is a possibility may cause the person and his family to go into a state of panic. This may result in the person grasping at straws and seeking help from someone who promises cure —the cancer quack.

When a person consults a cancer quack for diagnosis and treatment, he may be "cured" because he does not have cancer. Persons who do have cancer may lose valuable time or undergo treatments that spread rather than eradicate the growth. Persons who are in the terminal phase of cancer may experience an extended period of declining health. As the patient and members of his family observe his failure to respond to treatment, their anxiety increases as they wonder whether all that can and should be is being done. When they are told or read about a "doctor" who not only promises but is able to cure persons who are seriously ill with cancer by injections of a magic solution or rays of a mysterious light, they may be sorely tempted to consult him.

One form of protection of the patient and his family is the kind of supportive care that convinces them that all that can be done will be done. Among the values to patients who participate in studies of drugs and other treatments for cancer is that they are offered hope that they will be benefited in time. Perhaps at least as important is the interest that medical and nursing personnel express in their behavior and progress. Many patients take pride in knowing that they may die making a contribution to knowledge of the prevention and treatment of cancer.

To help people avoid cancer quacks, the American Cancer Society has prepared a group of criteria that the public can use in the selection or rejection of a doctor to diagnose and treat cancer. They are [76]

1. Be suspicious of a doctor who promises a sure cure when other doctors will not;
2. Beware of the doctor who says that he has an *exclusive method;*
3. Be on guard against the doctor who tells you that organized medicine is against him;
4. When in doubt about a man who says he is a cancer specialist, ask your family doctor to investigate.

The American Cancer Society and the local county medical society are sources of information about many quacks.

In addition to the role of the nurse in public education, the nurse also helps to prevent patients from seeking attention from quacks by the practice of her supportive role. Patients and their families desperately want to have something done that offers hope. They want evidence that something is being done. They want to feel that those who care for them care about what happens to them. The quack offers this hope and exploits the feelings of the patient and his family to his own ends.

In all phases in the life of the patient with cancer, the nurse contributes to the care of the patient through her use of her supportive and therapeutic roles. She has a part to play in prevention and in detection of cancer as well as in the phases in which the patient has overt disease. In whatever stage of illness, the nurse has much to offer the patient. This is true even, and particularly, in the care of patients who have widespread and progressive disease. To paraphrase Oliver Wendell Holmes's injunction to physicians, "Nurses participate in cure seldom, relieve often, and comfort always."

[76] "Cancer Quacks," *Cancer News,* 12:10 (Spring) 1958.

REFERENCES

BOOKS

Akerman, Lauren W., and del Regato, J. A.: *Cancer: Diagnosis, Treatment, and Prognosis,* 4th ed. (St. Louis: The C. V. Mosby Company, 1969).

American Cancer Society: *Cancer Management* (Philadelphia: J. B. Lippincott Company, 1968).

Bouchard, Rosemary: *Nursing Care of the Cancer Patient* (St. Louis: The C. V. Mosby Company, 1967).

Brauer, Paul H.: "Should the Patient Be Told the Truth?" In *Social Interaction and Patient Care,* James K. Skipper and Robert C. Leonard, eds.

(Philadelphia: J. B. Lippincott Company, 1965).

Busch, Harris, and Lane, Montague: *Chemotherapy: An Introductory Text* (Chicago: Year Book Medical Publishers, 1967).

Cancer Nursing: A Manual for Public Health Nurses (Washington, D.C.: U.S. Department of Health, Education, and Welfare, Public Health Service, Division of Chronic Diseases, 1955).

Cowdry, E. V.: *Etiology and Prevention of Cancer in Man* (New York: Appleton-Century-Crofts, 1968).

Engel, George L.: "Grief and Grieving" in *A Sociological Framework for Patient Care,* Jeannette

R. Folta and Edith S. Deck, eds. (New York: John Wiley & Sons, Inc., 1966).

Essentials of Cancer Nursing (New York: American Cancer Society, Inc., 1963).

Griffiths, John D., and Salsbury, Alan J.: *Circulating Cancer Cells* (Springfield, Ill.: Charles C Thomas, Publisher, 1965).

Haddow, Alexander, and Weinhouse, Sidney, eds.: *Advances in Cancer Research,* Vol. 10 (New York: Academic Press, Inc., 1967).

Herberger, Winfried: *Treatment of Inoperable Cancer* (Baltimore: The Williams & Wilkins Company, 1966).

Hickey, Robert C., ed.: *Palliative Care of the Cancer Patient* (Boston: Little, Brown & Company, 1967).

Nealon, Thomas, ed.: *Management of the Patient with Cancer* (Philadelphia: W. B. Saunders Company, 1965).

The Physician and the Total Care of the Cancer Patient. A Symposium presented at the 1961 Scientific Session of the American Cancer Society, Inc., Biltmore Hotel, New York, October 23–24, 1961 (New York: American Cancer Society, Inc.).

Recent Advances in the Diagnosis of Cancer (Chicago: Year Book Medical Publishers, Inc., 1966).

PAMPHLETS

Nursing Division

Memorial Hospital for Cancer and Allied Diseases Treatment Unit of Memorial Sloan-Kettering Cancer Center, New York:
"A Handbook of Nursing Care for Head and Neck Patients"
"A Handbook on Radiation for Nurses"
"Home Care for the Patient After Urological Surgery"
"Rehabilitation of the Colostomy Patient"

Pamphlets for Patients

American Cancer Society, National Headquarters, 219 E. 42nd St., New York, N.Y., 10017 (there are also local and state divisions; not all useful pamphlets are listed):
"After Mastectomy"
"Cancer of the Breast"
"Cancer of the Lung"
"Care of Your Colostomy"
"The Hopeful Side of Cancer"

PERIODICALS

Abrams, Ruth D.: "The Patient with Cancer: His Changing Pattern of Communication," *New Eng. J. Med.,* 274:317–22 (Feb. 10) 1966.

Ackerman, Norman B.: "Clinical and Experimental Uses of Radioisotopes in the Diagnosis of Cancer," *Amer. J. Surg.,* 115:653–56 (May) 1968.

Barckley, Virginia: "The Crises in Cancer," *Amer. J. Nurs.,* 67:278–80 (Feb.) 1967.

Barckley, Virginia: "Nursing the Patient with Cancer: An Exercise in Timing," *CA,* 17:126–27 (May–June) 1967.

Bard, Morton, and Sutherland, Arthur M.: "Psychological Impact of Cancer and Its Treatment. IV. Adaptation to Radical Mastectomy," *Cancer,* 8:656–72 (July–Aug.) 1955.

Bergel, F.: "Current Advances in Cancer Research," *Nurs. Times,* 63:1609–11 (Dec. 1) 1967.

Binger, C. M., et al.: "Childhood Leukemia: Emotional Impact on Patient and Family," *New Eng. J. Med.,* 280:414–18 (Feb. 20) 1969.

Bottomley, R. H.: "Problems Associated with Chemotherapeutic Agents," *Cancer Bulletin,* 20:29–30 (Mar.–Apr.) 1968.

Browne, M. Kennedy: "Malignant Melanoma," *Nurs. Times,* 65:135–37 (Jan. 30) 1969.

Cipollaro, Anthony C.: "Cancer of the Skin," *Amer. J. Nurs.,* 66:2231–37 (Oct.) 1966.

Copeland, Murray M., and Scott, Wendell G.: "Mammography," *Amer. J. Surg.,* 116:57–61 (July) 1968.

Crate, Marjorie A.: "Nursing Functions in Adaptation to Chronic Illness," *Amer. J. Nurs.,* 65:72–76 (Oct.) 1965.

Craytor, Josephine K.: "Talking with Persons Who Have Cancer," *Amer. J. Nurs.,* 69:744–48 (Apr.) 1969.

Crile, George J.: "The Natural History of Metastases in Lymph Nodes," *Amer. J. Surg.,* 116:1–2 (July) 1968.

"Current Concepts in the Management of Cancer," *Southern Med. Bull.,* 57:7–130 (Mar.) 1969.

Davis, Marcella Zaleski: "Patients in Limbo," *Amer. J. Nurs.,* 66:746–48 (Apr.) 1966.

Devlin, H. Brendan, and Plant, Josephine A.: "Colostomy and Its Management," *Nurs. Times,* 65:231–34 (Feb. 20) 1969.

Dulbecco, Renato: "The Induction of Cancer by Viruses," *Sci. Amer.,* 216:28–37 (Apr.) 1967.

Durant, John R.: "Immunology and Cancer," *Ann. Intern. Med.,* 68:252–53 (Jan.) 1968.

"Exploitable Molecular Mechanisms and Neoplasia," *CA Bull.,* 20:108–11 (Nov.–Dec.) 1968.

Feinstein, Alvan R.: "A New Staging System for Cancer and Reappraisal of 'Early' Treatment and 'Cure' by Radical Surgery," *New Eng. J. Med.,* 279:747–53 (Oct. 3) 1968.

Feinstein, Alvan R., et al.: "The Epidemiology of Cancer Therapy," *Arch. Intern. Med. (Chicago),* 123:448–61 (Apr.) 1969.

Fishbein, Morris: "History of Cancer Quackery," *Perspect. Biol. Med.,* 8:139–66 (Winter) 1965.

Folta, Jeannette: "The Perception of Death," *Nurs. Res.,* 14:232–35 (Summer) 1965.

Fox, Jean E.: "Reflections on Cancer Nursing," *Amer. J. Nurs.,* 66:1317–19 (June) 1966.

Fox, Shirley A., and Bernhardt, Louis C.: "Chemotherapy via Intra-Arterial Infusion," *Amer. J. Nurs.,* 66:1966–68 (Sept.) 1966.

Gauthier, Ruth A., Sr., and Hassels, Anna: "2000 Hospital Workers Answer Questions About Cancer," *Amer. J. Nurs.,* 68:2177–80 (Oct.) 1968.

Hall, Thomas C.: "Chemotherapy of Cancer," *New*

Eng. J. Med., **266**:129–34, 178–85, 238–45, and 289–96 (Jan.) 1962.

Harrop, Margaret, ed.: "Symposium on Nursing in Cancer," *Nurs. Clin. N. Amer.,* **2**:585–690 (Dec.) 1967.

Hart, Roger G.: "Selective Destruction of Cancer Cells," *Perspect. Biol. Med.,* **10**:592–600 (Summer) 1967.

Horsfall, Frank L.: "Some Facts and Fancies About Cancer," *Perspect. Biol. Med.,* **8**:167–79 (Winter) 1965.

Huck, P.: "Coping with Cancer," *Nurs. Mirror,* **126**:28–29 (Apr. 5) 1968.

Johnson, Ralph E., *et al.*: "Patient Tolerance to Extended Irradiation in Hodgkin's Disease," *Ann. Intern. Med.,* **70**:1–6 (Jan.) 1969.

Johnston, R. N.: "Lung Cancer," *Nurs. Times,* **65**:73–75 (Jan. 16) 1969.

Karnofsky, David A.: "Cancer Chemotherapeutic Agents," *CA,* **18**:72–79 (Mar.–Apr.) and 232–34 (July–Aug.) 1968.

Keating, J. L., Yonemoto, Robert H., and Byron, Ralph L.: "Cytotoxic Drug and Hormone Therapy After Adrenalectomy for Advanced Breast Cancer," *Surg. Gynec. Obstet.,* **127**:538–42 (Sept.) 1968.

King, Joan M.: "Denial," *Amer. J. Nurs.,* **66**:1010–13 (May) 1966.

Knock, Frances E.: "Chromosomal Residual Protein: SH Groups in Cancer and Gene Control," *Perspect. Biol. Med.,* **10**:310–13 (Winter) 1967.

Koenig, Ronald, Levin, Saul, and Brennan, Michael J.: "The Emotional Status of Cancer Patients as Measured by a Psychological Test," *J. Chronic Dis.,* **20**:923–30 (Nov.–Dec.) 1967.

Lacher, Mortimer J.: "Long Survival in Hodgkin's Disease," *Ann. Intern. Med.,* **70**:7–17 (Jan.) 1969.

Lemon, Henry M., and Foley, John F.: "Cytotoxic Agents," *Practitioner,* **200**:158–66 (Jan.) 1968.

Levitan, Alexander A., and Perry, Seymour: "The Use of an Isolator System in Cancer Chemotherapy," *Amer. J. Med.,* **44**:234–42 (Feb.) 1968.

Linden, George: "The Influence of Social Class in the Survival of Cancer Patients," *Amer. J. Public Health,* **59**:267–74 (Feb.) 1969.

Livingston, Barbara M.: "How Clinical Progress Is Made in Cancer Chemotherapy Research," *Amer. J. Nurs.,* **67**:2547–54 (Dec.) 1967.

McFadyen, Iain R.: "Choriocarcinoma," *Nurs. Times,* **64**:793–94 (June 14) 1968.

MacMahon, Brian: "Epidemiologic Aspects of Cancer," *CA,* **19**:27–35 (Jan.–Feb.) 1969.

Moore, George E.: "Cancer: 100 Different Diseases," *Amer. J. Nurs.,* **66**:749–57 (Apr.) 1966.

Moore, George E.: "The Importance of Biopsy Procedures," *JAMA,* **205**:917–20 (Sept. 23) 1968.

Morgan, Sir Clifford Naunton: "Treatment of Cancer of the Rectum," *Amer. J. Surg.,* **115**:442–48 (Apr.) 1968.

Oettle, Alfred George: "Cancer Epidemiologist," *Cancer Bull.,* **20**:102–105 (Nov.–Dec.) 1968.

Payne, Edmund C., and Krant, Melvin J.: "The Psychosocial Aspects of Advanced Cancer," *JAMA,* **210**:1238–42 (Nov. 17) 1969.

Perez-Tamayo, Ruheri: "Lack of Communication and Motivation: The Iron Curtain of Curable Cancer," *Cancer Bull.,* **21**:3 (Jan.–Feb.) 1969.

Pritchard, Deirdre Y.: "I'm Afraid It May Be Cancer," *Nurs. Times,* **64**:1128–30 (Aug. 23) 1968.

Radley, Robin A.: "Total Clearance of Pelvic Organs for Carcinoma," *Nurs. Times,* **64**:1749–51 (Dec. 27) 1968.

Schulz, Wilford D.: "Radiation Therapy in the Clinical Management of Cancer," *CA,* **19**:18–26 (Jan.–Feb.) 1969.

Seargeant, P. W.: "Management of a Colostomy," *Nurs. Times,* **64**:36–38 (Jan. 12) 1968.

Smith, Richard T.: "Tumor: Specific Immune Mechanisms," *New Eng. J. Med.,* **278**:1207–14 (May 30), 1268–75 (June 6), 1326–31 (June 13) 1968.

Spratt, John S.: "Cancer Detection: Curability of Symptomatic and Advanced Cancer," *Cancer Bull.,* **21**:7–14 (Jan.–Feb.) 1969.

Stoker, M. G. P.: "Effects of Tumor Viruses on Growth Regulation in Cultured Cells," *Lancet,* **1**:362–65 (Feb. 15) 1969.

Svoboda, Emma H.: "The Child Under Treatment," *Amer. J. Nurs.,* **68**:532–35 (Mar.) 1968.

Traenkle, Herbert L.: "Symposium—Management of Skin Cancer: Basal Cell Epithelioma. Roentgen Therapy," *New York J. Med.,* **68**:863–65 (Apr. 1) 1968.

Ujhely, Gertrude B.: "What Is Realistic Emotional Support?" *Amer. J. Nurs.,* **68**:758–62 (Apr.) 1968.

Vernick, Joel, and Lunceford, Janet L.: "Milieu Design for Adolescents with Leukemia," *Amer. J. Nurs.,* **67**:559–61 (Mar.) 1967.

Verwoerdt, Adriaan, and Wilson, Ruby: "Communication with Fatally Ill Patients, Tacit or Explicit?" *Amer. J. Nurs.,* **67**:2307–2309 (Nov.) 1967.

Viola, Michael V.: "When to Hospitalize for Metastatic Carcinoma," *Hosp. Practice,* **4**:29–35 (Dec.) 1969.

Wangensteen, Owen H., and Sosin, Henry: "How Can the Outlook in Alimentary Tract Cancer Be Improved?" *Amer. J. Surg.,* **115**:7–16 (Jan.) 1968.

Welsh, Marian S.: "Comfort Measures During Radiation Therapy," *Amer. J. Nurs.,* **67**:1880–82 (Sept.) 1967.

Whitmore, Willet F., Jr.: "Wilms' Tumor and Neuroblastoma," *Amer. J. Nurs.,* **68**:527–32 (Mar.) 1968.

Wilson, J. B.: "Malignant Disease in the Home," *Nurs. Times,* **63**:1607–1608 (Dec. 1) 1967.

15

Nursing the Patient Having a Problem Resulting from Disorders in Regulation

Living things, including people, go to a considerable amount of trouble to stay alive. Some of the work and effort involved in staying alive is expended at the level of consciousness, but fortunately much of it is carried on autonomatically under the direction of the two great communication systems of the body—the nervous system and the endocrine system. In any multicellular organism which consists of cooperative clusters of highly differentiated cells there are systems of signals and mechanisms for the transmission of messages from one part of the organism to another.[1]

PART A
Chemical Regulation

Overview

What are the nurse's responsibilities in caring for a patient with regulatory dysfunction?

The Transmission of Hereditary Information

What are the genes and how do they act?

How is a knowledge of the sources of enzymes employed in the diagnosis of disease?

Communication Mechanisms

How do hormones act?

What are the causes of endocrine disorders?

What are the nurse's responsibilities in caring for a patient with adrenal dysfunction?

What are the nursing objectives in caring for a patient with hyperthyroidism?

Overview

The mechanisms regulating and integrating physiological and psychological processes are only begining to be understood. This should not be surprising, as regulation takes place on many levels and is highly complex. The general function of regulation is to enable the organism to modify its behavior so that it adapts to its environment and/or adapts the environments to its needs. Most adaptive behavior is of one of the following types: (1) the defensive escape, and avoidance reactions that serve to protect the organism from injury; (2) the reactions that are concerned with providing materials for energy, for the maintenance of protoplasm, and for growth; and (3) the responses that are

required for the perpetuation of the species. In a broad sense all these reactions contribute to the maintenance of intracellular as well as extracellular homeostasis. Any disturbance in homeostasis acts as a stimulus that initiates activity resulting in its restoration.

Adaptations to the environment involve all aspects of function from those taking place within individual cells to the integrated functioning of the organism as a whole. Within the cell, literally thousands of different biochemical reactions occur simultaneously. They are regulated so that controlled amounts of energy are released and the structure and function of the cell are maintained within limits. This is accomplished despite differences in the supply of nutrients and the demands placed on the cell by the organism. Metabolic activities are regulated so that anabolism and catabolism are kept equal. If equilibrium is disturbed, adjustments are

[1] Jay Tepperman: *Metabolic and Endocrine Physiology,* 2nd ed. (Chicago: Year Book Medical Publishers, Inc., 1968), p. 15.

made so that balance is restored. Proteins are synthesized to maintain the protoplasm of the cell. The growth potential of the cell is controlled so that cells grow and divide only in response to specific stimuli.[2] Growth ceases when the need of the organism has been met. The physical and chemical structure of the cell is maintained. Despite the fact that each individual originates from a single cell formed by the union of two germ cells, genetic activity is so regulated that cells differentiate into different types of tissues, some of which have highly specialized functions. Intracellular regulation is probably as complicated as the regulation of the whole individual. Adaptations of multicellular organisms depend on structures and physiological processes whereby messages are communicated from one area of the body to another. Activities in which the entire organism participates to a greater or lesser degree include those involved in the maintenance of physiological and psychological homeostasis, locomotion, sensation, and psychic processes. All these activities depend on the function of individual cells, tissues, organs, and systems, but no part of the organism functions independently of other parts. There is an amazing unity of biological control at all levels of organization. Through regulation, structure and function of the parts are maintained within limits, so that the needs of the entire organism are met. Priority is usually given to basic needs. When the basic needs are met more or less automatically, attention can be devoted to higher needs.

Regulatory agencies are of two general types —chemical and neurochemical, or neurohumoral. Formerly the regulation of intracellular activities was thought to be entirely chemical. Recent findings support the belief that the nervous system probably also participates. Chemical regulators within the cell include genes, enzymes, and vitamins. Products of metabolism, such as carbon dioxide, also influence the activity of the cells; consequently, they are regulatory. Two types of agencies are involved in the communication of messages from one part of the body to another. The older and more primitive type is the hormones; the other is the nervous system.

Before discussing specific regulatory structures and functions and the effects of injury or disease of specific structures, the general implications of disturbances in regulation will be presented. To reiterate, regulation enables the organism to maintain the function of cells, tissues, organs, and systems within the central range described as normal. Regulatory mechanisms prevent the excessive excursions of func-

tion that are incompatible with the safety and survival of the individual. They do this despite changes in the internal or external environment. A change in the internal or external environment acts as a stimulus that sets into motion a change or series of changes that correct the effects of the disturbance, or remove the individual from it.

Etiology of Disorders in Regulation

Some general causative agents that produce malfunction, injury, and disease of regulatory structures include infectious agents, autoimmune responses, trauma, vascular disturbances, poisons, neoplasms, developmental defects, and psychogenic disorders. Particularly in the brain, disturbance in the blood supply is a frequent source of injury. Traumatic injury to the brain and other parts of the nervous system is not infrequent. Neoplasms involving endocrine glands differ from those in other parts of the body inasmuch as they sometimes secrete the hormone of the parent gland, thus causing signs and symptoms of hyperfunction. Regulatory facilities are also subject to defective development that may be of genetic origin, or they may result from a lack or excess of required materials or injury at a critical point in the process of development. Disturbances may also result from the failure of a target cell to respond to agencies controlling its function. For example, in some instances hyperactivity of the adrenal cortex appears to result from the failure of the gland to respond to the governing influence of the adrenocorticotropic hormone (ACTH). Diabetes mellitus may be caused, in some instances, by loss of sensitivity of cells to insulin.

Disturbances in regulation with alterations in physiological or psychological behavior may arise out of the manner in which the individual perceives his situation. Thus harmless things or situations may be the source of malfunction. Six-year-old Bobby Tears presented an extreme example of disturbed function caused by a harmless event. When he was two years old, he had been knocked down by a dog. Except for an abrasion on his elbow, he was not hurt physically. However, for years, if even the most sedate and harmless old dog approached him, he became terrified and developed nausea and vomiting, followed by prolonged anorexia. In contrast, disturbances in regulation can result in effects that are interpreted as being of psychological origin when they actually have a physical basis. As a result, they may be ignored or misinterpreted. For example, Mr. Heron had physiological manifestations that were thought to be of psychological origin but that were actually caused by a neoplasm causing pressure

² Renato Baserga and Walter E. Kisieleski: "Autobiographies of Cells," *Sci. Amer.*, 209:103–10 (Aug.) 1963.

on his spinal cord. One of the major manifestations experienced by Mr. Heron was a lack of desire to void until his urinary bladder contained approximately 3,000 ml of urine. The nurse can contribute to the identification of the nature of the patient's medical problem by careful description of her observations including the circumstances under which the signs and symptoms presented by the patient occur.

General Results of Failure of Regulation

The general consequence of failure of regulation is an inability of the organism to adapt appropriately to its environment. Except at the time of death, failure of adaptation is not complete, but there is an inability to maintain one or more functions within the central range referred to as normal. Function may be hypo-, hyper-, or disorganized. Because most important physiological processes are subject to more than one regulatory mechanism, a disturbance in one is likely to unbalance others. Sometimes this is useful to the organism; at other times it may be harmful. Depending on the nature of the offending agent and the site of its action, the condition may be temporary or permanent. When a disturbance is of limited duration, the care of the patient is directed toward protecting him from the effects of his adaptive failure until such time as he is restored to health. When a disability is of a long-term or permanent nature, the patient and his family require instructions and support so that the patient can learn how to live as fully as possible within the limits imposed by the disorder. Because a long-term illness involving one member of a family usually affects the lives of the others, any assistance to the patient is likely to have a beneficial effect on the family as well.

What are the nurse's responsibilities in caring for a patient with regulatory dysfunction?

The nurse has an important role in the care of patients with disturbances in regulation. Attention should be given in the nursing plan of care to modifying the environment of the patient so that the effect of the regulatory disability is minimized. This may be done by modifying the environment of the patient so that his needs are met with a minimum of effort on his part, or by supporting a defective adaptive mechanism. For example, Mr. Olena is admitted to the hospital in an unconscious state as the result of a cerebrovascular accident. His capacity to protect himself from injury is minimal. His survival depends on identifying the sources of injury and protecting him from them. One of the most immediate and serious threats to his well-being is the inability to maintain a clear airway. Measures must be instituted and carried out regularly to promote drainage of the tracheobronchial tree and to prevent aspiration of pharyngeal and gastric secretions. Because Mr. Olena is unable to protect his tissues from the effects of pressure, this must be done for him. His future recovery also depends on his extremities being maintained in good alignment and position, so that joint and muscle function is preserved. Passive exercise of extremities is essential to preserving joint and muscle function.

In contrast to Mr. Olena, whose survival depends on others modifying his environment so that his needs are met, Mr. Esbo requires care directed toward supporting a failing adaptive mechanism. Mr. Esbo, who is obese, secretes insufficient insulin to utilize normal amounts of glucose. If his requirements for insulin can be reduced, his own insulin-secreting capacity may be adequate to his needs. One of the objectives in his care is, therefore, to lessen the demands on his islet cells to secrete insulin. The methods employed are a diet limiting the quantity of carbohydrates as well as the number of calories. By reduction of the carbohydrates in his diet, his insulin requirement is lessened. The reduction in his calories should lead to a loss of weight and, with it, a decrease in his insulin requirement. Should these measures be inadequate to maintain the level of glucose in his blood within physiological limits and to prevent the excessive use of fat and protein for fuel, insulin may be prescribed to supplement his own supply.

Following the preceding overview of some of the general aspects of regulation, attention will be directed first to a brief summary of the roles of genes, chromosomes, and enzymes in regulation of intracellular activities and to some of the results of failure of these regulators. A more detailed presentation of the role of hormones and the nervous system in integration of body processes will be made.

The Transmission of Hereditary Information

DNA

Modern genetics can be traced back to the work of Mendel. In 1866 Mendel published his work in which he demonstrated that certain characteristics of peas are transmitted in an orderly and predictable pattern from parent to progeny. Despite the accuracy of his observations, Mendel did not know how or by what means hereditary characteristics were transmitted. In 1869, Miescher isolated a substance from the nucleus of the cell that he called nuclein; today this nuclein is called DNA. He knew that it contained nitrogen and phosphorus, but he had no idea about what it was or how it functioned. The specific question "What are genes and how do they act?" has been asked for about 50 years. Since approximately 1913 it has been known that genes—the individual units of heredity—are strung along chromosomes, which are threadlike structures in the nucleus of the cell. In 1953 James D. Watson and Francis H. C. Crick first described the information-giving part of the cell as a giant molecule of deoxyribonucleic acid, or, as it is commonly called, DNA.[3]

From studies made over the past few years DNA has been demonstrated to be present in the nuclei of all cells. Small amounts have been found in mitochondria. It is the chemical control system that governs heredity. Not only does it transmit information from one generation to the next, but it directs all the processes within the cell. Although most of the DNA remains in the nucleus of the cell, it regulates the activities of all its parts. It has the capacity to divide into two parts in such a way that each new part is an exact copy of the original.

The DNA molecule is a double helix that is sometimes described as a coiled ladder or spiral staircase. A single helix is composed of four kinds of nucleotides.[4] Each nucleotide is connected to the next by a phosphate bridge between the deoxyribose sugars.[5] These alternating units of deoxyribose and phosphate form the backbone of the DNA molecule. The nucleotide bases of one helix are hydrogen-bonded to those of a second helix and may be thought of as forming the rungs in a ladder. Adenine is normally bound to thymine and cytosine to guanine. Although the bases are attached at regular intervals, their order is not regular. It is the sequence of the bases that is believed to carry the genetic message. More specifically, the order in which the bases are attached to the backbone of the nucleic acid determines the sequence of the amino acids in the proteins. They therefore code whether the protein that is synthesized is that of a man, mouse, or tree. In an individual the sequence and arrangement of the amino acids within the DNA molecule determine whether the protein synthesized is

muscle or insulin or whether either is formed at all. Proteins contain most or all of the 20 common amino acids. Each amino acid is directed to its proper place in the protein chain by the sequence of bases in the DNA molecule. When the fact that a typical protein molecule contains approximately 200 subunits linked together in a specific sequence is considered, the possibilities for mistakes in sequence would appear to be large.

DNA, which is present in the nucleus as well as the mitochondria of all cells, normally transfers information by three mechanisms, duplication, transcription, and translation.[6] DNA can also transfer information in a few species of bacteria, and possibly in other species, by a process of transformation.[7]

Duplication. A process whereby DNA provides exact copies of itself for transmission from one generation to the next. The language and the alphabet are the same in the copy as in the original.[8]

Transcription. A process whereby a copy is made of the original. The copy resembles but is not the same as the original. The language is the same, but the alphabet differs slightly. The copy that is called RNA is located in the nucleus and in the cytoplasm. It is of two types, messenger or template RNA and transfer RNA. RNA has two main functions. It carries the genetic information from the nucleus to the ribosomes and acts as the pattern or template for the synthesis of polypeptides. DNA directs the formation of mRNA. The sugar in the RNA molecule is ribose instead of deoxyribose and uracil is substituted for thymine.[9]

Translation. A process whereby one language is rendered into another. In this instance the 4-element language of RNA is translated into the 20-element language of the proteins.[10]

Transformation. A process whereby DNA penetrates a cell and becomes incorporated into the genetic apparatus of the cell. Transformation has been demonstrated in only a few species of bacteria. The significance of transformation may extend beyond bacteria, however, because viruses enter cells of higher plants and animals, as well. Although genetic combination of viral DNA with cellular DNA has been hypothesized, until recently support has been lacking. Dulbecco and his associates

[3] J. D. Watson and F. H. C. Crick: "Molecular Structure of Nucleic Acids: A Structure for Deoxyribose Nucleic Acid," *Nature*, 171:737–38 (Apr. 25) 1953.
[4] F. H. C. Crick: "The Genetic Code," *Sci. Amer.*, 207:66–74 (Oct.) 1962.
[5] Nucleotides are formed from a combination of a purine or pyrimidine base with a sugar and phosphoric acid. In DNA, the sugar is deoxyribose. The four bases in the DNA molecule are the purines, adenine and guanine, and the pyrimidines, cytosine and thymine.

[6] S. Spiegelman: "Hybrid Nucleic Acids," *Sci. Amer.*, 210:48 (May) 1964.
[7] Alexander Tomasz: "Cellular Factors in Genetic Transformation," *Sci. Amer.*, 220:38–44 (Jan.) 1969.
[8] Spiegelman, *op. cit.*
[9] *Ibid.*, p. 48.
[10] *Ibid.*, p. 48.

report evidence that a fragment of viral DNA attaches itself at one or multiple sites to the cell's own DNA and becomes a part of the genetic message that is duplicated each time the cell divides. Furthermore, it prevents the cell from responding to normal controls, thus changing it into a cancer cell.[11]

Further support for the possibility that viral DNA induces some forms of cancer comes from studies of DNA isolated from mitochondria. Although its function is not known, small amounts of DNA are found in the mitochondria. The first DNA to be studied came from the laboratory strain of human cells called HeLa cells. Later in three patients with leukemia there were found similar chains of mitochondrial DNA in their leukocytes.[12]

RNA

Because DNA is localized in the nucleus of the cell, some means is required to transfer its instructions to sites of synthesis in the cytoplasm. Ribonucleic acid (RNA) is required for this purpose. Brachet[13] states that DNA directs the formation of RNA, and RNA, which is present in both the nucleus and the cytoplasm, acts as an intermediary arranging the amino acids in the proper sequence in the synthesis of protein. There are actually three kinds of RNA. The first is messenger, or template, RNA. It specifies the sequence of amino acids in the protein to be synthesized. The second RNA, transfer RNA, transports the amino acids to the proper sites on messenger RNA. The third type is ribosomal RNA which in conjunction with specific proteins forms the ribosomes. According to Nirenberg[14] for each of the 20 naturally occurring amino acids there is a specific enzyme; each cell contains a specific enzyme that functions to attach a specific amino acid to its particular transfer RNA.

In the synthesis of a polypeptide chain or protein, mRNA attaches itself in the cytoplasm to groups of ribosomes called polysomes. The ribosomes move along the mRNA, reading the base code, removing one amino acid from one of the twenty transfer RNAs, and bonding sequentially one amino acid to the next by peptide linkage until the chain is complete. Three nucleotide bases code for one amino acid. The functions of DNA and RNA in the synthesis of

protein have been compared to those of the architect and contractor or builder. The DNA is the architect who makes the blueprints or plans for the building. The RNA is the contractor who, following the directions of the architect, constructs a building of bricks and mortar. The size and function of the building depend on the original directions and how they have been executed.

Nirenberg[15] states that the number of proteins required by a typical cell to perform its functions is not known, but it is probably several hundred. Most, if not all, proteins act as enzymes to direct the hundreds of chemical reactions going on continuously within each cell. As a consequence of the lack of or the presence of an abnormal protein or enzyme, there may be a failure in one or more chemical reactions in the cell that can result in the synthesis of an abnormal substance or the failure to use one or more metabolites.

Chromosomes

Chromosomes are giant molecules consisting of protein, deoxyribonucleic acid and a small amount of ribonucleic acid.[16] Each human adult cell contains 46 chromosomes. There are 22 homologous pairs called autosomes and two sex chromosomes. Females have two X chromosomes and males one X and one Y. To prevent the doubling of chromosomes in each germ cell or gamete, the diploid number is reduced to a haploid number of chromosomes, by a process known as meiosis. Each gamete contains either an X or a Y chromosome. The ovum normally contains one X chromosome. The sperm may contain an X or a Y chromosome. The sex of the individual depends on whether the sperm fertilizing the egg carries an X or a Y (sex) chromosome. Although the X chromosome carries many genes other than those determining sex, the Y chromosome carries little other genetic material.

DISORDERS CAUSED BY ABNORMAL CHROMOSOMES

The chromosomes may also be responsible for congenital malformations. Despite the involvement of the material of inheritance, they are not hereditary in the usual sense of the word. Neither are these disorders environmental. They arise from a defect in the mechanism by which the hereditary material is transmitted from parent to offspring.

Chromosomal abnormalities include the following: (1) Inversion—a disorder in which

[11] "Science and the Citizen: Subversive DNA," *Sci. Amer.*, 219:56 (Nov.) 1968.
[12] "Science and the Citizen: Interlocked DNA," *Sci. Amer.*, 218:46–51 (Jan.) 1968.
[13] Jean Brachet: "The Living Cell," *Sci. Amer.*, 205:52 (Sept.), 1961.
[14] Marshall W. Nirenberg: "The Genetic Code: II," *Sci. Amer.*, 208:83 (Mar.) 1963.

[15] *Ibid.*, p. 80.
[16] F. H. C. Crick: "The Structure of the Hereditary Material," *Sci. Amer.*, 191:54 (Oct.) 1954.

genetic material crosses over in a single chromosome. As a result, the genes are arranged in an abnormal order. (2) Deletion—a piece of a chromosome is broken off and lost. (3) Translocation—parts of two dissimilar chromosomes are broken off and relocate. Translocation is similar to inversion, except that chromosomal material is relocated in a different chromosome. (4) Nondisjunction—the failure of two homologous chromosomes to segregate during meiosis. A number of disorders have been demonstrated to be caused by nondisjunction. (5) Crossing over—the exchange of genetic material between two homologous chromosomes. Crossing over occurs during meiosis.

A number of disorders have been demonstrated to be caused by one or the other of the preceding. Mongolism usually results from the fertilization of an ovum containing two number 21 chromosomes (a small somatic chromosome). The resulting zygote contains three chromosomes, instead of a normal pair. Most patients with Klinefelter's syndrome who have been studied have two X chromosomes in addition to one Y chromosome. The resulting individual is a male who is tall, has enlarged breasts, and produces few, if any, sperm. In this instance, the individual may inherit the abnormality, that is, nondisjointed chromosomes, from either his father or his mother. In another chromosomal disorder, males with an XYY karyotype are said to be abnormally aggressive and to be more frequently involved in crimes of violence than normal XY males.

There are a number of other disorders known to result from a failure in the process whereby the hereditary material is passed from the parent to his child. The type of resulting abnormality depends on the nature of the defect. These disorders are not hereditary nor are they environmental in the usual sense of these terms. They may result from the effect of an illness or a drug at a critical stage in the development of a gamete. Examples include certain virus infections. A number of drugs, including LSD, have been believed to damage chromosomes. In mongolism the age of the mother appears to be a predisposing factor, for the incidence of mongolism rises steeply as the age of the mother increases. The nurse may be able to reinforce the assurance given by the physician that anomalies caused by an abnormality in the process of meiosis are not hereditary. Children born later are likely to be normal.

What are the genes and how do they act?

The gene, a part of a DNA molecule, is defined as the unit of hereditary material. The genome is the total of all the genes in the cell. Each gene directs the synthesis of a polypeptide chain. When it is considered as the smallest unit of genetic material directing the synthesis of a specific polypeptide it is sometimes called a cistron. Each gene is derived from a pre-existing gene. Genes are self-reproducing inasmuch as they copy themselves when they divide. Each gene has a specific position, or locus, on a chromosome. The gene occupying the same relative position on a corresponding chromosome is known as an allelomorph, or allele. Although a gene usually stays on the same chromosome, it may exchange with its allele by a process known as crossing over. Crossing over makes the recombination of genes possible. Chromosomes can also break and recombine. Damage to a chromosome can occur and be repaired.

If both genes of a pair influence a given trait in the same way, the individual is said to be homozygous for that characteristic. If one member influences a character differently from the other, the individual is said to be heterozygous. For example, if both genes influence growth in such a way that tallness results, then the individual is said to be homozygous for tallness. If, however, one gene is for tallness and the other is for shortness, then the individual is heterozygous for height. The trait exerting its influence over the other one is said to be dominant. The one that is hidden is recessive. Thus if the person is heterozygous for height and at maturity he is tall, tallness is dominant over shortness. Dominance may or may not be complete. For example, sickle cell anemia is a disorder in which a defective gene produces an abnormal form of hemoglobin. The person who has one normal gene and one sickle cell gene synthesizes two kinds of hemoglobin, one normal, or hemoglobin A, and the other abnormal, or hemoglobin S. Through the use of appropriate methods both types can be identified. Whether the person evidences sickle cell disease depends on the proportion of normal to abnormal hemoglobin. Only a slight excess of abnormal to normal hemoglobin is sufficient to cause sickle cell disease. Persons who have some abnormal hemoglobin but who do not have sickle cell disease are known as carriers. Although they do not have the disease, they can transmit the tendency to their offspring. The gene for sickle cell anemia illustrates a point made earlier; that is, genes direct the synthesis of proteins, and the specific character of a protein depends on the instructions relayed to the ribosomes by a specific gene. Sickle cell hemoglobin differs from normal hemoglobin in only one respect; the amino acid valine is substituted for glutamic acid at a specific point in the hemoglobin molecule. Hemoglobin S, when deoxygenated, tends to form crystalloid aggregates which cause distortion of the erythrocytes.

LINKAGE

When genes for different traits are carried by the same chromosome, this condition is known by the term *linkage*. Linkage is the basis for certain hereditary disorders that are associated with sex. The X chromosome carries genes for traits other than those that affect sex differentiation. Because the Y chromosome carries little genetic material some of the genes on the X chromosome may not be matched by a corresponding gene on the Y chromosome. If the unopposed gene is defective, its effect will be evident in the individual. As a consequence of linkage, the genes for sex-linked diseases such as hemophilia pass from father to daughter. Because the daughter has two X chromosomes, the defective gene is opposed by a normal allele and the daughter carries the trait for, but does not develop, the disease. The affected father's sons are free from the defective gene because they get their Y chromosomes from him and their X chromosomes from their mother. The sons of the carrier mother run a 50:50 chance of receiving a defective gene and her daughters have the same chance of becoming carriers. A famous example of a female carrier of a sex-linked disease is Queen Victoria. Several of her great grandsons were hemophiliacs because her granddaughters were carriers of the gene for hemophilia.

MUTATION

A gene may change in character, or mutate. Mutations may be spontaneous or induced by radiation or chemicals. Plant and animal experiments have demonstrated that the higher the dose of irradiation the larger the number of mutations produced. Moreover there is no minimum dosage of irradiation below which mutations do not occur. A wide variety of chemicals have been shown to induce mutations in experimental animals but very little is known about their effects in man.

Although mutations are generally harmful, they do not have to be. Mutant strains that are resistant to specific diseases or more productive than old strains have been developed in plants and animals. As examples, turkeys with broad breasts and a high proportion of white meat, and alfalfa that is resistant to drought have been developed as a result of selective breeding. In man, desirable mutations are less likely to be noticed than undesirable ones and may therefore be overlooked.

Another point is that a gene may favor survival under one circumstance and be detrimental under another. As examples, carriers of the sickle cell trait are more resistant to malaria than persons who are not so endowed. Because hypoxia increases the tendency toward red cells sickling, a sickle cell carrier is at a disadvantage at high altitudes.

Neel[17] calls the gene (genes) for diabetes mellitus the "thrifty gene" and postulates that at one time it may have favored survival. Growth is accelerated and the menarche is early in the diabetic child. Thus a girl's chances of reproducing during her short life-span are improved. Furthermore, the tendency of the diabetic toward obesity may have protected her during periods of famine.

In some instances when a gene no longer endows individuals with a selective advantage, its frequency may decrease. As an example, in certain parts of Africa about 4 per cent of the population have sickle cell anemia and as high as one in three are carriers. In the United States, the frequency of the gene is falling in each generation. Presently less than 10 per cent of the Negro population are carriers.[18]

From the discussion of the sickle cell gene, it would appear reasonable to conclude that recessive genes will eventually disappear. In fact, in small isolated populations either dominant or recessive genes can be increased in frequency. In large randomly mating populations, however, dominants do not increase at the expense of the recessives. In other words, the relative proportion of different genotypes remains unchanged.

Types of Genetic Disorders

The observation that some diseases occur in some families more frequently than in others is not new. Increased biochemical and physiological knowledge of the nature of heredity has made it possible to identify the reason in some instances. At this time genetic disorders are classified as (1) common disorders of complex etiology, (2) disorders caused by a mutant gene or simply inherited disorders, and (3) disorders caused by abnormal chromosomes.

COMMON DISORDERS

Many common disorders, such as hypertension, allergy, peptic ulcer, some types of neoplastic disease, as well as others, have a genetic component in their etiology. Possibly there is a direct or indirect genetic component in most, if not all, diseases.

[17] James V. Neel: "Diabetes Mellitus: A 'Thrifty' Genotype Rendered Detrimental by 'Progress'?" *Amer. J. Hum. Genet.*, 14:355 (Dec.) 1962.

[18] Alan E. H. Emery: *Heredity, Disease, and Man* (Berkeley: University of California Press, 1968), p. 167.

DISORDERS CAUSED BY A MUTANT GENE OR
SIMPLY INHERITED DISORDERS

A large number of disorders, some of which occur frequently and others infrequently, are caused by a mutant gene. Among them are the hemoglobin abnormalities such as sickle cell anemia and thalassemia. Also in this group are the inborn errors of metabolism.

As carriers of the hereditary characteristics of the individual, genes have an important influence on the health potential and longevity of the individual. There is some evidence to support the belief that heredity determines the reserve capacity of the tissues and organs of individuals and, as such, has a positive aspect. It also predisposes individuals to diseases such as the ones previously mentioned. Whether certain other diseases, in which heredity appears to be a factor, develop depends on the interaction of the individual with his environment. For example, a person who inherits a limited reserve of insulin-secreting cells may protect himself from diabetes mellitus by avoiding obesity. Conversely, a combination of a hereditary tendency, overeating, and underexercising favors its development. It is probably safe to say that, directly or indirectly, heredity plays a role in most disease states.

Because genes direct the synthesis of proteins and proteins act as enzymes or catalysts in chemical reactions, an abnormal gene may result in the failure to metabolize some substance. For example, phenylketonuria results from the failure of the individual to metabolize one of the common amino acids, phenylalanine, because of a deficiency in the enzyme, phenylalanine hydroxylase. In the absence of this enzyme, phenylalanine accumulates in the blood and the other body fluids. Unless the defect is discovered early in infancy, the phenylalanine injures the brain, causing mental retardation. If the condition is discovered early enough in the life of the child, the damaging effects to the child can be prevented by a diet low in phenylalanine. There is one negative aspect: Any offspring of an individual with phenylketonuria will carry the trait.

Heredity and Drugs

The discovery that there is a relationship between genetic constitution and the effects of some drugs has implications in drug therapy. One drug that has been studied is isoniazid (INH). Some individuals have been identified who inactivate INH quickly; others inactivate it slowly. As might be expected, those who inactivate INH quickly have a less satisfactory response to a given dosage than do those who inactivate it slowly. Barbiturates and certain other drugs are highly toxic to persons with a relatively mild hereditary disorder known as porphyria variegata.

Genetic Counseling

One of the problems facing the individual who may be a carrier or who has a hereditary defect is whether or not he should marry. Despite the inability of the nurse to give the patient a definite answer to his questions, she can be of help by encouraging him to seek advice from his physician. In some instances the family physician will be able to provide the person with the desired information. In others, he may be referred to a physician who specializes in medical genetics.

Five types of knowledge help the physician to predict whether or not a genetic disorder is likely to be inherited and what the chances are that it will be: (1) the manner in which the defective gene is inherited, (2) the ability to identify abnormalities in the absence of disease, (3) the frequency of the defective gene in the population, (4) the character of the gene and the age at which the disorder manifests itself, and (5) the hereditary background of the individual seeking advice.

As an example of the first, sons of a father with a sex-linked disease such as hemophilia will not have hemophilia unless they develop a mutant gene. His daughters will carry the gene, but are not likely to develop hemophilia. It is possible to identify carriers of the sickle cell anemia trait by subjecting their erythrocytes to hypoxic conditions in a test tube; abnormal cells undergo sickling. Some genes such as those for galactosemia occur infrequently. Knowledge of such factors as (1) whether the disorder is caused by a single gene or several; (2) whether or not the gene is dominant, incompletely dominant, or recessive; and (3) the age at which the disorder is manifested is extremely important to making a satisfactory prediction. As an example, a dominant gene is responsible for Huntington's chorea, but the disorder does not usually develop until after the person is 50 years of age. Finally, the gene for cystic fibrosis is recessive, but occurs quite commonly in the population. If two people with a history of cystic fibrosis in the family marry, the possibility of their having children with cystic fibrosis is as high as one in four. Because children with cystic fibrosis are now living to be adults, all of their children can be predicted to be carriers.

Prevention and Therapy

The prevention of genetic disorders is not

easy. Theoretically diseases in which carriers can be identified could be eliminated in one generation by preventing them from reproducing. The elimination of thalassemia is being attempted in Italy. Persons with diabetes in both families are discouraged from marrying.

Therapy of genetic disorders is often difficult. As stated previously, the damaging effects of PKU may be limited by a diet low in phenylalanine. Diabetes mellitus may possibly be prevented by the prevention of obesity and controlled so that the individual can live a more or less normal life.

Summary

Genes, as the units responsible for the hereditary characteristics of the individual, may transmit abnormal as well as normal traits. Although a person carries one or more abnormal genes, he is not certain to develop a hereditary disorder. A variety of factors influence the expression of hereditary diseases. These include (1) the character of the gene—dominant or recessive, (2) the effects of heredity on the reserve capacity of tissues or organs, and (3) the conditions in the environment of the individual. Each of these points has been discussed and illustrated.

Despite a lack of knowledge of the mechanisms for the control of genes, in differentiated cells they must be regulated. Almost all cells contain the same genes (genomes), yet these cells behave differently one from another. As an example, muscle cells and nerve cells are presumed to have the same genes, but they differ both in structure and function. Although smooth muscle and striated muscle have some common characteristics, they differ in some respects. Apparently some genes are active while others are inactive. Why this is so is being explored, but there are no certain answers.[19]

Although there are still many unanswered questions in genetics, knowledge has been greatly expanded since the discovery of DNA. Basic to reading the literature is an understanding of the vocabulary and of the processes of meiosis and mitosis.[20]

Enzymes

Enzymes are proteins that are synthesized under the direction of the genes. Enzymes within cells are organized into teams that function as organic catalysts in biochemical reactions. Like inorganic catalysts, they do not initiate, but they enter into, intermediate stages of chemical reactions. They affect the speed of chemical reactions without themselves appearing in the final product. Organic catalysts have the advantage of being effective at lower temperatures than inorganic catalysts. During a chemical reaction in which catalysts are involved, they combine momentarily with the substance whose reaction they are speeding. In the absence of enzymes or other catalytic agents, the rate at which many chemical reactions occur at body temperature is so slow that life could not exist. The actions of most enzymes are specific; that is, they act on a single substance or a closely related group of substances. Some enzymes are concentrated in a particular type of tissue. For example, among the enzymes found in the cells of the lung are those that catalyze the conversion of the bicarbonate ion to carbon dioxide. Enzymes in the kidney catalyze the reabsorption of glucose and the excretion of urea. The synthesis of enzymes is common to all living cells. Some of the products of bacteria, such as exotoxins, may be enzymes. One factor in bacterial resistance to penicillin is that bacteria synthesize an enzyme, penicillinase, that destroys penicillin. Frieden[21] quotes the biochemist Ernest Borek as follows: "We live because we have enzymes. Everything we do—walking, thinking, reading these lines—is done with some enzymic process." And in the words of Frieden himself, "Life is essentially a system of cooperating enzyme reactions."

Only a few of the many thousands of biochemical reactions catalyzed by enzymes in human beings are illustrated by the following reactions: (1) the hydrolysis of foods in the alimentary canal; (2) the movement of substances across cell and other membranes; (3) the transformation of carbohydrate, fat, and protein into energy; (4) the synthesis and storage of glycogen and fat; (5) the synthesis of proteins; (6) the synthesis and degradation of hormones; (7) the formation of a blood clot; and (8) the digestion of tissue and other debris associated with inflammation. The preceding list of body processes in which enzymes are involved is in no sense complete, for all biochemical processes in the body require the presence of enzymes. Anything interfering with the activity of one or more enzyme systems can be expected to have widespread effects.

As knowledge of the nature and actions of enzymes has grown, interest in them as causative agents in disease as well as in its diagnosis and treatment has been stimulated. In the last

---

[19] Roy J. Britten and Eric H. Davidson: "Gene Regulation for Higher Cells: A Theory," *Science,* **165:** 349 (July 25) 1969.

[20] For a glossary of terms see Emery, *op. cit.,* pp. 225–33 or A. McGehee Harvey *et al.: The Principles and Practice of Medicine,* 17th ed. (New York: Appleton-Century-Crofts, 1968).

[21] Earl Frieden: "The Enzyme-Substrate Complex," *Sci. Amer.,* **201:**125 (Aug.) 1959.

30 years or so, knowledge of enzymes has increased at a phenomenal rate.

As indicated earlier, the presence of a mutant gene may deprive the organism of an enzyme required by the cell to catalyze a step in a biochemical reaction. This can result in the accumulation of partly utilized materials in the tissues or in the formation of an abnormal or defective protein. It can result in failure to digest or to absorb nutrients or in failure to clot blood. It also suggests the possibility that enzymes may be involved in disorders of growth. One recurring and as yet unsubstantiated theory relating to cancer is that the enzyme pattern in malignant neoplasms differs from that of healthy tissue. What actually happens in the absence of an enzyme depends on the process that is blocked by the lack of the required enzyme. Because all biochemical processes are dependent on enzymes, the variety of disorders having their origin in some disturbance in the enzyme system appear to be great.

Because enzymes appear to be dependent on the physical and chemical conditions in their environment, many disorders may have adverse effects on the functioning of enzyme systems. Most enzymes function at a narrow range of temperature and hydrogen ion concentration. The injury to tissue in hyperpyrexia may result from the effect of elevated temperature on enzyme systems. Failure to convert the hydrogen atom to water when oxygen is deficient may be the cause of death in shock.

Certain poisons, such as salts of cyanide, are highly lethal because they inactivate respiratory enzymes. Without respiratory enzymes, oxidation-reduction reactions proceed at such a slow rate that insufficient energy is released to carry on the activities of the cell. Death occurs within a matter of minutes.

The removal of a glandular organ either by disease or by surgery may also be responsible for a deficiency of one or more enzymes. For example, when the pancreas is surgically removed in the treatment of cancer, enzymes secreted by the pancreas are not available for the digestion of fats, proteins, and carbohydrates. Because the pancreas is the principal source of lipase (fat-digesting enzyme), the individual has a problem in the digestion of fat unless lipase is replaced. The most serious problems that arise following pancreatectomy do not stem from a lack of insulin, but from the absence of the digestive enzymes secreted by the pancreas.

How is knowledge of the sources of enzymes employed in the diagnosis of disease?

Knowledge of the action of enzymes is employed in the diagnosis and treatment of disease. Their use in diagnosis is based on the hypothesis that enzymes produced by a cell remain in the cell until the cell disintegrates, or until there is sufficient alteration in energy-producing pathways to alter the cell membrane and increase the permeability of that membrane to the point where enzyme leakage occurs. As the cell breaks up, enzymes are released into the blood. Through the use of appropriate laboratory tests, the increase in the level of the particular enzyme in the blood serum can be demonstrated. Some examples include the elevation of serum amylase in acute pancreatitis, the elevation of the serum *acid* phosphatase in cancer of the prostate, and the elevation of lactic dehydrogenase in acute myocardial infarction. In all these disorders cell membrane permeability may be increased, or cells undergo necrosis and the cell membrane is disrupted, releasing enzymes into the blood.

ENZYMES IN THERAPY

Not only are enzymes useful in establishing the presence and sometimes the site of a disease process, but they have a variety of uses in therapy. They may be administered to replace enzymes that are deficient or to modify the effect of a disease or treatment. For example, pancreatic enzymes may be given to the patient who has had a pancreatectomy. Hyaluronidase, an enzyme that digests hyaluronic acid, may be administered with subcutaneous fluids or local anesthetics to facilitate absorption. Agents containing protein-digesting enzymes are sometimes applied to wounds to aid in their débridement. An enzyme, fibrinolysin, has been studied to determine its effectiveness and safety in the treatment of intravascular clotting.

Besides the introduction of enzymes into the body, treatment may involve the inhibition of enzymes already present. For example, a number of modern diuretics are effective because they block an enzyme system. The organic mercurial diuretics are believed to interfere with the enzyme systems that are required for the reabsorption of sodium and fixed anions. Water loss is secondary to the loss of electrolytes. Acetazolamide (Diamox) inhibits carbonic anhydrase, an enzyme catalyzing the hydration of carbon dioxide. As a result, hydrogen ion is not available to substitute for sodium and potassium ions. These cations are excreted in the urine as bicarbonate salts. When the excretion of sodium increases, water is excreted.

The special problems of patients who have a deficiency or lack of essential enzymes are related to the fact that many of these disturbances have a genetic basis and continue throughout the life of the individual. In these conditions the capacity of the individual to adapt on the biochemical levels is in some way deficient. In some instances, as in phenylketonuria, the nature of the disturbance is known and, if discovered early enough, can be controlled. In others, control is not yet possible.

The objective relating most specifically to the nursing of these patients is to assist the patient and his family to gain the knowledge and skill required to control the progress of his disease, when this is possible. When the course of the disease cannot be altered, the nurse should direct the attention of the patient and his family toward living as full a life as is compatible with his disorder and toward preventing unnecessary disability. For the nurse to be of maximum assistance to the patient and his family, she should have some understanding of the cause and nature of disorders of enzyme systems, and be familiar with the objectives and means of therapy. Because of the nature and prognosis of these disorders, she will undoubtedly require competence in the expressive role of nursing.

The field of enzymology and its applications to health and disease is rapidly expanding. The literature in the field is enormous. Because enzymes function in regulation at the biochemical level, their effects are widespread and profound. By their action or lack thereof, they influence the capacity of the organism to adapt to its environment. Lack of, or alteration in, the activity of enzymes may be the cause of disease. Likewise, disease may alter the activity of enzymes. Without enzymes, life cannot exist.

Communication Mechanisms

In large multicellular organisms, the activities of cells and the structures of which they are a part must be integrated and coordinated so that each accomplishes its functions and has its needs met. Basic elements in a regulatory mechanism are (1) receptors or sensors sensitive to changes in the environment—gain, loss, or expenditure; (2) a means of communicating information (structural or humoral); (3) centers for the reception and interpretation of messages from the receptors; (4) centers for the initiation of messages as well as for the detection and correction of errors; and (5) a means of communication to effector or target cells which receive and respond to the message.

There are two agencies for communicating information from one part of the body to another—the nervous and endocrine systems. In the past, these systems were considered independently of each other. Because of the many interrelations between them, a specialty in neuroendocrinology has developed. Directly or indirectly, secretion of most, if not all, hormones is under the control of the nervous system. Conversely, the level of most hormones directly or indirectly affects the functioning of the central nervous system.

There are many overlapping functions between the nervous and endocrine systems. The adrenal medulla is part of the sympathetic nervous system and its products, epinephrine and norepinephrine, are secreted by other portions of the system as well. Tepperman [22] compares the two systems to a wireless communication system and a telegraph system. Endocrine glands form chemical substances that are distributed by the blood to all parts of the body. They have their effect on target or specialized cells that are especially responsive to them.

Hormones

A common definition is: Hormones are chemical regulators synthesized by specialized organs, the endocrine glands. They are carried by the blood and other body fluids to the cells of the body. Specific structures on which they have a marked effect are called target tissues, or organs. Despite seeming specificity, the action of hormones is not limited to their target organs; rather they all probably have widespread effects. The actions of hormones influence the rate not only of energy metabolism, but of mineral metabolism, as well as the growth and development of the organism.

TISSUE HORMONES

Although some scientists define hormones as chemicals secreted by specialized cells and delivered to distant sites by the extracellular fluids, others include in the definition chemicals having their effect in the tissues where they are released. As an example, the kidney is able to regulate its own blood flow. One of the chemicals involved in its regulation is the renin-angiotensin system. According to McGiff,[23] angiotensin is a hormone formed in the blood in response to renin, which is found in the juxtaglomerular apparatus in the kidney. Although angiotensin can elevate the systemic blood pressure, it is not believed to reach sufficient levels to do so very frequently. Its principal effect is on the blood vessels within the kidney itself, probably on the efferent arterioles.[24]

In addition to its influence on blood flow

[22] Jay Tepperman, op. cit., p. 15.
[23] John C. McGiff: "Tissue Hormones: Angiotensin, Bradykinin and the Regulation of Regional Blood Flows," Med. Clin. N. Amer., 52:264 (Mar.) 1968.
[24] Ibid., p. 265.

through the kidney, the renin-angiotensin system may also stimulate the release of aldosterone by the adrenal cortex. A renin-like substance has been isolated from the pregnant uterus. It is believed to regulate blood flow through the placenta.

CLASSIFICATION OF HORMONES

Classified according to their chemical structure, they are steroids, proteins and polypeptides, and amines. The sex hormones and the adrenocortical hormones are steroids. They are secreted by glands having their origin in the mesenchymal zone in the embryo. There are some overlapping functions of adrenocortical and sex hormones. As as example, women patients receiving or secreting large quantities of adrenocortical hormones undergo masculinizing changes.

Hormones from the adenohypophysis, pancreas, and parathyroid are proteins or large polypeptides. Those secreted by the thyroid, adrenal medulla, and neurohypophysis are amines. Although most naturally occurring hormones are more effective when administered parenterally, proteins and polypeptides must be administered by injection; otherwise they are destroyed by digestion.

Rasmussen [25] lists 35 hormones. There are 19 polypeptides, 10 releasing factors including the steroids, and 6 amines. Of these hormones, all except relaxin have been purified and the structures of 21 of them are known.

How do hormones act?

The mechanism(s) by which hormones act is largely unknown. However there is some support for each of four theories that have been proposed to explain their actions: (1) they regulate the activity of enzymes, (2) they act on membranes, (3) they alter the activity of genes, and (4) they bring about the release of ions or other small molecules within cells.

CONTROL OF ENZYME ACTIVITY

The first and oldest theory is that hormones control the action of enzymes. This theory was proposed after the discovery was made that vitamins enter the cell and act as coenzymes. A hormone may enhance or inhibit the action of an enzyme or the order in which enzymes act. Some hormones have been shown to interact with specific enzymes in the test tube, but thus far this action has not been demonstrated in living organisms.

ACTION ON MEMBRANES

Despite evidence that hormones do act on membranes, this theory is not firmly established. As an example, insulin does increase the quantity of glucose entering muscle and fat cells, but this is not unique for exercise and hypoxia have a similar effect. Whether or not the mechanism of action is the same is not known.

ACTION OF GENES

A third theory proposed to explain some of the actions of hormones is that they alter the activity of genes. One factor in achieving maturity is that genetic information comes into play in the correct order and at the proper time. Karlson [26] states that, because hormones reach all the tissues, they may well act as timing devices for the development of peripheral organs.

Davidson [27] cites evidence supporting the hypothesis that hormones regulate the activity of genes. This hypothesis may explain some of the puzzling features of hormone activity such as the time lag between the administration of some hormones and the appearance of their effects. As an illustration, within 10 to 15 minutes after the administration of thyroxin, new messenger RNA is synthesized and within an hour synthesis of all classes of RNA has been stimulated. Within ten hours, RNA-DNA polymerase has been increased. This is followed later by a general increase in protein synthesis.

RELEASE OF IONS OR SMALL MOLECULES

Sutherland and his associates [28] introduced a concept of hormone action that they call the "second messenger concept," the first messenger being hormone. According to this concept, as a result of the action of the hormone at or near the cell membrane, a second messenger, a chemical known as cyclic 3' 5'-AMP (adenosine monophosphate) is released within the cell where it mediates a variety of hormonal responses. There may well be other second messengers that react with one or many proteins and enzymes.

Sutherland et al.[29] have demonstrated that epinephrine acts by causing liver cells to release cyclic 3' 5' AMP, which in turn causes glycogen

[25] Howard Rasmussen: "Organization and Control of Endocrine Systems," *Textbook of Endocrinology*, 4th ed. Robert H. Williams, ed. (Philadelphia: W. B. Saunders Company, 1968), p. 7.

[26] Peter Karlson: "New Concepts on the Mode of Action of Hormones," *Perspect. Biol. Med.*, 6:208, (Winter) 1963.

[27] Eric H. Davidson: "Hormones and Genes," *Sci. Amer.*, 212:36 (June) 1965.

[28] Earl W. Sutherland, G. A. Robinson, and R. W. Butcher: "Some Aspects of the Biological Role of Adenosine 3',5' monophosphate (cyclic AMP)," *Circulation*, 37:300 (Feb.) 1968.

[29] E. W. Sutherland, I. Øye, and R. W. Butcher: "The Action of Epinephrine and the Role of Adenyl Cyclase System in Hormone Action," *Recent Progr. Hormone Res.*, 21:628–29, 1965.

to be converted to glucose. Other hormones believed to act in a similar manner are ACTH on the adrenal cortex and vasopressin on the kidney. The end products of the reaction are different in the three target organs. In the liver, glucose is released; in the adrenal cortex, glucocorticoids are released; and in the kidney there is a change in the permeability to water.

As more is learned about the regulation of intracellular homeostasis, the action(s) of various hormones will be clarified. To date, efforts have tended to be concentrated on finding a single action for each hormone. It may be that a hormone has more than one fundamental action in a given cell. It may also be that it acts differently in one cell than in another.

PERMISSIVE ACTIONS

Certain hormones have what is referred to as a permissive action. They condition the animal to adapt to or respond to his environment. In other words, they affect the manner in which the organism responds under a given set of circumstances. To illustrate, the adrenocortical hormones are essential for the organism to respond to any form of stress, be it physical, chemical, or emotional. In other words, a minimum level of adrenocortical hormones is required for adequate cell and tissue functioning. In the human being, the thyroid hormones sensitize the individual to epinephrine. The patient who is hyperthyroid is hypersensitive to epinephrine. A therapeutic dose of epinephrine may induce ventricular fibrillation in such a person. Hypothyroidism increases the sensitivity of the nervous system to depressant drugs such as codeine, morphine, and meperidine. A single dose of any depressant drug may result in profound depression of the nervous system. The actions of other hormones are also determined by conditions in the body. In hyperthyroidism, the possibility of liver injury can be reduced by an adequate intake of the vitamin thiamine.

Hormones may also be classed as those essential to life and those required for normal growth and development. For example, the adrenocortical hormones are necessary to life. The same is true for insulin. Although the thyroid hormones are required for normal growth and development and for healthy physical and mental functioning, their absence does not result in the death of the individual.

SOME GENERALIZATIONS

Some hormones act on all or most cells, whereas others have more limited effects. It may be that there are receptor sites in cells that are specific for particular hormones. Thus all cells are believed to respond to thyroxin and the growth hormone. Insulin is required by muscle and fat cells to utilize normal amounts of glucose, whereas nerve and brain cells do not require it. Some of the releasing hormones act only on their target glands. As an example, the thyrotropic hormone causes the thyroid gland to release its hormones.

Some hormones, such as the steroids and thyroxin, have specific carrier proteins. It is not known whether the polypeptides do.

The half-life of hormones varies. For some it is only a few minutes; for others it is a matter of days. Epinephrine has a short half-life, and thyroxin's is long. When hormones are used in therapy, one factor determining the frequency with which they are administered is their half-life.

Hormones are not believed to initiate functions. They alter the rate of reactions, usually by enhancing them, but, in some instances, by limiting them. Thus the cells metabolize glucose in the absence of insulin. In the presence of insulin, the rate at which glucose is removed from the blood is accelerated.

Another characteristic of hormones is that none is secreted at a precisely uniform rate. Some hormones, such as the adrenal steroids, are secreted according to a daily (diurnal) rhythm. Others, such as the gonadotropins and the female sex hormones, maintain a cyclical rhythm. Still others, such as insulin, are secreted in response to the level of a constituent in the blood. Some, such as insulin, are secreted somewhat in excess of the quantity required. As a consequence, after the blood glucose is raised, its level in the blood may drop slightly lower than it was before glucose was ingested. It then returns to normal.

Hormones are effective in relatively small amounts. The effective dose of tri-iodothyronine and aldosterone is in the microgram range. Because of the minute quantities of hormones found in the plasma, direct measurement is difficult.

Hormones are continuously lost from the body either by excretion or by metabolic inactivation, and they must be replaced. Inactivation occurs in the target organ or liver. Excretion is by the kidney. Effects of hypersecretion may, therefore, be caused by oversecretion by a particular gland or by failure of a mechanism by which a particular hormone is inactivated. For example, aldosterone is inactivated by the liver. One of the factors in edema in diseases in which there is functional failure of the liver may be an elevation in the level of aldosterone.

For some hormones, a latent period exists between their administration and the time effects become apparent. In the case of epinephrine or insulin, the length of the latent period is relatively short. Thyroxin, on the other hand, has a long latent period, taking from 8 to 14 days to act. After absorption thyroxin immediately combines in the blood with a plasma protein from which it is slowly released to the cells. This accounts for the long half-life of thyroxin.

For reasons that are not understood, individuals tend to be hypersensitive to hormones that they lack. The patient who is hypothyroid requires a smaller dosage of thyroxin to cause symptoms of hyperthyroidism than the one who is euthyroid. Persons with the growth-onset type of diabetes mellitus are very sensitive to exogenous insulin.

There are a number of other generalizations that may be made about hormones. Each hormone has widespread effects on the organism. Few, if any, functions are exclusively dependent for regulation on one hormone. Most functions are dependent on a number of hormones in adequate balance and sequence. Several hormones may act at the same time or in a series. A hormone may oppose or supplement the action of another. For example, insulin lowers blood sugar; the adrenal glucocorticoids, epinephrine and glucagon, oppose the action of insulin by elevating it. The growth and thyroid hormones have synergistic effects on growth. Some hormones have overlapping actions. Oxytocin and vasopressin have long been known to have some common pharmacological properties. This is also true of the mineralo- and glucocorticoids secreted by the cortex of the adrenal gland. Their actions are quantitatively, but not qualitatively, different. Because hormones do not initiate functions, but only modify them, other elements may be responsible for disturbances in functions regulated by particular hormones. To illustrate, growth depends not only on adequate secretion of thyroid and growth hormones, but also on the genetic background and nutrition of the individual. A serious or prolonged illness at a critical period in the life of a child may also stunt growth. Although thyroid hormones regulate the rate of energy metabolism, other factors contribute to it. This is demonstrated by the fact that, in the absence of the thyroid gland, the basal metabolic rate falls about 35 per cent. Expressed in the usual terms for reporting, the metabolic rate of an individual without a thyroid gland is about −35. Other factors are responsible for the remaining 65 per cent of the metabolic rate.

In health, the level of each hormone is maintained within physiological limits, as well as in a state of equilibrium with other hormones, by at least two types of regulatory mechanisms. One type is a negative feedback relationship between the regulator and the target gland. (In negative feedback, there is a regulatory relationship be-

tween two factors or elements in which the increase in one results in an increase in the activity of the second, but the increase in the activity of the second results in a decrease in the activity of the first.) In the other type, no feedback relationship between two glands has been demonstrated. Rather, stimulation or depression of secretion results from the level of a component of the blood such as glucose, water, or the sodium cation. An example of a negative feedback is the relationship of the anterior pituitary to the adrenal cortex. The level of production of the adrenal glucocorticoids is increased by adrenocorticotropin (ACTH) from the anterior pituitary. As the concentration of the glucocorticoids rises, the secretion of ACTH is depressed. As the level of the glucocorticoids falls, the secretion of ACTH rises. Superficially, the preceding relationship is true. It is now known that the release of ACTH and other tropic hormones requires the intervention of the releasing factor from the hypothalamus. Where no feedback mechanism is known to exist, the rate of hormone production is presumed to be controlled by some mechanism at the site of the formation of the hormone. This may be nervous, chemical, or physical in origin.

Little doubt exists at the present time that the release of a number of hormones is under the control of the nervous system. Regulatory mechanisms can be viewed as parts of one system, organized in a hierarchy with the nervous system as the head. In some instances the exact means by which the nervous system controls the secretion of hormones is not clear. In others, the relationship of the chemical regulator to its neural counterpart is so intimate that they appear to be part of the same mechanism. For instance, the relationship between the sympathetic nervous system and the adrenal medulla, which has been described earlier, is so close that some authorities speak of them as the sympathoadrenal system. There is an embryological, anatomical, and functional basis for this hypothesis.

The neurohypophysis (posterior pituitary) is generally described as an anatomical and functional extension of the nervous system. Like the adrenal medulla, the neurohypophysis originates from embryonic structures in common with the nervous system. There are also clearly defined nerve pathways between nuclei (groups of cells) in the hypothalamus and the neurohypophysis. The hormones released by the posterior pituitary, vasopressin and oxytocin, are believed to be synthesized in nuclei in the hypothalamus, after which they travel down to the gland, where they are released on stimulation.[30]

[30] Tepperman, *op. cit.*, p. 28.

No discussion of the functions of the endocrine system is complete unless the relationship between the nervous system and the secretion of hormones is emphasized. The hypothalamus stands in a key position between the nervous and endocrine systems. Either directly or indirectly the hypothalamus serves as a center for the exchange of messages between higher centers in the nervous system and endocrine glands. The hypothalamus receives and relays messages from the higher centers to the appropriate endocrine gland. It also sends messages to the higher centers apprising them of conditions within the organism.

PROCESSES REGULATED BY HORMONES

As implied above, hormones participate in the regulation and integration of all important body activities. The functions in which hormones play a significant role are summarized as follows:

1. Hormones are important to reproduction and all the activities related to it.
2. Hormones are essential to growth and to structural and biochemical differentiation.
3. Hormones participate in the regulation of intra- and extracellular homeostasis.[31]

Although it would be appropriate to do so, this chapter does not include a discussion of the role of hormones in reproduction. The content of the chapter will be limited to points two and three, with particular emphasis on three.

The variety of metabolic (biochemical) reactions regulated by hormones include (1) energy metabolism—that is, the rate of oxidation-reduction reactions in the mitochondria in the cytoplasm of cells; (2) calcium-phosphorus balance between body fluids and bony structures; (3) water balance; (4) electrolyte balance; and (5) metabolism of carbohydrates, proteins, and fats and the rate of transport of materials across cell membranes. Not only are these reactions regulated in relation to supply, but they also are regulated in relation to conditions in the internal and external environments. Furthermore, hormones not only modify the rate of body functions in health, but they also integrate many responses of the organism to injury or threats of injury. They also modify the course of some diseases. For instance, some breast cancers appear to be dependent on ovarian and adrenocortical hormones for their growth. In hormone-dependent cancers of the breast, regression of the growth may follow removal of the ovaries and adrenal glands. In contrast, the growth of some malignant neoplasms is inhibited by the adrenocortical hormones. Some children with acute leukemia im-

prove for a time when they are treated with adrenocortical steroids.

What are the causes of endocrine disorders?

Endocrine glands are subject to the same types of pathology as other structures in the body. Structures and function are impaired when a gland is deprived of its blood supply. Infection and autoimmune disorders may have a similar effect. Unfavorable genetic and/or environmental conditions may result in an absence of, or insufficient, tissue to secrete an adequate supply of a hormone or hormones. Failure to control the growth potential of the secreting or supporting cells of a gland may result in a benign or malignant neoplasm. When secreting cells are involved, alterations occur in the level of secretion of the hormone(s) elaborated by the affected gland. Either hypo- or hypersecretion may result. The effects of neoplasms as space-occupying and metastasizing lesions depend on the location of the gland involved. A neoplasm of the thyroid gland may obstruct breathing or swallowing.

A disturbance in the functioning of an endocrine gland may result from malfunction in the regulating mechanism or from failure to respond to regulation. To illustrate, Cushing's syndrome is a disorder resulting from hyperactivity of the adrenal cortex. The hyperplasia of the gland, along with its hypersecretion, could be the result of excessive stimulation caused by oversecretion of ACTH or to failure of the adrenal cortex to respond appropriately to controlling mechanisms. Thus it continues to secrete despite a decrease in the secretion of ACTH. Other endocrine disorders may be caused by failure of end organs to respond appropriately to a hormone. Inappropriate secretion of a hormone (one is ADH) occurs in certain types of malignant neoplasms and a variety of other disorders not of endocrine origin.[32]

Because hormonal disturbances are usually characterized by the hypo- or hypersecretion of a hormone or result from the imbalance between or among hormones, the first objective in the therapy of patients with hormonal disturbances is to restore hormone balance. When a disorder is characterized by hypofunction, one or more of the following approaches may be used to maintain function. The first and most frequently employed is the replacement of the deficient hormones. In some instances, the individual's requirements for the hormone may be lessened. Finally, measures may be utilized to stimulate the production of the hormone by the individual. For example, among the factors in

[31] Tepperman, op.cit., p. 17.

[32] Robert D. Utiger: "Disorders of Antidiuretic Hormone Secretion," Med. Clin. N. Amer., 52:381–91 (Mar.) 1968.

the etiology of diabetes mellitus is a deficiency in insulin supply. Diabetes may be treated by replacing the deficient insulin, by reducing the individual's insulin requirements, or, if he is middle-aged or older and his diabetes is not too severe, by stimulating his islet cells to release insulin.

In patients with conditions characterized by hyperfunction, therapy is directed toward returning secretion to normal levels. This may be accomplished by the surgical removal of all or a part of the secreting tissue or by blocking the production of the hormone. When all the tissue is extirpated, or destroyed, the individual is treated by the same general methods employed in the therapy of persons with hypofunction.

When patients require continued therapy with hormones, they should be observed for symptoms and signs indicating over- and underdosage. They should also be taught why they require the hormone, what effects are to be expected, and what to do should untoward symptoms develop; sensitivity to hormones differs from person to person and in the same person from time to time. Symptoms of overdosage are comparable to those found in disease states characterized by hyperfunction. In addition to the factors mentioned, patients also should be instructed about how to administer their own medication and why a regular schedule is required. Some endocrine disorders make it necessary for the person to modify one or more aspects of his life. Emphasis in the instruction should be on helping the patient to develop the knowledge and competence that he requires to manage his disease. Success in management of some of the more common endocrine diseases frequently depends on the willingness and ability of the patient and his family to assume responsibility for the management of the disease. Physicians and nurses can and should act as teachers and consultants. Instructional plans should, therefore, help to prepare the patient to assume the necessary responsibility. To be successful, the instruction should take into account what the patient can and will be able to do. Some patients respond better to a structured program, while others do better when responsibility is delegated to them. A highly elaborate teaching plan may not be effective unless it makes provision for the individual patient's home and work situations.

To summarize, hormones are essential for the communication of information from one area of the body to another. They are produced by the glands comprising the endocrine system. Each gland in the system is an individual organ. There exists, however, among the endocrine glands a complicated relationship and a complex yet uni-fied working together toward a common goal—the maintenance of homeostasis.

Although there are many disorders involving hormones, only diabetes mellitus, hyper- and hypothyroidism, and hyper- and hyposecretion of the adrenal cortex will be presented in detail. For detailed information about other disorders of the endocrine system consult the References at end of this chapter.

METHODS UTILIZED IN DIAGNOSIS OF ENDOCRINE DISEASE

1. Laboratory tests
   a. Direct measurement of the concentration of the hormone in the plasma, blood, or urine
      (1) Immunoassay
      (2) Chemical assay
   b. Indirect methods
      (1) Tests to determine the blood or plasma level of a metabolite influenced by the hormone
      (2) Capacity of the gland to respond to an increased load
      (3) Intake or output of a metabolite or product of metabolism
      (4) Capacity of end organs to respond
2. Nonspecific tests—water test
3. Clinical manifestations—signs and symptoms

It would appear that the way to establish the nature of an endocrine disorder would be to measure the level of a specific hormone in the blood. Because of the exceedingly small quantity of hormones as well as for other reasons, not all hormones in the plasma can be measured. Hormonal secretion may be estimated by measuring the amount of the hormone or its degradation products in the urine.

From the measurement of plasma or urinary hormone levels, the physician may be able to determine (1) the quantity of hormone secreted, (2) the rhythmicity—normal or abnormal—of secretion, and (3) how the gland responds to various types of stimuli, inhibitory as well as excitatory. Stimuli may be physiological. For example, glucose is a physiological stimulus for insulin secretion, while tolbutamide is a pharmacological stimulus.

Even when it is possible to measure the level of a hormone in the blood, other tests may be required to establish the nature of a disorder. Failure may not be caused by inadequate secretion but by inactivation of the hormone or failure of the end organ to respond. As an example, in the growth-onset or juvenile diabetes, insulin output is inadequate or even absent. In the maturity-onset type, the individual may have elevated plasma insulin levels. This type is sometimes referred to as high output failure. The difficulty lies not in the quantity of insulin secreted but in one or more of the following possibilities: (1) the secretion of inactive insulin, (2) the inactivation of insulin by an antagonist, or (3) the failure of the muscle and fat cells to respond to insulin in a normal manner.

One of the common methods utilized in the diagnosis of endocrine disorders is the determination of the level of one or more metabolites regulated by a particular hormone in the blood or urine. As examples, hyperglycemia and glycosuria are both present in diabetes mellitus. Low sodium combined with elevated potassium is found in adrenal insufficiency.

Abnormalities found in some disorders may not be evident under all circumstances. In some instances the reserve capacity of a gland can be determined by placing stress on its capacity to adapt to an increased load. To illustrate, in some individuals the blood glucose is within normal limits unless the glucose-regulating mechanism is taxed. The glucose tolerance, i.e., the reserve capacity to secrete insulin, can be tested by comparing the quantity of glucose in the blood before and after a meal or the ingestion of 100 g of glucose. Further strain may be placed on the capacity to utilize glucose by cortisone.

In the patient with a mild adrenal insufficiency, signs and symptoms can be precipitated by withholding sodium chloride. Because the patient will continue to lose sodium chloride in the urine, acute adrenal insufficiency may be precipitated. Careful observation and immediate reporting of (1) any drop in blood pressure, (2) nausea and vomiting, (3) diarrhea, (4) weakness, (5) restlessness, or (6) irritability must be included in the plan of care.

Some abnormalities seen in endocrine disorders are nonspecific. All the preceding signs and symptoms occur in many other types of disorders. The interpretation of indirect laboratory tests is complicated by the fact that hormones are not solely responsible for any one function. The basal metabolic rate is an example. Under normal conditions the thyroid is responsible for about one third of the total rate. Other factors are responsible for the other two thirds. Moreover, basal conditions are difficult to achieve during the performance of the test. For most indirect laboratory tests a single negative result is not generally relied on, especially when there is reason to believe that the patient has an abnormality.

USES OF HORMONES

Naturally occurring hormones and their synthetic analogues are used (1) to correct a deficiency, (2) to aid in diagnosis of an endocrine or metabolic disorder, and (3) as a drug. Thus insulin is administered in the therapy of diabetes mellitus. ACTH may be used to determine the secretory ability of the adrenal cortex. Finally, some hormones are administered for their pharmacological effects. Large doses of cortisone or one of its relatives may be administered in the treatment of very different disorders, such as septic shock, acute lymphoblastic leukemia, and rheumatic fever.

ANTERIOR PITUITARY (ADENOHYPOPHYSIS)

The anterior pituitary in man is a small structure, about the size of a pea, and it is located along with the neurohypophysis just below the center of the brain in the sella turcica. It is controlled by the hypothalamus by way of a venous portal system. Despite its small size, the anterior hypophysis secretes at least six important hormones. These hormones control growth, sexual development, reproduction, adrenocortical and thyroid activity, and they have an important effect on the general response of the body to stress.[33] Among the hormones secreted by the anterior hypophysis are the growth hormone (GH), adrenocorticotropin (ACTH), the two gonadotropins—the follicle-stimulating hormone (FSH), the luteinizing hormone (LH), the thyroid-stimulating hormone (TSH), and the melanocyte-stimulating hormone (MSH).

The hormones secreted by the anterior pituitary induce their effect in two different ways. They affect tissues directly and they regulate the output of hormones of other glands, such as the adrenal cortex, thyroid, and gonads (ovaries and testes). Although the function of the tropic hormones was formerly believed to be limited to their target glands, these hormones can produce effects in the absence of their target glands.[34] Because of the difficulty of discussing the tropic hormones without also including the hormones secreted by their target glands, they will be considered with the gland that they stimulate. The general relationship of the hypothalamus, the anterior tropic hormones, and the target glands is illustrated in Figure 15-1.

THE GROWTH HORMONE

Secretion of the growth hormone is regulated by the hypothalamus. Somatotropin-releasing factor is thought to be formed in the paraven-

[33] Choh Hao Li: "The ACTH Molecule," *Sci. Amer.,* **209**:46 (July) 1963.
[34] *Ibid.,* p. 46.

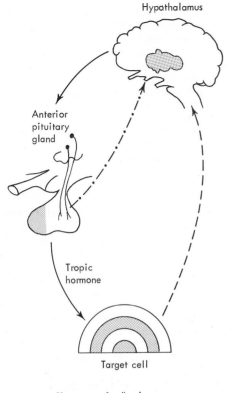

Hypothalamus

Anterior
pituitary
gland

Tropic
hormone

Target cell

—·—·— Short neg. feedback
— — — Long neg. feedback

FIGURE 15-1. Feedback relationships among the hypothalamus, the anterior pituitary gland, and the target cell. *Dashed line,* long negative feedback; *dashed-dotted line,* short negative feedback. (After a drawing by Leola Hogan.)

tricular nuclei and delivered to the anterior pituitary via the hypothalamic-hypophyseal portal vessels. Not all the factors influencing its release are known. Among those that increase its release are the lowering of blood glucose; the administration of amino acids, particularly arginine; exercise; and certain types of excitement. The corticosteroids lessen its release.

In man, the human growth hormone has three metabolic effects: (1) anabolic, (2) lipolytic, and (3) diabetogenic. In its anabolic effect it stimulates the rate of growth, particularly of muscles and epiphyseal cartilages. It stimulates all aspects of protein metabolism. These effects are evident when there is a plentiful supply of nutrients and insulin is present. Absence of the growth hormone before maturity is accompanied by a marked slowing of the rate of growth. Factors other than the lack of the growth hormone also contribute to failure to grow.

The lipolytic and diabetogenic effects of the growth hormone are similar to those seen in starvation. Among these are an increase in the mobilization of free fatty acids, an increase in fat in the liver, loss of body fat, ketonemia, decreased peripheral utilization of glucose, and resistance to insulin.

From animal experiments and the observation of patients with disorders of growth hormone secretion, the interdependence of hormones becomes clearer. Among the hormones interacting metabolically with the growth hormone are insulin, adrenal glucocorticoids, thyroid hormones, and glucagon. Diabetes mellitus in pancreatectomized animals is mild if the animal is also hypophysectomized. Growth retardation is frequently observed in children receiving large doses of the adrenal glucocorticoids. In animals that are hypothyroid and lack the growth hormone, both hormones must be replaced for growth to proceed normally.

HYPERSECRETION

Hypersecretion of the growth hormone in an immature animal leads to overgrowth of the skeleton, or giantism. Hypersecretion after growth has ceased leads to a condition known as acromegaly. A characteristic feature in acromegaly is an enlargement of flat bones, such as those of the hands, feet, and head. The lower jaw enlarges and the face takes on a coarse appearance. There is also an enlargement of all viscera except the brain. Acromegaly may be accompanied by symptoms of hyperthyroidism and of diabetes mellitus. Many patients can be cured by irradiation of the pituitary gland. The skeletal changes are permanent, however.

PANHYPOPITUITARISM

In a strict sense the anterior hypophysis is not essential to life. Hypophysectomized animals not given any hormone substitution therapy may live for months or years provided they are protected from environmental stress. They must be kept in a warm, air-conditioned room, protected from infections and from very much physical exercise. In panhypopituitarism, whether induced by disease or by the complete removal of the gland, the manifestations result from a deficiency of the antidiuretic, the thyroid, the adrenocortical, and the gonadal hormones.[35] Of these the first three are of the most significance to survival and health, and they must therefore be replaced. Because the thyroid gland contains a supply of hormones, after hypophysectomy a patient may not require an exogenous supply of thyroid hormones for as long as three months. The other hormones, however, are necessary

35 The antidiuretic hormone is released by the posterior hypophysis.

immediately. In most instances the patient will require hormone replacement therapy for the remainder of his life.

POSTERIOR PITUITARY (NEUROHYPOPHYSIS)

Modern theory postulates that antidiuretic hormone (ADH) or vasopressin and oxytocin are synthesized by the neurons of the supraoptic and paraventricular nuclei. They are stored in and released by the neurohypophysis. The principal effect of ADH is to increase reabsorption of water by the renal tubules. In massive hemorrhage, ADH has a blood pressure–raising effect. The stimulus to secretion is an increase in the osmolality of the blood.

The disorder with which the hypofunction of the neurohypophysis is most commonly associated is diabetes insipidus. The characteristic effect is a large volume of urine of low specific gravity. There may be as many as 15 to 28 liters of urine per day, and its specific gravity ranges from 1.001 to 1.005. With this large loss of water, hypovolemia with dry skin and intense thirst occur. The polyuria is not lessened by depriving the patient of water, nor is the specific gravity of the urine increased. Polydipsia is secondary to the polyuria. Thirst may be so intense that, unless the patient is continuously supplied with water, he will drink whatever fluid is available including, in extreme cases, his own urine.

When the cause of polyuria and polydipsia are in doubt, the patient may be deprived of water for a period of time. When water is withheld from a patient, he should be closely observed for signs indicating the development of hypovolemia. Changes in the rate and volume of the pulse as well as any decrease in the blood pressure should be reported immediately. Because polyuria and polydipsia may have psychogenic causes, the patient should also be observed to be sure that he does not have access to water and other fluids.

The treatment of diabetes insipidus has two aspects. When a pituitary lesion is responsible, it is corrected. Until this is done and in those persons who have a permanent loss of function, replacement therapy with ADH is indicated. This usually is required throughout the life of the individual. The antidiuretic hormone may be administered by subcutaneous or intramuscular injection or by nasal insufflation. In the latter, a solution containing pituitary hormones may be applied by placing small cotton pledgets that have been soaked with a solution containing the hormone against the nasal mucosa or by snuffing posterior pituitary powder into the nares. When replacement is in the form of vasopressin tannate in oil, it is administered intramuscularly.

It is best given at night to prevent polyuria and thus to insure the patient of a good night's sleep. The patient (or nurse) should be instructed to warm the vial of vasopressin tannate and to shake it repeatedly and thoroughly, because the active material has a tendency to precipitate out of the oil.

Disorders arising from hyperfunction of the neurohypophysis have not been described. Although hypersecretion of the neurohypophysis can occur, when it does it is an appropriate or inappropriate response to injury or threat thereof. Secretion returns to normal when the crisis is past. As an example, some authorities ascribe the retention of water after major surgery or a serious injury to an increase in the secretion of the antidiuretic hormone. A factor in edema in heart failure may be the inappropriate secretion of the antidiuretic hormone. Neither of the above can in any sense be considered to be caused by a disordered function of the neurohypophysis.

In addition to disorders caused by abnormal secretion, tumors of the pituitary gland are occasionally responsible for pressure on related structures. The usual cause is an adenoma (tumor originating in gland cells). The most serious effect of enlargement of the pituitary gland is blindness as a result of pressure on the optic chiasm. The optic chiasm is formed by the fibers of the optic nerves that pass over the pituitary gland on their way to the visual areas in the occipital lobes of the brain. Fibers from the retina on the lateral side travel to the same side of the brain. Those on the inner, or nasal, side of the retina cross and go to the opposite side of the brain. As the lesion enlarges, pressure on the optic tracts leads to the loss of one or more fields of vision and eventually to complete blindness. Because of the proximity of the floor of the brain, there may be disturbances in vegetative functions. Depending on the nature of the lesion, removal may be by irradiation or by surgical means. Irradiation is used when at all possible, because of the difficulties involved in exposing the area.

THE ADRENAL GLAND

The adrenal gland consists of two parts, the medulla and the cortex. The medulla arises along with the sympathetic nervous system from the neural crest. It secretes two hormones, epinephrine and norepinephrine. The latter is also released at the nerve ending of the sympathetic nervous system. Both hormones are secreted continuously in small amounts. The adrenal medulla, along with the sympathetic nervous system, appears to regulate functions enabling the organism to adapt to emergency situations. It responds readily to stimulation by the sympathetic nervous system in a wide variety of conditions, with the result that a message borne by a preganglionic fiber of the sympathetic nervous system is converted to a blood-borne one. The release of the hormones epinephrine and norepinephrine by the adrenal medulla contributes to the widespread reaction following activation of the sympathetic nervous system. As emphasized previously, the action of the sympathetic nervous system and that of the hormones secreted by the adrenal medulla are similar. Emergency conditions activating the sympathoadrenal system include hemorrhage, hypoglycemia, hypoxia, pain, strenuous exercise, fear, and anger, as well as various pharmacological agents.

The physiological effects of the two hormones are different. Norepinephrine acts primarily on the alpha receptors. It increases both diastolic and systolic blood pressure by increasing the peripheral resistance. Epinephrine acts on both the alpha and beta receptors. Its actions are principally inhibitory and metabolic. It increases the contractility and excitability of the heart muscle, thereby increasing cardiac output. It facilitates the flow of blood to the muscles, brain, and viscera and increases the basal metabolic rate. It enhances the blood sugar by stimulating the conversion of glycogen to glucose by the liver and by decreasing the uptake of glucose by muscle. It inhibits smooth muscle contraction. The adrenal medulla is not necessary to maintain life but contributes to the ability of the organism to cope with stress.

HYPERFUNCTION OF THE ADRENAL MEDULLA

A neoplasm known as a pheochromocytoma is associated with hyperfunction of the adrenal medulla. A functioning pheochromocytoma is characterized by hypertension that may be either paroxysmal (periodic attacks) or continuous. The character of the hypertension depends on whether the tumor secretes constantly or intermittently. The clinical manifestations depend on whether the tumor secretes epinephrine or norepinephrine, or both. Mrs. Lanera presented a classic picture of a patient with the paroxysmal type of hypertension caused by pheochromocytoma. Between attacks she lay quietly in bed. During an attack she appeared to be acutely anxious. She said that she felt shaky and that her head ached. She thrashed about in bed and complained of her heart's pounding (palpitation). She felt nauseated, and vomited and perspired profusely. Her blood pressure rose to 200 mm Hg systolic and 135 mm Hg diastolic. She did not have paresthesia or tetany.

Because there is a possibility for cure and patients having this condition are frequently young, the diagnosis is important. The urine is examined for excessive catecholamines or their metabolites. In patients whose blood pressures are below 170 mm Hg systolic and 110 mm Hg diastolic, a drug such as histamine or methacholine hydrochloride may be administered to provoke symptoms. Following the administration of histamine the healthy person's blood pressure falls, his skin flushes, and he is likely to have a headache. In the patient with pheochromocytoma, the blood pressure usually, though not always, rises. Methacholine chloride likewise causes a rise in blood pressure. To prevent overreaction to methacholine chloride, atropine sulfate, 1 mg, may be administered before it is given.

In patients whose blood pressures are above 170/110, drugs that block the effect of norepinephrine on the blood vessels may be employed to establish the diagnosis. The best known is phentolamine hydrochloride (Regitine Hydrochloride). When a dose of 5 mg of phentolamine is administered intravenously to a patient with pheochromocytoma, the blood pressure falls immediately. The maximum decrease is reached in two to five minutes and lasts for ten minutes or longer. A fall of 35 mm systolic and 25 mm diastolic or more is considered to be positive; that is, it indicates the presence of pheochromocytoma.

The treatment of pheochromocytoma is the surgical removal of the tumor. Preoperatively the patient can be protected from severe hypertension by the regular administration of phentolamine. Because the manipulation of the lesion during the operative procedure may cause the release of epinephrine and/or norepinephrine, the blood pressure of the patient may rise to critical levels. Because the patient can be protected from an excessively high blood pressure by the administration of phentolamine, the blood pressure of the patient should be monitored continuously. In the immediate postoperative period the patient may have episodes of hypotension, and occasionally a patient suffers severe shock. Norepinephrine or phenylephrine hydrochloride (Neo-Synephrine Hydrochloride) may be prescribed by the physician to elevate the blood pressure. The blood pressure of the patient should be observed frequently until it is stabilized. Because stabilization may not occur for two or three days after surgery, the patient requires monitoring for a longer period than most postoperative patients. When the patient gets out of bed, he should be cautioned to change from the supine to the upright position slowly so that the blood vessels have time to adapt. Dizziness and a feeling of faintness are indicative of hypotension. Depending on the severity of these symptoms, the patient may have to be returned to bed. Certainly he should be protected from falling. In the absence of irreversible shock, patients usually make an uneventful recovery. Unless both adrenal glands are removed, adrenal steroid therapy usually is not required. Adrenomedullary secretions do not have to be replaced, regardless of whether one or both glands are excised. As far as can be determined, the adrenal medulla is not essential to life. When both adrenal glands are removed, the adrenergic response to stressing situations is somewhat lessened, but the sympathetic nervous system still reacts.

ADRENOCORTICAL HORMONES

The adrenal cortex is generally considered to be essential to life. In the absence of adrenocortical secretions the individual has difficulty in adapting to even mild degrees of stress. This includes all types—variations in temperature, exercise, changes in position, infections, burns, and emotional stresses. The degree of susceptibility varies somewhat from individual to individual. Exposure to severe stress, however, can be expected to induce a shocklike state characterized by prostration and peripheral circulatory failure. Death follows unless the deficient hormones are replaced. Life can be maintained in the absence of adrenocortical hormones if electrolytes and nutrients are carefully controlled.

Adrenocortical hormones are classified into three groups according to their major effects: (1) cortisol (glucocorticoids), (2) mineralocorticoids, and (3) adrenosterones (adrenal androgens). Examples of glucocorticoids are cortisone and hydrocortisone. In man the principal glucocorticoid is hydrocortisone. Mineralocorticoids are aldosterone and desoxycorticosterone. Aldosterone is secreted by the adrenal cortex; desoxycorticosterone is a synthetic analogue. The mineralocorticoids, as their name implies, regulate the reabsorption of the sodium cation and the excretion of the potassium cation by the renal tubules. All adrenal steroids affect sodium retention and potassium and chloride excretion to some degree. All these hormones have their origin in a common chemical, cholesterol. A lack of, or a decreased activity of, an enzyme catalyzing one hormone results in the increased formation of the others.

The glucocorticoids such as cortisone and hydrocortisone have a number of effects that are not exhibited to any degree by the mineralocorticoids. These include the following:

1. They reverse the delay in water diuresis seen in the adrenalectomized animal.
2. They enhance protein catabolism and inhibit protein synthesis.
3. They antagonize the action of insulin.
4. They affect the metabolism of glucose.
   a. They increase the synthesis of glucose by the liver—the source of glucose is mobilization of amino acids by the hormone from the peripheral supporting structures such as connective tissues. Amino acids are deaminized in the liver and converted to glycogen. The glycogen is converted to glucose, which is released into the blood, thereby elevating the level of glucose in the blood.
5. Glucocorticoids influence the defense mechanisms in the body. High concentrations act to suppress inflammation, inhibit the formation of scar tissue, and block certain allergic responses. They are also believed to have a significant role in adaptation to many kinds of stresses, such as traumatic injuries (surgical or accidental), burns, severe infections, and other similar challenges to the organism. The mechanisms by which the adrenocortical hormones participate in these complex events have not been elucidated. Other hormonal, neural, and nutritional factors also influence the response of the individual to injury. Current and future studies will undoubtedly contribute to an understanding of all the factors involved in the response of an individual to stress. Although some animals can be maintained on aldosterone, man requires hydrocortisone or corticosterone for his survival.
6. Hydrocortisone participates in the regulation of melanin metabolism.
7. The secretion of ACTH is regulated by the hypothalamus, which is regulated by the level of hydrocortisone in the blood.
8. The glucocorticoids appear to play a permissive role in metabolism. Many cells appear to respond to other influences such as neural or hormonal stimulation only when there is a certain basic level of adrenocortical hormones.
9. The glucocorticoids influence (directly or indirectly) emotional functioning. In adrenal insufficiency, patients are often depressed and anxious. By adequate replacement therapy, these effects are ameliorated. The long-term administration of large dosages of adrenal steroids in the therapy of patients with rheumatoid arthritis may result in euphoria (an unrealistic optimism or cheerfulness) or even in a frankly psychotic state in persons who are predisposed to this condition.

The secretion of cortisol fluctuates regularly according to a circadian rhythm. The highest levels are noted in the morning between 4 and 6 o'clock. The lowest levels are found in the evening. The secretion of cortisol and adrenal androgen is controlled by ACTH (adrenocorticotropic hormone), secreted by the anterior pituitary gland. ACTH also exhibits a diurnal rhythm. A decrease in the level of cortisol, either directly or by way of the hypothalamus, results in an increased release of ACTH. As the level of adrenocortical hormones rises, the production of ACTH by the anterior pituitary declines. Many environmental, chemical, and psychological factors influence the release of ACTH. Although ACTH may have some effect on the secretion of aldosterone, it appears to be regulated by the concentration of sodium and potassium in the body fluids. After the removal of the pituitary gland, secretion of aldosterone is maintained. In some instances, it is increased over prehypophysectomy levels.

Manifestations of disorders of the adrenal cortex result from the effects of hypo- or hypersecretion. Adrenal insufficiency may result from atrophy, destruction by a disease such as tuberculosis, hemorrhage into the gland, or surgical removal of both adrenal glands. It may be secondary to failure of the anterior pituitary gland. Although tuberculosis was formerly a more common cause of adrenal insufficiency than it is now, it still is responsible for a significant number of cases. Secretion of hormones by the adrenal cortex is depressed by the administration of exogenous hormones; withdrawal of hormone therapy may leave the patient in a state of relative deficiency. During the period immediately following withdrawal, the person is likely to be more susceptible to infection than usual. At one time adrenal insufficiency and other disorders of the adrenal cortex were believed to be extremely rare. Because of improved methods of diagnosis, disorders of the adrenal cortex are being identified with greater frequency. Whereas they were once believed to be rare, they can no longer be so considered. Most of the effects of adrenal insufficiency are caused by a deficiency of the mineralo- and glucocorticoids. Some of the signs and symptoms are caused by disordered electrolyte balance. Others stem from disordered metabolism of protein, fat, and carbohydrates.

The clinical manifestations of adrenal insufficiency were described by Thomas Addison more than 100 years ago and were as a result called Addison's disease. It was not, however, until the adrenocortical steroids were isolated and synthesized that marked progress was made in understanding their role in the regulation of body activities or in controlling the manifestations of the disease. Before the introduction of adrenocortical extracts, the prognosis of a person with Addison's disease was extremely poor. Since adrenocortical hormones have become available, it is much improved. The change in the outlook for the patient with chronic adrenal insufficiency is well illustrated by an uncle and his nephew, both of whom had Addison's disease. In 1926 John Seebon, aged 17, died from the effects of Addison's disease. Thirty years later his nephew, James, aged 14, developed symptoms that his mother recognized as being similar to those experienced by her brother. Medical examination revealed that her suspicions were justified. Twelve years later James is living and well. He works every day on his father's farm. In the interim a second brother has developed Addison's disease. In only four instances has Addison's disease been known to develop in two siblings.

Untreated adrenal insufficiency is characterized by weakness (asthenia), easy fatigability, and hypotension. Weakness is one of the most outstanding symptoms. In the beginning it tends to be worse on some days than on others. Eventually, it becomes so severe that the patient is confined to bed. Finally, even bed rest does not afford relief. Hypotension is also a common finding. The majority of patients have blood pressure readings of less than 110/70. In extreme cases it may be as low as 80/50 or even lower. A change in the color of the skin to brown, tan, or bronze is the most striking physical change that can be observed directly. The pigmentation may be diffuse, involving exposed and unexposed areas of the body, or it may appear in patches or freckles. Bluish black or slate gray discoloration of the mucous membranes may also occur. Disturbances in the function of the gastrointestinal tract may give rise to anorexia, nausea, vomiting, diarrhea, constipation, and abdominal pain. Weight loss is a common finding. As might be expected, mental changes may be prominent. Depression, irritability, lethargy, apprehension, and anxiety are common.

Methods used to diagnose the functional status of the adrenal glands include (1) direct measurement of the adrenocortical hormones or their degradation products in the plasma or urine, (2) response to ACTH stimulation (glucocorticoids), (3) plasma or serum levels of metabolites regulated by these hormones, (4) cellular elements in the blood, and (5) response to loading or withholding substances regulated by one or more hormones and the signs and symptoms presented by the patient.

Some of the commonly used tests to evaluate

TABLE 15-1

Diagnostic Tests Used to Evaluate Adrenocortical Status in Adrenal Insufficiency and Adrenocortical Hypersecretion

Adrenal insufficiency	Hypersecretion
1. Direct measurement of adrenocortical hormones or degradation products in the urine and blood.	
Low values for 24-hour excretion of 17-hydroxycorticosteroids and 17-ketosteroids.	Elevated 17-hydroxycortico-steroid (17-OHCS).
Low plasma 17-hydroxycorticosteroid.	
2. Response to ACTH stimulation. In panhypopituitarism, the administration of ACTH is followed by increased urinary excretion of adrenocortical hormones. In failure of the adrenal cortex, there is a minimum or no increase in the secretion of adrenocortical steroids. In a healthy person, the eosinophil count drops 70% or more.	Increased 17-OHCS when caused by adrenal hyperplasia. Decreased by dexamethasone administration.
3. Blood, plasma, or serum levels of metabolites regulated by hormones.	
Elevated serum potassium	Reduced serum potassium
Reduced serum sodium	Elevated sodium levels
Reduced CO_2 combining power	
Low fasting blood glucose	Hyperglycemia and glycosuria frequent
Hemoconcentration	
4. Cellular elements in the blood. Eosinophils elevated. Depending on the degree of insufficiency, values may range from low normals to marked changes in values. Does not drop in response to ACTH.	Eosinopenia Lymphopenia
5. Response to loading or withholding a substance regulated by one or more hormones. Water loading or withholding sodium. Seldom used.	

the secretory functions of the adrenal cortex are summarized in Table 15-1.

What are the nurse's responsibilities in caring for a patient with adrenal dysfunction?

Observation combined with a careful description of the emotional and physiological status of the patient cannot be overemphasized. When the adrenal cortex is stimulated by ACTH, the nurse should remember that ACTH is a polypeptide. Particularly in patients who lack endogenous corticoids, there is danger of an allergic response. A potent steroid such as 1 mg of fluorohydrocortisone may be prescribed to be given orally on the days when ACTH is administered to minimize the danger of a serious hypersensitivity reaction. The patient who has adrenal insufficiency is also predisposed to an acute febrile reaction when ACTH is administered in a solution of glucose and water.

COLLECTION OF 24-HOUR URINE SPECIMENS

When the urine is being collected, the patient, his relatives, and all nursing personnel should be instructed regarding the importance of saving all urine. The loss of even one voiding of urine can delay diagnosis, be responsible for unnecessary discomfort to the patient, and increase the cost of his illness.

Another less specific, but simpler, test of adrenocortical function is the response of the eosinophils in the blood before and after the administration of ACTH. In a healthy person, following the administration, the eosinophil count should drop 70 per cent or more. A lesser decline may indicate adrenal insufficiency.

THERAPY OF ADRENOCORTICAL INSUFFICIENCY

Despite differences in specifics, the general approaches to the treatment of patients with chronic adrenal insufficiency are similar to the treatment of diabetes mellitus. Hormones are available that can be employed to replace those that are lacking. Whether or not the patient is maintained in a satisfactory state of health frequently depends on himself. As in other disorders in which there is a permanent deficiency state, the patient must understand that he must continue therapy for the rest of his life. He must follow a prescribed routine and remain under medical supervision. Because he requires more hormones when he is under the stress of illness, he must understand this and know what to do. He should carry a card providing information such as his name, address, diagnosis, and the medications he is taking.

In some patients, adrenal insufficiency can be controlled by the administration of cortisol (5 to 15 mg three times daily) by mouth. In other patients a potent salt-retaining steroid as a fluorohydrocortisone or desoxycorticosterone acetate is required in addition to cortisone to maintain electrolyte balance. The first is administered orally in small dosages of from 0.1 to 0.3 mg daily. The administration of desoxycorticosterone is more complicated. The dosage is first established by determining the effects of daily intramuscular injections on blood pressure and serum electrolyte concentration. After the requirements of the patient have been determined, desoxycorticosterone may be administered by deep intramuscular injection once every three to four weeks or by intraoral tablets or buccalets placed in the mouth two or three times per day. Because absorption is less complete from the mucosa of the mouth than when the drug is administered intramuscularly, the daily requirement is two to three times that established for intramuscular injection. The patient who receives desoxycorticosterone should be instructed to weigh himself regularly because overdosage causes edema as a consequence of retention of the sodium cation. In marked overdosages of desoxycorticosterone, hypertension and congestive heart failure may be induced.

Adrenocortical failure secondary to failure in anterior pituitary function differs from primary adrenal insufficiency in that there usually are disturbances in thyroid and gonadal function as well. Disturbances in electrolyte balance, though present, are often less severe. As in primary adrenal insufficiency, the characteristic features are weakness, inability to cope with stress, poor resistance to infection, and the tendency to spontaneous hypoglycemia.[36] These effects can usually be controlled by small doses of cortisone.

The most serious event in chronic adrenal insufficiency is the development of acute adrenal insufficiency or crisis. In this condition all the signs and symptoms of adrenal insufficiency are intensified. Although prevention is to be preferred to therapy, the survival of the patient in acute adrenal insufficiency depends on prompt and vigorous treatment. Because an increased supply of adrenocortical hormones is required to cope with stress, any condition that makes extra demands on the individual can be anticipated to predispose to adrenal crisis. The dosage of hormones should be increased during infection, gastrointestinal upsets, trauma, surgery, and any other condition that is likely to increase the need of the individual for adrenal hormones. When the condition occurs, all signs and symptoms of adrenal insufficiency worsen. Unless it is corrected promptly, the patient goes into vascular shock and dies. The nurse should be alert to and report any evidence of an intensification of signs and symptoms, such as increasing weakness or a lowering of the blood pressure.

Therapy in adrenal insufficiency has three objectives: (1) to raise the level of adrenal hormones in the circulation, (2) to support the heart and vascular system, and (3) to control infection. To raise the level of hormones in the circulation, the patient is given 100 to 150 mg of hydrocortisone in 1,000 ml of 5 per cent glucose in physiological saline. The first 250 ml are administered quickly. The remainder is administered slowly over a four- to eight-hour period.

Objectives on which to base the nursing care plan include (1) to contribute to the accomplishment of the medical objectives, including the protection of the patient from infection, and (2) to maintain conditions of the physical, emotional, and social climate so that demands made on the patient to adapt are reduced to a minimum. The contribution of the nurse to the medical objectives includes the supervision of the treatments and observation of their effects on the patient. The patient should not be left alone. Observation of vital signs by the nurse or monitors and reporting of significant changes are important. Any drop in the blood pressure of the patient is likely to be significant because it may be at a critical level at the time treatment is initiated. Because hyperthermia is a problem in some patients, hourly recordings of temperature may be requested by the physician.

The importance of eliminating inasmuch as

36 Raymond V. Randall and Edward H. Rynearson, "Clinical Aspects of Anterior Pituitary Failure," *Postgrad. Med.*, **29**:25 (Jan.) 1961.

possible all form of stimuli is based on the fact that the patient who is in adrenal crisis is unable to adapt to even minor stresses. As a consequence, a situation that might be of no importance to a healthy person or one who is experiencing other types of illness may have an adverse effect. Attention should be given to details such as maintaining the temperature of the room between 70° and 75°F, protecting the patient from drafts and from bright lights, and providing a comfortable bed. The room should be quiet. Loud noises and talking should be avoided. Until the crisis is past, physical care should be kept to the minimum required for the comfort of the patient. He should do nothing for himself. Whatever care is required should be administered. This includes moving and turning as well as activities such as mouth care and feeding. When the patient is vomiting, he should be given assistance. Mouth care after an emesis is recommended. Conversation should be kept to the minimum required to give directions to the patient or for brief explanations of what is to be done. Persons with infections, including members of his family and hospital personnel, should be excluded from his environment. An environment that limits the demands made on him to adapt contributes to his recovery.

HYPERSECRETION OF THE ADRENAL CORTEX

The adrenal cortex secretes a number of hormones, each of which has different physiological effects. Consequently the clinical manifestations in disorders characterized by hypersecretion will depend on which hormones are oversecreted. In either hyperplasia or adenoma of the adrenal cortex, oversecretion of one hormone may predominate, or there may be a variable mixture of hormones. Three different clinical syndromes of hyperfunction are usually described. They are *Cushing's syndrome, adrenogenital syndrome,* and *primary aldosteronism.* Cushing's syndrome results largely from the hypersecretion of cortisol. Large doses of cortisol or one of its analogues, when administered over a time, produce effects similar to Cushing's syndrome. In primary aldosteronism, as the name implies, synthesis of aldosterone is excessive. The adrenogenital syndrome includes all the disorders of sexual development that can be attributed to abnormal adrenocortical function.

Cushing's syndrome is a state manifested by a group of signs and symptoms resulting from the inappropriate secretion of cortisol. The disorder may be caused by an adenoma, by a highly malignant neoplasm of the adrenal cortex of one gland, or by the diffuse hyperplasia of both glands. In some instances no abnormality of the adrenal gland is readily identifiable. Hyperplasia is usually caused by overstimula-

tion of the adrenal cortex by ACTH. In some instances the adrenal cortex may fail to respond to the regulating effects of ACTH.

The characteristic features of Cushing's syndrome are a peculiar type of obesity in which fat is distributed in pads between the shoulders —buffalo hump—and around the waist—girdle obesity; moonface; hypertension; easy fatigability and weakness; hirsutism; purplish striae over the obese areas; thin and fragile skin that is subject to ecchymosis; acne; a ruddy color of the face and neck; amenorrhea in women or impotence in men; edema; glycosuria as a result of disturbances in carbohydrate metabolism; osteoporosis; and increased susceptibility to infection. The patient is frequently irritable and changeable in mood. In addition to his clinical manifestations, almost all persons with this disorder have a high level of 17-hydroxycorticosteroid in the plasma and urine.

Medical therapy is directed toward reducing the level of adrenocortical secretion. Some patients respond favorably to irradiation of the pituitary gland. Others require surgical treatment. In addition, the patient requires potassium chloride, 4 to 6 g daily, to supplement that obtained in his diet. Potassium is given as enteric-coated tablets with meals, or as a 25 per cent solution of potassium chloride. Testosterone may be prescribed to facilitate the replacement of protein lost as a result of the disease.

After undergoing adrenalectomy, the patient's temperature, pulse, blood pressure, and central venous pressure should be monitored for 36 hours because cardiovascular collapse is a real possibility. Evidence that shock is developing, and in some instances disorders contributing to its development, includes (1) fever, (2) hypotension, (3) falling or rising central venous pressure, (4) tachycardia, and (5) nausea and vomiting. Patients undergoing total adrenalectomy must continue under competent medical supervision for the rest of their lives. A therapeutic plan identical to that of the patient with Addison's disease is indicated.

The objectives on which the nursing care plan is based include (1) to make observations that will be helpful to the physician in establishing accurate medical diagnosis and medical plan of treatment, (2) to provide the patient with a physical, emotional, and social climate that is safe and supporting, and (3) to assist the patient in acquiring the knowledge and skill that he will need to maintain physiological functioning should this be required.

One of the simplest and at the same time most difficult responsibilities in the care of the patient with Cushing's syndrome is the collection of urine specimens. Because adrenal hormones are excreted in the urine and some of the effects of the disease or its therapy are reflected in the composition and quantity of the urine, accurate and complete measurement and collection of all urine voided by the patient are important. Besides the collecting and recording of urine output, the intake of water and food should also be recorded. Despite the apparent obesity of the patient, he usually suffers from effects of the loss of protein and potassium, because an excess of adrenocortical hormones increases protein catabolism. Excessive potassium is lost in the urine and sodium is retained. The patient should be encouraged to eat the diet that has been prescribed for him. When a low-sodium, high-potassium diet is prescribed, the nurse should check the patient's tray to be sure that he receives the appropriate food.

The patient with Cushing's syndrome has a tendency toward emotional lability (fluctuation in mood). Depression and moodiness are common. The nurse should identify the types of situations that are disturbing and record them on the nursing care plan. The patient should be observed for evidence of depression, for suicide is not an uncommon occurrence. Some patients continue to be depressed after surgical removal of the adrenal gland. Observations made by the nurse indicating a depressed state should be reported promptly to the physician.

The tendency toward masculinization with hirsutism in women and obesity are frequent sources of emotional stress. Patients in whom the disorder is caused by a benign adenoma or hyperplasia of the adrenal cortices can be given reasonable assurance that following treatment they can expect to be restored to their former selves. Weakness, accompanied by the frustration of not being able to carry on their usual activities, is also distressing to patients. At times weakness is the most outstanding symptom. Friends, as well as members of the family, often have little sympathy for the patient. They do not see how anyone who is fat can be as weak as the patient says he is. The family should be helped to understand that weakness and obesity are, in fact, compatible. Nurses who meet these patients in the community should encourage them to seek medical attention.

Primary Aldosteronism

Another disorder caused by hypersecretion of the adrenal cortex is **primary aldosteronism.** It is usually an aldosterone-secreting tumor of the adrenal cortex. The principal features of this disorder are hypertension, renal and electrolyte abnormalities, muscle weakness, and an increase in the concentration of the salt-retaining hormone in the urine. Sodium is retained and potassium is lost from the body in excessive quantities. Aldosteronism is treated by surgical removal of the neoplasm. Recovery is complete when the tumor is benign. The nursing care of the patient is essentially that of any patient undergoing adrenal surgery.

To recapitulate, adrenocortical hormones have widespread effects on the metabolism of protein, carbohydrates, lipids, and the electrolytes sodium, potassium, and calcium. They also affect and are affected by hormones elaborated by other glands. They are essential to survival. In the absence—either absolute or relative—of adrenocortical hormones, the capacity to cope with stress of all types is lost. Hypersecretion of adrenocortical hormones leads to serious defects in the adaptive capacity of the individual. Clinical manifestations of disorders involving the adrenal cortex depends on which hormone predominates or is hypersecreted. The nursing of patients with disorders in which there are abnormalities in the secretion of the adrenal steroids should be based on the knowledge that they have difficulty in coping with stress of all types and that they have increased susceptibility to infection. Many of the most serious effects are caused by disordered electrolyte balance. Other nursing responsibilities include the making of observations contributing to the medical diagnosis and the carrying out of that part of the medical regime usually assigned to nursing. When the disorder experienced by the patient is incurable, the nurse has an important role in assisting the patient to acquire the knowledge and skills that he needs to maintain life and health.

THE THYROID GLAND

The thyroid gland synthesizes two hormones, thyroxin and tri-iodothyronine from the amino acid tyrosine and iodine. Together they are generally referred to as the thyroid hormone. The effects of thyroxin and tri-iodothyronine are similar. They differ inasmuch as tri-iodothyronine is three to five times more potent than thyroxin. Its action is more rapid but is less sustained than that of thyroxin. Thyroxin has a long latent period and a prolonged action. It takes about eight to ten days for it to cause its maximum effect and the effect lasts for five to six weeks.

REGULATION OF THYROID SECRETION

The thyrotropic hormone (TSH) secreted by the anterior pituitary regulates thyroid activity. TSH and the thyroid gland are in a negative feedback relationship with each other. As do other hormones secreted by the anterior pituitary, the hypothalamus secretes a thyrotropic releasing factor (TRF) that can increase the output of TSH. Thus changes in environmental conditions such as heat, cold, and emotional stress can alter thyroid activity. As is any function regulated by a negative feedback mechanism, the organism is protected from either hypo- or hyperactivity. The person is protected not only from endogenous hormone, but from exogenous hormone. Thus the euthyroid person who ingests thyroid hormone is, within limits, protected against thyroid excess. As the level of ingested thyroid hormone rises, his own production of thyroid hormone falls.

In addition to the regulatory effects of the thyrotropic hormone, the synthesis and release of the thyroid hormones involve at least six major enzyme systems. Preparatory to the formation of the hormone, the thyroid removes iodine, mostly in the form of iodine from the blood, and concentrates it in the gland. Specific enzymes are required to catalyze these reactions as well as those in the formation of the hormone proper. A defect in any one of these systems will interfere with the capacity of the organism to form hormones. Defects in one or more of the required enzyme systems are among the causes of congenital hypothyroidism.[37]

ACTIONS OF THE THYROID HORMONES

Although it is possible to describe many of the effects of the thyroid hormones as well as the consequences of a lack or excess, where and how they act are not known. Among the hypotheses that have been proposed and found wanting in one or more respects are that (1) they speed the rate of oxidation in cells, (2) they speed certain chemical reactions in the mitochondria, (3) they alter the permeability of the mitochondrial membrane and (4) they act through the genetic apparatus to speed the synthesis of proteins in some organs.[38]

The thyroid hormones affect the rate of metabolism of proteins, lipids, and carbohydrates, as well as of water, minerals, and vitamins. In physiological amounts, the thyroid hormones promote protein synthesis and fat breakdown. In hyperthyroidism the increased secretion of thyroid hormones is reflected by an increase in the loss of nitrogen in the urine and by a lowering in the level of cholesterol (a lipid) in the blood. In hypothyroidism the concentration of cholesterol in the blood rises. Thyroid hormones also have an influence on calcium metabolism,

for osteoporosis frequently accompanies severe hyperthyroidism.

The thyroid hormones are essential to the normal physical and mental growth and development of the child. A child who is born without functioning thyroid tissue or who develops this condition soon after birth fails to develop either physically or mentally. Maturation of his skeleton and other body structures is delayed. Hypothyroidism in a child results in a characteristic type of dwarfing known as cretinism. Normal growth is dependent on the presence of the growth hormone as well. Mental development is also retarded. Idiocy is common. In older children and adults hypothyroidism is evidenced by physical and mental slowing. These effects can, however, be reversed by the ingestion of adequate amounts of thyroid hormones.

DIAGNOSTIC TESTS OF THYROID FUNCTION

A wide variety of tests are available to assess different aspects of thyroid function. Many of these tests are altered in nonthyroid states or disorders. When there is doubt about the diagnosis, a test may have to be repeated several times or several different tests may be used to obtain a reliable picture. Four tests of secretory activity of the thyroid gland include (1) the basal metabolic rate (BMR), (2) the level of protein-bound iodine, (3) the thyroidal uptake of radioactive iodine, and (4) radioiodinated tri-iodothyronine erythrocyte or resin uptake (T_3).

Basal Metabolic Rate (BMR)

The basal metabolic rate is based on the observation that a healthy person of a given age, sex, and surface area utilizes a predictable amount of oxygen when he is well relaxed and fasting. The results of the BMR are expressed in the percentage of deviation from the norm which is no or zero deviation. Rates below the average are reported as minus; those above the average as plus. The normal range is from a −10 to a +10.

Ideally the patient who undergones a BMR should have a good night's sleep and not be disturbed in the morning. To ensure sleep some physicians prescribe a sedative such as secobarbital at the hour of sleep. The patient who is in the hospital is not disturbed in the morning before the test is performed. The outpatient is provided with an opportunity to rest before the test is started. Breakfast is delayed until after the test is performed. The patient should be told the purpose of the test and that he will be directed to breathe through a tube placed in his mouth. In addition to instructions about how the test is performed and how to prepare for it, pa-

[37] Lawson Wilkins: "The Thyroid Gland," *Sci. Amer.,* **202**:126 (Mar.) 1960.

[38] Robert Michels *et al.:* "Thyroxine: Effects on Amino Acid Incorporation into Protein in Vivo," *Science,* **140**:1417 (June 28) 1963.

tients who must be absent from work or employ a baby-sitter should be told about how long the test will take.

Since other tests of thyroid function have been introduced, the BMR is used less frequently than formerly. True basal conditions are difficult to attain; many conditions alter the BMR and a single BMR determination has only about a 50 per cent chance of being accurate.

Protein-Bound Iodine

Thyroid hormones are transported in an unstable combination with the globulin fraction of the serum proteins. The concentration of the thyroid hormones in the blood serum can be determined by precipitating the protein to which they are attached. The laboratory test by which this is done is known as the protein-bound iodine (PBI). The normal level is from 4 to 8 μg of protein-bound iodine per 100 ml of blood serum. In hypothyroidism the level may drop to less than 1 μg. In hyperthyroidism it may rise to as much as 20 μg. Although the PBI is a generally reliable test of thyroid function, abnormally high or low values can be found in a variety of conditions of nonthyroid origin.

Thyroidal Uptake of Radioactive Iodine

Another method of determining the functional activity of the thyroid gland is by the administration of a tracer dose of iodine, ^{131}I (radioactive iodine). The patient is given ^{131}I mixed with water to drink. The iodine is absorbed into the blood from the alimentary canal. As the blood circulates through the thyroid gland, ^{131}I is trapped in it. The rate at which ^{131}I is concentrated in the thyroid gland is measured by monitoring with a counter of radioactivity. The ^{131}I not trapped by the thyroid is excreted in the urine. Testing the functional capacity of the thyroid with ^{131}I is possible because the cells of the gland are unable to distinguish between radioactive and nonradioactive isotopes. Increased trapping of iodine occurs in hyperthyroidism and decreased in hypothyroidism. ^{131}I is valuable in identifying areas of hyper- and hypoactivity. Because the rate of uptake of iodine may be influenced by the previous ingestion of iodine by the patient, the physician will want to know whether the patient has been taking iodine-containing drugs before the test is undertaken. Drugs that depress thyroid activity also inhibit the removal of iodine from the blood and will therefore influence the outcome of the test.

Radioiodinated Tri-Iodothyronine

A test being used with increasing frequency determines the ability of serum to bind resins of tri-iodothyronine or erythrocytes labeled with ^{131}I. Serum from the patient is incubated with the labeled material. In thyrotoxicosis, binding is high. In hypothyroidism it is low. This test has the advantage of being simple to do. All that it requires from the patient is a sample of blood.

Other Diagnostic Tests

Many other diagnostic tests may be utilized to estimate thyroid function. In hyperthyroidism, blood cholesterol may be low; in hypothyroidism it is usually elevated. As indicated above, ^{131}I is excreted in the urine. An increase in the quantity excreted is to be expected in hypothyroidism. The response to drugs that normally suppress or increase thyroid activity may provide the physician with clues to the nature and site of the problem.

Like other disorders, those involving the thyroid gland may either be easily identified or require extensive investigation. Unfortunately no single test gives a uniformly valid answer. Often only when a number of tests are combined with the patient's history and observations of his behavior can the diagnosis be made.

DISORDERS OF THE THYROID GLAND

Disorders of the thyroid are manifested by changes in the size and structure of the gland and by an inappropriate increase or decrease in the production of hormones. The condition in which the size of the gland is increased is known as goiter. Goiter may be accompanied by normal, hypo-, or hypersecretion of thyroid hormones. Locally, as a space-occupying mass, a goiter may interfere with swallowing or breathing by causing pressure on the esophagus or trachea. In our culture, the enlargement of the neck is considered unsightly, and as such it may be a cause of psychological stress. In areas of the world where goiter is endemic and common, it has been accepted as evidence of health and beauty. In the Andean Mountains in South America, where goiter was the rule, dolls were made with enlarged necks like that observed in the person with a goiter.

As a result of epidemiological studies, scientists have learned that the incidence of goiter is high in the areas where the soil has been leached of its supply of iodine. Its incidence is low where the diet includes iodine-containing foods. For example, in mountainous and inland areas the incidence of goiter is high. In regions where the land is sprayed by seawater or where an appreciable part of the diet is from the sea, the incidence of goiter is low. Goiter may also have a genetic basis. A defect in any one of the enzyme systems involved in the synthesis of thyroxin may result from the presence of a mutant gene. As in other disorders, multiple factors influence whether or not goiter develops. It is much more common in females than in males. It is more likely to develop during those periods in the life of the individual when the iodine requirement is increased. Thus goiter is more likely to appear during puberty or pregnancy and in individuals whose protein intake is excessive. In some women who develop goiters during pregnancy, the condition disappears at the termination of the pregnancy. Infections in the gastrointestinal tract may contribute to the development of goiter by interfering with the absorption of iodine.

Goiters caused by a lack of iodine can be prevented by the regular intake of water or salt to which iodine has been added. When the addition of iodine to water or salt was first proposed, the furor was no less than it is today over the introduction of fluorides into public water supplies. Nurses have a responsibility to instruct homemakers to use iodized salt because it is one of the simplest forms of primary prevention available.

Types of Enlargement

Enlargement of the thyroid gland may be diffuse or nodular. Although not very common, goiter may also be caused by a malignant neoplasm. In all types of goiters, hormone production may be within normal limits, deficient, or excessive. The general effects resulting from disorders of the thyroid depend on the extent to which the output of thyroid hormones is below or above the normal range. Conditions characterized by hypofunction include cretinism and myxedema. Cretinism characteristically occurs in infants and young children, myxedema in older children and adults. Hypothyroidism may be present in the absence of either. In disorders characterized by alterations in the secretion of the thyroid gland, there is a tendency to classify them as hypo- or hyperthyroidism or thyrotoxicosis rather than by name, such as cretinism or myxedema. Hypothyroidism may be caused by failure of the thyroid gland to develop as a consequence of a genetic defect or from a pre- or postnatal immunological disturbance. Infection, surgical removal of the gland, or therapy with ^{131}I may reduce the quantity of tissue below that required for normal functioning. Hypothyroidism may be secondary to failure of the anterior hypophysis to produce TSH.

Conditions characterized by hyperfunction include exophthalmic goiter, or Graves' disease, and toxic nodular goiter. In exophthalmic goiter disease, the thyroid gland is diffusely enlarged. In nodular goiter, parts of the gland are increased in size. In exophthalmic goiter, the eyes protrude and the disorder is usually more severe than in nodular goiter. The question of why

the thyroid gland hyperfunctions has not been answered. All the signs and symptoms observed in hyperthyroidism except the exophthalmos can be produced by excessive dosages of thyroid hormones.

Authorities have believed that Graves' disease is caused by excessive stimulation of the thyroid gland by TSH. This hypothesis is being challenged because some investigators have found that although some hyperthyroid patients have elevated levels of TSH, others have normal or low levels. In some hypothyroid patients, TSH is elevated. These observations suggest that thyroid synthesis and release may be independent of the negative feedback system. The problem of what causes thyrotoxicosis is further complicated by the fact that two other factors have been found in the serum of some hyperthyroid patients. One is the exophthalmos-producing substance, EPS. The other is a long-acting thyroid stimulator, LATS.[39] LATS is an immunoglobulin G (IgG). There is some evidence suggesting that LATS is an antibody to thyroid antigens. Its origin is unknown and its role in Graves' disease is uncertain. When it is present the degree of hyperactivity and the level of LATS are correlated.

The other factor is the exophthalmos-producing substance (EPS). Some authorities have suggested that it is of pituitary origin. Its level in the blood correlates with the degree of exophthalmos. Because the onset of the hyperthyroidism is frequently precipitated by an event causing emotional stress, some authorities attribute it to emotional factors. One explanation of the relationship of emotion to hyperthyroidism is that persons who develop thyrotoxicosis are emotionally dependent individuals who become hyperthyroid at the time of an emotional crisis, particularly from the loss of a person who is important to them. Not all authorities agree, however. At least one study points to the emotional status of the patient being caused by, rather than causing, the disorder. Robbins and Vinson [40] discovered that thyrotoxic patients do not differ from patients with known structural and physiological changes in the brain. Moreover, when patients studied were adequately treated, they did not differ from normal controls. As a consequence of their studies, Robbins and Vinson define thyrotoxicosis as a "metabolic disease manifested by impaired psychologic integration, involving particularly the autonomic nervous system." This definition emphasizes

[39] Gerald Burke: "The Long-Acting Thyroid Stimulator of Graves' Disease," *Amer. J. Med.*, **45**:435 (Sept.) 1968.

[40] Leonard R. Robbins and David B. Vinson: "Objective Psychologic Assessment of the Thyrotoxic Patient and the Response to Treatment," *J. Clin. Endocr.*, **20**:120–29 (Jan.) 1960.

that there are changes in psychological and bio-chemical reactions of the individual. Many of the manifestations result from the alterations in the functioning of the autonomic nervous system, particularly of the sympathoadrenal portion.

The individual who is in a hypothyroid state has an inadequate capacity to adapt to changes in his environment. The individual with hyperthyroidism makes inappropriate adaptations to his environment. The hypothyroid individual complains bitterly when he is in a cool environment. The one who is hyperthyroid behaves as if it were hot even when the environmental temperature is cool as judged by a person who is euthyroid. Some of the differences between the effects of hypo- and hypersecretion of the thyroid hormones are summarized in Table 15–2.

To illustrate the problems of the patient who is experiencing severe hyperthyroidism, Mrs. Thinis, aged 28, sought medical attention after her husband gave her the alternative of seeing a physician or a lawyer. Patients with hyperthyroidism frequently find their way to an internist by way of a psychiatrist or a lawyer. For some time she had been increasingly irritable, tense, and jittery. She screamed at her husband and children at the slightest provocation, accused her husband of being unfaithful, and was upset for hours over insignificant things. Although she had always eaten moderately, she was continuously hungry. Despite eating huge meals and frequent between-meal snacks she did not gain weight.

During her visit to her doctor, Mrs. Thinis sat on the edge of her chair, jumped at a slight noise, and talked rapidly and in an excited manner. At one point she burst into tears. Mrs. Thinis told her physician that she was certain that her husband planned to leave her. On examination her hands were found to be wet, her pulse rapid, and there was some lid lag (the eyelid moves more slowly than the eyeball) and widening of the palpebral fissures of her eyes. She stated that her mother had recently commented about her looking popeyed.

After examining Mrs. Thinis, her physician decided to hospitalize her for further study and to initiate a plan of therapy. In less acutely ill patients, many of the diagnostic tests can be made in the clinic or office of the physician. In the instance of Mrs. Thinis, the physician felt that she needed to be placed in a quiet, non-stimulating environment where she could get as much rest as possible. He arranged for her to be in a private room for a few days and prescribed the following: (1) radioiodinated triiodothyronine test; (2) protein-bound iodine test; (3) diet—high-calorie, high-carbohydrate, and high in vitamins; (4) thiamine chloride; and (5) phenobarbital, 30 mg four times per day.

From the description of Mrs. Thinis and knowledge of the effect of hyperthyroidism, it was clear that her capacity to adapt to her environment was impaired in a number of respects. Among those that were of immediate importance in making the nursing care plan were disturbances in her capacity (1) to adapt to increases in environmental temperature, (2) to control her emotional and muscular responses, and (3) to maintain a food intake adequate in quantity and quality to her needs. Other factors to be considered in the making of the nursing care plan include the fact that Mrs. Thinis sweated continuously and her heart rate was rapid. Both sweating and tachycardia were adaptive. The sweating protected her from an excessively high body temperature by increasing the heat loss. Her heart rate also contributed to heat loss by circulating the blood through the skin. It served further to increase the supply of oxygen and nutrients to the cells and to remove the products of metabolism. The increase in the rate of metabolism and the associated tachycardia placed a burden on the heart. When tachycardia is continued over a long period of time or the patient has a previously damaged heart, it may precipitate heart failure.

What are the nursing objectives in caring for a patient with hyperthyroidism?

The objectives on which the nursing care plan for Mrs. Thinis were based were

1. To modify her physical and emotional environment so that her need to adapt was minimized.
2. To provide her with food adequate in quantity and quality to her needs.
3. To replace fluid lost from the body.
4. To provide the family with the knowledge and support they needed to be helpful to the patient.

The most important modifications of Mrs. Thinis' physical surroundings are those that were directed toward facilitating the loss of heat and preventing unnecessary stimulation. The radiator was shut off and the window opened. In hot, humid weather an air-conditioned room adds much to the comfort of the patient and reduces the strain on the heat-eliminating mechanisms. The severely thyrotoxic patient may be placed in an oxygen tent. He benefits not only from the higher than normal concentration of oxygen, but also from the low environmental temperature. Sponging the patient's face and hands and arms several times a day adds to his comfort.

Mrs. Thinis' bed was prepared by removing

TABLE 15-2

	Hypothyroidism	Hyperthyroidism
Conditions with which associated	Cretinism—infants, young children Hypothyroidism without myxedema (atrophy or destruction of the thyroid gland) Surgical extirpation Myxedema—older children, adults	Exophthalmic goiter, or Graves' disease Toxic nodular goiter
Basic physiological disturbance	Decrease in thyroid hormones at some stage of their production	Increased production of thyroid hormones and possibly other substances
Effects of alteration in level of thyroid hormones	1. Reduction in heat production 2. Failure of mental and physical growth in infants and children 3. Disturbances in the metabolism of proteins, lipids, carbohydrates, water, and minerals, with abnormal collections of water, salt, and protein in tissues	1. Production of heat rises 2. Deranged carbohydrate metabolism with glycosuria 3. May be increased use of fat and protein as fuel
Characteristic laboratory findings	Elevated blood cholesterol, 300–700 mg/100 ml	Lowering of level of blood cholesterol
Basal metabolic rate (BMR normal −20 to +15)	−20 to −40	+15 to +60
Uptake of ^{131}I in per cent of uptake	Less than 15%	Greater than 50%
Protein-bound iodine in μg per 100 ml	Less than 4	Greater than 8
Red cell count	May be severe anemia	
Signs and symptoms: Speech	Swelling of tongue and larynx—a halting, slurred, hoarse speech	Rapid and excited. May be hoarse from local pressure on recurrent laryngeal nerves.
Skin	Thick, puffy, dry	Warm, moist, and flushed. Increased sweating.
Hair	Dry, brittle, sparse. May be alopecia of outer third of eyebrows. May be premature graying.	Hair soft and silky
Nervous system and mental and emotional state	Often apathetic and lethargic. May be hyperirritable. Cerebration slow. In older children and adults intelligence is retained. Condition returned to normal when hormones are replaced. Patients with myxedema may develop psychosis, infants and young children, mental retardation.	Hyperactive. Emotionally labile. Tears are caused by trivialities. Hypersensitive, hyperirritable. Tense, jittery, restless. Has forebodings of disaster. Occasionally depressed, but is agitated and restless at the same time. Fine tremor of extended hands or tongue.

TABLE 15-2 (cont.)

	Hypothyroidism	Hyperthyroidism
Body fat and weight, appetite	Increased weight. Weight may not increase because appetite usually decreases.	Loss of weight depends on relationship of food intake to metabolic rate
Susceptibility to cold	Increased	Decreased—susceptible to heat
Circulatory system (includes heart and blood vessels)	Increased capillary fragility. Bruises easily. Heart may be enlarged and fail. Cardiac output decreased. Blood pressure decreased. Weak heart beat. Increased circulation time.	Tachycardia. Increased cardiac output. Palpitation. Increased systolic blood pressure. Decreased circulation time. Paroxysmal arrhythmia. Cardiac failure is not infrequent. Wide pulse pressure. Dyspnea.
Gastrointestinal tract	Constipation. Hypophagia. Low glucose absorption rate.	Anorexia, nausea, vomiting, and diarrhea. Hyperphagia.
Muscle	Weakness. Hypotonia.	Weakness. Muscle fibrillary twitching, tremors. Muscle wasting.
Eyes		Protruding eyeballs (proptosis). Infrequent blinking, lid lag. Failure of convergence. Failure to wrinkle brow on looking upward.
Immune mechanism	Infection-susceptible. Subnormal phagocytic capacity of leukocytes	Infection-susceptible
Menstruation	Prolonged	Oligomenorrhea. Amenorrhea.
Subjective symptoms	Vague aches and pains. Cramps, arthralgic pain. Some have constant rhinorrhea or coryza.	

Therapy	Thyroid U.S.P. or some other form of thyroid hormone	1. Inhibit the activity of thyroid tissue (lessen the synthesis of thyroid hormones) (goitrogens)
		
		  a. Propylthiouracil
		  b. Methylmercaptoimidazole (Tapazole*)
		  c. Iodine
		
		2. Reduce the amount of functioning thyroid tissue
		
		  a. Radioactive iodine (^{131}I)
		  b. Surgical removal

* Trade name.

the blanket and spread, leaving only the top sheet. The rubber sheet was removed. If this is contrary to hospital policy, the rubber sheet should be placed under the mattress pad. A contour sheet was placed over the mattress in order to facilitate keeping the bottom sheet free from wrinkles. The nurse suggested that Mrs. Thinis might find pajamas more comfortable than a gown, as a top sheet would be unnecessary should she be too warm. Because Mrs. Thinis was restless and perspired profusely her bed required straightening and changing rather frequently. Every effort was made to convey to Mrs. Thinis that these procedures were for her comfort.

Because Mrs. Thinis overreacted to emotional and physical stimuli her need for rest was greater than that of many patients. The nature of her illness contributed to the difficulty in providing conditions favoring rest. Every effort was made to prevent sudden and loud noises. Talking and laughing outside her room were avoided, because Mrs. Thinis tended to be suspicious. When she heard voices outside her room, she would get out of bed and go to the door to check on the talkers. The fact that the conversation had nothing to do with her did not alter her disquiet. Mrs. Thinis was found to be less restless and more relaxed in bed when she had some nonstimulating activity to do. Because she liked to knit, her husband brought her needles and yarn. She was encouraged to select a relatively simple pattern and to alternate periods of rest and activity. When rest is an important objective and the condition of the patient interferes with his resting, his program should be adapted so that he obtains as much rest as possible.

The fact that Mrs. Thinis was hyperirritable and easily upset for extended periods of time by minor incidents contributed to the difficulty in securing rest for her. Mrs. Thinis was given her bath and assisted with all aspects of her care despite her apparent ability to do many of these things for herself. Because Mrs. Thinis' frustration level was low, her light was answered promptly and every effort was made to get her medications to her on time. Topics that were disturbing to her were avoided in conversation, and this information was relayed to all the personnel in the unit. As is not infrequent, some of her visitors were upsetting to her. As a result all visitors with the exception of her mother and husband were asked not to stay more than ten minutes. The method of handling this problem differs with the wishes of the patient and his family. The objective is to protect the patient from unnecessary stimulation. The nurse who was responsible for Mrs. Thinis was well suited to her requirements. She had a quiet, low-pitched voice. Her manner was unhurried and relaxed. Because tension tends to be communicable, a tense nurse is likely to add to the tension of the patient. The same nurse was assigned to care for Mrs. Thinis over a period of time, which enabled her to learn what was important to the patient and to utilize this information in meeting her needs. The patient

also had an opportunity to develop confidence in the nurse. As the nurse identified Mrs. Thinis' needs and ways of meeting them, she recorded this information on Mrs. Thinis' nursing care plan so that it was available to others as required. Because of the severity of Mrs. Thinis' clinical manifestations and her need for rest, her physician ordered phenobarbital, 0.5 grain four times per day. Not all patients with hyperthyroidism need sedation. It is necessary only in those who are seriously ill.

One of the most important responsibilities of the nurse who cared for Mrs. Thinis was to make certain that all personnel—professional and nonprofessional—and the patient's family understood that Mrs. Thinis' behavior was part of her illness. Adjustments should be made by the person caring for the patient, rather than by the patient. If Mrs. Thinis' behavior was accepted as part of her illness, then attention could be given to modifying her environment in such a way that stimuli inducing the behavior were avoided. Reactions to the patient's irritability and hypersensitivity with anger or irritation only act to intensify her symptoms.

Mrs. Thinis was similar to many patients with hyperthyroidism in that her appetite was enormous. To satisfy it and to provide her with the extra calories she needed, she was given a diet high in calories, carbohydrates, and vitamins. The high-carbohydrate and high-vitamin content of the diet also help to protect the liver from damage. Liver glycogen tends to be depleted in hyperthyroidism. Mrs. Thinis ate well. She disliked soft-boiled eggs and became upset when they were served to her. Therefore her nurse made a point of checking her breakfast tray before it was served. Because she was hungry between meals, she was served sandwiches and milk mid-morning and afternoon and before retiring. Fresh ice water was kept at her bedside at all times.

Some years ago the author cared for a man with thyrotoxicosis who consumed a triple serving of food at each meal. Between-meal nourishments were distributed to the patients by the dietary department. In the evening these were left at the bedside of the patient soon after dinner was served. As soon as the patient received the food, he would begin to eat it. By bedtime the several sandwiches and the fruit would long since have disappeared and he would ask for a lunch. Needless to say, he did not lose weight. Neither did he gain any. The patient should be helped to understand that his food requirements are increased by his illness. Personal remarks about the enormity of his appetite may make the patient self-conscious and cause him to eat less than he needs.

Occasionally a patient has a poor appetite

despite hyperthyroidism. Under these circumstances, particular attention should be paid to increasing the patient's food intake. He should be provided with food that he likes. Between-meal feedings, unless they result in a decrease in appetite, may increase his intake of food.

THERAPY

In the selection of the method of therapy, the physician considered the degree of hyperactivity of Mrs. Thinis' thyroid gland and the status of her cardiac function, as well as her age and her personal preference. He also considered the possibility of each possible therapeutic method's effecting a cure, and what, if any, harmful effects it might have. Among the therapeutic methods to be considered were drugs suppressing the synthesis of thyroid hormone, surgical removal of the thyroid gland, and treatment with radioactive iodine. Because Mrs. Thinis was only 28 years of age and still of childbearing age, radioactive iodine was eliminated as a possible choice. In patients who are 40 years of age or older, iodine [131] (radioactive iodine) is frequently employed in the treatment of hyperthyroidism.

The plan finally decided on for Mrs. Thinis was to prepare her for surgical removal of a part of the thyroid gland at a later date. To decrease the synthesis of thyroid hormone, 100 mg of propylthiouracil and 10 minims of Lugol's solution were prescribed to be administered three times per day. To maintain the concentration of these drugs at a constant level they were administered at eight-hour intervals —8:00 A.M., 4:00 P.M., and 12:00 midnight.

The observation that iodine is useful in the treatment of disorders of the thyroid has been known since antiquity. During the Middle Ages, persons with enlargement of the neck were treated with burnt sponge or seaweed. Not until 1916 did the now classic experiments of Marine and Kimball prove that iodine could be used in the prevention of goiter. When it is administered to patients with hyperthyroidism associated with a diffuse enlargement of the thyroid gland (Graves' disease), the thyroid gland undergoes involution and the storage of colloid is promoted. Maximum effects are obtained 10 to 15 days after therapy is initiated. The effects of iodine on the thyroid gland are reflected in a lowering of the basal metabolic rate, as well as in the pulse rate and in an improvement in the general condition of the patient. The effects of iodine therapy are temporary, because the patient returns to his hyperthyroid state. In fact, the degree of hyperthyroidism may be intensified. The mechanism by which iodine acts in hyperthyroidism is not known.

The introduction of thiouracil, followed by its safer analogue, propylthiouracil, and other antithyroid drugs, made it possible to induce a more or less permanent remission of hyperthyroidism. According to Goodman and Gilman,[41] antithyroid drugs act by preventing the binding of iodine in the organic form; as a result the effects of hyperthyroidism are reversed. Therapy is initiated by administering 225 to 300 mg of propylthiouracil daily. The total dosage is divided into three so that the patient receives 75 to 100 mg three times during the 24 hours. Proper spacing is essential for effectiveness when the drug is given every 8 hours. After the patient becomes euthyroid, the dosage is reduced until the maintenance dosage is achieved. This may be as little as 25 mg daily. In about 50 per cent of persons treated for hyperthyroidism with propylthiouracil, a permanent remission of the disease is induced. In patients in whom remission does not occur, signs and symptoms diminish and the general state of health improves.

Mrs. Thinis responded rapidly after therapy was initiated. After three days of treatment she was discharged from the hospital with the expectation that she would continue drug therapy and a high-calorie diet for six or eight weeks. After her hyperthyroidism was controlled and her general health status was improved, she was to have a subtotal thyroidectomy. When she returned to the hospital eight weeks later her BMR was +2, her pulse was 74, and she had gained 10 lb in weight. She was more relaxed and less easily upset than she had been on her first admission.

Radioactive Iodine

Of the radioactive isotopes, ^{131}I is the most valuable in the therapy of disease. Because the thyroid gland removes iodine from the blood and concentrates it in itself, radioiodine is useful in the diagnosis and treatment of disease of the thyroid. Because iodine is readily absorbed from the gastrointestinal tract, it is administered by mouth. The amount of iodine concentrated in the thyroid gland can be tested with a Geiger or similar counter. In hypothyroidism little iodine will be concentrated in the gland. In hyperthyroidism the quantity will be excessive. Iodine not absorbed by the thyroid gland is excreted in the urine. Because the quantity of radioiodine used in diagnosis is very small, no precautions are required to protect the nurse or others giving care to the patient. Because larger quantities are used in therapy, the patient should be isolated. (See Chapter 4.) Therapy with ^{131}I has several important advantages. It is easy to

[41] Louis S. Goodman and Alfred Gilman: *The Pharmacological Basis of Therapeutics,* 3rd ed. (New York: The Macmillan Company, 1965), p. 1487.

administer and it results in the highest rate of cure of all forms of therapy. Although there may be some increase in symptoms on the fourth or fifth day, radioiodine is less likely to cause a serious exacerbation of the hyperthyroid state than other forms of treatment. The increase in the degree of hyperthyroidism is explained as follows: Radioiodine produces some degree of thyroiditis with necrosis of thyroid cells. With the disintegration of cells of the gland, there is an increase in the release of the thyroid hormone stored in the gland.

Radioiodine has three disadvantages. Because it requires special equipment for its storage and handling, it is available only in medical centers. It may have an adverse effect on the germ plasm, and it may be carcinogenic. To avoid the possibility of either of these effects, some physicians prefer not to treat patients younger than 40 or 45 years of age with ^{131}I. After evaluation of patients treated with ^{131}I, smaller dosages are now being used and are found to be effective.

Thyroidectomy

Although surgery is employed less frequently in the treatment of hyperthyroidism than it once was, it is still the treatment of choice for some patients. Furthermore, some of the hazards accompanying surgery on the thyroid gland have been lessened since introduction of the goitrogenic drugs, as most patients will become euthyroid after therapy with them. As a result of the use of the goitrogenic agents, there has been a marked reduction in the incidence of thyroid crisis following operation and a marked improvement in the mortality rate. Because these drugs reduce the metabolic rate and improve the general status of the patient, time can be taken to improve his nutritional state. Furthermore, emotional calm and confidence that his needs will be identified and met promptly have positive effects.

The basic principles underlying the care of the surgical patient are presented in Chapter 17. Following any operation, the site and nature of the operative procedure have an important bearing on the needs of the patient and the possible complications. On returning from the operating room Mrs. Thinis was placed in low semi-Fowler's position with her head well supported. In her preoperative preparation she had been taught that she should avoid either extending or flexing her head or her neck. She had also been taught to brace her head with her hands when she moved. This action served to prevent unnecessary pain and strain on the suture line. Until she was up and about she was turned every two hours. Deep-breathing and coughing were encouraged at the same

time. Her vital signs were checked every 15 minutes for 2 hours, then every 4 hours for 24 hours. She was helped out of bed the evening of the day of surgery. In preparation for getting up she was instructed to brace her head and assisted to the "dangling" position. After a few minutes she was assisted off the edge of the bed and helped to walk.

As soon as Mrs. Thinis was able to swallow, she was encouraged to drink high-carbohydrate fluids. She was given glucose in water intravenously. As is usual in patients following thyroidectomy, she complained of discomfort on swallowing.

COMPLICATIONS

Complications to which Mrs. Thinis was particularly predisposed were hemorrhage, paresis or paralysis of the vocal folds, tracheitis, parathyroid failure, and thyroid crisis or storm. The fact that the thyroid gland has a rich blood supply increases the possibility of hemorrhage. Although external hemorrhage is possible, bleeding into the tissues is more common and more dangerous. To detect external bleeding, dressings should be checked each time the patient is seen. Because water flows downhill, the back and lower portions of the dressings are likely to be stained first. To detect bleeding early, she was asked each time she was observed if her dressing felt comfortable. Had she had a feeling of fullness or tightness in her neck, the physician should have been called immediately. If hemorrhage is allowed to continue, the patient can be expected to become dyspneic and to have other symptoms indicating respiratory obstruction. When the symptoms progress rapidly, the nurse may loosen the dressing before the physician arrives. Because hemorrhage into the tissues surrounding the trachea can be expected to cause respiratory obstruction, a tracheotomy tray was placed in Mrs. Thinis' room before she returned from the operating room.

The recurrent laryngeal nerves that supply the vocal cords may be injured during the surgical procedure. When one nerve is injured, the sole effect is hoarseness, which improves with time. Should both nerves be injured or severed, a tracheotomy may be required for the relief of respiratory obstruction. Because of the possibility of traumatizing the recurrent laryngeal nerves at the time of surgery, some surgeons check the condition of the vocal cords immediately after the operation by observing them. When they are in good condition and the patient develops hoarseness within 24 to 48 hours after surgery, it is almost certainly because of swelling in the region of the glottis and can be expected to subside. Following thyroidectomy, hoarseness should be reported promptly to the surgeon.

A third complication following thyroidectomy is hypoparathyroidism. It may be caused by the removal of all or some of the parathyroid tissue or by the combined effect of edema and swelling of the remaining tissue. Evidence of this complication is not likely to be present before 24 hours or to develop after 48 hours.

Thyroid Crisis

A complication once common in patients who were severely thyrotoxic was thyroid crisis or storm. Thyroid crisis or storm can and does occur before surgical therapy, as well as in the immediate postoperative period. In either event, it is a serious condition and is accompanied by a high mortality rate. In thyroid crisis all the symptoms of hyperthyroidism are exaggerated. The pulse rate rises to 140 or 200 beats per minute. There is also a rise in the rate of respiration and in the body temperature. In severe thyrotoxicosis, the temperature-regulating center loses control of body temperature and the temperature continues to rise until the time of death. Treatment during thyroid crisis is directed toward supplying cells with oxygen and glucose and preventing hyperpyrexia. To accomplish these objectives the patient is placed in the oxygen tent and given fluids high in glucose by mouth and by intravenous infusion. Heat loss can be facilitated by continuous sponging with cool water or the application of ice packs. When a hypothermia blanket is available, it may be employed to increase the loss of heat. Whatever method is used must be sufficiently vigorous and continued long enough to prevent the exposure of the cells to the effects of prolonged hyperpyrexia.

The Scar

A source of stress for some patients is the scar resulting from the incision. Mrs. Thinis was concerned lest she be left with an unsightly scar. She was reassured that she could expect the scar would, after a time, be no more than a fine line. The incision is usually made so that it follows the lines of the neck. Some surgeons use skin clips to further decrease scarring. Although the newly formed scar can be expected to be red, it will shrink and fade with the passage of time. Women who wish to cover the scar may do so by wearing a necklace or scarf.

Exophthalmos

A complication accompanying hyperthyroidism in some patients is exophthalmos. It is associated with the disease and is not a complication resulting from surgical or other forms of treatment. In exophthalmos the eyeballs protrude or appear to do so. The mechanism that is responsible remains unsettled. Apparently the mechanism responsible for the seeming protrusion is not the same in all individuals. In some patients there is no forward displacement of the eyeball. In others there is. When there is true forward displacement, is is caused by edema and fibrosis of orbital tissues. It does not appear to be related to the severity of the hyperthyroidism nor is its progress affected by thyroidectomy. In fact, in some instances, exophthalmos seems to get worse following thyroidectomy. Although progressive exophthalmos is a self-limiting process, the eye may be lost before a remission occurs. If the eye is to be saved, it is imperative that the cornea be protected from drying. The patient should be taught to close his eyes consciously at regular intervals to moisten the eyeball with tears.

OTHER DISORDERS OF THE THYROID GLAND

One not uncommon disorder of the thyroid gland is simple goiter. In the early stages of simple goiter, the thyroid gland is diffusely enlarged. There is usually no change in function, though occasionally hypofunction occurs. Simple goiter is most likely to develop during periods when additional thyroid function is required, such as puberty or pregnancy. Although intake of iodine is inadequate and the enlargement tends to disappear, it may persist; it then almost always becomes nodular. When the gland is greatly enlarged, it may cause compression on the surrounding structures. Simple goiter is treated with thyroid hormone.

Mrs. Grivin, aged 50, illustrates fairly well the pattern by which simple goiter develops into a nodular goiter. She was born and reared in a large city in the Great Lakes region. Her mother had been thyrotoxic in 1918. At age 13, Mrs. Grivin had an enlarged thyroid gland that was diagnosed as a simple goiter of the iodine-deficiency type. She was treated with 15 drops of potassium iodide three times per day for three months. Although the gland decreased in size, she continued to have some asymmetrical enlargement of the gland. At age 30 her BMR was −17. At age 41 it was +1. At age 45 it was +3.

At the time of Mrs. Grivin's admission to the hospital for a thyroidectomy, she had an extensive nodular goiter. Study with ^{131}I indicated that thyroid function was normal. There was no clinical evidence of hyperthyroidism, though for the three months previous to her hospitalization her thyroid gland had been progressively enlarging. During the three weeks immediately preceding her admission to the hospital, she had had difficulty in swallowing and had been hoarse. Total thyroidectomy was performed to relieve pressure on the esophagus and the recurrent laryngeal nerves.

With the exception of developing parathyroid tetany, Mrs. Grivin made an uneventful recovery. The manifestations and treatment of hypoparathyroidism are discussed in relation to the parathyroid gland. Because its was necessary to remove all of her thyroid gland, she will have to take thyroid hormone for the remainder of her life. Should she neglect this for a period of time, signs and symptoms of hypothyroidism could be expected to develop.

Hypothyroidism

The clinical manifestations of hypothyroidism are summarized in Table 15-2. Not all persons with hypothyroidism develop a full-fledged picture of cretinism or myxedema. In mild hypothyroidism the patient may complain of mild aches and pains, easy fatigability, inability to control emotions, and, in women, menstrual disturbances. The patient may be pale in appearance. Because the symptoms experienced by the patient are common to many disorders, the fact that he is suffering from hypothyroidism may be missed. The most serious consequence of hypothyroidism is a type of heart failure known as myxedema heart. It can be prevented by continued and adequate dosages of thyroid hormone. Probably the most important reason for the correction of hypothyroidism and maintenance of the euthyroid state is that it is essential to the feeling of well-being and productivity of the individual. A patient who complains of symptoms or whose appearance suggests hypothyroidism should be encouraged to seek medical attention. Patients such as Mrs. Grivin should be helped to understand why they should take their medication every day for the rest of their lives. Because the effects of thyroid hormones are initiated slowly and continued for some weeks, the patient may feel well for a time after he discontinues his medication and conclude that he no longer requires it. The patient should be encouraged to continue under regular medical supervision.

When making a nursing care plan for the patient with hypothyroidism, the ways in which he fails to adapt to his environment should be identified. Plans should then be made to modify his physical and emotional environments. Unlike the patient with hyperthyroidism, the one with hypothyroidism is intolerant to cold. He is comfortable only when the temperature is relatively high. At night he sleeps in a flannel gown and bed socks and has three or four woolen blankets on his bed. If he has an electric blanket, the heat is turned on high. When in the hospital, despite the complaints of his roommates that the room is too warm, he desires several blankets on his bed.

Because the patient with hypothyroidism has a dry skin, soap should be used sparingly, and cream or oily lotion may add to his comfort. To prevent bruising the patient, care should be taken when handling him. Furniture should be placed so that the chance of bumping into it is minimized.

Although patients are often apathetic and lethargic, they may be hyperirritable, and their ability to maintain their emotional control may also be disturbed. As in the care of other patients, the nurse should adapt her behavior to the needs of the patient. When the patient is apathetic and lethargic, he cannot be hurried or stimulated to move quickly. When he is hyperirritable, this too is part of his illness. Fortunately, the patient can be approached with optimism. When he is treated with thyroid hormones, the condition can be corrected. Depending on the form of drug prescribed, improvement of the patient should not be expected immediately. It may take as long as ten days to two weeks for signs of definite progress to be evident. The dosage of hormone has to be adjusted to each patient. As stated previously, patients with a hypofunctioning gland are more sensitive to the thyroid hormones than are those with normally functioning glands. Signs and symptoms of overdosage are those of hyperthyroidism. One precaution relates to the increased sensitivity of hypothyroid individuals to drugs such as morphine or codeine. When they are prescribed by the physician, dosages should be lower than they are for persons who are euthyroid.

To recapitulate, the manifestations of disorders of the thyroid have their origin in the effects of the expanding lesion on the tissues in the vicinity of the thyroid and in alterations in the level of production of thyroid hormones. Mrs. Grivin illustrated two of the effects of a goiter on the surrounding tissue. She was hoarse (pressure on the recurrent laryngeal nerve) and she had dysphagia, or difficulty in swallowing. Had the condition been allowed to continue she might have developed respiratory obstruction.

She also exemplified one of the causes of hypofunction of the thyroid gland, because she had a total thyroidectomy. She should not develop signs and symptoms of hypothyrodism if she continues to take thyroid hormone for the rest of her life. The manifestations of hypothyroidism are the result of a lack of the thyroid hormones. The manifestations of hyperthyroidism, as exemplified by Mrs. Thinis, arise from an excess of thyroid hormones. Patients with either hyper- or hypofunction of the thyroid gland are unable to adapt appropriately to certain aspects of their environment.

PARATHYROID FUNCTION

Among the regulators of the stability of the composition of the internal environment is the parathyroid hormone that is also called parathormone. In man, this hormone is secreted by the four parathyroid glands lying behind the thyroid gland. This hormone has been separated from beef parathyroid glands by Rasmussen.[42] It is protein in nature. The molecule is rather small (a molecular weight of about 7000), though it is larger than insulin. Now that the hormone has been obtained in pure form, physiologists and biochemists are able to study its mode of action. For some time there has been a considerable body of knowledge about the effects of the parathyroid hormone. This knowledge was obtained by observing the consequences of disease or by removing the parathyroid glands and by administering crude extracts containing the hormone to animals. The parathyroid hormone regulates the level of calcium and phosphate ions in the body fluids so that their product is maintained constant. Calcium and phosphate ions are regulated so that when the level of one or the other rises, the other falls. A rise in the level of calcium ions in the blood, therefore, is accompanied by an increase in the excretion of the phosphate ions in the urine with the result that $Ca^{2+} \times HPO_4{}^{2=} = C$. Conversely, a rise in the level of the phosphate ions results in an increase in the excretion of the calcium ions.

In the past, scientists have not been agreed as to whether the effect of the parathyroid hormone is primarily on the kidney or on the bone. Those who supported the first view thought that the hormone regulated the rate of excretion of the phosphate ions in the urine and that other effects of its action were secondary. Others contended that its primary effect was to regulate the rate of release of calcium from bone.

According to Rasmussen [43] studies made with the purified parathyroid hormone show that it acts both on the bone and on the kidney and on absorption from the gut. It increases the activity of bone-destroying cells, or osteoclasts, with the result that calcium is released from the bone to be utilized elsewhere. The hormone also acts to increase the excretion of phosphate in the urine. Both actions are essential to the homeostasis of calcium and phosphate ions. By

the release of calcium ions from the bone, phosphate ions are also liberated. Without some mechanism for their removal, the level of the product of the two ions would be endangered. Recent studies using the purified hormone indicate that it also regulates the rate of exchange of calcium in the lactating mammary gland and in the gastrointestinal tract.[44] In brief, then, the level of calcium ions in body fluids as well as their relationship to phosphate ions is regulated by the parathyroid hormones. Parathyroid hormone increases the rate of release of calcium from the bones, the excretion of phosphate by the kidney, and the reabsorption of calcium by the kidney and absorption from the alimentary canal. This complicated regulating mechanism provides for both rapid and slow responses to changes in the level of the parathyroid hormone. The kidneys and the gastrointestinal tract are sensitive and respond rapidly to small changes in its level. Bone, on the other hand, is much less sensitive and responds slowly.

Unlike the thyroid hormones and certain other hormones, the secretion of the parathyroid hormone is not under the control of the anterior pituitary gland. Secretion is regulated by the concentration of calcium in body fluids. By a fall in the level of calcium in the blood, secretion is increased. Conversely, as the level of calcium rises, secretion of the hormone is decreased.

As in other homeostatic conditions, the concentration of calcium in body fluids is maintained by several regulatory agencies. The parathyroid hormone appears to regulate body processes so that the relationship of calcium to phosphate ions is maintained constant. The level of calcium ions in body fluids is also maintained constant. Vitamin D supplements the action of the parathyroid hormone in maintaining the constancy of calcium ions in the body fluids. As long as man wore few clothes, ingestion of vitamin D was unnecessary, because the skin manufactures vitamin D when it is exposed to sunlight. Since the time when most of the skin surface was covered with clothing, the addition of vitamin D from exogenous sources has been necessary. A relatively new hormone, thyrocalcitonin, secreted by the thyroid gland in response to hypercalcemia, lowers the blood calcium.

FUNCTIONS OF CALCIUM AND PHOSPHATE IONS

Calcium and phosphate ions are important in the formation of new bone. The source of these ions to the newly forming bone is the circulating fluids of the body. They are considered to be in simple equilibrium with the new bone; that is, calcium and phosphate ions move into and out

---

[42] Howard Rasmussen: "The Parathyroid Hormone," *Sci. Amer.*, **204**:56–63 (Apr.) 1961.

[43] Rasmussen, *op. cit.*, p. 59.

[44] *Ibid.*, p. 59.

of the bone depending on their level in the body fluids. When the level of vitamin D falls, the level of calcium and phosphate falls. These minerals are, therefore, unavailable for deposit in the collagen of the newly forming bone. As a consequence the bones stop growing and bend out of shape. The resulting disorder is known as rickets.

Other functions that are dependent on the level and ratio of calcium to phosphate include (1) the normal transmission of nerve impulses, (2) the contraction of muscles, and (3) the coagulation of blood. When the level of calcium and phosphate in body fluids falls below a critical level, the irritability of nerve and muscle fibers increases. The patient suffers from tetany, which is characterized by painful muscle spasms. An outstanding feature of the condition is carpopedal spasm. The muscles of the hands and feet contract powerfully and painfully. The hands assume a characteristic position. Spasms of the muscles of the face can be precipitated by tapping over the facial nerve. This is known as Chvostek's sign. Tetany can be relieved by the intravenous injection of calcium gluconate.

The action of digitalis is enhanced by calcium. The size of the dose and the rate of administration of calcium to a patient who is digitalized should be less than in those who have not been digitalized. Patients who have been digitalized and who are given calcium should be observed for evidence of digitalis toxicity.

Besides the parathyroid hormone and vitamin D, other hormones also play a role in the regulation of the calcium-phosphate balance. These include calcitonin, the sex and adrenocortical steroids, the growth hormone from the anterior pituitary, insulin, and the thyroid hormone.

The level of calcium and phosphate ions in body fluids depends not only on the integrity of the regulatory mechanisms, but also on the adequacy of the supply of calcium in the diet and the health of the gastrointestinal tract, the bones, and the kidney.

PARATHYROID DISORDERS

The parathyroid glands are also subject to disease and to injury; disturbances in the structure of the parathyroids may be accompanied by disordered function. Benign neoplasms are the most frequent cause of hyperparathyroidism. Inadvertent removal of the parathyroid gland during surgery of the neck, particularly thyroidectomy, and idiopathic atrophy are the most frequent causes of hypoparathyroidism. In both hyper- and hypoparathyroidism, homeostasis of calcium and phosphate is disturbed. Specific effects depend on the direction of the change in secretion.

According to Nordin,[45] the clinical manifestations of hyperparathyroidism are so diverse that they defy classification. This disorder, though by no means rare, is often discovered accidentally. Frequently the disturbance that causes the patient to consult a physician is bilateral renal lithiasis (kidney stones or calculi).[46] With the increased secretion of the parathyroid hormone, the activity of the osteoclasts in the bone is enhanced. If the quantity of calcium phosphate stored in the bone is decreased and the concentration of calcium in blood is elevated as calcium is removed from the bone, its density is reduced (osteoporosis). Occasionally the loss of mineral from the bone is so great that there are areas of cystic degeneration resulting in a disorder known as osteitis fibrosa cystica. With the demineralization of the bones, they become fragile, thus predisposing to fractures. Hyperparathyroidism can, however, exist without changes in the bones provided the intake of calcium is sufficient to prevent excessive demineralization of bone.

By an elevation in the level of calcium in the blood, its excretion in the urine is increased. When conditions such as concentration or alkalinity of the urine favor precipitation, stones form.

Symptoms experienced by patients with hyperparathyroidism include bone pain, particularly in the back; muscular weakness; anorexia; and vomiting. The high level of calcium and phosphates in the blood results in increased excretion of these substances by the kidney. Polyuria follows because water excretion increases with the loss of calcium. With polyuria, polydipsia is to be expected. A vast number of other signs and symptoms may occur, especially in patients in advanced stages of hyperparathyroidism.

When hyperparathyroidism is caused by a benign neoplasm, the disorder is cured by surgical removal of the neoplasm. Because the glands are small and the neoplasm may also be small, the surgeon may have difficulty in finding it. Hyperplasia of the parathyroid glands is a possible, though less frequent, cause of hyperparathyroidism. It may be either primary or secondary to some other disorder. For example, in advanced kidney disease in which the kidney no longer reabsorbs normal amounts of calcium, the parathyroid gland undergoes hyperplasia.

Much of the nursing of the patient with hyperparathyroidism is similar to that of any sick person who is undergoing diagnosis and possible

[45] B. E. C. Nordin: "Primary Hyperparathyroidism," *Postgrad. Med.*, 29:66 (Jan.) 1961.
[46] Hyperparathyroidism is not, however, the sole cause of this condition.

surgical treatment. In the care of patients in whom bone changes are evident, care should be taken to prevent placing stress or strain on bones when they are being moved either in bed or from the bed to the wheelchair. Attention should also be given to providing the patients with an adequate supply of water.

The management of patients with chronic hypoparathyroidism is directed to the goal of increasing the level of calcium in the blood and reducing the amount of phosphate ion. Parathormone may be used early to control tetany. After tetany is controlled, the calcium level may be maintained by vitamin D or Dihydrotachysterol (A.T. 10). The latter, a derivative of ergosterol, more closely simulates the action of the parathyroid hormone. To further reduce the level of phosphates in the blood, the patient may be placed on a low-phosphorus diet. Foods high in phosphorus include milk products, cauliflower, and molasses. Aluminum hydroxide, 0.6 g three times per day, may be administered to decrease the absorption of phosphates from the intestine.

In nursing the patient with acute hypoparathyroidism, or the one who is predisposed to it, attention should be directed toward detecting signs indicating increased neuromuscular irritability. Treatment should then be given promptly. Should the patient have a convulsive seizure, care of the patient during the seizure is no different from that of convulsions of other causes. The seizure can be terminated by the administration of calcium gluconate intravenously. This should, therefore, be done promptly.

SUMMARY

One of the important factors in the maintenance of each homeostatic condition is regulation of one or more processes. In order for regulation to be effective, a receptor, or sensing body must be affected by disturbances (such as changes in the concentration of a substance) in the environment of a cell or of an individual. Some means must be available to communicate information gained by the receptor to centers for interpretation, and finally to effector (muscle or gland) cells. One of the most important systems of regulation is the endocrine system. Hormones secreted by the endocrine glands are distributed throughout the body, where they regulate the responses of cells to changes in their environment. Some hormones, such as those secreted by the thyroid gland, alter the activities of all cells. Others appear to influence some but not all.

Although exactly how hormones act is not known, they all regulate activities having to do with the adaptation of the individual to his environment. In cooperation with the nervous system, hormones act to integrate the total behavior of the individual. Like other service facilities, endocrine glands are subject to disease and injury. Because they are regulating mechanisms, disturbances in endocrine structure and function are likely to be reflected by increased or decreased activities of cells or structures regulated by a particular hormone. Disturbances in the secretions of one endocrine gland are likely to lead to disturbances in the secretion of others. Often many, if not all, body functions are affected.

In nursing the patient with an endocrine disturbance, the nurse should have an understanding of the physiological effect of hormones as well as the effects of hyper- or hyposecretion. Because the patient with an endocrine disorder is unable to adapt to certain aspects of his environment, the nurse should be prepared to appropriately modify the demands made on him. In controllable, but not curable, disorders the nurse has a responsibility to assist the patient and the members of his family to learn to manage his disease.

REFERENCES

BOOKS

Bunning, Erwin: *Physiological Clock: Endogenous Diurnal Rhythm and Biological Chronometry,* 2nd ed. (New York: Academic Press, Inc., 1964).

Danowski, T. S.: *Outline of Endocrine Gland Syndromes* (Baltimore: The Williams & Wilkins Company, 1968).

Duncan, Garfield G., ed.: *Diseases of Metabolism,* 5th ed. (Philadelphia: W. B. Saunders Company, 1968).

Kalmus, H.: *Regulation and Control in Living Systems* (New York: John Wiley & Sons, Inc., 1966).

Lerner, I. Michael: *Heredity, Evolution, and Society* (San Francisco: W. H. Freeman and Company, 1968).

Lissak, Kalman, and Endroczi, E.: *Neuroendocrine Control of Adaptation* (New York: Pergamon Press, Inc., 1966).

Papazian, Haig P.: *Modern Genetics* (New York: W. N. Norton & Company, 1967).

Sawin, Clark T.: *The Hormones: Endocrine Physi-*

ology (Boston: Little, Brown and Company, 1969).

Williams, Robert H., ed.: *Textbook of Endocrinology,* 4th ed. (Philadelphia, W. B. Saunders Company, 1968).

Woody, Paul Amos: *Genetics of Man* (New York: W. W. Norton & Company, 1967).

PERIODICALS

Adams, H. D., and Murphy R.: "The Management of Primary Hyperparathyroidism," *Surg. Gynec. Obstet.,* **116:**45–52 (Jan.) 1963.

Ahyja, M. M. S.: "Parathyroid Function Tests: A Review," *Indian J. Med. Sci.,* **21:**439–49 (July) 1967.

Attinger, Ernst O., and Millendorfer, Hans: "Performance Control of Biological and Societal Systems," *Perspect. Biol. Med.,* **12:**103–23 (Autumn) 1968.

Avioli, Louis V.: "The Diagnosis of Primary Hyperparathyroidism," *Med. Clin. N. Amer.,* **52:**451–62 (Mar.) 1968.

Biglieri, E. G., *et al.:* "Hypermineralocorticoidism," *Amer. J. Med.,* **45:**170–75 (Aug.) 1968.

Bissell, Grosvenor, and Coseglia, Patrick: "Endocrine Emergencies," *Med. Clin. N. Amer.,* **46:** 495–505 (Mar.) 1962.

Brown, David M.: "Serum Measurements of Thyroid Function," *Postgrad. Med.,* **44:**37–40 (Aug.) 1968.

Burke, Gerald: "The Long-Acting Thyroid Stimulator of Graves' Disease," *Amer. J. Med.,* **45:** 435–50 (Sept.) 1968.

Butcher, R. W.: "Role of Cyclic AMP in Hormone Actions," *New Eng. J. Med.,* **279:**1378–84 (Dec. 19) 1968.

Childs, Barton, and Der Kaloustian, Vazken M.: "Genetic Heterogeneity," *New Eng. J. Med.,* **279:**1205–12 (Nov. 28), 1267–74 (Dec. 5) 1968.

Choh Hao Li: "Anterior Pituitary Hormones," *Postgrad. Med.,* **29:**13–23 (Jan.) 1961.

Clark, Brian F. C., and Marcker, Kield A.: "How Proteins Start," *Sci. Amer.,* **218:**36–42 (Jan.) 1968.

Coodley, Eugene L.: "Significance of Serum Enzymes," *Amer. J. Nurs.,* **68:**301–304 (Feb.) 1968.

Corney, Gerald: "Human Genetics: 1. General Principles," *Nurs. Times,* **64:**1199–1202 (Sept. 6) 1968.

Corney, Gerald: "Human Genetics: 2. Biochemical Aspects," *Nurs. Times,* **64:**1237–39 (Sept. 13) 1968.

Crick, F. H. C.: "Nucleic Acids," *Sci. Amer.,* **197:** 188–203 (Sept.) 1957.

Doughaday, William H., and Thomas F. Frawley (eds.): "Symposium on Endocrine Disorders," *Med. Clin. N. Amer.,* **52:**229–472 (Mar.) 1968.

Deiss, Wm. P., and Peake, Robert L.: "The Mechanism of Thyroid Hormone Secretion," *Ann. Intern. Med.,* **69:**881–90 (Nov.) 1968.

DiPalma, Joseph R.: "The Pituitary Hormones: Potential Wonder Workers," *RN,* **29:**65–72, 96–99 (Jan.) 1966.

Dobyns, Brown M.: "Goiter," *Curr. Probl. Surg.,* (Jan.) 1969.

DuBrul, E. Lloyd: "Pattern of Genetic Control of Structure in the Evolution of Behavior," *Perspect. Biol. Med.,* **10:**524–39 (Summer) 1967.

Ephrussi, Boris, and Weiss, Mary C.: "Hybrid Somatic Cells," *Sci. Amer.,* **220:**26–35 (Apr.) 1969.

Fierro-Benitez, Rodrigo, *et al.:* "Endemic Goiter and Endemic Cretinism in the Andean Region," *New Eng. J. Med.,* **280:**296–302 (Feb. 6) 1969.

Flink, Edmun B. (guest ed.): "Laboratory Procedures for Diagnosing and Managing Endocrine Disorders," *Postgrad. Med.,* **46:**72–177 (Nov.) 1969.

Gibson, John: "Mendel and Heredity," *Nurs. Times,* **63:**1456–58 (Oct. 27) 1967.

Goodly, William: "Outside and Inside Time," *Perspect. Biol. Med.,* **12:**239–53 (Winter) 1969.

Goodman, Harvey G., Grumbach, Melvin M., and Kaplan, Selna L.: "Growth and Growth Hormone," *New Eng. J. Med.,* **278:**57–68 (Jan. 11) 1968.

Greenblatt, Robert B., and Metts, James C.: "Addison's Disease," *Amer. J. Nurs.,* **60:**1249–52 (Sept.) 1960.

Hamolsky, Milton W.: "Radioisotopic Tests of Thyroid Function," *Lahey Clin. Found. Bull.,* **16:**313–19 (No. 4) 1967.

Harden, R. McG.: "What Is Goitre?" *Nurs. Mirror,* **126:**12–13 (Mar. 29) 1968.

Horowitz, N. H.: "Perspectives in Medical Genetics," *Perspect. Biol. Med.,* **9:**349–57 (Spring) 1966.

Ivy, Horace K.: "The Syndrome of Inappropriate Secretion of Antidiuretic Hormone," *Med. Clin. N. Amer.,* **52:**817–26 (July) 1968.

Kahil, Michel E., *et al.:* "Hyponatremia from Sustained Release of Antidiuretic Hormone," *Postgrad. Med.,* **44:**159–62 (Oct.) 1968.

Kalow, W.: "Pharmacogenetics," *Postgrad. Med.,* **42:**32–36 (July) 1967.

Katz, Fred H.: "Laboratory Aids in the Diagnosis of Endocrine Disorders," *Med. Clin. N. Amer.,* **53:**79–95 (Jan.) 1969.

Kriss, Joseph P.: "The Nature and Significance of the Long-Acting Thyroid Stimulator," *Advances Metab. Dis.,* **3:**209–30, 1968.

Lanes, Phyllis: "Primary Aldosteronism," *Amer. J. Nurs.,* **61:**46–47 (Aug.) 1961.

Levitsky, John: "Heredity and the Blood Dyscrasias," *Med. Clin. N. Amer.,* **46:**295–302 (Jan.) 1962.

London, D. R.: "The Corticosteroids," *Practitioner,* **200:**113–20 (Jan.) 1968.

McClintock, John C.: "An Appraisal of the Current Methods of Treatment of Toxic Goiter," *Surgery,* **65:**700–707 (Apr.) 1969.

McGirr, E. M., and Greig, W. R.: "The Treatment of Thyrotoxicosis," *Practitioner,* **200:**485–93 (Apr.) 1968.

McKusick, Victor A.: "Medical Genetics—1960," *J. Chronic Dis.,* **14:**entire issue (July) 1961.

McKusick, Victor A., and Rimoin, David L.: "General Tom Thumb and Other Midgets," *Sci. Amer.,* **217:**103–108 (July) 1967.

Marks, Charles: "Hypoparathyroidism and Its Clinical Effects," *Amer. J. Surg.,* 116:40–48 (July) 1968.

Mason, A. Stuard: "The Treatment of Thyrotoxicosis," *Nurs. Times,* 65:202–203 (Feb. 13) 1969.

Menguy, René, and Paloyan, Edward: "Symposium on Endocrine Surgery," *Surg. Clin. N. Amer.,* 49:1–206 (Feb.) 1969.

Mitchell, Robert Edgar: "Circadian Rhythms," *Postgrad. Med.,* 44:239–43 (Nov.) 1968.

Moffat, E. P.: "Hyperparathyroidism with Renal Failure," *Nurs. Times,* 65:9–11 (Jan. 2) 1969.

Mohler, Stanley R., *et al.:* "The Time Zone and Circadian Rhythms in Relation to Aircraft Occupants Taking Long-Distance Flights," *Amer. J. Public Health,* 58:1404–1409 (Aug.) 1968.

Monder, C.: "Stability of Corticosteroids in Aqueous Solutions," *Endocrinology,* 82:318–26 (Feb.) 1968.

Neel, James V., and Schull, W. J.: "On Some Trends in Understanding the Genetics of Man," *Perspect. Biol. Med.,* 11:565–602 (Summer) 1968.

O'Malley, Bert W., and Kohler, Peter O.: "Hypoparathyroidism, Part 1," *Postgrad. Med.,* 44:71–75 (Oct.) 1968.

Reich, Barbara Hoffman, and Ault, Leilee Powell: "Nursing Care of the Patient with Addison's Disease," *Amer. J. Nurs.,* 60:1252–55 (Sept.) 1960.

Reinberg, Alain: "The Hours of Changing Responsiveness or Susceptibility," *Perspect. Biol. Med.,* 11:111–28 (Autumn) 1967.

"RN Asks an Expert About Genetics," *RN,* 28:81–88 (May) 1965.

Rodman, Morton J.: "The Male Sex Hormones and Anabolic Steroids," *RN,* 30:41–46, 90 (May) 1967.

Selenknow, Herbert A., and Refetoff, Samuel: "Common Tests of Thyroid Function in Serum," *JAMA,* 202:153–54 (Oct. 9) 1967.

Simpson, D. P., and Vanderlaan, W. P.: "Treatment of Hyperthyroidism with Antithyroid Drugs," *Postgrad. Med.,* 29:86–93 (Jan.) 1961.

Smith, Stephen E.: "Drugs and the Thyroid Gland," *Nurs. Times,* 63:185–86 (Feb. 10) 1967.

Solomon, D. H., *et al.:* "Hyperthyroidism," *Ann. Intern. Med.,* 69:1015–35 (Nov.) 1968.

Stern, Curt: "Genes and People," *Perspect. Biol. Med.,* 10:500–23 (Summer) 1967.

Strong, J. A.: "Human Growth Hormone," *Practitioner,* 200:502–508 (Apr.) 1968.

Thorn, G. W.: "The Adrenal Cortex," *Johns Hopkins Med. J.,* 123:49–77 (Aug.) 1968.

Tompkins, Gordon M. *et al.:* "Control of Specific Gene Expression in Higher Organisms," *Science,* 166:1474–80 (Dec. 19) 1969.

Wagner, David H.: "The Function of the Parathyroid Glands and Their Disturbances," *Surg. Clin. N. Amer.,* 42:171–84 (Feb.) 1962.

Wagner, Robert P.: "Genetics and Phenogenetics of Mitochondria," *Science,* 163:1026–30 (Mar. 7) 1969.

Wiener, Harry: "External Chemical Messengers: IV. Pineal Gland," *New York State J. Med.,* 68:912–38 (Apr 1), 1019–38 (Apr. 15) 1968.

Wroblewski, Felix: "Enzymes in Medical Diagnosis," *Sci. Amer.,* 205:99–107 (Aug.) 1961.

Yanofsky, Charles: "Gene Structure and Protein Structure," *Sci. Amer.,* 216:80–94 (May) 1967.

PART B
Neural Regulation *

Overview

Organization of the Central Nervous System

Integration of Brain Function

Nursing Care of the Patient with Impairment of Neural Regulation

Overview

ANY complex multicellular organism requires means by which its activities can be controlled. Organisms with highly elaborate differentiated systems demand means for relating these to one another, for adjusting to varying demands. Part A of this chapter has discussed various regulatory systems that facilitate these adjustments. The nervous system, which will be the concern of this section, stands in position to integrate, direct, and control them all. With a mature and functionally perfect nervous system, the bodily life of the organism goes on smoothly, meeting exquisitely, in the environment to which it is suited, its needs as an individual. When there are defects in the nervous system, the organism may be handicapped only slightly and able to compensate quite satisfactorily, or, as is the case in any complex organization with a highly elaborate administrative system when departments are absent or ineffective, chaos can result.

The history of the nervous system reaches far back in evolution; and the basic patterns of the simpler forms of animal life have been used, built upon, and elaborated until it is hard to see in the healthy adult the simple beginnings of so complicated a structure. By returning to the early life of the embryo and following the first weeks of its development, it may be seen that certain principles of growth will hold as well for the nervous system within the body as for the body as a whole. Here is a single example: Growth proceeds in cephalocaudal direction.

The earliest aggregation of cells that will shortly be delegated to undertake the elaboration of the nervous system is seen first at the anterior dorsal part of the embryo. As develop-

ment proceeds, it is at the cephalic end that evaginations and foldings that indicate the primitive brain occur. The simpler cord, growing caudally, retains for some time an appearance reminiscent of the nervous system of segmented animals such as worms, the nerves growing out from it seeming to pursue the primitive muscles that develop earlier.

Organization of the Central Nervous System

There are other principles, less familiar than the preceding one, that are more specific for understanding the nervous system. They will be stated here and subsequently referred to or applied in discussion.

1. The more important an organ or system is to the economy of the body as a whole, the more provisions there are for protecting its structure and blood supply.
2. The more highly specialized a tissue, the less able it is to survive severe and sudden deficits in supply.
3. After destruction of nerve cells, those remaining are unable to replace those that are lost.
4. Within the nervous system there is a hierarchy of control. No single part functions separately from other parts.
5. The nervous system imposes regulation and control not only on organs and systems of the body but also on itself.
6. In general, higher centers inhibit lower, and phylogenetically newer parts inhibit older.
7. The later in embryonic life a part of the nervous system develops, the more susceptible it is to injury.

* This part of the chapter was contributed by Esther H. Read, Professor Emeritus of Nursing, College of Nursing, Wayne State University, Detroit, Michigan; and Visiting Professor, School of Nursing, Universidad del Valle, Cali, Colombia. Miss Read acknowledges her gratitude to Dr. John Stirling Meyer, Professor and Chairman, Department of Neurology, Baylor College of Medicine, for his reading of the manuscript of this part of Chapter 15 and for his helpful suggestions.

As the system responsible for the control and regulation of all others, the economy of the body dictates that the nervous system be well shielded (Principle 1). Although this armor lies outside the nervous system, its structure needs to be appreciated nevertheless, because a break in the integrity of the protectors may constitute a threat to the nervous system they guard. Example: A compound fracture of the skull may be serious not so much on its own account as for the hazard of brain injury or infection it presents to the contents within.

The nervous system in man is well protected. The brain, after the period of rapid growth in infancy is over, is enclosed in a relatively rigid cranium of bone that is shaped by its inner tables to conform to and support the friable tissues that lie within the several fossae of the skull. In like manner, the spinal cord is guarded by a chain of vertebrae, rigid in themselves but held into a flexible tunnel for the cord by means of the heavy cartilaginous disks between their bodies and by powerful tendinous and muscle attachments. The safety of parts of the cord is enhanced by additional fixation offered by the shoulder and sacral girdles, although the thoracic section of the cord does not profit from such an additional shield.

Within the skull and vertebral column are three membranous coverings, the meninges. The outermost, the *dura mater,* is a heavy, relatively nonelastic tissue that forms a cloaklike covering for brain and cord and is reflected at these points to form deep folds: one, the *falx,* between the two cerebral hemispheres; the second, the *tentorium,* between the cerebral hemispheres and the cerebellum; and third, between the lobes of the cerebellum, the *falx cerebelli.* Like that of the skull, the protection offered by the dura is mechanical, and the partition erected by the falx tends to cut down on the transmission of pressure, or force, from hemisphere to hemisphere. The tentorium affords a comparable shield between the forebrain and the more vital structures of the midbrain and medulla below.

The second meninx, or *arachnoid,* is thin and made up of a delicate, fibrous, weblike tissue that both separates it from and joins it to the *pia mater,* the third membrane. Filling this mesh is the cerebrospinal fluid, which eventually will be returned to the blood by way of specialized structures of the arachnoid called villi, granulations, or the pacchionian bodies. See Figure 15-2.

The pia mater is also a thin membrane but tougher than the arachnoid, its connective tissue fibers being thoroughly interwoven. The pia is closely applied to the nervous system, helping to hold the very soft substance of brain in form and shape. In so doing, it follows the gyri and sulci and cuffs the blood vessels penetrating the surface of the brain. The thick mat

FIGURE 15-2. Diagrammatic coronal section through the head, including the layers of the scalp and the superficial cerebral cortex. This shows the emissary veins and the relations of the arachnoid villi to the dural sinuses. (Adapted with permission of the McGraw-Hill Book Company, Inc., from *A Functional Approach to Neuroanatomy,* by Earl Lawrence House and Ben Pansky. Copyright © McGraw-Hill Book Company, Inc., 1960.)

of blood vessels that are integral parts of the choroid plexuses is borne by the pia. Together they extend into the ventricles. This rich blood supply, and the action by which the pia seems to resist invasion by microorganisms, a matter that will subsequently be discussed briefly, as well as its apparently purely mechanical function of support, qualify the pia as a protector of the central nervous system. The pia and arachnoid together are referred to as the *leptomeninges*.

Cerebrospinal Fluid

The *cerebrospinal fluid* found circulating in the subarachnoid space has its origin largely in the choroid plexuses in the ventricles of the brain. These are fluid-filled cavities that serve as another means for absorbing shock. The ventricular system is rather like a short series of little lakes, spring-fed, that are connected to one another by canals of greater and less width to reach a marsh that spreads wide to cover the brain and eventually drains, by way of the arachnoid granulations, into the great channels

of the dural sinuses. Thus the brain floats on a fluid cushion; and because the specific gravities of the brain and cerebrospinal fluid are about the same, a blow to the head moves all the cranial contents together so that contortion is at a minimum. See Figure 15–3.

In the analogy, the "springs" are the choroid plexuses, which are little clusters of blood vessels covered by the pia mater and a single layer of cuboidal epithelial cells, the whole rather resembling a raspberry, that project into the lateral, third, and fourth ventricles. Cerebrospinal fluid is extravasated from them continuously at a rate estimated to be about 500 ml per day.[44] Nothing is found in cerebrospinal fluid that is not found in blood, but the concentrations are quite different, which implies that the fluid is a secretion rather than a filtrate. (See Table 15–3.)

The secreted fluid passes from the lateral ventricles through their foramina (of Monro) into the third ventricle, where continuation of the

[44] Arthur C. Guyton: *Textbook of Medical Physiology*, 3rd ed. (Philadelphia: W. B. Saunders Company, 1966), p. 461.

Figure 15-3. Diagram showing relationship of brain and cord to meninges. The choroid plexus forms the cerebrospinal fluid. (Modified with permission of The Macmillan Company from *The Principal Nervous Pathways*, 4th ed., by Andrew T. Rasmussen. Copyright © The Macmillan Company, 1952.)

TABLE 15-3

Average	Blood Plasma	Cerebrospinal Fluid
Protein, mg per 100 ml	7,500	20
Na, mEq per liter	137	141
Cl, mEq per liter	101	124
K, mEq per liter	4.9	3.3
Glucose, mg per 100 ml	92	61

choroid plexus contributes to the volume that passes through the aqueduct of Sylvius into the fourth ventricle where still more fluid is formed. In the fourth ventricle are two foramina (of Luschka) placed laterally and one (of Magendie) in the mid-line that permit passage of fluid into the *cisterna magna* and out into the subarachnoid spaces, the "marsh" over the brain. Only a small amount of cerebrospinal fluid is required to float the spinal cord and *cauda equina,* that cluster of spinal nerves that supplies the lower part of the body and that was seemingly left to drag behind by the uneven rate of growth, in early life, of cord and spinal column. It is this slender column of fluid in the lumbar spinal subarachnoid space that the physician taps when he seeks to determine the present chemical or bacteriological composition of his patient's cerebrospinal fluid or to determine the intracranial pressure.

The arachnoid granulations protrude through the venous walls and permit easy return to the blood of water and electrolytes as well as small protein molecules, for the osmotic gradient favors this. The amounts of fluid secreted and absorbed daily are normally the same, and this is some four times the total volume of the cerebrospinal cavity.[45] Circulation is maintained because the pressure in the capillaries at the point of secretion is greater than in the area of absorption.

Blood-Brain Barrier

The fourth protector of the nervous system is determined more by inference than by vision: This is the *blood-brain barrier.* All substances that circulate freely in the blood stream and pass into interstitial spaces of the body cells will not pass into the cerebrospinal fluid or brain parenchyma under normal circumstances. Whatever the nature of this barrier, it tends to protect the central nervous system from being affected by many agents that are potentially harmful. Although the circumstances that lower this barrier and permit molecules ordinarily excluded to

[45] *Ibid.*

pass through have been extensively studied, there is still no consensus of opinion on this point. The student who wishes to read further on the subject is referred to the references listed at the end of this chapter. The presence of the barrier is important to appreciate in drug therapy. When a drug is prescribed to treat an infection in the nervous system, meningococcic meningitis, for example, it is necessary to use one that penetrates the barrier, such as sulfadiazine; many other forms of sulfa do not, and would be ineffective.

Blood Supply of the Brain

The tissue of the nervous system, which will be discussed subsequently, is the most specialized of any tissue of the body and as such demands and receives a rich blood supply, about 750 ml per minute.[46] This is provided both by the carotid arteries, which enter at the base of the skull and divide to form the middle and anterior cerebral arteries, and by the two vertebral arteries, which branch off the subclavian artery and enter through the foramen magnum to form the basilar artery. These great vessels deliver to the brain blood which has only recently left the heart and is rich in oxygen and nutrients. Both the carotid and vertebral arteries variously coalesce, branch, and subdivide to assure excellent blood supply to all areas, the smallest arteries eventually forming capillaries from which veins arise that return to the subarachnoid spaces, and finally to the dural sinuses through which the brain is drained at last into the internal jugular veins that return to the superior vena cava.

A test frequently performed in the course of a diagnostic spinal tap illustrates some points discussed in the foregoing paragraphs. With a manometer attached to a lumbar-puncture needle inserted into the spinal canal, the cerebrospinal fluid will be noted to oscillate in direct relation to both the patient's pulse and respiration. If pressure is then applied to the patient's neck over the jugular veins, there will be a prompt rise in the column of cerebrospinal fluid in the manometer. Partial occlusion occasioned by jugular-vein compression has temporarily interfered with blood leaving the cranium, but the arterial inflow continues. This increases the volume of the intracranial blood and hence increases the intracranial pressure, which is reflected at once in the height of the fluid column in the manometer.

Cerebral Metabolism

It will be well to discuss in some detail the

[46] *Ibid.,* p. 322.

histological structure of the nervous system. Brain tissue demands much for its nourishment and respiration to meet its large energy requirements. Cerebral oxygen utilization is about 3.5 ml per minute for each 100 g of brain.[47] In the absence of oxygen, cerebral function can be supported for only ten seconds before symptoms result. Glucose consumption of the brain is 5.4 mg per minute for each 100 g of brain. The brain can survive for only one to one and one-half hours in the absence of glucose, before symptoms of hypoglycemia appear. (Principle 2: The more specialized a tissue, the less able it is to survive severe and sudden deficits in supply.) Although nerve cells have certain features in common and are quite unlike cells of other tissues—muscle, bone, and blood, for instance —these nerve cells vary greatly from one another, for they are well adapted in form to the special activities they carry on. In discussing "a typical nerve cell," one needs to understand that many nerve cells will be structurally quite different in appearance from the "typical" one used for illustration.

MICROSCOPIC STRUCTURE OF BRAIN

A nerve cell and all that is contained within it together with the processes of the cell are termed a *neuron,* the structural unit of nerve tissue. The processes that convey impulses to the cell are termed *dendrites* and referred to as *afferent processes* (*ad* meaning "to," *ferre* meaning "to bring"). Those that convey impulses away from the cell for delivery to a muscle or gland or to the dendrites of another nerve cell are *axons* and are referred to as *efferent processes* (*ex* meaning "from"). When an axon of one cell delivers its message to the dendrites of another, the point of transfer is a *synapse* (*syn* meaning "together," *aptein* meaning "clasp"). It is believed that the synapse offers some resistance to passage of nerve impulses and that the frequency with which impulses are sent along a pathway may influence this resistance so that it is reduced, a factor that may well be a part of perfecting manual or mental skills. Certain drugs, of which strychnine is an example, act at the synapse to speed up or delay transmission.

Inside the nerve cell will be found all the activities of any cell, with the exception of those having to do with cell division and replication. Because nerve cells cannot replace themselves, there will be no centrosome and no mitotic activities to be seen. (Principle 3: After destruction of nerve cells, those remaining are unable to replace those that are lost). *Nissl bodies,* seen only in nerve cells, appear as heavily stained granules scattered plentifully about in healthy nerve cells. They are nucleoprotein in nature, are concentrations of RNA (see page 665), and respond promptly to illness of the cell by breaking up and largely disappearing, a situation referred to as *chromolysis.* This is a reversible process, and if the cell recovers, the Nissl substance returns as before. Mitochondria are very numerous, as would be expected in a type of cell with vigorous metabolism.

STRUCTURE OF NERVE

The description of nerve fibers that follows applies both to afferent and efferent fibers of the peripheral nerves and to efferent fibers within the central nervous system. The only difference that needs to be mentioned is that nerve fibers within the central nervous system lack a *neurolemma* (sheath of Schwann), the outer cellular sheath of the peripheral nerve that permits sucessful regrowth after destruction of the fiber within, a privilege not accorded to nerve fibers lying within the central axis. Nerve fibers, acording to Elliott, are simple in structure, being tubes of plasma, containing elongated protein molecules.[48]

The *myelin* coat that covers many fibers serves to insulate the fiber and speed conduction along it. Myelinization is the work of the cell of the neurolemma sheath, the Schwann cell, and may involve the neuron itself as well.[49] The process begins in fetal life and continues actively until the individual is about two years old and, to a lesser extent, into adolescence. The developing *structure,* with the appearance of myelin, can be seen to correlate with the control of *function* in the maturing organism; e.g., it is useless to expect conscious control of bowel and bladder by a child before the age of about two years, when myelinization has proceeded to a point where this is possible for him. It is myelin that names the *white matter* of the nervous system, for nerve cells, or *gray matter,* have no glittering fatty covering to reflect light.

There are progressive diseases of the nervous system that are known as demyelinizing diseases. Of these, *multiple sclerosis* is probably most well known. The nurse will recall the slow, hesitant, inaccurate activity of patients with multiple sclerosis manifested in speech as well as in gross and other fine motor skills. This inadequacy demonstrates the loss of the rapid discrete conduction that their previously well-insulated nerve fibers had accorded them.

Inside the central nervous system where

[47] *Ibid.,* p. 323.

[48] H. Chandler Elliott: *Textbook of Neuroanatomy* (Philadelphia: J. B. Lippincott Company, 1963), p. 36.
[49] *Ibid.,* p. 42.

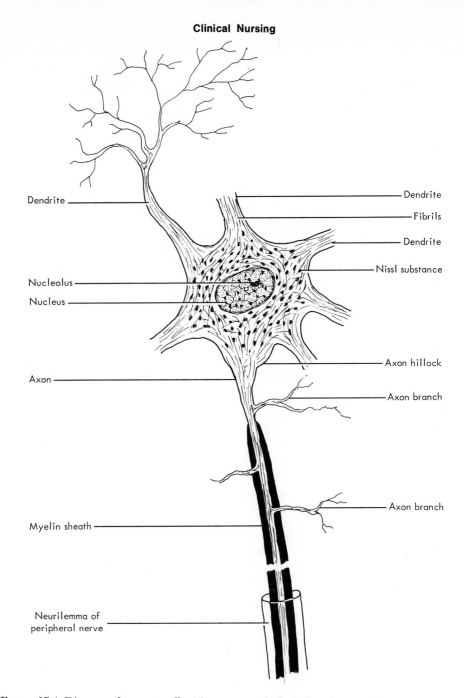

Dendrite

Dendrite
Fibrils
Dendrite

Nissl substance

Nucleolus
Nucleus

Axon hillock

Axon

Axon branch

Axon branch

Myelin sheath

Neurilemma of
peripheral nerve

FIGURE 15-4. Diagram of a nerve cell with processes. (Adapted with permission of Holt, Rinehart and Winston from *The Living Body*, 4th ed., 1958, p. 508, by Charles H. Best and Norman B. Taylor.)

nerves are without a neurolemma, the process of myelinization depends on certain of the *neuroglial cells*. The neuroglial cells are accessory to the cells of the nervous system and may be likened to connective tissue cells in the body as a whole, in that they support both structure and functions of other tissues. These cells are of several types, *astrocytes, oligocytes, microcytes*. Unlike nerve cells, they are possessed of centrosomes and are capable of reproducing themselves. More than half of intracranial neoplasms are tumors of the neuroglia.

Figures 15-4 and 15-5 show that the nerve fiber itself emerges naked from the cell but, as it proceeds, is very soon wrapped in myelin and covered over by a thin neurolemma. The myelin sheath, however, is broken at short intervals, and the neurolemma appears to be nipped in at this point. Each interruption is termed a *node of Ranvier*. The continuity of the nerve fiber and that of the neurolemma remain; only that of the myelin is broken. Because myelin acts to insulate the contained fiber, nerve fibers that conduct rapidly and for which discreteness of function is important, as, for instance, that of discriminating touch, are heavily insulated by myelin. The neurolemma of each node of Ranvier has a single flattened cell that is vital to repair of a damaged fiber, a process that, when comprehended, will make clear some points of importance for the care of patients who have suffered damage to peripheral nerves.

When rapidly growing, skinny Sarah stumbles up the back steps, she trips, falls, and knocks over a milk bottle. As she and the bottle tumble down the steps, the bottle breaks and Sarah cuts her forearm deeply on a fragment of the heavy glass bottle. In addition to incising skin, blood vessels, and muscle, Sarah severs the radial nerve, which is a *mixed peripheral* nerve that supplies a part of her hand. It is a *peripheral* nerve because it lies outside the central nervous system and supplies peripheral areas, and it is *mixed* because it contains, bound up in its structure, many nerve fibers with and without myelin, each with a neurolemma, some of which carry information from Sarah's hand to her spinal cord and brain (afferent fibers) and some of which, the axons of cells located in her spinal cord (efferent fibers), are responsible for delivering directions for action to the muscles and glands of her hand. The mixed nerve is like a telephone cable in some respects, containing many insulated wires, each with assigned work to perform.

In such an injury, the patient cannot feel anything in the parts once supplied by the now severed nerve: the area supplied is *anesthetic,* or without feeling. The afferent fibers are cut. She cannot move the parts either, and, very shortly, the muscles will begin to atrophy. If an appropriate electric current is supplied, there will be a failure to respond to galvanic current although there continues to be a response to faradic current: the so-called *reaction of degeneration*. This paresis of the parts must follow the break in continuity of the efferent fibers. The muscles are present but they have now lost their innervation: they are *denervated* and cannot act.

Sarah has excellent surgical care, no infection, and good health. Her well-repaired wound heals cleanly. She is careful to follow the direc-

FIGURE 15-5. Diagram of nerve regeneration. **A.** A normal neuron with its axon enclosed in myelin and a neurolemma sheath. Two nodes are shown. **B.** A neuron two or three days after section of the axon. Retrograde degeneration back to first node proximal to cut; swelling and chromolysis of the cell body, with displacement of the nucleus. Wallerian degeneration in the distal stump; the axon disintegrates, the myelin breaks down into droplets, and only the neurolemma survives. **C.** Beginning of regeneration. The axon sprouts into profuse branches. The cell body reverts toward normal. If a branch of the axon reaches the surviving neurolemma sheath of the distal stump, it will grow down it and restore functional continuity. (Adapted with permission of the J. B. Lippincott Company from *Textbook of Neuroanatomy*, 1963, Fig. 4-9, p. 47, by H. Chandler Elliott.)

tions given her to protect the partly anesthetic hand from thermal or mechanical injury and, a few months later, notes curious prickly sensations, pain, and tingling in her hand. These abnormal sensations, or *paresthesias,* continue to herald the fact that nerve repair is progressing, and eventually Sarah may regain much of what she lost when the radial nerve was severed by the fragment of glass.

The process of reinnervation of the partly denervated hand can be understood by following what goes on in a single fiber of the patient's radial nerve. This fiber originates as the axon of a motor cell in the anterior horn of the spinal cord. It is a very long fiber and was cut well toward the end. After such an injury, the distal fragment of the axon becomes swollen, the myelin disintegrates, and both are disposed of by phagocytosis. The neurolemma remains and survives. On the proximal side of the cut nerve as well there are changes. The cell body within the cord may demonstrate profound shock because of the damage to its process far away. The Nissl substance undergoes chromolysis, and the nucleus of the cell itself loses its central position. At the cut end of the axon, degeneration occurs comparable to that which is happening in the distal fragment, but this proceeds only as far as the next node of Ranvier. In a few days' time, when the cell has recovered its normal healthy state and the injured fiber fragments have been carried away, new little nerve fibrils begin to emerge from the node. They wave about seeming to seek guidance and a path. There are many of them, but it is obvious that only a few will find the waiting neurolemma of the distal stump that is essential both to guiding them to the muscles they should supply and also to provision of myelin needed for efficient performance.

Many of the new fibrils find no way and eventually disappear. If the break between proximal and distal fragments is great, more than a few millimeters, the regenerating fibrils will not find the distal neurolemma at all and, although they will continue to grow for some time, will ball themselves up in a little matted tumor, or *neuroma,* that can be a source of pain. The hand will, of course, remain without innervation and the part will be useless.

The most favorable outcome possible from a peripheral nerve injury such as the one described is not by any means the commonest and depends on circumstances only partly subject to control. At the time of the injury great care must be taken to prevent overvigorous application of a tourniquet. Blood lost can be replaced if it is necessary to do so—a little free bleeding is an effective douche to wash the damaged parts—but compression of the nerve higher up with resulting hypoxia to the entire arm from a tight tourniquet will seriously insult already damaged tissues.

Sarah's mother took a smoothly ironed linen guest towel, laid Sarah's forearm on it, and bandaged the whole forearm from wrist to elbow very firmly with a strip torn from an old sheet, before driving her to the hospital. The towel was reasonably clean, having been ironed and stored in a linen drawer probably free of pathogenic bacteria. Firm pressure exerted over the length of the forearm checks but does not stop bleeding and in no way interferes with arterial supply. The emergency treatment provides gentle pressure to the bleeding points locally and does not cause additional pain to the patient and thereby increased demand on her mechanisms for adaptation to stress that the original trauma has already activated. (See Chapter 6.)

Infection cured but with resultant scarring may leave a barrier that no newly regenerating axon fibril can cross. It is, therefore, important for everyone to do everything possible to prevent infection from occurring. Everyone needs be his brother's keeper; and although the gentlest and most skillful surgery is indicated, it will not bring the best possible results if there has been a lack of respect by anyone for bacteria, for the vulnerability of injured tissue, or for the person of the injured patient.

The second principle given at the beginning of the chapter stated that the more highly specialized a tissue, the less likely it is to survive deficits in supply. A neuron, nerve cell and fiber, has been described, and the effects of injury discussed. Although all nerve tissue is specialized, the specialization varies in degree. We have seen in the foregoing that even the most homogeneous part of the neuron, the fiber, suffers actual dissolution at its point of injury for a measurable distance toward its cell (up to the next node of Ranvier), and that the sensitive cell itself, though many inches away, reflects the shock when serious injury to the fiber is sustained. However, recovery of the shocked cell is prompt, as is the cell's immediate attention to repair its fiber. But this regeneration is not a simple process even in the fiber. It is one that demands no interference with the prescribed sequence and is possible only in the peripheral nerves.

Functional Unit of the Nervous System

As the neuron is the unit of nerve structure, the *reflex arc* is the unit of function. Because nervous structures exist to direct, control, and integrate all parts of the organism, discussion of the reflex arc involves end organs and nerves as well as neurons. In the broadest sense, these are a structure to receive a stimulus and one to react to a stimulus, which may be referred to simply as *receptor* and *effector* end organs. Thus, in simplest form, one may see the reflex arc illustrated when the patellar tendon, the receptor end organ, is stretched by a sharp blow on it, and the leg, the effector end organ, extends in response. This reaction implies the presence of an afferent nerve to convey the impulse to the spinal cord, intact synapses within the cord, and an efferent nerve to take the message for contraction out to the muscles of the leg. All parts of the circuit are needed. Any break in the circuit results in loss of the reflex. Each reflex, whenever elicited, is invariably repeated in the same pattern. It represents a pathway that has become useful to the animal over generations and, as it were, brooks no interference with its habits. A little thought will recall many familiar reflexes: the blink of the eye in response to threat, withdrawal of the finger from a flame, etc. In the case of peripheral nerve transection described previously, both afferent and efferent fibers were cut by the injury, so the hand was neither aware of the injury nor could it move to react. In poliomyelitis, however, the reflex will be lost because the motor cell in the spinal cord is destroyed by disease; and although the message from the struck tendon can be conveyed to the cord, there is no longer a motor cell within to activate an impulse to be conveyed out to the muscle of the leg.

This cell in the anterior horn of the spinal cord has many dendrites. All directions for the control of motion that are coming down from the brain by way of the descending tracts will eventually end at the synapses on these dendrites. This cell with its processes is therefore called the *lower motor neuron*. The axons that proceed from it to form the spinal and then peripheral nerves are called the *final common path*. In other words, all motion, consciously planned or not, must in the end be effected through these large motor cells and be carried out through these axons, a pathway that, though it may begin as far away as the cortex of the brain, is the last segment in the road on the way to the effector end organ (muscle or gland), and is common for all travelers. The name is a good one; it is the final pathway, to be used by all.

The simple cord reflex used to illustrate a reflex arc requires no planning on the part of the individual, but ordinarily he is aware that it has occurred. He may see it; he may be aware of the coldness or heat of the instrument that struck his knee; he may even inhibit the reflex by an elaborate play of higher activities on these simple ones that have not actually required any involvement of his brain at all.

Spinal Cord

Because this chapter is concerned with the over-all administrative system of the body, it is necessary to understand more than the last and simplest unit of action, to appreciate the main channels of communication, some of the lower and higher administrative branches, and how they influence one another. The discussion has referred already to the spinal cord and structures within it, the motor cells with their many dendrites around which axons synapse, bringing impulses from the brain above. Much of the cord is devoted to conveying information up and down its length and also to delivering some of the messages at appropriate stops along the way. The remainder of the cord is concerned with its relations to the periphery of the body. Structurally, the cord reflects these functions. Only slightly larger in diameter than a pencil, it is somewhat elliptical in shape with some increase in size at the thoracic and sacral enlargements. Neatly suspended in the spinal foramina of the vertebrae, two roots emerge on each side, one dorsal and one ventral, and pass through foramina in each vertebra. These roots presently join, and from this point on belong to the peripheral nervous system, which has just been discussed briefly in considering the reflex arc.

Looked at in cross section, the cord shows a central, H-shaped portion made up of cells, or gray matter, lying within a heavy border of fiber masses, or white matter. Many of the cells are those of neurons that are responsible for intercommunication within the cord: these are connectors that constitute a large part of the bulk of nervous tissue and are termed *internuncial* neurons. The white matter or nerve fibers of the cord tend to be grouped according to function; each group of fibers that is fairly discrete is called a *tract* and has a name. The form of the name usually indicates the direction of the tract, the point of origin being stated first and the destination, second. Thus, the *spinocerebellar tract* names a group of nerve fibers that conveys from the spinal cord to the cerebellum, which may be required to act on this knowledge, information about the state of contraction of muscles. A tract, then, represents a group of nerve fibers all of which have the same function.

ASCENDING TRACTS

The first neuron implicated in conveying a sensation to the brain is the neuron whose cell is located in a small swelling in the dorsal root just outside the spinal cord, called the posterior or *dorsal root ganglion* (see Figure 15-6). The

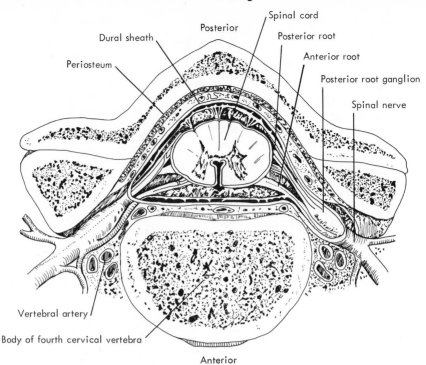

Posterior

Spinal cord

Dural sheath

Posterior root

Periosteum

Anterior root

Posterior root ganglion

Spinal nerve

Vertebral artery

Body of fourth cervical vertebra

Anterior

FIGURE 15-6. Cross section of vertebral column at the level of the fourth cervical vertebra, showing spinal cord in position. (Adapted with permission of the J. B. Lippincott Company from *Basic Physiology and Anatomy*, 1964, Fig. 136, p. 203, by Ellen E. Chaffee and Esther M. Greisheimer.)

processes of this cell extend in two directions; the shorter one centrally to enter the cord in the dorsal part and the other extending to the periphery to end in muscle, in skin, or around a hair follicle. This process extending to the periphery should be recognized as a single afferent unit in the cable of the peripheral nerve. It will terminate in one or another of a specialized nerve ending, peculiarly adapted to its place and function. Fibers that carry pain are naked and end in little brushes that cover a considerable surface, a square centimeter,[50] and may overlap one another, whereas touch, for which the animal requires far more discrimination than for pain, is provided with a myelinated fiber and three different kinds of specialized endings. Cold, heat, pressure—each is represented by its own ending adapted to meet the need. (See Figure 15-7.) Each specialized ending, on stimulation, sends the message along the sensory nerve fiber to the cell in the dorsal root ganglion whence it proceeds into the dorsomesial part of the cord. If this sensation is one of pain or temperature, the fiber, on entering the cord, ascends a segment or two and ends on

[50] *Ibid.*, p. 118.

the dendrites of a second neuron that immediately *decussates* (crosses over to the other side), to travel in the *spinothalamic* tract in the lateral part of the spinal cord to the thalamus. (See Figure 15-8.)

The *proprioceptive* pathway accounts for the conveyance of those sensations that are peculiarly one's own, within oneself (*proprio* meaning "own"). These are the muscle-tendon-joint sensations and vibration. It is by means of these columns that one is aware of his position in space. It is not, for example, necessary to look at one's foot to know where it is and whether or not the knee is bent. These fibers enter the cord by way of the dorsal root and sweep upward into the great wedge-shaped columns that occupy the whole dorsum of the cord. These columns are variously named, and the student should recognize *dorsal* or *posterior columns, fasciculus gracilis* and *fasciculus cuneatus,* and *dorsal fasciculus* as terms that indicate these tracts that proceed without decussation to the medulla, where the fibers end on secondary neurons. These fibers decussate at once and proceed as the *medial lemniscus* to the thalamus.

Reference has been made previously to the spinocerebellar tract, another afferent pathway

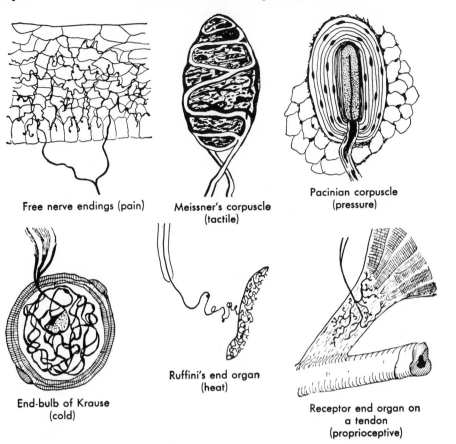

Free nerve endings (pain)   Meissner's corpuscle   Pacinian corpuscle
                                        (tactile)   (pressure)

End-bulb of Krause   Ruffini's end organ   Receptor end organ on
     (cold)   (heat)   a tendon
                                                                  (proprioceptive)

FIGURE 15-7. Specialized nerve endings. (Adapted with permission of The Macmillan Company from *Anatomy and Physiology*, 14th ed., Fig. 169, p. 202, by Diana Clifford Kimber, Carolyn E. Gray, Caroline E. Stackpole, and Lutie C. Leavell. Copyright © The Macmillan Company, 1961.)

of the spinal cord, but this one goes to the cerebellum. This tract lies at the periphery of the cord in two distinct divisions. The fibers conduct with great rapidity and are heavily myelinated. They ascend for a considerable way before they synapse with secondary neurons that are scattered along in the dorsal columns. Because the cerebellum is responsible for rapid adjustments of posture it requires quick and accurate information. The spinocerebellar tract keeps the cerebellum continuously informed of the state of contraction of muscles and of any change in tension. A disease that is not commonly seen today, tertiary syphilis, may result is degeneration of the dorsal columns which, it will be recalled, convey also part of touch as well as proprioception and vibration. Patients with this disease suffer many disabilities, of which loss of position sense, *ataxia* (without order), and awkward, faulty coordination (cerebellar adjustment) are conspicuous. This condition is called *tabes dorsalis* (*tabes* meaning "decay," *dorsalis* meaning "of the back").

Ascent of the sensation of touch is less simple to detail, and no attempt will be made here to do so to any extent. Some of the touch axons ascend in the dorsal columns and others end on the secondary neurons that decussate and form the ventral spinothalamic tract. The whole inflow of touch is widespread, an arrangement that permits considerable damage to the spinal cord in one area or another without utterly obliterating this extremely important sensation.

It will be noted by now that (1) sensations all land in the thalamus, and (2) all afferent pathways, with the possible exception of the spinocerebellar, have decussated once on the way to the brain. Knowledge of where that decussation occurs is helpful on occasion to understanding a patient's symptoms and complaints. If Mr. Samuelson has a lesion that has obliterated the function of his spinal cord at a

POSTERIOR

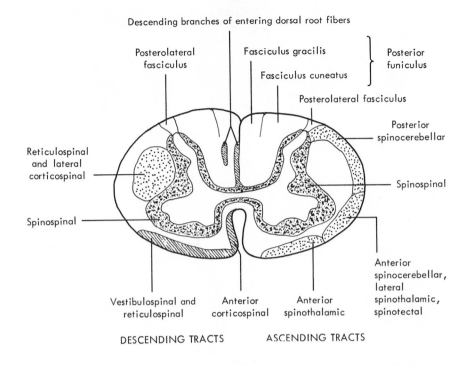

Descending branches of entering dorsal root fibers

Posterolateral fasciculus

Fasciculus gracilis

Fasciculus cuneatus

Posterior funiculus

Posterolateral fasciculus

Posterior spinocerebellar

Reticulospinal and lateral corticospinal

Spinospinal

Spinospinal

Anterior spinocerebellar, lateral spinothalamic, spinotectal

Vestibulospinal and reticulospinal

Anterior corticospinal

Anterior spinothalamic

DESCENDING TRACTS   ASCENDING TRACTS

ANTERIOR

FIGURE 15-8. The main tracts of the spinal cord. Afferent, ascending tracts on the right side; efferent, descending tracts on the left. It must be remembered, however, that both ascending and descending fibers are present on each side. (Adapted with permission of the W. B. Saunders Company from *Fundamentals of Neurology*, 4th ed., 1963, Fig. 128, p. 223, by Ernest Gardner.)

low thoracic level on the right side, one may expect that he will lose sensations of heat and cold and pain on the opposite side of the body, his "good," or left, side, below the level of the lesion; that he will lose the sensations transmitted by the dorsal columns, muscle-tendon-joint and vibration, on the right side; but that he will retain some awareness of touch, however defective, on both sides. The nurse who is aware of the patient's sensory deficit will recognize the hazards involved in mechanical or thermal damage to Mr. Samuelson's legs and also to his peace of mind if he notes the defective perception in his "good," left leg.

Up to this point we have considered these structures in the spinal cord—the afferent pathways and the neurons that convey messages within the cord—and we have mentioned the large motor cells of the anterior horn of spinal cord gray matter that form, with their processes, the *lower motor neuron* and whose axons are the *final common path*. A third cell found in the *thoracolumbar* part of the cord belongs to the efferent system of the *sympathetic nervous system*. The axons of these cells emerge from the anterior, or motor, root of the cord along with those of the anterior horn cell, and most of them have a synapse with dendrites of cells in the sympathetic chain lying paravertebrally outside. The cells of the *parasympathetic nervous system,* or *craniosacral* division of the autonomic nervous system, are quite differently placed. The cells of the cranial division are found in the brain stem and those of the sacral division in the sacral cord, in two compact masses and some scattered cells. The autonomic nervous system has been discussed to some extent in Chapter 6 in respect to the responses of the body to injury. There will be here no further extended consideration, but a few reminders to the student. Hormones are chemicals, and chemicals act diffusely; even chemicals that act quickly may not be at hand at the right moment unless there is something authoritative that reacts quickly to call them forth. The autonomic nervous system and the other regulators, hormones, enzymes, etc., work closely together, but it is the nervous system that responds promptly when, for instance, there is a need to speed up the heart in an emergency, and that sees to it that epinephrine is produced promptly and a supply maintained.

The remaining parts of the spinal cord consist chiefly of the descending or efferent tracts. These tracts constitute the rest of the white matter of the cord. They are concerned with bringing to the lower motor neuron the results of the concerted and integrated work of the higher centers: the cortex, various sub-cortical cell masses, and the cerebellum, which have worked and planned together on the information presented to them by the afferent pathways. These tracts are now bringing the result of the brain's planning to deliver to the anterior horn cell. This cell will send it out by way of the peripheral nerves to the final performers, the muscles and glands. It will be simpler, because the student has by now the outlines of the circuit traced, to learn about these descending tracts from their sites of origin in the brain. Therefore, discussion of the descending tracts will be delayed for the present.

Integration of Brain Function

It is now time to re-examine the cranial cavity to discuss the brain, which is itself responsible for originating much of what is carried out by the cord and peripheral nerves as well as all that goes on in respect to the special senses, vision, hearing, etc., and everything that we think of as "brains," e.g., higher thought, emotion, learning, and memory.

As the brain developed in higher animals from the simple linear structure seen in worms, and tended to concentrate at the anterior end of the animal, it bent back upon itself, and, in higher mammals and man, developed and enormously enlarged certain parts, notably the cerebral hemispheres. These great hemispheres, that bubble over and obscure almost all else seen by the casual viewer, cover up the evidence that remains of the curves and bends in the structure of the brain, which is finally crammed into a space and maintained at a weight (1,400 g) that a man can support and still not be top-heavy. Study of the brain's development in the embryo does demonstrate these changes, and even in the cut adult brain one can easily note that the lower parts, *medulla oblongata,* or *bulb,* and *midbrain,* are in direct linear continuity with the cord and are smaller and less complicated in physical form than are other much larger, evolutionarily newer, parts. These newer parts, some of the cerebellum, and the cerebral hemispheres show, even on gross examination, much greater bulk than bulb and midbrain, and reveal an enormous surface area that has been achieved by wrinkling and folding of the surface layers. Even a cursory view of the cut brain should demonstrate two other points that are helpful in looking at the structural basis for control and integration of function from a developmental point of view and that recall principles stated in the beginning of the chapter. (Principle 4: Within the nervous system there is a hierarchy of control. No single part functions separately from other parts. Principle 5: The nervous system imposes regulation and control not only on organs and systems of the body but also on itself. Principle 6: In general, higher centers inhibit lower centers and phylogenetically newer parts of the brain inhibit older or lower centers.)

On examination of the brain, two things are striking: (1) Heavy bands of white matter are evident running between parts recognizable as gray matter, and (2) although it is obvious that the surface of cerebrum and cerebellum is gray matter, e.g., made up of nerve cells, there are a good many other masses of cells lying embedded in white matter paired up along the central axis. These clumps of gray matter, literally covered up, and to an extent metaphorically as well, by the cerebral hemispheres, are referred to as *nuclei.*[51] They were present and more completely dominant in simpler animals before the cerebral cortex developed and overwhelmed them. We shall make frequent reference to these cell masses from now on, for although in man they are by no means at the top of the hierarchy of control, they are of great importance to him, and when any of these structures are damaged directly or thrown out of kilter by being poorly informed, integrated performance is handicapped.

What one sees, hears, smells, tastes, or feels must involve anatomically many parts if it is to be physiologically useful. One must not simply see or hear the car coming round the corner but retreat to the curbing to avoid being struck, an act that utilizes many nervous connections from the instant the eye or ear perceives the threat until the muscles of trunk and leg effect the life-saving backward steps. This activity involves sense organs, the cerebral cortex, the cerebellum and subcortical cell masses, reticular formation in the brain stem, and efferent tracts in

---

[51] This use of the word *nuclei* may confuse the student. The term as used in this paragraph, and as used considerably in the text that follows, means a group of nerve cells and does not refer to the central structure of a single cell. Examples: (1) The *red nucleus* (group of cells) is in the midbrain. (2) The two major divisions of a cell are the *nucleus* (the central organizing part of a single cell) and the *cytoplasm.*

the cord. All these will be considered in their turn. Before going further it may be well to review, restate somewhat differently, and add a bit.

Above the cord, the relatively simple form of an H-shaped mass of cells surrounded by fiber tracts becomes modified. Centrally, from bulb to thalamus, there is the reticular formation, a loose-appearing network of cells and nerve fibers in which some quite discrete cell masses are seen. From the bulb to the *pons* (bridge) the pairs of cranial nerves branch off; the cells of these nerves form nuclei that are embedded in pairs along the way. (See Figure 15-9.) Still larger masses of cells are to found as one moves upward, and all are surrounded by the great masses of white matter, tracts carrying their messages from one area to another, connecting,

projecting, and associating the work of their cells. The greatest bulk of white matter will be found in the cerebral hemispheres, and there, too, are the greatest number of nerve cells, spread in the thin wrinkled layers of the *cerebral cortex* (*cortex* meaning "bark"). It is these millions of cells that initiate; and it is their fibers, their axons and dendrites (some so short that they run only between cells of the cortex itself and some so long that they pass all the way to the spinal cord) that make possible those activities that are most characteristically human—complex thinking, memory, judgment, and highly developed learned skills. These cells are at the top of the hierarchy: they are newest in evolutionary and embryological development. Although the most human, they are least vital in a biological sense and the most intolerant of

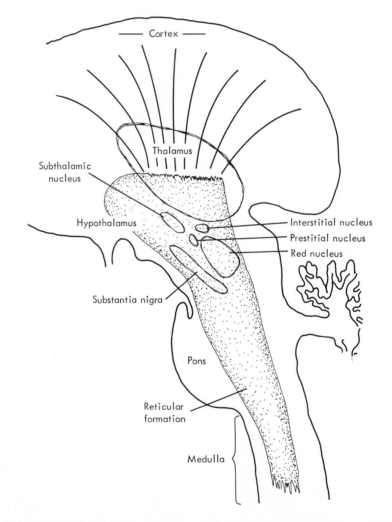

FIGURE 15-9. The reticular formation and its relationship to adjacent structures of the brain stem and cerebrum. (Adapted with permission of the W. B. Saunders Company from *Textbook of Medical Physiology*, 3rd ed., 1966, Fig. 629, p. 785, by Arthur Guyton.)

hypoglycemia and anoxia. (Principle 7: The later in embryonic life that a part of the nervous system develops, the more susceptible it is to injury.)

Looking at the nervous system from a developmental point of view and at the cerebral hemispheres as very late comers, one will realize that control and integration of everything of a biological nature must have been possible for the organism before the cerebrum was there at all. These structures, which are both dominated by the cerebrum in man and yet important to the integrity of cerebral function, are the vestibular nuclei belonging to the eighth cranial nerve, thalamus, cerebellum, basal ganglia, reticular formation, and a number of cell masses enclosed within it.

Reticular Formation

Some of these cell masses, or nuclei, just referred to, seem in the course of evolution to have condensed from a more diffuse-appearing substance made up of scattered cells and fibers that extends along the central axis from the bulb through the pons to the posterior part of the hypothalamus and into the ventral thalamus. This diffuse nerve cell–fiber system is called the *reticular formation* (*reticulum* meaning "net"). The reticular formation has become a subject of intense interest to neurophysiologists relatively recently. Although there is still much to be learned about this interesting area, nevertheless, certain contributions of the reticular formation at different levels throughout its length have been determined.

Functionally the reticular formation of the brain stem corresponds to the internuncial neurons of the spinal cord, neurons that work like the U.S. Senate page boys, taking information from one committee of the legislature to another, committees that will facilitate or inhibit action. In this formation, a vast number of reflex connections are made, all those for the cranial nerves and many others, some of which will be noted in discussion of the basal ganglia. Stimulation of parts of the reticular formation excites muscle activity, whereas stimulation of other parts inhibits it—a sort of brake-and-throttle action.

An important part of the life of any animal is sleep; and for animals that must respond quickly to the advent of danger or the presence of approaching prey, a ready change to alertness is as vital. The anterior part of the reticular formation alerts the whole cerebrum. This is accomplished by connections to the hypothalamus, to the thalamus, and thence to both the cortex and basal ganglia. The brain, thus made alert, is quickly cleared for action whether this be for the sleeping cat to waken and run across the lawn and leap into the grape arbor to escape the collie dog, or to develop a strategy and adjust its entire muscular system in order to catch a field mouse in the meadow in the evening.

In disease, the effect of this reticular activating system on the cortex as a whole can be illustrated by two examples. In an attack of *grand mal* epilepsy, it can be shown electrically that this part of the reticular formation is excessively stimulated. An electorencephalogram will demonstrate that the entire cerebral cortex is experiencing extreme neuronal activity during the convulsion.[52] On the other hand, when this area is destroyed, either by disease or by mutilation, of which encephalitis and gunshot wounds are examples, the patient presents the appearance of being asleep and cannot be wakened.

Already, from previous chapters, the student has become familiar with the neurophysiology of respiration (respiratory center) and with factors that affect arterial pressure (vasomotor center). These are parts of the reticular formation. The needs of the body for more or less pulmonary ventilation are mediated through connections in the reticular formation, as are other homeostatic mechanisms; so are the sympathetic and parasympathetic control of the heart and vascular system, and relays from the hypothalamus for control of temperature and other affairs of metabolism.

Thalamus

Anatomically, the *thalamus* lies above the brain stem and beneath the cortex, seeming to push up against the floor of the lateral ventricles. It is bounded on its sides and below by the fibers of the internal capsule that are wedged between the thalamus and basal ganglia. Although the most primitive part of the thalamus has no connections to the cortex because it developed in simple animals that had none, the rest of the thalamus is organized into large nuclei, cells onto which specific sensory tracts discharge and from which the information they bear is sent on to the cortex to be associated with different information coming from other thalamic sources, and is appreciated, integrated, and acted on. The cerebral cortex, in turn, reports to the thalamus. The trip by the sensations to the cortex and back seems by some means to have modified and refined the traveler, for the thalamus itself has a sort of coarse, undisciplined, conscious awareness that can be demonstrated when the cortex of an animal is removed. The creature reacts excessively: The decorticated cat will spit and snarl in response to a

[52] Guyton, *op. cit.*, p. 846.

stimulus at which a normal cat would simply rise, stretch, and walk away. The cat with the mutilated nervous system has no means by which to evaluate the stimulus: if it is of a noxious nature, no matter how minor, he "gives it all he has" in response. The normal cat, on the other hand, has all his integrating mechanisms intact and, evaluating the minor nature of the annoyance as just that, he simply moves away and conserves himself for a real emergency.

Absence of the cortex results in dementia with impaired memory, speech, judgment, and insight and *intensity of affect* (an emotional response out of relation to the stimulus). This intensity of affect is caused by loss of the disciplining effect of the intact cortex on the thalamus and is an illustration of the sixth of the principles stated at the beginning of Part B of this chapter: that higher centers inhibit lower and phylogenetically newer parts inhibit older.

The thalamus has connections to all the subcortical cell masses that have been mentioned, the hypothalamus, basal ganglia, red nucleus, etc., and to the cerebellum. It is a most important correlation center that must have its material in order before presenting it to the cortex and that must then take an active part—as an intermediary to be kept informed—in order that no details of the performance that is ordered by the cortex, on the basis of information received, should go astray.

Although the thalamus is to be thought of chiefly as sensory, the basal ganglia, also large cell masses situated nearby, are parts of the motor system. See Figure 15-10.

Basal Ganglia

These large cell masses or nuclei lie slightly caudal to the thalamus and on the outside of the wedge of the internal capsule. The nomenclature of these bodies is difficult. The term *corpus striatum* (striped body) can be used almost synonymously with basal ganglia. Separately, these cell masses are the *caudate* (tailed) nucleus, *putamen,* and *globus pallidus* (pale body). In reading, the student will come across other terms as well, such as *neostriatum* and *paleostriatum.* In this chapter the parts will be discussed simply as a unit and called the basal ganglia, but the student should recognize the other terms and also realize that not all parts of the basal ganglia have identical functions.

In general terms, the basal ganglia are concerned with the control of automatic associated movements of the body (e.g., the swing of the arms in alternation to the legs in walking). They work together with the cerebellum, thalamus, and cortex and have many connections with the reticular formation. The red nucleus in the

FIGURE 15-10. Vertical transverse section through the brain. (Adapted with permission of Holt, Rinehart and Winston from *The Living Body,* 4th ed., 1958, Fig. 12-16, p. 538, by Charles H. Best and Norman B. Taylor.)

reticular formation of the midbrain is the origin of a main efferent descending tract, the *rubrospinal,* which carries directions for control to the lower motor neuron and thence to muscles or glands.

Some of the motor tracts originating in the brain stem are short and completely contained within the brain itself (e.g., for eye movements), while others run in close proximity to the voluntary motor tract, the pyramidal, whose origin is cortical. All these tracts decussate and therefore exert control on the side of the body opposite their origin. The student can easily determine their origins and destinations simply by their names: reticulospinal, reticulobulbar, etc. Their great responsibility for the perfection of motor control can be grasped best by observing the problems of those who have disease in any of the nuclei from which they rise.

When there is injury or disease referable to the basal ganglia and nearby nuclei in the reticular formation, the individual is greatly handicapped. Depending on the part involved, he not only loses his automatic associated control but also is beset with a variety of nuisance movements that plague him, and also by alteration in muscle tone, a rigidity that makes every move more difficult. The student can easily learn to recognize these aberrations.

Athetosis is a writhing, wormlike squirminess. In *chorea,* there are contractions of muscles occurring without control so that the sequence of movement is interrupted and the patient accomplishes nothing effectively, for he is repeatedly thrown off by jerks of interrupted patterns. The *tremor* of basal ganglia disease is most obvious in the hands, which tend to be held pointing medially, fingers rather close, moving against the thumb in what is called a "pill-rolling" tremor. *Hemiballismus* is a violent jerking of large parts of the body. Like other abnormal movements of basal ganglia disease, hemiballismus may be provoked or made worse by voluntary efforts for controlled movement on the part of the patient. The rigidity seen in damage to basal ganglia is of a plastic type. When the individual is quite at ease, he may seem free of it, but on effort or with anxiety, the stiffness returns to resist the smooth accomplishment of every act. Parkinson's disease and some types of cerebral palsy are diseases wherein the basal ganglia are affected.

Vestibular Nuclei

That portion of the eighth cranial nerve that comes from the vestibular, or labyrinthine, portion of the ear and is concerned with informing the brain of the position and change of direction of the head in order that appropriate adjust-ments can be made to maintain equilibrium is called the vestibular portion of the eighth, or auditory, nerve. It has four nuclei in an irregular line along the floor of the fourth ventricle at the level of the caudal portion of the pons and upper portion of the medulla oblongata. As the vestibular fibers coming from the peripheral sense organ, the ear, enter the central nervous system, they bifurcate. Some of the branches go to a fifth vestibular nucleus in that part of the cerebellum that is phylogenetically the oldest, having arisen in animals (fishes) whose most important problem in coordination is maintaining appropriate swimming position. (You will recall noting that the dying goldfish keeps losing this position and slips over onto its side.) The other branches go to one or another of the four pairs of vestibular nuclei more centrally located. The bulk of the fibers of secondary neurons collects to form a tract, the vestibulospinal, that descends in the cord and ends on cells many of which control extensor muscles of the limbs.[53]

The whole vestibular apparatus, from ear to brain stem to cerebellar nuclei to efferent cell in the cord, helps to keep the animal on an even keel. When the horse is galloping round the ring, his legs on the inside must take up more sharply or he will topple on the curving track. The horse's vestibular apparatus contributes to maintaining perfection of gait even though this demands continuous adjustment because of the constant curve of the riding ring.

Cerebellum

This is the largest division of the brain after the cerebral hemispheres. Situated posterior to the central axis, it is connected by three large masses of white matter, the cerebellar peduncles, to the pons, midbrain, and medulla oblongata. The cerebellar cortex consists of two layers whose cells are provided with an enormous number of processes. The Purkinje cell, which is the effector cell, has so extensive a provision of branching dendrites that it looks like a microscopic Japanese barberry bush. The cellular structure and arrangement of the cerebellar cortex is such that incoming stimuli will excite a wide cortical area. (See Fig. 15-11.)

The cerebellum has evolved with the increasing complexity of the animal, as has the rest of the brain, and several divisions can be recognized that are correlated with phylogenetic age.

[53] When the brain stem is cut across just above these nuclei, the decerebrated animal goes into a state of *extensor rigidity.* This state may be seen in human beings when, through disease, the brain stem and cord are functionally cut off from control of higher parts, as with any large intracerebral mass that compresses the upper brain stem. This is called in man *decerebrate rigidity.* (See Principles 5 and 6.)

FIGURE 15-11. Purkinje cell with branching dendrites, greatly enlarged, in the cerebellar cortex.

We have spoken of one, the most primitive, that is simply an outgrowth of the vestibular system, but shall here, as was done in the case of the basal ganglia, discuss briefly the function of the cerebellum, not in parts, but as a whole.

In reviewing the material to this point the student will recall that

1. The afferent tracts to the cerebellum report to it the existing state of contraction of muscles and changes in tension; that the fibers are heavily myelinated and conduct with great rapidity.
2. The basal ganglia, concerned with control of associated movement and acting on information received from thalamus and cortex, report to midbrain centers.
3. The reflex connections of the cranial nerves, vestibular included, whose nuclei are in bulb and pons, take place in the reticular formation.
4. There are connections of these structures to thalamus and cerebral cortex.

It must, then, be evident, with mention of the large peduncles of white matter that bind the cerebellum to all these structures by way of their connections to the brain stem, that the cerebellum works with them all, and this is the case. Its work is in association with others, not independent. There is, for example, no tract running from cerebellum to cord. In its function the cerebellum illustrates especially well the second parts of the fourth and the fifth principles. (No single part of the nervous system functions separately from other parts. The nervous system imposes regulation and control not only on organs and systems of the body but also on itself.)

CEREBELLAR FUNCTION

Specifically, the cerebellum accepts on many dendrites the motor impulses discharged from the various centers we have just reviewed and spreads them widely in the cerebellar cortex. Although these incoming impulses, which represent a plan for action to be undertaken, have already been organized to some extent, they need a final revision with correction of errors. This is the work of the cerebellum. If more impulses for a given movement have been initiated than will be required, the cerebellum can arrange to have them cut down; if too great speed has been undertaken, this will be inhibited by instructions to the motor cortex to excite antagonist muscles and inhibit agonists. The revisionist activities of the cerebellum are accompanied by very efficient and extremely rapid feedback mechanisms which Guyton, terming them servomechanisms, compares to the control

system of an automatic pilot in an airplane. (See Fig. 15-12.)

When the cerebellum is diseased and this servomechanism breaks down, the individual no longer is able unconsciously to make the necessary corrections. He does not predict very well how a sequence of planned motions will come out, and the faster the motions, the worse the results. A common test of this is to ask the patient to rotate the forearm and hand rapidly. It is a simple thing to do with an intact cerebellum, but results in a futile jumble of uncoordinated moves when there is cerebellar disease. This inability to perform rapidly coordinated movements is called *adiadochokinesia*. Talking demands rapidly coordinated sequential movements. When these cannot be effected, speech may become nearly unintelligible. Some syllables are too loud or too soft, held too long or not long enough, and the patient is said to have *dysarthria*. Cerebellar disease results also in *dysmetria*, a faulty ability to measure. The individual over- or undershoots his mark when he reaches for something. *Asynergia* is also a problem for the patient with defective cerebellar function. The student will recognize the meaning from remembering its use in pharmacology. Synergistic drugs work together effectively to enhance one another; but the cerebellar patient's activity is asynergic—nothing works together. Hypotonia, tremor, nystagmus, and ataxia may all be noted in disease of the cerebellum. The patient, being competent intellectually, will make conscious attempts to compensate for errors that his previously intact cerebellum would not have permitted. Some efforts are more successful than others. He can make his ataxic gait safer by walking with his legs far apart, thrusting his pelvis forward, and holding onto the furniture. No amount of intelligence, conscious planning, or years of experience in the act will enable him now to perform neatly an act such as cracking and emptying a soft-boiled egg.

This is, perhaps, a good place to stop and illustrate in a small way a basic reason for a professional nurse's having some understanding of the nervous system. One learns that, ordinarily, a patient should be permitted to undertake independently or with assistance all the activities of daily living that he can. This is better for his morale than having them done for him. It may help him to recover. Like all generalizations, this one must be accepted with wariness, and the knowledge that generalizations have their exceptions. The nurse who understands the basis for the awkwardness of her cerebellar patient knows that he will be nothing but worse off for the attempt to open his own eggs, being left frustrated, humiliated, and

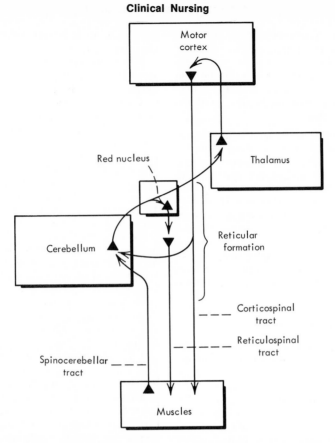

FIGURE 15-12. Pathways of cerebellar "error" control of voluntary movements. (Adapted with permission of the W. B. Saunders Company from *Textbook of Medical Physiology,* 3rd ed., 1966, Fig. 645, p. 811, by Arthur Guyton.)

hungry. She will see that this and similar little services are performed for him.

Cranial Nerves

Previously the statement was made and has since been referred to that the reflex connections for cranial nerves were centered in the reticular formation; little, however, has yet been said about the cranial nerves themselves other than the vestibular portion and nuclei of the eighth, and a statement that the nuclei of the cranial nerves are paired along either side of the center, in bulb and pons. There are several points by which it is interesting to compare cranial with peripheral nerves. (1) They are specialized, in that some are sensory, some motor. Although some have both a sensory and a motor component, these have their own nuclei and are quite discrete. (2) Their fibers are without neurolemma and cannot regenerate. They seem in some respects rather more like tracts than nerves. The cranial nerves are very frequently referred to by number instead of

name in speaking and in designation on the patient's chart. It is convenient to know the names that belong to the Roman numerals, but some persons find the task of learning them difficult. There is a mnemonic that has helped students for generations to learn the names.[54] A brief discussion of arrangement may also help, especially if the student will keep in mind the arrangement of features in the head of an animal such as a dog. The sense organ right out in front in animals is the snout; so the *olfactory* nerve is the most anterior, number I. Eyes come next; so *ocular* is II, large nerves whose fibers cross at the optic chiasm above the pituitary and proceed as *optic tracts* to the visual cortex. These two cranial nerves are sensory. But eyes need to be moved; and III, *oculomo-*

[54] On   Old   Olympus'   Topmost   Top
olfactory optic oculomotor trochlear trigeminal
A   *Finn*   *And*   *German*   *Viewed*
abducens facial auditory glossopharyngeal vagus
Some   *Hops*
spinal accessory hypoglossal

tor, IV, *trochlear,* and VI, *abducens,* provide this control. III includes parasympathetic fibers to constrict the pupil of the eye. Eyes are set in a face that is both above and below them; the Vth nerve, *trigeminal,* emerges between IV and VI. This great nerve, with three branches, is sensory (pain, temperature, touch, proprioception) to face and scalp and motor to muscles of mastication. The slender VIIth nerve, the facial, supplies motion to the muscles of expression of the face and taste to the anterior two thirds of the tongue. It pursues a circuitous route intracranially and fans out to supply a large area extracranially, and not infrequently is damaged either centrally or peripherally. Sadly collapsed muscles of the face result. Ears are double organs set to deal with hearing and to assist with balancing. Cranial nerve VIII has two divisions, auditory and vestibular, each coming from the appropriate portion of the ear. Not much below the ears, the throat begins where one finds IX, the glossopharyngeal (tongue-pharynx), which is largely sensory, supplying taste to the posterior third of the tongue and feeling to the upper pharynx. X is the vagus, the main outflow for the cranial division of the parasympathetic fraction of the autonomic nervous system. It is sensory to auricle, pharynx, larynx, and viscera of chest and abdomen, and motor to pharynx, larynx, base of tongue, and autonomic ganglia of chest and abdomen. The maintenance of homeostasis (see Chapter 3) depends heavily on the activities of the parasympathetic, and the largest bulk of fibers of the vagus goes to visceral organs that are assisted by its activity to maintain their normal vegetative functions or to regain these when they have been disturbed by stress on the animal. The XIth is the spinal accessory nerve, motor supply to the pharynx and palate and to the trapezius and sternomastoid muscles, and the hypoglossal, or XIIth cranial nerve, provides the motor supply to the tongue and muscles of the neck.

Long before this point the student must have become clearly aware of the validity of Principle 4, the interdependence of various parts. Everything that has been described or illustrated so far, however, has been concerned with patterns of activity, mostly with immediacy, not with individuality or originality. We are human beings, and although other animals share with us ability to store experiences, to learn, and to modify behavior in terms of learning, this is limited and more stylized than for man. Only in man can the life experiences of one individual or group be transmitted to the next generations so that they can be appreciated and used. However great the genius of an individual, even though he may be a true innovator, in a sense, his works are never completely his own creation.

His human heritage, the effects on his consciousness of work and techniques of artists who preceded him, have been received and integrated. Although what he builds, paints, or composes may seem to be quite unlike anything that has been done before, the unique product of the creative genius of one man, it could not have been built or painted so had other artists not left him their buildings, paintings, musical scores, and poetry.

In this respect, the oriole's nest hanging in perfect level and balance from the elm branch is different. We admire it and say, "It is a work of art." But the beautiful structure perfectly adapted to the needs of orioles would not satisfy all definitions of a "work of art" for, exquisite as it is, the nest of one is like that of another, like that of the parent, and of the next generation. The characteristics the nest has are those of the bird's species or class, not of itself as an individual builder; one oriole's nest will provoke neither more nor less admiration from us than that of another.

With these last notes on structure and function of the nervous system we have reached the top of the ascent from the cord and peripheral nerves and shall remain at this height long enough to gain a view, though cursory, of the activities of the human cerebral cortex. Then, with a quick descent on the motor tracts, the circuit will be completed.

The Cerebral Cortex and Its Function

The activities of the cerebral cortex are intimately and inextricably tied to the thalamus. The connections in both directions, thalamus to cortex and cortex to thalamus, are innumerable, constituting most elaborate feedback situations whereby impressions arriving at the thalamus by way of afferent pathways are relayed to appropriate parts of the cortex for analysis. Because analysis may demonstrate the need of appreciation from other parts of the cortex before final actions are taken, this factor may require another trip to the thalamus and relay by still other neurons to different parts of the cortex. These corticothalamic relays may have both immediate and long-lasting effects, relatively simple and quite complex. The sensory stimulus may cause a *motor response,* and the total experience may provoke new thoughts and also be stored in *memory,* perhaps to be useful in the future, three results differing from each other considerably but all necessary for men.

The student who wishes to learn any considerable amount of what is known today of the functions of the cerebral cortex is referred to a contemporary medical or neurophysiology text. The knowledge is incomplete at best, and the following text is but an over-all summary. Structurally, the cortex is a very thin, layered structure, the thickest part not more than 4 mm. The area is enormous, however. If one could flatten out its convoluted surface, it would cover more than two square yards. Considering the size of a single cell, this surface, even though only a few millimeters deep, provides a large acreage for a human being to manage and direct the work of his body, to think, plan, act rationally or not, communicate with others, and develop cultural and ethical behavior. This thin sheet of cells shows, histologically, six layers. Seen in microscopic section, the cell processes form a veritable mat, providing communication with cells in all layers, passing to more distant areas in the same or opposite hemispheres, or being themselves parts of the afferent and efferent systems to the brain and cord below.

The cerebral cortex looks quite homogeneous, yet certainly there are parts that are specialized in function. Considerable areas seem not to have a single function but only to reinforce by presenting wider areas for association. Figure 15-13 shows broad areas of cortical localization. One of the most interesting of these for human beings is the surface of the temporal lobe at the angular gyrus. This small region bears responsibility for interpreting sensory experience from whatever source. Complex and elaborate memories are stored here,[55] and any damage to the

[55] Guyton, *op. cit.*, p. 852.

area has serious effect on intellectual competence. Even though the entire visual and auditory apparatus from eye and ear to visual and auditory cortex may be intact, if there is loss of the interpretive area no proper use can be made of the sensory experience; it will not be integrated with previous experiences and so is valueless. For example, on walking toward a railroad crossing the individual might see the flashing red light and hear the noise of the approaching train but even though, before his damage occurred, the meaning of this sight and sound was clear to him and his behavior appropriate in terms of the correct interpretation and recollection, now he walks on, for the signals are meaningless and have no value to him anymore.

The most anterior parts of the cerebrum in front of the motor areas are termed the prefrontal lobes. There are connections from these to the hypothalamus that evoke responses associated with anger and distress and other responses mediated by the autonomic nervous system. For the most part, however, the prefrontal lobes seem to have a disciplinary function to perform. Without specialized function themselves, they provide a considerable area for reinforcement. In their presence, the individual has the means to work at complicated problems, resist distraction, deal with abstract thought, and weigh the relative merits of one line of behavior against another. If they are cut off from their influence on the rest of the brain, the individual

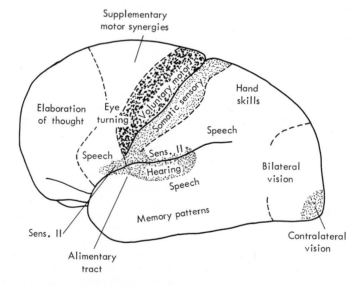

FIGURE 15-13. Functional areas of the human cerebral cortex as determined by electrical stimulation of the cortex during neurosurgical operations and by neurological examinations of patients with destroyed cortical regions. (Adapted with permission of The Macmillan Company from *The Cerebral Cortex of Man*, Fig. 117, p. 221, by Wilder Penfield and Theodore Rasmussen. Copyright © The Macmillan Company, 1950.)

is unable to discipline himself to any of these complex activities. He is incapable of abstract reasoning although he can follow concrete patterns of behavior. He may perform correctly the arithmetical tasks involved but be unable to solve a problem that presents no interesting challenge to him, for he is too easily distracted to grasp its import. His social behavior may be quite unorthodox and unsatisfactory to others, for he responds directly to his impulses without evaluation of consequences. This apparent isolation of the braking, inhibiting, or disciplinary effect of the frontal lobes is sometimes one of the unfortunate consequences of encephalitis, an inflammation of the brain.

Human beings can talk; it is their most important means of communication. They read and write and use symbols to express themselves by these means. These activities are very complicated, utilizing many areas of the cortex, some highly specialized. These are sometimes selectively destroyed by hemorrhage, tumor, or disease, and the patient may have any of the following disabilities resulting: He may be unable to form words although he knows what he wants to say—*motor aphasia;* he may be unable to comprehend by word or gesture what is said to him—*sensory aphasia;* one variety of sensory aphasia is an inability to attach meaning to words heard—*auditory agnosia,* or *word deafness;* and there may be a similar problem with words read—*visual agnosia,* or *word blindness.*

It is common knowledge that in right-handed persons the left hemisphere has ascendency over the right after early childhood. Motor speech for these persons is largely handled by the appropriate area—low in the premotor cortex—of the left hemisphere. One of the frequent and most trying disabilities of those who suffer a cerebral accident or *stroke* resulting in damage to this hemisphere is not the weakness of arm and leg so much as the maddening inability to express, in words, the thought that the mind can formulate. The student has probably noted that, in right-handed persons, the stroke that occurs in the right hemisphere does not have this unhappy result.

Mention of these difficulties with communication brings us at last to the parts of the cortex concerned with the control of motion and appreciation of sensations. There are large areas of the surface of the brain that, when stimulated, will result in movement of one or another group of muscles. These must all be included under the term *motor cortex* although some parts considerably overlap areas that are sensory (see Figure 15-14). The cortical region right around the central sulcus is purely motor. The number of cells that are present and responsible for initiating voluntary control of a part relate to fineness of control expected of that part; thus there are more cells in the cortical area concerned with voluntary control of the fingers that can be trained to operate with great dexterity than in the region devoted to control of the muscles of the thigh where voluntary control of muscles to any great degree is unnecessary.

Figure 15-13 demonstrates the considerable surface devoted to sensory functions, the special senses, and body sensations. Although, for example, the primary auditory cortex recognizes sounds, and bilateral oblation of this area of

Motor cortex

FIGURE 15-14. Areas of the cerebral cortex from which corticospinal fibers originate. (Adapted with permission of the W. B. Saunders Company from *Textbook of Medical Physiology,* 3rd ed., 1966, Fig. 636, p. 802, by Arthur Guyton.)

cortex will result in deafness, the sounds are not analyzed into useful forms until they have undergone switchbacks to the brain stem and again to the cerebrum where, in the angular gyrus of the temporal lobe, they are correctly interpreted, having been correlated with other experiences, and can be intelligently acted on. For example, the auditory motor cortex is stimulated by the train whistle, the sound coming to it from the eighth nerve by way of the thalamus. Switchback to the reticular formation results in alerting the necessary cortical areas so that when the angular gyrus and other parts of the cortex put everything together, the man will note the flashing red lights and stop his car. (Sound was used here as an example. A like process occurs with other sensations.)

A curious example of sensory defect is not uncommonly seen in children who have cerebral palsy with spastic hemiplegia of a type wherein there is cortical damage that includes the somatosensory areas just posterior to the central sulcus. These children have an *astereognosis,* an inability to identify a familiar object by the feel and form in the affected hand. With eyes closed they will accept a key and say that it is cold and that it has weight, but until they open their eyes they cannot identify the key. Such damage can occur later in life but it is not then so much of a handicap as to the child, who is so active a learner.

In the beginning of Part B of this chapter, under discussion of the cerebellum and cell masses in the brain stem, something was said about the coordination of unconscious muscle activity and automatic associated motion and the efferent tracts that arise from these nuclei. With this brief discussion of the cerebral cortex, there has been mention of voluntary control. It will be evident now, if we regard critically a simple activity of daily living, that these systems work together. The motor systems of the brain are very complex and, as yet, by no means completely understood or worked out.[56] In a very general way the *pyramidal, or corticospinal,* system is largely concerned with the control of voluntary motion, and those pathways that have to do with the coordination of unconscious adjustments and with the control of automatic associated movements are termed *extrapyramidal* or *extracorticospinal* (*extra* meaning "outside of"). A perfectly executed "voluntary" act implicates not only the pyramidal and extrapyramidal but sensory systems as well. The student is asked here to seat himself in a chair from a standing position while paying the most alert attention he can to all that goes on. Although he will not note everything, he will nevertheless realize that the strictly voluntary, conscious-

ly willed part of the act is only a small fraction and that the sensory awareness of his initial position and the shifts that were made as he neatly lowered himself to the chair were coordinated and adjusted with an exactness impossible for him had they depended on conscious planning alone.

The voluntary part of the controlled act of sitting down originated in cells of the motor cortex just anterior to the central sulcus. There are large cells there, the cells of Betz, whose heavy axons form a conspicuous fraction of the pyramidal tract. But the entire sensory motor cortex contributes to this tract whose fibers gather together first in the *internal capsule.* (The internal capsule is a massive band of white matter that contains the bulk of all fibers running to and from the cortex. It forms a sharp angle and appears to be squeezed in between thalamus and basal ganglia.) The fibers of the descending pyramidal tract give off collaterals to basal ganglia, reticular formation and nuclei therein, and indirectly to the cerebellum, as they continue through the pons to the medulla oblongata. Here they appear on the surface, and, as they continue caudally, most of the fibers decussate. The few that do not are found in the ventral part of the spinal cord, but the major number that decussate form the lateral *pyramidal tracts* that occupy a considerable fraction of the lateral white matter of the cord, running just anterior to the important extrapyramidal tract, the rubrospinal. As the text indicates, these two systems, pyramidal and extrapyramidal, are repeatedly in communication with each other through brain stem nuclei. The term *extrapyramidal* is not a good one; the interplay is too close. As is the case with all efferent tracts, the termination is on the lower motor neuron (anterior motor neuron in the spinal cord). It is the anterior horn cell there that will send the impulse to muscle or gland along the final common path. Interference with the tract at any point or with the cortical cells from which it arises will necessarily result in some measure of weakness and inadequacy of voluntary control, especially in fine discriminative movements.

The origin of the pyramidal tract is higher than that of the extrapyramidal pathways, and Principle 6 reminds us that higher centers tend to inhibit lower. When a patient has damage to the pyramidal pathway, these inhibiting forces are released and one sees activity that the wholly intact nervous system has under disciplined control after babyhood. There is constantly increased muscle tone, spasticity, with increased tendon reflexes and a marked tendency to develop contractures, absence of surface reflexes (abdominal and cremasteric), and the

[56] Elliott, *op. cit.,* p. 251.

Babinski reflex is present (upturning of the big toe and fanning of the others when the plantar surface of the foot is gently stimulated). Any number of pathological states in the nervous system will in some way encroach on the pyramidal tract so that testing for its integrity by eliciting abdominal reflexes and a normal plantar response (clenching of the toes and withdrawal on plantar stimulation) are commonly part of any general physical examination. If the person's responses to these are normal and he has no obvious signs of central nervous system disease, the physician will often assume that no further neurological testing is necessary.

Nurses may observe the signs of involvement of the pyramidal tract in the course of daily care of a patient after a cerebrovascular accident, or stroke. The abnormal reflex responses are demonstrated in the course of the bath, and the others will be noted during range-of-motion exercises.

By the act of sitting down in the chair perfectly performed, we have involved nearly everything that has been discussed in this section on the nervous system. An effort has been made to increase the student's knowledge of the nervous system beyond that gained in her basic course in anatomy and physiology and so to provide a basis for understanding difficulties patients may have that relate to involvement of the nervous system. Then it is easier to observe intelligently, to analyze the patient's needs for nursing care more specifically, and thereafter to meet them wisely. The nervous system is not a thing apart even though shut up in a bony box. It is nourished by the same blood supply and suffers insults from many of the same agents that injure the rest of the body. Whatever types of patients the nurse cares for, she will inevitably find some with complications involving the nervous system. Often, it is the nurse who is present when these signs first manifest themselves, and the professional nurse should be prepared to recognize their import. The remaining paragraphs of this chapter offer suggestions for rational care to meet the needs of patients troubled by some of the everyday problems of neurological origin that one encounters in nursing.

Nursing Care of the Patient with Impairment of Neural Regulation

Care of Persons with Increased Intracranial Pressure

In the adult, there is no potential for expansion of the skull when the need arises. The skull has many foramina in it provided for the entry or emergence of blood vessels and nerves, but they are well sealed off. The fontanels have long been closed, and the suture lines are too tight to be split open again. There can be no increase in bulk of any element within the head except at the expense of something else (Monro-Kellie doctrine).[57] Therefore, increase in intracranial pressure must occur with increase in intracranial bulk from any cause, and if this is long continued, there will be cell death.

Increased intracranial pressure may develop slowly, as in the case of a tumor growing above the tentorium, or very rapidly after a head injury with intracranial bleeding that frees a high-protein fluid eager to attract and hold water in a box that is already full. Intracranial pressure rises in inflammatory diseases of the nervous system such as encephalitis. In any condition where there is arteriolar spasm, the volume of blood circulating in the capillaries is reduced, and they become highly permeable. This sometimes occurs in acute nephritis and in malignant hypertension, and results in an edematous brain. Anything that blocks, partly or completely, the normal course of cerebrospinal fluid will cause pressure to rise. This could be a tumor that presses on the channels, gluey inflammatory exudate from meningitis that seals the foramina of Magendie and Luschka or absorptive areas in the meninges over the cortex. Whatever the cause, the patient is likely to demonstrate some characteristic signs. Although some signs may be caused by local pressure, they depend much more on the fact that the more crowded the nonexpansible space becomes within the cranium, the more limited will be the blood supply, and hence the oxygen, to each cell. The point of no return for the cells of the cerebral cortex in respect to lack of oxygen comes quickly, and for the cells of the brain stem a little later, but none can stand starvation for long, and the patient's symptomatology reflects their faltering.

Persons with increased intracranial pressure have headache. They need to have their heads elevated somewhat and often to be given acetylsalicylic acid compounds and caffeine. Elevation assists venous return from the head and caffeine is a cerebral vasoconstrictor agent and so decreases the headache. The nurse will find no orders to give opiates that decrease respiratory rate and efficiency, already depressed by the disease process. As congestion increases, the blood pressure will rise and the rate of pulse will slow down, because of ischemia of vasomotor centers. The patient, who may have been restless and irritable earlier, becomes lethargic and slow in his verbal responses. Later he may be stuporous. In stupor the individual is not alert to the stimuli to which he would ordinarily respond, but can be roused with some effort. As

[57] Elliott, *op. cit.,* p. 402.

pressure continues, respirations may become arrhythmical with periods of apnea, and the patient falls into a coma from which he cannot be roused; and at last, unless relieved, the hard-pressed bulb can no longer send forth stimuli to produce any respiration.

At any point in this sequence of events the nurse may note signs referable to involvement of cranial nerves other than X and should be alert to these and report them: A dilated pupil that fails to constrict on exposure to a light, drooping of one eyelid (III), and facial weakness (VII) should not only be recorded, but also the time at which these signs were first observed. These signs, and others, are not necessarily results of the increased intracranial pressure itself but are indicative of changes going on and of further involvement that the nurse, being present, may be the first to note.

Patients with increased intracranial pressure are required to have pulse, respiration, and blood pressure recorded frequently and regularly. Whoever may be assigned the task, it is the professional nurse's duty to know the trend of the record so that the physician may be notified if this trend becomes adverse. A record of vital signs that shows a consistent slowing of pulse and respiration accompanied by a rising blood pressure should be called to the physician's attention and not just left for him to find for himself.

When patients have surgery for some difficulty that lies intracranially below the tentorium and within the confines of the posterior fossa, the bone that is removed is not replaced. Often the dura is not resutured at the end of the operation. Several blood vessels will have been clipped during the surgery, and the blood supply may be temporarily somewhat less than normal. Edema may build up in the area in the hours after operation and endanger the patient's respiration temporarily, for he may be subjected to considerable compression of the bulb thereby. It is safest always with patients who have had craniotomies of this sort to keep the head in alignment with the body at all times including those moments when he is being turned. The rules are simple: (1) Have as many persons as are necessary to turn the patient without twisting him, and (2) leave him supported on his side so that his nose is in line with the xiphoid process. If the patient is an infant, one nurse can accomplish the turning safely alone; but if he is a man, this may require four nurses, with one person whose sole duty is control of the head. The infant's large head and narrow shoulders usually permit lining up nose and xiphoid very simply, securing the position by a small folded pad under the side of the chin. A child's head, being relatively smaller in relation to his shoulders than the infant's, will need one or two folded pillowcases; and the athlete with heavy, broad shoulders will need to have considerable height to the support under the head to bring it in line. When the work of adjusting the patient's position has been well done, he should be so perfectly balanced that there is no need for a pillow at his back although there is no objection to this, if the patient wants it, after correct position has been attained.

Care of Patients Subject to Seizures

Many times disease in the nervous system is accompanied by seizures, convulsions, or fits, three terms that should be equally useful, although the shortest one seems, nowadays, to be regarded as undignified. Until the nurse has had some experience with patients who are subject to seizures, she may fail to recognize those of a minor nature (*petit mal*) that often have no, or only a slight, motor component. The experienced person will recognize the momentary lapse of focus, the fading out of the voice, and the little meaningless movements of a part as manifestations of a seizure, and will record the occurrence. No one can fail to note or recognize a major convulsion, but the inexperienced nurse may be frightened and rendered incompetent when first seeing one. Fear reduces effectiveness, and the patient who has seizures may need some assistance from his nurse. His physician too, may need a careful description of the attack.

Although the patient may be in bed when the attack starts, it is quite likely that he may not and that he will fall down wherever he is. In a large percentage of major (*grand mal*) attacks, the person is immediately unconscious and in a state of generalized tonicity, with teeth clenched, body stiff, and no respiratory exchange occurring at all. Although this phase lasts only a few seconds, it is long enough for the face to become very turgid in appearance and for saliva to collect in great quantity. Shortly, the fit shifts to rhythmical jerking, the clonic phase; the patient breathes adequately, and his color clears. This clonic phase lasts from moments to many minutes. Gradually, the rhythmical jerking becomes slower and slower and finally stops, and the patient shows signs of returning consciousness, often making random movements accompanied by attempts at verbalization, but he seems confused and still incompetent. Complete recovery from the attack is usual after he has slept for a period, although headache for a few hours is not uncommon.

Because, at the onset of the attack, clenching of the jaws occurs at once, there is no possible way to prevent the patient's biting his tongue if it was between his teeth when they clamped together. Neither is there any way to prevent the patient from "turning black in the face and foaming from the mouth," for he is not breathing. No attempt should be made to force a wedge between the teeth. To do so results in bruising the gums and has been known to break a tooth. These few moments can be employed more usefully in loosening the collar and belt. After this, one cannot do better than to drop to the floor, kneeling at the patient's head, and, taking it firmly in hand, prop it either on one's own thighs or on a jacket or sweater placed underneath it, turning the head so that saliva can run out and the tongue drop forward away from the airway. It is now possible to insert a padded wedge, but this is rarely useful. By this time the convulsion will be in the clonic phase and one can protect the patient's head from pounding up and down on the floor or pavement throughout the attack. While a postseizure headache may be the rule, it is certainly not made less severe by preventable banging. It is neither useful nor advisable to restrain the patient during the attack other than to control the head. Urinary incontinence often occurs during the seizure and sometimes fecal, as well. No attempt should be made to move the patient until the seizure is over unless attendant circumstances make this imperative. Furniture or other encumbrances should be moved away from him. When the attack is over, he should be helped to a quiet place and permitted to sleep until he wakes, when he may resume his activities as before, if he feels able.

Certain convulsions are focal in nature. They start at a point and spread. This type of seizure may indicate a localized lesion in the brain and is often immediately preceded by paresthesias in the part that will shortly begin to twitch. Patients subject to such attacks often have time to walk to a bed and lie down and even to put a wadded face cloth or handkerchief between their teeth before the attack begins. They are usually conscious for the early part of the seizure, but, when it spreads to become generalized, are likely to go unconscious briefly.

These attacks should be carefully and completely described by the nurse, especially if one has not already been observed by the patient's physician. This is not easy to do the first time, and a nurse should not be chagrined if she has failed to note everything, so long as she is sure that she is accurate in reporting what she has seen. The following will illustrate a description.

Patient came to me looking scared and said, "Rub my left hand." I did so and walked with her to her bed where she lay down, and immediately the fingers of the left hand began rhythmical twitching. This spread to involve wrist, whole arm, and then left leg, and then the whole body. The patient seemed to watch the jerking until the attack became generalized, at which time she was apparently unconscious. I did not time the attack but estimate it to have been altogether about a minute and one half, with the period of unconsciousness about 15 seconds. The patient was alert again shortly after the attack. Her left-hand grip was weak and remained so for an hour.   [Signature]

Care of the Patient Who Is Subjected to Lumbar Puncture, Pneumoencephalogram, and Ventriculogram

These diagnostic procedures are not always accorded the seriousness they deserve and are needlessly uncomfortable. One who is to have a lumbar puncture should be helped to the appropriate position on his side with thighs flexed on the abdomen, back bowed, but with the lumbar spine kept parallel to the edge of the treatment table. The patient must keep his "up" shoulder from falling forward or his spine will rotate. If the nurse slips her arm under the patient's neck, stoops and opposes her shoulder to the patient's, it will make this easy for the patient, and secure the shoulder.

Patients who are to have air or oxygen injections into the ventricular system either directly through a burr hole in the skull or by the lumbar subarachnoid space should have forewarning of postprocedure headache and know that they will be asked afterward to turn from side to side. The injected air, being light, tends to pocket in the uppermost ventricle. There is no mechanism for absorption in the ventricle; the gas will have to go the regular route (see page 705). Recovery from the procedure is slow if the patient refuses to roll, and rolling over hurts for the first day.

Both these procedures have hazards. Gases such as air or oxygen are foreign bodies to these tissues and produce cellular reaction. Sudden withdrawal of considerable fluid from below may cause dislocation downward of the medulla into the foramen magnum and respiratory death; therefore, encephalogram is not done when there is any considerable increase in intracranial pressure. It is especially hazardous if the cause of pressure lies below the tentorium, as in cerebellar tumor. If visualization of the ventricles is important, the ventriculogram may be safer, for the tentorium provides a roof between, and the pressure changes incurred by the procedure are less likely to produce medullary compression. Uncomfortable and unfavorable responses may occur in response to these air injections whether or not the report is "negative." Every patient subjected to these examinations deserves intelligent observation and thoughtful care, which will necessarily include watching for signs of generalized increase in intracranial pressure, as a response to the irritation from the injected gas, and, especially, for depressed respirations.

Nutrition: Care in Feeding the Physically Dependent Patient

In normal healthy existence, one ordinarily swallows while in a sitting or standing position when the head is in line with the body. It is not difficult, however, to swallow when the head is slightly flexed forward, as one does in using a drinking fountain; but to twist the head sharply to the side and eat is so difficult that one always returns his head to the midline, or nearly, before swallowing. Persons who are recumbent in bed are therefore at a disadvantage in respect to ease of swallowing. The position is unnatural. If the nurse remains aware of her own behavior in respect to this normally automatic act, she will be careful to make eating as easy as it can be for the patient in bed. This will always include having the patient's head in line with his body and, unless specifically contraindicated, somewhat elevated. If this elevation cannot be allowed, the patient should be carefully placed in a side-lying position for safety, because it is very difficult for a small nurse to assist a large patient, who is lying perfectly flat on his back, quickly enough to avoid serious aspiration if he chokes in an attempt to swallow. If the patient has a neurological problem, he may be trying to cope not only with a position that is mechanically unfavorable but with an organic difficulty in the act of swallowing, too.

In some clinics, after craniotomy no patient is permitted anything by mouth until "tested for swallowing" by the surgeon. The observant nurse will note that the doctor who is doing this has put the patient well over on his side, has made sure the patient's mouth is clear, and has the suction tip in one hand and a teaspoon of water in the other. The doctor then introduces the water carefully and watches intently to see how successfully this act of swallowing is completed. If swallowing is impossible for the patient at this time, it is easy for the doctor to suction the fluid back. Even when a patient is permitted feedings after a successful test, the nurse should appreciate his recent difficulties, and act to make eating as safe and as easy as it can be.

Neurological patients often have trouble with vomiting, both those with lesions in the appropriate areas in the brain stem and those with generalized intracranial presure. If the reasons for this vomiting cannot be remedied promptly, the individual's nutrition suffers. Careful obser-

vation of time and circumstances that provoke emesis is needed. The patient's observations about himself in this regard may be helpful and should be sought. There are often patterns of serving food to the patient that will result in more calories being retained than just by giving the three meals a day in the routine manner at the routine hours. If, for instance, radical change of posture provokes trouble, it may be advisable to get the patient out of bed before breakfast so that the episode will be over some time before breakfast is served. If the man has had trouble after his regular full meals but manages successfully a dry ham sandwich at three-thirty every afternoon, it will be worth trying to give him only solids at meals and his fluids in between. There are no rules for guidance except those of careful observation, resourcefulness, and concern for the patient's welfare. Remember that the patient's trouble is in his brain and not his digestive tract; and if the nurse either withholds food because of vomiting or fails to meet the basic nutritional needs of the patient through supplying again the calories he loses—and chlorides along with them—there may arise problems of electrolyte balance to add to those already present. (See Chapters 9 and 12.)

Care of the Patient with Acute Spinal Cord Damage

Chapter 18 considers rehabilitation of the patient with spinal cord damage. Because, in these days of street accidents, many persons suffer injury to the spinal cord, nurses not infrequently have such patients to care for during their acute phase on general wards. There are few patients who so promptly and devastatingly reveal poor care as these; but, on the other hand, nurses who can maintain in good shape the bodies and spirits of their patients with pathology in the spinal cord may justifiably feel great satisfaction.

Everything one has learned of the structure and function of the spinal cord and peripheral nervous system can be put to use. Everything one knows of normal development of the personality and the effects of sudden helplessness on it will be invaluable knowledge to the sensitive nurse. If transection is functionally complete, one knows that afferent impulses cannot ascend from below the level of the lesion to the brain or efferent impulses descend to parts below the break in continuity of the cord. There will be paralysis, necessarily, and there will be anesthesia and vasomotor instability of the body beginning a little higher up than the level of the lesion (see pages 711–15). The patient will be unaware of his distended bladder and unable to empty it or his bowel voluntarily. Sooner or later he will be aware of inadequacy of sexual function. If the lesion is in the thoracic cord or above, his breathing will be affected and his weak chest movements will keep him continuously in danger of pneumonia. Only isolated cord reflexes, cut off from any inhibiting control from above, remain. These, if they occur, have nuisance value only. (See Chapter 18.)

The helpless patient lies dead weight in gravity position on his bed and quickly begins to develop contractures and foot drop. The muscles, whose nerves are no longer supplied by axons coming from anterior horn cells that are being constantly excited by stimuli coming from above, lose tone and will atrophy. A soft atrophic muscle supports poorly; the veins are not well pumped by vigorous muscle contractions any more, so the circulation is not brisk and the patient's tissues are prepared to break down easily.

If the patient has a badly fractured spinal column, he may have to be immobilized. But if the cord is damaged either traumatically or by disease without significant fracture of bone, effective nursing care seems to hinge largely on cleanliness and movement. A good rule for the nurse to have for herself is: "I must see every square inch of this patient's body every day."

There are mattresses which are made in cells and are inflated by circulating fluid so that the pressure is continuously changing under the weight of the motionless body and limbs of the patient. These are excellent, but one may not always have such a mattress and, even with one, there is need for meticulous care.

The patient should be washed with soap and plenty of water daily, rinsed with clear water, and dried by brisk friction with a Turkish towel. This, in itself, exercises the tissues as well as cleans the skin. The clean, dry patient needs a perfectly smooth, dry bed. He will not feel the wrinkle or the bread crumb that injures the skin of his buttock. The supports of his flail feet must be kept clean and smooth as well as those pads arranged to prevent hyperextension of his knees. All the movement that can be provided is to his advantage: joints stay mobile; skin and muscle, which is of poor tone, are relieved of pressure; vital capacity remains higher than otherwise; the often cheerless and disheartened person gets a little change of view.

Although drugs for control of urinary tract infections are excellent today, the paralyzed patient is at risk. High fluid intake that provides for a copious output of dilute urine is less likely to become infected and to burn tissues than the meager output of concentrated urine of the dehydrated incontinent. Whatever may be the eventual pattern of bowel and bladder evacuation of the chronic patient with a damaged spinal cord, it is not established at once. The newly incontinent invalid demands great sensitivity on the part of his nurse, and this includes awareness that prevention of fecal impactions is accomplished best through knowing what is taking place from day to day and seeing that this preventable complication does not occur. The fluid fecal seepage that keeps the bed damp and soiled indicates both impaction and inattentive nursing, and will be followed by tissue breakdown.

Skin surfaces that lie on top of one another are not shifted in the paralyzed. Moving the patient tends to separate the skin surfaces, remove pressure, and permit air to bathe them. Often a patient, even one acutely ill, can be moved about a good deal if the nurse understands the advantages of it. A litter provides different pressures on the body from those of a mattress on a bed; a wheelchair has a firm surface, and an upholstered chair a more resilient one. These little changes are helpful and supplement the absolutely essential ones of daily complete bath and toweling repeated at night for back, sacrum, and buttocks at least. Moving, shifting body position, and providing a high water intake are things that can be done to try to prevent renal caculi, which so frequently occur when bones decalcify as a result of continuing immobility. These renal stones compound the danger of stasis in the urinary tract.

A mere "ounce of prevention" is not enough in nursing the patient with spinal cord injury; there are too many issues at stake. Each one of them, the integrity of lungs, skin, urinary tract, and joints, needs its own ounce if the patient is to be accorded even a chance for his "pound of cure."

Sensory Stimulation and Deprivation Concerns of Nursing

Living things gain their knowledge of how to adapt to life through sensory experience. The body of the sea anemone is stimulated by the incoming tide and puts forth its tentacles to catch food that the fresh inflow of water will bring. The intelligent, highly trained and practiced college youth sights the football coming his way and runs to place himself in position to complete a play, the strategy of which he fully comprehends, and to which he can make a number of adaptations. Bruner, who is quoted in J. A. Vernon's monograph on experiments in sensory deprivation, says, "We deal with our environment by a set of models or expectancies that have been gradually acquired since birth.

They are based on previous experience." [58] The needs and experiences of the sea anemone and of the college football player are widely different, but for both, the essential elements are present. The coelenterate will not act appropriately without the stimulus of the changing environment, nor will the man.

The sense of touch has been referred to earlier as all-important and it is of considerable significance to nurses. The animal has means for receiving touch just about everywhere on the surface of his body and a variety of tracts by which it ascends to his brain. He has, in the reticular formation, means for alerting wide areas of his cortex and for involving his cranial nerves: in his cerebellum and basal ganglia he has means for completing the integration and plan for control. Tracts descending in his spinal cord inform his muscles by way of the neuron of the final common path, and activity takes place.

Stimulation of the body surface of the newborn animal by the mother's tongue as she licks it dry is followed by defecation and the getting underway of its digestive tract. If deprived of this or comparable stimulation by mechanical means, digestive activity does not occur and the baby animal dies. The child who is born deaf or blind has a devastating handicap because of his sensory deprivation and will need extraordinary incitements to learning by the stimulation of his remaining major senses, sight or hearing and touch, if he is to come eventually to respond adequately to life. When a previously well person suffers illness or mutilation of any considerable degree, his environment changes, his own body image may be considerably modified, and his life as a patient may markedly change the sensory inflow on which so much behavior is based. It is only this last that will be considered here in reference to some common nursing situations.

The baby girl who at a few months of age is noted to have congenitally dislocated hips has fully half of her body, about which she has been learning since birth, encased in a rigid plaster for many months. She no longer has the experience of kicking, hitting her legs together, and learning to play with her feet, thereby getting to know all about this half of her body, because it is no longer available to her. She does not gain experience in reciprocal motion, in learning the feel of textures and of varying weights and pressures upon her legs. The environment of the lower half of her body is homogeneous, receiving few stimuli, offering her little to evaluate and therefore little from which she can learn.

From these facts arise two situations of concern to the nurse. This very young child who has necessarily suffered deprivation of sensory experience will have very little knowledge to go on when she is released from her cast, mechanically sound, and undertakes the task of learning to walk. Her performance cannot be compared to that of her three-year-old contemporary who happens to break a leg, is in a cast for a few weeks, and is running around again without difficulty shortly after being released. Although the sensory and motor deprivations are serious, they are unavoidable under the circumstances, and the child's nurses will do everything they can to stimulate her senses in other areas, giving her toys she must manipulate, food to handle, stories to listen to, people to talk to, and a change of environment by moving her from place to place.

Furthermore, as Vernon points out, the human being finds a homogeneous situation unendurable and will strive to change it in any way available. If he cannot build a new environment he will rid himself of the old in order to effect some sort of change, and the change the individual can most easily make is to fall asleep.[59] The nurse will recognize that for this child, or for patients of any age, 2-hour naps morning and afternoon and 12 hours of sleep at night are indications not for keeping curtains down but for raising them both literally and figuratively.

Early sensory deprivation prevents the formation of adequate models and strategies for dealing with the environment, as illustrated in simplest form by the foregoing example of the baby with dislocated hips who is deprived before she has had much chance to learn. Normal adults, however, who were experimentally deprived by isolation in a dark room, demonstrated marked upset of their ordinary discriminative and evaluative abilities. Bruner found that these men failed to identify common foods or to enjoy eating. They gauged time poorly, they slept to excess and dreamed beyond their usual patterns, and suffered various hallucinatory phenomena. All these men knew that the confinement was temporary and that change and normal life would return, yet when sensory input was sharply reduced, integration was inadequate and the behavior faulty or bizarre.[60]

The sick individual, more or less sensorily deprived, may not be confident that everything will be all right again in the future and, being

[58] Jack A. Vernon: *Inside the Black Room* (New York: Clarkson N. Potter, Inc., 1963), p. 200.

[59] *Op. cit.,* pp. 201–202.

[60] J. S. Bruner: "Cognitive Consequences of Early Sensory Deprivation," paper No. 13 in *Sensory Deprivation: A Symposium Held at Harvard Medical School* (Cambridge: Harvard University Press, 1961), pp. 195–207.

sick, does not have normal forces to help him make the best adjustments. He needs the help of others, certainly of his nurses.

An elderly man who has recently had a stroke with resulting hemiplegia and aphasia has lost what once he had opportunity to develop fully. Recovery of useful motion and speech will be hard and will advance very little with nurses who handle him as little as they can and who give their meager care in silence. Unless there is sensory input there will be little output. "Mr. Abdou, I am washing your arm and hand. Now I am bending your wrist up. I'd like you to help me to do this and I'll tickle it a little so you will feel it better." The stroke has deprived Mr. Abdou, and his nurse knows that his hand and arm can become increasingly remote from him and thereby harder to rehabilitate without stimulation and continued awareness. The fact of deprivation creates a situation that "upsets the balance of the regulating system, namely, the ascending reticular arousal system (ARAS). (See p. 717.) When this happens perception is disrupted, attention gives way to distractibility, and interest to boredom. Behavorial performance is either held in abeyance or becomes highly stereotyped and not adaptive." [61]

The man who has had the stroke will be helped to regain lost motor patterns as well as more subtle interests and abilities by appropriate sensory stimulation and other therapy. But it is not only deprivation that results in poor or undesirable responses but also what Lindsley calls sensory distortion and sensory overload. All represent disturbances within the ARAS by which the higher parts of the brain are poorly informed and do not integrate and respond normally.

There are diseases during which one aims to reduce sensory stimulation for the very reason that there is hyperesthesia. With hyperesthesia, undesired and harmful motor responses occur from any kind of sensory stimulation. Tetanus is one such disease, and acute meningitis, another. Certainly, too, there are times when tactile stimulation can be damaging or make it hard for the patient. Inconsequent sensory stimulation can result promptly in dramatic emotional disturbance.[62] Examples of the sad truth of this crowd the mind: the sudden change of affect to one of withdrawal or seemingly unprovoked weeping by the patient who has overheard what was not meant for his ears (inconsequent auditory input), and the anger and

increased agony of the one who, being in great pain, has been severely jarred when his bed is knocked by a passing portable x-ray machine. In Chapter 16, another aspect of this nursing responsibility is touched on in the discussion of the adolescent male patient, but this is a somewhat special circumstance. It is in daily routines of care that nurses often needlessly fail their patients. To darken a room simply because the patient is ill is as thoughtless as it is totally irrational, the more so if he is chronically or progressively ill. It is not uncommon for someone to darken a room for the patient's afternoon rest and then never re-enter it again to raise the shades. The patient, awakening from his postprandial nap to a dreary twilight, makes no effort to move or undertake any occupation and so slips farther down the slope toward apathy. Human beings seek light from early infancy throughout life: when they are ill, it should not be denied them.

With increasing years and attendant diminution of sensory perception, acuity of sight and hearing especially, one may expect less accuracy in interpretation than formerly. This is especially the case when there are concomitant arteriosclerotic changes in the brain. In general, people in their own homes or familiar surroundings adapt satisfactorily to these gradual losses as they have to other changes within themselves throughout life. With illness and transfer to an unfamiliar environment in a hospital where they are attended by many persons who are strangers and are subjected to procedures and a daily mode of living that is foreign, often in noisy surroundings, the elderly become the victims not only of the illness that has put them in hospital but also of the effect of the altered environment on sensory systems less acute than they used to be, and, therefore more prone to provoke inaccurate or false integration and response.

Some elderly patients struggle with the confusion, asking for repetition of what they do not hear or understand, complaining and demanding frequently, and refusing to be conquered by circumstances with which they need help. These patients are not really difficult; one has only to give the help and to respond to the demands and clarify what is irritating or confusing. One can identify the shadows of the waving branches outside that make queer patterns on the wall, and explain the meaning of the squawking loudspeaker that is so offensive and sounds like Donald Duck calling the doctors.

Patients who have no courage or energy to struggle are those whose needs are greater and who demand much more acuity on the part of those who care for them. In childhood, in old

---

[61] D. B. Lindsley: "Common Factors in Sensory Deprivation, Sensory Distortion and Sensory Overload," paper No. 12 in *Sensory Deprivation, ibid.*, p. 177.

[62] Austin H. Riesen: "Excessive Arousal Effects of Stimulation after Early Sensory Deprivation," paper No. 3 in *Sensory Deprivation, ibid.*, p. 40.

age, and at any age in time of severe illness, common sensory experiences may become distorted and terrifying. We expect this in childhood and are prepared for it; with the aged and severely ill, the possibility of confusion is not to be forgotten and can be anticipated. "Mrs. Elder, do you enjoy watching the play of the shadows of those lilac branches on your wall or does it annoy you? I can move your chair so you can see them more easily or not at all." "Mr. Olds, I think that the loudspeaker that calls the doctors has been bothering you. It distorts voices dreadfully, I know, but it will soon be turned off for the night."

The elderly patient, being often worn and tired, easily deals with his altered environment by withdrawal from it. He sleeps, he dozes when urged out of bed, he accepts everything wanly, he does not seem to seek to communicate at all. From such a patient, already withdrawn, breeziness and chatter will rarely receive a favorable response. One must work from a more basic level than that of verbal interchange. Often, the nurse's best approach is through touch. Physical care of a simple kind given with dignity and gentleness conveys feeling to the patient and is a means of communication of an elemental and very fundamental nature. By acceptance of this feeling, the patient is stimulated to respond, perhaps not with speech but by some change of position made to assist the nurse in her care of him. This move is her satisfaction and her success; she has comprehended her patient's needs, can now formulate plans for working to meet them, and by this slight response from the patient, she sees that she has already achieved her first goal.

Stimulus, receptor, arousal system, integrator, and effector: If any are absent or weak the response is lacking or poor. Good nurses on any level recognize that they are in position to enhance or weaken the force of the circuit and they accept that responsibility with good will and understanding.

REFERENCES

BOOKS

Bogoch, Samuel (ed.): *The Future of the Brain Sciences* (New York: Plenum Press, 1969).

Crosby, Elizabeth C., Humphrey, Tryphena, and Lauer, Edward W.: *Correlative Anatomy of the Nervous System* (New York: The Macmillan Company, 1962).

Elliott, H. Chandler: *Textbook of Neuroanatomy* (Philadelphia: J. B. Lippincott Company, 1963).

Gardner, Ernest: *Fundamentals of Neurology*, 4th ed. (Philadelphia: J. B. Lippincott Company, 1963).

Grinker, Paul C., and Sahs, Adolph L.: *Neurology*, 6th ed. (Springfield, Ill.: Charles C Thomas, Publisher, 1966).

Guyton, Arthur C.: *Textbook of Medical Physiology*, 3rd ed. (Philadelphia: W. B. Saunders Company, 1966).

Hooper, Reginald: *Neurosurgical Nursing* (Springfield, Ill.: Charles C Thomas, Publisher, 1964).

Horwitz, Norman H., and Rizzoli, Hugo V.: *Postoperative Complications in Neurological Practice* (Baltimore: The Williams & Wilkins Company, 1967).

Konorski, Jerry: *Integrative Activity of the Brain* (Chicago: University of Chicago Press, 1967).

Lewin, Walpole: *The Management of Head Injuries* (London: Baillière, Tindall & Cassel, Ltd., 1966).

McAlpine, Douglas, Lumsden, Charles, and Acheson, E. D.: *Multiple Sclerosis: A Reappraisal* (Baltimore: The Williams & Wilkins Company, 1965).

Mayo Clinic: *Clinical Examinations in Neurology*, 2nd ed. (Philadelphia: W. B. Saunders Company, 1963).

Sinclair, David Cecil: *Cutaneous Sensation* (New York: Oxford University Press, 1967).

Solomon, Philip, ed.: *Sensory Deprivation: A Symposium Held at the Harvard Medical School* (Cambridge: Harvard University Press, 1961).

Vernon, Jack A.: *Inside the Black Room* (New York: Clarkson N. Potter, Inc., 1963).

PERIODICALS

Ballantine, H. Thomas, and Prieto, Alberto: "Early Recognition and Management of Neurosurgical Emergencies," *Surg. Clin. N. Amer.,* **46**:527–38 (June) 1966.

Boegli, Emily H., and Steele, Mary S.: "Scoliosis," *Amer. J. Nurs.,* **68**:2399–403 (Nov.) 1968.

Bonner, C. D., *et al.*: "The Team Approach to Hemiplegia," *Postgrad. Med.,* **40**:708–14 (Dec.) 1966.

Brocklehurst, J. C.: "Cerebrovascular Disease," *Nurs. Times,* **63**:880–82 (July 7) 1967.

Butts, C., and Canney, Vesta E.: "The Unresponsive Patient," *Amer. J. Nurs.,* **67**:1886–88 (Sept.) 1968.

DeBakey, Michael E., *et al.*: "Surgical Treatment of Cerebrovascular Disease," *Postgrad. Med.,* **42**:218–30 (Sept.) 1967.

Diamond, I. T., and Hall, W. C.: "Evolution of the Neocortex," *Science,* **164**:251–62 (Apr. 18) 1969.

Fairburn, B.: "Neurosurgery Today. 6. Spinal Cord

Surgery," *Nurs. Times,* 63:249–51 (Feb. 24) 1967.

Floodmark, S., and Steinwall, O.: "A Method for Study of the Interrelation Between EEG and Blood Barrier Phenomena," *Acta Physiol. Scand.,* 2:112–19 (Dec.) 1968.

Gardner, M. Arlene: "Responsiveness as a Measure of Consciousness," *Amer. J. Nurs.,* 68:1034–38 (May) 1968.

Geldard, Frank A.: "Body English," *Psychol. Today,* 2:43–47 (Dec.) 1968.

Glassman, Alexander: "Brain Barrier to 5-HTP," *New Eng. J. Med.,* 278:281 (Feb. 1) 1968.

Greenhouse, Arnold H.: "Modern Concepts in Cerebral Vascular Disease," *GP,* 35:99–105 (May) 1967.

Guerrieri, Belga O.: "Survey of the Knowledge of the Nurse in Direct-Care Services Concerning Proper Bed Positioning of the Patient with Hemiplegia," *Nurs. Res.,* 17:157–59 (Mar.–Apr.) 1968.

Haynes, Una A.: "Nursing Approaches in Cerebral Dysfunction," *Amer. J. Nurs.,* 68:2170–76 (Oct.) 1968.

Knapp, Miland E.: "Spinal Cord Injury. Part 1," *Postgrad. Med.,* 42:A95–A99 and Part 2, A111–A116 (Aug.–Sept.) 1967.

Kurze, Theodore, and Pitts, Frederick W.: "Management of Closed Head Injuries," *Surg. Clin. N. Amer.,* 48:1271–78 (Dec.) 1968.

Langan, E.: "Nursing Care of Neurosurgical Patients: Post-Operative Care," *Nurs. Times,* 63:111 (Jan. 27) 1967.

Locksley, Herbert B.: "Hemorrhagic Strokes," *Med. Clin. N. Amer.,* 52:1193–1212 (Sept.) 1968.

McHenry, Lawrence C., and Jaffe, Marvin E.: "Cerebrovascular Disease. Part I: Diagnosis," and "Part II: Management," *GP,* 37:88–101 (Mar.) and 37:98–106 (Apr.) 1968.

Mannarino, Emanuele, and McLaurin, Robert L.: "Management of Head Injuries," *Surg. Clin. N. Amer.,* 48:723–36 (Aug.) 1968.

Plummer, Elizabeth M.: "The MS Patient," *Amer. J. Nurs.,* 68:2161–67 (Oct.) 1968.

Rahman, A. N., and Luttrell, C. N.: "Pathogenesis of Meningoencephalitides: Enhancement of Viral Penetration into the Brain," *Bull. Johns Hopkins Hosp.,* 112:1–14 (Jan.) 1963.

Ramey, Irene C.: "The Stroke Patient Is Interesting," *Nurs. Forum,* 6:273–79 (Summer) 1967.

Robertson, J. D.: "The Membrane of the Living Cell," *Sci. Amer.,* 206:64–72 (Apr.) 1962.

Smith, Aron: "Neurological Aspects of Stroke," *Stroke,* 2:9–13 (Fall) 1967.

Smith, Samuel Walker: "Subdural Hematoma in Adults," *Postgrad. Med.,* 42:A59–A64 (Aug.) 1967.

Talbot, Herbert S.: "Adjunctive Care of Spinal Cord Injuries," *Surg. Clin. N. Amer.,* 48:737–57 (Aug.) 1968.

Therrien, Barbara, and Salmon, James H.: "Percutaneous Cordotomy for Relief of Intractable Pain," *Amer. J. Nurs.,* 68:2594–97 (Dec.) 1968.

Tizard, J. P. M., Paine, R. S., and Crothers, B.: "Disturbances of Sensation in Children with Hemiplegia," *JAMA,* 155:628–72 (June 12) 1954.

Travener, Deryck: "Trigeminal Neuralgia," *Nurs. Times,* 64:514–16 (Apr.) 1968.

Treherne, J. E.: "Transfer of Substances Between the Blood and Central Nervous System in Vertebrate and Invertebrate Animals," *Nature,* 196:1181–83 (Dec. 22) 1962.

Udall, John A.: "Anticoagulant Therapy for Progressing Strokes," *Postgrad. Med.,* 42:212–17 (Sept.) 1967.

16

The Relationship of Illness to the Maturational Level of the Individual *

There is a tide in the affairs of men
Which, taken at the flood, leads on to fortune;
Omitted, all the voyage of their life
Is bound in shallows and in miseries.
Julius Caesar IV: 3, Shakespeare

Overview: Man as a Complex Whole

How can the laws of growth be used in understanding human development?

Reactions to Illness at Various Maturational Levels

How can knowledge of human development help the nurse in her day-by-day care of the adult patient?

Overview: Man as a Complex Whole

IN the preceding chapters man has been presented from many views: his basic needs, physiological, psychological, and sociological; his major systems, such as the circulatory system as the transporter, and the nervous and endocrine systems as the coordinators and integrators of all levels of response from the simplest to the most complex. Every human being has these major systems, minor systems, organs, tissues, and cells that present needs that must be met so that the total body may function harmoniously in health. They may be altered in illness, with all the protective and adaptive mechanisms coming to the fore to re-establish a harmonious balance or homeostasis and restore man to health. In this chapter the nurse is asked to keep all those factors to which she has been introduced previously in mind but to regard them now synthesized as they are in one complex whole—a human personality whatever his age or constitution may be.

The complexity of the human organism is so great that in order to understand its different aspects, systems, organs, and needs each must be studied separately. As one part, system, or need is studied, it becomes readily evident that even study of one system is difficult because it does not function alone. Each part is dependent on every other part if it is to survive and accomplish its functions. Furthermore, no part is static, but it is changing, moving, growing, or developing. Thus, too, the whole is an ever-changing, dynamic, moving force. John Henry Cardinal Newman put it more aptly when he said, "Growth is the only evidence of life."

Let us begin at conception, wherein man is endowed with a complex of genetic potentialities or constitution. One accepted definition is:

Constitution is currently conceived as the sum total of the structural, functional, and psychological characters of the organism. It is in large measure, an integral of genetic potentialities influenced in varying degrees by internal and external environmental factors. It is not a biological given, a structure destined to function in a predetermined manner. Rather it is a process, a series of operative questions that even by the time of birth have not become final declarative answers.

What is given is the genotype, the complex of genetic potentialities with which the organism is endowed. Each individual's genotype is a unique physicochemical system comprising particular kinds of potentialities that have definite limits. . . . The genes, self-duplicating giant protein molecules of great complexity, are organic catalysts that accelerate essential chemical reactions, the original builders of the body, which they serve to differentiate according to the type of medium or other conditions that surround them in their interactive chemical relations. . . .

---

* This chapter was contributed and revised by Jane Frances Ronan, Associate Professor of Nursing, College of Nursing, Wayne State University, Detroit, Michigan.

The manner in which the genotype functions depends in part on the environment in which it undergoes development. . . . Heredity, accordingly, is not constituted merely by the genotype, but by the genotype as modified by the environment in which it has developed. It is the resultant of the dynamic interaction between the two.[1]

From the definition it is clear that this complex of genetic potentialities is not static but ever changing and developing according to the environment, internal and external, in which man lives. Therefore, throughout life man reflects both his constitution and his environment through his total being. Consequently, if we are to look at a human being, child or adult, at a given time we must consider his genetic endowment and his total experiences from conception as well as those of the present.

Laws of Growth

In this great complex and ever-developing organism with its dynamic interrelationship of activity there is not chaos but great order. Laws have been identified that govern the growth and development of man. They are [2]

1. Growth is both quantitative and qualitative.
2. Growth is a continuous orderly process.
3. The tempo of growth is not even.
4. Different aspects of growth develop at different rates.
5. Both rate and pattern of growth can be modified from within and without the body.
6. Each child grows in his own unique way.
7. Growth is complex—all of its aspects are interrelated.[3]

The preceding laws, more specifically the implication of them, apply to full maturity of the organism and continue to govern and affect the development of the organism throughout the life-span. For example, growth is a continuous and orderly process. What happens to the fertilized ovum in utero affects the individual positively or negatively throughout his life. Another example of this same law is the following: The relationship that the mother and child establish in early infancy is the individual's basis for making relations with all persons the rest of his life. Granted the individual's relationships with others can be changed or modified

[1] Helen Witmer and Ruth Kotinsky: *Personality in the Making* (New York: Harper and Brothers, 1953), p. 30.
[2] Marian Breckenridge and E. Lee Vincent: *Child Development* (Philadelphia: W. B. Saunders Company, 1955), p. 4.
[3] For further study of the laws of the growth, see Marian E. Breckenridge and E. Lee Vincent: *Child Development* 4th ed. (Philadelphia: W. B. Saunders Company, 1960), Chap. 1.

to some extent by later experiences, nevertheless the early mother-infant relationship is the basis or the raw material the infant has for the development of relationships with others throughout his life. One other example is the immunological competency that the individual establishes in infancy and early childhood. This is the basis for his ability to handle or cope with pathogenic organisms the rest of his life. It is also related to his ability to accept or reject homo transplants, i.e., skin, cornea, kidney. The law that reads "Both rate and pattern of growth can be modified from within and without the body" is very evident in molecular diseases with reference to the degree of expressivity of the genetic defect. An example of this is the hemolytic phenomenon seen in the individual with the defect of deficiency of the enzyme glucose-6-phosphate dehydrogenase. If he does not ingest specific agents, i.e., sulfanilamide or fava beans, he has no difficulty; if he does, hemolytic anemia results.

How can the laws of growth be used in understanding human development?

The laws governing growth and development are simply stated, but their implications are far-reaching. In studying and contemplating these laws it becomes evident that age alone means little. There are norms of development available that are stated in terms of age alone, e.g., a baby sits at 6 months. These norms are averages; they do not imply that an individual is not within the range of normalcy if he has not reached this specific developmental level at this given age. Evaluation of developmental progress must be made in terms of normal range rather than the precise age norm. The use of ranges in preference to ages is cumbersome, but the individuality of man is greatly maligned if ranges are not used. A baby 7 months old may or may not be able to sit alone, or a woman of 48 may or may not be going through the menopause. Whether the infant is sitting or the woman has reached the maturational level of menopause will depend in part on the law of individual difference. A given individual may be on a fast or slow developmental schedule based on the dynamic interrelationship of his constitution and his past experiences. Although each individual grows and develops in his own way, each goes through a life cycle of development that, in a broad framework, is similar to that of all other human beings. Therefore, human development is generally predictable passing from one state or level of development into the next from conception to death. Consequently it is more meaningful to ask in which stage of development is this individual rather than to ask how old is this individual.

In perusing the literature one can find examples of the great authors defining different stages of development of man. Probably the most classic examples are those found in the Bible and in the works of Shakespeare. These two examples will be given because they are interesting to read and to compare with the contemporary scheme of development that will be presented. Both are in some aspects akin to twentieth-century living.

In Shakespeare's *As You Like It,* he says:

. . . All the world's a stage
And all the men and women merely players.
They have their exits and their entrances,
And one man in his time plays many parts,
His acts being seven ages. At first the infant,
Mewling and puking in the nurse's arms.
Then the whining schoolboy with his satchel
And shining morning face, creeping like snail
Unwillingly to school. And then the lover,
Sighing like furnace, with a woeful ballad
Made to his mistress' eyebrow. Then a soldier
Full of strange oaths and bearded like the pard,
Jealous in honor, sudden and quick in quarrel,
Seeking the bubble Reputation
E'en in the cannon's mouth. And then the justice,
In fair round belly with good capon lin'd,
With eyes severe and beard of formal cut,
Full of wise saws and modern instances:
And so he plays his part. The sixth age shifts
Into the lean and slipper'd pantaloon,
With spectacles on nose and pouch on side;
His youthful hose well sav'd, a world too wide
For his shrunk shank, and his big manly voice,
Turning again toward childish treble, pipes
And whistles in his sound. Last scene of all,
That ends this strange eventful history,
Is second childishness and mere oblivion—
Sans teeth, sans eyes, sans taste, sans everything.[4]

Ecclesiastes III (Verse 1–8) reads:

For everything there is a season
and a time for every matter under the heaven:
A time to be born, and a time to die;
a time to plant, and a time to pluck up
what is being planted;
A time to kill, and a time to heal;
a time to break down, and a time to build up;
A time to weep, and a time to laugh;
a time to mourn, and a time to dance:
A time to cast away stones, and
a time to gather stones together;
A time to embrace, and a time to refrain
from embracing;
A time to seek, and a time to lose;
a time to keep, and a time to cast away;
A time to rend, and a time to sew;
a time to keep silence, and a time to speak;
A time to love, and a time to hate;
a time for war, and a time for peace. . . .

[4] Scarlett, in his article (see References), presents excerpts from other works of Shakespeare that expound on each of these stages.

This chapter was introduced by a quotation from Shakespeare:

There is a tide in the affairs of men
Which, taken at the flood, leads on to fortune;
Omitted, all the voyage of their life
Is bound in shallows and in miseries.

This quotation is identical in essence to Havighurst's definition of a developmental task, which reads: "A developmental task is a task which arises at or about a certain period in the life of the individual, successful achievement of which leads to his happiness and to the success with later tasks, while failure leads to unhappiness in the individual, disapproval by the society, and difficulty with later tasks." [5] Shakespeare's observation and Havighurst's definition are similar to that which Erik Erikson, in his ground plan of the life cycle of man, describes as the central tasks or core problems of each developmental stage. (The student may well be reminded of the same concept from her study of embryology: Each organ has its time of origin; if missed, not only is the organ doomed as an entity, it endangers the whole hierarchy of organs.)

Erik Erikson's thesis of human development will be the contemporary one presented in this chapter.[6] His scheme of development was chosen because it shows clearly the flow of development during the entire life-span. It gives the beginning student the major stages of human development and how each stage is built on the previous ones and is at the same time the foundation stone for the successive ones. From this approach the student is able to grasp an over-all view of development from birth to death. As the student grows in personal and professional life her grasp of human development will take on greater meaning. She then will be able to add depth and understanding to this broad framework learned as a beginning student.

Erikson divides the life cycle of man into eight stages, each with a core problem or crisis that the individual struggles to master during these specific stages. Each core problem or central task has a positive and negative component, e.g., trust-mistrust, that must be fought through successfully by the individual so that he can move to the next stage. As part of the matrix of these central tasks are innumerable other tasks (developmental, e.g., walking, talking) to master. Each is distinct in itself but, when mastered, aids in the accomplishment of

[5] Robert J. Havighurst: *Human Development and Education* (New York: David McKay Company, 1953), p. 2.
[6] Erik Erikson: *Childhood and Society* (New York: W. W. Norton & Company, Inc., 1963).

the central task, or problem. For example, the core problem of the toddler age is autonomy, the mastery of self and his environment. Some of the developmental tasks of this maturational level are walking, talking, and bowel and bladder control. It is easy to see how these play an important role in the over-all task of autonomy.

Although Erikson's schema is primarily a psychosocial development of man, much more is included. Concerning this factor Erikson [7] says, "For the eight stages of psychosocial development are, in fact, inextricably intwined in and derived from the various stages of psychosexual development that were described by Freud, as well as from the child's stages of physical, motor, and cognitive development. Each type of development affects the other and is affected by it." The following is an overview of Erikson's eight stages of the life cycle of man.

The Eight Stages in the Life Cycle of Man

"Personality," Erikson has written, "can be said to develop according to steps predetermined in the human organism's readiness to be driven toward, to be aware of, and to interact with a widening social radius, beginning with a dim image of a mother and ending with an image of mankind. . . ." Following are the steps he has identified in man's psychosocial development, and the special crises they bring. In presenting them, he has emphasized that while the struggle between the negatives and positives in each crisis must be fought through successfully if the next developmental stage is to be reached, no victory is completely or forever won.

I. INFANCY: TRUST VERSUS MISTRUST

The first "task" of the infant is to develop "the cornerstone of a healthy personality," a basic sense of trust—in himself and his environment. This comes from a feeling of inner goodness derived from "the mutual regulation of his receptive capacities with the maternal techniques of provision"—a quality of care that transmits a sense of trustworthiness and meaning. The danger, most acute in the second half of the first year, is that discontinuities in care may increase a natural sense of loss, as the child gradually recognizes his separateness from his mother, to a basic sense of mistrust that may last through life.

II. EARLY CHILDHOOD: AUTONOMY VERSUS SHAME AND DOUBT

With muscular maturation the child experiments with holding on and letting go and begins to attach enormous value to his autonomous will. The danger

[7] Kathryn Close: "Youth and the Life Cycle," *Children,* 7(2):45 (Mar.–Apr.) 1960.

here is the development of a deep sense of shame and doubt if he is deprived of the opportunity to learn to develop his will as he learns his "duty," and therefore learns to expect defeat in any battle of wills with those who are bigger and stronger.

III. PLAY AGE: INITIATIVE VERSUS GUILT

In this stage the child's imagination is greatly expanded because of his increased ability to move around freely and to communicate. It is an age of intrusive activity, avid curiosity, and consuming fantasies which lead to feelings of guilt and anxiety. It is also the stage of the establishment of conscience. If this tendency to feel guilty is "overburdened by all-too-eager adults" the child may develop a deep-seated conviction that he is essentially bad, with a resultant stifling of initiative or a conversion of his moralism to vindicativeness.

IV. SCHOOL AGE: INDUSTRY VERSUS INFERIORITY

The long period of sexual latency before puberty is the age when the child wants to learn how to do and make things with others. In learning to accept instruction and to win recognition by producing "things" he opens the way for the capacity of work enjoyment. The danger in this period is the development of a sense of inadequacy and inferiority in a child who does not receive recognition for his efforts.

V. ADOLESCENCE: IDENTITY VERSUS IDENTITY DIFFUSION

The physiological revolution that comes with puberty—rapid body growth and sexual maturity—forces the young person to question "all sameness and continuities relied on earlier" and to "refight many of the earlier battles." The developmental task is to integrate childhood identifications "with the basic biological drives, native endowment, and the opportunities offered in social roles." The danger is that identity diffusion, temporarily unavoidable in this period of physical and psychological upheaval, may result in a permanent inability to "take hold" or, because of youth's tendency to total commitment, in the fixation in the young person of a negative identity, a devoted attempt to become what parents, class, or community do not want him to be.

VI. YOUNG ADULTHOOD: INTIMACY VERSUS ISOLATION

Only as a young person begins to feel more secure in his identity is he able to establish intimacy with himself (with his inner life) and with others, both in friendships and eventually in a love-based mutually satisfying sexual relationship with a member of the opposite sex. A person who cannot enter wholly into an intimate relationship because of the fear of losing his identity may develop a deep sense of isolation.

VII. ADULTHOOD: GENERATIVITY
VERSUS SELF-ABSORPTION

Out of the intimacies of adulthood grows generativity—the mature person's interest in establishing and guiding the next generation. The lack of this results in self-absorption and frequently in a "pervading sense of stagnation and interpersonal impoverishment."

VIII. SENESCENCE: INTEGRITY
VERSUS DISGUST

The person who has achieved a satisfying intimacy with other human beings and who has adapted to the triumphs and disappointments of his generative activities as parent and co-worker reaches the end of life with a certain ego integrity—an acceptance of his own responsibility for what his life is and was and of its place in the flow of history. Without this "accrued ego integration" there is despair, usually marked by a display of displeasure and disgust.[8,9]

In studying the stages of development of man whether stated in a classic or contemporary form it becomes evident that each stage with its problem must be mastered by the individual himself. Meaningful people in his environment assist him in his development. The members of his immediate family are the persons who generally are the most meaningful, but the nurse is in a very singular position to assist the patient in his development regardless of the level of his maturation. It is also evident that these problems in mastery take considerable effort and time on the part of the individual to accomplish.

Reactions to Illness at Various
Maturational Levels

Although there are definite and progressive stages of development, how the individual develops will depend on his genetic endowment and his environment. Environment includes the culture in which he lives, the age in which he lives, and how his own family views the development of their own children in accordance with their own philosophy. It includes as well how he, as an individual, perceives his own growth, his own family, and the society and the age in which he is living.

It is interesting to note that nowhere in the schemes of development presented or in other developmental schemes is there an allotted time for illness. (One of the verses from Ecclesiastes

[8] From "Youth and the Life Cycle," an interview with Erik Erikson by Kathryn Close, Mar.–Apr. 1960 issue of *Children*, interprofessional journal published by the Children's Bureau, Department of Health, Education, and Welfare.

[9] For further study see Erik Erikson, *op. cit.*

might be interpreted by some to mean illness.) In reality man does become ill and illness does demand much energy and effort on the part of the individual to return to health. The individual's total being is affected by his illness and he uses his total development to overcome his illness.

How can knowledge of human development help the nurse in her day-by-day care of the adult patient?

The reader at this point may well be saying, "This chapter is all about the growth and development of children—even Erikson's scheme of development deals more with childhood than adult life. We'll learn that in the nursing care of children. Now, we want to learn about the nursing care of adults." These stages of development are not just acquired for the individual to have permanently—they must be reinforced or reaffirmed throughout life. An example will help to clarify this. Mr. Smith comes into the hospital to have elective surgery, i.e., a herniorraphy. Mr. Smith, like most people, was reared in a family that encouraged the development of trust in other people, but Mr. Smith has lived some three decades and has learned that all people are not to be trusted. He must, therefore, discover if his nurse and the other hospital personnel are trustworthy. Until he is assured of this, his relationship with his nurse will be tentative and superficial. He must develop faith in her. He does this in the same ways that he used to establish his basic sense of trust, i.e., testing, questioning, looking for behavior that says to him, "She thinks I'm worthy, she respects me as a human being, she knows I'm demanding but she likes me anyway; she will comfort me." What happens to Mr. Smith's sense of autonomy at this time? When he is given a general anesthesia, he surely loses his autonomy and his ability to control himself and his environment because he loses all consciousness and therefore all control over himself. To survive and go on to full recovery, he must reaffirm his autonomy. How does the nurse help him to gain self-control? Think of the toddler and how he acquires autonomy. His stock answer to most things is "No!" Another statement he uses frequently is "Me do!" These are ways the toddler tells of his desire and need to be in charge of himself and his environment. Frequently, when the adult patient is in a stressful situation, i.e., asked to cough or ambulate postoperatively, he replies with a negative statement. And just as the toddler says "Me do," the adult patient desires to be a participating member of the health team—not just a blank entity on whom procedures are being performed by many people. If the nurse permits him to participate and to really be an active member of the team, she will find she has more time for actual care because it takes less time to win his confidence and cooperation in his care. A cliché that is heard around sick people too often is "He seems to have no will to live." How is this related to these central tasks of trust and autonomy that we have been talking about?

The other two stages of development dealing primarily with childhood, i.e., initiative and industry, could be explored and shown to play important roles throughout life. A very practical manner of studying and learning in these areas is to observe and study children as they go about their daily activities and then compare their behavior with the behavior exhibited by adults. Watch especially how preschool children establish relationships with each other. Watch, too, how the school-age child initiates conversation with his peers and then with persons in authority. The student will find that much of the behavior is in essence the same—perhaps a bit more veneer or social tact on the part of the adult but basically the same.

The first four phases of development, trust, autonomy, initiative, and industry, have been discussed on the preceding pages. They are primarily tasks of infancy and childhood. These tasks, like all others in life, are not simply acquired at specific times in one's life and therefore a permanent acquisition for the rest of the individual's life; they continue to be threatened and must be reaffirmed if the individual is to maintain his homeostasis. Take an example of a developmental task; around a year an infant learns to walk, but if as an adult he is confined to bed or chair over an extended period of time because of illness, he must struggle again through the steps in learning to ambulate independently just as he did when he was a small child. If this is true in this elementary task, it is equally true in the entire realm of development; the human being strives to maintain the growth he has gained and continues to further its development.

Adolescence

The next stage of human development is the period of adolescence. In years this period extends over a longer period than do any of the first four. Therefore, it is usually divided into three phases, prepubescence, pubescence, and postpubescence, each of these phases contributing to the total growth and each initiating specific needs. It is the time in life when the youngster moves from being a child to being a man or a woman. This is the time when sex differences begin to play a major role in the total developmental patterns of the human being.

Adolescence is not a gray vague interim but a period of accelerated growth and development in all areas, physical, social, emotional, intellectual, and spiritual. Postnatally, it is the period of most rapid growth with the exception of infancy. There are tremendous physical changes accompanied by great hormonal changes that introduce new and demanding biological urges. At the same time the psyche is undergoing an upheaval so that the adolescent may move from childlike reactions to adult reactions that society demands of its mature citizens. Is it any wonder that the adolescent is continuously complaining of one trouble or another? Equally true, it is easy to understand why so many adults stereotype the adolescent as the chronic hypochondriac. Adolescents are not hypochondriacs; they are simply asking, "Is this normal?" With the tremendous changes going on in their bodies they do not know what is normal and what is abnormal. They are asking for help to understand the rapid change in their bodies and psyches. With so much growth in so short a period, many things can go wrong. It is the adolescent's birthright to have an excellent evaluation of his total health.

The central task of this developmental stage is identity. The development of the sense of identity points up many questions the adolescent must meet and answer if he is to develop a sense of who he is. Some of the more obvious questions are: Who am I? Where am I going? What is the purpose of life? Where do I fit in society? Will I be able to select, win, and hold a mate for life? Will I be able to be a parent? Will I be able to get a job—to hold it? The negative component of this stage of development is diffusion. This is seen in all adolescents as they struggle for identity—they are erratic and vacillating, unable to grasp or take hold. If they receive help from meaningful adults, the positive component, identity, takes over and they are less and less diffuse in their actions and beliefs.

With all these bodily changes and psychic upheaval that are going on, the adolescent is struggling valiantly to establish his identity. Add to this struggle an illness such as diabetes mellitus, or a fractured leg when he has just made the varsity team, or the orthopedist's decision at this time to correct the scoliosis that resulted from a vertebral infection in childhood. What effect does one of these conditions have on this individual youngster and his struggle for identity? He overreacts to all stimuli very much like the toddler in the period of autonomy. He probably is the most demanding, erratic, vacillating patient to be found. Right in the middle of a procedure he may change from adult behavior to childlike behavior, demanding, questioning, resisting, screaming, and crying. Today he may be very knowledgeable about his condition and have a sound approach to his illness. Tomorrow he may be able to use very little of his knowledge and have an entirely different idea of what this illness is, why he has it, or what it means to him. Will you punish him for his behavior by demanding that he act as an adult or even that he act as a child? Or will you use your knowledge of this developmental stage and support him through this illness?

Regression is a common companion of illness or great stress at any age. This intensifies the problems to be met in illness perhaps more —at least more dramatically in the adolescent than for any others. All too often we find the adolescent or youth in the adult hospital ward. Remember he is no longer a child, but he is not yet an adult. An example will be helpful. The female adolescent patient may well be as big as or bigger than the nurse; the male adolescent may well be 6 ft and weigh 180 lb. Physically they are more adult than child, but under this frightening stressful situation of illness and hospitalization they may well regress and act very much like the toddler. The behavior of a toddler is understandable and acceptable; you simply pick up the youngster and cuddle him, show you love and accept him, and help him with his own controls. Physically you cannot pick up this big adolescent; furthermore, it would be inappropriate behavior. How do you, the nurse, show your affection, acceptance, and love for this adolescent? You can recognize his valiant efforts toward achieving identity and support them, or you can avoid this patient as much as possible because his behavior is so aggressive. You can meet his aggression with aggression, thus increasing his anxiety and guilt feelings with resulting increase in pulse, respiration, and blood pressure, or through your understanding of his struggle, you can help him to achieve at least a small measure of identity through his relationship with you.

Another factor plays an important role here, especially with the male adolescent. Around 16 to 18 years of age, or in postpubescence, the male youth experiences stronger sexual drives than he will throughout the remainder of his life. Most nurses are female. Keep this in mind when you come in close physical contact with your young male patient; do not add burdens to his already great struggle for control by unwitting but nevertheless seductive behavior. This factor demands that you use your ingenuity and imagination to the utmost when you are seeking ways to comfort and support this young male as he experiences stressful situations, for he must borrow from your strength to maintain himself through the experience.

It is not only the adolescent who is struggling for identity; all adults, sick or well, continue this struggle in a more or less intense manner the rest of their lives. They continue to seek their place in the flow of history, to realize themselves as individuals. For the adult who is critically ill or who is hospitalized over a long period of time the intensity of the struggle for maintaining his identity is heightened by simply being cut off from normal family life, job situation, and normal social intercourse with peers. The struggle may be heightened because of the illness itself, loss of control over bodily functions, loss of privacy, procedures that involve exposure of the body, and intrusion into bodily orifices and cavities. It may be heightened by the attitudes and behavior of the nurse and other hospital personnel, i.e., failure to gain the explicit consent of the patient, autocratic treatment, depersonalized care, or failure to prepare the patient for what to expect and what is expected of him. An empathic attitude in the nurse will do much to help the patient maintain his identity and be a more contributing member of the health team and better prepared to resume his place in the family, job, and society.

Young Adulthood

In our culture when the individual has reached physical maturity and has developed a considerable sense of identity, a relatively consistent pattern of reactions to stimuli that meets with society's approval emerges, and we say this individual is now an adult. The central task or problem of this stage of development is intimacy. If the individual has met and resolved the conflicts inherent in the other stages of development as he grew up, he is now ready to move into this stage. When the young person is quite sure of his identity (who he is—where he fits into society), he seeks friendships of a closer or more intimate nature. He desires to know himself better and share the essence of his being with others on a reciprocal basis. This eventually leads to a love-based, mutually satisfying sexual relationship in marriage. The culture in which the individual lives affects the stages of development: The American culture, on the whole, does quite well in contributing to the earlier stages of development, but it gives little help even in its literature and music to the development of this stage of intimacy. Our family life and its institutions, including the church and school, give little help to the young adult striving for a mature sense of intimacy. Youngsters coming through our school systems are reared on an age-grading system, and essentially the same pattern is carried on at home, e.g., the ten-year-old can stay up an hour later in the evening than the eight-year-old. The young adult soon becomes aware that the adult society functions on a social status system and not on an age-grading system. He soon realizes he stands alone and is expected to function as a full-fledged adult as soon as he embarks on his life's work. He needs help, but he is also acutely aware that there are not many resources to help him; he must depend on his own inner strengths. Owing to the mobility of our society, many young people do not even have the emotional support that comes from living close to one's family. It is as though this period of young adult life were the final examination for his childhood.

In all phases of development society has specific expectations for the individual; e.g., during late childhood, in the period of industry, society expects the child to learn his basic intellectual skills. Society has specific expectations for the young adult too. The tasks or expectations that society dictates are the establishment of oneself in a career and in marriage. These are two very demanding tasks closely related to the central task of intimacy—the ability to commune with oneself and relate effectively to others in a job situation as well as in a more personal way in courtship and marriage. And yet society really offers little help to our young adults.

These tasks are demanding not only physically but also psychically. They are demanding financially too, at a time in the life of the individual when he has had little time to accrue much in the way of savings. What does it cost physically, psychologically, and financially to establish oneself in a profession such as pharmacy, or to start a small business, or to furnish the first home following marriage? All of this puts great stress on the person. Here society fails too. We offer little to the young male in the way of adequate, much less excellent, medical supervision. The young female in our society, in a way, is better cared for medically because these are her childbearing years, and she is under the care of a physican more often than her spouse or the rest of the young male society. We know these people do succumb to illness as they are seen on the hospital wards. What does illness mean to them—separation from their spouse, an interruption in their career, a missed chance for advancement, a pay check or two lost, a sizable debt incurred, a baby cared for by someone other than its mother? The implications of these questions are great, but do we

think about this as we see the young adult on the ward or do we think and act toward him as we do toward the 50-year-old adult who is likely to be established in his career and marriage?

The student might have difficulties in relating to this young adult patient. She is in the same developmental stage, struggling with the same problems; therefore, the tendency is to identify with this patient. The identification may be so strong that it prevents effective nursing. Unless the nurse understands this phenomenon, she may lose patience when he fails to conform to her expected norm of behavior. With help she may be able to be supportive to this young patient but be of less assistance to his spouse, thereby preventing her from supporting her young husband.

There is another factor about young males that is of importance to those in the health fields. The young male (18 to 25 years of age) overreacts to illness. Given the same illness, the same virulence of organism, the young female adult will usually return to health more quickly with fewer sequelae than her male counterpart. Clinical evidence supports this well, but there is less scientific support for this observed phenomenon. We do know that in convalescence there is a less pronounced metabolic and endocrine change in the female than in the male. It is thought to be related to the smaller tissue mass in males; it may well be sex-associated.

What do illness and hospitalization do to the young adult male or female who is struggling for the attainment of intimacy over isolation? Do we give him an opportunity to relate to us, thus providing a very good opportunity for him to release tension? Or do we treat him in a formal, stereotyped manner, encouraging isolation by our formal stand-off manner?

As the young adult increases in his sense of intimacy, he has more and more meaningful relationships and experiences in the adult world. As a result of positive experiences in adult society, the young adult's concerns and interests gradually move from the present to what he will contribute to the next generation. He then moves into the next stage in the life cycle of man, which is the period of generativity, or the development of the parental sense. He is not only concerned about having children of his own but about nurturing or caring for the children of others. He is ready to take on greater responsibilities—not just those of providing for himself and spouse but of guiding a new life to maturity. He is able now to give of himself in a more profound way. The parental period of development extends over a span of many years. It flows out of intimacy and extends up to senescence.

Adulthood

Society expects much of the individual as he goes through this period of his life. For most people it is their entire period of productivity —the years they make a place for themselves in the flow of history. The two tasks that society expected of the individual in the period of intimacy are brought to fruition—he matures in his career and he watches his children grow in wisdom and strength. This, too, is a very demanding and taxing stage of development. To succeed in one's career, and to be a good spouse and a good parent demands great energy and effort on the part of the individual. It means giving of oneself and in turn being able to receive much from colleagues, spouse, and children. Society demands not only that he succeed in his career and his family life, but also that he have energy, creativity, and interest left over so that he can serve the community on a voluntary basis. At the beginning of this period and during the preceding period he was establishing himself in the adult world; now he is helping to run the adult world and shape history for the oncoming generations.

This is not only an age of great activity, but because most people in this developmental period hold responsible positions, many other persons are dependent on them in a variety of ways, i.e., for emotional support, for financial support, and for important decisions. Think for a while what it means to this individual who recognizes and accepts these responsibilities to be hospitalized for a week, a month, or longer. Reflect on what it means to the hospitalized female patient who has four school-age children at home. She may well be anxious, demanding, or depressed or perhaps have a rise in blood pressure around 3 o'clock in the afternoon. These behaviors may well be caused by her feelings of responsibility to these children and not by the disease process per se. Also consider the effects of this mother's hospitalization on her children and her spouse.

The positive component of this maturational level has been stressed. As in all other stages of development there is a negative component here. This component is self-absorption. Coping with illness, profound or even minor if aggravating, takes much energy on the part of the individual. It is easy to see how the patient slips into self-absorption. Reflect for a moment on the patient who has a myocardial infarct. This is a fear-provoking experience. It demands that pressing responsibilities be lessened or perhaps eliminated entirely for a period of time. It also demands a rather prolonged period of convalescence. How does he cope with not meeting his responsibilities to his wife, children, colleagues, and society? Is it any wonder then that the patient exhibits a good deal of self-absorption? Or take a less profound condition but persistent in its presence, i.e., the polyneuritis of adult lead poisoning. This individual will undoubtedly continue to meet his job responsibilities, but this may be all he can do. The continuous nagging pain from the neuritis prevents him from discharging his other responsibilities fully.

There are many cartoons depicting the busy executive frantically answering the three or four telephones that are on his bedside table as the attendant stands patiently waiting to take him to surgery or x-ray. Funny, yes! Sad, yes! Perhaps his subordinates need this kind of help and support from him to function and he knows it. Perhaps not! This may well be his way of saying to you, "Don't take my autonomy from me!" "Don't let me lose my identity in this maze of strange and frightening activity; I'm frightened." "Help me!"

Late Adulthood

One of the major health concerns in the early part of this period, and extending as far back as late adolescence, is that this is the period of life when many of the chronic degenerative diseases (e.g., multiple sclerosis) begin to manifest themselves. What does the diagnosis of multiple sclerosis mean to the young man just established in his profession? What does it mean to the young woman who has just married or perhaps has been married for five years and has three preschool children? What does it mean to the spouse of this patient? What does it mean to the small children of this parent? Let your imagination work for you. Chronic degenerative diseases are not curable but only manageable. These individuals and their families (colleagues, too) need much help to understand and resolve the conflicts surrounding a diagnosis such as multiple sclerosis, tuberculosis, or diabetes mellitus. It is not only the immediate adjustment that causes strain on personal and family relationships but the continuing adjustment that is required as the disease process progresses. Families or individuals not only need help to adjust psychologically to this kind of condition but need very practical kinds of help, i.e., equipment, household help, nursing care, and financial help. Do you know the resources in your community so that you can refer them to the right people? Or do you say, "That's none of my business; I can't afford to get involved." Isn't it? Can't you?

At the end of the generativity period, a biological maturational task occurs that is of concern to all people in the health fields: that is, the climacteric. A very simple explanation of the climacteric is an altered hormonal balance primarily concerned with reduction of gonadal function. In the male this is a very slow, gradual process beginning as early as 30 years of age in some males and later in others. There is usually no sharp demarcation of beginning or end as there is in the female. In fact, if men experience acute overt manifestations of the climacteric (e.g., vasomotor symptoms, emotional instability), it is taken out of the realm of normality and considered pathological. In females it is different. It is one of the three fundamental biologically determined maturational crises in womanhood. The other two are puberty and pregnancy. These three maturational crises are different from other maturational tasks. The difference lies in the intense and specific interdependence between the psychological and the biophysiological changes and the fact that they are all remorselessly irreversible. In all three of these periods, a number of new, specific libidinal and adaptive tasks confront the individual. Often these tasks are diametrically opposed to the central tasks and activities of the preceding stage. Each one of these stages seems to revive and unsettle psychological conflicts of earlier development, each one requiring new and different solutions. In all three the mastery of this biologically initiated phase depends on the solution and maturational reorganization of this disequilibrium, i.e., adulthood in puberty, motherhood in pregnancy, and aging in menopause. It is this factor that adds to the adaptive process the quality of the inevitable, emphasizing it as the point from which there is no return. Once an adolescent you cannot be a child again; once a mother you cannnot be a single unit again; and once beyond the menopause you cannot bear a child again. The demands, psychological and biophysiologic, that are placed on the woman's body as she goes through this maturational task are surely important factors to consider when caring for a patient at this stage in development. These demands affect the management of her diabetes mellitus, hypertension, or convalescence from a thyroidectomy. They also affect how she perceives herself as a feminine being and her role in society—now. Then, too, the time of menopause frequently coincides with the time when children are leaving the family home to begin careers, to marry, and to have children of their own. Reflect how all these factors may influence the women's ability to cope with the negative component, self-absorption, in this stage of development.

The final stage in the development of the human being is old age or the development of the sense of integrity. It is the culmination and integration of his entire development. The child and youth who has come through the various maturational levels satisfactorily is ready and eager for adulthood. The adult who has enjoyed the intimacies of the adult world with his spouse and colleagues, who has enjoyed and adequately met the responsibilities of parenthood and also his work responsibilities, arrives at the end of his life with ego integrity. Erikson describes this as follows:

Integrity thus means a new and different love of one's parents, free of the wish that they should have been different, and an acceptance of the fact that one's life is one's own responsibility. It is a sense of comradeship with men and women of distant times and of different pursuits, who have created orders and objects and sayings conveying human dignity and love. Although aware of the relativity of all the various life styles that have given meaning to human striving, the possessor of integrity is ready to defend the dignity of his own life style against all physical and economic threats. For he knows that, for him, all human dignity stands or falls with the one style of integrity of which he partakes.[10]

The adult in senescence who has not or does not develop integrity is the adult who feels he has been cheated in his life and wishes he could relive it. If you carry this to the extreme, he is the adult who experiences despair and disgust. Despair conveys the feeling that life was too short to develop integrity; he has been cheated! Disgust is a cover-up for despair, chronic complaining of how poorly life is run. The sense of integrity is a part of human nature that must be reaffirmed over and over with the help and comfort of faith, the arts, and wisdom which offer proof of the integrity of humanity.

Although aging begins at birth (the aorta is the body structure to show initial aging) and continues very gradually throughout life, senescence is the period of life when the greatest amount of the aging process takes place. Today with the great strides in all health fields, we have more and more people living to old age.

The laws of growth that were presented earlier in this chapter seem to deal primarily with the growth and development (anachronobiology) of the organism, but they are also applicable in the aging process (catachronobiology). For example, each child grows in his own way —each adult ages in his own way—some fast, some slow. Another example, the tempo of growth is not even—the tempo of the aging process is not even; some of the structures of the body age rapidly and others more slowly. The law that states that growth is a continuous, orderly process is one of which we see clinical evidence every day on hospital wards—the 85-year-old woman's hip does heal; the suture line

[10] Witmer and Kotinsky, *op. cit.,* p. 25.

of the operation in the 80-year-old man does grow together. Probably the fact that all aspects of growth are interrelated is seen most dramatically in the elderly person. It is quite easy to relate his emotional, social, psychological, and physical needs to his illness. He may well be ill because he was physically or financially unable to nourish himself or just not interested in eating or too lonely to eat. The interrelatedness of the body brings problems of duplicity and multiplicity to illness in the aged. For example, poor nutrition leads to poor resistance, which may lead to contracting pneumonia, which may lead to cardiac difficulties, which may lead to renal failure. Another related problem in illness in the aged is the chronicity of the illness.

The period of senescence is long for a good many people. The aging process itself varies with individuals. These two statements are very much related to nursing care. Just because a patient is 65, 75, or 85 years old does not mean that he cannot hear, think adequately for himself, or be a contributing member of the team that is engaged in his health care. His total behavior will dictate his nursing needs.

The material in this chapter was presented to help the nurse bring into sharp focus her knowledge of human development and to show how she can relate this knowledge to her day-by-day care of her patients. It was presented to remind the young student that each patient is an individual member of society, each struggling to further his development in order that he may be a better or more complete human being, thus fulfilling his destiny as he understands it, to remind the student, too, that each of her patients is an individual, with his own genetic endowment, his unique past and present experiences, as well as an individual with a pathological condition.

It is hoped that, from reflecting on the material presented, the student may see the art in nursing as well as the science. Generally a young person comes into nursing more knowledgeable and interested in the art rather than the science of nursing. She comes in wanting to commit or dedicate herself to the nurturing of mankind through the practice of nursing. It is hoped that through practicing nursing as presented in this chapter she may further develop her appreciation and knowledge of the art and bring it into sharp focus with her knowledge of nursing science, thereby gaining greater satisfactions for herself and better care for her patients. Only as the nurse is able to fuse the art and science of nursing will she be able to give excellent care, because man has a psyche as well as a body—each of which needs to be nurtured.

Examples of Reactions to Pathologic Conditions and Surgical Procedures at Various Stages of Development

In the following paragraphs a common medical condition and a simple surgical procedure will be explored to show how they affect an individual at various phases of his development. The medical condition to be explored is simple diarrhea and the surgical procedure is circumcision.

DIARRHEA

Diarrhea is a common condition at any age. In the newborn and in early infancy it is a dread disease accompanied by severe fluid and electrolyte problems. Unless the infant is treated promptly by physicians who understand the significance of fluid and electrolyte balance in infancy, he may well die. Most infants, well treated, go on to live with few sequelae even to their development of trust because they are hospitalized such a short time.

Diarrhea in the toddler age (period of autonomy) is physiologically not a severe disease. The greater problem of diarrhea to this child is psychological (precisely with his psychosocial and psychosexual development). He has just acquired bowel and bladder control, which is very much a part of his total autonomy or his will to control himself and his environment. With diarrhea the toddler has little or no control over bowel evacuation. The toddler's intellectual development is not such that he has any appreciable concept of time or ability to understand diarrhea; consequently, he cannot say to himself, "Oh, this will only last a few days and I'll be in control again." He can only think, "I've failed! Will Mama scold? Mama doesn't love me anymore. That's why I'm here." (Of course his language development is not this great—but his thinking and feeling are.) His loss of control, so hard-won, and his separation from his mother are overwhelming problems to the small child and must be taken into consideration when planning and giving his nursing care. Diarrhea may cause the same problems for the child in the next period of development, preschool, but this child has a bit more intellectual and ego development to help him.

From this stage of development until late in senescence, diarrhea is more a nuisance than anything else. In the elderly person again the problem arises of fluid and electrolyte balance. He may need to be hospitalized. In the elderly, hospitalization or any profound change in daily living is a threat to his total functioning. A well-functioning elderly person may become confused with the stress of illness and hospitalization with all of the hustle and bustle of today's hospitals. Like the young child, he too, may experience separation anxiety. He and his wife may have been married 50 or more years. With mutual support they function well, but without each other one or both may become confused and disoriented. Provisions are made for the mother to stay with the hospitalized young child, but no comparable provision is made for the elderly patient. With more people living into the seventh, eighth, and ninth decade, nurses need to think of the kind of care that will support the elderly patient's total well-being and not just cure or manage the pathology he exhibits.

CIRCUMCISION

Regarding the surgical procedure, circumcision in the newborn period is a very safe, simple surgical procedure. The baby is not upset by the procedure in the least. An infant a little older will object strenuously while the procedure is being performed but then is not bothered by it.

Circumcision in the toddler age (one to three years old) is something different. Ordinarily the child is given a general anesthetic and experiences considerable discomfort and pain following the procedure. It is ordinarily done in a hospital setting, and this often means separation from his mother. This is the age when the child is struggling for autonomy. The discomfort is quite localized to his penis and becomes very clearly related to control of his bladder. Separation is one of the most threatening experiences a toddler or a preschool child can experience. It can have a very real effect on his total development.

As the child moves from a toddler to a preschooler (three to six years old), he is sure he is a separate person in his own right. He spends considerable time and effort exploring the various kinds of people there are in the world. This is the period that the youngster learns whether he is a boy or she is a girl and what it means to be a boy or a girl. He is developing considerably in his self-image and is threatened by activities concerned with bodily mutilation. It is very easy to understand, from a child's point of view, that circumcision represents mutilation of his body. What does it do to his self-image? Do not be surprised if the child wonders whether he is still a boy. This age child, too, will be given a general anesthetic and hospitalized, which often means separation from his mother.

Let us move to the period of adolescence with all of its turbulence surrounding sexual growth accompanied by new and powerful biological drives. What does a circumcision mean to a youngster aged 13 or 15? In his quest for identity he is questioning all authority. Two powerful authority figures, i.e., parents and physician, say he must have a circumcision now. It is not just a medical or surgical treatment but a procedure closely related to his masculinity. What is his reaction to this? How will he react to this at the time of the surgery?

Compare the adolescent to the young adult aged 23 or 24 who is preparing for marriage and whose physician recommends that he be circumcised before marriage. Difficult as it is for the young male, it is his choice. The decision to have surgery holds tangible rewards.

A surgical procedure in the older adult male that evokes similar stress is a prostatic resection. It, too, is viewed as a mutilating procedure and therefore as a threat to his self-image, especially that which is related to his concept of being a virile, masculine person. This stress may be no different for the 40-, 50-, or 60-year-old male.

Many other medical conditions or surgical procedures could be explored to point up the significance of the relationship between reactions to illness and the stage of development of the patient. Some are anatomical in nature, such as the short, thin omentum in infants and small children, which is ineffectual in walling off intra-abdominal infections. Others are related to physiological reactions, i.e., the encephalopathy (usually followed by mental deterioration) in the lead poisoning of children as compared to polyneuritis commonly found in adults. One of the major physical factors to keep in mind when dealing with an adolescent who is growing with great rapidity is that growth must always be considered with maintenance, whether it be in nutrition or with a long-term drug such as insulin. Maintenance alone is not sufficient. Still others are more related to the psychological, e.g., the differences in reaction to a radical mastectomy for a malignancy in a newly wed young woman, a young matron of 30 years, and a woman 65 years old.

This phenomenon is equally true with respect to invasion of the body by particular organisms, e.g., hemolytic streptococcus: A toddler overreacts with a temperature of 105°F, which may well be accompanied by convulsions; an adult is sick but rarely develops such exaggerated symptoms. Specific kinds of illness are common at certain levels of maturation; e.g., infections and anomalies in infants and children, chronic degenerative diseases in the middle years, and in the aged progressive reduction in the ability of the organism to function brings duplicity and multiplicity to most pathologic conditions.

It is evident from the preceding discussion that individuals react to illness differently at various maturational levels. Clinically this is seen daily. The more the nurse knows and understands human development, the more able she is to recognize the relationship of the patient's reactions and responses to illness to his maturational level. Although such relationships are well documented in health care literature about children, there is a scarcity of this kind of research with sick adults. One such research study was done with male patients having coronary artery disease. These patients ranged in age from 35 to 67. It is interesting to note that the 50-year-old males (especially those from 50 to 55 years) had more difficulty in coping with the psychological stress than did the 40- or 60-year-old groups. More of the 50-year-old group were depressed, manifested overt anxiety, and were uncooperative with the medical regimen. Concerning this, Rosen and Bibring state:

Men in their 50's appear to encounter a period of crisis, reminiscent of adolescence, in which there is open conflict over the shift from the active orientation of youth to the passive position of later years. These men still cling to achievement-autonomy goals, feeling they must push on; yet they have begun to doubt their ability to reach these goals, and while some are no longer certain that the rewards of striving are so desirable, they are reluctant to retreat from the struggle.[11]

If the nurse is to meet the individual patient's needs, she must consider his genetic endowment, his total life experiences (maturational level), and the pathology of his illness.

[11] Jacqueline Rosen and Grete Bibring: "Psychological Reactions of Hospitalized Male Patients to a Heart Attack: Age and Social-Class Differences," *Psychosom. Med.*, **28**:808–21 (Nov.–Dec.) 1966.

REFERENCES

BOOKS

Breckenridge, Marian, and Murphy, Margaret: *Growth and Development of the Young Child*, 7th ed. (Philadelphia: W. B. Saunders Company, 1963).

Breckenridge, Marian, and Vincent, E. Lee: *Child Development*, 5th ed. (Philadelphia: W. B. Saunders Company, 1965).

Clark, Margaret, and Anderson, Barbara: *Culture and Aging: An Anthropological Study of Older Americans* (Springfield, Ill.: Charles C Thomas, Publisher, 1967).

Duvall, Evelyn: *Family Development*, 3rd ed. (Philadelphia: J. B. Lippincott Company, 1967).

Engle, George: *Psychological Development in Health and Disease* (Philadelphia: W. B. Saunders Company, 1962).

Erikson, Erik: *Childhood and Society*, 2nd ed. (New York: W. W. Norton & Company, 1963).

Haimowitz, Morris, and Haimowitz, Natalie (eds.): *Human Development, Selected Readings* (New York: Thomas Y. Crowell Company, 1960).

Hansen, P. From (ed.): *Age with a Future: Proceedings of the Sixth International Congress of Gerontology* (Philadelphia: F. A. Davis Company, 1964).

Havighurst, Robert: *Developmental Tasks and Education*, 2nd ed. (New York: David McKay Company, 1952).

Neugarten, Bernice (ed.): *Middle Age and Aging* (Chicago: University of Chicago Press, 1968).

Rose, Arnold, and Peterson, Warren (eds.): *Older People and the Social Order—The Sub-culture of the Aging* (Philadelphia: F. A. Davis Company, 1965).

Vedder, Clyde (complied by): *Problems of the Middle-Aged* (Springfield, Ill.: Charles C Thomas, Publisher, 1965).

Witmer, Helen, and Kotensky, Ruth (eds.): *Personality in the Making: The Fact Finding Report of the Midcentury Whitehouse Conference on Children and Youth* (New York: Harper and Brothers, 1952).

PERIODICALS

Donovan, Helen: "Creativity and the Nurse," *Hosp. Prog.*, **45**:98–102 (June) 1964.

Ferlic, Anne: "Existential Approach in Nursing," *Nurs. Outlook*, **16**:30–33 (Oct.) 1968.

"Hypothesis: Effector Mechanism in Immunity," *Lancet*, **1**:25–58 (Jan.) 1969.

Janeway, Charles: "Progress in Immunology," *J. Pediat.*, **72**:885–903 (June) 1968.

Levine, Rhoda L.: "Disengagement in the Elderly —Its Causes and Effects," *Nurs. Outlook*, **17**:28–30 (Oct.) 1969.

Meyer, Herbert: "Predictable Problems of Hospitalized Adolescents," *Amer. J. Nurs.*, **69**:525–28 (Mar.) 1969.

Mickley, Barbara: "Space and Place in Patient Care," *Amer. J. Nurs.*, **68**:511–16 (Mar.) 1968.

Rosen, Jacqueline, and Bibring, Grete: "Psychological Reactions of Hospitalized Male Patients to a Heart Attack: Age and Social Class Differences," *Psychosom. Med.*, **28**:808–21 (Nov.–Dec.) 1966.

Scarlett, E. P.: "Doctor out of Zebulum: The Case

History of Man," *Arch. Intern. Med.,* 113:769–72 (May) 1964.

Skipper, James, Togliacozzo, Daisy, and Mauksch, Hans: "Barriers to Communication Between Patients and Hospital Functionaries," *Nurs. Forum,* 2:14–28 (Winter) 1963.

Smoyak, Shirley: "Cultural Incongruence—The Effect on Nurses' Perception," *Nurs. Forum,* 7:234–47 (Summer) 1968.

"A Symposium on the Elderly," *Practitioner,* 200:761–92 (June) 1968.

Tryon, Phyllis: "Patient Participation vs. Patient Passivity," *Nurs. Forum,* 2:48–61 (Spring) 1963.

Van Slambrook, Marilynn: "Boredom and Loneliness in Growing Old," *Geriat. Nurs.,* 4:7–10 (Apr.) 1968.

"Viewpoint: Discrimination Against the Elderly Is a Major Problem," *Geriatrics,* 24:40–46 (Mar.) 1969.

"Viewpoint: Rejection of Old Age May Be the Best Attitude," *Geriatrics,* 24:46–50 (Feb.) 1969.

Walker, Lorraine: "Every Patient Is Unique," *Nurs. Outlook,* 16:39–43 (Sept.) 1968.

17

The Requirements of Patients Treated Surgically

"Notice"

As of today, May 15, 1847, every doctor or student who comes from the dissecting room is required, before entering the maternity wards, TO WASH HIS HANDS thoroughly in a basin of chlorine water which is being placed at the entrance. This order applies to all, without exception.

I. P. Semmelweis, M.D.[1]

Overview

What elements should be considered when planning the nursing care of a patient who is treated surgically?

The Preoperative Period

What can be done to minimize anxiety of patients?

What are some of the important activities the nurse may undertake to prepare the patient for surgery?

What are the responsibilities of the nurse in the immediate preoperative period?

The Operative Period

What are the objectives of the surgical team during the operative phase?

The Immediate Postoperative Period

What preparations are made for the patient who is in the immediate postoperative period?

What are the causes of shock in the surgical patient?

What is the basis for blood grouping?

What are the manifestations of a transfusion reaction?

What are some of the disturbances in gastrointestinal function that may occur postoperatively?

The Later Postoperative Period

How can wound infection be prevented?

What are the responsibilities of the nurse when wound dehiscence or evisceration is impending or has occurred?

What is the nature of pain?

How does surgical therapy threaten the self-concept of the patient?

Overview

WITH the development of modern surgery, many conditions that have plagued man since the beginning of time have been brought under control. Although the list is much too long to enumerate, examples include such conditions as acute appendicitis, cholecystitis, hernia, compound fractures, and even defects in the structure of the heart. Much of the knowledge on which modern surgical treatment of disease is based has been acquired in the last 100 to 150 years. Since the early nineteenth century the science of surgery has developed so that an increasing number of surgical procedures can

now be performed with reasonable safety and benefit to the patient.

The treatment of disease and injury by surgical methods probably goes back to the beginning of mankind. The earliest records of surgical procedures left by man are primitive tools found in burial grounds. Other early records include writings and drawings on stone tablets and on the walls of caves and houses. Records may also have been made on perishable materials such as bark or bamboo, but if they were, they have been destroyed by the elements and are no longer available.

History of Surgical Procedures

A variety of surgical procedures were performed by primitive man including the setting

---

[1] Jurgen Thorwald: *The Century of the Surgeon* (New York: Pantheon Books, Inc., 1957), p. 234.

of broken bones and the treatment of wounds. Trephining, a procedure in which a hole is made in the skull, was performed by primitive surgeons in many parts of the world. Skulls, eight to ten thousand years old, have been found bearing marks of trephination in France and other parts of Europe. In the New World, Peru is the site where trephining was practiced most extensively, but it was performed as far north as Alaska. As far back as 4000 B.C., the Egyptians did circumcisions as well as ophthalmic surgery. The Homeric legends refer to regimental surgeons as fighters and physicians.[2] Histories of other civilizations contain reference to surgical treatment, but much of the early surgery was both cruel and crude. Its use was hampered by inadequate knowledge of effective and humane ways to control pain, hemorrhage, and infection. Some of this surgery was done not for the purpose of removing diseased tissue or of correcting anatomical defects but to allow evil spirits to escape. By modern standards, making an opening in the skull to provide an avenue for the escape of a demon seems strange, but in relation to the knowledge of the time it was logical.

Some of the knowledge essential to the practice of surgery was discovered and then lost, to be reintroduced at a later time. For example, the use of ligatures was known and described by Celsus shortly before the beginning of the Christian era. Since their use by Ambroise Paré (1510–1590), ligatures have been used as the method of choice in hemostasis.

Phases in the Development of Surgery

Modern surgery has gone through two phases in its development. In the first, the objective was to make surgery safe and humane. In the second, the objective was to make the patient safe for surgery. Both are important to the welfare of the patient. The first phase has its origins in the sciences of anatomy, chemistry, bacteriology, psychology, sociology, and anthropology.

The three elements that are essential to safe and humane surgery are hemostasis, asepsis, and anesthesia. Without an adequate method to control bleeding, the patient may die from hemorrhage. Before the development of the science of bacteriology, he frequently died from infection. Since anesthesia made possible the prevention of pain, the surgeon can take the necessary time to handle tissues gently and perform the surgical procedures carefully and accurately. Knowledge of anatomy and the factors

that influence wound healing was important to the development of surgical methods.

CONTROLLING BLEEDING

Because man has always been faced with bleeding, the methods of stopping the flow of blood were developed early. Methods used to control hemorrhage developed in three stages. As might be anticipated, pressure was the first to be used; the second was the cauterization of wounds; and the third was use of some type of material to tie the ends of blood vessels. As in many other fields of knowledge, the introduction of new methods did not entirely replace the old, but each new procedure increased the ability to control hemorrhage. All these methods are still used today. The causes, effects, and treatment of hemorrhage will be discussed later in the chapter.

MODERN ASEPSIS

The modern concept of asepsis is based on two premises, neither of which is really new. One is that the environment contains something that, when it is introduced or it enters into a wound or individual, can cause harm. The other is that something can be done to prevent the harmful agent (spirit or microbe) from entering the body or its harmful influence can be nullified. As an example, some primitive people isolated the sick by placing them outside the village walls or abandoned their houses when someone died in them. Others made loud noises or practiced some kind of ritual to frighten the evil spirit or immobilize him.

Asepsis as it is known today developed in three stages: the first was the stage of isolation and cleanliness; the second was the stage of antiseptic surgery; and the third and present stage is the stage of asepsis. The value of isolation and cleanliness was demonstrated in the 1840's by Semmelweis, a young Hungarian physician who practiced in Vienna.[3] Despite lack of precise knowledge of microorganisms, Semmelweis instituted measures that were successful in the prevention of puerperal fever. These measures were based on the observation that the incidence of puerperal fever was much lower in a ward where the women were delivered by midwives than in a ward where the women were examined by medical students who had come from autopsy rooms where they had handled tissues of women who had died of puerperal fever. Next he instituted techniques to control the factor he believed to be responsi-

---

[2] Otto L. Bettmann: *A Pictorial History of Medicine* (Springfield, Ill.: Charles C Thomas, Publisher, 1956), p. 15.

[3] About the same time Oliver Wendell Holmes published an essay, "On the Contagiousness of Childbed Fever."

ble. He insisted that physicians and medical students wash their hands before they examined patients. Despite active opposition to this rule, the lives of many mothers were saved by it. Semmelweis died a depressed and disappointed man; although he had proved over and over the soundness of his ideas, they were not rapidly accepted by his colleagues. As happens even today, there was a considerable lag between the development of knowledge and its acceptance and use in practice.

The work of many men, some who preceded Semmelweis and some who followed him, contributed to the development of modern aseptic surgery. Among those usually mentioned is the seventeenth-century Dutch lens grinder, Leeuwenhoek. He is credited with being the first to see bacteria. It was not until 1850–1865, or nearly 200 years later, that the foundation was laid for antiseptic and, soon thereafter, aseptic surgery. A French chemist, Louis Pasteur, was employed by the wine growers of France to identify the cause of the souring of wine and to devise techniques for preventing it. As a result of his work the theory of spontaneous generation was disproved for all time and the germ theory of disease was established. According to the germ theory, disease is caused by a living agent. After it is introduced into an individual, the agent establishes itself, grows, multiplies, and may cause disease.

Other men, notably Lister and Koch, added to the body of knowledge that contributed to the acceptance of the germ theory. Lister, a physiologist and surgeon, read reports of the studies made by Pasteur on the cause and prevention of the souring of wine. If microorganisms present in the air caused wine to sour, might not microorganisms infect wounds? To remove microorganisms from the air, Lister had the operating room sprayed with a dilute solution of carbolic acid previous to the start of the operation. Following the operation he placed a disinfectant bandage over the incision. He had some success with the latter, for he found that he could prevent the infection of compound fractures, that is, fractures in which the skin is broken and there is a direct communication between the broken bone and the external environment. Compound fractures treated in this manner healed as well as simple ones, that is, those in which the skin remained intact. Lister reported his experiments and clinical trials in 1867.

The third stage, or the stage of asepsis, quickly followed the stage of antisepsis. In 1877 Robert Koch published *The Cause of Infection in Wounds*. In what has come to be known as Koch's postulates, he stated the conditions that must be fulfilled for a microorganism to be es-

tablished as the cause of a disease. The work of Semmelweis, Pasteur, Lister, Koch, and others demonstrated that the pus that was formed in a wound resulted from the introduction of an outside agent and was not an essential part of the healing process. With this knowledge as a basis, methods were developed to prevent microorganisms from gaining access to the wound.

Previous to these discoveries, wounds were so regularly infected that pus was considered an essential aspect of wound healing. The type and quantity of pus present in a wound depended on the infecting microorganism and often provided a clue to the prognosis. Thus abundant, creamy pus with little or no odor was usually associated with recovery and was therefore called laudable pus. A thin, watery, or malodorous pus is characteristic of hemolytic or anaerobic streptococcal infection and implied a poor prognosis. Presently, it is known that any type of infection in a wound delays healing and may threaten the life of the individual.

Despite a large body of knowledge acquired over the last 100 years or so indicating that the external environment contains microorganisms capable of causing disease, wounds continue to be infected. Among the elements contributing to infections are a lack of understanding of existing knowledge and failure to follow prescribed techniques. For example, Miss Smith, a nurse in the operating room, awakens in the morning with a sore throat or a boil on her neck. A heavy operative schedule is planned for the day. Should she go to work or should she remain at home? If she goes to work, she may be able to rationalize her behavior by saying, "I'm not very sick. I'll wear a mask. It's on the back of my neck. I'm needed." But she will be demonstrating that she does not know what, as an operating room nurse, she should know or that she does not accept her knowledge as having validity. Other considerations take precedence in influencing her behavior. Among the additional elements contributing to the continued problem of wound infection are susceptibility of the host and the ecological balance between or among microorganisms. It is likely that there are others as well.

Fundamentally, the practice of asepsis depends on two factors:

1. Knowledge of the factors to be controlled and development of suitable techniques.
2. The conviction of practitioners that the knowledge is valid and that the techniques are practical and will accomplish their purpose.

Semmelweis failed not because his observations or techniques were unsound but because his colleagues refused to accept them as valid, practical, and necessary.

ANESTHESIA

The third element required, if surgery is to be safe and humane, is some means of preventing pain during the performance of surgery. Prior to the middle of the nineteenth century, surgery was limited to emergency procedures or those absolutely essential to life. Agents that were used to prevent painful sensations were limited to belladonna, hemp, opium, and alcohol. Most of these drugs lessened the patient's perception of pain or his memory of it. In some instances the patient was rendered unconscious by a blow on the head. When the condition of the patient was believed to contraindicate the administration of large doses of alcohol or opium, the patient was held or tied and the operation performed with all possible speed. After the introduction of safe and effective anesthetic agents, time and speed were no longer the prime considerations.

Thus the discovery and acceptance of a variety of safe chemical agents have been important to the development of surgery. The chemical discovery of the anesthetic agents preceded their actual use by many years. The first anesthetic, nitrous oxide, was discovered in 1776 by Priestly. In 1799 Sir Humphry Davy reported that it prevented pain and suggested that it might be used in surgical operations. Although others experimented with nitrous oxide and ether, the first recognized use of anesthesia for a surgical operation did not come about until Morton, in October 1846, successfully anesthetized a patient with ether at the Massachusetts General Hospital.

Today a great variety of anesthetic agents are available. Some are suitable for inducing unconsciousness; others may be used to anesthetize a region of the body or a small area of the skin or mucous membrane. Methods used in their administration are also varied and are related to the state in which the agent occurs. For example, gaseous anesthetics are administered by way of a face mask or through a tube introduced into the trachea. Liquid anesthetics that evaporate rapidly can anesthetize the skin by freezing it. Other liquids produce anesthesia when applied to mucous membrane. Liquids may also be injected into the skin, sensory nerves, and spinal canal and even intravenously. Because of the variety of agents now available, an anesthetic agent can be selected that suits not only the desired method of administration but also the condition of the patient.[4]

[4] For detailed information about various anesthetic agents, the student is referred to the References.

Previous to the discovery of effective and safe anesthetics, speed was one of the essential features in the performance of a surgical procedure. As a consequence, incisions were often crudely made and tissues suffered unnecessary damage. One of the most significant contributions to modern surgery was made by Halsted, who correlated surgical technique with wound healing. He emphasized the careful handling of tissue. For hemostasis, he clamped only the blood vessels with as little of the surrounding tissue as possible. He used a fine ligature that was tied just tight enough to approximate the tissues without strangulation. The care taken by the surgeon in making and closing a surgical incision is one of the important factors in recovery of the patient.

What elements should be considered when planning the nursing care of a patient who is treated surgically?

As the preceding accomplishments have become a reality, and knowledge of psychology, biochemistry, and physiology are advancing, surgeons are directing their attention toward making patients safe for surgery. Knowledge of physiological and biochemical processes has led to the discovery of methods that can be used to support patients during prolonged surgical procedures. As the relationship between the capacity of the patient to adapt physiologically and psychologically and his recovery has come to be appreciated, methods to evaluate his status and to correct abnormalities have been developed. With greater understanding of the physiological needs of people and the effects of surgery on structure and function, the care of the patient can be better regulated, so that recovery is facilitated.

Among the elements to be considered is that every patient is an individual. For most persons some aspect of surgical therapy is tantamount to a crisis situation. The psychological, social, and physiologic behavior of the patient can be expected to be similar to his behavior in any other highly stressful situation. (See Chapter 7.) Because of their familiarity with the risks and other aspects of surgical treatment, physicians and nurses may not be sufficiently aware of the uniqueness of the experience to each patient. Furthermore, their perception of the proposed procedure and its consequences may be quite different from that of the patient. Unless they are aware of the possibility of differences in perceptions and are alert to clues indicating the emotional state of the individual, they may not be as helpful as they should.

As an illustration, 15-year-old Jesse is to have a wart removed from the sole of his foot. Although his physician has tried to reassure him that removal of the wart is a relatively simple procedure, Jesse fears that he will lose his leg or at least his foot. Physicians and nurses know that a removal of this wart is a minor procedure, and they cannot understand why Jesse continues to turn on his light and to make unnecessary demands for service. About 3 o'clock in the morning, when the night nurse was answering his light for the fifteenth time, she said, "Jesse, you are having trouble getting to sleep, aren't you? It's hard to sleep when you are away from home. Would you like me to stay with you for a little while?" She sat quietly beside his bed. In a few minutes Jesse asked, "Are they going to cut my foot off tomorrow?" When the nurse knew what was troubling Jesse, she was able to reassure him by saying, "My goodness, no," and then explained what was planned.

Besides the individuality of the patient, a variety of other factors should be considered. In each phase of therapy—preoperative, operative, postoperative, and convalescence—definite objectives are to be accomplished and the patient is exposed to a variety of risks or threats to his well-being. As a basis for planning nursing action, additional factors should also be known: *the site of the incision, the function of the organ or tissue,* as well as the *disease or condition being treated.* For example, to remove the thyroid gland an incision is made in the neck. The location of the scar and its possible appearance is a possible source of psychological stress. Extension of the neck causes strain on the incision, as well as pain. The patient's head, therefore, should be supported in such a way that it is kept in a relatively normal position without strain on the incision. Because the thyroid gland is a highly vascular organ, it is important to observe the patient for evidence of bleeding in the tissue surrounding the operative side. Because the parathyroid glands are located in the region of the thyroid gland, they may be accidentally removed (a relatively rare event) or damaged. Consequently, the patient may experience parathyroid deficiency (see Chapter 15, Part A). One of the more common complications is caused by the anatomical relationship of the thyroid gland to the recurrent laryngeal nerves and trachea. Breathing can be impaired if the recurrent laryngeal nerves are damaged. The resultant paralysis of the laryngeal muscles causes the vocal folds to fall together and obstruct or greatly reduce the space between them, thereby changing the patient's voice or obstructing his breathing. The trachea itself may be occluded by edema from excessive movement or retraction of the trachea or by pressure from accumulated blood. Knowledge of the state of thyroid function is important in all phases of surgery. Although less frequent today than in the past symptoms of hyperthyroidism may be intensified during the immediate postoperative period resulting in thyroid storm or crisis. The prognosis of the patient and his future needs will depend on many factors such as the nature of the disease and whether or not enough, and not too much, tissue was removed to secrete adequate quantities of thyroid hormones.

Although the example cited is limited almost entirely to the factors to be considered during the postoperative phase, the same general points have relevance to the other phases of surgery. To summarize and to emphasize the points to be considered in planning nursing care, the nurse should give attention to the following:

1. The patient as an individual person.
2. The risks to which the patient is exposed before, during, and after surgery.
3. Problems related to the incision and approach to the organ or tissue.
4. The functions of the involved organ or region of the body and their effect on functions of other areas of the body.
5. The disorder under treatment and the effects of therapy.
6. The patient's perception of the nature of his disorder, the therapy, and his prognosis.

The Preoperative Period

The preoperative period may be defined as the period of time beginning with the moment it is recognized that surgery is needed and ending when the patient arrives in the operating room. During this period the nature of the patient's illness is determined and a therapeutic plan is made. For example, Mr. Thome has had symptoms of indigestion periodically for the last six months. For the most part, his symptoms have been mild and he has been able to explain them to his satisfaction and secure relief by taking antacids. One morning he awakened feeling nauseated and with a pain in his upper abdomen. He reviewed what he had eaten during the last 24 hours to determine what might be responsible for his symptoms. He took two anti-indigestion pills. Instead of his feeling relieved, however, the symptoms increased and he began to feel frightened. His wife suggested that she call a doctor, who determined that he needed surgery. Mr. Thome had entered the preoperative period, which did not end until he was transferred to the operating room, where he expected to have a partial gastrectomy for the removal of a portion of his stomach.

During the early preoperative period the nurse may act as a case finder and a health educator by encouraging the patient who is in the

"Is it or isn't it" stage to seek medical attention. Delay in the treatment of some disorders increases the danger of serious complications and may lessen chances for recovery. As an illustration, acute appendicitis, when operated on early, is accompanied by only a small risk. The death rate following appendectomy is less than 0.3 per cent when the operation can be performed before perforation. The complication rate after perforation has been shown in at least one study to be seven times that of the preperforation rate.[5]

At the time Mrs. Thome called the family physician, he entered the phase of diagnosis. He still had moments of "Is it or isn't it." He also felt relief that at last he was under medical care, but his relief was mixed with anxiety about the nature of the cause of his symptoms and the treatment that would be required. At this time Mr. Thome was subjected to a series of investigations directed toward answering two questions: What was the nature and extent of his illness? What was his physiological and psychological status? Answers to the first question determined whether or not surgery was indicated in his treatment and the type of procedure that would be of benefit to him. Answers to the second question provided information about any abnormalities that required correction before he was operated on and his capacity to adapt to surgical therapy.

Psychological Stress

Many of the sources of psychological stress are similar to those to which any sick person is likely to be exposed. There are some, however, that are peculiar to, or more likely to occur among, surgical patients. During the period of diagnosis, the patient may be subjected to a variety of procedures some of which are strenuous, embarrassing, and even painful. At the time surgery is performed, the diagnosis may be uncertain or the patient may believe that it is. Even when the diagnosis has been established as something relatively benign, it is not unusual for a patient to fear that he may have cancer. The patient may not understand the nature of the procedure to be performed or believe that it will be more extensive than it is actually planned to be. Uncertainty about the diagnosis and required treatment can be the source of severe stress. Jesse was under psychological stress because he did not understand the extent of the planned surgical procedure. Another example is Mrs. Thomas, who had a small

lump in her breast. Although her physician tried to assure her that the tumor was almost certainly benign, Mrs. Thomas was sure that it was malignant and that she would have a radical mastectomy. Previous to the removal of the tumor for examination, she was in a state of near-panic. During the period of recovery from the anesthetic, she wept and referred over and over to loss of her breast. Not until she was fully recovered from the anesthetic could she be assured that her breast had not been removed.

Among other sources of concern to some patients are the anesthetic, its effect, and its effectiveness in preventing pain, as well as the possibility that they may behave in an embarrassing manner. Mr. Thome wonders whether he will be awake or asleep during the operation. He has heard that people sometimes reveal secrets or say foolish or embarrassing things as they go to sleep. The man in the room next to him was awake while he was operated on, but he is not sure that he would like that either. Is it really possible to prevent pain when one is awake? How does one lie awake and allow someone to cut into one's abdomen? If he is awake, will the time of the operation pass quickly or will it be endless and seem to go on and on? Will he have pain after the operation?

In some types of surgery, organs having special meaning to the patient may have to be removed. Although any organ can have some special significance to a given individual, certain ones are more likely to have special meaning than others. Because the heart is essential to survival, surgical procedures on the heart are especially likely to be associated with anxiety and fear of death. Surgery on the organs of reproduction may affect the individual's self-concept, so that he or she feels that he or she is less a man or woman. In the American culture, the breast is a symbol of femininity. A woman may therefore feel less a woman after losing a breast. When a surgical procedure either temporarily or permanently prevents a husband and wife from having sexual relations, it may affect the stability of the marriage or the individual may fear that it will. When the loss of a part of the body necessitates changes in the way of life of the patient or in his role at work or in the family, the patient usually experiences some degree of anxiety.

Another source of anxiety is the risk to which the patient exposes himself by undergoing surgical therapy. The nurse should be aware of the fact that every operation, no matter how minor, is accompanied by some risk. The risk may be slight or it may be great. When a new procedure or an exceptionally hazardous one is performed, the patient may be aware of the nature of the risk. He may also know that if surgery fails, his

[5] J. Garrott Allen: "Appendicitis and the Acute Abdomen," *Surgery: Principles and Practice,* 3rd ed. (Carl A. Moyer *et al.,* eds.) (Philadelphia: J. B. Lippincott Company, 1965), p. 968.

chances for living are negligible. Some of the preceding continue to be sources of anxiety during the period of recovery following the operation. Attention is given to provide the patient with sufficient care of good quality to assure him that his needs will be met. Possibly too little consideration is given to the effects of what the patient regards as too much care. For example, during the period when Mr. Norman was being prepared for, and immediately following, the introduction of an aortic prosthesis (artificial aortic valve), he received more attention than he had possibly experienced over his entire life-span. The effect was not to assure him but to frighten him, for he said, "Who am I to receive all this care? No one has ever cared this much about me before. Why should they do so at this time? I must be terribly sick, or people would continue to ignore me as they have in the past." Following the immediate postoperative period, Mr. Norman became deeply depressed. Although some depression is common, Mr. Norman was unusually depressed. During an interview with a psychiatrist, he expressed his feelings. The nurse who cared for him before and immediately after the operation remembered that he had made a similar comment to her but she had not recognized its significance. Possibly, if he had had an opportunity to express his feelings previous to surgical therapy his depression would have been less severe.

What can be done to minimize anxiety of patients?

Despite the virtual impossibility of eliminating all psychological stress, much can be done to minimize it. Among the various factors contributing to a lessening of psychological stress is a climate in which the patient feels that nurses and doctors are concerned for his welfare. Some of the actions that contribute to this include: (1) being kind and courteous, (2) respecting his rights as an individual, (3) protecting his patterns of modesty, (4) preparing him for what to expect and for what is expected of him, (5) determining his level of knowledge and what he wants to know, (6) personalizing his care by modifying those aspects of his care that are important to him insofar as these modifications do not interfere with his recovery, (7) attending to his physiological and physical needs, and (8) utilizing other sources of support for him, such as arranging for him to talk with his spiritual advisor or a social worker.

Most of the points enumerated above are discussed in Chapter 7. Essentially their implementation does not differ for the patient undergoing surgical therapy from that required by any seriously ill patient.

In most situations, stress can usually be minimized by creating a climate in which the patient feels free to raise questions that are troubling him. To help to prevent misconceptions and misunderstandings, the patient requires information about the nature of the illness, why the surgery is needed, and what can be expected from the anesthetic and the surgical procedure and experience. He should be provided with information about hospital routines, the recovery room, and postoperative procedures. The patient wants to be assured that those who are responsible for his care are competent and will be available when he needs them. Although some of the preceding are the responsibility of the surgeon, nurses are frequently faced with questions that the patient asks for information and reassurance. Even when the surgeon provides the patient with a detailed explanation, the patient may be so overwhelmed and confused by the fact that surgery is necessary that he comprehends very little of what he is told. In addition, the patient may stand in awe of the surgeon and hesitate to ask questions. Later, when the patient has had an opportunity to think about his situation, he may have questions that should be answered. The nurse has an obligation to secure answers to the question or questions the patient is asking. Whether she answers the questions herself or refers them to the physician and how she answers those that she does not refer depends on the nature of the questions and her own competence.

When the patient has questions that the nurse cannot or is not permitted to answer, she can still be helpful to the patient. She can express her interest in the patient by listening to him and, if required, initating action. Someone who is willing and able to listen may be all the patient wants or needs. She can also help the patient to clarify his questions and can encourage him to ask the surgeon for information. She can also determine the urgency of the need of the patient to have his question answered. Miss Elder had been in the hospital for some weeks for the treatment of a fractured hip. The fracture was treated by open reduction, following which Miss Elder was encased in a double spica cast. About a week previous to the incident related below, she had been told that she might go home on the following Tuesday and all the arrangements had been made. The day before she planned to leave the hospital, the surgeon made a window in the cast in order to examine and dress the wound. After the required equipment was delivered to the room, the surgeon explained what he was going to do. Because Miss Elder was unprepared for the procedure, she heard nothing. Although her wound was healing nicely, she quickly concluded that it was not healing and that she would not be discharged from the hospital. She was so upset that she could not ask the surgeon for an explanation. Shortly after the surgeon left, a nurse found Miss Elder in tears. Although the nurse knew that Miss Elder was to be discharged as planned, she was sure that reassurance of the patient depended on direct word from her physician. She immediately called him and he assured her that Miss Elder was to be discharged the following day. This information was relayed to Miss Elder so that she could relax and complete her plans for leaving the hospital.

In some hospitals the problem of what patients can be told about the nature of their illness, why surgery is needed, and what can be expected during all phases of illness is met by the preparation of two types of manuals that the patient may be given to read and the nursing staff given to use as a guide in answering questions. One type includes essential information about the nature of a particular disease and its therapy, or its content may deal primarily with the surgical aspects of therapy. For example, one manual might cover the disease diabetes mellitus and its treatment. Another might be prepared for the use of the patient having a colostomy or thoracic surgery. These manuals emphasize what the patient needs to know to help himself recover and give answers to frequently asked questions. They are usually prepared by a committee of physicians and nurses.

A second type of manual provides information about hospital routines such as admission procedures, visiting hours, and special facilities such as the recovery room. The guide may also include suggestions about how the patient and his visitors can help to facilitate the recovery of the patient as well as what they can expect from the hospital personnel. It may be given to the patient before admission by the physician or at the time he is admitted. Any material preparing the patient for what to expect and for what is expected of him should be helpful. In addition to well-prepared written explanations, the patient needs oral instruction as to what to expect. Admission to the hospital is accompanied by emotional stress and, at the time, the patient is likely to be more or less confused. Some attention should be given to the family of the patient. Relatives should know the time the patient is expected to be taken to the operating room and whether or not he is expected to return to his room immediately after his operation or will be cared for in a recovery room or an intensive-care unit. For example, a patient may remain in a recovery room only until he has regained consciousness and major physiological derangements have been corrected, or he may stay in an intensive-care unit for 24 to 48 or more hours. Whatever the practice is, the patient and his family should be prepared for what to expect. They should know that the recovery room or intensive-care unit is a service provided for the welfare of the patient.

The psychological status of the patient is an important factor in his capacity to withstand the stress imposed by surgery. How the patient regards the surgical procedure that is to be performed, as well as its possible effects, influences his chances for survival and for recovery. The nurse may be helpful to the patient and to his family by providing a climate in which the patient feels free to express his feelings and in which he feels accepted and esteemed as an individual human being. She can also be helpful to the patient by relaying any concerns that he has to the physician, so that the physician can more accurately assess the psychological status of the patient and plan to correct his misconceptions and misinformation. To paraphrase Fielding (see Chapter 3), when fears are hidden, they grow until they become overwhelming, but when they are taken out and examined, they can be put into their true perspective and confined.

Physiological Status

Just as surgical therapy places a strain on the capacity of the patient to maintain emotional homeostasis, it also places a burden on his capacity to maintain physiological homeostasis. An important aspect of making the patient safe for surgical therapy is, therefore, the evaluation of his physiological status as a basis for prevention or correction of any abnormalities. The investigation includes (1) an evaluation of all homeostatic conditions with particular emphasis on his nutritional state, (2) the identification of any diseases or disorders that increase the risk of surgical therapy, and (3) an estimation of the capacity of the patient to tolerate additional stress and to respond favorably. All the preceding are interrelated.

AGE

Because there is a relationship between age and the capacity of the individual to maintain physiological homeostasis under stress, the age of the patient has some bearing on the risks to which he is exposed during surgical therapy. Very young children tolerate the trauma of surgery remarkably well and recover quickly. They are, however, easily upset, and they are particularly sensitive to chilling, exposure, and rough handling. Gius [6] states that the loss of an ounce of blood by an infant may be equivalent to the loss of a pint of blood by an adult. The infant should therefore be closely observed for evidence of blood loss, because seemingly small losses represent a relatively large part of his blood volume. He must also be protected from conditions in the environment predisposing to chilling. These include a low environmental temperature, drafts, and wet clothing. With proper care, an infant survives surgical therapy very well.

At the other end of the life-span, the elderly patient has generally been believed to tolerate surgical therapy poorly. Although modern surgical management has greatly reduced the hazards of surgery to the elderly patient, some surgeons have known for many years that old age, by itself, is not a contraindication to surgical therapy. One surgeon who is frequently quoted on this point is Sir James Paget.[7] He wrote

Years, indeed, taken alone are a very fallacious mode of reckoning age: it is not the time but the quantity of a man's past life that we have to reckon. . . . The old people that are thin and dry and tough, clear-voiced and bright-eyed, with good stomachs and strong wills, muscular and active, are not bad; they bear all but the largest operations very well. But very bad are they, who, looking somewhat like these, are feeble and soft-skinned, with little pulses, bad appetites, and weak digestive powers; so that they cannot in an emergency be well nourished.

Moyer,[8] in a summary of a review of the literature on the influence of age on operative mortality, concludes that (1) the operative mortality is higher among the aged in disorders accompanied by pus formation or other complications such as perforation of a viscus, (2) the operative mortality rate is the same for all groups in disorders that are seldom accompanied by complications, and (3) the death rate from burns is higher among the aged than among younger persons.

In more general terms, the elderly person's capacity to respond to the stress of a single surgical procedure of short duration is satisfac-

tory, but he is less able to tolerate prolonged stress and multiple stresses than are younger persons. The elderly person is less able to tolerate disorders accompanied by prolonged physiological disturbances. Because he has less reserve than the younger person the old person's capacity to maintain and to restore homeostasis in the presence of continued strain is less than that of a younger person. He is more likely to have one or more chronic diseases that decrease his reserve or place a burden on his capacity to adapt. When the strain placed on his adaptive capacity is within his reserve, he responds favorably. As in the care of the very young, attention should be given to preventing unnecessary demands on the adaptive capacity of the elderly person.

When planning and implementing the nursing care of the elderly patient, the nurse should be mindful of the fact that as people age, their renal, cardiovascular, and pulmonary reserves diminish. As a consequence, these structures are less able to cope with conditions placing stress on their functional capacity, and they are more likely to be sites of complication than they are in young persons. Among the elderly, the exact chronological age of the patient is of less significance than his outlook and physiological status. A hopeful, optimistic attitude combined with a good nutritional status and reasonable cardiovascular, renal, and pulmonary reserve makes an elderly person quite safe for surgery.

Any disorder that reduces the capacity of the individual to adapt and to maintain homeostatic conditions increases the risk of surgery. Among the many disorders increasing risk are shock; hemorrhage; disorders in water and electrolyte balance; acidosis and alkalosis; anemia; pulmonary, cardiac, and renal disorders; undernutrition; hypoproteinemia; obesity; adrenal insufficiency; alcoholism; hyperthyroidism; diabetes mellitus; disease of the liver; and psychic and emotional disturbances. All these disorders lessen, in some manner, the capacity of the individual to maintain homeostasis. Some, such as disturbances in water and electrolyte balance, indicate impairment of one or more homeostatic conditions. Most of the disturbances increasing surgical risk are discussed elsewhere. The comments that follow will be limited to the relationship of a few of the preceding to surgical risk. When the life of the patient is not immediately threatened, surgical treatment is usually delayed until the physiological and psychological condition of the patient is improved as nearly as possible to the optimum condition. In the investigation of the patient, the surgeon is interested in uncovering any condition that will either make the development of a compli-

[6] John Armes Gius: *Fundamentals of General Surgery,* 3rd ed. (Chicago: Year Book Medical Publishers, Inc., 1966), p. 272.

[7] Sir James Paget: *Clinical Lectures and Essays* (London: Longmans, Green & Co., Ltd., 1877) quoted in U. H. Eversole: "The Anesthetic Management of the Elderly Patient," *Surg. Clin. N. Amer.,* 34:622 (June) 1954.

[8] Carl A. Moyer: "The Assessment of Operative Risk," *Surgery: Principles and Practice,* 3rd ed. (C. A. Moyer *et al.,* eds.) (Philadelphia: J. B. Lippincott Company, 1965), pp. 220–22.

cation more likely or reduce the capacity of the person to adapt to stress.

NUTRITION

Among the important factors influencing response to surgery is the nutritional state of the patient. Because the various factors in nutrition have been covered in Chapter 12 they will not be reviewed here. Among the nutritional factors that are of greatest significance to the surgical patient are undernutrition, with or without hypoproteinemia, and obesity. Adequate nutrition is essential to the general response of the patient and to wound healing. The nutritional elements that are of the most importance in wound healing are protein and vitamins B and C.

Of the patients who are treated surgically, some are more likely to be undernourished than others. Chronically ill and aged persons are more likely to be malnourished than are previously healthy children and adults. Persons who have disturbances in the functioning of the alimentary tract are predisposed to malnutrition. These disturbances result from failure to either ingest, absorb, or retain food in the alimentary canal long enough for it to be digested and absorbed. The patient who has had a chronic loss of protein-containing body fluids, including blood, is likely to suffer from hypoproteinemia. One often neglected aspect relating to nutrition is the effect of diagnostic examinations that require the withholding of food and purging. For example, examinations of the alimentary canal are usually preceded by withholding of food and fluids, sometimes for an extended period of time. This may create serious problems in the already dehydrated and undernourished patient. Unless contraindicated, food and fluids should be served at the completion of a diagnostic test. Between meal and bedtime snacks can be added to increase the patient's intake. If the patient is losing excessive amounts of fluid or is not taking in proper amounts of food or liquids, the physician should be notified so that he may order supplemental feedings of intravenous fluids. All these measures require a thoughtful concern for the welfare of the patient and appropriate planning. All the measures suggested in Chapter 12 may be required to improve the nutritional status of the patient sufficiently to make him safe for surgery.

Some disorders that are associated with undernutrition are also responsible for the loss of water and electrolytes. In addition to insufficient water and/or electrolytes, water may accumulate in body cavities or in the interstitial spaces in the form of edema. Because water and electrolyte balance is treated in another chapter, it will not be further discussed other than to say that it is a significant factor in surgical risk.

OBESITY

Obesity is also a problem in many patients. Because it cannot be corrected quickly, excessively obese patients should be placed on a weight-reduction regimen and whenever possible surgery delayed until the patient reaches a satisfactory weight. Obesity burdens the patient with a number of handicaps. Because fat has a poor blood supply, these patients are more susceptible to infection. Fat is more difficult to approximate than other tissues. Large amounts of fat also increase the difficulty of exposing organs in the abdominal cavity and may reduce the pulmonary vital capacity by pressure on the diaphragm. The problems associated with weight reduction have been presented in Chapter 12.

PULMONARY STATUS

Because conditions in the lung and tracheobronchial tree affect and are affected by the response of the patient to anesthesia, unconsciousness, and bed rest, correcting or minimizing the effects of abnormalities in these structures is imperative. X-ray examination of the chest is an essential part of the assessment of the status of the respiratory system. It is useful in detecting tuberculosis and emphysema as well as many other disorders of the lung that may not be found during a routine history and physical examination. Among the disorders that aggravate the problem of cleansing the airway in the immediate postoperative period are tracheobronchitis and emphysema. Tracheobronchitis is more common in persons who smoke than in nonsmokers. When tracheobronchitis is present and the person smokes, he should be encouraged to stop or reduce the amount he smokes. Smoking definitely increases the likelihood of respiratory difficulty during and after any type of surgery.

The patient who has a large accumulation of secretions in the tracheobronchial tree may be instructed to perform postural drainage. This has been described in Chapter 8. The patient who has a disorder that makes keeping the tracheobronchial tree clean more difficult will require more attention to this function in the immediate postoperative period than the patient who has no such disorder.

CARDIOVASCULAR STATUS

In the evaluation of the cardiovascular system, the condition and reserve capacity of the heart and blood vessels are investigated. When there is evidence of pathology, the physician then tries to estimate the adequacy of the cardiac reserve; this helps him to determine if the patient will be able to tolerate the strain of surgery. Contrary to popular opinion, the patient may have considerable cardiovascular pathology and the heart may still be able to tolerate certain surgical procedures with little or no difficulty.

In the evaluation of the state of the blood vessels, two factors are reviewed. One is the capacity of the body to adapt the diameter of the blood vessels to the changing needs of the organism. The other is the adequacy of the blood supply to the tissues that will be operated on. The level of the blood pressure of the patient provides information about the first factor. In a patient with a blood pressure below 90 systolic or above 120 diastolic, the capacity to adapt to the stress of surgery is likely to be inadequate or greatly diminished. The patient with an excessively low systolic blood pressure may be suffering from a variety of fluid and electrolyte problems, cardiovascular disease, or adrenal insufficiency. The patient with the high diastolic pressure is especially likely to develop or already have significant impairment of renal function. Because healing is dependent on the adequacy of the blood supply, an estimation of the capacity of the heart and blood vessels to deliver sufficient blood to the tissues is essential. Pallor and coldness of extremities and blanching on pressure with slow return of color are indications that the amount of blood being delivered to the tissue is greatly reduced.

The capacity of the circulatory system to deliver adequate amounts of oxygen, glucose, and other metabolic necessities to the tissue depends not only on the competence of the heart as a pump and the adaptability and patency of the blood vessels but on the quantity and quality of the blood. After an acute hemorrhage both the quality and quantity of the blood may be diminished. With long-standing nutritional deficiencies or chronic loss of blood, the quality of blood may be poor. The most commonly used measures of the quantity of blood in relation to the size of the vascular system are blood pressure, pulse, and central venous pressure. Blood volume determinations may also be of value. The quality of the blood in relation to its red cell content may be measured by either the hematocrit or the hemoglobin content, or both. A reduction of either indicates a decrease in the oxygen-carrying capacity of the blood. Because the adequacy of the oxygen-carrying power of the blood and the blood volume both directly affect the chances of the patient for survival, surgery is seldom sched-

uled until arrangements have been made to replace needed blood. If the surgical procedure is one entailing a large loss of blood, additional blood may be required to replace that which is lost at the time of the operation.

RENAL FUNCTION

In any condition in which the body is placed under increased physiological stress, the capacity of the kidney to function is of great significance. It functions in homeostasis to eliminate or conserve water and electrolytes and it eliminates the wastes of protein metabolism. In the absence of evidence to indicate that the kidney reserve is limited or that the kidney is diseased, the urine is tested for sugar, acetone, and albumin. The presence of sugar and acetone in the urine are not tests of kidney function but they are important because they may indicate that the patient has diabetes mellitus. Albumin in the urine usually indicates the presence of kidney disease or some condition that limits its blood flow. In a woman, albuminuria may not be significant unless the urine specimen is obtained by catheter. To estimate the adequacy of kidney function, the level of the creatinine, urea, or nonprotein nitrogen in the blood is determined. Other tests of kidney function include the capacity of the kidney to concentrate phenolsulfonphthalein in the urine or to increase its specific gravity when water is withheld.

Evaluation of renal function is important not only because it influences operative risk but because it affects the capacity of the patient to handle the parenteral fluid and electrolytes administered during the postoperative period. Although output should be compared with intake in all patients, these measurements are especially important in patients with renal disease.

What are some of the important activities the nurse may undertake to prepare the patient for surgery?

AMBULATION

During the preoperative period, disorders affecting operative risk are identified and treated so that their effect can be minimized. In addition to corrective therapy, attention is paid to preventive care, one aspect of which is ambulation. Attention to ambulation is most important for the patient who is admitted to the hospital for diagnosis and preparation for surgery. Patients who remain at home during the period are less likely to be able to remain in bed. Although the patient was once kept in bed because it was thought that rest conserved strength, studies indicate that bed rest results in a loss of strength as well as of proteins and other nutrients. Exercise within the limits tolerated by the patient improves his psychological as well as his physiological status. When the patient feels unwell, he may have to be encouraged to be up and about; on the other hand, the patient who feels reasonably well may require some protection from overactivity. The patient should have the help that he needs to get out of bed and to walk. To make certain that he does ambulate, there should be a plan to ensure it. Because most people eat better when they are out of bed the plan may include getting the patient into the chair for his meals. Depending on how the patient feels, he may then have a rest period followed by a bath and then another rest period followed by a walk down the hall. When he is in bed, he should be encouraged to do deep-breathing exercises and to flex and extend his feet and legs. By alternating periods of activity with rest, the patient builds up his strength and is at the same time protected from overactivity.

PREPARATION OF THE GASTROINTESTINAL TRACT

In addition to the general psychological and physiological preparation, which may take several days or longer, the gastrointestinal tract and the skin are prepared one or two days preceding surgery. Regardless of whether the gastrointestinal tract is directly involved, preparation of the patient for surgery often includes emptying this tract. Food and fluids are withheld and the lower bowel is emptied by the administration of one or more enemas. Preparation for colon surgery may involve several enemas and laxatives for three or more days. Intravenous fluids may also have to be given to elderly patients, especially if there is any evidence of dehydration or hypovolemia.

In the past, to make sure that the stomach was empty at the time of surgery, food and fluids were withheld from midnight until the surgery was performed the following day. Many surgeons have modified this procedure in terms of the time it takes the stomach to empty, for prolonged abstinence from food and fluids is of no general value and increases the likelihood of dehydration. Unless there is an obstruction, food usually remains in the stomach six hours or less. Liquids leave the stomach even quicker. In fact, liquids may pass immediately from the esophagus to the duodenum. To make sure that the stomach is empty, food intake is restricted for at least eight to ten hours, and fluids are prohibited for four or more hours before surgery. The nerv-

ous adult or older child may have food sit in his stomach for many hours. This is less likely to occur in infants and children, and fluids should be restricted in the latter as little as possible. An empty stomach is important, because it reduces the likelihood of the patient's vomiting and aspirating gastric juice into the lung; when gastric juice is inhaled, it produces a very serious type of pneumonitis. However, dehydration of the patient is not necessary to prevent aspiration.

In preparation for many major abdominal operations such as gastric surgery, a nasogastric tube may be used to empty the stomach. When the patient has an obstruction of the intestinal tract, decompression of the bowel may be necessary before he can be operated on with safety. The cause and effects of obstruction of the alimentary canal are presented in Chapter 12. Gastric or intestinal intubation with suction often is employed during the postoperative phase of surgery to reduce vomiting and gastric or intestinal dilatation from swallowing air. Gastrointestinal activity is often greatly reduced or even paralyzed (ileus) after surgery, especially if the stomach, intestines, or colon was involved. Failure to keep this inactive bowel decompressed may result in distention of the abdomen with increased stress on the abdominal incision or impairment of respiration. The bowel that is extremely distended also tends to remain paralyzed for longer periods of time.

Decompression is accomplished by the introduction into the stomach or intestine of a tube to which suction is applied. Removal of fluids and gas from the stomach can be accomplished by a single-lumen Levin tube. Removal of the contents from the jejunum or ileum requires a long intestinal tube with either a single or double lumen. A bag or balloon is often added to the end of the tube to facilitate its movement after it enters the duodenum. When a single-lumen tube is used, a bag filled with mercury is attached to the tip before it is inserted. When a double-lumen tube is used, one lumen opens into a balloon that is distended with water, air, or mercury; the other lumen provides for the removal of fluid and gas. Either type of tube is passed through a nostril, the pharynx, and the esophagus into the stomach. After the short tube (Levin) reaches the stomach, it is taped to the face. No tube should be taped to the nose and above the eye, because when the tube is taped in this position it presses on the underside of the nostril and may cause pressure necrosis. It should either be taped to the upper lip or anchored in the position that it takes naturally. See Figures 17-1, 17-2, and 17-3.

FIGURE 17-1. This technique for anchoring nasal tubes with tape should not be used because it will soon produce pressure necrosis on the underside of the nostril.

The long tube is passed from the stomach through the pylorus and into the duodenum. The passage of the tube through the pylorus may be facilitated by having the patient lie on his right side. After the tube enters the duodenum, the physician inflates the balloon; peristalsis, if present, may carry the balloon and tube through the intestine. To hasten the movement of the tube toward the site of the obstruction, the physician may leave an order for the nurse to advance the tube a specific distance at regular intervals of time. If the patient is able, he can assist in this by swallowing as the tube is pushed forward. The act of swallowing also helps to suppress the gag reflex. During the procedure the physician can check the location of the tube by x-ray or by fluoroscopic examination. When the tube reaches the desired site, it is then taped in the manner previously described.

After either the short or long tube has reached the stomach, suction is applied. There are a number of methods for producing suction. The method that is selected depends on the wishes of the physician and the equipment provided by the hospital.[9] Whatever method is utilized to secure suction, the force should be

⁹ For students who wish an extensive review of intubation and drainage of the alimentary canal, see Bertha Harmer and Virginia Henderson: *Textbook of the Principles and Practice of Nursing*, 5th ed. (New York: The Macmillan Company, 1955), pp. 823–39.

gentle, usually not in excess of 1.5 lb of negative pressure. When excessive suction is applied, the mucosa lining the intestine or stomach may be sucked into the opening in the tube, damaging the mucosa and occluding the tube. The injury to the mucosa is similar to that induced in the mucosa lining of the trachea and bronchi by excessive suction. To secure suction, the system must be airtight and the device should be checked at intervals to be sure that it is working. However, because secretion is not constant, fluid does not flow continuously from the tube. Should there be doubt as to whether or not the system is operating, the tube leading to the stomach can be irrigated with a small amount of saline. If fluid returns when the apparatus is connected, then it is operating satisfactorily. Frequent irrigations of the tube or the use of large amounts of water should be avoided, as water and electrolytes required by the body are removed in the process. However, gastrointestinal secretions contain solid particles that may accumulate and obstruct the tube. The tube should, therefore, be irrigated at regular intervals and frequently enough to keep it patent. Occasionally when a tube is irrigated, the fluid runs in, but an obstruction to its return acts as a ball valve. In this event the fluid intro-

FIGURE 17-2. A suggested technique for anchoring nasal tubes with tape. When this technique is used, adherence of the tape must be checked frequently; when the patient perspires, the upper lip becomes moist, and the tape is dislodged.

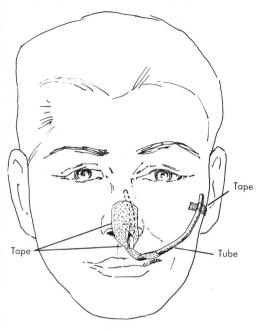

FIGURE 17-3. A suggested technique for anchoring nasal tubes with tape. When this technique is used, adherence of the tape to the nose must be checked frequently. Perspiration and skin oils cause the tape to loosen. The tape is split half its length, and the split ends are wrapped securely in opposite directions around the tube after the broad end has been taped to the nose. The free end of the tube can then be taped over the zygomatic arch or secured to the clothing of the patient to prevent pulling on the tube.

duced into the stomach contributes to further distention of the stomach. Sometimes the obstruction of the tube can be eliminated by changing the position of the patient or the tube. If this does not relieve the obstruction, the physician should be notified. To prevent the loss of fluids and electrolytes, some surgeons prescribe the use of air to check the patency of the tube. Smaller amounts of air can be introduced, and thus distention avoided. If one places a stethoscope just below the xiphoid process and listens, he will hear the muffled "woosh" that accompanies the passage of air through a patent gastric tube. The amount of air required varies with the length and diameter of the tube; with a Levin tube, for example, 15 to 25 ml are usually adequate.

When the outlet of the stomach is obstructed, a large tube with multiple openings may be required to remove the food particles and other debris that accumulate. Cleansing of the stom-

ach may be furthered by pouring water or saline into the tube and then sucking out the fluid. The procedure is repeated until the solution that returns is clear. Because of the size of the tube, it is passed through the mouth and is removed at the completion of the procedure.

PREPARATION FOR GASTROINTESTINAL INTUBATION

Gastrointestinal intubation often causes some psychological stress in the patient. Many patients regard this as one of the most disagreeable aspects of the entire hospital or operative experience. Mrs. Repeat illustrates this point very well. Two years ago, she had abdominal surgery. She says, "The thing that I dread the most is having all those tubes. Worst of all is that tube they put into my stomach." When gastric intubation is a part of a patient's preoperative preparation, he should be helped to understand how intubation contributes to his recovery. He should also understand how the tube is passed and what he can do to help and what will be done to assist him. He should know that the tube will be lubricated to make it pass more easily. He should also know that he will be able to help by swallowing as the tube is passed and that he will be reminded to swallow at the appropriate times. The patient who has had the symptoms of obstruction may welcome the relief that the introduction of the tube brings.

Although the physician usually passes the tube, the nurse may be required to learn to do it. Before the nurse does this, she should prepare herself by studying the anatomy of the area and acquaint herself with the possible difficulties she may encounter. In addition to preparing the patient for what to expect and for what is expected of him, she also prepares the patient physically. The patient may be in either the recumbent or the sitting position. In either event, the head should be hyperextended until the tube is in the esophagus. The head may then be lowered in order to facilitate swallowing of water. Because the patient is likely to gag and may vomit and secretions are increased, a supply of paper tissues and an emesis basin should be within easy reach. The required equipment and supplies should be at hand and in working order before the procedure is started. Thorough lubrication of the tube makes for ease in passing it. If oil is used, any excess should be removed to decrease the danger of aspiration of oil into the lungs. Because of this possibility, some physicians prefer to use glycerine or a water-soluble substance to lubricate the tube. As the tube is passed the patient should be reminded at appropriate intervals to swallow. Some patients find swallowing easier if they are allowed sips of water as the tube is passed. Patients should be kept appraised of the success of their efforts and they should know when the tube reaches the stomach. The nurse should be mindful of the fact that it is difficult to pass a tube through the upper alimentary canal without the cooperation of the patient who is conscious. The patient should know what his role is and be helped to carry it out.

The mouth of the patient with gastric or intestinal decompression requires the same or more care than that of a patient who is not taking food and fluid by mouth. The patient should have an opportunity to brush his teeth and rinse his mouth with mouthwash three or four times a day. Mouthwash, if not overused, is refreshing. Too frequent rinsing of the mouth contributes to dehydration by loss of saliva. The flow of saliva may be stimulated by encouraging the patient to chew gum or to suck lemon or orange slices or sour lemon balls. The saliva helps to keep the mouth moist and clean. It also washes out the ducts leading from the parotid gland and decreases the possibility of surgical parotitis. Free drainage from any gland is essential to its health. Blocking of the duct from a gland favors the development of infection in the gland. After the mouth has been cleansed, the tongue and other mucosa may be coated with a milk of magnesia substrate. If the patient is unable to perform his own oral hygiene, a half-strength solution of hydrogen peroxide (3 per cent) should be applied to all surfaces of the tongue, teeth, mucosa, and palate every four hours. The foam is promptly removed and the mouth should be rinsed with water.[10]

When the tube is left in place for some days, the throat may be irritated by it. The patient may be allowed sips of water or anesthetic troches to relieve the soreness. When he is allowed water, attention should be given to limiting the amount of water taken to that prescribed by the physician. Any water that is taken returns through the tube, bringing with it electrolytes that are secreted into the stomach. The relief that the patient obtains is therefore at the expense of his body's electrolytes. Some surgeons remove the tube after two or three days and allow the patient to have a period of rest. The tube is then reinserted 12 or 18 hours later if the patient continues to require it. After the tube has been removed, the nurse should observe the patient for signs and symptoms that indicate that the gastrointestinal tract is not

functioning. These include distention, a feeling of fullness, nausea, or vomiting. The sensation of fullness is often the earliest symptom to indicate that the stomach is not emptying properly and along with any other symptoms should be reported promptly. To detect developing distention the abdomen may be measured with a tape. One way to test the function of the alimentary canal without removing the tube is by clamping it for a period of time. When the tube is clamped, the patient should be checked for the symptoms listed. Later the tube is unclamped, and the amount of fluid escaping from the tube is measured. Any accumulation of fluid indicates that gastrointestinal function has not yet been restored.

Because the nostril through which the tube is passed may be irritated by the tube, it may be passed through the opposite nostril when it has to be reintroduced. However, sometimes structural abnormalities make it difficult if not impossible to use the other nostril. Tubes in the nose and pharynx stimulate increased local secretions which may be aspirated or interfere with ventilation. This must be seriously considered in patients with any pulmonary difficulty or complications.

As long as the tube is in place, the nurse should observe the amount and character of fluid that is returned through it. Any abnormality of color or odor is important. Because the effectiveness of the procedure depends on the equipment being in working order, the nurse must check at regular intervals to make sure that the system is airtight and operating.

As peristalsis resumes or the obstruction is relieved, the surgeon removes the tube or clamps it. The removal of a tube from the stomach is relatively simple. The removal of the long tube is more complicated. If the tube has passed the ileocecal valve, the surgeon may cut the tube and allow it to progress through the gastrointestinal tract, as the forcible return of the tube and balloon through the valve may damage it. The tube should not be released at the nose until it has been secured below. Otherwise a laparotomy may be required to retrieve the tube. The patient may need to be reassured that the tube will progress through the alimentary canal just as the normal contents do. When the tube is returned through the mouth, the doctor pulls gently and allows the intestine time to release its attachment to the tube.

When gastrointestinal fluids and electrolytes are removed by suction, the oral fluid intake of the patient is restricted and fluids must be administered by intravenous infusion. To have a basis for determining the adequacy of the fluid intake of the patient, his urine output and the

[10] Joyce Y. Passos and Lucy M. Brand: "Effects of Agents Used for Oral Hygiene," *Nurs. Res.,* **15**:196–202 (Summer) 1966.

other fluids should be measured accurately as long as the gastric or intestinal tube is in place.

PREPARATION OF THE LOWER ALIMENTARY TRACT

In addition to the preparation of the upper alimentary canal for surgery, the colon and rectum are often emptied by the administration of one or more enemas. The reason generally advanced is that this practice lessens the possibility of soiling the peritoneal cavity if the bowel is entered during surgery; there also may be less difficulty with constipation postoperatively. Not all surgeons, however, agree that enemas are either necessary or desirable. Harbison [11] condemns the routine practice of giving an enema in the preoperative preparation of patients. He states that because most people defecate early in the day, an enema is unphysiological and it also subjects most people to unnecessary psychological stress. When the intestine itself is the site of surgery, it is cleansed to lessen the likelihood of spillage of fecal contents into the peritoneal cavity. In surgical procedures involving organs in the pelvic cavity, an empty bowel is essential to the exposure of the operative site and to its protection from injury. When barium studies have been made of the gastrointestinal tract, the barium should be removed by enemas or laxatives, if necessary, in order to prevent it from forming an impaction postoperatively. In some disorders such as acute appendicitis, enemas are contraindicated; the fluid introduced into the intestine can raise the pressure within the intestine and stimulate peristalsis. When the solution contains soap or some other irritating agent, peristalsis is further intensified, and the danger of perforation of the appendix is increased.

In surgery on the large intestine, prevention of contamination of the wound and the peritoneal and pelvic cavities by feces requires that special measures be taken to lessen the volume of feces. Bacteria are responsible for more than half the weight of the dried stool. These organisms are harmless and may even be helpful as long as they remain in the intestine. However, when they escape into the peritoneal or other body cavities, they may cause serious morbidity. By using antibiotics and chemical antiseptics that are not absorbed from the intestine, the bacterial count in the intestine can be greatly reduced. Many physicians do not use these nonabsorbable antibiotics because of the chance of developing superinfections. Most surgeons, however, agree that the colon should be cleansed mechanically if the surgery will involve the left side of the colon.

[11] Samuel P. Harbison: "Unnecessary Routine Orders," *JAMA,* **152**:396 (May 30) 1953.

PREPARATION OF THE SKIN

An important aspect of the immediate preparation of the patient for surgery is the thorough cleansing of the skin. Both the skin and mucous membranes have large numbers of bacteria on their surfaces. These organisms are usually harmless unless they are provided with a portal of entry, such as a break in the skin. Despite differences in details or routines, the objective toward which the preparation of the skin is directed is to reduce the number of microorganisms on it to a minimum and at the same time protect it from injury. The skin must be thoroughly cleansed but not broken or damaged in the process. In some hospitals, patients who are able to do it are asked to shower or take a tub bath, and those who are not able to are given a bed bath. In other hospitals, only those patients whose skins can be seen to be dirty are bathed. When showering or bathing is part of the preoperative preparation, the patient should understand that this requirement is not a reflection on his standard of cleanliness or hygiene. When a sudsing agent containing a germicide is employed, the germicide must have time to act. Varco [12] suggests that part of the skin preparation should be repeated sudsing of the skin with an agent containing hexachlorophene. The suds should be left on the skin for at least five to ten minutes. He [13] also states that, in theory, the skin should not be shaved the day or evening before the operation is scheduled, because if the skin is broken, bacteria have an opportunity to enter the lesion and to multiply. If the incision crosses the area where bacteria have entered the tissue, they may be carried deep into the wound.

Whether or not the entire body is showered or bathed, the region surrounding the site of the surgery should undergo special cleansing to remove microorganisms and materials that may harbor microorganisms. Two procedures, washing with a sudsing detergent and shaving, are usual. When cationic surface-active agents such as benzalkonium chloride solution (Zephiran Chloride) [14] are employed in preparation of the skin, soap should not be used as the lathering agent previous to the operation. Because soap is anionic [15] it antagonizes the action of the cationic agents. Care should be taken to remove

[12] Richard L. Varco: "Principles of Preoperative and Postoperative Care," *Christopher's Textbook of Surgery,* 9th ed., Loyal Davis, ed. (Philadelphia: W. B. Saunders Company, 1968), p. 184.
[13] *Ibid.,* p. 185.
[14] Trade name.
[15] Don W. Esplin: "Antiseptics and Disinfectants, Fungicides, Ectoparasiticides," *Pharmacological Basis of Therapeutics,* 3rd ed., Louis S. Goodman and Alfred Gilman, eds. (New York: The Macmillan Company, 1965), p. 1042.

all the hair and to avoid nicking the skin. The size of the area to be shaved depends on the nature of the proposed surgical procedure and the directions of the surgeon. Crile and Shively [16] state that pubic hair should be shaved only when necessary. The discomfort suffered by the patient as the hair grows outweighs any advantage of its removal. For this reason some surgeons do not require the pubic hair to be shaved preceding a dilatation of the cervix and curettage of the uterus. Harbison [17] states that larger areas are often shaved more than is necessary. He agrees that the pubic hair does not require removal previous to abdominal surgery. Eyebrows should not be removed. Although Harbison blames outdated nursing texts for extensive skin preparation, some surgeons are of the opinion that it is necessary. Because some questions have been raised about the validity of some of these routine practices in preoperative preparation, nurses and physicians should examine what they do more carefully in terms of its value and effects.

Because of the serious nature of bone infections, some orthopedic surgeons order that the skin be specially prepared. The skin is shaved and then washed with a detergent and covered with sterile towels; this washing may be repeated twice daily for several days. Particular attention should be given to preventing nicks in the skin. The towels should be anchored so that they stay in place and the equipment and materials used should be sterile. Attention should be closely paid to all principles involved in the maintenance of asepsis.

Preparation of the scalp for a surgical incision also requires some modification of the ordinary procedure. Before the hair can be cut and the scalp shaved, a permit from the patient or a responsible member of the family is usually required. As a rule, arrangements are made to have a barber cut the hair and shave the scalp. Particularly for women, the removal of the hair is a source of considerable psychological stress. Members of the family, such as the husband or mother, may also be understandably distressed. For a not inconsiderable number of women, their hair is truly their crowning glory. Before the hair is removed, the nurse should make sure that the patient is not facing a mirror and that a head scarf or cap is ready to cover the head as soon as it is shaved. Some hospitals provide wigs for female patients. The hair should be placed in a paper bag and given to a relative. When a woman or girl has long hair, she may want to have a headpiece made from

it. Headpieces and fancy caps are now available to disguise the head and should be used whenever possible.

SEDATION BEFORE SURGERY

To ensure that the patient sleeps well and to reduce apprehension, the surgeon usually prescribes a sedative for the patient the night preceding and the morning of surgery. The specific drug selected varies with the surgeon but is often one of the barbiturates such as pentobarbital (Nembutal), 0.05 to 0.1 g, or secobarbital (Seconal), 0.1 to 0.2 g. Occasionally this has to be repeated later in the night. When the patient has been prepared for sleep, he should know whether or not the nurse expects to visit him during the night. Nothing can be more frightening to a person who sleeps in a room by himself at home than to go to sleep and to be awakened by someone opening the door and coming into the room. For example, Miss Tee was admitted to the hospital in the late afternoon for diagnostic surgery the following day. About 9 o'clock in the evening she was given secobarbital (Seconal), 0.2 g, and prepared to sleep. The door to her room was closed. At midnight an aide opened the door and entered her room to remove the water glass. Miss Tee awakened frightened, and, needless to say, she had difficulty returning to sleep.

The morning of surgery the same drug that was administered the preceding night may be repeated. In addition, morphine, 8 to 15 mg, or meperidine hydrochloride (Demerol), 50 to 100 mg, may be administered an hour before the operation is scheduled. Currently, there appears to be disagreement among physicians about the necessity and desirability of using either morphine or meperidine hydrochloride preoperatively. Some surgeons are of the opinion that they serve no useful purpose because, previous to the operation, patients do not have pain and the barbiturates are at least as effective as morphine in relieving preoperative apprehension. In addition, these drugs may have some undesirable effects. In some patients, they cause nausea and vomiting. They can also depress respiration, the cough reflex, and the activity of cilia in the tracheobronchial tree because they can increase the tone of the tracheobronchial musculature. In man, they can be harmful in the patient who is asthmatic. All these effects decrease the capacity of the patient to cleanse the tracheobronchial tree and aerate the lung. The influence of morphine on mechanisms for cleansing the tracheobronchial tree is particularly undesirable in patients having thoracic and upper abdominal surgery.

Certain disorders or circumstances alter or

[16] George Crile, Jr., and Franklin L. Shively, Jr.: *Hospital Care of the Surgical Patient,* 2nd ed. (Springfield, Ill.: Charles C Thomas, Publisher, 1946), p. 125.
[17] *Op. cit.,* p. 397.

increase the patient's response to morphine. For example, the patient with hypothyroidism often becomes stuporous and suffers respiratory depression following relatively small doses of morphine. Infants and children can usually tolerate morphine quite well if the dosage is adjusted to their body weight. In contrast, there is evidence that elderly persons may be extremely sensitive. Because morphine depresses the respiratory center and increases the cerebrospinal fluid pressure, it is contraindicated in patients who are undergoing brain surgery or who have had surgery on the brain; in such patients it is contraindicated after, as well as before, the operation.

To further reduce anxiety of the patient toward his surgery and to counteract the tendency toward increased tracheobronchial secretions, atropine sulfate or scopolamine hydrobromide is frequently prescribed to be administered to the patient about one hour before the operation is scheduled. When the tranquilizing effects are desired, scopolamine is more likely to be selected than atropine because of its increased tendency to cause drowsiness, amnesia, euphoria, and fatigue. Occasionally it produces excitement, talkativeness, restlessness, and even delirium and hallucinations. The patient who is given scopolamine when he is in pain is more likely to respond with excitement than if given it when he is free of pain. The nurse should anticipate this possibility when a patient who is in pain is given scopolamine. The more important action of both atropine and scopolamine is the depression of the effector cells of organs enervated by postganglionic cholinergic fibers with a resultant decrease in secretions in the tracheobronchial tree. Because one of the actions of these drugs is dilation of the pupil, these anticholinergic drugs are contraindicated in patients who have glaucoma.

What are the responsibilities of the nurse in the immediate preoperative period?

In most hospitals the patient or a responsible relative signs a permit for the patient to undergo the contemplated surgery. The nature of the operation and its risks should be explained prior to the signing of the permit. This should generally be done the day prior to surgery; moreover, the patient should sign it before he receives his preoperative medication. Practice varies as to whether the nurse or the physician secures the signature of the patient. Even when the physician is responsible, the nurse should ascertain whether or not the permit has been signed before administering the preoperative medication.

To prevent distention and possible injury to the urinary bladder during the operative period, the urinary bladder should be emptied just before the patient is transferred to the operating room. To facilitate exposure of pelvic organs and to reduce the possibility of injury to the bladder during surgical procedures in the pelvic cavity, an indwelling catheter is usually introduced prior to surgery in this region.

Because of the danger of aspiration into the airway of dentures or removable bridges, they should be removed before the patient is transferred to the operating pavilion. Occasionally a patient has very strong feelings about having others see him without his teeth. In rare instances, when the psychological stress created by removing dental prostheses is very great, the nurse should explore the possibility of the patient keeping them in place until he arrives in the operating room. They can then be removed and returned to the patient's room or ward. Care should be taken to prevent the loss of dentures. Their loss or damage subjects the patient to inconvenience and psychological stress and may be an added expense to the hospital and patient.

If the patient does not already wear some form of identification such as an identification bracelet, an identification tag should be prepared and attached to him before he is transferred to the operating room. On it should be his full name, his hospital number, the name of the surgeon, and any other pertinent information. The chart of the patient should be complete. The following should be included: (1) morning temperature, pulse, and respiration; (2) results of the blood tests, hematocrit or hemoglobin, and urinalysis; (3) drugs that were administered preoperatively; and (4) any significant observation that relates to the patient's emotional or physiological status. Should any of the preceding be found to be abnormal, the abnormality should be drawn to the attention of the physician.

Although the practice varies from hospital to hospital, the patient may be transported to the operating room in his bed, on a cart, or in a wheelchair. Even if an orderly is responsible, when possible, the nurse should accompany the patient. In some hospitals relatives are encouraged to accompany the patient as far as the entrance of the operating suite. Throughout the entire preoperative period every effort should be made to convey to the patient and his family that: (1) the welfare of the patient is the prime consideration in his care, and (2) all persons who participate in his care are competent and trustworthy.

In the preoperative preparation of the patient, the care of the patient is planned and organized to meet the following objectives: (1) to prepare the patient psychologically, (2) to prepare him physically, and (3) to prepare him physiologically for the operative experience. The time available to accomplish each of these may vary from one day to several weeks or months. Unless emergency surgery is contemplated, the patient who is in the hospital for only a short period of time receives much of the preliminary preparation for his operation in the physician's office and/or clinic. The way in which nurses in the office or clinic treat him and his problems contributes to his preparation for his hospital experience. Courtesy and thoughtfulness on the part of everyone from the doorman to the nursing personnel contribute to the feeling of the patient that he is welcome and that everyone is interested in his welfare.

The Operative Period

The operative period begins the moment the patient is anesthetized and ends when the last stitch or dressing is in place. During this time the needs of the patient are met by a team of individuals each of whom has a well-defined role and tasks and on whom other members of the team depend. Some members of the team are removed from direct contact with the patient, but every member acts in behalf of the patient. The surgeon is the leader of the team, but certain circumstances may make it necessary for him to temporarily relinquish his leadership role.

The Surgeon

Throughout the operative phase the surgeon also gives attention to the prevention of serious physiologic disturbances. He ties blood vessels before or immediately after he cuts them. He may reduce excessive loss of fluid by covering exposed organs with moist towels. He handles organs and tissues gently. He estimates blood loss, or when procedures are long and there is the possibility of considerable loss of blood, he has the sponges weighed. He takes time to identify structures so that the blood supply to the tissues in the area is maintained and injury to important structures is prevented. He also attends to the nature of the response of the patient and modifies the surgical procedure in terms of the reaction of the patient. During the operative phase, the complications that are most troublesome and frequent are those of hemorrhage, shock, and hypoxia. Because these complications may also be problems in the postoperative phase, they will be discussed later. During the operative phase of surgical therapy, the purposes of the operation are, hopefully,

accomplished, and the dangers to which the patient is exposed are controlled. Many of the problems encountered by the patient during the postoperative phase depend on the care and attention the patient received during the operation or in earlier phases of treatment.

The Anesthetist

A second member of the surgical team is the anesthetist. In some hospitals, the anesthetist visits the patient the day or night prior to surgery and acquaints him with what to expect from the anesthetic. During the operative procedure the anesthetist has several important responsibilities. One is to induce a sufficient degree of anesthesia to prevent the patient from having pain and another is to secure the degree of relaxation necessary to the performance of the operation. The anesthetist is also concerned with the observation and maintenance of the physiologic status of the patient. He pays particular attention to maintaining

1. A clear or patent airway. In addition to the usual problems encountered in the maintenance of an open airway, the patient must be protected from aspirating secretions from the gastrointestinal tract. The danger of aspiration is increased in patients who have emergency surgery, because time may not be sufficient to have the stomach emptied properly.
2. Adequate breathing and exchange of gases (oxygen and carbon dioxide) in the lungs.
3. The systemic circulation.

Throughout the entire operative period the anesthetist is charged with the responsibility of observing the general condition of the patient and reporting the results of his observation to the surgeon. He observes and records the pulse, respiration, and blood pressure of the patient at regular intervals. When the surgery is associated with a large loss of blood, he may also monitor the central venous pressure, especially in poor-risk patients. Should an abnormality occur, he calls this to the attention of the surgeon so that appropriate measures can be taken.

The Nurse

The third member of the surgical team is the nurse and her assistants. The nurse has two general responsibilities. One is to anticipate and meet the needs of the surgeon for instruments and supplies during the operative procedure. The other is the general management of the operating room so that all those who are participating in the surgical procedure have what they need and the safety of the patient is protected. Obviously, these two different functions require two nurses. The first nurse is usually called a scrub, or instrument, nurse because she scrubs her hands and arms before donning a sterile gown and gloves; the second is called the circulating nurse. Although the activities of the nurse who handles instruments may appear to be the more difficult and responsible role, it is not. The circulating nurse has multiple responsibilities, as she must anticipate and plan to meet the needs of each member of the operating team; she must be alert to threats to the patient's safety; she watches for breaks in technique or for conditions that, if allowed to continue, will lead to a loss of asepsis; she saves and counts discarded sponges and instruments; she controls the number and behavior of visitors in the operating room; and she reminds the surgeon and others that the patient is awake when this reminder is necessary. In general she manages the environment of the patient, so that the progress of the procedure is furthered and the safety of the patient is protected. Few activities of the circulating nurse are glamorous or exciting. Yet the smooth running of the operating room depends on having a circulating nurse who has initiative and intelligence and who exercises sound judgment. All members of the team are important. Each member of the team contributes to the success of the surgical procedure.

What are the objectives of the surgical team during the operative phase?

The objectives of the surgical team during the operative phase are (1) to achieve the purpose of the surgical therapy, (2) to keep the patient safe during the operative procedure, and (3) to keep the surgery safe for the patient. Each of these objectives is important. Failure to achieve any one of them may result in injury or death to the patient.

The Purposes of Surgical Intervention

The purposes for which surgery is performed are several. One is to observe the gross or microscopic structure of an organ or tissue. When tissue is removed for the purpose of microscopic examination, the procedure is called a biopsy. The word *biopsy* comes from the Greek. *Bio* is derived from *bios,* which means life. *Opsy* comes from *opsis,* which means sight or vision. The term *biopsy* means not only the taking of tissue but also its microscopic examination. Biopsy is useful in confirming diagnosis, estimating prognosis, and following the course of disease and the effectiveness of treatment. To illustrate, Mrs. Stubby has a lump in her breast. The surgeon removes the lump and the pathol-

ogist examines it microscopically. He reports to the surgeon that the tumor is benign or that it is malignant. Should it be malignant, the surgeon removes the breast and surrounding lymph nodes. From the examination of the breast tissue and the lymph nodes, the nature of the neoplasm can be determined and the extent to which it has spread can be estimated. If the lesion is benign, Mrs. Stubby's prognosis is excellent and she should make a complete recovery. Should the lesion be malignant, both the nature and extent of spread will be important in predicting her chances for recovery.

Tissue may be removed for study by various methods. The method used depends on the nature and location of the lesion. In the instance of Mrs. Thomas, her breast tumor was removed by surgical excision. A patient with a tentative diagnosis of myelogenous leukemia has bone marrow removed from his sternum by means of a punch. A punch is a hollow instrument similar in appearance to a large needle; it is introduced into, and removes, a piece of tissue. Tissue may also be obtained by aspiration, a method useful when the lesion contains fluid or when fluid is formed in a serous cavity. Tissue may be procured by a number of other methods, which include (1) curettage, or the scraping of the surface of a lesion; (2) dragging of a sponge over the surface of tissue, usually a mucous membrane; (3) irrigation or washing of a serous cavity; and (4) examination of cells in sputum or other secretions. The last, which is known as the Papanicolaou technique, is based on the fact that cells are shed into secretions. (See Chapter 14.)

After the surgeon removed the tumor from Mrs. Thomas, it was sent to the pathological laboratory for examination. The pathologist examined its gross appearance and then he gave it to a technician who prepared slices of tissue from the tumor for examination by two different methods. One is called a frozen section and the other a paraffin or permanent section. Each has its advantages and disadvantages. In this instance the surgeon wished to have an immediate report and a frozen section was made at once. Later another portion or the rest of the tumor was placed in paraffin after it had been fixed in a suitable preservative. Although the latter method is more accurate, either method can be utilized with good results by experts. When the results obtained by frozen section indicate that the patient requires additional surgery, it can be instituted without delay.

Besides biopsy, exploratory surgery with or without the removal of tissue may be performed for the purpose of establishing diagnosis. At times, despite the best efforts of the physician and the use of modern diagnostic devices, a diagnosis cannot be confirmed or rejected, nor can the extent of a disease process be known for sure. For example, Mr. James has bronchogenic carcinoma. His surgeon is not certain whether the tumor can be cured with resection. One way of determining this is to examine the mediastinum through a small incision in the neck. If the procedure, called a mediastinoscopy, shows that there are no involved lymph nodes in the mediastinum, then the chances of the surgeon curing the patient are greatly increased. Mrs. Smith has had periodic attacks of severe pain in her abdomen. Despite inconclusive evidence as to its cause, the surgeon operates and finds the source of her pain, which is corrected.

In addition to its use in the diagnosis of disease, surgery is performed to effect a cure by the removal of diseased tissue or a diseased organ. Organs such as the kidney or lung may be removed provided the other organ of the pair is healthy. Some organs such as the stomach or large intestine may be removed in part or in entirety. The resection of most or all of the stomach is often followed by some impairment in nutrition and/or health. A tumor may be removed with or without the removal of surrounding tissue. Cure can sometimes be effected by the drainage of an abscess that is well walled-off. Following the removal of the contents of the abscess, the surrounding tissues are then able to complete the process of repair.

During surgery the normal functional relationships or normal continuity of structures may be disrupted following the removal of an organ or a part of the organ. For example, when Mr. Brave had the distal two thirds of his stomach removed following repeated hemorrhage from a peptic ulcer in the duodenum, a new connection between the remaining portion of the stomach and the intestine was required. Following fractures in which the ends of the bone are displaced, surgery may be required to restore and maintain the normal alignment of the bones. In the treatment of hernia, the contents that have escaped from a body cavity are replaced and the opening through which they escaped closed. Deformities resulting from failures in development or from disease may be corrected. One of the major triumphs of modern surgery is that, in the abnormal heart, openings may be closed, valves opened or reconstructed, and blood vessels rerouted so that the effects of deformities are overcome.

Surgery may also be performed to relieve symptoms, even when there is no expectation that the patient can or will be cured. Operations that are performed to relieve symptoms and to increase the comfort of the patient without any definite attempt at cure are said to be palliative. Palliative surgery is of several types. Infected and necrotic tissue may be removed in order to lessen odors and to relieve pain, detours may be established around obstructing neoplasms, pressure on vital structures may be relieved, and pain may be eliminated. For example, in advanced cancer of the breast in which ulceration of the skin and superficial tissues has occurred, the breast may be removed, not because the removal of the breast is expected to cure the patient, but to relieve the pain and remove the infection that accompanies ulceration.

In conditions accompanied by obstruction of any tubular structure such as the intestines, bile ducts, ureters, or bladder, surgery may be performed so that the contents of the tube are rerouted around the obstruction. For example, in cancer of the head of the pancreas, the common bile duct may be obstructed by the expanding neoplasm. The obstruction can be relieved by connecting the gallbladder or a portion of the common duct to the duodenum or jejunum. In cancer of the urinary bladder, the ureters may be transplanted into the ileum or sigmoid colon or opened onto the abdominal wall. A colostomy may be performed to relieve an obstruction of the transverse, descending, or sigmoid colon or rectum. A gastroenterostomy, a new opening between the stomach and jejunum, may be made to relieve the symptoms accompanying the blocking of the pyloric end of the stomach. Many of these same procedures are also used in the treatment of disease in which the outcome is expected to be curative. Any treatment whose primary objective is to relieve symptoms rather than produce a cure is palliative.

Expanding lesions in the cranial cavity or spinal canal can cause symptoms by pressing on the brain, spinal cord, or nerve tissue and by increasing intracranial pressure. Relief of symptoms can sometimes be secured by removing a portion of the skull or part of a vertebra. In the latter instance, the lamina and the spinous process of the vertebra are most likely to be removed.

Under certain circumstances the nerve supply of an organ or part may be interrupted to relieve muscle spasm or pain. In some patients whose spinal cords have been transected, muscle spasms may be severe. By cutting the motor nerve root to the involved muscles, a spastic paralysis is converted into a flaccid, or limp, one. In patients with severe and intractable pain, such as that associated with trigeminal neuralgia, sensory nerve fibers may be cut or destroyed by injection of certain chemicals, such as alcohol, into or around the nerve. Occasionally a patient suffering from advanced cancer may have severe pain that is not relieved by the usual methods. The surgeon may then cut the lateral spinothalamic tract in the spinal cord; the fibers in this tract carry pain impulses from the affected part to higher centers. When any tissue is deprived of its sensory nerve supply, it loses one of its most important defense mechanisms; therefore the involved area should be inspected regularly for redness, pallor, and other evidence of impending tissue injury. When they occur, measures should be instituted to protect the area from further damage. For example, the eye of a patient who has had the ophthalmic branch of the trigeminal nerve interrupted is deprived of its sensory nerve supply. He should be taught to protect his eye from dust and other foreign bodies and to inspect it regularly for redness, especially after he has been out of doors or in a dusty area. The patient who has a transection of the sensory pathways in the spinal cord should be instructed to change his position regularly and to keep his bed and clothing free from crumbs and wrinkles. He should also inspect the involved areas regularly. When the patient is unable to do these things for himself, they should be done for him. Unless these points receive special attention, a decubitus ulcer may develop, especially over bony prominences.

As indicated, when the patient arrives in the operating room, the surgical procedure that has been planned can be expected to accomplish one or more purposes. It may establish the nature and extent of his illness or how well he is responding to therapy. It may effect cure or relieve symptoms.

Safety During the Operative Procedure

At the time the patient arrives in the operating suite he is likely to be awake but drowsy. Operating room personnel should keep the fact that he is awake foremost in their minds and constantly remind each other of this fact. Conversation other than that directed to the patient should be avoided. He should be greeted by the surgeon or told that the surgeon will arrive shortly. Until he is anesthetized, he should be apprised of what to expect, and he should be protected from physical harm. Because he is drowsy, he should not be left alone on a cart in a corridor or in the operating room.

After the patient arrives in the operating room, he is transferred from the cart or bed to the operating room table. (He may or may not have been previously anesthetized.) The position in which he is placed on the table after he is anesthetized depends on the organs to be exposed during the operation. Sometimes the position in which the patient is placed during the operation contributes to his discomfort in the postoperative period. To prevent the patient from moving and/or from falling during the period of surgery, he is strapped to the table. The straps should be well padded and loose enough to allow adequate circulation to the extremities. The elbow should be padded, especially on the inner or medial side, to prevent ulnar nerve palsy. Care should be taken not to let the arms of the anesthetized patient dangle over the side of the table. The table should be well padded. These points are of particular importance during a lengthy operation.

Another important aspect of protecting the patient as he is prepared for surgery, as well as during the operative phase, is the maintenance of asepsis. In fact, the preparation of an aseptic environment and materials forms a large part of the preparations that are made before the patient arrives in the operating room. Because of its importance, every member of the team is responsible for securing and maintaining asepsis in all phases of surgery.

Making the Surgery Safe for the Patient

WOUND INFECTION—BASIS OF PREVENTION

As in the prevention of any infection, the following types of information are essentials: (1) the reservoirs of sources of microorganisms, (2) the vehicles by which they are spread, (3) the resistance of the microorganisms to environmental conditions including their susceptibility to physical and chemical agents, and (4) the conditions favoring the spread and growth of the microorganism.

The reservoirs or sources of microorganisms are usually people who are carriers of or are infected by the offending organism, but they may be animals or contaminated objects or materials. Not only are other persons possible sources of microorganisms, but the skin and mucous membrane of the patient may be. Vehicles for the transmission of microorganisms from the reservoir to the wound include the hands, air, instruments, linens, sutures, and any other material coming in contact with the wound. In the practice of asepsis, attention is given to preventing contact between any reservoir and the patient and to ridding vehicles of any microorganism. The methods employed depend on the character of the object to be disinfected and the susceptibility of the microorganism to destruction.

Because the incision through the skin or mucous membrane provides a portal of entry for microorganisms into the underlying tissues, measures are instituted to prevent the introduction of bacteria into the incision. The site of the incision is thoroughly cleansed. When time permits, cleansing procedures are usually initiated some time before the patient is transferred to the operating room. In the operating room the final skin preparation is made and the area is draped with sterile materials. Recently developed plastic materials, such as "Vi-drape," which adheres to the skin, have been especially helpful in preventing contamination of the wound by bacteria from an adjacent skin area.

To isolate members of the surgical team from the wound, they remove clothing worn in the other areas of the hospital or on the street and don special clothing. The hair is covered with a cap or turban and the mouth and nose are covered with a mask. The mask should be discarded before it becomes wet. For a mask to be effective, it must be dry. The maximum length of time the mask is protective is from 60 to 90 minutes. After this time, the effectiveness of the mask rapidly decreases. The purpose of the mask is to prevent the spread of microorganisms from the nasal and pharyngeal mucosa to the wound of the patient. Even when masks are properly constructed and worn, they do not trap all the microorganisms carried by the droplets of moisture during talking. Because masks are only partly effective, all but the most necessary conversation in the operating room should be discouraged.

After the thorough scrubbing of the hands and arms, a sterile gown is donned and rubber gloves are placed on the hands. The gown and gloves act as a barrier between the member of the surgical team and the wound. Before gloves were introduced, various chemicals were utilized to reduce the number of microorganisms on the hands. Semmelweis dealt with the problem by insisting that persons examining patients wash their hands in a solution containing chlorine. Lister introduced the use of carbolic acid, or phenol. Interestingly, rubber gloves were introduced by Dr. William Halsted, who had them made to protect the hands of a nurse who assisted him. She had developed a mercury dermatitis that made working in the operating room impossible. Because he valued her services, he had a pair of rubber gloves made for her. Later, other members of his operating team wore them, first to protect their hands and then later to protect the wound.

In addition to the preceding, all materials and instruments coming in contact with the wound are sterilized before they are used in the operative procedure. A variety of physical and chemical agents are now available for this purpose. They can be selected not only on the basis of being effective against organisms in either the vegetative or spore state but according to the type of material to be sterilized.

Maintenance of asepsis is one of the important elements in making surgery safe for the patient. Each and every member of the surgical team is responsible not only for his own conduct but for that of other team members. Thus the nurse reminds the surgeon that he is in danger of, or has, contaminated his gloves, gown, a drape, or an instrument. The surgeon likewise reminds the nurse. Every team member is asepsis-conscious and acts to protect the safety of the patient.

ANESTHESIA

Before the operative procedure is begun, the patient is anesthetized. The type of anesthetic used and the method by which it is administered will depend on the type and length of the procedure to be performed, the condition of the patient, his preferences, the equipment available, the skill and the training of the anesthetist, and the preference of the surgeon. When an operation is performed under local or spinal anesthesia, everyone in the operating room should be fully aware that the patient is awake. Conversation that may be disturbing to the patient should be avoided.

The Immediate Postoperative Period

The postoperative period begins the moment the surgeon completes the last stitch and continues until the metabolic and tissue changes resulting from the surgical procedure have returned to normal. This may require several days, weeks, or months. One of the major goals during this period is to anticipate, prevent, and, if necessary, treat postoperative complications. When this goal is accomplished, the patient has the greatest chance for optimal recovery. Whether or not complications are prevented frequently depends on the quality of nursing that the patient receives. Many nurses enjoy the care of patients in the postoperative phase of surgery because the results of their efforts are immediately evident. The patient fulfills the expectations of the nurse by getting well promptly. Changes indicating progress toward recovery can be seen from one day to the next and are sources of satisfaction. There are some disappointments, because not all patients get well and some develop complications.

To anticipate and prevent complications, the nurse requires knowledge of (1) the effects of anesthesia on the capacity of the patient to function, (2) the site of the incision and its effects on function, (3) the organ and tissue operated on and the general nature of the surgical procedure, and (4) knowledge of the manner in which the body responds, locally and generally, to trauma. This knowledge will influence (1) the preparations that are made for the patient in the immediate postoperative phase, (2) how he is transported from one area to another, (3) the care he receives in the period that follows the completion of the operative procedure until he is ambulating, and (4) the care he receives until he is fully rehabilitated. The psychological and physiologic status of the patient are not only important in the preparation of the patient for his operation and in assessing his ability to withstand the actual procedure, but they influence his recovery from the operation. His age predisposes him to, or protects him from, certain hazards. Personal habits, such as smoking, make him more vulnerable to certain complications, particularly those involving the tracheobronchial tree.

A few generalizations that can be used as guides in the care of the patient during the early postoperative phase of surgical treatment are (1) the periods of induction and recovery from anesthesia are the most critical of the operative experience, (2) the patient can be expected to have some disruption or depression of his defense mechanisms, (3) his capacity to adapt physiologically or psychologically is lessened, (4) the functions of organs and systems may be stimulated or depressed, (5) disturbance in one function can be the cause of disturbances in others, and (6) therapeutic measures may have adverse effects.

As stated, the periods of induction and of recovery from anesthesia are the most critical in the entire operative experience. Gius [18] compares the induction and recovery from anesthesia to the take-off and landing of an aircraft. In both situations human and mechanical failures occur. Many of the hazards to the patient and the circumstances contributing to accidents are known and should therefore be preventable. The principal complications during the period of anesthesia are circulatory collapse, cardiac arrest, respiratory complications, and injury or death caused by fire and explosions. During the period in which the patient recovers from the effects of the anesthetic, the problems in his care continue to be (1) the maintenance of a clear airway, (2) the prevention of the aspiration of saliva and gastric secretions, and (3) the maintenance of cardiovascular stability. Obstruction of the airway, shock, and hemorrhage are the principal complications occurring during the immediate postoperative period. The

[18] Gius, *op. cit.*, p. 314.

nurse shares in the responsibility for the care of the patient during both periods, but the extent of her responsibility is usually greater during the period of recovery. Nowhere, however, are the identification and control of unsafe acts more important than in the care of the patient who is in one of the stages of anesthesia.

When the operation is completed, the patient is transferred to the recovery room, the intensive-care unit, or to his own room. The recovery room has the advantage of having a trained and experienced staff who know what to expect in the postoperative period and how to prevent and treat conditions predisposing to complications. The recovery room is also specially equipped to meet any emergencies that may arise. It should be located in or adjacent to the operating suite so that equipment from the operating room is readily available. Physicians are also more likely to be nearby should their services be required. To prevent obstruction of the tracheobronchial tree and aspiration of gastric secretions and saliva while the patient is being transported from one area to another, all personnel should be constantly on the alert for any signs indicating obstruction of the airway. Because the period immediately following the operation is a hazardous one, the patient should be accompanied by a professional person.

What preparations are made for the patient who is in the immediate postoperative period?

Preparations for the care of the patient following surgery should be begun as soon as he is transferred to the operating room. The bed or frame on which he is to be placed should be secured and prepared. In preparing the bed three criteria should be met. First, the bed should be made so that the patient can be easily transferred into it. In general, the transfer of the patient is facilitated if the top bedding is not tucked in at the foot but placed neatly folded to one side. Second, the mattress and pillows should be protected from emesis and drainage as necessary. For example, for a patient having a general anesthetic or a procedure involving the gastrointestinal tract or the head and neck, the pillow under the head should be protected by a plastic cover. However, the patient who has had a local anesthetic and the drainage of an abscess of his leg is not likely to stain the pillow under his head. The mattress and pillow under his leg are in danger of being contaminated by drainage from his leg and should therefore be protected. Last, there should be some consideration of any special equipment or positions that may be required. To illustrate, if the patient is expected to have a general anesthetic, or to have his eyes bandaged following eye surgery, or is elderly, side rails should be placed on the bed to remind the patient of where the edges of the bed are and to reduce his chance of falling out. A patient having surgery on his back may be placed on a frame so that turning from face to back is facilitated. If the patient is to be encased in a cast, a board may be placed under the mattress to provide a firm support for the cast. Although most hospitals are now equipped with beds having Gatch frames to elevate the head of the bed, few have the type that facilitate elevation of the foot of the bed.[19] The necessity for elevating the foot of the bed should be anticipated when the patient goes directly from the operating room to his room following a prolonged and difficult operation or when there is any other reason for anticipating that he may be unconscious or in shock. Some surgeons prefer to have their patients in a slight Trendelenburg position to facilitate drainage of secretions from the airway and to prevent the aspiration of vomitus or other liquids.

In the past the warming of the bed was considered to be essential. Although warming of the bed probably does no harm, unless the room and bed are cold, it probably is unnecessary. If hot-water bottles or other heating devices are used, they should be removed before the patient is transferred to the bed to protect him from burns and/or overheating. Overheating may cause sweating and may contribute to the dehydration of the patient. The aim should be to maintain the temperature of the room so that the patient is comfortable.

In addition to the preparation of the bed, equipment and supplies that will be required in the care of the patient should be assembled. The equipment and supplies used will depend on the kind of anesthetic used and the nature of the surgical procedure. Because the number-one problem in the immediate postoperative period for patients having a general anesthetic is the maintenance of adequate ventilation and the prevention of obstruction of the tracheobronchial tree, provisions should be made to remove oral and tracheobronchial secretions and to prevent saliva and vomitus from being aspirated. With some patients this can be accomplished by positioning the patient, but suction apparatus should always be available. Suction apparatus must also be available and in working order for patients who have gastric or other tubes.

A tracheostomy tray should be placed at the bedside of patients who have undergone head and neck surgery, including thyroidectomy, in anticipation of the possibility of acute obstruc-

tion of the airway. Other equipment should be obtained and prepared as required. This might include equipment for administering oxygen, drainage or irrigation sets, and solutions. Because practice varies, no attempt will be made to list all the types of equipment or supplies that may be required in the care of the patient; however, whatever is necessary should be obtained and tested to make certain that it is in working order before the patient is returned to his room.

The First Six to Eight Hours

Since most of the problems of the unconscious patient are similar whether he is being transported from one area to another or he is in bed, they will be discussed here.

Some of the more important problems in the care of the patient during the first six to eight hours following the completion of the surgical procedure include: maintaining a clear airway, preventing aspiration of vomitus, maintaining blood pressure, and preventing injury caused by falling. Depending on the type of anesthesia used and the stage of anesthesia he is in, the patient may be deeply unconscious or fully awake. During the first six to eight hours after surgery, the patient's cardiovascular system does not adapt well to rapid changes in position. Even when his blood pressure is stable at the completion of the surgical procedure, movement or jarring of the patient is likely to cause it to fall. Care should be taken to handle him slowly and gently and to avoid bumping the cart or bed.

POSITIONING THE PATIENT

To prevent obstruction of the respiratory tract by secretions and aspiration of saliva and gastric juice, the patient should be placed in a position favoring drainage. Although some surgeons recommend that the unconscious patient be transported on his side, this is seldom done except with children or if the patient is vomiting. The patient may be transported with his head and shoulders slightly lower than the legs and buttocks. Excessive lowering of the head, however, increases the pressure of the viscera on the diaphragm, reduces ventilation, increases intrathoracic pressure and may actually decrease blood flow to the brain by initiating reflex constriction of the carotid arteries. The head should be turned to one side, in order to keep the posterior portion of the tongue and soft tissues from blocking the glottis. This position not only favors the drainage of fluid from the tracheobronchial tree and the mouth, but it also reduces stasis of blood in the lower extrem-

[19] Some carts or stretchers used in recovery rooms are adjustable and a patient can be placed in almost any position desired.

ities. Return of fluid and blood to the general circulation is important for maintaining cardiac output. During the period that the patient is unconscious and well relaxed by the anesthetic, an oropharyngeal airway placed in the mouth may be helpful in keeping the tongue and soft tissues from falling back into the pharynx. In the event that the airway becomes obstructed, the mandible should be raised and moved forward. If the mouth can be opened, the tongue can be grasped with a gauze square and pulled forward so that the obstruction of the airway is relieved.

Until he regains consciousness, the head should be lowered slightly and/or turned to the side unless there is some reason contraindicating it. The child who has had a tonsillectomy under general anesthesia is usually placed face down. Because blood and saliva will drain from the mouth by gravity, aspiration of these materials into the tracheobronchial tree is avoided and the extent to which the patient is bleeding can be determined. The patient having intracranial or head and neck surgery is not placed in the head-down position. No matter where a part is located, if it is placed in a dependent position, gravity decreases venous return from it and increases the chance of swelling and bleeding. The position of the patient may also be modified by the presence of other disorders. The obese or emphysemic patient should be placed in a sitting position to facilitate breathing. The patient with a spinal anesthetic should usually be kept relatively flat in bed. Because spinal anesthesia lessens the ability to adjust the diameter of the blood vessels to position changes, it predisposes to severe postural hypotension (the blood pressure falls when the individual rises to sit or stand). A less dangerous effect is headache (spinal headache), which is thought to be caused by a reduction in the pressure of the cerebrospinal fluid. To prevent either or both of these complications, the patient is usually kept in the supine or recumbent position for a longer time than the patient having a general anesthetic.

When placing the patient on his side, the nurse should keep two points in mind. One is that the weight of the body should not be allowed to rest on the dependent arm. The other is that the weight of the body should be distributed so that the body holds itself on the side. To prevent pressure on the arm, the body may be turned on the side with the lower arm parallel to the side. The arm on the dependent side is then pulled through so that it lies posterior to the trunk. The nurse then stands behind the patient and places one hand under the iliac crest and the other under the trochanter of the femur and pulls his body

toward herself. The upper leg and thigh may be flexed at the knee and be carried forward over the dependent leg. The side-lying position not only facilitates the drainage of secretions, but it helps to maintain the tongue and soft tissues forward so that they do not block the pharynx or larynx.

RECOVERY FROM THE ANESTHETIC

When the patient arrives in the recovery area, he may be fully awake or in any one of the various stages of anesthesia. If he is unconscious, he may have an oropharyngeal airway in place. It should not be removed until the swallowing reflexes of the patient return and the patient tries to remove it. The oropharyngeal airway should not be confused with an endotracheal tube. As may be deduced from its name, an endotracheal tube is placed in the trachea and its primary purpose is to administer an inhalation anesthetic. It should only be removed after the patient is awake and can ventilate adequately. Some physicians and anesthetists measure the patient's tidal volume before removing the endotracheal tube. Patients who have had chest surgery are often placed on a respirator for a few hours or even days before the endotracheal tube is removed. The endotracheal tube should always be removed by a physician because it may have to be reinserted if the patient does not breathe adequately without it. A laryngoscope should be available in case the tube has to be reinserted.

STAGES

As the patient recovers from the effects of a general anesthetic, which takes about six to eight hours, he passes through the same stages that he did in its induction, except that the order is reversed. In the induction of the anesthetic, the concentration of the anesthetic gas or mixture of gases is higher in the alveoli than it is in the blood. Therefore, the gas moves from the alveoli into the blood at a more rapid rate than it moves out of the blood into the alveoli. When the desired level of anesthesia is reached, the amount of gas inhaled by the patient is adjusted so that the amount entering the blood equals that leaving the blood. At the termination of the operation or at some suitable point previous to it, the administration of the anesthetic gas is terminated. In the period of recovery, the process is reversed. As the patient inhales air or oxygen, the concentration of the anesthetic gas in the alveoli is diluted and, as a consequence, its partial pressure is reduced. With the reduction in the partial pressure of the gas in the alveoli, the gas in the blood escapes into the alveoli, where it is mixed with inspired air and exhaled. This process continues until all the gas is removed from the body.

The degree of general anesthesia may be divided into four stages. During stage IV respiratory paralysis of central origin occurs. This depth of anesthesia is seldom seen except in the operating room when large amounts of anesthesia may be used. Death occurs unless ventilation is maintained by the anesthesiologist.

Stage III is known as the stage of surgical anesthesia. The patient is unconscious and reflexes are repressed or paralyzed. This stage is divided into four planes, according to the degree to which reflexes are repressed or paralyzed, with plane 1 being the lightest and plane 4 the deepest. Most surgical procedures are carried out in plane 2.

As the patient eliminates the anesthetic, he goes into the second stage of anesthesia or the stage of excitement or delirium. This stage, as the name implies, is accompanied by a number of hazards to the patient. Although the patient becomes unconscious in stage II, there is great variability in the degree of excitement manifested by patients as they pass through this stage. Some remain relatively quiet, whereas others may be so disturbed that they are difficult to control. As a result of the use of modern drugs and anesthetics, the length of the stage of excitement has been shortened and decreased in severity. The nurse should, however, be alert to the possibility of the patient's becoming excited. She should take appropriate steps to decrease the likelihood of his becoming excited and to protect him from injury if he does. Bedside rails should be raised, and someone should be in constant attendance on the patient. The environment of the patient should be regulated so that all sources of stimulation such as noise, drafts, and loud talking are eliminated. The patient should be handled gently. In the past, efforts were sometimes made to increase the rate at which the patient regained consciousness by stimulating him, by shouting at him, or shaking him. Because the rate of the recovery of the patient depends on the rate at which the anesthetic agent is eliminated, these procedures cannot be counted on to be very effective, and they may be harmful. In addition to increasing the likelihood of the patient's becoming excited during stage II, the capacity of the patient to adapt the functioning of his cardiovascular system to rapid changes in position is reduced and as a result his blood pressure may fall.

During stage I, the patient is drowsy. He can be awakened and will respond to questions, but then he lapses back into sleep. He may waken and complain of pain and in a moment or two return to sleep. At this time the nurse must assess the need of the patient for a pain-relieving medication. She must estimate the severity of the pain experienced by the patient and the extent of his recovery from the anesthetic and preanesthetic medications. Questions the nurse should be able to answer before she administers an analgesic medication include the following: Has the patient recovered sufficiently from the effects of the anesthetic to require a pain-relieving medication? Is the respiratory status of the patient such that it is safe to administer a drug to him that depresses respiration? What evidence indicates that the patient does or does not require an analgesic? The objective is neither to give nor to withhold medication; too great delay in the administration of an analgesic can cause as much harm to the patient as administering one too soon. The objective should be to minimize the pain experienced by the patient and at the same time protect him from the hazards of overmedication. For example, the author recently spent the afternoon with a friend who had had a general anesthetic earlier in the day. She was drowsy and slept for extended periods of time. At one point she roused and complained of pain. In a moment or so she went back to sleep and continued to sleep for an hour or more. When she awakened at this point, she again complained of pain. This time she did not go back to sleep and she was obviously uncomfortable and restless. Because her respiratory rate was within normal limits and there were no other contraindications, she was given a pain-relieving medication. It should be emphasized that restlessness may also be caused by hypoxia. The administration of a narcotic to a hypoxic patient will cause further respiratory depression and may result in death.

MAINTENANCE OF A CLEAR AIRWAY

As stated earlier, equipment should be available to remove secretions from the mouth and pharynx as they appear. The patient should be observed for signs that may indicate some airway obstruction, such as noisy respirations and/or labored breathing. The movements of the chest as well as the use of the accessory muscles of respiration should be observed and abnormalities reported. Cyanosis is a relatively late sign of oxygen deficiency or hypoxia, as it depends on the presence of 5 g or more of reduced (unoxygenated) hemoglobin in the capillary blood. Thus cyanosis may not become evident in an anemic patient until just prior to death. If evidence of obstruction is ignored until the patient becomes cyanotic, the patient's condition has been allowed to deteriorate to an unacceptable degree. Treatment should be promptly instituted to prevent and to relieve obstruction and to lessen the possibility of a serious degree of hypoxia. (See Chapter 8 to review the effects of a lack of oxygen to the brain and other tissues.)

Should the unconscious patient develop signs indicating any respiratory obstruction, the nurse should check the tongue to make certain that it is not responsible. In prolonged unconsciousness, obstruction can be caused by the lodging of a foreign body transversely in the oral pharynx. One source of foreign bodies is crusting, which frequently develops on the hard palate of patients who breathe through their mouths. This crust may subsequently become dislodged and cause obstruction. Conscientious mouth care and an adequate fluid intake can prevent this complication. The condition of not only the anterior but of the posterior part of the mouth should be regularly determined. Movement of the patient from side to side may promote coughing and expulsion of a mucus plug from the tracheobroncial tree. In the patient who has had head and neck surgery, including thyroidectomy, the area around the incision should be checked for signs of hemorrhage. When the obstruction cannot be relieved by procedures within the province of nursing, the physician should be notified immediately so that the cause of the obstruction can be determined and the appropriate remedy initiated. The therapy prescribed by the physician will be determined by the factors contributing to the hypoxia and the severity of the hypoxia.

When laryngospasm is responsible for obstruction of the airway, action must be taken promptly to relieve it or the patient will die from the effects of hypoxia. The nurse can recognize this condition by the characteristic crowing sound occurring during respiration. The sound is caused by the movement of air through the narrow space between the vocal folds, which are tightly adducted because of laryngeal muscle spasm. The patient appears to be struggling to breathe, especially during inspiration, and uses his accessory muscles of respiration. Although the simplest method used to treat laryngospasm is to administer oxygen under pressure by way of a tight-fitting mask placed over the face, laryngospasm can also be relieved by the introduction of an endotracheal tube by a physician. A nurse must *never* attempt this procedure. The administration of oxygen under pressure is usually successful. Enough oxygen gets by the adducted vocal folds to reduce the degree of hypoxia sufficiently to cause the folds to relax. When the proper equipment is not readily available, a tracheotomy may have to be performed to establish an open airway. Other indications for tracheotomy such as pressure on the trachea and excessive secretions, as well as

the care of the patient with a tracheotomy, are discussed in Chapter 8.

The patient should be turned at regular intervals from side to side. As soon as he responds, he should be encouraged to perform deep-breathing exercises and to cough at hourly intervals or until he has cleared his lungs of any secretions. An upright position increases the effectiveness of coughing and the vital capacity. Slight pressure over the incision by the nurse may reduce the pain of coughing or make the patient feel more secure about his incision. When the condition of the patient permits, some surgeons direct that the patient be placed in the sitting or standing position to cough and to do breathing exercises. Although either position increases the effectiveness of mechanisms for cleansing the tracheobronchial tree, the patient who has so recently experienced a major operation may become very anxious when the suggestion is made that he is to sit up or get out of bed. He should, therefore, be given appropriate psychological and physical support.

Reactions of the Cardiovascular System to General Surgery

VITAL SIGNS

In addition to the observation and maintenance of respiratory function, the nurse should check all the vital signs. These include the pulse and blood pressure as well as the depth, rhythm or pattern, and rate of respiration. Vital signs should be checked every 15 minutes for the first 4 hours and then hourly until they are stable. Frequent measurements of central venous pressure enables one to evaluate how well the heart is handling the volume of blood in the cardiovascular system. The response to a fluid load rather than the absolute level gives the most accurate information. When evaluation is made of the condition of a patient, all evidence should be taken into consideration. The fact that the blood pressure of a patient is within the range expected for the patient should not cause the nurse to discount other evidence that the patient is in trouble. As a matter of fact, accumulation of carbon dioxide may cause the blood pressure to be higher than it would be otherwise.

What are the causes of shock in the surgical patient?

A relatively frequent complication occurring during the operation and early postoperative phase of surgery is shock. In serious states of shock, life may be threatened unless the disorder is treated promptly and effectively. As defined elsewhere, shock is an abnormal physiological state characterized by inadequate cellular metabolism. This may be caused by poor tissue perfusion or other factors. Postoperatively it is often caused by a serious discrepancy between the capacity of the blood vessels and the circulating blood volume. Any disorder resulting in a marked increase in the capacity of the blood vessels or noticeably decreasing the volume of circulating blood can cause shock. One effect of the disparity between blood volume and the capacity of the blood vessels is a fall in the blood pressure. The consequence, in terms of cells, is failure to deliver enough oxygen and other substances to maintain adequate metabolism.

In a closed system such as the vascular system, the pressure of the fluid within the system above simple hydrostatic pressure is maintained by three factors: (1) an effective pumping mechanism, (2) fluid to pump, and (3) appropriate resistance in the pipes or vessels. Although any abnormalities of one of these factors may be involved in development of shock in the surgical patient, the last two are probably the most frequent. In the patient who is treated surgically or who suffers serious physical trauma or is burned, fluid volume is decreased by loss of blood and the loss of body fluids. Dehydration may be an initiating or sustaining factor in shock because it contributes to a reduction in circulating blood volume. Shock caused by the reduction in the circulating blood volume is classified as hypovolemia.

HEMORRHAGE

As indicated, hemorrhage is one of the more common causes of shock. Moreover, it is a possibility in all phases of surgery. In the instance of Mr. Brave, bleeding from an eroded blood vessel located in a peptic ulcer caused him to seek medical attention. Mrs. Smith lost approximately 3 pints of blood during the removal of her uterus (hysterectomy), and Sunny Day bled profusely from the tonsillar fossa in her pharynx after tonsillectomy. Johnny Hopper suffered an open or compound fracture (a break in a bone in which one or more fragments protrude through the skin) when he fell from a tree. In all these patients the primary factor causing hemorrhage was a disruption in the continuity of one or more blood vessels.

Although physical injuries are usually responsible for breaks in the continuity of blood vessels, the condition of the wall of the blood vessel influences its ability to withstand trauma or chemical destruction. Examples of disorders weakening the walls of blood vessels include arterial aneurysms or venous varicosities. In an arterial aneurysm, the wall bulges as a result of disease or structural defect. As it bulges, the

wall thins and becomes less resistant to the pressure of the arterial blood. Furthermore, the tension against the wall of a vessel increases with its diameter (Laplace's law). Sooner or later it is likely to rupture and result in arterial hemorrhage. When varicosities—elongated, tortuous, thin-walled veins—are located in the esophagus, food passing over may cause erosion of the already thin wall and cause serious hemorrhage. In addition to localized areas of weakness in the walls of blood vessels, deficiency of vitamin C is accompanied by a generalized fragility in the walls of capillaries.

Following injury to a blood vessel, the body responds to protect itself from an excessive loss of blood. Among these responses are the self-sealing mechanism, the elevation of interstitial fluid pressure created by the escaping blood, and the immobilization of the injured area by muscle spasm. In the self-sealing mechanism, the muscle in the cut end of the blood vessel contracts and thereby reduces the diameter of the lumen. Muscle contraction occurs whether the blood vessel is large or small and may be sufficient to control bleeding, even from large arteries. Sealing of the remaining lumen is accomplished by the formation of a blood clot within the terminal portion of the cut end of the blood vessel. As the clot matures, it, too, contracts and forms a tight plug in the end of the blood vessel. The self-sealing mechanism is usually successful in limiting blood loss from small wounds and from areas where the surface tissue has been removed, as in an abrasion or burn.

When a large area of tissue has been denuded or for some other reason the self-sealing mechanism is ineffective, sufficient blood may be lost to form a soft clot over the site of bleeding. The clot, instead of contracting and sealing the underlying blood vessels, remains soft and the vessels behind it continue to bleed. Before blood loss can be checked, the soft clot must be removed.

To illustrate, after the surgical removal of the tonsils, the surgeon dries the denuded area by gently patting the surface with a sponge. He continues this process until the cut ends of the blood vessels have constricted and the blood has clotted within them. Should bleeding recur, a clot forms external to cut ends of the blood vessels and bleeding continues underneath it. One theory advanced to explain continued bleeding is that the blood clot probably releases fibrolysin, which prevents clotting in the ends of the blood vessels. Control of bleeding usually requires that the soft blood clot be removed and that the area again be dried. Pressure is often applied to control bleeding until the self-sealing mechanism becomes effective.

Following prostatectomy, bleeding from the lining of the bladder usually occurs. Because of its anatomy, pressure over the bleeding sites is difficult, if not impossible, to apply. Continued bleeding is usually the result of a soft clot adhering to the lining of the bladder and interfering with the formation of clots within the disrupted blood vessels. Bleeding can usually be prevented or stopped by the removal of blood and clots from the bladder by irrigation. When irrigation of the bladder is prescribed following prostatectomy, sufficient fluid should be introduced to remove blood and blood clots, and the procedure should be performed frequently enough to prevent clot formation within the bladder lumen.

Besides the self-sealing mechanism, blood loss into a closed space is opposed by the rise of tissue pressure caused by blood accumulating in the space. As tissue fluid pressure rises, it exerts pressure against the wall of the bleeding vessel. Blood flow ceases when the interstitial pressure exceeds the blood pressure. Conversely, bleeding into a body cavity where blood can escape is more likely to be severe because the blood is removed from the cavity. Thus bleeding from the nose or into the alimentary canal or other hollow organs is more likely to be profuse. Muscle spasm in an affected part contributes to immobilization and may also increase the pressure exerted against the exterior of the involved blood vessels. All these factors may combine to lessen the quantity of blood lost.

Hemorrhage has one effect: It lessens circulation of blood by decreasing blood volume. When a large quantity of blood is lost quickly, the blood pressure falls. As much as 10–20 per cent of the blood volume can be lost without any appreciable effect on the blood pressure, especially if it is lost slowly. A rapid loss of 30 per cent or more is usually associated with a considerable drop in blood pressure. As stated, if the fall in blood pressure is not too great, it may help to produce hemostasis by reducing blood flow through the severed blood vessels. The effect of the decrease in the blood volume is counteracted by (1) the constriction of blood vessels, thereby reducing the size of the vascular bed; (2) constriction of the arterioles, which increases peripheral resistance; and (3) transfer of fluid from the interstitial and cellular spaces to the blood. All these mechanisms help to maintain perfusion of the heart and brain by reducing the disparity between the size of the vascular bed and the blood volume.

In addition to a decrease in the volume of circulating blood, hemorrhage causes a reduction in the oxygen-carrying capacity of the blood caused by a loss of erythrocytes and hemoglobin. Serious as the loss of hemoglobin

is, it is not of as much immediate importance in acute hemorrhage as it is later on in chronic blood loss. The effects of the loss of hemoglobin are discussed in Chapter 10.

When arteries are disrupted, a third problem is created because the tissues supplied by the artery are partly or completely deprived of their blood supply. For example, in an accident with an electric saw, Jim Green's lower leg was severed, so that only about one fourth of the tissue remained intact. Whether or not his foot can be saved will depend in part on whether the arterial blood supply is sufficient or, if not, whether it can be re-established. Interestingly, it is often the integrity of the veins that is more crucial. Lack of adequate venous drainage may result in severe congestion and death of the involved organ or limb.

SIGNS AND SYMPTOMS OF HEMORRHAGE

Besides the signs and symptoms caused by the effects of hypoxia and reduction of blood volume, the site of hemorrhage influences some of the other effects of hemorrhage. The site of bleeding determines whether blood increases pressure within an organ or tissue or escapes to the outside. In tissues or organs where the escaping blood is trapped, such as in the cranial or spinal cavity, the signs and symptoms may be caused primarily by increased pressure on the brain or cord or by the irritation of the brain or nerves by the blood. Although some blood is lost, the quantity is not sufficient to affect the blood volume.

When bleeding is in an organ or tissue from which it can escape to the outside, blood as well as the consequences of a reduction in blood volume can be observed. Blood escaping from an artery is bright red and comes in spurts; blood from a vein generally has a dusky hue and flows steadily; and capillary bleeding is characterized by seepage.

TREATMENT OF HEMORRHAGE

In instances in which bleeding is not self-limiting, therapy of hemorrhage is directed toward two objectives. The first is to stop the hemorrhage. The second depends on the extent of blood loss and the effects of the accumulation of blood on involved structures. When the loss of blood is sufficient to affect the blood volume, a second objective is to replace the blood volume. When blood has accumulated in a tissue or organ in sufficient quantity to impair its function, then an objective is to remove the blood or to relieve the pressure created by it. Before bleeding can be treated, it must be detected. Any patient who is predisposed to hemorrhage by the nature of his illness or treatment should be under an intelligent program of surveillance. Dressings should be inspected regularly for evidence of fresh blood. Like other fluids, blood runs downhill; parts inferior to the dressing should be inspected. Fluids drained or discharged from affected organs should be examined for blood. When the incision or injury is in an organ or tissue from which blood cannot escape, the patient should be observed for signs and symptoms indicating pressure on the organ or surrounding tissues.

Although bleeding may occur in any incision, it is most likely to take place in large wounds, in those in which the operated surface is exposed, and in highly vascular areas. Internal bleeding may also result from the failure of a ligature to hold a large artery severed during the operative procedure; large amounts of blood can be lost in a very short period of time. Traumatic injuries are a frequent cause of hemorrhage, and certain blood dyscrasias are associated with a tendency to bleed. Formerly operations on patients with obstructions in the biliary tract were likely to be associated with hemorrhage because of failure to absorb vitamin K. Now, many of these patients can be prepared so that they are not subject to any special hazard.

In some surgical procedures the tendency of the patient to bleed can be controlled by appropriate care. As previously indicated, patients having intracranial and head and neck surgery are usually placed in a position with the head and back up. In patients who have surgery on an extremity, the limb is elevated to improve the venous return and to lessen the tendency to bleed into the wound. Occasionally, a special tourniquet is applied to a limb so that surgery can be performed distally in a bloodless field. This may be done safely for up to one to one and a half hours at a time. The extremity is also immobilized until the danger of hemorrhage has decreased. As discussed earlier following prostatectomy, bleeding from the bladder is controlled by bladder irrigation. In the control of bleeding from any organ, the location of the structure and the nature of its functions have to be considered. In general, measures are used to immobilize the part, overcome the force of the blood pressure, or support or to assist the self-sealing mechanism.

One of the most common methods (perhaps the oldest) of controlling hemorrhage, particularly in the emergency situation, is the application of *pressure*. The points at which bleeding may most easily be stopped by applying pressure are those where large blood vessels overlie bony prominences. The vessels that meet this criterion include the temporal, facial, carotid, brachial, and femoral arteries. Pressure

should be applied with the cleanest available material. Although tourniquets have long been used to control bleeding from an extremity, they often do more harm than good. Their use is not advocated. If a tourniquet is applied, it should be tight enough to prevent blood from entering the affected limb and it should be left in place until the patient is examined by a surgeon. If the tourniquet is not tight enough to occlude the arterial flow but does occlude venous return, blood loss distal to the tourniquet will be greater than without any tourniquet at all. The patient should be treated as soon as possible to protect the tissue that is deprived of its blood supply. A properly applied tourniquet should be left in place only one or two hours; if prolonged, this method of hemostasis in itself may cause severe tissue injury.

Hemorrhage from an accessible organ or cavity such as the uterus or the nares may sometimes be controlled by packing the organ with sterile gauze. The gauze is usually left in place until the self-sealing mechanism controls bleeding. Occasionally, bleeding is renewed after the packing is removed, and the packing may have to be replaced. Patients should always be observed following the removal of packing for evidence of recurrent hemorrhage.

Although the application of pressure is frequently life saving when utilized to control bleeding from a large artery or vein, large vessels often must be ligated before hemorrhage is actually checked. Otherwise the bleeding starts again as soon as the pressure is removed. The self-sealing mechanism is usually successful in curbing blood loss from small vessels. Pressure applied over an area in which there is bleeding from small vessels may be of value until the self-sealing mechanism is effective in controlling bleeding.

Another old, but probably newer, method of controlling the loss of blood is *cauterization* of the wound. In its earliest use, cauterization was not the carefully confined and controlled application of heat to a limited area of tissue that it is today. One old method of cauterizing tissue was to pour boiling oil into the wound. Styptics, astringents, or a hot iron were also used. Although the techniques used in cauterizing wounds have changed and cautery is less frequently utilized than it once was, it still has its uses. Many surgeons now use electric cautery with fine tips to control bleeding during surgery. Not only is it useful in controlling hemorrhage, but it may also be employed to destroy tissue. For example, it is used in brain surgery to both destroy tissue and prevent bleeding. Cautery is often employed to open colostomies; in this procedure a loop of the colon is brought above the surface of the skin and allowed to remain closed until the second or third day after the initial surgical procedure. This procedure is not painful because the tissues of the intestine do not have nerve endings that are sensitive to heat. The patient may be frightened, however, because he does not believe that it will not hurt. To lessen his fear, his eyes should be covered with a small towel and he should be informed about the successful progress of the procedure. Through the use of heat enough tissue is destroyed to provide an opening into the intestine, and the blood vessels in the affected tissue are sealed.

Although pressure and cauterization are of value in hemostasis, neither method provides an adequate means of controlling the loss of blood during a major operative procedure. It was not until materials were available that could be used to tie the ends of blood vessels that the prevention of blood loss during surgery became a practical reality. Early materials to be used in tying off blood vessels were silk or linen thread. As noted earlier, *ligatures* have been known for centuries, but their regular use is of relatively modern origin. Today the surgeon has the choice of many materials, some of which are absorbable and some of which are not. During an operative procedure he also has instruments, hemostats, that he can use to close the ends of vessels before he severs them or to grasp them after they are cut.

A variety of methods are available to prevent and to limit the loss of blood. The method selected depends on a variety of factors. Among them are the urgency of the situation, the rate at which blood is being lost, the extent to which blood volume has already been diminished, the site of bleeding, as well as the facilities at hand. As in shock, the safety of the patient depends on the rapidity with which hemorrhage is detected and appropriate measures are instituted.

In addition to stopping the bleeding, treatment should restore blood volume if it has been significantly decreased. When the loss of blood is within the limits to which the patient is able to adapt, no special measures may be required, but when the loss of blood seriously threatens the blood volume, measures such as intravenous fluids, plasma, volume expanders, and blood transfusion may be required.

TRANSFUSION

Although attempts have been made to transfuse blood for at least 400 years, the ability to transfuse blood with reasonable safety to the patient is an accomplishment of the twentieth century. In some of the early experiments, blood taken from one dog was successfully transfused into another. Transfusion of human blood from one person to another was less suc-cessful and at least half of the recipients died. Because of the frequency with which death occurred, laws were passed prohibiting blood transfusions in England, France, and Italy. Before blood can be safely transferred from one person to another, three factors must be considered: (1) the blood groups and the Rh-Hr system, (2) calcium and blood clotting, and (3) diseases transmitted by blood.

What is the basis for blood grouping?

In 1900 Landsteiner made an observation that was to serve as the basis for the discovery of why at least one half of those who were transfused with the blood of another died. He noted that when the red blood cells of one person were exposed to the serum of another, they sometimes clumped or agglutinated. During the next two years Landsteiner and his associates investigated this phenomenon more fully. From these studies they learned that all human beings could be placed in one of four blood groups. The blood group to which any individual belongs is determined by the presence or absence of one or both of two antigens or iso-agglutinogens in his erythrocytes. Landsteiner called these antigens A and B. Persons whose erythrocytes contain neither antigen A nor antigen B were classified as belonging to blood group O, the most common blood group among Caucasians, as 40 to 45 per cent of the population have type O blood. Those who have iso-agglutinogen A in their erythrocytes belong to blood group A; this is the next most frequent type, as about 40 per cent of the population belong to group A. Those who have isoagglutinogen B in their erythrocytes belong to group B; about 10 per cent of the population are in group B. About 4 per cent of the population have both isoagglutinogen A and B in their erythrocytes and are in group AB.

Agglutination depends on the presence in the serum of an antibody, agglutinin, that reacts with the antigen in the erythrocyte. The agglutinin reacting with isoagglutinogen A is named anti-A and the one reacting with B is called anti-B. The blood serum of a person does not contain the agglutinin that reacts with the iso-agglutinogen in his red cells. Thus type A blood contains anti-B but not anti-A agglutinin. Persons in blood group O do not have either antigen A or B in their red cells, but they do have both anti-A and anti-B in their serum. Persons in blood group AB have antigens A and B in their erythrocytes, but they do not have either agglutinin in their serum. Because the blood of the donor is diluted as it enters the blood of the recipient, there is relatively less concern about the effect of the antibodies in its serum on the red blood cells of the recipient.

Some authorities question the dilution factor as an explanation of why the donor's isoagglutinins do not agglutinate the erythrocytes of the recipient. Whatever the reason, the antibodies in the donor's serum do not usually adversely affect the recipient's red cells. Because erythrocytes of group O blood do not contain either antigen, they can be transfused into persons with other types of blood. For this reason a person with group O blood is said to be a universal donor; theoretically his blood can be transfused into all other individuals. Although group O blood can often be transfused into persons of other blood groups without causing a reaction, it can cause a reaction, especially if there is a high titer of anti-A and anti-B in the serum of the donor. When the titer of antibody is high, the agglutinin in the blood serum of the donor can react with the iso-agglutinogen of the recipient to produce hemolysis of the erythrocytes of the recipient. Persons with group O blood must be transfused with group O blood. Despite their ability to give to other groups, they can take only from their own group.

Because antibodies are absent from the serum of persons with group AB blood, they can theoretically receive blood from persons of all blood groups, and, therefore, these persons are known as universal recipients. They can give blood only to persons with type AB blood. Because not all persons react as expected on receiving blood, cross matching is an essential part of the preparation for blood transfusion. In cross matching, the erythrocytes of the donor are exposed to the serum of the recipient and the erythrocytes of the recipient are exposed to the serum of the donor.

As Landsteiner and his associates studied the factors influencing the agglutination of erythrocytes, they learned that there were more antigens and isoagglutinogens than A and B. Perhaps the most important of these other iso-agglutinogens are those belonging to the Rh-Hr system. Six cell characteristics have been identified with this system. These factors have two sets of names, the American and the British. They are Rho, rh', rh", Hro, hr', hr". The corresponding British nomenclature is D, C, E, d, c, c_1. The red cells of each person contain at least one member of each of the three groups of antigens. In some persons the red cells contain four, five, or six of them. The number of possible combinations is therefore great. In general, if the patient's red cells have D antigens, he is considered to be Rh positive. More recently, however, the presence of both C and E has also been considered to be Rh positive. As a consequence, more exact Rh typing and matching is being done, especially in potential mothers.

Rh-Hr antigens differ from A and B antigens in that the antibody that acts against them is not normally found in the blood serum. It is formed when an Rh-negative person is given Rh-positive blood. This happens under two circumstances. In one, a person who is Rh-negative is transfused with Rh-positive blood. Although there is no obvious reaction, the individual reacts by producing antibodies in his blood serum against the Rh factor. Should this person receive a transfusion of Rh-positive blood at a later date, a serious reaction occurs. In the second situation an Rh-negative woman who is pregnant with an Rh-positive child is sensitized to the Rh factor. Usually nothing obvious occurs during the first pregnancy, and often during the second pregnancy, to indicate that the woman is becoming sensitized to the Rh factor. In many instances a number of normal children can be borne before the mother becomes sensitized to the Rh factor. Apparently, the sensitization comes about because the red cells of the Rh-positive baby escape through the placenta and stimulate the production of anti-Rh antibodies in the mother. These antibodies pass from the mother through the placenta into the blood of the baby, causing hemolysis of the red cells of the baby. The condition in the baby is known as erythroblastosis fetalis. If these babies are born alive, they may still suffer severe brain damage from the high levels of bilirubin that can develop in the fetus because of the hemolysis. If the condition is not too severe, their lives may be saved and brain damage prevented by an exchange transfusion in which the blood of the baby is removed and replaced by Rh-negative blood.

Many different agglutinins have been discovered since recognition of the ABO and Rh factors and have been referred to as Kell, Duffy, Kidd, and others. In 1926 an especially interesting type of agglutinin was described by Landsteiner and Levine.[20] This agglutinin in the blood plasma of an individual coagulates his erythrocytes when the temperature of the blood plasma is reduced below normal body temperature. Because the activity of the agglutinins depends on temperature, they are called cold agglutinins. Cold agglutinins are present more frequently in the blood of Negro donors than in Caucasians. They are also frequent in persons who have cirrhosis of the liver, severe anemia, hemolytic anemia, and many other chronic diseases. Cold agglutinins were not of much significance when blood was administered soon after it was drawn. It has assumed more importance now that blood is stored under refrigeration in

[20] K. Landsteiner and Philip Levine: "On the Cold Agglutinins in Human Serum," *J. Immun.*, **12**:441 (Dec.) 1926.

blood banks. When patients are known to have cold agglutinins, blood is warmed before it is administered. After the blood is warmed, its temperature may be maintained at 37°C (98°F) by passing the tubing through a blood warmer. Some commercial blood warmers are now available and are used in many of our larger operating rooms, especially if there may be a need for massive transfusions. Because blood proteins can be altered or denatured by heat, care should be taken not to overheat the blood. Any mixing of the blood should be gentle, as hemolysis of red cells is increased by mechanical stress. Because of the increased possibility that the blood plasma of the patient with chronic illness may contain cold agglutinins, when he is transfused with cold blood he should be observed carefully and frequently for symptoms indicating hemolysis of cells. Hemolysis may result from the action of cold agglutinins in the serum of the donor on the red cells of the recipient or from the action of cold agglutinins in the serum of the recipient on the red cells of the donor.

Besides the antigens and antibody systems just presented, there are other rare antigens that may be present in erythrocytes. In certain diseases, such as hemolytic anemia, the red cells of the person become sensitized to an antibody in his own serum. The cells of these patients, as well as those of persons who are Rh-negative and who have been sensitized to the Rh factor, react with Coombs' serum. Coombs' serum is prepared from the serum of rabbits exposed to human globulin. The rabbit serum then contains antibodies that will react with any human antibodies that are globulins. If the human red blood cells have any antibodies attached to them, the antihuman globulin will cause the red cells to agglutinate. Because Coombs' serum reacts only with the red blood cells that are sensitized in the living organism, and have antibodies (globulin) attached to their red blood cells, the test is useful in determining the presence of hemolyzing antibodies in the blood serum of the patient. One of the important uses of the Coombs' test is in determining the presence of antibodies against the Rh factor in a person with Rh-negative blood. When the test is performed by treating blood cells from the individual with Coombs' serum, it is called a direct Coombs' test. In the indirect Coombs' known cells are exposed to the patient's serum in order to identify antibodies in the patient's serum.

Second in importance to the discovery of blood groups was that sodium citrate was safe in certain circumstances and could be used to prevent the clotting of blood. The citrate ion combines with the calcium ion. Ionized calcium is necessary for the clotting of the blood. Before this discovery, blood had to be transferred immediately from one person to another, usually by direct transfusion. When sodium citrate is added to blood, it prevents blood clotting and simplifies the transfer of the blood from the donor to the recipient.

STORAGE OF BLOOD

A more recent innovation, the development of methods for the refrigeration and storage of blood, has made even greater delay possible. Because the life span of erythrocytes is from 100 to 120 days, the oxygen-carrying capacity of blood continues for some time. However, blood that is three weeks old or older is considered to be too old. White blood cells and platelets die within a few hours after blood is drawn. Therefore, when their action is desired, the blood must be freshly drawn. Freshly drawn blood can be used to restore any of the elements of the blood. Stored blood is satisfactory for restoring the blood volume, erythrocytes, and the blood proteins, but it is of no value in the replacement of platelets or leukocytes. In the seriously undernourished patient, blood is sometimes administered for its nutritive value. For example, each pint of blood contains approximately 35 g of protein in the form of plasma protein. Cellular elements are further sources of protein and other nutrients.

An average of 1 person in 80 will require a blood transfusion within the next year, and some of these individuals will require as many as 40 pints of blood. In fact, a patient who is dialyzed weekly on an artificial kidney may use as much as 416 pints during a year. Where does all this blood come from and how is it obtained? In the past, most of the blood was donated, but because too few people donated their blood, more and more blood has to be purchased. In addition to the cost and the possibility of the price rising greatly, blood that is purchased from a commercial agency is much less reliable than donated blood; people who sell their blood are more likely to misrepresent ttheir medical histories. Blood-borne diseases for which there is no ready method of identification include hepatitis and malaria. The protection of the patient depends on the honesty of the potential donor in admitting he has had either or both of these diseases.

Blood is obtained by two different types of agencies; one is voluntary and the other commercial. Voluntary agencies include the Red Cross, hospital blood banks, and community blood banks. Commercial blood banks, located in large cities, collect, process, and distribute blood for the purpose of making a profit. They depend on paid donors for blood, and the risk that the blood will carry organisms of one or more of the blood-borne diseases is therefore greater.

BLOOD DONATIONS

There are a number of explanations for the decrease in blood donations, despite an adequate number of persons who meet the criteria for blood donors. According to *Changing Times,*[21] if every eligible person gave blood, the supply would be ten times the need. That there are actually more people who are eligible to give blood than are needed is demonstrated by the experience in Delaware where there is a nonprofit blood-replacement program covering 40 per cent of the people of the state. Persons participating in this plan agree to donate blood when they are called upon. Although this plan has been in operation for eight years, some persons are now only being asked to contribute their second pint of blood. Through the organization of the community, the needs of persons requiring blood have been met without any individual being required to make a great sacrifice.

Multiple factors, mostly psychological and cultural, account for the failure of people to donate blood in proportion to the need and their capacity to give. In some communities two or more agencies may work cooperatively or vie with each other to collect blood from willing and available donors. The Red Cross is the largest single agency collecting blood, but it does not have centers in some communities and does not completely fill the need in others.

Many persons who have not donated blood hesitate to do so because they fear the consequences to themselves or the unpleasantness of the procedure. There are altruistic and selfish reasons for donating blood. There is no more personal way of helping one's fellow man than by donating blood. Many voluntary agencies encourage individuals to donate blood by promising that should they or a member of their families need blood within a specified period of time, it will be available. In terms of safety, a healthy person who is between the ages of 18 and 59 can give blood every eight to ten weeks for an indefinite period of time without his health being threatened.[22]

[21] "The Blood Bank Mess," *Changing Times,* 17:26 (July) 1963.
[22] The Red Cross has a well-organized plan for blood donors. They accept as a donor any healthy adult 18 through 60 years of age who weighs at least 110 lb. Those under 21 years of age must have written consent of a parent or guardian, unless they are married. Unmarried minors may be donors without written consent of a parent or guardian if they are living away from home and are self-supporting or if they are members of the armed services. Donors are allowed to give blood every eight weeks but not more than five times in a calendar year.

In the previously cited article in *Changing Times,* a manager of a nonprofit blood-collecting agency is quoted as saying that giving blood is not a status symbol. In factories, proportionately more blood is donated by the men on the assembly line that by union stewards or office personnel, and the executive class gives least of all. Because blood for transfusion is essential to save lives, nurses have a responsibility to help to interpret to the public why it is needed and why the donation of blood is safe and is a source of satisfaction to the donor.

HAZARDS IN BLOOD TRANSFUSION

As indicated, blood transfusion can be a source of danger as well as benefit. The dangers may result from (1) transmission of blood-borne diseases, (2) transfusion of incompatible blood, and (3) too rapid infusion of blood into the individual. Under appropriate circumstances all of the above can be life threatening.

Diseases Transmitted

Of the diseases that may be transmitted through blood transfusions, those that are of the greatest concern are syphilis, malaria, and homologous serum jaundice (serum hepatitis). Persons who have syphilis can be identified by one of a number of serological tests. Each of these tests is named after the man who originated it (Kline, Kahn, and Hinton). These tests depend on the presence of an antibody-like substance (sometimes called reagin) in the blood serum. It appears in the patient's blood serum soon after the onset of the disease. Those who have a history of having had malaria or who have been in a malarious area within a two-month period are not used as blood donors.

Although persons having a history of jaundice are not used as blood donors, a person can have hepatitis without apparent jaundice and thus be unaware that he can transfer the hepatitis virus when his blood is transfused into a recipient. In the United States, hepatitis is probably the most common disease to be transmitted by transfusion. Because of the possibility of serum hepatitis, some physicians avoid the administration of blood unless it is absolutely essential. Serum hepatitis may develop up to 120 days after transfusion and is associated with a high mortality and morbidity rate. For example, four months ago Mrs. Seven was delivered by cesarean section of a 6-lb baby boy. She required a blood transfusion. Two months after delivery she became ill. Because she was acutely ill and jaundiced, she was admitted to the hospital for diagnosis. Although her progress was satisfactory, she had to spend six weeks in the hospital. Until there are methods of identifying carriers of the virus that produces jaundice, this condition will remain one of the major risks that occur with the transfusion of blood.

Infusion of Incompatible Blood

A second danger, the infusion of incompatible blood, is present in every blood transfusion. That it does not happen more often is a tribute to the care that is taken from the moment the blood is taken from a donor until it is infused into a recipient. As indicated, the transfusion of incompatible blood results in the agglutination and hemolysis of the erythrocytes of the donor by isoagglutinins in the blood plasma of the recipient. Should the blood plasma of the donor have a high titer of isoagglutinins, the erythrocytes of the recipient can also be agglutinated. Such cells tend to be hemolyzed more readily than normal. Signs and symptoms are caused by the blocking of blood vessels by agglutinated cells or hemolysis of cells. Among the usual signs and symptoms are back pain, icterus, tightness in the chest, or a sensation of burning of the face. There may be some degree of collapse, chills, fever, and a rapid pulse. Hemoglobin may appear in the urine and anuria may develop. This anoxia may be caused by a blocking of the renal tubules by hematin that is released on hemolysis of red cells and/or reduced blood flow through the kidney.

Although not all transfusion reactions caused by the infusion of incompatible blood are accompanied by serious effects, they may be. In addition, mild reactions in seriously ill or depleted patients may have grave consequences. To make sure that the patient receives properly matched blood, hospitals have rules regulating the collection and labeling of blood, the removal of blood from the blood bank, and the identification of the patient who is to receive the blood. All of these regulations are for the purpose of protecting patients from receiving mismatched blood. They should be meticulously followed.

All labels for blood taken from a patient for typing and cross matching should include the full name of the patient, diagnosis, the name of his physician, and his hospital or clinic number. This information should be printed or written legibly. The possibility always exists that two patients with identical names and diagnoses may be present in the hospital at the same time. An added precaution to the complete labeling of all slips is to have the slips made at the bedside at the time the blood is drawn. In some hospitals only the physician is allowed to remove blood from the blood bank. As a further precaution, only one unit may be removed at a time. Blood taken from the blood bank should be labeled with the names of the patient and the donor, the date the blood was drawn, the blood group, and the hospital where the blood is to be administered. The safety of the patient depends on all persons paying strict attention to details, so that unsafe acts are prevented.

What are the manifestations of a transfusion reaction?

Despite the precautions instituted to protect the patient from incompatible blood, transfusion reactions do occur. Any time a patient has any of the signs or symptoms attributable to incompatible blood, the transfusion must be discontinued at once. Even small amounts of mismatched blood can cause a serious reaction. The remaining blood should be saved and returned to the blood bank where it is rechecked for incompatibility and for bacterial contamination. Following a transfusion reaction the urine output of the patient should be measured and the first specimen should be saved. If the patient develops any renal failure, he should be weighed daily and his fluid intake adjusted to his output. (See Chapter 9.)

Infusions of blood are frequently administered by a "double setup." One tube is attached to the bottle of blood and another to a bottle of physiological saline or glucose in water solution. The two tubes join leading to the patient by means of a Y tube. The flow of blood or fluid into the patient can be regulated by opening or closing the tubing leading from one or the other of the bottles. If glucose is to follow a transfusion, the tubing should first be rinsed with saline to prevent blood clotting.

Another hazard to the patient is the too rapid infusion of the blood. Too much blood or blood given too rapidly may cause heart failure, which may be severe enough to produce pulmonary edema. Judgment as to the rate at which blood is to be administered is the responsibility of the physician. At times, when a large volume of blood has been lost in a short period of time, the life of the patient may depend on blood volume being restored rapidly. Almost continuous monitoring of the central venous pressure is vital in such patients. In other instances, blood must be administered slowly to protect the circulation from overload. Occasionally, when danger of overload is especially great, most of the plasma is removed and only the packed red blood cells are transfused. The responsibilities of the nurse are two: One is to maintain the rate of flow as prescribed by the physician and the other is to observe the patient for evidence indicating the development of any type of reaction to transfusion—in addition to the rate of flow of blood; vital signs including temperature, pulse, and respiration; and symptoms reported by the patient such as apprehension, feeling overly warm, or back pain. Although the temperature is not routinely checked during the administration of a transfusion, a rise in temperature frequently occurs earlier than most other signs and symptoms. Should any of these signs or symptoms occur, blood flow should be terminated until the physician has had an opportunity to check the patient. The physician should be notified immediately.

Besides the dangers already cited, the blood or equipment used may contain a variety of substances that cause varied types of reactions. Before the introduction of plastic disposable sets, the tubing used for blood transfusion sometimes contained pyrogenic materials capable of causing a febrile reaction. This type of reaction is not usually serious, though it may be a problem in debilitated patients. Urticaria sometimes occurs during a transfusion reaction. Although the cause is usually not found, it may be caused by the sensitivity of the patient to some untested substance in the blood of the donor.

Certain patients are more likely to develop transfusion reactions. For example, some blood dyscrasias, as well as repeated blood transfusions over a period of time, appear to predispose to reaction. Although all patients should be conscientiously observed during blood transfusion, those who are predisposed to reaction should be even more carefully observed.

In addition to the transfusion of whole blood, some fraction of the blood such as plasma, packed erythrocytes, or platelets may be administered. Plasma or a plasma expander is utilized when the requirements for blood replacement are very large, when blood is not immediately available, or when the plasma portion of the blood is diminished out of proportion to the red cells. For example, Mrs. Norman has second- and third-degree burns over two thirds of her body. She received these burns when she attempted to light a wood stove by throwing gasoline on some smoldering wood. The fire blazed up and ignited her clothing. Shortly after she was admitted, her hematocrit was elevated to 60 per cent. The increased concentration of her blood was the result of the loss of plasma into the burned area. Saline and blood plasma were then infused in an effort to restore her plasma volume. Plasma and plasma expanders are more effective than solutions of glucose or electrolytes because they remain in the blood vessels longer and contribute to the osmotic pressure of the blood. If the osmotic pressure falls too low, fluid tends to leave the vascular system and the patient becomes edematous. Because blood is pooled in the preparation of plasma, plasma is more likely to be contaminated with the virus of hepatitis than is whole blood. Storage of plasma at room temperature for six months usually removes any risk that hepatitis will be transmitted by the plasma. Packed red cells are administered to increase the oxygen-carrying power of the blood without causing a comparable increase in the blood volume.

THERAPEUTIC USES OF BLOOD

In addition to the previously cited uses of blood in therapy, blood transfusion makes certain forms of treatment possible. Many surgical procedures could not be performed today were it not for the availability of human blood and the ability to transfuse it safely. Many patients undergoing prolonged surgical procedures require from 2 to 10 pints or more of blood to maintain an adequate blood volume and oxygen-carrying capacity. The more extended the operation and the greater the loss of blood, the more blood is needed. Some surgical procedures could not be started without blood. Although the newer types of pumps used in heart surgery require little or no blood for priming, a large quantity of blood may be used before the procedure is completed. As much as 500 to 700 ml of blood are required to prime an artificial kidney. Some treatments such as total-body irradiation could not be performed were it not for the ability to replace the cellular elements of the blood.

The uses of blood transfusion, whatever the nature of the patient's illness, can be summarized as follows:

1. To restore blood volume.
2. To restore red blood cells.
3. To provide platelets or other factors important in clotting.
4. To provide protein and/or other nutritive elements.

Of the preceding, the first two are the most common purposes of blood transfusion. The need for either may arise out of conditions that are treated medically or surgically. Despite the frequency with which blood transfusions are administered, they are always attended by the possibility of a serious complication. The patient should always be under the surveillance of a doctor or a nurse.

By virtue of the nature of surgical treatment, the patient almost always loses some blood. The significance of the bleeding, in terms of its threat to the survival of the patient, depends on the degree to which the circulation to the cells is maintained. Although shock can and does exist in the absence of blood loss, hemorrhage increases the ease with which a patient may go into shock from any cause.

Surgery and the Gastrointestinal System

Not only are the functions of the respiratory and circulatory systems threatened by the various aspects of surgical therapy, but the functioning of the gastrointestinal system is also affected. As emphasized earlier, the gastrointestinal tract is very sensitive to the state of health of an individual. Furthermore, the sympathoadrenal system, which is activated by the physical and psychological stress of surgery, depresses the activity of the alimentary canal. Some disturbance in the functioning of the alimentary canal is, therefore, to be expected in patients who have been anesthetized and have undergone surgical treatment. The effects are usually manifested as anorexia, nausea, and vomiting. These effects may persist for several hours or days. Because of the inactivity of the alimentary canal, bowel sounds are usually absent for at least several hours after general anesthesia.

In patients who have surgery on the gastrointestinal tract, function returns more slowly. It usually takes two or three days for the patient to be able to tolerate fluids and for the normal bowel sounds to appear. All the preceding effects are normal accompaniments of surgical treatment and do not constitute complications unless they are prolonged or unusually severe. To prevent overdistention of the bowel and to increase the comfort of the patient whose gastrointestinal functioning is expected to be slow in returning, nasogastric suction may be instituted. Because the responsibilities of the nurse in the care of the patient treated with nasogastric suction were discussed earlier in the chapter, they will not be repeated here. After nasogastric suction has been discontinued, symptoms such as a feeling of fullness and nausea indicate that the gastrointestinal tract of the patient is not ready to tolerate fluids. As indicated earlier, developing abdominal distention can be detected early by measuring the abdomen with a tape measure.

When the bowel sounds are returning, but before water is tolerated, other fluids such as ginger ale or a similar carbonated beverage may be tried. Some patients find tea more acceptable than water or coffee. Dry crackers or toast may be better tolerated than fluids. Sitting the patient upright is sometimes helpful in preventing vomiting. Simple nursing procedures such as providing the patient with mouthwash after he vomits and emptying and washing the emesis basin promptly help to increase the comfort of the patient. Because suggestion sometimes plays a part in the continuance of vomiting, the emesis basin, although placed within easy reach, should be out of sight. When vomiting continues and there does not appear to be an organic basis for it, the physician may order a drug such as dimenhydrinate, U.S.P. (Dramamine), or chlorpromazine (Thorazine). Just as the character and amount of fluid removed in gastric suction should be observed and recorded, the characteristics of emesis such as odor, color, consistency, and the type or description of solid particles should be noted and recorded. Choking or a paroxysm of coughing during or after vomiting indicates the possibility of aspiration of vomitus. Evidence of aspiration should be reported to the physician. The circumstances under which the patient vomits are sometimes significant and should be observed. Should vomiting continue longer than is expected, a search should be made for its cause.

Because nausea and vomiting are frequent accompaniments of disease, by themselves these symptoms mean little more than that the patient is sick. Nausea and vomiting in the postsurgical patient can be caused by a great variety of disorders. These disorders may include idiosyncrasy to drugs, emotions, pain, shock, uremia, disturbances in water and electrolytes or acid-base balance. If the nausea and vomiting are persistent, it is more likely to be of serious surgical significance and is often associated with a physiological or mechanical obstruction somewhere along the alimentary canal.

Perhaps the simplest cause of vomiting in the postoperative patient is idiosyncrasy to a drug. An observant nurse may note that the vomiting occurred after the administration of a drug, such as morphine or meperidine hydrochloride. It is most severe soon after the drug is administered and recedes as the time for the next dose approaches.

Discomfort from gas pains following major surgery or trauma is not uncommon. Gas pains differ from vomiting in that they indicate that gastrointestinal function is returning but that its activity is not yet coordinated. Since the introduction of nasogastric suction and early ambulation, few patients have severe gas pains. When a patient does have severe gas pains, the insertion of a rectal tube or a small enema may provide relief. Both must be prescribed by the physician. The patient should be encouraged to be active and to walk. Because analgesic drugs such as morphine reduce the activity of the alimentary canal, they favor the development of gas pains. They should therefore be administered only as required to prevent pain in the postoperative patient.

What are some of the disturbances in gastrointestinal function that may occur postoperatively?

Although disturbances in gastrointestinal

function are more likely to be prolonged when a surgical procedure involves the gastrointestinal tract, peritoneum, or abdominal organs, they may follow any operative procedure. The three most serious gastrointestinal complications are acute gastric dilatation, paralytic ileus, and mechanical obstruction of the intestine. Both acute gastric dilatation and paralytic ileus may result from inadequate or abnormal peristalsis and/or abnormal swallowing of air. Obstruction may result from functional failure, or it may be the consequence of organic changes involving the wall of the digestive tube. Obstruction may occur soon after surgery or years later. Functional disturbances along the gastrointestinal tract tend to be self-perpetuating; that is, they act like a positive feedback system. As the motility of the digestive tube decreases, secretions and air accumulate, causing distention. Distention further inhibits motility. With the distention of the wall of the stomach or intestine, the wall thins and lessens the capacity of blood vessels to deliver blood. A vicious circle ensues: decreased motility → distention → thinning → decreased blood supply → decreased motility. When functional disturbances are accompanied by vomiting or the need for continued suction, they may also lead to hypovolemia and serious disturbances in water and electrolytes unless appropriate quantities of fluids and electrolytes are given intravenously.

Symptoms indicating that the function of the gastrointestinal tract is not returning as expected include (1) nausea and vomiting more than 12 to 24 hours after surgery (this may persist longer in patients having surgery on the gastrointestinal tract or in those with peritonitis), (2) distention of the abdomen, (3) pain in the abdomen (gas pain), (4) absent bowel sounds, and (5) evidence of obstruction on x-ray. High-pitched, tinkling bowel sounds often indicate a mechanical obstruction of the bowel. Postoperatively, this is usually caused by a poorly functioning anastomosis, adhesions, or a hernia.

ACUTE GASTRIC DILATATION

In the patient who develops an acute gastric dilatation, prodromal symptoms may include a feeling of fullness, hiccoughs, and retching. Overflow vomiting may also occur. The patient vomits small amounts of dark-colored, foul-smelling fluid. Gastric dilatation may develop rapidly and present a picture of acute shock. Unless the stomach is emptied and kept empty until function returns, death is a possibility. The nurse assists in the prevention of acute gastric dilatation by maintaining the function of the gastric suction apparatus and by regulating the

amount of fluid that the patient ingests orally until the capacity of the gastrointestinal tract to tolerate fluids has been tested. The nurse also helps to prevent the gastric dilatation from becoming serious by reporting early signs and symptoms indicating that gastrointestinal function has not been re-established.

ADYNAMIC ILEUS

In adynamic ileus the motor activity of the gastrointestinal tract is not strong or coordinated enough to maintain normal peristalsis. As a result the normal bowel sounds do not return as expected. Loops of small and large intestine fill with gas, but neither gas nor feces are passed by rectum. Gastric suction and the insertion of a rectal tube may relieve the symptoms. When distention is not relieved by gastric suction, a long tube may be necessary to decompress the more distal small bowel.

MECHANICAL OBSTRUCTION

Although it does not usually cause difficulty during the first hours after surgery, fecal impaction is another problem that arises from disturbances in the function of the gastrointestinal tract. It may result when barium is introduced into the alimentary canal and incompletely removed prior to surgery. As the water is absorbed from the barium, it forms a hard mass similar to a plaster cast. Barium impactions can usually be prevented by the removal of the barium within one to two days after the x-ray examination is completed. This can be accomplished by the administration of a mild laxative and/or cleansing enemas. Both of these must be prescribed by the physician. Identification of the need for such a prescription is a responsibility of the nurse. She should also be alert to signs and symptoms indicating that a barium impaction has been formed. Should the enema fail to remove the barium, this should be reported and recorded. Aged patients may also develop fecal impactions either following surgery or in the course of an illness. Symptoms that suggest the presence of an impaction include painful defecation, a feeling of fullness in the rectum, pain in the rectum, and constipation or a diarrhea-like stool. A rectal examination reveals a hard mass that may have to be broken up before it can be passed.

To lessen the possibility of fecal impactions, some surgeons prescribe mineral oil for the patient the day before surgery and for a few days after gastrointestinal function is resumed. Some surgeons also prescribe an enema for the patient on the second or third day postsurgery or after there is evidence that gastrointestinal activity has resumed. Others do not believe that enemas are necessary. When enemas are given, the extent of their effectiveness should be reported. Especially in elderly patients, not only should the fact that feces were evacuated be noted but also the size of the stool should be described. Symptoms indicating the possible development of a fecal impaction should be reported and recorded.

As soon as the gastrointestinal tract begins to function normally, as evidenced by the presence of bowel sounds, absence of abdominal distention, and/or the passage of feces or gas per rectum, fluids and food may be ordered by the surgeon. The length of time that oral food and fluids are withheld varies with the nature of the surgical procedure, the type of anesthetic used, and the response of the patient. Usually patients having operations on the alimentary canal are not able to tolerate food as early as those having surgery on other parts of the body. When fluids are first administered, the volume may be restricted to 15 to 30 ml per hour and increased gradually to fluids as desired. Fluids should be discontinued and the physician notified if the patient vomits, becomes distended, or complains of a feeling of fullness. (See Chapter 12.)

When a patient was reasonably healthy before surgery, his appetite can be expected to return within a few days. Except in those patients who have special requirements, patients are returned to a full diet as soon as they are able to tolerate it. Patients having surgery on the stomach usually require some reduction in the volume of food eaten at one time. The consistency may also be modified by reducing the amount of roughage contained in it. The objectives are to prevent distention of the stomach with strain on the sutures and to meet the nutritional requirements of the patient. Thus the patient is fed four to six small meals each day. Foods having a high cellulose content, such as cabbage and cucumbers, are eliminated.

All patients require an adequate intake of protein and vitamin C. Because the nutritional requirements of persons undergoing severe stress are discussed in Chapter 12, they will not be further elaborated on here.

Surgery and Renal Function

In the period immediately following surgery, or a traumatic injury, the formation of urine by the kidney is depressed. Oliguria is generally believed to be caused by an increase in the production of the antidiuretic hormone (ADH) by the posterior pituitary gland. Accompanying the retention of water is sodium retention, which may be the result of an increase in the production of the adrenal cortical steroids. Because of this tendency to retain salt and water after injury (surgery), the urine output of the patient is likely to be decreased below normal levels for the first 12 to 24 hours after operation. This oliguria may be prevented to a certain extent by infusion of adequate amounts of fluid before, during, and after surgery. Following a period of oliguria, the patient may have a period of diuresis. In patients who have been in severe shock for an extended period of time, oliguria or even anuria may continue for days or even weeks. Unless the fluid intake of the patient with renal failure is balanced against his fluid output, he may die from overloading with water. Because of the possibility of continued suppression of urine following surgery, the accurate measurement and recording of the urine output and the fluid intake for the first days following surgery are of great importance. Measurement of the specific gravity and/or osmolality of the urine is also important. Small quantities of urine with a high specific gravity are usually indicative of dehydration, hypovolemia, and/or poor renal perfusion. If the specific gravity is low, the diagnosis is more difficult and the oliguria may be at least partially related to renal disease or failure.

URINARY RETENTION

In addition to the possibility of oliguria or anuria, a considerable number of patients experience retention of urine; that is, they are unable to void during the early postoperative period. Retention of urine can be a troublesome condition. In some patients who undergo surgery in the region of the bladder, such as gynecologic surgery, or in operations on the large bowel or rectum, the ability to empty the bladder is often temporarily depressed.

Another cause of urinary retention is that some patients cannot void in bed. The position is abnormal and psychological conditioning against it may be very strong. In surgical patients the frequency of urinary retention has been reduced by early ambulation. Patients who are not allowed to be out of bed may be permitted to stand beside the bed or to use a bedside commode. One or more of a variety of nursing measures can sometimes be employed successfully to induce voiding when a patient finds it difficult. Because tenseness of the patient aggravates the problem, the approach to the patient should be relaxed and the patient protected from anxiety-provoking situations. A screen around the bed or in front of the door will help to shield the patient from unexpected visitors. A warm bedpan is a necessity. Relaxation is sometimes encouraged by placing the feet of the patient in warm water. Suggestion sometimes works. Water is allowed to run from the tap, or warm water is poured over the vulva of a woman. When the bladder is not overly full, the patient may be urged to try to void and, if he is not able, to try at a later time. One thing to be avoided is to encourage the patient to try too hard, as he then becomes overly tense and is unable to relax the sphincters in the urethra.

CATHETERIZATION FOR THE TREATMENT OF URINARY RETENTION

When other measures are ineffective in encouraging the patient to void, or the nature of the surgical procedure is such that the bladder should not be allowed to become distended, catheterization may become necessary. When catheterization is required, it must be prescribed by the physician, and he makes the decision about whether the patient is to be catheterized when the bladder is full, at regular intervals, or whether an indwelling catheter be inserted. Two objectives should guide the nurse in her preparations for, and performance of, catheterization. The first is to remove urine from the bladder. The second is no less important than the first and is more difficult to achieve. It is to prevent infection of the urinary tract. To prevent infection, all equipment and materials should be sterile, the procedure itself should be clean, and trauma to urethra and bladder avoided. To prevent trauma to the bladder, it should not be permitted to become overdistended. Overdistention predisposes to breaks in the continuity of the mucosa and diminishes the blood supply to the wall of the bladder. The danger of trauma to the bladder and urethra by the catheter can be lessened by using the smallest possible catheter, lubricating it well, and encouraging the patient to relax. The lubricant lessens friction by preventing the catheter from coming in direct contact with the wall of the urethra. Relaxation can usually be achieved by asking the patient to take a deep breath at the moment the catheter is introduced. The patient should have been prepared for what to expect and he should be adequately covered, so that his modesty pattern is observed. Should an obstruction to the passage of the catheter be encountered, the catheter should not be forced. It will usually slip into the bladder if the pressure on the catheter is reduced and the patient is asked to take a deep breath. When the catheter is in place, it must be held there, as the pressure of the urine in the bladder is likely to carry it out. Should the catheter escape from the urethra, another sterile catheter must be introduced.

To minimize the number of microorganisms introduced into the bladder, a number of precautions should be taken. The catheter and lubricant should be sterile; and the catheter should be well lubricated. The area around the meatus should be well cleansed with a bacteriostatic agent. To prevent pushing bacteria normally present in the terminal meatus into the urinary bladder, the urethra may be irrigated by inserting a sterile Asepto syringe about three fourths of an inch into the urethra and irrigating it with 1 ounce of 1:1,000 aqueous benzalkonium chloride solution, or an antibacterial lubricant may be used.

To adequately expose the meatus, the patient should be in the recumbent position, with the knees flexed and the legs separated. A good light placed to illuminate the area is essential. Unless the patient is in a position that permits adequate exposure of the meatus, the nurse cannot see what she is doing, the catheter is likely to be contaminated before it is introduced, and urethral trauma is more difficult to prevent. If the catheter becomes contaminated before it is introduced, another sterile catheter should be obtained.

Unnecessary discomfort to the patient should be prevented. In patients who have surgery on the perineum, exposure of the meatus may be painful. This discomfort can be minimized by preparing the patient for what to expect and by assuring the patient that every effort will be made to handle the tissues with gentleness. When the patient to be catheterized is a male, the female nurse should still provide the same instruction and precautions for him as she does for a female patient. In relation to the procedure itself, she is responsible for setting up the equipment and obtaining a doctor, a nurse, or a qualified male attendant to catheterize the patient. Catheterization can usually be performed with a minimum of distress to the patient. Time must be taken to prepare the patient for what to expect and for what he or she can do to assist the nurse. Another precaution is that urine should not be drained off too fast from a greatly distended bladder. Sudden rapid decompression of the bladder may cause shock or hemorrhage from the bladder.

CARE OF AN INDWELLING CATHETER

When an indwelling catheter is left in place, attention should be given to the maintenance of continuous free drainage. The tubing should be free of kinks, twists, or bends, and from pressure of resting body parts. It should be arranged so that the urine flows downhill into the drainage bottle. When prescribed by the physician, the catheter should also be irrigated at regular intervals to ensure its patency; this procedure should be carried out according to strict surgical aseptic principles. One way to irrigate the catheter, which is equally as effective and which eliminates the possibility of introducing microorganisms, is to make certain that the patient has an adequate fluid intake. Ansell [23] suggests that, when possible, the fluid intake should be sufficient to produce a flow rate of 50 ml of urine an hour, thus preventing the upward migration of motile bacteria in the collection tubing. He further urges the use of "bacteriologically sealed drainage systems with antiseptic in the collecting bottle to prevent growth of any possible contaminant." Because cranberry juice helps to keep the urine acid, it may be offered to patients who find it acceptable; acid urine inhibits bacterial growth.

When the patient has an indwelling catheter, a sterile closed drainage system with an antiseptic added to the collecting container should be used. Disposable collecting systems are available and are safer and more convenient than glass bottles. A rigid collecting container should be used for ambulatory patients. The tubing leading from the bladder should be below the level of the bladder but above the level of the urine. (See Figure 17-4.) The area around the meatus should be washed at least twice daily with a bacteriostatic agent such as pHisoHex or 1:1,000 aqueous benzalkonium chloride solution.

After the catheter is removed, the quantity of each voiding should be measured accurately so that retention with overflow is detected should it occur. Frequent voiding of small amounts of urine may be indicative of retention with overflow. In the care of patients who are catheterized for retention of urine, the bladder should not be allowed to become overdistended, as overstretching of the mucosa predisposes to breaks in its continuity and diminishes the blood supply to the wall of the bladder. Both disorders predispose to infection of the urinary bladder. This applies especially to patients who are catheterized for retention with overflow. The overstretching of the muscle wall may also delay the return of normal function.

Urinary tract infection is a possibility in any patient who is subject to repeated catheterization or in whom the bladder is allowed to become overdistended or in whom urine is retained. Preventive measures include an adequate intake of fluids and prevention of overdistention of the bladder with urine. When catheterization is necessary, attention should be given to ". . . defend the drainage system's three portals of entry: the urethra, and urethral meatus, the connection between the catheter and the tubing, and the end of the drainage

tube." [24] Trauma to the urethra and bladder should also be avoided. Some physicians prescribe an antibiotic such as acetylsulfisoxazole (Gantrisin acetyl [25]) as a prophylactic measure for patients who have an indwelling catheter or who are subject to repeated catheterization. Others may prescribe, either alone or in conjunction with antibiotics, acidifying agents such as methenamine mandelate (Mandelamine [25]). Drugs should not, however, be considered a substitute for cleanliness and maintaining effective drainage.

The Later Postoperative Period

Not all complications following surgery occur in the immediate postoperative period. Two that are likely to be manifested later are venous thrombosis and pulmonary embolism. Pulmonary emboli usually result from venous thrombi that break off and block a portion of the pulmonary artery bed. Like complications occurring after surgical procedure, thromboembolic phenomena are not unique to the postsurgical patient. They may develop in any patient in whom the nature of the disorder or some other factor favors intravascular clotting. The capacity of the blood to clot under appropriate circumstances is a valuable defense against the loss of blood. In health, the factors causing the blood to clot are controlled so that its fluid state is maintained. Although the reasons for the formation of blood clots within blood vessels are not well understood, three factors are believed to contribute to the possibility: (1) a roughening of the vascular endothelium lining the blood vessel by a microorganism or a chemical or physical agent, (2) a stasis or slowing of blood flow, and (3) changes in the composition of the blood that increase its tendency to coagulate.

Venous Thrombosis

In health, damage to platelets and other elements in the blood is minimized by the smoothness of the vascular endothelium. Further protection is offered by the probability that a single layer of negatively charged molecules of protein repels negatively charged platelets and prevents the platelets from coming in contact with the vascular endothelium. Incident to surgery, as well as to disease, the vascular endothelium can be injured by microorganisms, trauma, or chemical agents with the result that

---

[23] Julian Ansell: "Some Observations on Catheter Care," *J. Chronic Dis.,* **15**:676 (July) 1962.

[24] Delores Santora: "Preventing Hospital-Acquired Urinary Infection," *Amer. J. Nurs.,* **66**:793 (Apr.) 1966.

[25] Trade name.

Body

Bladder

BEST

Bladder

Body

NO

Tubing
lower than
collecting
device

Bladder

Body

NO

Patient
lying on
tubing

FIGURE 17-4. Gravity bladder drainage systems. (After a drawing by Leola Hogan.)

it becomes roughened. The roughened surface increases the likelihood of thrombocytes being broken down. When the wall of a thrombocyte is ruptured, it releases thromboplastin, which, in the presence of calcium ions, reacts with pro-thrombin to form thrombin. Thrombin then interacts with the blood protein, fibrinogen, to form fibrin. The fibrin forms a network of long, sticky threads or strands that entraps, in a manner similar to sticky flypaper, platelets (thrombocytes) and red cells and forms a blood clot.

The second factor favoring the formation of blood clots in blood vessels is stasis, or slowing of the flow of blood. Inactivity combined with the supine or sitting position favors stasis in the veins of the legs. With a normal rate of blood flow, cells are concentrated in the center of the blood vessel and are separated from the intima by a layer of plasma. As the rate of blood flow slows, cells tend to leave the center core and move toward the periphery, where they come in contact with the intima. Thus stasis of blood is believed to increase the likelihood of venous thrombosis in patients who are predisposed by other factors to it.

One aspect of the response to surgical or other trauma and to disease is an increase in the tendency of the blood to clot. Inasmuch as this response contributes to the effectiveness of the self-sealing mechanism, it is homeostatic. Like other homeostatic mechanisms, it can also be the source of problems. A number of changes in the blood contribute to its increased tendency to clot. Thrombocytes increase in number and become sticky. Instead of repelling each other, they tend to adhere one to another. Leukocytosis also occurs. When dehydration is allowed to develop, all the solid elements, including platelets and fibrinogen, increase in proportion to plasma and further increase the tendency of the blood to clot. In the absence of an adequate clotting mechanism, the individual faces the possibility of hemorrhage. When it is too active or clotting occurs in inappropriate sites, the clotting mechanism is also a source of danger to the individual.

As stated previously, knowledge of why intravascular clotting occurs following surgery or trauma is incomplete. Although blood clots may form in any vein, deep veins in the lower extremities are most commonly affected. Something, perhaps a roughening of the endothelial lining of the vein, causes blood platelets to accumulate in that area. They release thromboplastin, which initiates the process of blood clotting. After a clot is formed, it continues to grow, provided the clot does not obstruct the flow of blood. The continued growth of the clot depends on blood flowing over it to provide the materials from which the clot is formed. Growth usually ceases when the clot reaches a site where the vein in which it is formed joins another vein. The rate of blood flow is increased at the point where two vessels unite; the thromboplastin in the blood from the vein containing the thrombus is diluted and its clotting effect is reduced. Clots formed in the deep veins in the calf of the leg may propagate into the femoral and iliac veins.

As the clot forms, the fibrinogen within the clot is converted into fibrin. If there are throm-

bocytes in the clot, the fibrin threads within the clot fold and pull the clot together, resulting in clot retraction. The clot is also invaded by macrophages that digest the red blood cells and release their hemoglobin into the body fluids. Later, fibroblasts enter and organize the clot, so that within a few weeks it becomes a firm, fibrous mass. After a period of months, all that may remain of the thrombus is a small fibrous band.

Although the factors responsible for intravascular clotting are not entirely clear, stasis seems to play a major role. Two of the benefits of early ambulation after surgery is the improvement in venous return from the legs and the reduction of thromboembolic complications. Many authorities disagree about the relationship of phlebothrombosis and thrombophlebitis. Some believe that these two conditions are phases of the same condition. Others state that they are two different conditions. Be that as it may, the predominating feature in phlebothrombosis is the formation of a blood clot. In thrombophlebitis the predominating characteristic is inflammation of the wall of the vein, which may extend to the surrounding tissue and involve lymphatic channels as well. In phlebothrombosis, the problem is to prevent the detachment of a portion of the clot. The floating clot, or embolus, in a vein is dangerous because it can block the flow of blood through the pulmonary arteries or its branches.

Pulmonary Emboli

Clots originating in the leg veins reach the right atrium and ventricle of the heart by way of the inferior vena cava. From the right ventricle, the embolus enters the pulmonary circulation via a pulmonary artery. It continues to move forward until it obstructs an artery through which it cannot pass. If the clot is large enough to obstruct more than half of the pulmonary circulation, the patient may die without warning or go into a severe shocklike state. Smaller clots move into the pulmonary circulation until they reach arteries too narrow for them to pass. They then obstruct the flow of blood to the area supplied by the occluded artery. This tissue, deprived of its blood supply, may die or become infarcted.

The symptoms and signs that accompany small emboli vary. The patient may have pain in the chest similar to the pain of pleurisy and described by the patient as a "catch in his chest" when he breathes. Hemoptysis (blood in the sputum) occurs in only a small percentage of patients. When there is hemoptysis, the sputum is brick red at first, but later it becomes dark red or brownish black. Small clots may also be expectorated. Although the patient usually has some fever, it rarely exceeds 101.5°F and lasts only four or five days. Most patients with pulmonary emboli may have only a relatively sudden onset of dyspnea. Any patient who suddenly becomes short of breath, especially 10 to 14 days after surgery, should be considered to have a pulmonary embolus until proved otherwise. The treatment of pulmonary embolism is basically that of treating the phlebothrombosis or thrombophlebitis that causes it.

Unlike phlebothrombosis, a massive embolus is not likely to be formed in thrombophlebitis. Thrombophlebitis is more likely to be followed by disturbances in venous drainage with the development of incompetent venous valves and chronic stasis of blood in the feet or legs.

PHLEBOTHROMBOSIS—SIGNS AND SYMPTOMS

Although patients with phlebothrombosis may have little in the way of signs or symptoms to indicate the presence of a clot, they may have a slight increase in temperature over normal levels. In some patients the temperature remains slightly elevated longer than is usual and there may be a small elevation in the leukocyte count. One of the most common symptoms is leg pain, usually in the calf. Should the patient mention the pain, he is likely to ascribe it to the fact that he is wearing slippers with heels that are lower than those to which he is accustomed. The patient may suffer only mild symptoms and go on to complete recovery or he may develop a severe form of thrombophlebitis or a pulmonary embolism. Only about half of the patients with pulmonary emboli have leg symptoms at the time of embolus.

THROMBOPHLEBITIS—SIGNS AND SYMPTOMS

In the patient who has a thrombophlebitis, symptoms may range from mild to exceedingly severe. At the site of the thrombus, the cardinal signs of inflammation may be marked. The concern of the surgeon in the care of the patient is the prevention of the changes that may lead to chronically dilated leg veins with insufficient valves.

As with other complications, prevention is preferred to cure. Authorities, however, do not agree as to the value of the various methods that are employed in prevention. With few exceptions, the following are stressed: early ambulation, leg exercises while the patient is in bed, avoidance of pressure against the leg and thigh by a pillow or knee roll, maintenance of sufficient fluid intake to prevent dehydration, and prevention of hypotension.

THERAPY

For the patient who is predisposed to intravascular clotting or who has already developed phlebothrombosis or thrombophlebitis, the physician may prescribe an anticoagulant such as heparin or bishydroxycoumarin or one of its substitutes. The action of heparin in preventing coagulation of the blood involves at least four interrelated effects: (1) It acts as antiprothrombin to prevent the conversion of prothrombin to thrombin. (2) It antagonizes the action of thromboplastin, by a mechanism not fully understood. (3) It prevents the conversion of fibrinogen to fibrin. (4) It prevents the agglutination or clumping of platelets. Bishydroxycoumarin produces its effect by inhibiting the synthesis of prothrombin. Because heparin interferes with the action of substances already present in the blood, its action is prompt. Because bishydroxycoumarin inhibits the synthesis of prothrombin, its maximum effect does not occur for from two to four days and its action continues for some days after it has been discontinued. There is little or no question about the effectiveness of heparin when it is given properly; the bishydroxycoumarin-like substances, on the other hand, have had conflicting reports on their ability to prevent or retard clotting. In patients in whom the anticoagulant effect is immediately required, heparin may be administered by intravenous or deep intramuscular injection until the bishydroxycoumarin has had an opportunity to be effective. Bishydroxycoumarin is almost always administered orally. All patients who are being treated with anticoagulant therapy should be observed for evidence of bleeding. Should it occur, the condition should be reported immediately. The physician may discontinue the drug or decrease the daily dosage. To reduce the danger of hemorrhage in the patient who is receiving bishydroxycoumarin or one of its substitutes, the prothrombin time is initially checked either daily or every other day. The objective is to keep it between 25 and 15 per cent of normal.

ELEVATION OF THE LEG

Bed rest with elevation of the affected leg is usually prescribed for the patient with thrombophlebitis. Although elevation of the leg is a simple procedure, its effectiveness in promoting venous return and the comfort of the patient depend on its being properly done. Because water runs downhill, distal parts should be higher than proximal parts. Support of the leg should extend along its entire length. Pillows should be placed so that they form a firm base under both the leg and thigh, and after they are in place, the muscles of the leg and thigh should appear to be relaxed. The pillows should look as if they were supporting the leg rather than the leg the pillows. Moreover, pillows have a way of becoming disarranged. Any position, no matter how comfortable at the beginning, becomes tiring. The obvious conclusion is that the nurse should check the patient regularly. He should have an opportunity to change his position and to have the supporting pillows rearranged, so that they continue to be supporting.

The physician may prescribe heat to be applied locally to the area. When warm, moist packs are used, they should be kept warm and some method should be employed to keep the bed dry. Chilling increases vasospasm and aggravates the condition.

Should the patient develop signs and symptoms indicating the possibility of a pulmonary embolism, the doctor should be notified immediately. In addition to anticoagulant therapy, the patient is placed on absolute bed rest and oxygen therapy is usually prescribed. Drugs to relieve the apprehension of the patient and to relax smooth muscle spasm may also be ordered. These include morphine, atropine, and papaverine. The development of a pulmonary embolism, especially a large one, is a frightening event for the patient, his family, and those responsible for his care. An embolism may occur during sleep or it may be associated with some ordinary activity such as getting out of bed or using the bedpan. Should the patient be out of bed at the onset of symptoms, he should be returned to bed and supported in a comfortable position. Should he be short of breath, he is likely to be more comfortable in a sitting than in a supine position. If at all possible, someone should remain with the patient until he is comfortable and his acute symptoms are relieved.

How can wound infection be prevented?

Perhaps the most nearly unique aspect of the surgical patient is the incision that is made to approach the organ to be operated upon. Many additional aspects of wound healing are discussed in Chapter 6. As emphasized earlier in this chapter, the incision disrupts one of the individual's most important defenses against infection. All patients who have surgery run a certain risk of developing an infection in the wound or operative site.

The prevention of wound infection depends to a great extent on the application of the principles of asepsis from the moment the patient is admitted to the hospital until the time of his discharge. Other factors contributing to its prevention include a proper state of nutrition. Not only does starvation with inadequate proteins and vitamins hinder wound healing and increase the chance of infection, but obesity also predisposes to wound infection. Adipose tissue is more vulnerable to infection than many other tissues because it has relatively poor blood supply and is difficult to approximate properly. The problem of wound infection is further considered in the section on wound healing.

Wound Disruption

Disruption of the wound is one of the serious sequelae of impaired wound healing. Separation of the wound may occur at any time following the closure of the incision. It may occur immediately after the wound is closed and before the patient has been transferred from the operating room or at some later time. A common time is about the seventh day. The degree to which the wound separates varies. When the skin as well as the underlying tissue separates and the contents of the abdominal cavity extrude, the condition is known as evisceration. Although disruption of any wound may occur, the most common site is in midline abdominal incisions.

Although wound disruption is possible in any patient, certain conditions in the various phases of surgery predispose to it. In the preoperative phase, obesity, undernutrition particularly of protein and vitamin C (ascorbic acid), conditions associated with metabolic disorders such as diabetes mellitus, Cushing's syndrome, and uremia, and advanced cancer or liver disease appear to predispose to impaired wound healing. Weight reduction, when a patient is obese, and attention to the nutritional status of patients during the preoperative period are important preventive measures. During the operative phase, many of the activities of the surgeon are directed toward making and closing the incision in such a manner that wound healing is favored or, conversely, is protected from disruption. Thus attention is given to the site and direction of the incision. Wound healing is a consideration in the selection of sutures and in the suturing technique. Careful hemostasis and the maintenance of asepsis are also important. With the exception of asepsis, all the preceding preventive measures are mainly the responsibility of the surgeon.

During the postoperative phase a variety of conditions predispose to separation of an abdominal incision. Perhaps the most frequent cause is some disorder that places strain on the incision by increasing intra-abdominal pressure. Thus separation of the wound is associated with abdominal distention, retching, unrelieved coughing, sneezing, hiccoughs, or uncontrollable motor activity. When any of these disorders exist, attention should be directed toward their relief. The nurse has a responsibility to report any of the disorders to the physician and to carry out measures for their relief. Should the surgeon believe that the patient is seriously predisposed to wound disruption or that separation of the wound is imminent, he may use special "retention sutures" that encompass all layers of the abdomen for 1 to 2 inches on either side of the incision and apply a binder to the abdomen of the patient.

SIGNS AND SYMPTOMS OF WOUND DISRUPTION

Staining of the dressing over the incision with a serosanguineous material, which looks very much like cherry soda, is a warning sign that wound disruption will possibly occur. At the time the wound separates a large amount of serosanguineous material may escape. The patient may feel something give or burst. He may call attention to the fluid by saying that the area around the wound felt as if warm water had been poured over it. He may have pain in the wound, which may be severe. In addition, he may vomit and develop signs of shock. When evisceration occurs, coils of intestine may protrude from the wound or escape into the bed, an extremely hazardous situation.

What are the responsibilities of the nurse when wound dehiscence or evisceration is impending or has occurred?

When there is evidence that wound dehiscence or evisceration is impending or has occurred, the physician should be immediately notified. At best, these sequelae to impaired wound healing are extremely serious. As little time as possible should be lost between the event and the initiation of treatment. The patient should be instructed to lie quietly on his back in a horizontal position. If coils of intestine can be seen, they should be covered with sterile towels or other sterile materials, which are kept moist with physiologic saline. Because wound disruption predisposes to shock, the patient's blood pressure should be determined and his pulse and respirations counted. When at all possible, a nurse should remain with the patient until he is seen by his physician. To assure the patient that all is being done that can be, he should be told that the physician has been notified and is coming. For most patients who are suddenly faced with a serious threat to their physical well-being, evidence that measures are being taken to correct the condition is in itself reassuring. They rightly interpret action as the appropriate activity. Preparations should be made for the physician. A nasogastric tube and suctioning equipment should be secured and the tube should be ready to insert. Because retching increases intra-abdominal pressure, a local anesthetic should be ready for use to anesthetize the pharynx. A mask and a sterile gown and gloves, as well as sterile towels, should be obtained for the surgeon. Sterile saline should be warmed and available. If intravenous fluids are not running they should be made available for starting by the physician. When the surgeon arrives, he will decide on the place and type of therapy. When the condition of the patient permits, most surgeons prefer to have the patient transferred to the operating room for treatment. In the process of transferring the patient, enough help should be available to move the patient without increasing his intra-abdominal pressure. Depending on the extent to which the tissues are separated and on the condition of the patient, the surgeon may support the incision by taping the abdomen or return the patient to surgery for a secondary closure.

Other Signs and Symptoms of Surgical Trauma

In addition to the signs and symptoms already discussed in relation to the effect of surgical trauma, pain, fever, and hiccough must also be mentioned. Although pain and fever always occur, severe hiccoughs are uncommon.

PAIN

One of the most common manifestations of illness is pain and fear of pain. In the minds of many people some illnesses, such as cancer, as well as certain treatments, such as surgery, are practically synonymous with pain. The nurse has a siginficant role in both the prevention and relief of pain. She should be able:

1. To make the observations necessary for deciding whether or not a patient is in pain.
2. To institute appropriate action to prevent or to alleviate pain.
3. To observe the effects of measures used to relieve pain.

To fulfill her role with understanding, the nurse requires some knowledge of (1) the nature of pain, (2) the anatomy and physiology of pain, (3) what constitutes the pain experience, (4) the factors increasing the suffering caused by pain, (5) the physiological and emotional responses to pain, (6) signs or other evidence of pain, and (7) the measures useful in the therapy of pain.

What is the nature of pain?

The fact that pain is a private and personal experience is not to be denied. No one except the person who is in pain knows how much pain he has, or its exact nature, or what the pain means to him. There is a poverty of words in the English language to describe pain. The words used by the patient to describe his pain are chosen on the basis of what he thinks is happening. He uses words such as crushing, boring, burning, prickling, or gnawing. For many centuries and until recently, pain was not classified as a sensation but as the antithesis of pleasure. Despite extensive study, pain had never been defined to the satisfaction of all scientists. Most definitions, however, include the following points: (1) pain is a sensory perception; (2) pain has a psychic component; (3) pain is unpleasant; (4) pain, even when it is localized, involves the whole person; and (5) pain is useful to the extent that it causes the individual to seek help in determining its cause and in securing relief. On the other hand, fear of pain may cause a person to delay seeking necessary treatment.

THE ANATOMY AND PHYSIOLOGY OF PAIN

Knowledge of pain as a sensation has come about during the last hundred years or so. Keats and Lane [26] state that most of the progress in the treatment of pain has been made in the therapy of specific pain. Nonspecific pain is one of the unsolved problems in clinical medicine. To illustrate the magnitude of the problem the *Physician's Desk Reference* for 1968 lists approximately 64 different systemic analgesics. Until relatively recently the anatomy of pain has been described in terms of specific pain receptors, pain fibers, and pain centers in the central nervous system. Melzack [27] states that the modern view of pain is not that it is a single sensation but that it is a complex experience that involves the total individual. The anatomy of the sensory perception of pain is fairly well known; that of the complex experience is just beginning to be identified. Knowledge of the latter is at the point where there is sufficient knowledge to make hypotheses but not enough to be sure that the hypotheses are correct. Haugen [28] states that there are two pathways that carry pain impulses to the central nervous system, one conducting impulses rapidly and the other conducting them slowly. Like other sensory perceptions, pain impulses are transmitted from receptors to spinal tracts by way of mixed peripheral nerves. Keats and Lane [29] also state that pain impulses are transmitted over two sets of nerve fibers, both of which are present in all peripheral nerves. In one system, known as the A delta fibers, the fibers are large and myelinated. They conduct impulses rapidly.

In the other, or the C fibers, the fibers are small and unmyelinated and they conduct pain impulses slowly. The two systems contribute somewhat differently to the pain experience. The A delta fibers alert the individual to the presence of pain and localize it. The C fibers contribute to the suffering in pain. Keats and Lane summarize the pain pathways as shown in Figure 17-5. The A delta fibers, which are myelinated, pass more or less directly to the thalamus and the sensory areas in the cerebral cortex. The collateral system connects with the reticular formation and provides for slower conduction than does the main pathway. In addition, it has many diffuse connections with many centers in the brain. These fibers are unmyelinated. The suggestion has been made that the role of the collateral system is to integrate information from many sources and to modify the reaction of the individual to pain. Melzack [30] states that fibers have been identified that go from the brain to message-carrying nerve pathways in the spinal cord. These fibers modify impulses coming into the spinal cord over sensory fibers. As a consequence, impulses may be suppressed and never get beyond the level of the spinal cord, or be altered so that the message that is delivered is different from the one that originated the impulse. According to Melzack,[31] a portion of the sensory nerve impulse entering the spinal cord or brain stem passes over a dense network of interconnecting internuncial neurons. Although not proved, this may be the point at which memory, thoughts, and emotion modify sensory messages after injury. There is experimental and psychological evidence to support the assumption that higher centers in the brain do modify sensory nerve impulses at various lower levels. In time, the pathways whereby higher centers influence lower centers will undoubtedly be identified.

Sensation of any type requires not only pathways for the conduction of impulses and centers for their interpretation and integration but receptors that are sensitive to painful stimuli. Formerly it was believed that there were specific pain receptors in the skin. The current view is that the skin contains widely branching bushy networks of receptors that overlap one another and are stimulated by noxious stimuli, including stretching of the tissue. When the stimulus approaches the point of tissue damage, the resulting sensation is interpreted as pain. The point at which the individual interprets sensory stimulation as pain is known as sensory pain perception. In our present state of knowledge, the thalamus appears to function in the awareness to pain. The thalamus has, however,

[26] Arthur S. Keats and Montague Lane: "The Symptomatic Therapy of Pain," *DM*, p. 3 (June) 1963.
[27] Ronald Melzack, "The Perception of Pain," *Sci. Amer.*, **204**:49 (Feb.) 1961.
[28] Frederick P. Haugen: "Current Concepts of the Pain Process," *J. Chronic Dis.*, 4:9 (July) 1956.
[29] *Op. cit.*, p. 4.
[30] *Op. cit.*, p. 44.
[31] *Ibid.*

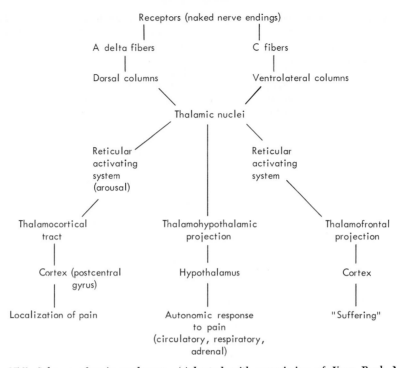

FIGURE 17-5. Schema of pain pathways. (Adapted with permission of Year Book Medical Publishers, Inc., from "The Symptomatic Therapy of Pain," *Disease-A-Month*, June 1963, p. 7, by Arthur S. Keats and Montague Lane.)

connections with many areas of the brain. The cerebral cortex is presumed to function in the localization of pain and in the recognition of its nature, severity, and significance.

THE PAIN EXPERIENCE

The integrity of sensory mechanisms is essential to the perception of pain. Occasionally a child is born who lacks pain and temperature receptors in his skin. Although this deficit does not interfere with the survival of the child, he lacks one of the mechanisms for learning to protect himself from injury. More common is the individual who, because of disease, injury, or therapy, is deprived of structures or functions enabling him to perceive or interpret pain sensations. The individual then must learn how to protect the tissues thus deprived from injury and to inspect them for evidence of injury. For example, Melvin Gale suffered a transection of his spinal cord at the level of the first lumbar vertebra. He was completely paralyzed below the point of injury. For the remainder of his life, measures must be instituted for the protection of the paralyzed parts of his body from the effects of pressure and other injury. As soon as his physical condition permitted, he was taught the importance of moving and turning himself

regularly, of checking the temperature of bath water with his hand or a thermometer, and of inspecting his skin for evidences of pressure or injury. In contrast, Mr. Roberts, who was paralyzed as a result of acute anterior poliomyelitis, did not have this problem. Despite his flaccid paralysis, he was sensitive to painful stimuli. In fact, during the acute stage of his illness, his skin was so sensitive that his nurse was frequently reminded of the princess who could feel a pea though it was covered by seven mattresses.

A third example is that of Mr. Westwind, a 68-year-old man with trigeminal neuralgia. As a result of this disorder, Mr. Westwind suffered paroxysms of excruciating pain. To relieve him of his pain, the surgeon cut all the sensory branches of the trigeminal nerve. The trigeminal nerve is sensory to the skin and mucosa of the head, to the teeth, and to the cornea of the eye. Mr. Westwind was therefore deprived of the ability to detect foreign bodies in, or injury to, the eye, or to detect stimuli indicating the possibility of injury to the skin of his head or to the buccal mucosa. In his care, provisions were made to protect the structures thus deprived of sensation and to teach Mr. Westwind what he needed to know and do to protect himself from injury. Part of his instruction was to inspect his eye at least three times a day for evidences of irritation. He was also taught to inspect the inside of his mouth and tongue after each meal for food remaining in his mouth and for evidences of injury and to protect the affected side of his face from overexposure to cold. Fortunately most patients with trigeminal neuralgia do not require that all branches of the trigeminal nerve be cut for relief of pain. The branch supplying the cornea of the eye can usually be saved, and when it is, special protection of the eye is unnecessary.

Mr. Gale and Mr. Westwind have been used to illustrate some of the problems that arise when an individual is deprived of his sensory nerve supply. Tissues are no longer warned that they are being exposed to noxious stimuli. Plans for the nursing of the patient should include provisions for the protection of the tissue from injury and for the instruction of the patient in how to protect himself. The basic protective measures are those that prevent injurious agents from coming in contact with the tissue or that limit the length or degree of exposure. Because there is always a possibility of injury the affected area should also be regularly inspected for evidence of inflammation.

THE PSYCHIC COMPONENT

In addition to the perception of pain, the pain experience has a second aspect, or the psychic component, which is also known as the reaction to pain. It includes what the person thinks and feels about his pain as well as what he does about it. Interest in the psychic component in the pain experience has been stimulated by the observation that, despite similar bodily injuries, the degree of pain varies from individual to individual or even in the same individual at different times. Melzack[32] illustrates this point by quoting the studies of Beecher. During World War II, Beecher was surprised to find that among seriously injured soldiers admitted to a combat hospital, only one in three complained of pain severe enough to require morphine. Moreover, many of these men denied having any pain at all. After the war, he studied a group of civilians who had incisions similar to the wounds received by the men in battle. In this group, four out of five stated that they had severe pain and wanted something to relieve it. From these findings, Beecher concluded that factors other than the extent of the wound determine the degree of pain experienced by an individual. One of the most fundamental factors is the meaning that the pain has for the person. The soldiers were grateful for having escaped from the field alive. In contrast, civilians regarded their situations as a serious mis-

[32] *Ibid.*, p. 42.

fortune or even a catastrophe. Instead of being saved from death, they were facing the possibility of serious injury, pain, and even death. On the battlefield, injury results in the relief of anxiety. The patient facing surgery or some other painful experience has an increase in anxiety. In the words of Crowley,[33] three factors contribute to the production of anxiety in the patient in pain: "They are the threat to the self, the loneliness of pain, and the element of the unknown in pain."

Contributing to the meaning that a pain-eliciting situation has for an individual are his past experiences and his memories of them. Apprehension, with the resulting tension, is likely to be increased when a patient fears that he is going to be hurt. The tension resulting from fear and anxiety can be expected to increase the degree of pain suffered by the patient. When the patient knows that those who are responsible for his care will be gentle, that they will not allow him to suffer unnecessarily, and that when pain is unavoidable he will be warned so that he can prepare himself, he is less likely to be unnecessarily apprehensive.

FACTORS INFLUENCING BEHAVIOR OF A PATIENT IN PAIN

Since culture influences the way in which people view the various events in life, it also influences what the individual regards as painful and how he reacts to pain. Mark Zborowski's studies of the cultural components in responses to pain were cited in Chapter 7. In the United States, the group of people who place a high value on health regard pain as an indication for seeking medical attention. They expect that the cause of the pain can be determined and the condition treated successfully. The behavior of the patient in pain is in part attributable to culture and training. In many American families, girls may cry when in pain, but boys are told that men do not cry and that they should bear pain like a man. In some cultures, such as certain tribes of American Indians, children are taught from infancy to bear pain without giving evidence of suffering. Procedures such as hypodermic injections that cause the ordinary child to cry out are tolerated without any display of emotion. Other patients are also seen who, as a result of culture and training, bear pain silently. The only evidence that they are in pain may be a drawn facial expression, beads of perspiration on the brow, or a quickened respiratory or pulse rate. Others express their pain for all to hear and see.

Patients with deep religious faith may tolerate conditions that are ordinarily associated

[33] Dorothy M. Crowley: *Pain and Its Alleviation* (Berkeley: University of California, 1962), p. 61.

with severe pain with little evidence of pain. This is explained by the meaning that the religious faith of the patient gives to his pain. He may believe that pain has a spiritual purpose and that suffering should not be wasted. Care should be taken to make sure that patients who have pain receive attention. Patients who do not express their pain freely may be overlooked. Those who are noisy and demanding may also be neglected, because of the tendency to regard them as overdemanding, neurotic, or childish.

Pain is increased by anything that focuses attention on it. Conversely, any condition or event that distracts the attention of a patient, tends to lessen his pain. Hundreds of examples ranging from the trivial to the dramatic could be used to illustrate this point. The pain of minor burns and scratches in children is relieved by a kiss, a dab of colored antiseptic, or a tape bandage. A small child that has fallen and bumped his head may pick himself up and start to play again only to start crying when his mother, looking anxious, asks him where he hurt himself. Athletes, soldiers, and even ordinary laymen may, at the time of an emergency, carry out a necessary activity and completely ignore or be oblivious to the pain of serious injuries. Mr. All, who was burned, is a good example. Despite serious burns, he returned to his apartment to rescue his son. After his son was safe, he fainted. The pain-relieving effect of distraction and activity is quite often seen in patients. When the nurse enters the room, the patient complains of pain and general discomfort. By the time the nurse has bathed him, placed him in a comfortable position, and administered whatever care is required to improve his general comfort, he may be experiencing very little pain. A similar effect of distraction frequently is seen in elderly people who spend much of their time alone. When a visitor first arrives, Mrs. Cotton complains of the pain in her joints and other discomforts. By the time the visitor is ready to leave, her pain may be all but forgotten. The nurse frequently uses distraction to lessen a patient's pain or discomfort. She talks to him during a procedure or instructs him to do something such as to take a deep breath or to squeeze her hand.

When the pain experienced by the patient is mild or moderate, diversions such as music, reading, visiting, or crafts may serve to distract the attention of the patient from pain. This is not meant to be a universal prescription, however. In the patient who is suffering severe pain, attempts at diversion may increase the tension of the patient. Diversion should be employed when it is indicated and avoided at other times. In general, patients who are acutely ill, including those who have recently undergone major

surgery, should be protected from overstimulation and fatigue. What they need is a quiet, calm, and restful atmosphere combined with a feeling that they can trust those responsible for their care to meet their needs. Less acutely ill patients, and most particularly those with long-term illness, may be benefited by diversional activities that are suited to their state of health and personal interests. These patients should also be protected from overfatigue, as fatigue lowers the tolerance of the patient to pain.

The fact that the effectiveness of analgesic drugs is increased by telling the patient that the drug will relieve his pain has been demonstrated by experimental study. In some patients pain can be relieved by the assurance that the injection or pill he is receiving will relieve his pain. This is known as the placebo effect. This does not mean, as it is generally interpreted to mean, that the patient does not have pain. By reassuring the patient that something is being done for his pain, his attention is distracted from the pain and his apprehension is relieved. A nurse is appropriately utilizing the placebo effect when she says to the patient as she administers a pain-relieving medication, "I have something (a hypodermic or pill) that will relieve your pain." Occasionally, the physician prescribes an injection of water or saline for its placebo effect, but a nurse should never make the decision to give a patient a placebo without such an order. Psychological factors are of importance in all patients who have pain. They should be utilized to the benefit of the patient.

Another factor in the suffering caused by pain is the feeling of the patient that he has or does not have some degree of control over his pain. To provide the patient with a feeling that he has some control over his pain, some physicians allow certain of their patients to keep analgesics, such as acetylsalicylic acid, at the bedside. When the patient is in pain and the nurse is responsible for the administration of an analgesic drug, she can add to the sense of security of the patient by administering it promptly.

When movement aggravates pain, as it is likely to do, every effort should be made to prevent unnecessary pain. Attention should be given to minimizing both the sensation of pain and the fear of pain. The first step is to prepare the patient for what to expect and for what is expected of him. For example, "We have come to turn you to your other side. We will use the turning sheet. You can help by holding your spine as 'stiff as a poker.'" Suggestions made by the patient should be treated with kindness and respect. Therefore, when the patient says, "I always keep my neck from moving by placing my hands on each side of my face," the nurse responds by saying, "Fine, we will tell you when we are ready and then you can help." The nurse should use discretion in following the suggestions of the patient; one that is harmful should not be followed. The patient should be told why his suggestion is rejected in such a way that his self-esteem is maintained. Courtesy and tact should be characteristics of the behavior of the nurse at all times.

The patient who has been, or is, in pain is frequently reluctant to move. Whether or not movement of the patient is essential at a particular time depends on the needs of the patient and of the situation. If harm is likely to result to the patient unless he is moved, then he should be encouraged to move or to permit himself to be moved. Often allowing a patient to wait for a short time in order to give him an opportunity to mobilize his resources will lessen his reluctance. He should be assured that enough competent assistance is available so that he will be moved with a minimum of discomfort. The number of persons required to move a patient is not always the deciding factor. One or two skillful nurses who are trying to do what must be done gently may be all that is required. Finally, the patient should know why he should move or be moved at this particular time. Sometimes the reluctance of the patient results not so much from his lack of acceptance of what has to be done but from the fact that he is ill.

The patient's fear of pain can be minimized by providing his care in such a manner that he knows that those who are giving him care will do their best to protect him from unnecessary pain. All care should be characterized by gentleness, steadiness, and smoothness. Force, haste, or rough, jerky movements have no place in the care of the patient in pain. Noise, confusion, and ineptitude are disturbing to the patient in pain and should therefore be eliminated. In patients who have a painful illness, expressions of negative feelings are common. The nurse should try to accept these as part of his illness and continue to treat the patient with kindness and consideration. Undue levity and boisterousness should be avoided. Although the nurse does not help the patient by being as depressed by the pain as he is, neither is he aided by excessive cheerfulness. What is generally beneficial is a combination of acceptance of the fact of the suffering of the patient and an air that implies that something can and will be done to lessen it.

PHYSICAL ASPECTS OF PAIN

Attention to the physical aspects of pain is also important in its prevention and relief. All body structures should be maintained in anatomical alignment. Support should be provided as needed to achieve positions that will eliminate strain on parts. Basic to securing good alignment and to preventing strain on muscles is a firm mattress. When a patient is heavy, a board under the mattress may be required to achieve a firm surface. In some institutions a nurse may place a board under the mattress when it is required; in others a prescription from a physician must be secured. In the prevention of strain, the body and any of its parts should be moved as a unit. In moving the torso, the patient can assist by trying to keep his spine straight and stiff. The movements of all who participate in the turning should be synchronized so that everyone moves together. Counting "one, two, three, go" is helpful. Devices such as casts, braces, and corsets may also be utilized to keep the spine and other joints immobile.

To move an extremity, the general principles already enunciated apply. The part should be supported so that strain is minimized and unnatural movements are avoided. Both hands may be used, supporting the part on the palms of the hands, or the extremity can be supported by placing the hand and arm under its length. Pressure should be avoided over painful areas. Here again, movement may be made less painful by the use of a splint, brace, cast, or even a pillow to support the painful part while it is moved.

In postoperative patients with incisions through the chest or abdominal wall, coughing causes more or less pain. The patient should be taught that coughing is part of his postoperative management and how to cough. He should also know that the discomfort in his incision can be decreased by supporting the wound when he coughs. Whether the nurse or the patient provides the support depends on the location of the incision and the wishes and the capability of the patient. In patients who cough in excess of that required to maintain the patency of the tracheobronchial tree, a binder may be required to provide continuing support for the incision.

When immobility of the trunk or thigh is required, or movement is accompanied by excessive pain, the desired result may be attained by placing the patient on a Foster, Stryker, or Bradford frame. They also facilitate the giving of patient care.

Swelling, particularly in tissue surrounded by a bony wall or encased in a circular bandage or cast, is painful and may be dangerous. The most effective treatment for this is to reduce the swelling by utilizing the force of gravity to remove the excess fluid. Mrs. Erie offers a good example. She was admitted for the reduction of a fractured tibia, which was followed by the application of a cast. Several hours after the cast was applied, she called and asked to have something for her pain. Her toes on the affected side were slightly swollen. Instead of getting Mrs. Erie an analgesic, the nurse elevated her leg on pillows and told Mrs. Erie that, as soon as the swelling was relieved, her pain would disappear. An hour or so later Mrs. Erie said that she was free of pain and was able to eat breakfast. If the toes were cold or cyanotic, the cast should immediately be cut or bivalved by a physician.

ANALGESICS

Nurses also administer medications to relieve pain. The means by which different drugs relieve pain differ. They act by (1) removing the cause of pain, (2) decreasing consciousness, (3) lessening the conduction of impulses over pain fibers, (4) raising the threshold for pain perception, and (5) lessening the awareness, or appreciation, of the significance of pain. To illustrate, pain in the patient with a peptic ulcer increases when the hydrochloric acid is undiluted by food or fluids. Relief of the pain is afforded by alkali or bland foods such as milk. These substances do not attack the basic cause of the ulcer, but they are effective in relieving the immediate cause of the pain.

The drugs most commonly used to suppress consciousness are the general anesthetics. Although they can be utilized to suppress pain of all types, their use is limited almost entirely to the operative period of surgical therapy. Local anesthetics are most frequently employed to prevent pain during a surgical procedure, but they may also be used to relieve pain that does not respond to the more usual methods of treatment. Procaine, when injected into a nerve, interrupts the transmission of nerve impulses. The procedure is known as a nerve block and is employed to prevent pain incident to making a surgical incision or in the treatment of painful diseases. In the instance of Mr. Westwind, a patient with trigeminal neuralgia, alcohol injected into his gasserian ganglion relieved the pain for about a year.

Drugs commonly utilized to relieve pain are known as analgesics. Modell [34] classifies analgesic drugs as the greater, or addictive, analgesics and the lesser, or nonaddictive, analgesics. The most important member of the first group is morphine. Its substitutes, such as meperidine hydrochloride and methadone hydrochloride, are also useful. The lesser, or nonaddictive, drugs fall into four groups. They are the salicylates, antipyrine, the coal tar derivatives, and cinchophen. Drugs that are not of

[34] Walter Modell: *Relief of Symptoms,* 2nd ed. (St. Louis: The C. V. Mosby Company, 1961), pp. 86–100.

themselves analgesics may contribute to the relief of pain when combined with an analgesic by decreasing the capacity of the patient to evaluate pain and the meaning of pain. Thus a patient may be given acetylsalicylic acid (aspirin) in combination with phenobarbital or one of the so-called tranquilizers, such as chlorpromazine. Acetylsalicylic acid is believed to raise the threshold to pain, or the point at which the patient experiences pain. As a result of the action of chlorpromazine or some other tranquilizing drug, the patient is less concerned with the significance of his pain. For specific information about various drugs, the reader is referred to a textbook on pharmacology. Morphine appears to have both effects, as it is effective in allaying the apprehension of the patient as well as in lessening his perception of pain. In fact, there is experimental evidence that morphine diminishes pain only when the level of anxiety is high.[35]

In the selection of an analgesic for a patient, the physician considers a number of factors: the nature and location of the pain, the elements contributing to the pain, the length of time that the patient can be expected to have pain, the probable outcome of the patient's illness, and the effects of the drug itself. For example, morphine or one of its substitutes is likely to be prescribed for the patient who has just had abdominal surgery and who can be expected to require pain relief for a period of not more than 48 hours. Under these circumstances the danger of addiction is minimal. In fact, in any condition in which pain is severe, addiction is not as likely to develop as when the pain is mild. By way of contrast, when pain is mild or moderate and/or the patient is expected to require relief for a long period of time, the physician usually prescribes the mildest drug in the smallest dosage that can be expected to afford relief. The selection of the medication and the interval at which it is given is the prerogative of the physician. The nurse administers the medication within the framework of the prescription of the physician. When the physician prescribes the medication at stated intervals, the drug must be given at the times prescribed unless the patient develops signs of depression of the respiratory or nervous system or other toxic effects. When the prescription left by the physician permits the nurse to use her discretion, then she may give the drug as often as required. Usually the prescription or the policy of the agency sets some limits on the maximum frequency with which a drug can be administered. This is usually every three to four hours. Generally, the patient gets more benefit from the drug if his pain is not allowed

[35] Melzack, *op. cit.,* p. 43.

to become too severe. There is some evidence to support the observation that patients who can count on having their pain relieved promptly suffer less pain than those who cannot. Dickman made a study to determine the effect of knowing or not knowing on the quantity of drug required by postoperative patients for comfort. Patients who knew that they could have a pain-relieving medication required less medication than those who did not know.[36] Most patients tolerate painful or unpleasant procedures better if they have their medication before the procedure is performed. During the first 48 hours after surgery or immediately after the development of a painful disorder, such as a myocardial infarction, addiction is not very likely to develop.

CONDITIONS LESSENING PATIENT'S ABILITY TO TOLERATE PAIN

Pain that is long continued reduces the capacity of the person to tolerate pain. Miss Smart illustrates this point very well. She was a middle-aged woman with a diagnosis of subacute bacterial endocarditis; the bacteria causing the infection showed a high degree of resistance to available antibiotics. To try to control the infection, Miss Smart was given one or another antibiotic by intramuscular injection every two hours around the clock. Before too long, Miss Smart's body was studded with painful spots. Her ability to tolerate pain and discomfort was reduced to the point that she screamed at the slightest touch or jarring of her bed. Fatigue, sickness, debility, and repeated painful procedures reduced her tolerance to pain to an exceedingly low level. After the injections were discontinued and her condition improved, she was able to tolerate pain as well as most people.

Pain is a subjective experience. Because every person is different, each patient can be expected to behave in an individual maner when he is in pain or in a pain-provoking situation. There is abundant psychological and experimental evidence to indicate that psychological factors are of great importance in the pain experience. To prevent and relieve his pain, the way the patient feels and thinks about his pain must be taken into account. The nurse cannot always know why one patient has more or less pain than does another, but she can assume that there is a reason. She can modify the care of the patient so that unnecessary pain is avoided. Pain cannot always be eliminated, but it can be made more bearable by kind and thoughtful care.

[36] Helen Mae Dickman: *A Pilot Study of Pain in the Postoperative Patient* (Detroit: unpublished Master's Essay), 1959.

The nurse has another responsibility to the patient who is in pain, that is, to observe pain and its effects. Pain may originate in superficial or visceral structures or in the central nervous system. Superficial pain is initiated by the effect of an injurious agent on the skin. The points at which tissue damage and pain occur have been demonstrated to be very close. Sensitivity of the skin to painful stimuli varies from anesthesia, to hypesthesia, to hyperesthesia. In anesthesia, the skin is insensitive to painful stimuli. In hypesthesia, a greater than normal stimulus is required to evoke pain. In hyperesthesia, the skin is abnormally sensitive. Anesthetic and hypesthetic skin lacks the normal protective mechanisms against heat, cold, pressure, and trauma. Depending on the extent and location of these areas, protective measures may be required in the protection of the patient. Hyperesthesia is common in acute febrile diseases and in neuritis. In the latter condition the skin may be exquisitely painful over the affected area. Stimuli that would not ordinarily cause any discomfort may result in severe pain. The area may even have to be protected from the weight of bed coverings by a cradle. Hyperesthesia of the edges of a wound is common, and when it occurs, the patient can be assured that it is expected and will disappear in time.

With severe superficial pain, certain defense mechanisms of the body are mobilized. There is an increase in the activity of the sympathetic nervous system and in the production of epinephrine, with a resultant tachycardia and peripheral vasoconstriction. With the increase in the heart rate and vasoconstriction, the blood pressure can be expected to rise. In patients who do not express their discomfort either verbally or by a change in facial expression, the nurse may have to depend on evidences of increased sympathoadrenal activity, such as sweating, tachycardia, and a rise in blood pressure, to detect pain. A generalized increase in muscular tension may also indicate pain.

Pain can be deep, such as that occurring in bones or viscera. Pain in bones is often dull, aching, and localized. Pain in the viscera is usually dull and diffuse. Pain impulses arising in deep muscles and in the viscera are often mediated by nerves that also convey sensations from various areas of the skin or other viscera. This contributes to difficulty in identifying the origin of the pain. For example, difficulty may be encountered in distinguishing between the pain of cholelithiasis, peptic ulcer, and myocardial infarction. A type of sensation often called referred pain may accompany pain in the viscera. This referred pain occurs in the superficial structures supplied by the same sensory apparatus as the organ that is diseased or injured. The explanation usually given is that the brain is unable to locate the specific origin of the pain and therefore projects it to the skin. The following are illustrations of disorders characterized by referred pain. In tuberculosis of the hip, pain is frequently referred to the knee. In myocardial infarction, pain may be referred to the neck, the shoulder blades, and the left arm. The patient may have so much pain in his shoulder that he hesitates or refuses to move his arm and, as a result, develops a frozen shoulder. In subphrenic abscesses, the pain is often referred to the top of the shoulder.

Severe deep pain differs from superficial pain in that it is more likely to cause failure in homeostatic defense mechanisms. Weakness, hypotension, pallor, sweating, bradycardia, and nausea and vomiting are common. These signs and symptoms can be observed in patients with a variety of thoracic and abdominal conditions. Examples include myocardial infarction, perforations of abdominal viscera, and biliary or renal colic.

Central pain is a type of pain that is perceived in the mind of the individual and for which there is no peripheral cause at the time the pain is experienced. The classic example is phantom limb, a condition in which a patient has pain and other sensations in an amputated limb even when he can see that the limb has been removed. For example, one patient asked to have a pillow in his bed to support his amputated leg. He had the feeling that he had to hold his leg up off the bed. Such a sensation can occasionally be relieved by placing a pillow in the bed where his leg would have normally rested. Many patients have sensations that appear to originate in the amputated extremity. Although these sensations usually eventually disappear, occasionally they persist for years, and they may be so severe that the person is incapacitated.

The manner in which pain is elicited differs with different types of tissues. The skin is sensitive to cutting, burning, pricking, and trauma. Severe pain is induced in skeletal muscles by ischemia. This is the basis for Mr. Elderly's pain during exercise. He has severe atherosclerosis that limits the ability of the arteries to increase the blood supply to his legs during exercise. When he walks for a block or so, he develops a severe cramplike pain, which is known as intermittent claudication in the calf of his leg. Pain in the skeletal muscles can also be caused by prolonged contraction and by the injection of irritating substances into them. Ischemia is also the cause of pain in the heart muscle. The ischemia may be relative or absolute. In atherosclerosis or as a result of arterial spasm, the capacity of the coronary arteries to

deliver blood to the heart muscle may be inadequate. When Mr. Plump increases his activity, he develops a cramplike pain in his chest. Essentially Mr. Elderly and Mr. Plump have a similar problem. Both of them have pain because their arteries are unable to deliver sufficient blood to maintain muscular activity. In both, pain is protective inasmuch as it acts as a warning. With the onset of pain they stop whatever they are doing; they rest and allow their muscles to recover. They also learn to avoid activities that precipitate the pain. When an artery supplying a muscle is obstructed, pain continues for some time. It is not relieved by rest or by drugs that dilate arteries and increase the blood supply.

Pain in the gastrointestinal tract may be caused by trauma to the mucosa and by stretching or spasm of smooth muscle. The intestine and stomach can be cut or burned without giving rise to pain. Stretching or spasm of smooth muscle in the biliary and urinary tract usually causes severe pain. Arteries also give rise to pain when they pulsate excessively as in migraine headaches or in arteritis.

Observation of the patient is necessary to the collection of information on which the nurse bases her judgment that the patient does or does not have pain of sufficient degree to require relief. From her observations of the patient, the nurse also decides on the course of action that she will take to treat the pain experienced by the patient. The first step is to determine whether or not the patient is in pain. When a patient is asleep or resting quietly, he is not likely to be in pain. When he is aroused he may complain of pain and then lapse back into sleep. The belief that all postoperative patients and patients with cancer have pain is erroneous. Keats[37] cites a study of another investigator who found that 44 per cent of 237 patients did not complain of pain after operation. In his own series he found that 21 per cent of 104 patients who had either a gastrectomy or colectomy received no more than one dose of an analgesic during the entire postoperative period. Some of these patients received none. Despite the preceding, it is invalid to conclude that a patient who does not complain of pain is comfortable.

When the patient complains of pain, he should be asked to indicate its location and to describe it. The patient may be asked to point to the painful area. Leading questions should be avoided as they may result in the patient giving misleading information. The question should be phrased so that the cause of the discomfort experienced by the patient can be

[37] Arthur S. Keats: "Postoperative Pain: Research and Treatment," *J. Chronic Dis.,* **4:**72–73 (July) 1956.

determined. The resulting answer may indicate that the patient is in pain or that he is sleepless; is suffering from discomfort from a nasal oxygen catheter; has a sore throat, headache, or backache; is in an uncomfortable position in bed; has an overdistended bladder; or has some condition other than pain from an operative incision or relating directly to his disease. The selection of the method of treatment should be based on the cause of the discomfort. Information should be elicited about any situation or condition that provokes or relieves the pain. For example, Mrs. Robin continued to complain of pain five or six days after a gastroenterostomy. Her nurse noted that the pain was always precipitated by Mr. Robin's visit. About the same time, Mrs. Robin also made the comment that she always felt so good after she had a "hypo." Both facts were reported to her physician. As Mrs. Robin was showing early signs of addiction to morphine, the drug was discontinued and other therapy prescribed.

The quality of the pain and other characteristics of the pain should be noted and recorded, preferably in the words used by the patient. The mode of onset of the pain, its duration, severity, and time of onset are all important. When the character of the pain experienced by the patient changes or pain appears in a new or unexpected area, this information should be reported to the physician. Whether this is done immediately or delayed until the next regular visit of the physician depends on the possible significance of the pain. Severe pain or pain and other symptoms and signs indicating involvement of the viscera should usually be reported before an analgesic drug is administered, as the drug may mask the patient's pain and thus eliminate an indispensable factor in helping the physician to identify the nature and location of visceral involvement.

OTHER INDICATIONS OF PAIN

In addition to the description of the pain by the patient, there is usually other evidence to indicate that a patient has pain, for example, restlessness, discomfort indicated by facial expression, hands pressed over the painful area, moaning or other sounds indicating pain, irritability, refusal to move or moving carefully, perspiration, and anorexia. When the pain is severe, the blood pressure may be elevated or depressed and the pulse and respiratory rate altered. Not all these effects are unique to pain. Restlessness is also common in hypoxia, and it is important to rule out the possibility of respiratory difficulty before any analgesic, especially a narcotic, is given. Anorexia occurs in many types of illness. When pain is long continued, it contributes to the debility of the patient by decreasing his food intake. In just a few weeks, Mr. Westwind (trigeminal neuralgia) lost 25 lb. Each time he tried to eat, a paroxysm of pain was precipitated. Therefore he refused to eat. Pain, even when it is not induced by food, is so all-encompassing that everything else becomes unimportant.

Observation of the patient should continue after measures have been taken to relieve pain. Observation should be directed toward determining the success or failure of the treatment and any undesired effects. Some of the drugs used to relieve pain depress the respiratory and other centers in the brain. Patients with borderline cardiovascular function or hypovolemia may go into shock soon after intramuscular or intravenous narcotics are given. Such patients should be given narcotics only in small amounts or not at all. A patient may have an idiosyncrasy to any one of these drugs. When the patient exhibits unusual behavior shortly after a drug is administered and his behavior improves after a period of time, the probability is that there is a relationship between his behavior and his reaction to the drugs. Examples have been cited earlier in the chapter. Patients who have severe pain are often afraid that the pain will continue or return or that the pain indicates they have a serious illness from which they will die. They are afraid to allow themselves to relax and to go to sleep. When they are under the watchful eye of a nurse whom they trust to meet their needs, they have less need to remain alert. The external environment of the patient should also be controlled so that the therapy has an opportunity to be effective. A quiet, cool, but not cold environment is usually conducive to rest. For some patients the feeling of safety is increased by having a relative or good friend sit quietly at the bedside. The relative may require some instruction as to how he should behave and some recognition of the value of his contribution to the patient. Furthermore, the nurse should continue to assume the responsibility for the care and supervision of the patient. The relative should supplement, not replace, the nurse.

Pain and fear of pain are common to most illness. The extent to which each aspect predominates varies with the individual and with the cause of his illness. Pain is useful because it serves to warn the individual that something is wrong and spurs him into appropriate action. It is harmful when it frightens him so much that he avoids action or when it exhausts his physical and psychological resources.

The nurse's responsibilities in the care of the patient as they relate to pain are summarized in the following objectives:

1. To care for the patient so that preventable pain is avoided.
2. To evaluate the nature and cause of the patient's pain, so that appropriate measures may be instituted.
3. To convey to the patient that he can count on or trust the nurse (nurses) to meet his needs.
4. To continue to offer comfort and support to the patient whose pain persists despite the best efforts of all concerned.

As an addendum, at a number of points in the discussion of pain, reference was made to the necessity for the nurse to evaluate the degree of pain experienced by the patient. The author is haunted by a patient who was selected by a student for the purpose of studying her nursing care requirements. The patient, who was approximately 40 years old, had been an actress as a child but was now destitute. She was divorced and lived with her mother. She had developed a severe proctitis as a consequence of large doses of radiation in the treatment of cancer of the cervix. Because of her dependent behavior, she was seen by a psychiatrist who described her as being immature and childlike. Despite her pleas for relief of what is known to be an exquisitely painful condition, pain-relieving medications were unfortunately withheld until she became mentally disorganized. Although Mrs. Child Actress is an extreme example, the incident is uncommon only in degree. When a patient says he has pain, his complaint should be treated seriously. Insofar as possible, the causes should be determined and appropriate treatment undertaken.

FEVER

A symptom that may also be of great importance during the recovery of the patient is fever. For the first two or three days postoperatively a slight elevation of temperature and of leukocyte count may be expected because of the tissue damage. A marked increase in body temperature during the first 24 to 72 hours, however, frequently indicates a developing atelectasis. Later elevations may be caused by thrombophlebitis or an infection in the operative site or urinary tract.

HICCOUGH

Hiccough (singultus) is an annoying, though not usually dangerous, symptom. It results from a paroxysmal and intermittent contraction of the diaphragm. It may be the result of chemical or mechanical irritation of the peritoneum or pleura that invests the diaphragm. Hiccoughs will often respond to simple measures—a drink of water, something that startles the person, a cough, a change in position. Other procedures that may be prescribed by the physician include rebreathing air in a paper bag, carbon dioxide inhalation, gastric lavage or suction, and sedatives. In extreme cases in which hiccoughs are prolonged and do not respond to other treatments, crushing the phrenic nerve may be required. Severe and continuous hiccoughing is exhausting because it interferes with rest and the ingestion of food and fluid.

How does surgical therapy threaten the self-concept of the patient?

In the discussion of the preoperative phase of surgical therapy, some mention was made of the psychological aspects of surgery as a threat to the survival of the individual. Many aspects of surgical therapy can provoke anxiety. This anxiety may be further augmented by the disease, or what the person perceives to be the disease, that makes surgery necessary. Many aspects of the total surgical experience threaten the self-concept of the individual. During the operative phase of his treatment, the patient loses complete control over what happens to him. He is utterly dependent on the surgeon, the anesthetist, and the assistants to the surgeon. The patient faces, and then experiences, pain and fear of pain. Throughout the entire experience, from the day he becomes aware that he is ill until he has completed his convalescence, the unknown plays a part in his reactions. Was surgery necessary? Was it successful? Was the cause of his illness cancer? Was it all removed? Has the doctor told him the truth?

The surgical treatment of disease frequently threatens his self-concept, by actual fact or by the perception of the individual. These are the persons who, though they make a full physiological recovery, have some change in their anatomy that threatens their self-concept. Full psychological recovery depends on their accepting the change in themselves as necessary and for their welfare. This involves a change in self-concept without a prolonged period of depression or other evidence of failure to accept reality.

Types of surgery that place the greatest strain on the adaptive capacity of the individual are those involving the loss of a part of the body (1) that is obvious to others, such as an eye or an extremity; (2) in which the patient has an emotional investment; or (3) that involves an obvious change in function, such as a colostomy, ileostomy, or cystostomy. The patient can and should be expected to experience some grief and anger. He may also feel a certain degree of shame or guilt. The psychosocial aspects of illness are discussed in some detail in Chapter 7, and the reader is referred to it for a more complete discussion of this very important aspect of the care of the surgical patient.

Exercise and Rest

One aspect of postoperative care that has changed greatly over the last 20 or 25 years is the shift in emphasis from rest to exercise. As recently as 25 years ago, any patient who had major abdominal surgery was kept in bed for from ten days to two weeks postoperatively and then he was permitted to gradually resume activity over a period of six weeks to three months.

The rationale on which bed rest was based in the postsurgical treatment of patients was that rest was conducive to healing and that the wound was liable to disruption should strain be placed on it. Men such as Dr. Daniel Leithauser noted that patients who refused to stay in bed did as well as or better than those who remained in bed and that the incidence of wound disruption was no greater. Although the practice was recommended by Reis more than half a century ago, early ambulation did not receive widespread acceptance until Leithauser [38, 39] reintroduced it.

The earliness with which surgical patients are ambulated varies with the surgeon, the surgical procedure, and the patient. Leithauser, who was one of the more vigorous proponents of early ambulation, advocated that patients be ambulated as soon as they had recovered from the depressing effects of the anesthetic. The only exceptions were patients who were in shock, experiencing severe uncontrolled hemorrhage, or in thyroid crisis.[40] Some surgeons add sepsis to this list of exceptions because exercise can promote the spread of an infection.

When early ambulation was first introduced, patients, nurses, and physicians were fearful that harm might come to the patient. They had been indoctrinated with the belief that bed rest was necessary to the healing of the wound and that exertion by the patient was dangerous. Patients who entered the hospital expecting to have good rest were surprised and somewhat frightened because they were forced to get out of bed and walk. Today patients are mentally better prepared to ambulate. They know that the neighbor across the street was out of bed a few hours after he returned from the operating room. Despite previous warning, however, the patient who gets out of bed for the first time after undergoing a major surgical procedure is frequently frightened and anxious.

BENEFITS OF EXERCISE

The reader will find a more extensive discussion of the nervous, hormonal, and metabolic response of the individual to stress in Chapter 6. However, one of the immediate responses to acute injury or threat of injury is activation of the sympathoadrenal medulla system. Many of the effects of its increased activity, such as increased sweating, vasoconstriction, and inactivation of the alimentary canal, have been previously described. According to Leithauser, this response is intensified and prolonged by bed rest and can be minimized in degree and shortened in length by the early mobilization of the surgical patient.

Following surgery, the patient undergoes metabolic changes similar to that of the general response to injury. It is more pronounced in the young healthy individual than it is in the debilitated and elderly and it is intensified by bed rest. In the early stages, it is characterized by increased catabolism of protein and a negative nitrogen balance.

Among the positive effects of exercise following surgery is the reduction in the loss of nitrogen. According to Coller and DeWeese,[41] simple bed rest leads to a loss of nitrogen and a depression in the appetite. It also leads to a loss of muscle tone and to muscle weakness. Excessive rest results not only in nitrogen loss from muscles but also calcium loss from bones. In active healthy young persons, especially young men, who are suddenly and completely inactivated, loss of calcium may be so great that it forms kidney stones. This tendency can be counteracted to a certain extent by exercise and a high fluid intake. Return to physiologic functioning of the respiratory, circulatory, gastrointestinal, and nervous systems is earlier in patients who exercise.

Although exercise out of bed is more beneficial, exercise in bed can also be beneficial and has its indications. Exercise improves the psychological status and morale of the patient. To the extent that exercise is accompanied by relaxation of the patient, it lessens pain, and, as a consequence, less postoperative medication is required. Mrs. Hammer illustrates the latter point. During a recent pregnancy Mrs. Hammer was found to have a marked elevation of her

[38] D. J. Leithauser *et al.:* "Prevention of Embolic Complications from Venous Thrombosis After Surgery," *JAMA,* **147:**300–303 (Sept. 22) 1951.

[39] Daniel J. Leithauser: "Early Ambulation," *Amer. J. Nurs.,* **50:**203–206 (Apr.) 1950.

[40] Leithauser, *op. cit.,* p. 301.

[41] Frederick A. Coller and Marion S. DeWeese: "Preoperative and Postoperative Care," *JAMA,* **141:**644 (Nov. 5) 1949.

blood pressure. At the time of delivery, she went into hypovolemic shock as a result of severe hemorrhage. Despite reasonably prompt replacement of blood loss, she became anuric and remained so for about ten days. After this time her urine output began to increase but her renal function was still very poor, as evidenced by the low fixed specific gravity of her urine and the rising blood levels of potassium and urea. When potassium and urea levels rose to a critical level, peritoneal dialysis was initiated and Mrs. Hammer was instructed to lie still. What the physician meant was that Mrs. Hammer should not toss about or get out of bed. What Mrs. Hammer perceived was that she must not move a muscle. In fact, she was so fearful and held herself so rigidly that she developed muscle soreness that persisted for a week.

Because Mrs. Hammer was being "specialed" by a physician, she was given little attention by a nurse. When a nurse finally asked her how she felt, she said, "Awful. Nobody does anything for me, no one even talks to me." The nurse gave Mrs. Hammer a bath and, as she did, she put her extremities through their normal range of motion. She showed Mrs. Hammer how she could wiggle her toes and exercise her arms and legs without disturbing the tubing. Except for giving directions and instructions, the nurse did not talk very much. When she had completed Mrs. Hammer's care, she asked her how she felt. At this time Mrs. Hammer said, "Oh so much better. I had just about given up." Although there were other factors in Mrs. Hammer's improvement, exercise was one.

For the purpose of this discussion exercise following surgery will be considered under three headings: (1) mobilization or exercise of the patient in bed, (2) mobilization or exercise of the patient out of bed, and (3) exercises for the restoration of specific functions. All types of exercise have a common goal, the restoration of function. The effects of exercise can be summarized as a law of nature: Parts, especially muscles, develop in proportion to the stresses and strains placed on them.

Many of the exercises performed in bed have been previously presented in other chapters. Mobilization and exercise are essential for patients who for some reason cannot get out of bed. These exercises are essential for the protection of respiratory, circulatory, and joint function and to prevent the loss of muscle strength and tone. Depending on the condition of the patient, exercise can be passive, that is, performed by the nurse, or it can be active, that is, performed by the patient. Exercise can also be assistive, with the nurse helping the patient to exercise.

EXERCISES TO IMPROVE RESPIRATORY FUNCTION

The exercises performed by the patient to protect respiratory function have been discussed in some detail in Chapter 8. These include turning from side to side, deep-breathing, and coughing. Deep-breathing exercises can be made more effective by exhaling against resistance. A simple device for this purpose is a set of blow bottles. (See Chapter 8.) As a result of these exercises, the patient cleanses his airway, improves his vital capacity, and strengthens his respiratory muscles. Complications such as atelectasis and postoperative pneumonia are less likely to develop.

EXERCISES TO IMPROVE CIRCULATORY FUNCTION

Not only do the exercises that have been described improve respiratory function, but they also aid in promoting circulation. With inspiration the pressure within the thoracic cavity falls. Blood in the veins of the abdomen, head, and extremities moves toward the area with lower pressure, that is, in the thoracic cavity. Circulation in the lower extremities may be further stimulated by foot and leg exercises, which should be taught to the patient during the preoperative period. Contraction of the muscles of the feet and legs squeeze on the deep veins in the legs and push the blood toward the heart. The valves in the veins support the column of blood so that it can move only in the direction of the heart. Inactivity allows blood to stagnate or pool in these veins. This venous stasis tends to occur in anyone who sits quietly for an extended period of time. Examples include the person who takes a long bus ride and the elderly person who sits in a chair from morning until night without moving. Stasis of blood in leg veins also occurs during the operative and early postoperative phases of surgery. This is particularly marked in spinal anesthesia which causes complete paralysis of the muscles of the legs for up to several hours. Because of the tendency for blood to pool in the lower extremities during anesthesia, some surgeons wrap the lower extremities from the toes to the knee or to the groin with elastic bandages.

Unless there is a specific contraindication, patients undergoing surgical procedures should perform foot and leg exercises regularly. These exercises consist of dorsiflexion alternating with hyperextension of the feet. The knee and the thigh should also be flexed and then extended. The movements of the leg and thigh are often referred to as bicycle exercises, because the movements are similar to those used in riding a bicycle. Although foot and leg exercises are more beneficial when the patient is able to perform them himself, they may also be performed by the nurse as passive exercises. Until the patient is up and walking, they should be initiated at one- or two-hour intervals, depending on the condition of the patient and the prescription of the surgeon. As with the deep-breathing exercises, most patients require some reminding, encouragement, and assistance.

Many physicians discourage the use of pillows or rests under the knees for two reasons. One is that the localized areas of pressure where the legs rest against the pillows tend to interfere with the venous return from the lower extremities and predispose to venous stasis and thrombosis. Pillows or knee rests also tend to reduce the mobility of the patient, because they help to hold the patient up in bed. Without the pillow or the knee rest, the patient slides down in bed. When he becomes uncomfortable, he boosts himself up in bed to increase his comfort and in the process stimulates his circulation, respiration, and muscle activity.

For patients who are confined to bed for more than a day or two, a variety of simple devices are available to increase the mobility of the patient as well as enable him to assist with his own care. One such device is the overhead swing, or "monkey bar," which, when used, strengthens the arm muscles, enables the patient to move about in bed, and allows him to assist with his care. A rope or sheet tied to the foot of the bed may be used by the patient to pull himself into a sitting position. The arms and shoulders may be strengthened by the patient placing his hands palms down on the bed and raising his buttocks from the bed. This exercise is useful in the preparation of the patient for crutch walking.

Exercise should be an integral part of the care of virtually all patients. When a patient is treated by bed rest, the nurse should include range of motion exercises as part of the morning and evening care. When the patient is able, he may perform these exercises himself. As the term *range of motion* implies, extremities are moved at the joints within the limits of the usual range of motion for the patient. One precaution should be observed in the performance of these exercises: The nurse should never force a part beyond the point at which it moves freely or causes pain. This is especially important after any trauma at or near a joint.

Although exercises mobilizing the patient in bed are valuable, they are not as effective as getting the patient out of bed. The term *to ambulate* means to walk, not to get up and sit in a chair. This is a point emphasized by Leithauser in his writings and lectures about ambulation. In fact, he stresses the point that patients should be discouraged from sitting in a chair. They should either be walking or in bed. Lei-

thauser opposes the sitting position because the dependent position of the legs and the weight of the body on the thighs interferes with venous return from the legs. Venous stasis predisposes to the development of thrombophlebitis, which, in turn, may lead to pulmonary embolism. Venous stasis in the legs of some elderly patients may be so severe that, if they sit for a long time, hypotension may develop. The benefits to the patient from ambulation include less pain in the operative site, earlier disappearance of pain, a protein-sparing action, reduction in certain postoperative sequelae, improvement of the patient's morale, and earlier discharge from the hospital.

A METHOD FOR GETTING THE PATIENT OUT OF BED

The first step in getting a patient out of bed is to have enough competent assistance available to assure the patient that he will not be allowed to fall. He should also be assured that his wound will not suffer from the activity. When a patient is large or heavy, a male nurse or orderly can make a real contribution to the actual physical safety and confidence of the patient. In the process of getting out of bed, the patient should be allowed sufficient time to adjust to each change in position.

If the method suggested by Leithauser [42] is followed, the patient starts from the supine position. Preparatory to getting the patient out of bed, the bed should be lowered. Then the patient turns on his side and, as he starts to sit up, swings his feet over the edge of the bed. By the time he is in the upright position, his feet are over the edge of the bed. At this point the patient may wish to rest with his hands on the edge of the bed or on the shoulders of a nurse standing in front of him. Then the patient should be assisted to the standing position. In those hospitals where the height of the bed is fixed, the simplest way to get the patient out of bed is to let him slide off the edge of the bed until his feet touch the floor. He should be supported and encouraged to cough, so that secretions are eliminated from the tracheobronchial tree. He should then be encouraged to walk to the foot of the bed and return to the center of the bed. He is then assisted back into bed. If he is short and the bed is high he may step on a stool six to eight inches high before getting into bed. After a period of rest, he is again encouraged to get up and walk. With each successive period out of bed, his strength and courage usually improve.

Following chest surgery, ambulation offers some difficulties but these are not insurmount-

42 Leithauser, *loc. cit.,* p. 206.

able. If the patient has chest drainage tubes, attention should be given to preventing tension on them. If the bottles are moved, they should be kept below the point where the tubes enter the thorax so that fluid will not be sucked back into the pleural cavity. Suction is discontinued and tubes are clamped only when prescribed by the physician. Ambulation of the patient receiving intravenous fluids can be accomplished if the arm with the needle is stabilized. When the needle is introduced into a vein over a joint, the joint must be immobilized with a splint. Attention should be given to the prevention of any tension on the tubing. In patients with indwelling catheters, the catheter can often be clamped while the patient is up and about. If there is some contraindication to clamping the catheter or the patient is to be up for some time, then the catheter may be attached to a bag strapped to a leg or the bag may be carried with the patient.

Although exercise is important in the care of the patient, adequate rest must also be emphasized. Despite Leithauser's contention that patients will not overexert themselves, some patients do require protection from overactivity. As the patient begins to recover, he may feel that he is farther along in his convalescence than he actually is. He should be encouraged to exercise to moderation and stop before he becomes fatigued.

Another source of exhaustion of patients is the number of procedures performed on them. Frail or seriously ill patients are sometimes exhausted by the continuous activity, especially in intensive-care units. Mr. Watts had open heart surgery and his diseased aortic valve was replaced with a prosthesis. For the first three days postoperatively, he was in borderline shock. On his first postoperative day, he was to be turned from side to side, to do deep-breathing exercises, and to cough each hour. All the preceding are required to prevent postoperative atelectasis and to promote the re-expansion of the lung. However, because Mr. Watts was frail and unable to cooperate well, each maneuver took the better part of an hour. At one point when his care had just been completed and he was prepared to rest, the surgeon and his assistants came in. The patient was then raised to a sitting position and moved so that his chest could be examined. Shortly after the physicians departed, the patient vomited without any warning and soiled the bed with emesis. The bed required changing, further depriving Mr. Watts of rest. His nurse felt that there was another requirement—that is, some planning between the surgeon and the nurse so that the visit of the physician could be substituted for one of his exercise periods. The nurse has the responsibility for taking initiative to protect the patient

from too rigorous exercise and to make sure that he gets needed rest. This lack of needed rest may be especially important after heart surgery or any extended stay in an intensive-care unit. Severe psychosis or depression may result in 1 to 2 days if the patient is awakened every 15 to 60 minutes and is not allowed adequate sleep or rest.

A third type of exercise is prescribed to protect or restore the functions of a specific structure or part. For example, the loss of muscle tone in an extremity can be reduced by the performance of muscle-setting exercises. To prevent the loss of strength in a leg encased in a cast the physician sometimes prescribes special exercises that require contraction of the quadriceps muscles. The nurse can practice performing this exercise on herself as preparation for teaching patients. As the quadriceps muscles shorten, the kneecap can be felt to move. Before encouraging a patient to exercise a muscle or muscles in an extremity that has had surgery, the nurse should consult with the physician about when the exercises may be started.

Following a radical mastectomy, exercise of the arm and shoulder on the affected arm may be prescribed by the physician to maintain joint motion and muscle tone in the area. Surgeons' opinions differ as to the time exercises should be started. When the resection has been extensive, closure of the wound may be difficult and proper healing of the wound may depend on immobilization and rest of the area. The nurse should always consult with the surgeon before initiating any exercises that may affect the operated area. Specific exercises that are used are described in Chapter 14.

When patients are treated by physical therapy, the nurse should know what the purpose of the therapy is and how she can assist the work of the therapist. Although this discussion has been related to the needs of the postsurgical patient, it is also important in the care of any bedfast patient, regardless of his diagnosis or treatment. The proper amount and kind of exercise are important factors in restoring any patient to health. Whether the exercise is performed in bed or out of bed, it improves the psychological as well as the physiologic status of the patient. Although a program of exercise is begun in the early postoperative period, it continues to be important in all phases.

Summary

In the last century, surgical therapy has become a reality; diseases in all parts of the body are now treated by surgical methods. In its development, surgery was first made safe for the patient by the development of techniques of hemostasis, asepsis, anesthesia, and increased skill in incising and treating tissues. More recently, advances in knowledge have made it possible to give proper attention to making the patient safe for surgery. As a result, most patients are restored to health and vitality after surgery with a minimum of discomfort and disability. This is true of patients in all age groups and even those who have extensive surgery. Some of the complications that may delay recovery or cause death have been indicated.

Despite numerous possibilities for difficulty in the postoperative period, most patients have what is called an uneventful recovery. In those who do develop a complication, signs and symptoms are usually detected early so that procedures are promptly instituted to correct the problem. Much of the credit for the reduction in operative morbidity and mortality can be given to the application of knowledge of physiology, microbiology, and psychology to the care of the patient in all phases of his operative experience. Credit must also be given to nurses who carry out, or assist patients in carrying out, procedures to protect and support bodily processes. Because of the amount of time nurses spend with patients, they also are in a position to observe and report early signs and symptoms that indicate a complication is developing. Despite the united efforts of the patient, nurse, and doctor, complications do occur. Many of the possibilities have been indicated in the preceding discussion. Surgery places stress on physiological and psychological functioning. Even in minor surgery, the combination of the effects of an anesthetic and a surgical procedure may result in depression or disorganization of function. If continued, some disturbances in function are self-perpetuating or lead to more serious changes that are difficult to correct.

Complications that develop in the postoperative period can be summarized as having their origin in (1) abnormal function of one or more systems—respiratory, gastrointestinal, urinary, or cardiovascular; (2) stress that exceeds the adaptive capacity of the individual—shock, hemorrhage, psychological disturbances; (3) failure to heal the wound; and (4) sepsis—wound infection or infection of other structures such as the urinary bladder, leg veins, peritoneum, or lungs.

The complications that have their origin in the respiratory system have been discussed in Chapter 8. They are believed to have their origin in obstruction of portions of the tracheobronchial tree by accumulated secretions and inadequate coughing or ventilation. Occasionally, aspiration of salivary and/or gastric secretions may play a role. These problems are best prevented by proper preoperative study and preparation and maintenance of the adequate ventilation during and after surgery. Failure to clear the lungs of accumulating secretions may result in a vicious cycle, with the secretions reducing ventilation, the inadequate ventilation allowing more secretions to accumulate, and so on.

During the postoperative period the objective in the care of the patient is to enable him to return to optimal physiological and psychological functioning as rapidly and safely as possible. The surgical procedures, including the incision, the anesthetic, the pain-relieving medications, and excessive bed rest, combine to depress and to disorganize bodily functions. An important part of the patient's care is to anticipate, protect, and maintain the functions that are disrupted. To do this effectively requires some understanding of physiology and how function can be maintained until the patient can carry it on himself. In assessing the needs of the patient in the postoperative period, the nurse should try to determine the functions with which he requires assistance. Individual factors, such as age and personal habits, that may influence the prognosis of the patient should be given consideration. For example, the elderly patient usually has a lowered capacity for responding to stress. His respiratory reserve decreases with age and he is more susceptible to respiratory complications than he was earlier in his life. The patient who has chronic bronchitis as a consequence of heavy smoking over a period of years is especially predisposed to respiratory complications. In addition, the fact that he has a chronic cough renders him more liable to wound disruption. Both these patients, then, require more than the usual attention toward keeping the tracheobronchial tree clear of secretions.

Only a small part of the patient's convalescence is spent in the hospital. As soon as the requirements of the patient can be met at home, he is likely to be discharged from the hospital. Plans for the discharge of the patient should include instruction in those aspects of his care that require some modification of his daily patterns of living. He should know when he should visit his physician, how much rest and exercise he should take, any modifications of his diet that are required, and when he can anticipate returning to work. Even when the patient has made what is called an uneventful recovery, the nurse should ask herself the question, will this patient and his family be able to meet his needs after he leaves the hospital? If the answer is yes, as it will be in many instances, then nothing more needs to be done. If the answer is no, then the next question is, what kind of help does he or his family require? And then, what are the resources in the community that can be utilized to provide the help the patient and

his family require? What steps should be taken to secure continuing care for the patient?

REFERENCES

BOOKS

Ackerman, Lauren V.: *Surgical Pathology,* 4th ed. (St. Louis: The C. V. Mosby Company, 1968).

Beal, John M., and Eckenhoff, James E. (eds.): *Intensive and Recovery Room Care* (New York: The Macmillan Company, 1969).

Betschman, Lucille I.: *Handbook of Recovery Room Nursing* (Philadelphia: The F. A. Davis Company, 1967).

Cannon, Walter Bradford: *Bodily Changes in Pain, Hunger, Fear, and Rage* (Boston: Charles T. Branford Company, 1929).

Committee on Pre and Postoperative Care, American College of Surgeons: *Manual of Preoperative and Postoperative Care* (Philadelphia: W. B. Saunders Company, 1967).

Franklin, Benjamin: *A Dissertation on Liberty and Necessity, Pleasure and Pain* (reproduced from the 1st ed.) (New York: Facsimile Text Society, 1930).

Hale, Donald E. (ed.): *Anesthesiology,* 2nd ed. (Philadelphia: F. A. Davis Company, 1963).

Marshall, Henry Rutgers: *Pain, Pleasure, and Anesthetics* (New York: The Macmillan Company, 1894).

Nardi, George L., and Zuidema, George D. (eds.): *Surgery,* 2nd ed. (Boston: Little, Brown & Company, 1965).

Sadove, Max, and Cross, James H.: *The Recovery Room* (Philadelphia: W. B. Saunders Company, 1956).

Storer, Edward H., Pate, James W., and Sherman, Roger T.: *The Science of Surgery* (New York: McGraw-Hill Book Company, Inc., 1964).

Tichener, James L., and Levine, Maurice: *Surgery as a Human Experience* (New York: Oxford University Press, 1960).

Welch, Claude E. (ed.): *Advances in Surgery,* Vol. 3 (Chicago: Year Book Medical Publishers, Inc., 1968).

White, James C., and Sweet, William H.: *Pain: Its Mechanisms and Neurosurgical Control* (Springfield, Ill.: Charles C Thomas, Publisher, 1955).

Wohlgemuth, A.: *Pleasure-Unpleasure* (New York: Cambridge University Press, 1919).

Wolff, Harold G.: *Stress and Disease,* 2nd ed. (Springfield, Ill.: Charles C Thomas, Publisher, 1968).

Wolff, Harold G., and Wolf, Stewart: *Pain,* 2nd ed. (Springfield, Ill.: Charles C Thomas, Publisher, 1958).

Zimmerman, Leo M., and Levine, Rachmiel (eds.): *Physiologic Principles of Surgery,* 2nd ed. (Philadelphia: W. B. Saunders Company, 1964).

PERIODICALS

The Preoperative Period

Brownsberger, Carl N.: "Emotional Stress Connected with Surgery," *Nurs. Forum,* 4:46–55 (No. 4) 1965.

Carnevali, Doris L.: "Preoperative Anxiety," *Amer. J. Nurs.,* 66:1536–38 (July) 1966.

Cassady, June R., and Altrocchi, John: "Patients' Concerns About Surgery," *Nurs. Res.,* 9:219–21 (Fall) 1960.

Dumas, Rhetaugh G., and Anderson, Barbara J.: "Psychological Preparation Beneficial: If Based on Individual's Needs," *Hosp. Top.,* 42:79–81, 124 (May) 1964.

"Forum on the Progress in Surgery," *Nurs. Forum,* 4:3–108 (No. 3) 1965.

Healy, Kathryn M.: "Does Preoperative Instruction Make a Difference?" *Amer. J. Nurs.,* 68: 62–67 (Jan.) 1968.

Jones, Genevieve P. (ed.): "Symposium on Orthopedic and Surgical Nursing," *Nurs. Clin. N. Amer.,* 2:379–569 (Sept.) 1967.

Moore, Charles B.: "Evaluation and Preparation of Cardiac Patients for Thoracic Operations," *Surg. Clin. N. Amer.* 46:1381–87 (Dec.) 1966.

Peitchinis, Jacquelyn: "Psychological Care of Patient Important to Surgery's Outcome," *Hosp. Top.,* 43:113–19 (Nov.) 1965.

Perry, John F.: "Surgery in the Aged," *Postgrad. Med.,* 41:414–17 (Apr.) 1967.

Quint, Jeanne C.: "Communications Problems Affecting Patient Care in Hospitals," *JAMA,* 195:36–37 (Jan. 3) 1966.

Surgical Treatment of Specific Entities

Ajemian, Sylvia: "Bypass Grafting for Femoral Artery Occlusion," *Amer. J. Nurs.,* 67:565–68 (Mar.) 1967.

Colcock, Bentley P.: "Surgical Aspects of Thyroid Disease," *Postgrad. Med.,* 42:A85–A89 (Nov.) 1967.

Devlin, H. Brendan: "Abdominoperineal Resection of the Rectum," *Nurs. Times,* 64:1364–68 (Oct. 11) 1968.

Ehrenhaft, J. L.: "Femoral Bypass," *Surg. Clin. N. Amer.,* 46:1293–1310 (Oct.) 1966.

Keiser, Robert: "Treatment of Scoliosis," *Nurs. Clin. N. Amer.,* 2:409–18 (Sept.) 1967.

Mielke, John E., and Kirklin, John: "Renal Function During and After Surgery," *Med. Clin. N. Amer.,* 50:979–83 (July) 1966.

Morton, John H.: "Surgical Transfusion Practices," *Surgery,* 65:407–16 (Mar.) 1969.

"Observations, Investigation and Indications for Operation," *Nurs. Times,* 61:353–56 (Mar. 12) 1965.

"Operations on Arteries, I," *Nurs. Times,* **61**:387–90 (Mar. 19) 1965.

"Operations on Arteries, II," *Nurs. Times,* **61**:418–22 (Mar. 26) 1965.

Plant, Josephine A., and Devlin, H. Brendan: "Ileostomy and Its Management," *Nurs. Times,* **64**:711–14 (May 24) 1968.

Rains, A. J. Harding: "Arterial Surgery for Nurses: Historical, Introduction and Types of Arterial Disease," *Nurs. Times,* **61**:276–78 (Feb. 26) 1965.

Rains, A. J. Harding: "Care After Arterial Operations," *Nurs. Times,* **61**:454–56 (Apr. 2) 1965.

Rienhoff, William F., Jr., *et al.:* "Surgical Treatment of Hyperparathyroidism," *Ann Surg.,* **168**: 1061–74 (Dec.) 1968.

Wasserman, Reuban R.: "Management of Patients with Lower Extremity Amputations," *Mod. Treatm.,* **4**:416–41 (Mar.) 1967.

Welch, Claude E.: "Abdominal Surgery," *New Eng. J. Med.,* **280**:358–63, 419–25 (Feb.) 1969.

The Postoperative Period

Bergstrom, Nancy I.: "Ice Application to Induce Voiding," *Amer. J. Nurs.,* **69**:283–85 (Feb.) 1969.

Berne, Clarence J., and Rosoff, Leonard (eds.): "Symposium on Trauma," *Surg. Clin. N. Amer.,* **48**:1185–1414 (Dec.) 1968.

Breslau, Roger C.: "Intensive Care Following Vascular Surgery," *Amer. J. Nurs.,* **68**:1670–76 (Aug.) 1968.

De Veber, George A.: "Fluid and Electrolyte Problems in the Postoperative Period," *Nurs. Clin. N. Amer.,* **1**:275–84 (June) 1966.

Ambulation

Kottke, F. J.: "The Effect of Limitation of Activity upon the Human Body," *JAMA,* **196**:825–29 (June 6) 1966.

Leithauser, Daniel .: "Early Ambulation," *Amer. J. Nurs.,* **50**:203–206 (Apr.) 1950.

Leithauser, Daniel, Gregory, Louis, and Miller, Stella M.: "Immediate Ambulation After Extensive Surgery," *Amer. J. Nurs.,* **66**:2207–2208 (Oct.) 1966.

Pain

Barnard, Jan: "Understanding and Treating the Patient in Pain," *RN,* **30**:73–78 (May) 1967.

Black, Stephen, and Friedman, Max: "Effects of Emotion and Pain on Adrenocortical Function Investigated by Hypnosis," *Brit. Med. J.,* **1**: 477–81 (Feb. 24) 1968.

Blaylock, Jerry: "The Psychological and Cultural Influences on the Reaction to Pain: A Review of the Literature," *Nurs. Forum,* **7**:262–74 (No. 3) 1968.

Eckenhoff, James E. (ed.): "Symposium on Pain and Its Clinical Management," *Med. Clin. N. Amer.,* **52**:1–225 (Jan.) 1968.

Gates, Marshall: "Analgesic Drugs," *Sci. Amer.,* **215**:131–36 (Nov.) 1966.

Goshen, Charles E.: "The Placebo Effect: For Whom?" *Amer. J. Nurs.,* **66**:293–94 (Feb.) 1966.

Haugen, Frederick P.: "The Autonomic Nervous System and Pain," *Anesthesiology,* **29**:785–92 (July–Aug.) 1968.

Hinton, John: "Sedatives and Hypnotics," *Practitioner,* **200**:93–101 (Jan.) 1968.

Hodges, William F.: "Effects of Ego Threat and Threat of Pain on State Anxiety," *J. Personality Soc. Psychol.,* **8**:364–72 (No. 4) 1968.

Lasagna, Louis, and Werner, Gerhard: "Conjoint Clinic on Pain and Analgesia," *J. Chronic Dis.,* **19**:695–709 (June) 1966.

Macaffery, Margo, and Moss, Fay: "Nursing Intervention for Bodily Pain," *Amer. J. Nurs.,* **67**: 1224–27 (June) 1967.

"Pain. Part I: Basic Concepts and Assessment," *Amer. J. Nurs.,* **66**:1085–1108 (May) 1966.

"Pain. Part II: Rationale for Intervention," *Amer. J. Nurs.,* **66**:1345–68 (June) 1966.

Prescott, L. F.: "Analgesics," *Practitioner,* **200**:84–92 (Jan.) 1968.

Therrien, Barbara, and Salmon, James H.: "Percutaneous Cordotomy for Relief of Intractable Pain," *Amer. J. Nurs.,* **68**:2594–97 (Dec.) 1968.

Wound Healing

Abt, Arthur F., and VonSchuching, Susanne: "Aging as a Factor in Wound Healing," *Arch. Surg.* (Chicago), **86**:627–32 (Apr.) 1963.

Calnan, J., and Davies, A.: "The Effect of Methotrexate (Amethopterin) on Wound Healing: An Experimental Study," *Brit. J. Cancer,* **19**: 505–12 (Sept.) 1965.

DeVito, R. V.: "Healing of Wounds," *Surg. Clin. N. Amer.,* **45**:441–59 (Apr.) 1965.

Dunphy, J. Englebert: "The Fibroblast: Ubiquitous Ally for the Surgeon," *New Eng. J. Med.,* **268**:1367–77 (June 20) 1963.

Efron, G.: "Abdominal Wound Disruption," *Lancet,* **1**:1287–91 (June 17) 1965.

Goldin, Elliot G., and Joseph, Norman R.: "The Role of Connective Tissue Ground Substance in Wound Healing," *Surg. Forum,* **16**:87–89, 1965.

Pories, Walter J., *et al.:* "The Measurement of Human Wound Healing," *Surgery,* **59**:821–24 (May) 1966.

Ross, Russell: "Wound Healing," *Sci. Amer.,* **220**: 40–50 (June) 1969.

Complications

Glenn, Frank, and Beal, John M (eds.): "Symposium on Immediate Postoperative Complications," *Surg. Clin. N. Amer.,* **44**:303–564 (Apr.) 1964.

Isler, Charlotte: "Most Post-op Pulmonary Complications Are Preventable," *RN,* **29**:65–72, 92–93 (Nov.) 1966.

Peltier, Leonard F.: "Some Complications of Fractures," *Curr. Probl. Surg.,* pp. 2–44 (May) 1967.

"Symposium on Postoperative Complications," *Amer. J. Surg.,* **116**:325–406 (Sept.) 1968.

18

Nursing in Rehabilitation *

An optimist is a person who sees a green light everywhere. The pessimist sees only the red light. But the truly wise person is colorblind.

Albert Schweitzer

Overview

Rehabilitation Nursing

Specific Rehabilitation Situations

What are the nurse's responsibilities in rehabilitation?

Overview

REHABILITATION has become an often used and vital word. We are made constantly aware of objects, buildings, areas, and people being rehabilitated. Rehabilitating a beautiful old home in the city can be more of a status symbol than owning a sprawling modern home in suburbia. The rehabilitation of whole countries or cities, although overwhelming, does seem possible. The word *rehabilitation* connotes many things to society. What was of value previously will be retained. Broken and unnecessary components will be taken away. Emphasis is placed on eliminating those qualities that detract from beauty or function. The entity will have not only new life but will be better able to justify its existence. No one would expect, for example, a rehabilitated state park to be less beautiful than it once was or to attract less people than it once did. Society's a priori assumption here is that with time, effort, and money, rehabilitation will be successful. Planning the rehabilitation of a permanently disabled person is done on the basis of his eventual return to this society.

Certainly the word *rehabilitation* will continue to be used many ways; however, those who work with the permanently disabled as well as the disabled person himself have as a result an even greater task presented to them, for we have come to expect useless elements of rehabilitated entities to be replaced, but we do not always remember that the total ramification of a permanent disability of a human being cannot be removed.

Types of Disabilities

Illnesses and disabilities are traditionally classified as being either acute or chronic. An acute disorder is one having a rapid onset, severe symptoms, and a short course, progressing either to death or recovery. Chronic disorders are those that cannot be cured, do not go away, and are long and drawn out. These terms, *acute* and *chronic,* are not entirely functional classifications. Indeed the increasing use of the terminology "chronically ill and elderly" could not possibly be meant to be functional. The sheer number of disorders that the term *chronic illness* envelops is enough to inflict negative psychological stigma. The chronically ill seem to be a helpless lot. Their situations are overwhelming and irreversible. Little or nothing is seen to be done. Moreover, there seems to be no reason to try to do anything. Not uncommonly, as the chronically ill decline, slowly but steadily, the term *custodial care* accompanies the term *chronicity.* The negative aspects of each grow to form an unmanageable, deplorable, hopeless state.

It is for these reasons that a different classification has been suggested—the classification of temporary, progressive, and permanent illness or disability. Although *temporary* and *acute* can have similar meanings, the terms *progressive* and *permanent* dissect chronicity and

---

* This chapter was contributed by Nancy Martin, Director, Nursing Department, Rehabilitation Institute of Chicago, Chicago, Illinois.

thereby acknowledge that different types of stressors contribute to long-term physical and psychological illnesses. It is exactly because there are different types of stressors that persons in the paramedical disciplines are able to formulate specific approaches for meeting the needs of the ill and disabled.

To structure a frame of reference for this classification, an illness or disability can be defined as an event that either temporarily, permanently, or progressivly interrupts an individual's physiological, psychological, and, secondarily, social equilibrium. In a temporary illness or disability, one of two things may occur: (1) The illness or disability may be so severe as to cause death; if, however, death does not occur, then (2) whatever the disrupting or altering factor was, it will be removed. The individual will return to the type of life he possessed premorbidly. After the illness or disability has been treated and recovery occurs, there will be little if any residual effects on the person. Examples of temporary illness or disability are acute anxiety state, fractures, and appendectomy. The length of time necessary for the individual to return to his former physical and psychological state may vary, as, for example, the difference in the length of time required for discharge from a hospital following appendectomy from the length of time required for a fracture to heal. Nevertheless, if there is no fear of impending death, temporary illnesses and disabilities are fairly easily managed by patients and those around them. There is relatively little threat to the body image or the person's self-concept. Temporary illnesses and disabilities are familiar and can and do happen to everybody without serious sequelae. The important point here is that it is well known both by the patient and by those around him that he will return to his normal productive social role.

In permanent illness or disability the individual will physically never again be as he was premorbidly. Whatever physical changes occurred are irreversible. This person cannot be cured—he cannot be made whole. The lost function or part will not be restored. Although in some cases it is possible to substitute for the loss in such manner as to allow the person to lead "a normal life," the disability remains. The obvious and permanent physical change that has occurred necessitates a drastic and painful revision of the individual's concept of self. Such conditions as blindness, deafness, amputation, paraplegia, quadriplegia, cerebrovascular accident with organic brain damage, paresis or paralysis, and cerebral palsy fall into the category of permanent disabilities.

Progressive illness or disability differs from the other two in that the individual will be in a state of flux physically and psychologically, relative to the alteration that continues to progress until the disorder is permanent or until the individual dies. Again, as with permanent illnesses or disabilities, progressive disorders are not curable, although various therapeutic measures may lessen the effect of the disorder on the individual. Examples of progressive disorders are multiple sclerosis, muscular dystrophy, and myasthenia gravis. Instead of altering the concept of self once, as in the case of a permanent disorder, the person with a progressive disability or illness must continuously revise his concept of self as his disease progresses.

Essentially this chapter will consider rehabilitation of persons with permanent neuro-muscular-skeletal disorders. It is well to remember that in both progressive and permanent disorders the individual will be unable to function as he did premorbidly and that he will, therefore, be disabled to whatever physical or psychological extent that alteration implies for that person. Although remaining physical abilities may be increased and strengthened, the patient must, at some point, learn to accept and to live with his disability. Return of function does not occur and all rehabilitation goals must be formulated with this as the basis.

Need for Rehabilitation

Interest in rehabilitation was fostered in this country primarily because of the disabled servicemen who received their injuries during World Wars I and II. From the expansion of the field of rehabilitation has come the physiatrist, or physician who practices rehabilitation and physical medicine (the nursing student is urged to explore the writings of Howard Rusk, Henry Kessler, and Paul Magnuson, who were involved in the evolution of this specialty). That there is an ever greater need for rehabilitation of the physically disabled is obvious. The growing population as well as the increasing contact of more persons with high-powered machinery, such as automobiles, cannot help but produce greater numbers of permanently disabled persons. To meet the total needs of the permanently disabled, many specialties, or disciplines, have combined their services and function as a team. The team generally consists of physician, nurse, social worker, physical therapist, occupational therapist, psychologist, vocational counselor, nutritionist, recreational therapist, and speech pathologist. This team can function either in a general hospital or as a separate rehabilitation center.

Immediately following injury or illness, the disabled person will receive care in a general hospital. The services of these institutions are not limited to care of the patient with a neuro-muscular-skeletal condition. The type of care and how it is given are extremely vital factors during the acute stage of the disability, as a foundation for future rehabilitation begins when the patient is admitted to the first agency. Following the acute period of illness, the patient may be admitted to another institution or to another division of the same hospital for more lengthy treatment. These agencies are the re-habilitation centers, and their philosophies are directed toward rehabilitation or upgrading of the patient. It should be noted that initially emphasis was placed primarily on private and separate rehabilitation centers. However, ever-increasing numbers of general hospitals are pro-viding rehabilitation units within their own con-fines.

The combined services of these institutions alone cannot meet the total needs of physically disabled persons. Other official and nonofficial agencies should be an integral part of the re-habilitation process. More often than not a local, state, or federal agency will be involved, e.g., Visiting Nurse Association, Division of Services for Crippled Children, and Office of Vocational Rehabilitation.

Concepts and the Process of Rehabilitation

When beginning our study of rehabilitation of the physically disabled, we are confronted by a series of questions that should be con-sidered before further investigation will be fruit-ful. When does rehabilitation begin for the patient? When does it begin for paramedical disciplines? Are there differences in how each see it; if so, why does this occur? Why is not rehabilitation always successful? What happens when it is? What happens when it is not success-ful; and if it "has not worked," who says so? When goals are set, for whom are they set? Why, when we encounter rehabilitation in the literature, does it seem we already know what the author has to say? Yet, why then is it so hard to pull this rehabilitation gossamer into a meaningful, functional whole? Why can the process of rehabilitation seem so elusive when we are easily and constantly reminded of the immediacy of the disability, with all that the disability means to the patient and his family?

When you talk about rehabilitation you are talking about a concept. And concepts are pub-lic domain in that we arrive at what something means to us all by ourselves. We do this be-cause of our attitudes, values, beliefs, and ex-periences. Everyone has his own concept of rehabilitation. The area of rehabilitation itself is full of concepts—independence, dependence,

help, goal—all of these are words that are used freely and often. When each of us hears these words or uses them, they are perceived accord-ing to our own conceptualization of them, and our actions flow from our perceptions. When we think about rehabilitation we do so on a conceptual basis, but when we are involved with people in rehabilitation it must of necessity also become a viable process.

It is helpful to consider how the word *reha-bilitation* is used as a means of differentiating the concept from the process. In the literature we encounter the classic definition of rehabilita-tion as assisting the patient to his maximum level of functioning; usually this definition in-cludes the words *physical, emotional, voca-tional, independence,* and, sometimes, *social.* Rarely is the word *avocational* used, and even more rarely is the ultimate level of functioning stated in terms of what the patient desires or the degree of independence the patient is able or motivated to achieve. Rehabilitation is also defined as being the third stage of medicine. How much easier our roles would be if it were no more complex than that. Certainly it is true that there are techniques and approaches that medicine and the paramedical disciplines use, but these are techniques and approaches and nothing more.

Moreover, the nursing profession has tended to view rehabilitation in a somewhat nebulous way. We, too, have set it aside as a specialty, although often our curricula indicate that it is important enough to be a basic, continuing thread in the education of nurses, along with nutrition and patient and family teaching. Too often we have seen rehabilitation solely in terms of the patient who needs a footboard or range-of-motion exercises. We have thought of it in terms of physical therapy consultations and pa-tients ambulating between parallel bars. We have viewed rehabilitation in terms of the equipment that occupational therapy brings to the patient. Not uncommonly this equipment only clutters the patient's already cluttered bed-side table and hardly ever is used. Usually this is because we do not know how to use the equipment or exactly what it is supposed to do. Furthermore, we know that there are official and nonofficial health agencies, but their serv-ices are rather vague to us, and even more obscure is how and when they enter the patient situation. We have also thought of rehabilita-tion in terms of how the patient leaves the hospital, and he usually goes in one of two ways. He may go in his new wheelchair with all of his potted plants (rehabilitation was suc-cessful here), or he is placed on an ambulance stretcher and is taken to a nursing home (re-habilitation was not successful here).

Rehabilitation has been elusive to nurses in that we are never really certain when it starts and when it is supposed to stop. If asked when rehabilitation should start we automatically respond, "At time of admission." Yet we are also aware that it starts at a later time, such as when the physician who has managed the acute stage does not have anything else to do for, or to, the patient. The beginning of rehabilitation then becomes a very direct thing when this physician sends the patient to a specific place where he will "get rehabilitation" or "be rehabilitated." Therefore as each of us, according to our own concept, sees rehabilitation starting at a different time, perhaps we should look for that time when rehabilitation begins for the patient.

If we use as a definition of rehabilitation a relearning of old skills, then rehabilitation for the disabled starts before admission at the time the disability occurs. It starts at the time the disabled person becomes aware he can no longer move or feel or say what he could before. The old skills that must be relearned or upgraded are the activities of daily living. These words mean far more than meaning how to walk and dress again or how to transfer from a bed to a wheelchair, although these things are very important. Activities of daily living mean such things as relearning what one's role in one's family is, relearning how to view oneself realistically, and relearning how to cope as successfully as possible with the stresses of life. These are the things that make rehabilitation a process, or a series of events, and it becomes a process for the disabled person from the beginning. It becomes his process and what we must learn to do is not only operate on our own concept of rehabilitation for a specific patient but operate equally in his process of relearning.

When nurses operate solely on their own concepts of rehabilitation, they will be involved in the patient's rehabilitation process only at those particular times when their "concept" happens to occur within the patient's "process." We can see, then, that it would be entirely possible for the nurse to be completely uninvolved in a patient's rehabilitation process; for example, if the patient suffered a stroke, with resultant mild hemiparesis and severe language disorder, he will need little, if any, retraining in the areas of ambulating and dressing. But he will need much assistance in relearning to communicate. When the nurse in this situation views rehabilitation as a series of physical activities, which of course are no problem for this particular patient, then the patient's real needs can hardly be met because they are only barely recognized.

Not only then do we need a comprehensive view of the patient's rehabilitation process but we must examine clearly and carefully his entire disabling condition, and this can be a very difficult task, for, regardless of our interviewing skill, wealth of information about the patient premorbidly, and awareness of his total diagnosis, we can know only a part of those things that trouble him, cause him anxiety, and eventually alter the manner in which he copes with his disability, as well as the reactions of the able-bodied to him.

The situation facing the disabled person, and those assisting him in his relearning process, has essentially three components. The first two, the physical and psychological, in turn affect the third component, the sociological aspect. In fact, appropriate management of the first and second components is for the achievement of a satisfactory social adjustment. Strange indeed is the lack of attention we give the eventual social adjustment of our patients. At best we are concerned that adequate placement after discharge occurs, and our efforts usually indicate some acknowledgment of this factor. However, how often do we consciously or unconsciously ignore the obvious. For example, one needs only to witness the confusion and uncertainty that can arise when the paramedical team is made aware of the probability that a young, male paraplegic, who has not yet accepted his disability, will turn again to narcotics. His former use of narcotics was known to the team, as was the obvious fact of his depression and nonacceptance of paralysis. Yet, somehow the connection between the attractiveness of such release to this person and the ease of his obtaining narcotics when he returns home for weekend visits was not made. For some reason this natural turn of events for him was not anticipated. Rather, he had to tell us. A few of our members might say, "Well, this was his premorbid pattern—obviously little can be done." And yet he told us, and by telling us, asked for help. How clinically aware we can be of the psychological picture, as well as the patient's exact physical status—but how truly negligent and naive are our abilities at grasping the total circumstances. Our restricted vision into the needs of the disabled, although often innocent, is far from acceptable.

Wherever, then, does one begin with the severely physically disabled? Science has taught us much about their physical needs. That we can now keep physically disabled persons alive longer is an infinitesimal feather for our caps if we cannot help them manage the rest of their living. One useful point of departure is to be aware of how the disabled are viewed by the able-bodied. This not only involves all the able-bodied of society but indeed the person with the newly acquired disability, for how this disabled person now views himself postmorbidly is attributable at least in part to how he viewed the disabled premorbidly.

The altered physical appearance of the disabled is a stimulus that triggers our reaction. Having perceived the obvious and negative difference, it is difficult to halt or alter the series of events that follow. The physically "discreditable" persons of whom Goffman [1] writes are those the normal stigmatize. The stigmatization process, or perception of the negative stimulus that flows to color other attributes of the disabled's being, is instantaneous. Delegating the physically disabled to minority status is obviously not done on a rational basis, but this process is swift and can be permanent. The initial contact with physically disabled persons usually occurs in childhood. The shock that accompanies this type of introduction can be lessened somewhat by an understanding adult. Far more often, however, the child is left to work alone with his unaltered impression, be it fear, pity, repulsion, curiosity, or a combination of these. He may always retain these initial impressions whether his contact with the disabled is great or infrequent.

Not a small part of the task presented the paramedical team, therefore, is dealing with already formed prejudice and rejection of permanently or progressively disabled conditions by the able-bodied and disabled.

Rehabilitation Nursing

As stated before, the disabled person who goes to a separate rehabilitation facility will initially have received care in a general hospital and will usually be followed eventually by a community nursing organization. All nurses who work for agencies giving care to the disabled person are involved in and have responsibility for his rehabilitation program. Although the purpose of the agency will indicate fairly clearly what the prime objectives of his care at that time should be, it is necessary for each nurse to understand the total rehabilitation needs of the patient, and consequently she should know what nursing intervention has already occurred and, to some degree, what will follow. There is no doubt that the more direct and comprehensive the communication between nurses in these agencies, the better the nursing carry-over.

The nurse in a general hospital must direct her attention toward keeping the newly admitted patient alive. She must be aware of the physiological reactions that occur as a result of of a neuromuscular-skeletal disability. For ex-

ample, she must know that the person who has sustained an injury resulting in a severed spinal cord will not perspire below the level of his injury. The remaining innervated areas of the body must now assume the entire responsibility for the insensible water loss mechanism. If the injury to the spinal cord is in the region of the cervical vertebrae, the only remaining innervated areas will be the head, neck, and shoulders, and these become, therefore, the only body areas capable of perspiration. The nurse should anticipate an extremely high temperature elevation and be prepared to institute measures to assist the body in lowering the temperature.

At this time the most diligent, consistent, and strict attention must be given to preventing any torsion on the spinal cord. For if the cord is not totally transected, and there is any chance at all for return of function, further insult to the cord can entirely preclude such return. This means that any movement of the patient must be done in the most careful manner. If there is any possibility that a patient brought to the emergency room has sustained spinal cord damage, he should be seen by a physician before being transferred from the ambulance stretcher. All transfer activities must be done by sufficient personnel to assure that the patient's entire body is moved at once. The personnel should accompany the patient wherever transfers are involved, e.g., x-ray department, surgery, or patient unit.

The initial atmosphere in which the patient finds himself will have much bearing on his entire rehabilitation program. It is essential to remember the great physical and psychological shock these patients experience immediately following a neuromuscular-skeletal injury and address our efforts accordingly. An intelligent regimen must begin early or difficulty will be encountered in enlisting not only the patient's cooperation but his consent. For example, attempts at instituting a turning regimen for a lower extremity amputee only several days after surgery may be met with refusal by the patient. It is imperative that the patient have confidence in the nurse's ability. Unless the nurse is capable of meeting the patient's physical needs, and meeting them well, her efforts in other areas of concern (emotional, social) will be of little value. If the complexity of these problems is not anticipated and met, the patient's progress will be hindered and may result in no rehabilitation being possible. The great responsibility of helping to create this introductory atmosphere is that of the nurse in the general hospital.

The function of the nurse employed in a rehabilitation setting will to some degree be determined by the philosophy of that institution and

[1] Erving Goffman: *Stigma* (Englewood Cliffs, N.J.: Prentice-Hall, Inc., 1963), p. 41.

the number of other disciplines represented. She may be responsible for teaching the patient dressing techniques or for communicating his dressing progress to the discipline responsible for the initial teaching. She may follow the teaching program outlined by a part-time speech pathologist or she may primarily be responsible for observing whether the patient utilizes the retraining the speech pathologist feels he has accomplished. Certainly one of her most important responsibilities will be to communicate the patient's progress, when on the patient unit, to the other disciplines. It is essential that she observe and communicate not only his increased physical capabilities but his interactions with staff, other patients, and his visitors.

In addition the nurse has areas of teaching responsibility that are unique. Bodily needs and functions such as bowel, bladder, skin care, hygiene, diet, fluids, rest, and sleep that have been altered by the disability are of concern to nurses in all settings. In the acute stages of an illness or in the case of a temporary disorder these areas are taken care of for the patient until the time he again can do them himself. The emphasis in a rehabilitation setting, however, is on teaching the patient and/or his family new methods of managing these bodily functions. These new methods then become permanent components of living for the disabled person. If, for example, a non-brain-damaged male paraplegic will always need a retention catheter, he must know how to care for it, e.g., irrigating, inserting, sterilizing irrigating equipment, cleansing of leg urine collecting bags, as well as what to do for catheter blockage. The over-all goal here is for the disabled person to invest again in maintaining his own body integrity, to care about his body, and to know how to take care of it. Much of what he now must do is repugnant and unnatural. Activities of daily living such as digital stimulation for evacuation or examining one's body with a long-handled mirror for new pressure areas are not easily or quickly accepted. Therefore the manner in which the nurse goes about her teaching and the support she gives are as important as the teaching plan she has formulated.

Coordinating the patient's 24-hour day is a tremendously difficult nursing responsibility. In addition to what she must teach, the nurse must help the disabled person utilize and make a part of his life all that he is learning in other departments. It does no good to learn one means of transferring from bed to wheelchair in physical therapy if it is done another way on the patient unit. Relearning to dress in the occupational therapy department by using adaptive devices will be to no avail if nursing personnel dress the patient. Relearning to com- municate in speech pathology cannot be of value if the patient is communicated with in an inappropriate way outside of therapeutic sessions.

The nurse who works in rehabilitation settings obviously must learn a large and relatively new body of knowledge. If she is to assist the patient in implementing what he is learning elsewhere, she must be thoroughly aware of the goals and methods of other departments. Furthermore, it is essential that she look for the kinds of data other therapists need to know in order to evaluate the effect of the teaching the patient has received.

After a taxing day in the various therapies, the patient will be physically and emotionally exhausted. The patient unit is his "home," and the atmosphere must be conducive to relaxation. The nurse should be sensitive to his expressions of feelings of his progress. He should be told that she realizes these days are exhausting. There could be no better time for well-chosen words of realistic encouragement. The rehabilitation process is a slow and difficult one, and its day-by-day progress only makes more apparent to the patient the full meaning of his disability.

To the visiting nurse or public health nurse goes the responsibility of observing the results of efforts accomplished during the acute and chronic periods of care. No amount of rehabilitation activities instituted in either of the two former agencies will be of any value if the patient is not prepared to function outside their protective environments. Besides determining his physical status and abilities, the visiting or public health nurse must be alert to the entire complex of the patient's reactions on returning to his home. Although his activities may not be so extensive as before his disability, she must ascertain if he is participating to his fullest potential—and if not, why not.

Hospitals of all kinds tend to protect patients, and the impact of coping again with the outside environment—now with a disability—is overwhelming. This pertains to the family as well as the patient. The nurse can help to resolve many of the problems faced by the patient. Some, such as inability to find employment, she cannot help to resolve. Her only recourse then is to listen and give realistic support and encouragement. The public health nurse's role is to help the patient and family cope with the reality of the consequences of the disability in the community.

When the visiting or public health nurse is a member of the team, at least in the final period of the patient's hospitalization, the knowledge and guidance of the team are carried into the home. The combined efforts of nurses in the two hospitals and in the public health agency have immeasurable value to the total rehabilitation of the person afflicted with a neuromuscular-skeletal disability. Their activities are of equal importance and carry equal responsibility. Each stage is a vital part of the whole. If in any of the three areas the nurse does not strive to assist the patient to reach his optimum potential, she is answerable to herself, the patient, and her colleagues.

The Rehabilitation Process

DETERMINATION OF NEEDS

A comprehensive approach to the patient's needs is essential. Permanent disability involves much more than physical limitations. Psychosocial, vocational-economic, and physical needs can best be determined by the team of specialists. The number of team members involved in an individual patient situation corresponds to the specific needs of that patient. For example, if, as a result of a cerebrovascular accident, a patient has sustained severe organic brain damage, there is little need for the services of a vocational counselor. On the other hand, if the patient can utilize the services of the entire team and benefits from spiritual guidance, his clergyman may become an active team participant. It is the task of the rehabilitation team to determine how the needs of the patient may best be met. Their efforts are directed toward increasing his assets and substituting new methods for achieving old activities. Frequent team discussions, during which their observations are shared, inform them all of his progress.

More often than not, positive or negative signs will have been noticed by at least two disciplines. For example, John, a high school senior, sustained paraplegia as a result of a football injury. Three months after the accident he was admitted to a rehabilitation center. When the team first discussed possible goals for John, all departments reported he was greatly depressed and withdrawn. Furthermore, he appeared to have no interest in increasing his abilities and refused to do much of what he was then capable. This situation continued throughout the first month. At a team conference one and a half months after admission it became apparent that his attitudes and desires were changing. The nurse reported that John was now a full participant in ward activities and was more concerned about his physical appearance. The physical therapist reported he had expressed beginning interest in transfer from bed to wheelchair. Two weeks later the vocational counselor told of John's asking if he could continue his schoolwork required for graduation. At the following team conference, all disciplines reported that John appeared to be actively and positively involved in his rehabilitation program.

By combining their skills and knowledge of the patient's gains, necessary revisions in goal setting are made. At times this means arriving at the decision that the patient is not a candidate for extensive rehabilitation and that other plans are necessary for him. This is always a difficult task and one arrived at only after extensive consideration of the entire patient situation. It is extremely unfair to continue to demand of the patient that of which he is incapable. Moreover, it is unfair to other patients if the team's time and energy are frustratingly exhausted.

The rehabilitation team must not only be positively involved in the patient's program but all members must be working together and all at the same time. Each discipline, as needed by individual patients, is responsible for a unique area, and, again, all these areas are needed for the whole. Usually, as in John's situation, the team must begin without the patient's cooperation as he may need to see the possibilities before becoming an active participant. Many complications arise and time is lost if a comprehensive program is not attempted. Furthermore, the experienced team anticipates both physical and emotional delays. The complexities of a permanent disability demand the utmost patience of all concerned.

VIEWING THE PATIENT AS AN INDIVIDUAL

All persons, able-bodied or disabled, must be viewed as individuals. We cannot predetermine either the patient's physical or emotional capabilities by knowing only his disability. A person having sustained an injury resulting in quadriplegia may be completely self-sufficient and may provide valuable service to his employer, colleagues, and family. Another, following traumatic amputation of both upper extremities, may refuse prosthetic devices and remain at home, providing no service to anyone.

We must not underestimate the capabilities of the disabled person. For example, seven-year-old Jimmy, diagnosed as having cerebral palsy, was admitted to a general hospital for an obturator neurectomy to relieve adduction contractures to his legs. He was unable to communicate verbally with the nursing staff. No information was available about his abilities, and, as his home was in a distant part of the state, none was obtained from his parents. Complete custodial care was given this boy. Jimmy was fed, diapered, and allowed to remain totally inactive. Because he was unable to talk, no other means of communication were explored. When he was discharged to his parents, the nursing staff was shocked to learn that before admission Jimmy was completely toilet-trained and could communicate by using a word board. Many months of frustrating work by both the boy and his mother were undone by persons not attempting all possible means of communication with him and not viewing Jimmy as the individual he was.

SUCCESSFUL REHABILITATION PROGRAM

If a patient can be described as being success-fully rehabilitated, then one may assume all goals have been met. Only by determining and accomplishing short-term goals can the ultimate realistic goal be reached. Whether this ultimate long-term goal is partial self-care or returning to the community as a full participant does not alter the necessity for all concerned to strive for the possible—not probable—way of life for the patient. No excessive desire for unobtainable goals by any person involved can bring them about. Just as we must accept the patient's abil-ities, so, too, must we recognize his limitations. Achieving goals within the realm of possibility is difficult enough. Unrealistic goals and false encouragement can frustrate the patient to the point of rendering him incapable of achieving that which is possible. However, this is not to say that any patient's potential may not be greater than first believed. Caution and discre-tion are wise when initially informing the pa-tient and his family of long-term goals. Changes in their lives caused by the disability are trau-matic; having to tell them at a later date that the initially stated potential cannot be met is even more damaging.

Appropriate timing is necessary for a success-ful rehabilitation program. Positive patient and family motivation as well as the program out-lined by the rehabilitation team is needed. Often these constituents are ready but at differing times; and although it is possible to proceed in this manner for a period, total rehabilitation will not occur until the patient, his family, and the team are all working toward the same goal —and at the same time.

The problems of the rehabilitation process do not stop when the patient returns to the com-munity. There are many reasons for the dis-appointments that often occur. The patient's former associates, both vocational and avoca-tional, are rarely prepared for the role they must assume with him. Are the patient and his family capable of assisting friends and asso-ciates in this adjustment? There is no better test of the comprehensive guidance given by the team.

Although able-bodied persons are aware that the disabled person does have a social role, they often do not know how this is accomplished. Moreover, society knows neither what nor how to assist or help—only that some assistance is expected.[2] All of this only compounds the final test of a successful rehabilitation program: Does the patient increase his abilities after dis-charge? He should reach his highest potential at home, not while hospitalized.

THE PATIENT WHO CANNOT BE REHABILITATED

If we state a patient cannot be rehabilitated because he lacks motivation, we are incorrect. Reaction and attitude are always a result of motivation. Insofar as the rehabilitation process is concerned, patient motivation may be posi-tive or negative. It is important to remember that he is motivated in some direction and will respond accordingly. Herein lies one of the frus-trations of rehabilitation.

The area of secondary gains from a disability is vast. The reader is urged to explore other works whose attention is directed to these con-siderations. In writing of "motivational conse-quences," Wright states

A disability may serve many purposes. The per-son may wish to insure continuing financial com-pensation that his disability provides; he may wel-come the dependency facilitated by his disability; his disability may satisfy a masochistic need for punishment; it may afford him social sanction for avoiding competitive striving, which he fears. . . . The point is a simple one. When a disability is sat-isfying for one reason or another, it becomes mag-nified through beliefs and expectations.[3]

Physical limitations may be the determining factors in the decision that a patient cannot be rehabilitated. Here again the situation is not an uncomplicated one. Often the determinant is a medical component. For example, if an elderly person has had bilateral lower extremity ampu-tation as a result of arteriosclerosis with accom-panying arteriosclerotic heart disease, the task of learning to walk with prosthetic devices may be considered too great a strain for the already weakened heart. Therefore, the best means of life for this patient would be from a wheelchair. It is necessary again to mention realistic goal setting. When the patient is unable to meet the stated potential because of lack of physical abil-ity, then the original plans and subsequent pro-gram were in error. Too frequently we view a

[2] G. Ladien, E. Haufman, and T. Dembo: "Studies in Adjustment to Visable Injuries: Evaluation of Help by the Injured," *J. Abnorm. Social Psychol.*, 42:169–92, 1947.

[3] Beatrice Wright: *Physical Disability: A Psycho-logical Approach* (New York: Harper and Brothers, 1960), p. 173.

rehabilitated person in terms of ambulation—with or without braces. If, however, the early decision had been wheelchair existence, much physical and emotional energy would have been spared.

When thinking of future employment possibilities, the issue becomes more complicated in proportion to the extent of physical limitation. A unilateral lower extremity amputee faces a relatively uncomplicated situation. The problems of the severely afflicted rheumatoid arthritic, paraplegic, or multiextremity amputee are quite another matter. An employer hiring a person with physical limitations understandably will choose the least afflicted. Employment of environmental facilities must be negotiable for the wheelchair-bound. Transportation to and from employment may become an insuperable barrier. Generally, the greater the intelligence, the greater are future employment possibilities. For example, a person afflicted with quadriplegia must now depend almost completely on his mind. If he does not possess the necessary mental abilities, there can be no realistic thought of vocational goals.

It must be clearly understood that the patient may not accept a proposed vocational change. An area of great concern to the vocational counselor is helping the disabled person to make the necessary adjustments. By using testing devices that determine the patient's mental and manual abilities, new vocational areas are made apparent. The decision to accept a vocational change involves the process the disabled person goes through in changing his identity of self. Someone, for example, who can no longer drive a bus, a job he performed for 20 years, may be physically able to work in the bus company garage; but if his concept of himself is that of a bus driver, he will not be able to see himself in any other role, whether associated with busses or not. The possibilities can only be presented; here again the decision is the patient's.

Rehabilitation of persons with permanent disabilities is extremely expensive. The expense of time and physical and emotional energy can be greater than financial expense. The complete rehabilitation process of a patient will not be possible if any of these basic requirements cannot be met. The rehabilitation team can work only with what remains after the disability, and the emotional response of the patient is often more important than his retained physical abilities. However, even the patient who does not emotionally accept his disability can be upgraded physically and should therefore be able to live better than before his partial rehabilitation. The most minor achievements rarely occur without great effort and understanding on the part of everyone involved in the rehabilitation program.

THE PATIENT'S ROLE

No matter how brilliantly conceived a rehabilitation program may be, it will be worthless unless the patient is involved. He must be motivated positively—and this is the essence of rehabilitation. Whereas the rehabilitation team is the body of the process, positive patient motivation is the soul. The driving force must come from within the patient even though the team makes evident his potential and provides continued teaching, support, and encouragement.

A revision of self-concept is demanded for a patient to become positively motivated. The patient is no longer the physical being he was. Until such time as he recognizes and comprehends this all-important fact, no changes in how he now views himself will occur. In too many instances we expect him to have had a secure and positive self-concept prior to his disability. The patient is what he was before his injury—only more so. If he was cognizant of his strengths and weaknesses, such an awareness will tend to continue. If, however, he had not found his role previous to his disability, it will be extremely difficult for him to do so now. The situation in which he now finds himself and his premorbid personality are essential factors in revising his self-concept. We cannot expect changes in self-concept or positive motivation to occur rapidly. This is a process that requires greatly differing lengths of time and that will depend on the individual. Determining whether or not a patient is positively motivated is a very difficult undertaking and cannot and should not be done by one person.

Just as we must anticipate a delay in motivation, so, too, should we be alert to pseudomotivation. If the patient regularly attends his therapies and, in all other ways, is following (seemingly) the plan we have provided, we tend to assume he is a part of his rehabilitation process. This is not necessarily the true situation. There is no better way to be unaffected or overlooked by others than to perform in the manner expected. For example, Mary Simmons, a 30-year-old paraplegic, always seemed eager to attend the occupational and physical therapy appointments. She left the patient unit early enough to assure arriving early for therapy. The physical therapist presented a view of Miss Simmons quite different from what the nursing staff imagined. Although Miss Simmons was willing to exercise and increase the strength of her upper extremities, she would not agree to learn ways of compensating for the lost function of her lower extremities, e.g., transfer from bed to wheelchair.

It is impossible for the able-bodied to realize the full psychological impact on a person who has suddenly suffered a stroke, traumatic amputation or sustained paraplegia. In the patient's eyes and in the eyes of many others he immediately loses the attributes making him the unique individual he was, and he becomes part of the nonspecific world of the crippled. Whether or not the full consequences are evident to him at once is of little import. He need only know he no longer can move, feel, or care for himself; in ways he never knew existed, he is dependent on others. The shock is profound and does not leave.

The stages of psychological shock, denial, depression, and anxiety usually precede acceptance of a permanent disability. Initially, the patient will be concerned with the loss of the body part or function. He just cannot believe what has happened to him. Psychological shock may be expected no matter what the disability. Even the person who has agreed to amputation of an extremity will usually experience a period of mourning for the lost body part.

The patient may express denial in numerous ways: refusing to enter into or to allow planning for rehabilitation; refusing needed surgical procedures; and outwardly accepting physical and occupational therapies, while inwardly believing the disability is not permanent. The patient's denial is not difficult to understand. If he believes the condition does not exist, the reality of the situation need not be faced. By assuming, as in Miss Simmons' case, that the disability is temporary, the patient will see no need for rehabilitation.

As the full impact of the disability becomes obvious to the patient, he enters into a stage of depression. The disability has not gone away; physical sequelae further insult his disabled body; family savings are fast being exhausted; he can never return to his former vocation; previous life plans no longer are attainable. He is constantly reminded of his lost manhood. If he is of no value to himself, how can he possibly be to those who formerly depended on him? Society, with its pressures and emphasis on increasing production, offers no place for him. There seem to be no solutions to his problems, and he becomes further depressed and withdrawn. Again, he may exhibit various behavioral patterns, refusing all care, food, and fluids; refusing to talk; or refusing to sleep or sleeping all the time with the sheet pulled over his head.

Those around the patient should be alert to expressions of anxiety. As he begins in his rehabilitation program, the slowness of his progress and inherent frustrations increase his anxiety. He may express overconcern about further physical harm to himself; he may be verbally abusive to those around him; he may suddenly take great interest in family affairs and become dogmatic over seemingly trivial matters. One person, or everyone in his environment, may be the recipient of his expressions. If this is not understood and managed correctly, irreparable damage will occur. The value to the patient of progressing through these agonizing periods is the eventual acceptance of his disability. He cannot ignore or deny the lost function; it is part of him. And viewing himself as a whole, he eventually may see his abilities and limitations. Ideally this is the point at which he joins the rehabilitation team in his program.

How much easier it would be for all concerned if we could predict the time needed for these stages. If only they could occur once— and in order! But this just does not happen. The length of time varies from days to months to years. The stages are mixed; there may be progression and regression. Only by observing his behavior and being sensitive to his expressions can we determine our approach. We cannot propel him through these stages as we wish. No matter how great our desire or efforts, he cannot and should not move forward in our predetermined way. And this is what is meant by seeing and accepting each person as an individual. We must remember he may stop and remain in any stage. As he belongs to himself and not to us, this is his right. However, he then cannot be viewed as a candidate for a successful rehabilitation program. When we perceive it otherwise, we fool only ourselves.

If we use one word to describe the nurse's approach, it should be *adaptable*. She must be alert to the patient's manner of expressing just where he is in his adjustment process. She must know when to move ahead with him and when to leave him alone. She must be aware of the time when he becomes an active participant. Or she must accept the decision that he is not a rehabilitation candidate. Only by being objectively observant can she appraise; only by being adaptable can she function.

Hopefully, throughout the stages of shock, denial, and depression, realistic potentials have been made apparent to the patient. Being so vitally concerned with self and his inability to meet former goals, he is easily overwhelmed by well-meant but indiscreet barrages of future possibilities. Therefore, making him aware of his positive aspects of his future should be done carefully and appropriately.

PSYCHOLOGICAL SITUATIONS WITHIN THE FAMILY

When viewing the family, again we are considering individuals. It is unrealistic and hazardous to assume all in the family group possess the same attributes and have the same relationship with the patient. For example, 20-year-old Tom sustained extensive flaccid paralysis as a result of poliomyelitis. The father perceived his son's paralysis as destroying his plans for Tom joining him in business, whereas the mother viewed the disability as a means of keeping Tom dependent on her. Had Tom wanted independence, planned to live alone, and never wished to join his father in business, the situation would be even more complex. The nurse must be alert to the separate manifestations by the individual family members and their effects on the patient. If the patient-family relationship was positive prior to the disability, the manner in which each accepts the disability will affect the other. The family will go through the stages of adjusting as did the patient. Their eventual interpretation of the disability will also depend on how the disability meets or thwarts their needs and desires—both for the patient and for themselves.

Untold benefits to the patient result from continued support, encouragement, and love given by the family. They are capable of sustaining him in ways not open to any outsider. He needs to feel he is still an integral family member. If he is led to believe his role is no longer essential, and, indeed, he is a burden, the effect can be devastating. We should remember he may well feel this under any circumstances, and even the slightest affirmation by a family member (or friend) can prohibit later attempts at bringing him into family matters.

It is usually a very sad state when a patient is rejected by one or more members of his family. Regression in his rehabilitation process is caused by such things as being ignored by his family, divorce proceedings, disposition of property, and the moving of his family to another area. The nurse may or may not know of these occurrences; it is difficult in either event. We must also realize that at times family rejection is understandable. When, for example, previous to his disability, the patient was a ne'er-do-well or a tyrant, creating and not solving family problems, the prospects of caring for him now may be more than the family can do or should be expected to do.

An ever-present problem that the nurse will encounter when working with the family is fear. The family may be able to express their fear, but more often than not they will attempt to conceal it, for they think this is what is expected of them. The family may be incapable of local-izing their apprehension or anxiety even if they wished to communicate. The initial explanation of the disability will be given the family by the physician. It is the responsibility of the nurse to ascertain if they are aware of what to expect when first visiting the patient. They will immediately be concerned about his physical condition. Such things as whether he will live or die and what equipment is being used are of prime importance to them at this time. Trauma when first seeing the patient, even after being told what to expect, is great. The range of concern here is wide, depending on the condition: coma, stertorous breathing, hemiplegia, side rails, Stryker frame, water mattress. Families can be extremely frightened by assistive breathing devices such as an oxygen tent, tracheostomy, or positive pressure machine. Before and after this first visit, the nurse must provide time for explanation and questions.

The patient's physical appearance frightens the family. Following a cerebrovascular accident the patient may drool or be incontinent —the arm and leg appear glaringly lifeless. The patient who has sustained a cervicovertebral injury can move only his arms and head, but even "his arms do not move right" and "his fingers don't move at all." Their fear of physical contact with him can be twofold: either repulsion because of his appearance or fear of causing further damage to him. They are frightened because they do not understand what has occurred, and yet they are afraid of knowing the truth. Just as the patient needs support, so does the family. Care must be taken to avoid inappropriate reassurances, for this is equally as damaging to the family members as to the patient.

Sufficient time must be provided the family for questions. As the patient's condition changes, so, too, will the family's interests and concerns. Although the nurse should expect repetition in what the family states or asks, she must be alert to the family's asking the same question of many persons. This may mean no one has discovered what is really being asked. For example, Mr. Walker was admitted to a general hospital following a cerebrovascular accident. Mrs. Walker visited her husband daily, and several times during each visit she would ask various members of the nursing staff if there were enough nurses on duty who knew how to give him the care he needed. When she continued to be concerned about this, the head nurse spoke at length with her. She found that Mrs. Walker was really afraid of not being able to care for him at home and was not at all worried about the care given Mr. Walker by the nursing staff.

When the family states their need for assistance that requires referral to another agency it is essential that the nurse know appropriate resources and methods for the referral. The decision to seek assistance is not one easily made. What to the nurse may seem to be an obvious and a routinely met need can be extremely embarrassing and degrading to the family. When families ask for help, the referral should be swiftly and tactfully accomplished. They must be given specific and correct information and should not be left with the awareness that their need may or may not have been heard but was not answered. The nurse will be well acquainted with services available in her own institution. The task of determining the proper assistance agency will be greatly decreased if there is a social service department within her institution. When there is none, she must be familiar with official and nonofficial agencies in the community. Usually it will be the function of one agency to provide information on services offered by all agencies in the community, and the nurse should utilize this agency. Larger cities have an index or sourcebook of community agencies.

There are increasing numbers of groups formed by families of persons afflicted with the same disability. The value of families sharing problems and goals with each other is obvious. For example, nothing may be more comforting to parents who finally accept that their child has cerebral palsy than meeting other parents who have experienced and coped with the multitude of ever-present problems and discouragements.

The family may be provided reading materials that are written for the layman, e.g., *Care of the Patient with a Stroke* by Genevieve Smith and *Episode* by Eric Hodgins. By reading about the condition their family member has, they may more readily understand the entire situation. Even the most dedicated medical and paramedical personnel cannot hope to cover all necessary areas when talking with families. Furthermore, the family cannot quickly assimilate all information given to them verbally. More often than not, the family will return with new and important questions.

The family should be helped to understand the behavior patterns and personality manifestations of the patient. So often the patient does not behave as he did before the disability. Such things as hostility or silence of the paraplegic and drastic mood swings and cursing by the patient who has had a cerebrovascular accident must be explained. The family cannot and should not be expected to encounter and cope with these manifestations alone.

PREPARING THE FAMILY FOR HOME CARE

The family is included in giving care gradually. Activities such as placing a pillow comfortably and correctly and pouring the amount of water that will enable the patient to hold the glass himself can begin when the family seems ready. Knowing when the family is ready is not always easy. Generally it is wise to begin when there no longer is grave concern for the patient's life. The frustrating feeling of utter uselessness can overcome the fear of physical contact. The physical care of a person afflicted with a neuromuscular-skeletal condition is complex. Besides the obvious weakness or loss of function of the body part or parts, many other physical problems occur. If professional persons become overwhelmed by the physical needs of these patients, they should be even more aware of their teaching responsibilities to the family. Not only does the family need to know why and how activities of daily living are accomplished but they must understand the even greater problem of how to allow the patient to do what he can for himself. How much easier it is to protect those we love by doing for them rather than seeing them struggle to do for themselves.

The nurse must carefully ascertain the effect on the patient caused by family members assisting him. If the assistance is gradual and matter of fact, and if the patient is allowed to do what he can, he will usually accept it. Although we often speak of promoting patient independence, we must not forget there will be times when the family will and should pamper the patient. The pressures of stressing independence, while seeing how terribly real the discouragements are, can become intolerable. Both family and patient can benefit and are supported by the sharing of humor, tears, and occasional overindulgence.

After a period of weeks many institutions allow patients to go home for weekend visits. With continuous teaching the family will know how all care for the patient is accomplished. Range-of-motion exercise, how to prevent further injury to the patient, transfer from bed to wheelchair—all should be comfortably understood. If the preparation of both patient and family has been comprehensive and gradual the technicalities of Foley catheter irrigations, brace applications, and dressing techniques should present few problems. Having the family progress with the patient has several advantages: They are a part of his rehabilitation; his progress in the realistic program is apparent; and they are being prepared for his return home.

The following example is too frequently

seen: Mrs. Hicks had suffered a cerebrovascular accident with subsequent right hemiplegia and severe expressive aphasia (inability to communicate verbally). Mr. Hicks visited his wife daily, and when he arrived, he usually found her in a wheelchair waiting for him. Not until the time he attempted to lift her into the car to take her home did he realize she had always been tied in the wheelchair to keep her from falling. It is imperative that the family know what the patient can do for himself and the length of time required for completion of activities. If one hour and a quiet environment are required for the patient to dress himself, then this should be provided. In the event the family will be unable to keep the patient at home, this information is required for selection of the proper nursing home.

When planning the physical environment for home care, the family should be discouraged from making early and expensive alterations in their home. The exact changes required can best be determined by occupational and physical therapists. Because of the financial strain disabilities bring about, their recommendations are geared to adapting what is presently in the home as opposed to purchasing expensive equipment. Furthermore, only toward the end of hospitalization can the need for all necessary environmental changes and devices be determined. Often very little in the way of alteration is required.

The Approach of Nursing Personnel

The nursing student cannot anticipate the personnel with whom she will eventually practice her profession. She knows there are full- and part-time professional nurses, nursing technicians, licensed and unlicensed practical nurses, aides, and orderlies and that they all have varying backgrounds and philosophies. The desired objective is for all to work together for the patient's benefit. The difficulties encountered and their solutions are not unique to caring for the patient with a permanent disability, but the need for teamwork and continuity of approach cannot be better demonstrated than by considering care of this type of patient.

Although the nonprofessional personnel may have had few educational experiences, it is not unusual to find them possessing great insight and enormous capabilities. Often they are the first to know that the patient is entering a new stage of adjusting to his disability. The following situation occurred in a large respiratory center. All the patients had severe paralysis as a result of poliomyelitis and required the assistance of either a respirator or a rocking bed. It came to the attention of the head nurse that

when a patient wanted to know if he would move or walk again, often he would first ask the cleaning lady from the housekeeping department. Several days later the question would be put to aides and orderlies. Practical nurses were next in succession; eventually the question came to the registered nurses. Length of time needed for this sequence ranged from days to weeks. Through team discussions the head nurse emphasized the importance of this question and how it should best be attended to. Thereafter, when the first questions began, they were reported to the head nurse, who, in turn, relayed the information to the physician and psychiatrist. At this time an explanation of the patient's future physical potential was given.

One must remember that the nonprofessional staff is subjected to as many, if not more, positive and negative experiences with patient and family as is the professional nurse. We cannot expect them to understand or accept manifestations such as hostility when those with specific preparation find it difficult. When the nurse becomes disappointed in the nonprofessional staff for not utilizing her instructions and demonstrations of proper positioning and prevention of deformities, she should address her attention to their total knowledge of the patient situation and to how they feel about it. Being able to work out feelings of fear, anger, or frustration about a severely disabled person alone is not to be expected of the nonprofessional person.

It is the view of the author that there is but one means of attempting an organized and comprehensive approach to the care of patients: the nursing team conference. Pertinent information obtained from the conferences should be formulated into a nursing care plan. If a patient card index is used in the institution, this is the most practical method of transmitting the plan. As the plan must change with the patient's progress, so too should the information on the care plan. An outdated or redundant written care plan is as bad as no plan at all. Involving all nursing personnel in planning care means far more than exchanging observations and knowledge. When all are informed of the patient's progress or regressions, all become active participants in his rehabilitation. Nurses who employ this approach know of its value to all concerned and are able to find the necessary time for conferences.

When considering what the nurse can do for the patient, one is easily overwhelmed. So much must be understood about the disability and its aftermath. Specific nursing techniques are modified to meet the needs of the patient, and yet these things "are done to him" because of his loss. The more involved the physical condition, the greater in number are the procedures. Sequelae are as physically and emotionally damaging as the initial disability. When they have no meaning to the nurse in terms of her approach and activities, she may be assured she is giving little more than custodial care. For example, as stated earlier, a person does not perspire in the areas that are not innervated. The consequent extreme perspiration from innervated areas may be frightening to the patient. The patient with a high vertebral injury may perspire so freely in the areas of head and neck that a bath towel will be saturated in five minutes. Not only must the patient be kept dry, but he obviously also must be told what is happening. It is essential that the nurse assist the patient in maintaining and modifying his identity. What she does is not so important as how and why she does it. An example is phantom sensation (the feeling of sensation in a part that has been amputated). When, following surgery, the amputee is not told these phenomena usually occur, he may question not only his own sanity but, indeed, that of the surgeon. If the patient has agreed to amputation of three toes and postoperatively he feels sensation in these toes, he may be afraid the surgeon has amputated the wrong toes. Furthermore, if he is unaware that phantom sensation is a common occurrence, he is unlikely to ask for medication to relieve pain in toes that supposedly no longer exist.

Specific Rehabilitation Situations

The Patient with a Spinal Cord Injury

The problems of the patient with a severed spinal cord are very numerous and complex. Some complications are preventable; some are not. Most do not happen early in the disability and, therefore, are an excellent example of why diligent concern on the part of the nurse must continue, just as the disability for the patient does. All nurses, no matter in what area they practice, are responsible for the prevention of complications. Often nurses in both the general hospital and rehabilitation agency and the public health or visiting nurse see the same patient with the same complication but in differing degrees of severity.

One such complication is spasms. Following the initial spinal cord injury, the patient enters a period known as spinal cord shock. During spinal cord shock the paralysis is flaccid. Spinal shock may last from weeks to months. Eventually, the lower motor neuron, or reflex arc, which has not been damaged, begins to function again. Because there is no longer central nervous system control or modulation of the reflex arcs below the level of injury, the paralysis becomes and remains spastic. Involuntary muscular contractions of the lower extremities will be observed. Very little stimulus is needed to set the reflex arc into action. Such things as jarring of the bed, pressure of a sheet on a leg, or merely touching of the leg can send the part into spasm. The patient will notice his leg "moves" or "jumps." It is not difficult to imagine the meaning of this event to the patient. Whereas his legs have been "dead," they now obviously have "come back to life."

The patient often is still in the general hospital, and the nurse in this setting should help him understand what is happening. It can be very difficult to assist the patient to accept the fact that this new event has nothing to do with regaining control of the paralyzed part. He may or may not ask what is happening; indeed, he may be too afraid to ask. Nevertheless, one can be quite assured he and his visitors are aware of the movement.

Spasms vary in severity from person to person. They may present no problem at all and, in fact, may be of physiological value. On the other hand, they may increase in severity to the point of producing permanent flexion contractures. Only as the months pass can their result be determined. The nurse in the rehabilitation setting will see the patient learning to live with his spasms. The constant tap-tap-tap of a shoe on a wheelchair footrest when the leg is in spasm is annoying at best. Spasms may increase to the point of preventing the patient from wearing long leg braces, thereby prohibiting ambulation. The accompanying discouragement is felt by all involved.

When the physiatrist feels that because of spasms no further rehabilitation can be accomplished, a chemical block may be offered to the patient. Accepting or refusing rhizotomy (section of the posterior roots of the spinal nerves) is another decision that can be made only by the patient. Rhizotomy will result in a permanent flaccid paralysis as it destroys the reflex arc, but it will enable him to continue his rehabilitation process. Rhizotomy removes the little but obvious life remaining in his legs and precludes the miracle of walking again. Few patients accept it immediately; some never agree to the procedure. Again, no amount of persuasion can or should speed the patient into making an affirmative decision. The rehabilitation team can only make apparent why rhizotomy is indicated. Theirs is not the final judgment. The patient may be discharged to his home to consider alternatives and make his decision.

This is the time the visiting or public health

nurse will visit the patient. She may or may not know why he is home; he may or may not tell her voluntarily. Her success in assisting him in this adjustment will be greatly increased if this patient's referral contains information essential for his comprehensive care at home. She must determine at what stage he is and remember what events led him to that stage. His attitudes, interests, and behavior are understandably related to the weight of his problem.

When the decision is in the affirmative, the patient returns to the general hospital for surgery. It is not uncommon for the same nursing personnel who cared for him when his spasms first began again to plan his care. He is the same person as before but now with more problems. Additional disappointments have altered his behavior, and the nurse must adapt her approach accordingly. Above all, it is imperative he be supported in the decision he has made.

Problems with Skin Breakdown

Skin breakdown is always a matter of grave concern to the paralyzed person. Able-bodied persons constantly shift their body weight to relieve and redistribute pressure. This is not possible for the paralyzed person. Because of lack of sensation, they are not aware when they have been in one position too long; and if they were aware, they could not move because of motor paralysis. Prolonged pressure, particularly over a bony prominence, causes a lack of circulation, which is the etiology of a pressure sore. Ischemia is the first stage in the formation of a pressure sore. This is noticed by a blanching of the skin. At this point strict measures to prevent formation of the pressure sore should be instituted at once. The second stage is termed hyperemia. The area will be red, raised, and warm to the touch. Cell destruction and hemorrhage have already occurred. This is the time most pressure sores are observed, and one notes a general flurry of activity to prevent further skin breakdown. In the nonparalyzed these efforts are often of value; however, it is extremely difficult to halt this process in the paralyzed person. The final stage is a break in the skin. No matter how small the area, it is now a pressure sore.

The anatomical areas most often affected are over bony prominences that receive the greatest degree of pressure. The sacrum, iliac crests, ischial tuberosities, greater femoral trochanters, and heels are common sites. Other sites are anterior tibial crests, knees, elbows, and scapulae. It will be noted that some of these areas normally are protected by fat pads. Both muscle and fat pad atrophy play an important part in the formation of a pressure sore. The necrotic process continues, and unless very carefully attended, the pressure sore proceeds below the subcutaneous fat and will require plastic surgery.

Prevention is the best treatment for a pressure sore. All areas of possible breakdown must be inspected frequently. This does not mean only during the morning bath or evening care but every time the nurse is in the patient's room. These areas should be washed with soap and water and receive circulation-stimulating massage. Nursing students are told of the importance of turning patients from the day they begin their education as nurses. It is repeated so often it at times assumes the character of the boy crying "wolf." But there is no other effective way of preventing pressure sores. For the paralyzed bed patient, turning is as essential to skin integrity as breathing is for life. All four sides are to be utilized, and the patient should be turned at least every two hours. If a turning schedule is not begun soon after the disability occurs, a pressure sore will form, leaving only three sides for positioning—and so the process goes. A pressure sore can occur in a matter of a few hours. Usually pressure sores can be prevented by establishing and carrying out a regular schedule of turning. Maintenance of skin integrity is almost completely the responsibility of the nursing staff. There should be no reason for the physician to write orders for these patients to be turned. Although pressure sores will occur in some instances in spite of diligent nursing care, most occur as a direct result of improper care.

No matter whether in bed or in wheelchair, it is imperative that the body weight be distributed evenly over as wide a surface as possible. The larger the area of weight distribution, the less the chance for ischemia to occur. It is important to remember the special problems of the paralyzed patient under 20 years of age. Like any paralyzed patient, they often lean to one side of the wheelchair. These young patients not only are prone to great skin problems but tend to develop scoliosis caused by incomplete bone ossification.

When a pressure sore does form, treatment will be as ordered by the physician. It is fairly safe to say there are almost as many methods of treatment as there are physicians. Beyond agreeing that the area should be kept clean, any number of treatments are seen. If infection is present, antibiotics will usually be given. Negative nitrogen balance can be expected as a consequence of the metabolic response to injury. A greater amount of nitrogen is excreted by the body than can be ingested. Because of protein loss caused by tissue breakdown, protein-sparing agents are sometimes given. Although it is not possible to reverse negative nitrogen balance in the period immediately following injury by a high dietary intake of protein, the patient must be encouraged to eat foods containing sufficient protein, vitamins, and minerals. After the catabolic phase is completed, protein foods are essential to an adequate anabolic response. Vitamins B and C (ascorbic acid) are also essential to wound healing.

A sterile dressing will usually be placed over the pressure sore. Never, under any circumstances, are doughnuts to be used, as they only serve to put increased pressure on the area juxtaposed to the pressure sore. The desired objective is to reduce pressure. Ideally, no pressure will be placed on the sore. If there are pressure sores in several areas, this may be impossible, and the sterile dressings over them should be covered with large, bulky pads.

When the pressure sore penetrates the subcutaneous fat, plastic surgery is usually necessary. In addition to performing a full-thickness skin graft the surgeon will often shave the underlying bony prominence until it is paper-thin. As the full-thickness graft cannot compensate for the former fat pad, a protruding bony prominence can penetrate the flap graft.

As soon as possible the patient should become involved in daily observation of his skin. To examine all his body surface, a long-handled mirror should be used. He should be taught how to shift his weight to relieve pressure in both wheelchair and bed, and he should do this every 30 minutes. He is to be warned about the danger of pressure areas developing on his legs; because he has no sensation, injuries from ill-fitting braces and burns can occur without his awareness.

Psychological trauma caused by the formation of a pressure sore can be great. If the patient is with others who have them he soon learns what they would mean to his own rehabilitation program. This new body insult is but another cause for increased dependence on others. Pressure sores are always unsightly and often draining and foul-smelling. The nurse should never be more tactful than when giving care to a pressure sore. Not infrequently, they progress to the point of prohibiting any activity other than bed rest. The patient is "grounded." He can no longer be in a wheelchair; all therapies must be accomplished from his bed. Again the rehabilitation process is at a standstill and cannot be resumed until the pressure sore heals. At this point the physical sequelae can complicate each other. For example, if a full-thickness flap skin graft is indicated, the plastic surgeon will probably not attempt the procedure if spasms are severe, because within a few hours extremity movement caused by spasms can destroy the graft. Therefore, rhizotomy may be essential before surgical repair of the pressure sore is considered. Once more a major decision must be made by the patient. Months may elapse before additional goals can even be attempted.

Problems with Elimination

Bowel and bladder problems also plague the patient with paraplegia. A regimen must be established for each as soon as possible or physical and psychological trauma will occur. Consideration here will first be given to urinary complications.

Bladder sensation and control are lost following complete transection, or cross section, of the spinal cord. Immediately after the injury the bladder becomes atonic, or without tone, and remains so throughout the period of spinal shock. When reflexes again affect the detrusor muscle, the bladder will empty itself. The amount of urine the bladder is capable of holding varies. If the bladder can accommodate 250 to 350 ml and then expel this urine, the patient is said to have an automatic or reflex bladder. Initially an indwelling catheter will have been inserted. When attempts are made to "train" the bladder, the catheter will be clamped for one to four hours and then unclamped for drainage. If, after a period of time, the bladder continues to empty itself, with residuals of 60 ml or less, the catheter will be removed. Hopefully the bladder will continue to hold and then expel its maximum amount of urine. When the reflex bladder is a reality, expulsion of urine will be mainly determined by the amount of fluid the patient drinks. He must carefully calculate his intake in order to know when to anticipate the expulsion of urine. In lesions involving upper motor neurons, expulsion of urine by the bladder may be facilitated by tactile stimulation of the areas innervated by the pudendal nerve. In lesions involving lower motor neurons, exertion of manual pressure over the bladder (Credé's method) or straining may be helpful in inducing urination.

The length of time required for training the bladder varies greatly. Some patients are never able to achieve a reflex bladder and therefore will need permanent indwelling catheters or cystostomies. The male patient may wear an external collecting device that will be attached to his leg. At this time there are no successful female collection devices; therefore, the female patient will usually wear sanitary pads as well as rubberized pants.

Urinary complications are a constant area

of concern to the paralyzed. Disuse osteoporosis brings about abnormal calcium deposits. Although they can occur at any place in the body, these calculi are often seen in the genitourinary tract. Oliguria, retention, and stasis of urine also precipitate stone formation and infection. Chills, temperature elevation, decreased urinary output, or hematuria may be the first sign of urinary complication.

It is imperative to keep in mind all the disorders that could occur and watch for their signs other than the patient's complaint of pain, as these patients may no longer feel any sensation. The absence of pain has significance not only for genitourinary complications but indeed for all medical disorders. The nurse must remember that these patients are as prone to develop internal disorders as are nonparalyzed persons, i.e., persons with appendicitis, cholecystitis, and peptic ulcer.

Autonomic hyperreflexia (disturbed or abnormal reflexes) can occur. When caused by a plugged catheter or bladder or urethral obstruction, tremendous backup of urine greatly distends the bladder. This constitutes a medical emergency and must be corrected immediately. Again, the patient cannot tell you his bladder is greatly distended. However, he will be extremely anxious and may complain of a severe headache. The reflexes sent by the distended bladder may be carried to all parts of the cord. Blood pressure will usually be elevated; it is not uncommon to observe a systolic reading of 300. Other signs are slow pulse, diaphoresis, pilomotor reflex, and temperature elevation. This complication will most often occur when an indwelling catheter is being utilized. The patient who has an automatic bladder should realize there is urinary retention at a time earlier than that required for such a urinary backup to occur. The nurse should determine whether the catheter is patent. This situation must be reported to the patient's physician immediately. It is imperative that a patent catheter be inserted.

Because most urinary bacteria thrive in alkaline media, attempts may be made to maintain an acidic medium. Mandelamine, or mandelic acid, may be given. The patient should also be encouraged to drink fruit juices that assist in maintaining the acidity of urine. Such fruits are cranberries, plums, and prunes. The most important single measure will be an adequate fluid intake. At least 3,000 ml daily must be taken; the significance of this amount cannot be overemphasized. As soon as possible the patient should assume responsibility for drinking the sufficient amount, as it will be a daily activity for him for the rest of his life.

After discharge the patient will be followed very carefully by the physician. Intravenous pyelograms and x-rays of the genitourinary tract will be done every three to six months. The patient must know the signs of urinary complications, such as oliguria and hematuria, and the importance of contacting his physician immediately when these signs occur.

The physical, social, and psychological problems that arise as a result of loss of bladder control are as important to consider as any others encountered in the rehabilitation of the permanently disabled. Obviously, genitourinary surgery as well as rhizotomy and plastic surgery can halt the rehabilitation program. Not infrequently all three surgical procedures are seen in the same patient. In relearning to manage urination the patient has much to learn from the nurse. Watching for sufficient output is as important to know as the amount and kind of fluid to ingest. Only knowing how to irrigate his catheter is not enough; as stated before, he must know total management of equipment. Indeed, he must know and be able to use all the nurse can possibly teach him.

Problems with evacuation of feces occur generally with nonambulatory patients. The additional complication of cord transection compounds this ever-present concern for nurses. For one of many reasons, the diet is usually not conducive to facilitating normal bowel movements. Until such time as the patient does eat a well-balanced diet, difficulties can be expected. Insufficient fluid intake also precludes formation of a bowel program. Greatly diminished physical activity lessens the possibility of regular evacuation. Furthermore, the patient no longer has sensory or motor functioning necessary for evacuation. Far too often constipation and subsequent impaction are the rule and not the exception for these patients. The work of nurses in rehabilitation centers would be substantially assisted if the patient's bowel program were established prior to discharge from the general hospital. This is another area where early attention, planning, and action can prevent unnecessary waste of time and energy and alleviate emotional disturbances.

The usual hospital treatments for constipation are enemas. This approach to the problem of evacuation for the patient with paraplegia will never suffice as a desirable bowel program. Repeated enemas decrease normal bowel tone, and in the instance of the paralyzed patient the highest degree of peristalsis possible must be maintained. Enemas should be utilized only as specific beginning steps in initiating a bowel program. They should never under any circumstances be considered the total solution to evacuation for the paralyzed person. Another often seen, but equally incorrect, method of approaching this problem is manual removal of feces. Again, this is indicated only when it is a component of a carefully prepared plan for setting up a bowel program. Overzealous attention to manual evacuation should be carefully avoided.

The initial step when setting up a bowel program is to determine the time of day most convenient for evacuation after the patient returns to his home. If he will need the assistance of others, obviously it must be a time when there are persons in the home. Generally the time chosen will be early morning or evening. Regulating the bowel function is accomplished by using stool softeners, prune juice, and suppositories. Determining the amount needed is done by the trial-and-error method. If 6:00 A.M. is to be the time for evacuation, 200 ml of prune juice are taken at the hour of sleep on the previous night. At 5:30 A.M., a suppository is given. Or the patient may require two stool softeners and a suppository, and action of the suppository may occur within five minutes. The important consideration here is to experiment with these three items until the most workable pattern is achieved. Once begun, the plan must be continuous; inattention on only one day can destroy weeks of effort.

When for any reason the patient is placed on bed rest, one should anticipate problems with the bowel program. It is difficult to understand how valuable any physical activity is to the establishment and maintenance of a successful program. Even something as apparently insignificant as a quadriplegic being up in a wheelchair six hours per day can positively affect the functioning of a bowel program. Bed rest for upper respiratory or minor genitourinary infection can adversely affect a well-working program. So, too, can effects of preparation for tests such as intravenous pyelograms.

Functional bowel programs are not achieved quickly. During the period before the schedule is achieved, bowel movements can occur at any time, thereby causing embarrassment and discouragement to the patient. Psychological trauma caused by evacuation during meals, during visiting hours, or at occupational or physical therapy is obvious. Through continued efforts, patience, and support to the patient, a workable bowel program will evolve. The patient does need a definite program for the rest of his life, and only by working toward evacuation at a specific hour can he control this function; there is no reason to delay its establishment. Optimism is in order, as a plan can be achieved with time. The value to the patient of once again "controlling" evacuation of feces is immeasurable.

The Patient Who Has Sustained a Cerebrovascular Accident

PREVENTION OF CONTRACTURES AND DEFORMITIES

When at rest or inactive for long periods of time, limbs tend to assume positions that, unless altered, produce deformity. Not only are flexors and adductors the stronger muscle groups, but assuming positions of flexion and adduction affords relief of pain. We can be assured deformities and contractures will occur in certain conditions, i.e., cerebrovascular accident and rheumatoid arthritis, unless preventive measures are begun early and are continuous. The nursing student is urged to examine her own position when supine. The importance of diligent attention may then be more apparent to her. She will observe that her feet are in plantar flexion and her legs are externally rotated. Not infrequently her arms will be adducted and flexed.

From the time of admission the body should be maintained in good physiological alignment. This is accomplished by the use of sandbags, pillows, trochanter rolls, and footboards. Far too often utilization of these devices is neglected by all concerned after the initial discussion in introductory classes. Furthermore, one often sees these devices in the patient's environment, but they are serving no useful purpose. One such example is the footboard. Indeed, it is on the bed; however, the feet of the patient are fully four inches from it and are demonstrating plantar flexion. Because of the great inflexibility of footboards and variances of patient's heights, some nurses have found it of value to fashion their own footboards. Sandbags, which provide stability, are placed in a cardboard box (such as the kind that contains intravenous solutions); the box is then covered with a small sheet. The position of this footboard may be altered according to the height of the patient. Nurses are also often faced with a lack of sandbags. This may be a suitable project for auxiliary groups working in or with the hospital. Five-, seven-, and ten-pound sandbags are relatively easy to make.

Only at such time as the physician orders active or passive range of motion for the patient should the indicated exercises begin. The length of time following the disability until range-of-motion exercises can be started will be determined by the patient's condition. For example, if a cerebrovascular accident has occurred as a result of thrombus or embolus, these activities may be indicated within 48 hours after the accident. If, however, the stroke was caused by hemorrhage, the physician may not allow activity for six to eight weeks. When exercises are indicated and ordered, the necessity of their daily occurrence cannot be overemphasized. Talking with the physician about when he wished exercises to begin is always in order.

In the event the nursing student has not taken an extremity through range of motion and consequently does not know how it feels to move another person's limbs, she is urged to practice on a colleague. The "patient" should present her with two situations: First, she should make the limb as limp and lifeless as possible; second, her limb should assume and maintain positions of slight adduction and flexion.

The nurse may anticipate tightness and resistance when working with patients who have been inactive for a period of time. Inactivity of only a few days' duration produces limitations of motion and pain on movement. One such example is the "frozen shoulder" seen in patients who have suffered a cerebrovascular accident; the pain can be excruciating. For this reason sometimes these patients are encouraged to use their unaffected arm for taking the affected arm through range of motion, as they will know better than anyone else their own degree of pain tolerance. Daily range of motion should show some degree of increasing joint mobility.

The patient who has had a stroke should have his affected arm supported by a sling when either sitting or walking. If the arm is not supported, subluxation or partial dislocation of that shoulder may ensue. When a sling is used, two considerations are important. First, the wrist must also be supported to prevent wrist drop. Second, the weight of the arm in the sling should not exert excess pressure on the cervical vertebrae. The knot should be lateral to the vertebrae, and a foam rubber or felt pad may be placed over the vertebrae to reduce the pressure.

The nurse must be alert to flexion contractures about the hip joint in addition to those at the knee and foot. The onset of hip flexion may be quite insidious. Elevation of the head of the bed, no matter to what degree, will have some effect on the hip joint. It is helpful for these patients to be in a flat position several times daily. The origin of external rotation of the leg is at the hip joint; therefore, sandbags should be placed along the outer aspect of the upper leg as well as along the lower leg. Before placing sandbags, one should attempt to position the extremity in some degree of overcorrection (i.e., internal rotation of the leg) so that with the stronger opposite pull or external rotation a neutral position may be achieved. The legs should be maintained in a neutral position, neither externally nor internally rotated. A small pillow may be placed under the lower legs to relieve pressure from the heels, thus preventing pressure sore formation in these areas. Care must be taken that the pillow does not cause knee flexion, which in turn would produce additional contracture.

Respiratory Complications

Respiratory complications plague the disabled. The reasons are as numerous as are the basic diagnoses. The patient with paralysis caused by poliomyelitis or traumatic quadriplegia may lack control of breathing and coughing mechanisms and therefore may require assistance with both. The patient who has suffered a cerebrovascular accident with resultant paralysis is also prone to hypostatic pneumonia. Following a stroke, expressive and/or receptive aphasia may be present. Nothing can be more frustrating to the nurse than telling such a patient to cough, or breathe deeply, and hear him repeat the word *cough* but no longer be able to comprehend what the word means.

These patients must be protected from possible respiratory infections. Every precaution must be taken to prevent contact with persons having upper respiratory infections. If the patient is at all capable of coughing and deep-breathing, he should do so hourly. Turning is also essential in reducing the possibility of pulmonary congestion. The sooner the patient may be in an upright position, the less are chances for respiratory complications to occur. Never under any circumstances should oral fluids be given until it has been clearly ascertained that the patient can swallow. Aspiration pneumonia occurs when well-meaning but unthinking persons give fluids to the unconscious or dysarthric (paralysis or weakness of speech, swallowing, or tongue musculatures) patient.

Additional Disorders of the Patient Who Has Suffered Cerebrovascular Accident with Organic Residual

Hemiplegia or hemiparesis is easily observable and presents definite indications for specific nursing care. However, equally important to the comprehensive care of the patient who has had a stroke is the area of communication, perception, and "inner thinking." The degree to which each of these abilities has been affected differs from patient to patient. This knowledge is essential to good nursing care. Ascertaining the extent of brain damage is difficult and requires specific testing by highly skilled persons. Often these services are not available in general hospitals; therefore, the nurse may not have exact information about difficulties in these areas. By being aware of commonly seen sequelae and reporting her observations, she can provide invaluable assistance to medical and paramedical disciplines. Moreover, all rehabilitation must be planned around the communication capabilities and limitations of the patient.

Aphasia

Before discussing the various types of aphasia, it would be well to consider language per se. Language is a set of symbols by which we make our thoughts known to ourselves as well as others. Expressive language is that language used to reveal our needs and thinking to other persons. Receptive language is the language each of us uses to understand what others communicate to us. Inner language is that language individuals use to think or talk to themselves. The patient who has had a stroke may have had damage of varying degree to any or all of these three types of language. Therefore, if a patient is said to have expressive aphasia, it does not mean that he cannot hear and understand what is said to him or said in his presence. This fact must be clearly and completely understood by all persons (staff, visitors, and other patients) coming into contact with patients who are unable to speak. When attempting to communicate with such a patient, the nurse should talk with him as if he does understand her. Above all it should never be forgotten how devastating and frightening it would be to the patient to have others discuss within his hearing the hopelessness of his condition.

Verbal communication is the desired objective. Early and continued attempts to determine whether or not an aphasic patient can communicate in this manner are essential. If the patient does not demonstrate the ability to communicate verbally, it must be ascertained if he understands what is being said to him. Following the onset of aphasia one of the earliest and most basic forms of communication is the use of *yes* and *no*. Whether or not the patient has a reliable yes/no response must be carefully ascertained. A verbal or physical yes response may be demonstrated, but the patient may respond to any or all questions in this manner. As soon as the patient uses any form of yes/no response he should be asked questions that require both yes and no answers. Questions asked by the nurse such as "Are you a man?" "Are you a woman?" "Is the sun shining?" and "Is it raining?" will give a fairly clear idea as to the yes/no reliability. The patient who appears to be expressively aphasic may be capable of responding nonverbally to questions asked him that require yes or no answers. When he does respond by shaking his head or blinking his eyes, he should use these devices appropriately. However, neither the patient nor those in his environment should be allowed to rely on nonverbal communication if verbal communication is possible for him.

Agraphia is the inability to write words on command or to formulate ideas in written expression, although copying may still be possible. The inability to solve mathematical problems is acalculia. Word blindness, or lack of reading comprehension, is alexia.

When the patient has total expressive and receptive aphasia he is said to be globally aphasic. Global aphasia results from severe organic brain damage; therefore, rehabilitation potential for these patients is quite limited.

Expressive or receptive aphasia does not mean the patient is incapable of producing word sounds. He may utter nonintellectual word forms in substitution for meaningful speech, such as "da da da da." These sounds may or may not be used with vocal inflection. If the patient has little or no self-monitoring ability, he may be assuming he is responding appropriately to those attempting communication with him. Another example is emotional utterance. This is demonstrated by such things as words of endearment or cursing. Previous to his stroke, the patient may have controlled the desire for saying these words, but because of damage to the higher centers of the brain he is no longer capable of this control. The patient may demonstrate automatic speech. He may repeat an entire song or prayer but have no awareness of its meaning. The patient may be capable of social speech, comprised in the main of common salutations. He may say "Good morning" or "How do you do." When social speech is uttered at an appropriate time one may easily overlook the presence of a basic aphasic problem. The nurse who makes daily morning rounds would do well to engage such a patient in other areas of conversation. Another example is serial content. Here the patient is capable of giving such things as the days of the week or months of the year in sequence, although he does not know the meaning of all or of individual words.

Perseveration is repetition with or without provocation on either a verbal or motor level. The word or act is meaningless, although initially it may have been appropriate for one response. If the patient demonstrates a yes or a no perseveration but is capable of other meaningful speech, he should be asked questions that cannot be answered with either of these words. Even though perseveration should be halted and a new activity begun, one must be discriminate, as this may be the patient's first attempts at communication.

Agnosia

Agnosia is the inability to comprehend sensations. A person with tactile agnosia cannot perceive an object by feel. Auditory agnosia is demonstrated by an inability to understand the meaning of environmental sounds such as the ringing of a telephone. Visual agnosia is the loss of comprehension of objects by sight. Patients demonstrating auditory agnosia will often also have visual agnosia.

Apraxia

Whereas agnosia is a sensory loss, apraxia is the inability to perform acts without motor loss. A nonverbal, or motor, apraxia is demonstrated by a patient picking up a comb but having no idea of its use. Although he may use the article automatically, he cannot do so on command. Persons with a verbal apraxia are unable to utilize the speech musculature for formation of appropriate words.

Flexibility is the basis of approach to the patient with the aforementioned problems. The nurse must have some idea of the language disorder demonstrated, but no issue should be made of the loss. Sentences should be simple and short. A soft but easily understood voice should be used. An excessively loud voice is to be avoided. When assuming the patient is unable to hear, the speaker shows a tendency to speak far more loudly than necessary. It is essential not to bombard the patient with questions. If questions come too quickly, his answers may be behind by several questions. In such event even though his answers are correct, they may appear inappropriate and/or incorrect. It is wise to anticipate the word a patient is attempting to say. Although he should not be supplied the word immediately, he also should not be forced beyond his frustration point. After the word is supplied for the patient, he should be encouraged to repeat it. Above all, his speech should not be interrupted or depreciated in any manner. Any speech the aphasic patient utters should be encouraged. If his speech is discouraged in any way he may make no further attempts at communicating.

Inner Thinking and Personality Disorders

When brain damage has occurred, it is not possible to determine the exact amount of "inner thinking" disturbance. We cannot completely know how the patient views himself or what he feels about his disability. His present state may be totally overwhelming, or because of severe inner thinking difficulty, he may be unaware of his condition. Accompanying personality disorders are often seen. Inappropriate behavior may be obvious to hospital personnel. Moreover, personality and behavioral changes will be observed and may be mentioned by the patient's family.

The patient is easily overwhelmed by excess environmental stimuli. He should be asked to concentrate on only one object or activity at a time. Overloading him with many requests, or even several areas of conversation, confuses him greatly. The patient who has suffered brain damage needs to have his environment controlled and structured for him whether or not aphasia is demonstrated. Unnecessary stimuli are to be eliminated, and the setting should be quiet and composed. All possible efforts at assisting him in adjusting to his present state must be made. These patients show tendencies toward rigidity and inflexibility. They cannot adjust to rapid and unfamiliar happenings. They may demand that their daily physical care be done in the same sequence. Such patients can become extremely agitated if objects in the room are not arranged in a specific order. By not following the pattern required by the patient, one may frustrate him to the point of making future adjustments impossible. Working with such a patient is often extremely trying, but the nurse must remember that the patient is attempting not only to exhibit some control over his environment but to communicate with it as well. And this is the desired objective. Moreover, it must be kept in mind that the extreme anxiety demonstrated when making his desires known may be quickly followed by a complete reversal in the patient's manner. Just as they are easily exasperated, so, too, are they pleased.

The patient should not be confronted with daily changes. A routine should be established and continued. When at all possible, the same person on each shift should care for him until he is capable of communicating comfortably. Only when it is demonstrated to the patient that he and his needs are understood will he feel comfortable and supported, and he will not be at ease if he anticipates a changing atmosphere. No long-term goals can be attempted until the patient is secure with those caring for him.

These patients are usually withdrawn, as they are unable to express themselves or cope with their environment. It is not unusual for them to exhibit no interest in what is occurring around them. This may be seen even in the nonaphasic patient. Furthermore, the patient may appear to be more alert at some times than at others. When these situations occur, the nurse should try to stimulate the patient in some way. The object is to assist the patient in communicating with someone or something other than himself. The areas the nurse may explore are limitless, and her efforts are to be continued until some means of reaching the patient are found. Often the family can be of assistance through either their presence or knowledge of his interests. Not infrequently an object that was dear to the patient may begin his interest. Bringing him such things as a picture of a family member or a family Bible can be of great value.

Because efforts are to be directed toward bringing him again in touch with reality, allowing him constantly to be absorbed in a non-participatory activity should be avoided. An example of this is looking at television or listening to the radio. It is quite possible to be in the presence of these media and to be completely uninvolved. This is not to say that under certain circumstances utilizing these media should not be attempted; i.e., the patient who was previously a baseball fan might benefit from watching a game on television. Indiscriminate use, however, may force the patient into further withdrawal.

Persons having sustained a cerebrovascular accident are highly prone to mood swings. Inappropriate laughing or crying is not necessarily provoked. For no apparent reason the patient may weep unconsolably and, just as strangely and suddenly, laugh. Even though this phenomenon is understood and accepted by family and personnel, it can be greatly disturbing. The important factor here is that those in contact with the patient (including other patients) know that they are not necessarily responsible for the mood swings.

When the patient begins doing activities for himself, various other problems arise. Incoordination and confusion more often than not lead to unsuccessful attempts, no matter what the activity. It is imperative that the patient be encouraged to continue these efforts. Often the nurse must demonstrate even the most rudimentary methods of self-care, and these demonstrations will have to be repeated. This is particularly true when dressing or other self-care activities are taught. In all things, it is important to remember that these people tend to demonstrate past and not recent recall. For example, the patient may remember where a shirt is worn, but not recall the previous day's instructions of how to get his paralyzed arm through the sleeve. The patient may well have difficulty in retention of anything taught to him, especially if the new material is presented in abstract terms.

Because of his awkward motions and inability to perform activities correctly, the patient may become more anxious and frustrated. Impulsivity is commonly seen as a result of frustration. This patient is unable to see the consequences of an act. An example is striking at and knocking over a pan of bath water into the bed because he is unable to wring out the washcloth. It is because of such impulsive acts and concreticism that a decision may be made that the patient cannot safely be alone by himself for any period of time. Furthermore, use of safety devices such as wheelchair straps may be necessary.

The patient should be encouraged to continue attempting an activity to his frustration point. Not uncommonly, he may at this point summon all his energies and be successful. The nurse must not forget that the overt demonstrations of his great anxiety will be followed by a smile of satisfaction.

If the patient is provoked (by himself or others) beyond his frustration point, a catastrophic response may ensue. This is a psychobiological response of the entire organism when successful completion of an activity is not possible.[4] Expression of catastrophic response ranges from wild thrashing about to unconsciousness. The nurse must take great care not to frustrate the patient to this extreme. When it does occur, her action must be swift and sure. Observing this reaction is extremely upsetting; the nurse needs to think clearly and calmly. As casually as possible, whatever activity the patient is demonstrating must be stopped, even if this means being stopped physically.

Often, as activities of daily living are begun, nursing personnel become aware of the patient's visual loss, as, for example, ignoring food on one side of his tray or continuously bumping into objects on the same side. Hemianopsia, or loss of one half of the visual field of one or both eyes, may be present without the patient's being aware of his loss. If the patient is able to read, having him read aloud is one means of determining hemianopsia. If this is present, words or groups of words will be omitted from each line of print. Patients are taught to compensate for the loss of visual acuity or the effect of hemianopsia by scanning, or rotating the head, so that the object being scrutinized may be fully seen.

Activities of Daily Living

Daily self-care for permanently disabled persons is far too individualized to state a panacea. Although ingenuity of the nurse may be taxed to the point of exhaustion, it is her responsibility to determine the most feasible and safe manner by which self-care can be accomplished.

[4] Jon Eisenson: "Therapeutic Problems and Approaches with Aphasic Adults," in *Handbook of Speech Pathology,* Lee Edward Travis, ed. Appleton-Century-Crofts, Inc., New York, 1957, p. 473.

And this is self-care for the patient after discharge—not for the convenience of the nursing
staff. Inherent in self-care is the understanding
by the patient and his family of how complications are prevented.

The problems involved are as basic as being
certain that all areas of the body will be washed.
Simple though it may sound, such a goal is not
without frustration. If the patient with paraplegia denies his legs are a part of him, he is
not going to wash them, long-handled sponge
or not. How does one ever teach a person to
place a washcloth in a positioned, paralyzed
right hand for washing the left axilla if this
person is unaware he has a right side? The
"body image" of the patient who has had a
stroke will determine what he washes and what
he ignores.

What are the nurse's responsibilities in rehabili-
tation?

No matter in what areas the nurse is responsible for patient teaching, regardless of the
place of teaching, the needs of the patient will
determine her plan. Teaching must be continuous and purposeful. Intensity and design of
the teaching plan is as important for the
multiextremity amputee as for the quadriplegic.
What is taught must be presented in a well-
defined and vital manner. If it is not, the patient
cannot be expected to recognize the significance
of what he needs to know.

What the Nurse Cannot Do

The old and true saying that a nurse is not
capable of being all things to all people cannot
be better emphasized than when considering
rehabilitation of the physically handicapped.
One person cannot possibly accomplish the
total rehabilitation of permanently disabled
persons alone. Of necessity, the needs of the
patient and difficulties encountered in meeting
them demand the attention of several highly
skilled disciplines. When, as still occurs, necessary team members are not available, goals for
the patient must be set accordingly.

Too frequently in hospitals nurses assume
overprotection of the patient. The patient "belongs" to the nursing personnel. He may spend
most of the day in x-ray or two hours in physical
therapy, but he returns where he belongs—to
the patient unit. Although this is not without
some benefit, nurses can be quite perplexed by
the all too obvious fact that the patient is not
hers alone. To begin with, the patient belongs
to himself. Moreover, it is shocking indeed to
learn that the patient is as valuable to the occupational therapist and social service worker
(and vice versa) as he is to nursing personnel.

Imposing Her Values on the Patient

Nurses must at all times refrain from imposing their own values on patients under their
care. Assisting the patient in his rehabilitation
program provides excellent opportunity for seeing in the patient that which the nurse desires
to see. The particular situations encountered
with the disabled patient are complex for more
than one reason. First, this type of patient is
usually hospitalized for far longer periods of
time than the nondisabled patient. Therefore,
her feelings of identification with the patient,
or nonacceptance of his manner of adjusting to
his disability, will have more time to develop.
It is extremely difficult to change one's opinion
of such a situation when the reasons for forming the opinion are constantly reinforced. With
contact of many weeks the situation becomes
increasingly trying for all. Her perception of
the patient will determine what goals the nurse
can visualize for him. The nurse who cannot
accept a patient because his reaction is not what
she imagines hers would be will possess neither
the patience nor the interest necessary for planning and working with him. Moreover, efforts
toward rehabilitation by such a nurse can only
be considered for unrealistic goals, as they will
be geared toward her incorrect perception of
the situation.

Nonobjectivity

Occasionally the tragedy of the situation becomes the prime concern of the nurse. In allowing herself to see only the disastrous effects of
the disability on one or more lives, she is
utterly of no value to the patient or her colleagues. Patients and families deserve positive
support and are quite without need for yet another weakness on the way back to the purposeful existence. It is the obligation of the nurse to
maintain an objective approach, and this is to
be accomplished by whatever means necessary.
Equally as damaging to all concerned is the
nurse who becomes so emotionally involved
with the patient that she feels no one else is
capable of giving the care needed. Thereby she
meets her own emotional needs and not those
of the patient. This nurse misleads only herself.

Female nursing students must be alert to
disabled male patients who attempt to form
romantic relationships with them. Nothing
could better prove the continued existence of
his manhood than having a young female ro-
mantically interested in him. The young paraplegic who becomes (or remains) a Don Juan
can provide an extremely difficult situation.
Nurses who do become thus involved need help
in determining their motivation for such attachments.

When for any reason the nurse realizes she is no longer capable of being objective in a patient situation, she should seek help and guidance. Maintaining a purposeful approach with patients is extremely difficult and not easily accomplished. Admitting to herself that she needs help and then seeking the necessary guidance are actions far more beneficial to the patient and herself than any others she could take.

Approach of the Nurse

As stated earlier, the nurse must be flexible, and she will receive her clues for this flexibility from the patient. Listening to him and understanding what he says will tell her how best to formulate her approach. Having knowledge of the classic picture of the disability and how the patient's condition is similar to it is not enough.

The fear of saying the wrong thing to the patient is great. Wondering when she will inadvertently mention an activity no longer possible for the patient may constantly plague the nurse. The nursing student must understand that at some time she will err in her choice of words or topic of conversation. Only when she does make what she considers to be a gross error will the nurse realize how groundless were her fears. More often than not the understanding response of the patient will control the situation. He, too, has anticipated such an occurrence and will be prepared. There is no more astounding and rewarding facet of human capabilities than unexpected strength, and physical disability does not necessarily negate emotional resources. Furthermore, after discharge the patient's associates cannot provide him the controlled environment found in hospitals; therefore, supposedly ill-chosen words could serve as a means of preparing him for what he will later encounter. The fact is, avoiding reference to his disability is often for the nurse's own benefit, and when this is the case neither the patient nor the nurse is moving toward acceptance of his disability.

Efforts necessary for assisting the patient to reach his highest potential are thwarted for many reasons. The work is not glamorous or dramatic—and not infrequently it is totally unrewarding. Attempts at realizing well-conceived plans are often met with complete nonacceptance and therefore will have been to no avail. It must be clearly understood that frustration is the rule and not the exception. How, then, should the nurse approach the patient with a permanent disability?

First and foremost, she must always remember she is responsible for neither the disability nor what eventually will be the fate of the patient and his family. What has happened to them *is not her fault*. There will be times when remembering this will be the only means of enabling the nurse to function as she must.

It is imperative that she examine the motives for her actions and operate for the patient's benefit, not her own. She must carefully gear her thinking about the patient to his physical and emotional state; she must be aware of where he comes from and to what environment he will return. Knowing all these factors separately is not sufficient; they must be combined and their effect on the patient—at that time—determined.

The nursing student can be assured that when goals are accomplished, the meaning to all is immeasurable—for this cannot occur unless both patient and those involved in his rehabilitation process work together to the extreme limits of their capabilities. The rewards for all are great.

REFERENCES

BOOKS

Barker, R. G., et al.: *Adjustment to Physical Handicap and Illness: A Survey of the Social Psychology of Physique and Disability* (New York: Social Science Research Council, 1953).

Buck, McKenzie: *Dysphasia: Professional Guidance for Family and Patient* (Englewood Cliffs, N.J.: Prentice-Hall, Inc., 1968).

Chusid, J. G., and McDonald, J. J.: *Correlative Neuroanatomy and Functional Neurology* (Los Altos, Calif.: Lange Medical Publications, 1964).

Committee on Prosthetic Research and Development: *The Geriatric Amputee:* Conference held in Washington, D.C., April 13–14, 1961 (Washington, D.C.: National Academy of Science, National Research Council).

Cruckshank, Wm., et al.: *Psychology of Exceptional Children and Youth* (Englewood Cliffs, N.J.: Prentice-Hall, Inc., 1963).

Garrett, J. F.: *Psychological Aspects of Physical Disability* (Washington, D.C.: U.S. Government Printing Office, 1952).

Garrett, J. F., and Levine, E. S.: *Psychological Practices with the Physically Disabled* (New York: Columbia University Press, 1962).

Goffman, Erving: *Stigma* (Englewood Cliffs, N.J.: Prentice-Hall, Inc., 1963).

Hamilton, K. W.: *Counseling the Handicapped in the Rehabilitation Process* (New York: The Ronald Press Company, 1950).

Hirschberg, Gerald, *et al.: Rehabilitation: A Manual for the Care of the Disabled and Elderly* (Philadelphia: J. B. Lippincott Company, 1964).

Hodgins, Eric: *Episode: Report of the Accident Inside My Skull* (New York: Atheneum Publishers, 1964).

Kellogg, Marjorie: *Tell Me that You Love Me, Junie Moon* (New York: Farrar, Straus & Giroux, Inc., 1968).

Khalili, Ali A.: "Pathiophysiology, Clinical Picture and Management of Spasticity" in *Clinical Anesthesia: Neurologic Considerations,* Merel H. Harmel, ed. (Philadelphia: F. A. Davis Company, 1967), p. 112–36.

Krenzl, Judith, and Rohrer, Lois: "Paraplegic and Quadriplegic Individuals" in *Handbook of Care for Nurses* (Chicago: National Paraplegic Foundation, Wallard Press, 1966).

Krusen, F. H., Kottke, F. J., Ellwood, P. M. (eds.): *Handbook of Physical Medicine and Rehabilitation* (Philadelphia: W. B. Saunders Company, 1965).

Licht, Sidney, *et al.: Rehabilitation and Medicine* (Baltimore: Waverly Press, Inc., 1968).

Litman, T. J.: "Self-Conception and Physical Rehabilitation" in *Human Behavior and Social Processes,* Arnold M. Rose, ed. (Boston: Houghton Mifflin Company, 1962).

Myklebust, H. E.: *Auditory Disorders in Children* (New York: Grune & Stratton, Inc., 1954), Chap. 7.

Ruge, Daniel, *et al.: Spinal Cord Injuries* (Springfield, Ill.: Charles C Thomas, Publisher, in press).

Smith, Genevieve: *Care of the Patient with a Stroke* (New York: Springer-Verlag, 1959), p. 148.

Super, Donald: *Appraising Vocational Fitness* (New York: Harper and Brothers, 1952), Chaps. 1, 4, 6 (pp. 86–104), and 15.

Taylor, Martha: *Understanding Aphasia: A Guide for Family and Friends* (New York: Patient Publication No. 2, The Institute of Rehabilitation Medicine, New York University Medical Center, 1958).

Travis, Lee Edward (ed.): *Handbook of Speech Pathology* (New York: Appleton-Century-Crofts, 1957), Chaps. 12, 13, and 14.

Wepman, Joseph: *Recovery from Aphasia* (New York: The Ronald Press Company, 1951), Chaps. 10 and 11.

Wright, Beatrice A.: *Physical Disability: A Psychological Approach* (New York: Harper and Brothers, 1960).

PERIODICALS

Abramson, A. S.: "Modern Concepts of Management of the Patient with a Spinal Cord Injury," *Arch. Phys. Med.,* 48:113–21 (Mar.) 1967.

Abramson, A. S.: "The Human Community in the Rehabilitation Process," *Arch. Phy. Med.,* 49: 59–65 (Feb.) 1968.

Betts, Henry, *et al.:* "Rehabilitation of the Rheumatoid Arthritic," *Illinois Med. J.,* 124:5–523 (Dec.) 1963.

Bland, John H. (ed.).: "Symposium on Rheumatoid Arthritis," *Med. Clin. N. Amer.,* 52:477–764 (May) 1968.

Busse, W. B., "Some Emotional Complications of Chronic Disease," *Gerontologist,* 2:153–56 (Sept.) 1962.

Carroll, Virginia B.: "Implications of Measured Visuospatial Impairment in a Group of Left Hemiplegic Patients," *Arch. Phys. Med.,* 39: 11–14 (Jan.) 1958.

Christophersen, Victor: "Role Modifications of the Disabled Male," *Amer. J. Nurs.,* 68:290–93 (Feb.) 1968.

Comarr, A. E.: "Practical Management of the Patient with Traumatic Cord Bladder," *Arch. Phys. Med.,* 48:122–25 (Mar.) 1967.

Frankel, A.: "Sexual Problems in Rehabilitation," *J. Rehab.,* 33:19–20 (Sept.–Oct.) 1967.

Goldbranson, Capt. F. L., *et al.:* "Immediate Postsurgical Fitting and Early Ambulation," *Clin. Orthop.,* 56:119–31 (Jan.–Feb.) 1968.

Halper, A. S., Baker, E. J., and Worcester, C. S.: "Communication Problems of the Stroke Patient," *Nurs. Homes,* 10:16–19 (Oct.) 1967.

Holliday, Jane: "Bowel Programs of Patients with Spinal Cord Injury: A Clinical Study," *Nurs. Res.,* 16:4–15 (Winter) 1967.

Keller, Nancy: "Care Without Coordination," *Nurs. Forum,* 6:280–323 (No. 3) 1967.

Ladieu, G., *et al.:* "Studies in Adjustment to Visible Injuries, Evaluation of Help by Injured," *J. Abnorm. Social Psychol.,* 42:169–92, 1947.

Levine, L.: "Some Observations Pertaining to the Socially Handicapped," *J. Rehab.,* 34:32–34 (Nov.–Dec.) 1968.

Litman, T. J.: "An Analysis of the Sociologic Factors Affecting the Rehabilitation of Physically Handicapped Patients," *Arch. Phys. Med.,* 45:9–16 (Jan.) 1964.

Marshall, John: "Helping the Grief Stricken," *Postgrad. Med.,* 45:138–43 (Feb.) 1969.

Martin, M. A.: "Nursing Care in Cervical Cord Injuries," *Amer. J. Nurs.,* 63:60–66 (Mar.) 1963.

Meyerson, Lee: "Physical Disabilities as a Social Psychological Problem," *J. Social Issues,* 4:2–10 (Jan.) 1948.

Olson, Edith (ed.): "The Hazards of Immobility," *Amer. J. Nurs.* 67:779–97 (Apr.) 1967.

Plummer, Elizabeth: "The M.S. Patient," *Amer. J. Nurs,* 68:2161–67 (Oct.) 1968.

Roeher, G. A.: "Significance of Public Attitudes in the Rehabilitation of the Disabled," *Rehab. Lit.,* 12:66–72 (Mar.) 1961.

Rothberg, June S.: "The Challenges for Rehabilitative Nursing," *Nurs. Outlook,* 17:37–39 (Nov.) 1969.

Rubin, Reva: "Body Image and Self-Esteem," *Nurs. Outlook,* 16:20–23 (June) 1968.

Shapiro, Leo N., and McMahon, Arthur W.: "Rehabilitation Stalemate," *Arch. Gen. Psychiat.*, **15**:173–77 (Aug.) 1966.

Skipper, James K., *et al.:* "Physical Disability Among Married Women: Problems in the Husband-Wife Relationship," *J. Rehab.*, **34**:16–19 (Sept.–Oct.) 1968.

Talbot, Herbert S.: "A Concept of Rehabilitation," *Rehab. Lit.*, **22**:358–64 (Dec.) 1961.

Visotsky, Harold M., *et al.:* "Coping Behavior Under Extreme Stress," *Arch. Gen. Psychiat.*, **5**:423–28 (Nov.) 1961.

Weiss, Aaron, and Diamond, David: "Sexual Adjustment Identification and Attitudes of Patients with Myelopathy," *Arch. Phys. Med.*, **47**:245 (Mar.) 1966.

Whitehouse, F. A.: "The Utilization of Human Resources: A Philosophic Approach to Rehabilitation," *Dis. Chest,* **30**:606 (Dec.) 1956.

Wright, B. A.: "Spread in Adjustment to Disability," *Bull. Menniger Clin.,* **28**:198–208 (July) 1964.

Wright, B. A.: "Some Issues Concerning Psychology and Rehabilitation," *Rehab. Lit.,* **22**:2–9 (Jan.) 1961.

UNPUBLISHED MATERIAL

Halper, Anita: "The Aphasic Patient." Lecture given at The Rehabilitation Institute of Chicago, Chicago, Illinois, 1962.

Kir-Stimon, William: "Psychological Aspects of Physical Disability." Lecture given at The Rehabilitation Institute of Chicago, Chicago, Illinois, 1962.

Neal, Richard: "Medical Aspects of Physical Disability." Lecture given at The Rehabilitation Institute of Chicago, Chicago, Illinois, 1960.

19

Epilogue

PART A
Patients with Diabetes Mellitus

Overview

  Why has life expectancy improved?

The Nature and Causes of Diabetes Mellitus

  What factors appear to predispose to diabetes mellitus in man?

  What other organs participate in the homeostasis of glucose?

  What are the mechanisms for elevating the level of glucose in the blood?

What are the mechanisms for lowering the level of glucose in the blood?

  What are the effects of insulin?

Nursing Responsibilities and Care of the Patient with Diabetes Mellitus

  Besides insulin, what drugs are useful in the control of the level of glucose in the blood?

  What should the patient be taught concerning general hygiene?

Overview

AFTER saying that a good play does not require an epilogue, Shakespeare adds one to *As You Like It*. Although an epilogue may not be necessary, some of the content previously presented has been selected and applied to patients experiencing two different types of disorders. In the first part, six patients who have diabetes mellitus and who experienced a variety of complications are described. Information basic to understanding their needs has been selected and applied. In the second part, Mr. Allen, a patient who has been burned, is described. Information required to understand and meet his needs is presented. These patients illustrate many of the problems commonly experienced by persons who are ill. In Part 3, a guide for assessing level of consciousness is outlined.

In the not too distant past one of the critical tests of the skill of a nurse was her ability to meet the needs of a patient with an acute infectious disease such as typhoid fever or pneumonia. When the patient recovered, the nurse could rightly take credit for having made an important contribution to his recovery. As infectious diseases have been brought under control, the incidence of chronic illness has risen so that they now account for a significant portion of morbidity and mortality. The challenges presented by patients who are chronically ill are no less great than they are with patients with acute infectious diseases. Chronically ill patients often have a wider range of problems and need a greater variety of services than are needed to meet the needs of the acutely ill. Restoration of the patient to his optimum status and prevention of progress of his illness often demands the continued efforts of the patient, his family, the nurse, the physician, and other health and welfare personnel as well as the members of the community. With patients in whom progress toward recovery is slow and in whom control or prevention of the progression of disease is the goal rather than complete recovery, the nurse may not be able to see immediate results of her efforts. Instead of a relatively brief and intense relationship in which the patient is dependent on the nurse, the nurse often has a more or less prolonged relationship with him. This relationship with the patient changes from time to time, from dependence to independence to interdependence. To meet the needs of the patient, the nurse should be able to identify clues indicating the type of relationship best suited to the needs of the patient at a given time and to adapt her behavior accordingly. She must also be able to accept failure of the patient to make dramatic progress toward recovery or even failure of the patient to accept what is regarded as being essential to his welfare.

Today the test of the skill of the nurse is her ability to meet the needs of the chronically ill patient. If a single disease were to be selected as the modern-day test of nursing knowledge and skill, diabetes mellitus would undoubtedly receive many votes. There are many reasons that this is true. Diabetes mellitus has a relatively high incidence. It affects all age groups. Its complications are many and serious. There are, however, effective means for its detection, diagnosis, and treatment. With modern methods of therapy, persons with diabetes mellitus can live almost as long as those who do not have diabetes. Even more important, they can have full and useful lives with few restrictions on their activities. Young men with diabetes mellitus have been Rhodes scholars, mountain climbers, tennis champions, and television stars. Young women with diabetes mellitus go to college, successfully complete programs in nursing or teaching, marry, bear and rear children, and otherwise lead successful lives.

Health programs, as they relate to diabetes mellitus, have two general objectives. The first is to prevent or, if this is not possible, to delay the onset of the disease. The second is to maintain the health and vigor of the individual throughout his life. In the achievement of these objectives the nurse has three general responsibilities. The first is to aid in the detection of persons who are predisposed to or in the early stages of diabetes mellitus. The second is to participate in the education of the patient, his family, and the community in the management of diabetes mellitus. The third is to meet the needs of the sick person for nursing. Frequently the nurse performs all these functions simultaneously.

No nurse should accept the responsibility for the care of the patient with diabetes mellitus unless she knows as much as the well-educated patient is expected to learn about his disease. She should also be willing and able to recognize that the patient may feel differently about having diabetes mellitus than she thinks he should. Not infrequently a patient is told that he is fortunate to have diabetes rather than some other disease. The advantages that diabetes mellitus has over diseases are expressed by physicians and nurses who do not have diabetes. In contrast, the patient compares diabetes with health. The feelings of the patient result from the implications diabetes mellitus has for him now and in the future. In the beginning the patient or his parents are likely to express disbelief and then grief. (See Chapter 7.) In the case of the child, the parents, especially the

mother, grieve over the loss of a healthy child. Generally, the earlier the disease develops and more severe it is, the greater the adjustment. Problems of adjustment are particularly difficult for the adolescent.[1]

The nurse can be helpful to the patient by accepting his feelings as having a cause and by creating a climate in which he is free to express them. Eventually, most patients come to accept their diabetes with a reasonable degree of equanimity. A sound program of instruction adapted to the individuality of the patient can be expected to make a positive contribution to his acceptance of his therapeutic regimen.

Six Patients

As a basis for discussing the knowledge that the nurse needs if she is to meet the needs of patients with diabetes mellitus, the histories of six patients will be summarized in Table 19-1. Some of the material was collected for other purposes so the details in all instances may not be complete. Selection of information is on the basis of what is most pertinent to this discussion. The content contained in the summary will be commented on in the appropriate sections. Of the six patients it will be noted that five are female and one is male. They range in age from 15 to 73 years. Two of these six persons are college graduates and were diabetic at the time they entered college. One of them, Miss Arthur, lived in a dormitory and ate in a college cafeteria throughout her years in college; she had no problems in the selection of her diet. Both Miss Arthur and Mr. Benedict are self-supporting, and he has thus far been able to support his family. Although these patients do not present all the problems faced by patients with diabetes mellitus, they do have many of the common ones. Because they have all had their disorder for some time, they do not illustrate all the problems of the patient who just learned that he has diabetes mellitus.

Had these six people lived 100 years ago, the probability is that only Mrs. Curry and Mrs. Delft would have survived more than a year or two after the onset of the disease. One hundred years ago the prognosis of the diabetic child was hopeless. His status was similar to, and probably no better than, that of the child who now has leukemia. After the diagnosis was established, few children lived longer than a year. For the most part, the child led a miserable existence until he died in diabetic acidosis. Many persons now live as long as or longer than the life expectancy for nondiabetics of the same age. The average diabetic, however, lives about

[1] Phillip L. Isenberg and Donald M. Barnett: "Psychological Problems in Diabetes Mellitus," *Med. Clin. N. Amer.,* **49:**1125–36 (July) 1965.

TABLE 19-1

Summary of Six Patients' Histories

Factor	Bonnie	Miss Arthur	Mr. Benedict	Mrs. Curry	Mrs. Delft	Mrs. Keen
Age	15	22	29	62	71	73
Age at onset	4	13	8	60	62	55
Years of known diabetes	11	9	21	2	9	17
Sex	F	F	M	F	F	F
Severity	Severe	Severe	Severe	Mild	Mild	Severe
Reason for present hospitalization	Acidosis (numerous admissions in the past)	Hypoglycemia with unconsciousness	Evaluation of diabetes and investigation of complications	Myocardial infarction	Possible cerebro-vascular accident	Control of diabetes preparatory to operation
Present signs and symptoms	Nausea Vomiting Abdominal cramps Lips and tongue dry and parched Kussmaul breathing Glycosuria Ketonuria	Blood sugar on admission 55 mg/100 ml Unconscious	Weakness Easily fatigued Blurring of vision	Onset with diabetic retinopathy	Poor vision Blurring Severe frontal headaches Nausea and vomiting	Glycosuria Hyperglycemia Increased blood cholesterol
Adequacy of control	Poor	Generally excellent	Recent years generally satisfactory	Good with diet	Satisfactory with diet	Poor
Family history of diabetes	Grandmother diabetic	No family history known	Father and sister diabetic	Mother diabetic	None known	Sister diabetic
Weight at onset	Average	Average	Average	Obese	Obese	Obese

842

Therapy						
Diet	CHO 150 Protein 90 Fat 120	Diabetic	Low salt Diabetic	Diet 1,200 calories	Controlled by diet	CHO 175 Protein 80 Fat 80
Insulin	38U/NPH daily	Protamine zinc insulin	NPH	0		Lente insulin 10 U daily at time of discharge
Tolbutamide	—	—	—	Started with current hospitalization	—	Attempted, unsuccessfully
Exercise		Plays golf and tennis	Drives a car 90 miles/day			
Complications and concomitant disorders	Acidosis and cystitis	Hypoglycemia	Diabetic retinopathy Early hypertension Nephrosclerosis	Myocardial infarction Diabetic retinopathy	Retinopathy Cerebrovascular accident	Cataracts Myocardial ischemia
Employment	School	Secretary	Office worker	Housewife	Housewife	Housewife
Responsibilities	Self	Self	Two young children	Husband	Lives with daughter	Lives with daughter

three quarters of the life expectancy of the nondiabetic. Of the three patients who developed diabetes as children, all have lived nine or more years. Two of the adults have lived longer than the average life-span for nondiabetics.

Why has life expectancy improved?

The factors contributing to the great improvement in the life expectancy of persons of all ages who have diabetes mellitus include (1) greater understanding of the nature of normal as well as abnormal energy metabolism, (2) more appreciation of the value of diet in the control of hyperglycemia, (3) the discovery of insulin and its use in therapy, (4) the discovery of oral hypoglycemic agents, (5) the recognition that the control of diabetes mellitus is the responsibility of the patient and his family, and (6) the development of educational programs to prepare the patient to assume this responsibility.

Incidence

According to available statistics, the incidence of diabetes mellitus is increasing. In 1900 diabetes mellitus ranked twenty-seventh as a cause of death. In 1967, it was fifth.[2] The total number of persons with diabetes mellitus, that is, the morbidity rate, is not known for certain. If, however, the findings of the study made in Oxford, Massachusetts, apply generally, there are about 3 million persons in the United States with diabetes mellitus. About 2 million are known diabetics, whereas approximately 1 million are unaware of its presence. These figures are based on the Oxford study in which 70 persons were found to have diabetes. Of these, 40 were known and 30 were unknown diabetics.[3]

In a study reported by Lipkind,[4] screening tests were made on hospital outpatients and blood donors, and 7,164 persons were screened for diabetes. Of these, 1.3 per cent were diagnosed as diabetic. In another program 15,535 persons were screened and 210, or 1.35 per cent, were found to be diabetic.[5]

Furthermore, the incidence of diabetes mellitus tends to rise with each decade through the fifth and sixth decades of life; the number of persons who have the disorder can be expected to rise as life expectancy increases. Eighty per cent of diabetics are 40 or more years old. Forty per cent are 65 years or older. Some studies show that large differences in the rate of diagnosis do not occur between sexes or in different races. The fact that diabetic children are living to maturity increases the number of diabetics who are alive at one time. Moreover, when they marry and have children, the number of persons carrying the diabetic trait is increased. The incidence is highest in the parts of the world where food is most available and the need for exercise least. In parts of the world where there is little or no medical care and the collection of statistics is in a primitive state, little accurate information is available about the incidence of any disease.

Joslin[6] summarizes the factors contributing to the reported incidence of diabetes mellitus by saying that the frequency is highest where (1) the average age is highest, (2) women predominate, (3) obesity is most frequent, (4) medical supervision is closest, (5) deaths are most accurately reported, and (6) the proportion of Jews is greatest. Some of these points will be discussed further later. As indicated, recent studies do not support all of the above.

Historical Review

Despite the increase in the importance of diabetes mellitus as a cause of morbidity and mortality,[7] it is not a modern disease. Nor is the disorder limited to human beings, for it appears in domestic dogs, cats, and cows and laboratory animals including mice, monkeys, and dolphins. It even occurs in families of animals.[8] The first recorded reference to diabetes mellitus is believed to be in the Papyrus Ebers, which dates back to about 1500 B.C.[9] The first description of the clinical manifestations of diabetes mellitus was by Aertaeus, who described it as a melting of the flesh into the urine. Urine was described in the fifth century by Susruta as honey urine. Some 1,200 years later, Thomas Willis reported that the urine from a patient with diabetes mellitus tasted sweet.

[2] Metropolitan Life Insurance Company: *Statist. Bull.,* **48:**11 (Aug.) 1967.

[3] Hugh L. C. Wilkerson and Leo P. Krall: "Diabetes in a New England Town," *JAMA,* **135:**209–16 (Sept. 27) 1947.

[4] Jason B. Lipkind: "Evaluation of Continuous Diabetes Screening in a Hospital Outpatient Department," *Public Health Rep.,* **78:**471–76 (June) 1963.

[5] Glen W. McDonald *et al.:* "Large-Scale Diabetes Screening Program for Federal Employees," *Public Health Rep.,* **78:**553–60 (July) 1963.

[6] Elliot P. Joslin *et al.: The Treatment of Diabetes Mellitus,* 10th ed. (Philadelphia: Lea & Febiger, 1959), p. 19.

[7] James Augustine (ed.): *Diabetes Source Book, Public Health Service Publication No. 1168* (Washington, D.C.: U.S. Department of Health, Education, and Welfare, May 1964).

[8] Albert E. Renold: "Spontaneous Diabetes and/or Obesity in Laboratory Rodents," *Advances Metab. Dis.,* 3:50, 1968.

[9] Ralph H. Major: *Classic Descriptions of Disease,* 3rd ed. (Springfield, Ill.: Charles C Thomas, Publisher, 1955), p. 235.

In 1775, Dobson identified the material in urine as sugar. Almost a century later the first reasonably accurate determinations of the quantity of glucose in the blood were made by Claude Bernard. He also discovered glycogen as well as the function of the liver in its storage. In 1869 Langerhans described the islet cells in the pancreas that now bear his name. About 20 years later Von Mehring and Minkowski demonstrated that diabetes mellitus was induced in a dog by pancreatectomy. In 1921 Banting and Best isolated insulin from the islet cells in the pancreas, and in 1922 they made insulin available for patients. Because insulin usually corrects the disturbance in carbohydrate metabolism, scientists believed that the nature of diabetes mellitus was understood. This belief was shaken in 1930 when Houssay [10] reported that the severity of diabetes mellitus following pancreatectomy in the dog could be ameliorated by the removal of the anterior pituitary gland. Later Long and Lukens [11] demonstrated that the same effect can be produced in the cat by adrenalectomy. Studies of the metabolism of fat show that insulin is necessary for the synthesis and storage of fat in fat depots. These and more recent studies indicate that the pathological physiology of diabetes mellitus is complex and probably not subject to a simple explanation. After more than ten years of study (1945–1955) Sanger [12] and his associates finally clarified the structure of the insulin molecule. It is a polypeptide consisting of two chains joined by three $-S-S-$ (disulfide) bridges. They were able to demonstrate the sequence of amino acids in the molecule, as well as the fact that the sequence of amino acids differs somewhat in different species. Human and whale insulin are most similar to each other, whereas beef and sheep insulins differ in certain respects. Although these differences do not appear to affect their action as insulin, they do affect the degree to which they are antigenic. Some patients who develop allergic responses to beef or sheep insulin are able to tolerate pork insulin.

Unanswered Questions

Many questions remain to be answered about diabetes mellitus. Among the unanswered questions are the following: (1) What is the nature

[10] B. A. Houssay: "Advancement of Knowledge of the Role of the Hypophysis in Carbohydrate Metabolism During the Last Twenty-Five Years," *Endocrinology*, 30:884–90 (June) 1942.

[11] C. N. H. Long and F. D. W. Lukens: "The Effects of Adrenalectomy and Hypophysectomy Upon Experimental Diabetes in the Cat," *J. Exp. Med.*, 63:465–90 (Apr.) 1936.

[12] F. Sanger: "Chemistry of Insulin," *Brit. Med. Bull.*, 16:183–88 (No. 3) 1960.

and cause of diabetes? (2) How and where does insulin act? (3) How are different tissues affected by insulin? (4) Do the abnormalities in glucose tolerance occurring among the aged indicate diabetes mellitus or are they a "normal" part of aging? (5) Do some diabetic patients maintain glucose metabolism by utilizing non-insulin-dependent metabolic pathways? (6) Is the level of glucose in the blood the best way of measuring the degree of control of diabetes or are there better methods? (7) How can the vascular and neurological concomitants of diabetes be prevented? (8) What kind of program is needed to assist the patient and his family learn to cope with diabetes mellitus? (9) What kind of follow-up is required if the patient is to manage his disease properly? The last two questions are of particular importance if nurses are to provide maximum assistance to patients.

The Nature and Causes of Diabetes Mellitus

The oldest definition of diabetes mellitus is based on the observation that certain persons have a disorder characterized by the excretion of an abnormally large volume of urine or polyuria. The term *diabetes,* which is derived from the Greek and means to pass through a siphon, was therefore applied to this condition. Mellitus—*mel* is Latin for honey—was added in the eighteenth century by Willis. Based on the current state of knowledge, diabetes mellitus is defined as a chronic hereditary disorder in which there is (1) a relative or absolute lack of insulin characterized by disturbed metabolism of glucose, fat, and protein and (2) changes in the structure and functions of blood vessels.

Types of Diabetes

Diabetes mellitus is of two types, the juvenile-onset type and the maturity-onset type.

JUVENILE-ONSET TYPE

Although it may occur later, the juvenile-onset type usually develops before age 15. It is characterized by a rapid onset with rapid progression to coma. In the early stage of the disease the patient has an increase in insulin-like activity substances in the plasma and the islet cells undergo hyperplasia and hypertrophy. After about three months of treatment about one third of the patients undergo a remission. Their insulin requirement diminishes and they respond well to sulfonylurea and/or phenethylbiguanide. Within three months to a year, they have a relapse and return to a diabetic state. They are then dependent, as are those who do not have a remission, on insulin for the control of their diabetes for the rest of their lives.

Bonnie, Miss Arthur, and Mr. Benedict all have the juvenile-onset type of diabetes. The age of onset ranged from 4 to 13 years. All have severe diabetes and require insulin. Two of the three patients have a known history of diabetes. Although a family history of diabetes is somewhat more common among juvenile diabetics than among older diabetics, the incidence of a positive family history is the same in our group. All three were of average weight.

MATURITY-ONSET TYPE

Although the maturity-onset type of diabetes may develop earlier, its onset is usually after 35 or 40 years of age. Among its characteristic features are (1) absence of ketosis, (2) association with obesity, (3) delayed release of insulin after ingestion of glucose, (4) relatively easy to control with oral agents and/or diet, (5) may or may not have symptoms, and (6) vascular complications are common. Individuals who do not know they have diabetes are likely to have the maturity-onset type. It can be noted that for three of the six patients the known onset was 55 years of age or older. In two of the three patients, the disease was mild and satisfactorily controlled by diet. All three were obese.

Etiology

ABSOLUTE OR RELATIVE LACK OF INSULIN

Despite a lack of definitive knowledge of the etiology of diabetes, many authorities accept as a working hypothesis that insulin is lacking in either amount or effectiveness. Historically, failure of the beta cells to secrete sufficient insulin has been given the most attention. With the discovery that diabetes mellitus may be present despite normal or even elevated immunoreactive insulin and/or insulin-like substances in the blood, a new hypothesis is required.

DELAYED RELEASE OF INSULIN

In some patients with the maturity-onset type of diabetes, the release of insulin is delayed in relation to the time of absorption of carbohydrate. Studies show that proinsulin, a substance with relatively little insulin activity, cannot be distinguished from true insulin by immunoassay methods. The questions that follow are "Do obese persons with the maturity-onset type of diabetes secrete an abnormally large amount of proinsulin? Do they lack an enzyme that is necessary to convert proinsulin to insulin?" [13] One question that has been asked for some time is, "Is insulin abnormal in some way?" Proinsulin may be the answer. Another suggestion has been made that the blood contains an insulin-binding substance. The fact is that diabetes mellitus may be present while the insulin-like activity of the splenic blood of the vein draining the pancreas is normal.

Much of the evidence that diabetes mellitus is caused by a deficiency in insulin supply is indirect. Until the introduction of immunoassay methods insulin in the blood could not be identified. Information was obtained from experiments on animals and from the observation that severe diabetes mellitus cannot be controlled without insulin. Permanent diabetes mellitus in animals can be induced in a number of ways: (1) the removal of nine tenths or more of the pancreas, (2) the destruction of the beta cells in the islands of Langerhans by a chemical such as alloxan, (3) the prolonged administration of crude extracts of the anterior pituitary gland or of purified growth hormone, and (4) the prolonged parenteral administration of glucose.

The last two experimental conditions appear to have a common element: They increase the demand for insulin by causing a persistent elevation in the blood sugar. Because the secretion of insulin is believed to be regulated by the level of glucose in the blood, a continued elevation in blood glucose places a strain on the beta cells in the pancreas. Eventually insulin-secreting cells are exhausted. After animals treated with the growth hormones or prolonged administration of parenteral glucose die, their beta cells in the pancreas are usually found to have undergone degeneration. At autopsy, some, but not all, diabetics are found to have experienced destruction of the beta or islet cells. Hyperglycemia can be induced temporarily in some persons by the administration of adrenocortical hormones and by excessive dosages of thyroid hormones. It disappears when these hormones are discontinued.

Disorders Inducing Diabetes Mellitus

Diabetes mellitus is induced in persons who are treated by pancreatectomy for the removal of a malignant neoplasm in the pancreas or who have chronic pancreatitis. It also occurs in a high percentage of patients who have hemochromatosis, a disorder of iron metabolism characterized by the deposit of iron in the pancreas and other tissues. Deposits in the skin lead to the characteristic coloring that gives the disorder its name, bronze diabetes. The deposits

[13] "Insulin and Proinsulin: Relations and Implications," *JAMA*, 207:552 (Jan. 20) 1969.

of iron in the tissues lead to irritation and fibrosis. With destruction of the beta cells in the pancreas, diabetes mellitus ensues. It commonly accompanies Cushing's disease, a disorder in which there is an increase in the secretion of adrenocortical steroids.

What factors appear to predispose to diabetes mellitus in man?

HEREDITY

Two and possibly three factors appear to be important in the development of diabetes mellitus in man. They are heredity, obesity, and possibly hormonal disturbances (other than insulin). A variety of stresses such as pregnancy, infection, and thyrotoxicosis may bring the diabetes to light, if the tendency is present. The relationship of heredity to diabetes mellitus has been observed since at least the seventh century A.D. Despite evidence that heredity is a factor in diabetes mellitus, it cannot be demonstrated in all persons. Statistics from different clinics indicate that from 20 to 50 per cent of diabetic individuals have a positive family history for diabetes. The failure to identify a hereditary factor in some individuals may be caused by the following: (1) The onset of diabetes, which may occur at any time during the lifetime of an individual but is usually after 40 years of age—a child may develop diabetes mellitus before it develops in one of his parents; (2) a potential diabetic, who may also die from some other cause before diabetes develops; and (3) whether or not some individuals develop diabetes appears to depend on the presence of some other predisposing factor, such as obesity. Knowledge of diseases suffered by earlier generations is often limited.

Although some authorities believe that diabetes is inherited as an autosomal recessive trait, not all agree. Inheritance of diabetes mellitus among experimental animals is by a variety of patterns—autosomal recessive, dominant, and multifactoral traits. Therefore it is possible that inheritance in man may be as varied.[14] An interesting view of the hereditary nature of diabetes is presented by Neel,[15] who suggests that in prehistoric times the diabetic gene enhanced man's chances for survival. The diabetic tends to have accelerated growth in childhood, early menarche, large families, and later a tendency toward obesity. Thus she was able to reproduce during her short life-span and obesity protected her against famine.

OBESITY

In older individuals, heredity may be a predisposing rather than a direct cause of diabetes mellitus. For it to develop some other conditions placing a strain on the pancreas must be present; one such condition is obesity. The exact role of obesity in the development of diabetes is not understood. Seventy-five to eighty per cent of older diabetics are, however, obese at the time of the onset of the disease. It has been suggested that obesity in diabetes is a result of preferential utilization of insulin for fat synthesis and storage; that is, muscle tissue may be unable to utilize insulin owing to certain anti-insulin substances in the serum and its action is concentrated on adipose tissue. Therefore, the diabetic may be obese because he is diabetic, not diabetic because he is obese. Three of the patients in our group, and all of these over 50 years of age at the time of onset, were obese. Some persons gain weight just preceding the onset of diabetes mellitus. In many patients a loss of weight is accompanied by an amelioration of the condition. During periods in history when food is scarce, as in Europe during World War II, the incidence of diabetes tends to fall. In regions of the world where food is scarce, diabetes is infrequent. Some of the features of diabetes among the obese are described with the maturity type of diabetes.

Children differ from adults inasmuch as obesity is not a factor in the development of diabetes mellitus. The onset in children frequently occurs during periods of increased linear growth. Despite considerable evidence implicating obesity as a predisposing factor in diabetes mellitus, the nature of the relationship remains uncertain.

AGING

It has been known for 50 years that the ability to adapt to glucose diminishes with aging. As a result some authorities question whether the same standards should be used for the glucose tolerance test in older persons as for young and middle-aged adults. Zeytinoglu and associates,[16] however, studied 40 healthy men and women (20 male, 20 female) ranging in age from 68 to 91 years. In 29 of the subjects, the glucose tolerance was similar to that seen in young diabetics. Furthermore, a much higher percentage of women than men had abnormal glucose tolerance tests. The findings of Metz and his co-workers were similar. Furthermore, the concentration of free fatty

[14] "Diabetes Mellitus in Man and Experimental Animals," *Ann. Intern. Med.,* **66**:227–30 (Jan.) 1967.
[15] James V. Neel: "Diabetes Mellitus: A 'Thrifty' Genotype Rendered Detrimental by 'Progress'?" *Amer. J. Hum. Genet.,* **14**:353 (Dec.) 1962.

[16] Ibrahim Y. Zeytinoglu, Constantin N. Gherondache, and Gregory Pincus: "The Process of Aging: Serum Glucose and Immunoreactive Insulin Levels During the Oral Glucose Tolerance Test," *J. Amer. Geriat. Soc.,* **17**:1–14 (Jan.) 1969.

acids in the blood was higher among persons with impaired glucose tolerance than in those with a normal glucose tolerance.[17]

HORMONAL FACTORS

A deficiency in the supply of available insulin in relation to the quantity required to prevent hyperglycemia is conceded to be the principal endocrine factor in diabetes mellitus. The possibility exists that disturbances in the functioning of other endocrine glands may in some instances play a significant role in its genesis. To date, proof is lacking that abnormal function of glands such as the adrenal cortex or anterior pituitary causes diabetes mellitus unless the reserve capacity of the beta cells is inadequate. The hormones secreted by the adrenal cortex or anterior pituitary may precipitate diabetes mellitus in persons who have a pre-existing tendency to diabetes mellitus. Evidence to support a possible relationship of other hormones to the development of diabetes mellitus is derived from animal experiments and the observation that persons with acromegaly,[18] Cushing's syndrome,[19] and hyperthyroidism sometimes manifest hyperglycemia and glycosuria. Some persons under treatment with adrenocortical hormones or adrenocorticotropin also develop hyperglycemia. Because of their capacity to provoke hyperglycemia and glycosuria in persons who are predisposed to diabetes mellitus, hydrocortisone and cortisone may be employed to identify persons who are in the latent ("prediabetic") stage of the disease.

Animal experiments, such as those previously cited in the review of the development of knowledge of diabetes mellitus, also implicate the anterior pituitary and the adrenal cortex in the pathogenesis of diabetes mellitus. The injection of large dosages of anterior pituitary extracts injures islet cells. The removal of the anterior pituitary or the adrenal glands reduces the severity of diabetes mellitus in previously depancreatized animals.

Studies such as the ones cited cannot, of course, be made on human beings. Diseases in which hyperfunction of glands occurs can, however, provide information not otherwise available. With the developments in biochemistry, methods are becoming available whereby the various hormones appearing in blood, urine, and other body fluids can and will be identified.

There are two sources of information about the effects of hormones and glucose metabolism in the living human being. Hormonal changes occurring during pregnancy have a diabetogenic effect.[20] Women who are predisposed to, but have not yet developed, clinical diabetes mellitus may have an abnormal glucose tolerance curve that returns to normal on the termination of the pregnancy. According to Joslin, 90 per cent of women whose babies weigh 13 lb at birth become diabetic.[21] Most authorities agree that giving birth to an infant weighing more than 9 lb is indicative of latent diabetes. Some believe that the large size of the infant is caused by hypersecretion of the growth hormone.

What other organs participate in the homeostasis of glucose?

Because the liver and a number of endocrine glands—including the anterior pituitary, the adrenal, and the thyroid—participate in the homeostasis of glucose, they may play a role in the development of diabetes mellitus in some patients. Some of the effects of other hormones are considered under predisposing factors.

The mechanisms of action by which hormones other than insulin predispose to the development of diabetes mellitus have not been proved. Several hypotheses have been proposed: (1) The hormone or hormones act in some manner to decrease the secretion of insulin; (2) the hormone or hormones antagonize, inhibit, or block the peripheral action of insulin; and (3) the hormone or hormones act indirectly by producing conditions that increase the demand for insulin.

In permanent diabetes the growth hormone can be shown to elevate the blood sugar. It impairs glucose tolerance and responsiveness to insulin. Its mechanism of action is not known. The adrenal steroids promote the formation of glucose (gluconeogenesis) by the liver and may decrease its peripheral utilization.

Other evidence supporting the hypothesis that hormonal imbalance influences the development of diabetes mellitus is that the incidence of the disease rises in women at the time of menopause. Before the age of 45 years, the incidence is about equal in both sexes.

From time to time reference is made in literature to the hormone glucagon, which has been extracted from the islet cell in the pancreas. When it is injected, it causes a transient elevation in the blood sugar similar to that caused by epinephrine. There is no convincing evidence at this time that it plays a role in the pathogenesis of diabetes mellitus. It is useful in the treatment of drug-induced hypoglycemia.

[17] Robert Metz *et al.*: "Glucose Tolerance, Plasma Insulin, and Free Fatty Acids in Elderly Subjects," *Ann. Intern. Med.*, **64**:1042–48 (May) 1966.

[18] A disorder caused by an eosinophilic adenoma of the anterior pituitary, which secretes an excess quantity of the growth hormone.

[19] A disorder characterized by hypersecretion of the glucocorticoids of the adrenal cortex.

[20] Joslin, *op. cit.*, p. 703.

[21] *Ibid.*, p. 14.

INFECTION

Despite the frequency with which the onset of diabetes is coincident with an infection, infection is believed to act as a precipitating rather than an etiological factor. In other words, infection acts as a nonspecific stress. The changes that occur during the infection serve to intensify the disorder so that the clinical manifestations become evident. Changes increasing the insulin requirement, during infection, include an increase in the secretion of adrenocortical steroids and an increase in the rate of metabolism as a result of fever. Fever also predisposes to dehydration and acidosis, which also tends to aggravate the diabetic state.

Diabetes mellitus also increases susceptibility to certain types of infections, particularly those of the skin. In preinsulin days carbuncles and furuncles were frequent and difficult to cure. After they developed, the diabetic state was intensified and with it the resistance of the skin to infection was further diminished. The author once cared for an elderly man, Mr. Samuel, who had a huge carbuncle involving the entire back of his neck. Until his diabetes was brought under control, the infection continued to spread. After treatment of the diabetes mellitus was instituted, the area healed rapidly. The control of the infectious process also had a beneficial effect on his diabetes. As the carbuncle healed, his insulin requirement dropped. Another patient, Miss Murphy, was treated for furuncles (boils) for over a year. When her urine was finally tested for sugar, she was found to have glycosuria. With the control of her diabetes, her boils healed. The difficulties of Mr. Samuel and Miss Murphy were in no way unusual. Infection has an adverse effect on diabetes mellitus, and diabetes mellitus increases the difficulty of curing certain types of infections.

THIAZIDE DIURETICS

Patients on long-term therapy with thiazide diuretics occasionally develop a mild degree of hyperglycemia.

GROUP DIFFERENCES

The fact that diabetes mellitus appears to be more common among certain groups of people than others merits some comment. The incidence is higher among those who live in urban areas than those who live in rural areas. This is probably caused by the fact that persons living in urban areas are frequently more sedentary than those living in rural areas. It is recognized that exercise decreases the demand for insulin. The possibility also exists that persons living in urban areas have more adequate and better quality medical care available, and a higher *apparent* incidence of diabetes may be shown.

Most authorities emphasize that the incidence of diabetes mellitus is higher among Jews than among non-Jews. Joslin attributes this finding to the high incidence of obesity among Jewish people.[22] Cohen [23] challenges the belief that the incidence is higher among Jews than non-Jews. He suggests that it is based on data collected in clinics patronized by a disproportionate number of Jewish people. In the study of the incidence of diabetes mellitus in Israel, Cohen found the incidence to be similar to that of people living in other countries. He also discovered that the Yemenites and Kurds, who traditionally have a very low incidence of diabetes mellitus, became diabetic at about the same rate as other Israelis when they adopted Western habits—food as well as habits of living and working.

Summary

To recapitulate, the manifestations of diabetes mellitus result from a relative or absolute lack of insulin. Some of the possible causes for this deficiency have been suggested. Heredity, obesity, and age appear to be associated with the development of diabetes mellitus.

Among other factors that may contribute to the diabetic state are anti-insulin antibodies, other hormones, and resistance of the peripheral tissues to insulin. Although insulin antibodies have been identified, they are found only in patients who have taken insulin. Among the hormones that antagonize the effect of insulin are the glucocorticoids, the growth hormone, epinephrine, and glucagon. What the role of each of these factors is in the genesis of diabetes mellitus is still in some doubt. The combination of optimum age, obesity, and hereditary tendency may be sufficient to induce diabetes mellitus. The tendency to develop the disease may be further increased by such factors as dietary excesses and too little exercise.

Natural History

An important step in understanding a disease is a description of its natural history. Depending on the investigator, diabetes is considered as developing in three to seven stages. Danowski [24] classifies diabetes mellitus in seven stages as follows:

[22] Joslin, *op. cit.,* p. 65.
[23] A. M. Cohen: "Prevalence of Diabetes Among Different Ethnic Jewish Groups in Israel," *Metabolism,* 10:50–58 (Jan.) 1961.
[24] T. S. Danowski: "Clinical Manifestations: In Newborns, Older Infants, and Children," in *Diabetes Mellitus: Diagnosis and Treatment,* Vol. I, T. S. Danowski, ed. (New York: American Diabetes Association, Inc., 1964), pp. 21–22.

Stage I is prediabetes, or prodiabetes, i.e., the phase preceding the appearance of any carbohydrate disturbance.

Stage II is stress diabetes. It is present only during a period of stress, and disappears completely after stress is removed.

Stage III is the most common undiagnosed form of diabetes mellitus in the adult but is less frequent in children. It is characterized by normal fasting blood glucose levels with undue postprandial or glucose tolerance test hyperglycemia.

Stage IV is the most common recognized form of diabetes mellitus in children as well as in adults. The fasting blood glucose is elevated, and of course, the two-hour postprandial or glucose tolerance test blood glucose concentrations are also unduly increased. In Stages III and IV, there is no ketosis. This cardinal feature sharply delimits these two stages from Stages V, VI, and VII, each of which is characterized by ketosis.

Stage V: ketonuria is present in addition to the fasting and postprandial hyperglycemia. There is however no significant accumulation of ketone bodies in the plasma.

Stage VI: ketonuria is more marked and is accompanied by ketone accumulation in the plasma and a reduction of the serum CO_2 content to the 20 to 10 mEq/L range. Slight to moderate decreases in serum pH (7.3 to 7.1) are present. Stage VI can be referred to as ketoacidosis. Tachypnea is common and overbreathing may develop.

Stage VII is diabetic acidosis-coma, with marked accumulations of ketone bodies in plasma and urine, decrease in serum CO_2 to less than 10 mEq/L, and reduction of serum pH to values as low as 6.8 or 6.9. Kussmaul overbreathing is almost always present.

At the time of diagnosis children are usually in Stages V, VI, or VII.[25] Most patients with the maturity-onset type are in Stages II, III, or IV when the diagnosis is made. Despite exceptions, few patients with the maturity-onset type develop ketosis. Vascular changes may be demonstrated in all stages, including Stage I.

CLASSIFICATION ACCORDING TO THERAPEUTIC
REQUIREMENTS

Diabetes mellitus may also be classified according to the therapeutic requirements of the patient. Thus Underdahl [26] places patients in four groups: A, B, C, and D. About 50 per cent of the patients have mild diabetes and are in group A. They can be controlled by diet. About 25 per cent of patients have moderate diabetes and are in group B. They require oral hypoglycemic agents plus diet to control their

[25] Ibid., p. 22.
[26] Laurentius O. Underdahl: "Classification of Diabetes Mellitus According to Therapeutic Requirements," in Diabetes Mellitus: Diagnosis and Treatment, Vol. 2, George J. Hamwi and T. S. Danowski, eds. (New York: American Diabetes Association, Inc., 1967), p. 75.

diabetes. Another 20 per cent have severe diabetes. They require insulin as well as diet to control their diabetes. Finally, about five per cent of the diabetics have what is variously called brittle, unstable, or labile diabetes. Diabetes in patients in group D is extremely difficult to control. Despite rigid adherence to the therapeutic regime, these patients fluctuate between hyper- and hypoglycemia. Most patients with the maturity-onset type of diabetes are in either group A or B.

Those with the growth-onset type of diabetes are in either group C or D. The onset of the disease is sudden and is manifested by polyuria, polyphagia, polydipsia, ketoacidosis and coma. The patient with the growth-onset type of diabetes mellitus is very sensitive to exogenous insulin. Early in the course of the disease his response to insulin is erratic. After two or three months of treatment, about one third of the patients undergo a remission. Their insulin requirement diminishes and they respond well to a sulfonylurea and/or phenethylbiguanide. Within a few months to a year, these patients have a relapse and require insulin to control their diabetes.

Pathophysiology

Although progress has been made in understanding the nature of the metabolic disturbances in diabetes mellitus, much remains to be learned. A brief review of glucose metabolism is included here. For further discussion, see Chapter 12. As defined earlier, energy metabolism is a process whereby the energy stored in food is gradually liberated by a series of stepwise chemical reactions for use in cells or is converted to a form in which it can be stored for future use.

Because glucose is not chemically a very active substance, glucose must be converted to the chemically active glucose-6-phosphate before it can be used at body temperature. This reaction requires the presence of the enzyme hexokinase and is the first step in the utilization of glucose, regardless of whether the glucose is converted to glycogen, utilized as energy, or converted to fat and stored. The entrance of significant quantities of glucose into the cell also requires a transport mechanism. After glucose enters the cell and is converted to glucose-6-phosphate, the cell is protected against too much energy at one time by the stepwise release of energy. Furthermore, different pathways are available in the utilization of glucose and many chemical reactions in the utilization of glucose are reversible. Not only is energy liberated and utilized, but it is fixed as chemically useful energy and stored in the form of high-energy bonds such as the high-energy phosphate bonds.

A number of conditions must be met for energy metabolism to proceed normally. In the first place appropriate metabolites in the proper form must be present. Some of these are supplied from exogenous as well as endogenous sources, and they must enter the cell at an appropriate rate, neither too slowly, nor too rapidly. For example, at least 100 g of glucose must be metabolized daily to prevent the utilization of fat at an excessively rapid rate. Most of this glucose comes from outside sources as the quantity of glycogen (a storage form of glucose) stored in the liver is sufficient to supply the glucose needed for about five hours. Some chemical reactions depend on the presence of certain metabolites that are formed during metabolism to provide the energy required for the reaction. For example, for glucose to be transfered into cells and converted into glucose-6-phosphate, high-energy adenosine triphosphate is required. In some chemical reactions a metabolite necessary to initiate the reaction is released or regenerated at the end of the reaction so that it is again available. For example, acetyl Co A and oxaloacetic acid combine at the beginning of the Krebs cycle to form citric acid. Oxaloacetic acid is regenerated at the end of the reaction.

In addition to the availability of appropriate metabolites at varying stages of metabolism, enzymes and coenzymes are required to catalyze the various chemical reactions involved in the release or storage of energy. Some of these are synthesized by the cells, whereas others, such as thiamine, must be ingested in the diet.

In the nondiabetic person, the factors tending to elevate the level of glucose in the blood are promptly counteracted by factors tending to lower it. The reverse is also true. As long as the rates at which glucose enters and leaves the blood are equal, the concentration of glucose in the blood is maintained within physiological limits. Any disturbance that interferes with the mechanisms for elevating or lowering the blood glucose may, depending on the direction of change, lead to hyper- or hypoglycemia. As an example, if the mechanisms for lowering blood glucose are ineffective and/or those for elevating it are hyperactive, hyperglycemia will result. Both of these factors are likely involved in diabetes mellitus. Despite the practice of discussing diabetes as if it were simply a disorder of glucose metabolism, it is not. Its pathophysiology involves all facets of metabolism.

What are the mechanisms for elevating the level of glucose in the blood?

In the regulation of the level of glucose in the blood, certain cells recognize the need of the

organism for glucose. When this need is sufficiently great, it is translated into the sensation hunger. Hunger motivates the individual to search for, find, and ingest food. There are three sources or routes by which glucose enters into the blood. The usual route of entry is by absorption from the alimentary canal. A second route of entry is the secretion of glucose by the liver. In time of need, the liver can maintain the level of glucose in the blood within normal limits, despite the absence of food intake. Although the liver is able to do this in the absence of hormonal factors, the rate at which glucose is secreted into the hepatic vein by the liver is modified by hormones. A third and less common route is by parenteral injection as by intravenous infusion. Parenteral injection is usually reserved for patients who are unable to ingest food into or absorb it from the alimentary tract.

GLYCOGENOLYSIS

The process by which the liver converts glycogen to glucose and secretes it into the hepatic vein is known as glycogenolysis. This is a rapid reaction occurring in a matter of minutes. The rapid conversion of glycogen to glucose is adapted to protect the individual in emergency situations against a drop in blood glucose. Because the total quantity of glycogen in the liver is limited (a 1,500-g liver probably contains no more than 60 g of glucose), glycogen cannot be expected to protect the level of glucose in the blood for more than a brief period of time.[27] The process is regulated by epinephrine and possibly glucagon.

GLUCONEOGENESIS

Glucose is also formed in the liver by a process known as gluconeogenesis. As the term implies, new glucose is created or formed from noncarbohydrate sources. In gluconeogenesis the liver converts amino acids after they have been deaminized (NH_2 removed) to glucose. The source of the amino acids is the muscles of the body. Gluconeogenesis differs from glycogenolysis in two respects. Rather than being a rapid and brief source of glucose to the blood, it is a slow and sustained reaction. It protects the level of glucose in the blood in disorders in which the supply of glucose is deficient or loss is excessive. Thus the level of glucose in the blood is maintained in starvation, despite a failure in the supply from exogenous sources. It is also maintained in disorders of the kidney in which excessive quantities of glucose are lost in the urine.

[27] Jay Tepperman, *Metabolic and Endocrine Physiology,* 2nd ed. (Chicago: Year Book Medical Publishers, Inc., 1968), p. 159.

Whereas the rate of glycogenolysis is regulated by epinephrine and glucagon, the rate of gluconeogenesis is regulated by glucagon and the adrenal glucocorticoids (Cortisol or hydrocortisone). The exact mechanism by which the adrenal steroids regulate the conversion of amino acids to glucose is not known. According to Tepperman,[28] the adrenal steroids are believed to "permit" the anabolism-catabolism equilibrium to be tipped in the direction of protein breakdown. The adrenal steroids may also facilitate the conversion of amino acids to glycogen in the liver.

In addition to protecting the level of glucose in the blood by making more glucose available to the blood, reduction in the utilization of glucose by peripheral tissues may also be a factor in the maintenance of the blood glucose. In starvation, tissues adapt in such a manner that they utilize less glucose than when the glucose supply is adequate. One factor in adaptation to starvation is a drop in total metabolism. On the basis of tissue culture experiments it is postulated that the muscles of starving animals utilize relatively more fatty acids than glucose.[29]

Similar to other aspects of glucose metabolism, hormones are believed to regulate the processes involved in blocking the peripheral use of glucose. These hormones, which are often called insulin antagonists, are the growth hormone (anterior pituitary) and the adrenal glucocorticoids. The nature of the action of these hormones in blocking peripheral glucose oxidation is not known.

One factor that may possibly contribute to the elevation of glucose in the blood is an increase in the rate of destruction of insulin. A number of tissues, especially the liver, have been demonstrated to inactivate insulin. The insulin-destroying mechanism in the liver has been referred to as insulinase, but the nature of the system has not been firmly established.

Another factor influencing the level of glucose in the blood is the state of hydration of the patient. In severe hypovolemia, the level of glucose in the blood tends to rise, as well as other constituents such as potassium and sodium. Dehydration is one factor in the marked rise in the level of glucose in the blood of acidotic patients.

What are the mechanisms for lowering the level of glucose in the blood?

A variety of factors contribute to the lowering of glucose in the blood. Just as the sensation hunger motivates food-seeking behavior, satiety (satisfaction) tends to depress it. The normal response to satiety is to cease ingesting food or

[28] Tepperman, *ibid.*, p. 159.
[29] Tepperman, *ibid.*, p. 160.

to decrease the supply of exogenous glucose. After absorption, glucose is distributed through the body water, thereby reducing its concentration in any compartment, including that of the blood. A third mechanism for lowering the blood glucose is exercise. Exactly how exercise affects the level of glucose in the blood is not well known. It is valuable in the treatment of diabetes mellitus as working muscle oxidizes glucose independently of insulin.

INSULIN RELEASE

Although a number of hormones regulate the mechanisms involved in elevating the level of glucose in the blood, the only hormone known to lower the blood glucose is insulin. The regulation of the release of insulin is highly complex. Among the factors that are believed to increase its release are (1) a rise in the level of glucose as well as the rate at which it rises in the blood; (2) a substance secreted by the jejunum, triggered by the absorption of glucose; (3) stimulation of the vagus nerve; (4) glucagon; and (5) amino acids. An observation supporting point 2 is that glucose placed in the jejunum causes a greater rise in insulin release than the same quantity given by infusion. This fact may be of some importance when glucose is given by intravenous infusion for the purpose of supplying calories. Presumably less glucose will be lost in the urine when the rate of administration is slow to moderate than when it is rapid.

Among the factors inhibiting insulin release are epinephrine and norepinephrine. Thus epinephrine promotes hyperglycemia by increasing the breakdown of glycogen and by inhibiting the release of the hormone that corrects hyperglycemia.

What are the effects of insulin?

Insulin promotes the removal of glucose from the blood by three principal effects. It facilitates the conversion of glucose to fat (lipogenesis) in adipose tissue and the liver. It speeds the conversion of glucose to glycogen, especially in the muscles, and the oxidation of glucose in insulin-sensitive tissues. It also affects the rate at which amino acids enter the cells and the rate of protein synthesis.[30] In the absence of insulin all these processes are depressed to some extent. How insulin produces all its effects is uncertain. Some hypotheses suggested include the following: (1) Insulin promotes the conversion of glucose to glucose-6-phosphate by binding mag-

[30] Ira G. Wool and Phyllis Cavicchi: "Insulin Regulation of Protein Synthesis by Muscle Ribosomes: Effect of the Hormones on Translation of Messenger RNA for a Regulatory Protein," *Proc. Nat. Acad. Sci. USA,* **56**:991–98 (Sept.) 1966.

nesium to hexokinase. Apparently magnesium is required for all the actions of insulin. (2) Insulin facilitates the rate of transport of glucose, potassium, phosphate, amino acids, and fatty acids across cell membranes. Some investigators are of the opinion that insulin stimulates the synthesis of glycogen, fat, and protein without affecting the permeability of cell membrane. (3) One of the newer hypotheses is that insulin acts through the genetic apparatus by stimulating the synthesis of DNA and RNA, especially messenger RNA. If this hypothesis proves to be true, it explains many of the effects of insulin. By its action on DNA and RNA, insulin may influence the synthesis of enzymes with specialized functions. Different types of cells may synthesize different enzymes or a varying proportion of enzymes. As examples, adipose tissue cells synthesize enzymes that catalyze the reaction whereby fatty acids are converted to fat. Liver cells synthesize enzymes catalyzing the conversion of glucose to glycogen.

From the discussion of the effects of insulin, it is clear that insulin has many metabolic effects. The consequences of a deficiency in the supply of insulin can be observed in all systems of the body. The functions of nervous, cardiovascular, respiratory, gastrointestinal, and renal excretory systems are all affected in one or more phases of the disease. In most patients the degree of severity can be modified by adequate treatment. In older obese adults the tendency to ketosis is usually absent, but vascular complications caused by atherosclerosis are a common problem. In older patients vascular disorders may precede or follow its development. Juvenile diabetics have a tendency to develop atherosclerosis at an earlier age than nondiabetics. Four of our six patients present evidence of atherosclerosis and other arterial disease. Despite numerous admissions to the hospital for the regulation of her diabetes, Mrs. Keen never was in ketoacidosis. Young lean adults and children are, in contrast to the older obese diabetic, subject to ketoacidosis. Bonnie has been in the hospital on numerous occasions for the treatment of this complication. As a child, Mr. Benedict was in ketoacidosis on several occasions. Except for one episode associated with the clinical onset, Miss Arthur has not developed ketoacidosis.

ADAPTATION TO STARVATION

Some understanding of the pathophysiological changes in diabetes mellitus can be gained by reviewing the adaptation of the cells to starvation. The alterations occurring in starvation and to some degree in diabetes mellitus have survival value inasmuch as they protect the cells

against a deficient food supply. In contrast, in diabetes mellitus, when these changes are too intense, they may predispose the individual to harm. In starvation as well as in diabetes, the individual cells substitute fat for glucose as fuel. The first change initiating acidosis is a decrease in the utilization of glucose by the peripheral tissues, accompanied by a mobilization of stored (depot) fat in the form of free fatty acids,[31] non- or unesterfied fatty acids.

Besides the mobilization of fatty acids, the rate of breakdown of tissue proteins is intensified. The resulting amino acids are deaminated in the liver and converted into glucose (gluconeogenesis). In starvation there is usually some ketonemia (elevation of ketone bodies in the blood) and ketonuria (excretion of ketone bodies in the urine). When the supply of food is inadequate, the shift from glucose to fat metabolism has survival value as it enables the individual to adapt to an insufficient supply of exogenous glucose. Adaptation is further supported by a lessening in the rate at which cells utilize glucose.

In the instance of Bonnie as well as among other diabetics, the failure in glucose utilization stems not from a lack of glucose but from a relative or absolute lack of insulin required for the utilization of glucose. Many older diabetics who were obese at the onset of their disease presumably utilize sufficient glucose, so that there is not an excessively rapid mobilization of fat. They may have sufficient insulin to keep their fat stores or to continue synthesizing fat. They are not predisposed to acidosis. In young and lean adults with a severe form of the disease, metabolic acidosis is a continuing possibility. Acidosis occurs when some event upsets the balance between the quantity of insulin required and that available. Although we do not know what the precipitating event was in the instance of Bonnie, she may have omitted her insulin or her insulin requirement may have been increased by a sudden stress. Among the common precipitating causes of acidosis are infection, physical trauma, and emotional stress. The onset of acidosis in Bonnie was nausea frequently marked by vomiting. It was not known whether the nausea and vomiting were associated with an acute gastrointestinal disorder or with the onset of acidosis. With their advent, she failed to ingest either food or fluids. Thus Bonnie was deprived of a supply of exogenous glucose.

Although the factors contributing to the development of acidosis in Bonnie are not known with certainty, they include the possibility of

---

[31] An ester is formed by the combination of an alcohol with an acid. In the process, water as well as the ester is formed.

one or more of the preceding, that is, (1) failure to take her insulin, (2) some disturbance increasing her insulin requirements, and (3) abstinence from food and fluids as a consequence of nausea and vomiting. From Bonnie's history, her diabetes can be presumed not to have been maintained under very good control. As a 15-year-old, emotional stress arising from her relationships with her parents, teachers, or peers as well as how she felt about herself and the fact of having diabetes mellitus may have contributed to an increased need for insulin. Changes in her hormonal balance at the menarche may have been another factor.

As a consequence of insulin deficiency, utilization of glucose by the peripheral cells is diminished, as in starvation, and the conversion of glycogen in the liver to glucose (glycogenolysis) is increased. Because the quantity of glycogen stored in the liver is small, it serves only as a temporary source of glucose. Although slower to be effected, a more sustained source of glucose is the formation of glucose by the liver from deaminated amino acids (gluconeogenesis). Because there is an imbalance between the factors tending to elevate the blood glucose and those tending to lower it in favor of those tending to elevate it, the blood glucose rises. The elevation in the blood glucose partly compensates for the lack of insulin inasmuch as it makes more glucose available to the cell.[32] With an elevation in the concentration of glucose in the blood, more glucose is available to, and is presumed to enter, the cell. Theoretically, a sufficient elevation in the blood glucose should make enough glucose available to supply required energy. Elevation of the blood sugar is in part limited by the renal threshold [33] that is, the point at which the glucose transport mechanism is no longer able to return all the glucose in the glomerular filtrate to the blood.

EFFECTS OF GLYCOSURIA

Loss of glucose in the urine has several undesirable effects. First, it is wasteful, and unless food intake is increased in proportion to loss, it will be associated with a loss in body weight and strength. Second, glucose is osmotically active. It holds water in the urine and thereby causes polyuria. With polyuria, not only water but electrolytes such as potassium and sodium

are lost. Thirst and an increase in fluid intake prevent dehydration, unless and until the individual develops nausea and vomiting. With dehydration, the blood becomes concentrated and blood volume falls; blood pressure drops and circulation to the tissues fails. As circulation to the tissues fails, generalized tissue anoxia causes a shift to anaerobic metabolism. Lactic acid appears in increasing concentrations in the blood and reflects an elevation of the hydrogen ions in the cell. Unless the condition is corrected by improving the supply of oxygen to the cells, death from heart failure ensues. The sequence of events resulting from the effects of a lack of insulin on carbohydrate metabolism is diagrammed in Figure 19-1.

The deficiency of insulin and diminution in the use of glucose have important effects on the capacity of the individual to synthesize, store, and maintain storage depots of fat. With a lack of insulin and failure to utilize normal amounts of glucose, large quantities of fat are mobilized from fat stores and are poured into the blood in the form of fatty acids. In the severely ill patient, such as Bonnie and Miss Arthur, fat may be mobilized from fat tissue.

The liver is inundated with fat, most of which it metabolizes only to the acetyl CoA stage. The

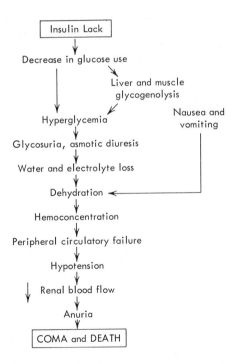

FIGURE 19-1. The effect of insulin lack on carbohydrate metabolism. (Adapted with permission of Year Book Medical Publishers, Inc., from *Metabolic and Endocrine Physiology*, 1968, Fig. 9-4, p. 165, by Jay Tepperman.)

[32] The effects of the raising of the blood glucose are an example in a living system of the law of mass action; that is, the speed of a chemical reaction is proportional to the molecular concentration of the reacting substances in a solution.

[33] The normal renal threshold is about 160 to 180 mg of glucose per 100 ml of blood. In patients who have long-standing diabetes mellitus the renal threshold is usually elevated, occasionally markedly.

two carbon atom fragments unite to form acetoacetic acid (diacetic acid and beta-hydroxybutyric acid), and an accumulation of these
acids in the blood results in metabolic acidosis,
one of the characteristic features of which is
Kussmaul breathing (deep and rapid breathing). In addition, as the production of ketoacids
exceeds the capacity of the kidney to reabsorb
them, they are excreted in the urine, and in the
process of excretion they take cations such as
sodium and potassium with them. Because electrolytes are osmotically active, they also require
water for their excretion. With the loss of sodium ions, the total quantity of sodium in the
body is diminished, and with the decrease the
water-holding power of extracellular fluid is
also reduced. With a loss of sodium, the total
volume of water in the extracellular fluid falls.
Blood volume drops and predisposes to peripheral circulatory failure. The effects of a deficiency of insulin on fat metabolism are summarized in Figures 19-2.

Not only does a lack of insulin impair the
use of glucose and fat, but it also affects protein
metabolism (Figure 19-3). With a deficiency in
the supply of insulin, protein synthesis, especially in muscles, is lessened and protein catabolism exceeds protein anabolism. The amino
acids released are deaminated in the liver, the
NH_2 fragment is removed, and the carbon-containing residues are converted to glucose or
fatty acid. Protein catabolism results in a loss
of nitrogen and potassium from the body and
thereby contributes to hypovolemia and its associated effects.

FIGURE 19-3. The effect of insulin lack on protein.
(Adapted with permission of Year Book Medical
Publishers, Inc., from *Metabolic and Endocrine
Physiology*, 1968, Fig. 9-6, p. 166, by Jay Tepper-
man.)

From the foregoing discussion, it should be
obvious that insulin influences the manner in
which carbohydrate, fat and protein are metabolized (Figure 19-4). Adequate supplies of insulin facilitate the use of glucose and favor synthesis and storage of fat. Inadequate insulin is
accompanied by impaired use of glucose, mobilization of fatty acids, in some instances triglycerides, and amino acids. As a consequence,
nutrition of the cells is reduced, water and
electrolytes are lost, and, unless these deficits
are corrected, circulation to the tissues is threatened.

*How is the presence of diabetes mellitus estab-
lished?*

Because hyperglycemia is accompanied by
glycosuria, diabetes mellitus is one of the easiest
of diseases to detect. The finding of glucose in
the urine is presumptive but not conclusive
evidence that a person has diabetes mellitus as
glycosuria can be present in a person who is
nondiabetic. Glycosuria occurring after the excessive ingestion of carbohydrates is known as
alimentary glycosuria. The person who has this
form of glycosuria may well be prediabetic.
Glycosuria also occurs in persons who have a
low renal threshold for glucose. The most frequent cause is, however, diabetes mellitus. The
presence of reducing substances in the urine
(mellituria) can also be associated with lactation (lactose lactosuria) and rare "metabolic
errors" (pentosuria, fructosuria, etc.). These
substances will give a positive reaction with
Benedict's solution and commonly used testing

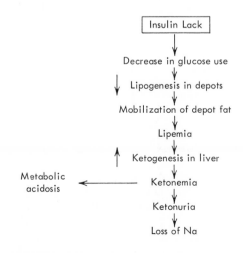

FIGURE 19-2. The effect of insulin lack on fat
metabolism. (Adapted with permission of Year
Book Medical Publishers, Inc., from *Metabolic and
Endocrine Physiology*, 1968, Fig. 9-5, p. 165, by
Jay Tepperman.)

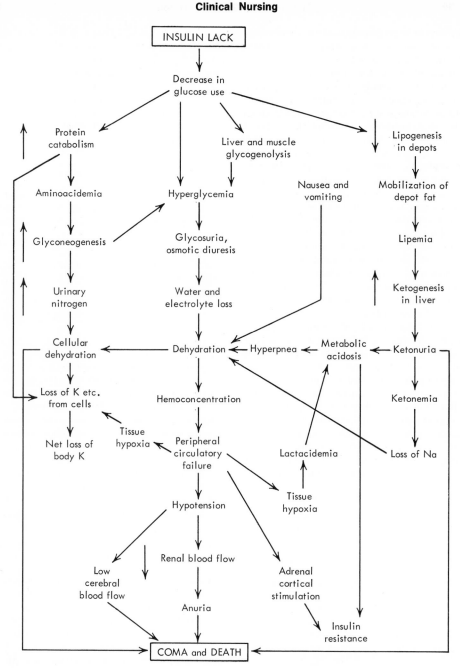

FIGURE 19-4. Composite summary of the pathophysiology of diabetic acidosis. Note particularly connections among the three general areas of metabolism. (Adapted with permission of Year Book Medical Publishers, Inc., from *Metabolic and Endocrine Physiology*, 1968, Fig. 9-7, p. 167, by Jay Tepperman.)

agents (Clinitest) but can be differentiated by test strips containing glucose oxidase (Testape, Clinistix). Glycosuria plus ketonuria is almost pathognomonic of diabetes mellitus. The diagnosis of diabetes mellitus is established by the presence of hyperglycemia in a person who is fasting or who cannot adapt at a normal rate to the stress produced by the ingestion of 100 g of glucose.

In many patients the diagnosis of diabetes mellitus is not established until the patient develops a complication. In some persons the disorder is discovered when they visit their physician for a medical examination. Other cases are discovered because an alert nurse encourages a patient with symptoms suggesting diabetes mellitus to seek medical attention. Still others are identified during community screening programs. These programs are usually sponsored by the American Diabetes Association through its local branches and the county medical society. Each fall these groups sponsor a Diabetic Detection Week. During the week materials are made available through the local pharmacies so that individuals can test their urine for glucose. An educational program is carried on at the same time to encourage individuals to avail themselves of this opportunity. The program is publicized by the various communication media. On specified days materials for testing urine are made available by the local pharmacies. Persons found to have glycosuria are referred to their physicians for diagnosis and, if need be, treatment.

Nurses have a number of opportunities to assist in the identification of persons who have diabetes mellitus. The suspicion of the school nurse should be aroused when a child develops polyuria and polydipsia. The public health nurse who visits in the home should be alert to the possibility of diabetes in family members. Recently a visiting nurse who was making a call to a mother with a new baby inquired about other members of the family. She learned that five-year-old Suzie was unusually irritable, that she was constantly "passing water," and that she drank large amounts of water, and was constantly hungry. The nurse obtained and tested a sample of urine. When she found that it was highly positive for glucose and acetone, she informed the mother that the child should see a physician as soon as possible. An appointment was made with the family physician, who examined Suzie and confirmed the fact that she had diabetes mellitus.

Some patients are discovered to have diabetes after they are admitted to the hospital. Most hospitals have a rule that before a patient can undergo any type of surgical procedure, his urine must be checked for glucose. In two instances known to the author, a nurse noted on the morning of surgery that the urine of a patient had not been checked for sugar. When the urine was tested, it was found to contain glucose. In both instances surgery was delayed until the patient's diabetes was brought under control.

In addition to opportunities for the nurse to participate in programs for the identification of persons who have diabetes mellitus, nurses have a role in the prevention of the disease. Because of the hereditary predisposition to diabetes mellitus, persons with diabetes are advised not to marry other diabetics or into families with a known history of the disease. Because of the frequency with which diabetes in the middle-aged person is associated with obesity, individuals are encouraged to avoid overweight by diet and exercise. About 10 per cent under the average weight is usually advocated for those over 30 years of age.

Onset

In the young, the onset of diabetes mellitus is likely to be rapid and acute, whereas in the middle-aged, obese adult, it is often slow. Among the latter, diabetes may be present for some time before the individual becomes aware of its manifestations. One estimate is that the middle-aged, obese adult is diabetic for about as many years before the disease is discovered as he survives after the diagnosis is made. Often, though not invariably, onset is precipitated by some physical or emotional stress.

The six patients whose histories are summarized in Table 19-1 illustrate the classic types of onset. In Bonnie, Miss Arthur, and Mr. Benedict, all of whom developed diabetes mellitus as children, onset was rapid. Although each of them had manifested polyuria, polydipsia, and polyphagia for an indefinite period, diagnosis was not established until they developed ketoacidosis. In retrospect Mrs. Arthur remembered that Miss Arthur had been eating very well, but she attributed Miss Arthur's appetite to the fact that her daughter was growing.

Among the three older diabetics, Mrs. Delft and Mrs. Curry were discovered to be diabetic when they sought medical attention for vascular concomitants. Mrs. Curry had blurring of vision from retinopathy. Mrs. Delft also had blurring of vision as well as dizziness and weakness on one side of her body. Mrs. Keen sought medical attention after observing that some urine that she had spilled left a shiny residue on drying.

In summary, in the young the onset is often more rapid and acute than in the mature, obese adult. Unless signs and symptoms are discovered early, acidosis is precipitated by some stress such as a respiratory infection and the individual becomes acutely ill. In the middle-aged, obese adult, onset is likely to be less acute. Diagnosis follows the discovery of glucose in the urine on a routine physical examination, or in association with an infection, or after a person seeks medical attention for the diagnosis and treatment of a related or unrelated disorder.

From the nature of the onset, the signs and symptoms manifested by patients at the time of diagnosis vary greatly. Not all adult patients are aware of any symptoms characteristic of diabetes mellitus. Discovery of glycosuria leads to an examination of the blood and the finding of hyperglycemia. Glycosuria is often, but not always, accompanied by polyuria, polydipsia, and polyphagia.

In women patients, glycosuria is frequently associated with pruritus—itching—of the vulva. The glucose in the urine may irritate the skin as it dries. It also serves as an excellent medium for the growth of *Candida*. Excoriation of the skin from scratching provides sites for the entrance of microorganisms. Prevention and relief of pruritus depend on the elimination of glucose from the urine by controlling the diabetes. Scrupulous cleanliness is also imperative.

Another result of glycosuria and the other metabolic disturbances in diabetes is loss of weight and weakness. In some patients, polyphagia is sufficient to compensate for the glucose lost in the urine. In severe forms of the disease, as much as a pound or approximately 500 g of glucose may be lost each day into the urine. In terms of calories, the person loses 4 calories with each gram of glucose excreted in the urine and as many as 2,000 calories may be lost each day by a person with severe diabetes. Mrs. Keen had enough glucose in her urine for it to be seen after the water evaporated. In the severe diabetic, weight loss is inevitable unless the disease is brought under control. When weight loss is accompanied by a loss of tissue proteins, weakness is to be expected. In the preinsulin days, loss of weight in the severe diabetic was often extreme and patients experienced marked weakness. Young emaciated diabetics are pictured as supporting themselves by leaning on a wall as they walk. Although weakness and weight loss are common complaints, they are not specific to diabetes mellitus, as they occur in any debilitating disease. Impotence is not infrequent in males.

To reiterate, not all adult patients have symptoms when they are found on medical examination to have diabetes mellitus. The chemical changes that are pathognomonic of the disease are hyperglycemia and glycosuria. With glycosuria, osmotic diuresis occurs and the patient becomes aware of voiding frequently in large amounts. Polyuria is followed by polydipsia and polyphagia. In women pruritus of the vulva is also associated with glycosuria. When the hyperglycemia is insufficient to compensate for the inefficient glucose metabolism, fat and protein catabolism are increased, which leads to an increase in the ketone bodies in the blood serum and urine. Despite increased appetite, loss of weight and strength occurs. Unless the diabetic condition is corrected, the individual with severe diabetes will go on to hypovolemia and possibly to heart failure and death.

Complications and Concomitants

Most of the complications resulting from diabetes mellitus were present in one or more of our six patients. They include hypoglycemia and acidosis, both of which require prompt and intensive treatment, and many of the disorders associated with long-standing diabetes mellitus. These include nephrosclerosis, diabetic retinopathy, cataracts, atherosclerosis, and peripheral polyneuropathies. None of our patients had tuberculosis, which occurs more frequently among diabetics than among nondiabetics.

The second complication of diabetes mellitus that is in the nature of an emergency is acidosis or ketoacidosis. Dr. Edward Rynearson, in his lectures to student nurses, emphasizes this point by saying that the patient in diabetic acidosis is to the physician what acute perforation of a viscus is to the surgeon. The point he is emphasizing is that the patient requires prompt and energetic treatment, if he is to survive. Joslin [34] states that the first few hours after therapy is started are most important to the recovery of the patient.

Before insulin became available, acidosis accounted for about two thirds of the deaths among young diabetics. Since the introduction of insulin, acidosis is generally less frequent and the prognosis of the patient is good, provided the patient is promptly and adequately treated. Acidosis is seen most commonly in the young at the onset of diabetes mellitus and among those who cannot or do not keep their diabetes under control.

Our teenager, Bonnie, presented a typical picture of the onset and course of acidosis. She was found to have diabetes mellitus at the age of four and has been admitted for the treatment of acidosis on numerous occasions. On one occasion she was comatose; that is, she could not be aroused. Details of each period of acidosis differed somewhat, but her present attack is reasonably representative. The day before she was admitted to the hospital she vomited throughout the day. During the night she developed abdominal cramps and her lips were dry and parched. When her mother brought her to the hospital, she walked into the emergency room but required a great deal of assistance from her mother. She was described by the admitting physician as lethargic. She had Kussmaul respirations; her skin and tongue were dry and her eyeballs were slightly soft, indicating marked tissue dehydration.

Constituents in her urine and blood were

[34] *Op. cit.*, pp. 371–72.

compatible with acidosis. Her blood sugar was elevated to 312 mg per 100 ml of blood serum. Serum acetone was present at a dilution of 1:20 but not at 1:40 and was indicative of a severe degree of acidosis. Carbon dioxide content was 15.2 mEq per liter. It was 20.8 mEq per liter when the test was repeated four hours after treatment was initiated. Three tests revealed increased concentration of her blood as a result of hypovolemia. Her leukocyte count was elevated to 19,500, her hemoglobin was 17.6 g per 100 ml of blood, and her hematocrit was 53 volumes per cent. Electrolytes, sodium, potassium, and chlorides were within normal limits. Normal values may, however, have been the result of loss of water from her blood. Had the normal volume of water in the blood been present, the levels of the electrolytes would probably have been depressed. At the time of admission Bonnie's urine was 4 + for both glucose and acetone.

The clinical picture presented by Bonnie is fairly typical of patients in acidosis. The effects were caused by the acidosis and the accompanying dehydration. The degree of hyperglycemia she experienced was not as great as sometimes occurs. Although not common, blood glucose levels of as high as 2,000 mg per 100 ml of blood have been observed. Moreover, acidosis does not always accompany a moderate elevation of the blood sugar. Despite a blood glucose of 276 mg and poor control of her diabetes, Mrs. Keen has presented no evidence of acidosis.

Bonnie lost water by three avenues: hyperventilation, vomiting, and in the urine. Within limits the kidney can compensate for the loss of water by other routes by concentrating urine.

Two factors prevented Bonnie's kidney from conserving water. Her renal threshold for sugar was exceeded, so that water was excreted passively due to increased osmolality of the glomerular filtrate. Second, the kidney plays an important role in the maintenance of acid-base balance by conserving or eliminating excess anions or cations. Elimination of either anions or cations requires water. In acidosis, cations are required to excrete the anions of the ketoacids. The mechanisms by which the kidney conserves cations, other than the hydrogen ions, also fail. (See Chapter 9.) Acidosis, therefore, contributes to the depletion of water and electrolytes. With the loss of water the hematocrit increases and the blood volume decreases. These changes, if severe and continued, predispose to failure of the cardiovascular system.

To accommodate the increase in anions of the ketoacids, the concentration of bicarbonate anions is lowered by hyperventilation (Kussmaul breathing; see Chapter 9), and sodium cations are made available to maintain electroneutrality. One result is a reduction in the carbon dioxide content as well as in the carbon dioxide–combining power of the blood plasma. The latter is the result of the sodium ion being unavailable to combine with the bicarbonate ion. On admission the carbon dioxide content of Bonnie's blood had been lowered to 15.2 mEq per liter. The normal range is from 21 to 30 mEq per liter.

Although the skin of the patient in acidosis is often florid, Bonnie was pale. She was less alert than usual, but she was not stuporous. Drowsiness followed by stupor, coma, and death can be expected unless the acidosis is corrected.[35] Some patients in acidosis are restless and thrash about and moan in bed. Until the patient is fully recovered, he should not be held responsible for his own safety. Side bars should be raised or placed on the bed. When the patient is excessively restless, they may need to be padded to protect him from injury. In some hospitals a nurse or physician remains with the patient until he is well on his way to recovery. It is essential that the patient be under intelligent and continuous observation.

Eventually, if the acidosis continues, the cardiovascular system fails. The pulse becomes weak and thready, and the blood pressure falls; anuria develops, and the patient dies. When adequate therapy is instituted early enough, recovery is the rule.

When Bonnie was admitted to the hospital, the immediate problem in her care was to correct the acidosis and its effects. The therapeutic and nursing plan that was initiated had three objectives: (1) to restore normal carbohydrate metabolism; (2) to replace water, minerals, and other substances lost in the urine and vomitus; and (3) to protect Bonnie from injury. All these objectives were carried out more or less simultaneously.

To restore the normal rate of carbohydrate metabolism, Bonnie was given insulin. Patients whose diabetes is long-standing are frequently resistant to insulin, and they are likely to require more insulin when they develop acidosis than do newly discovered diabetics. The longer the acidosis is allowed to persist, the more resistant the patient is likely to be to insulin. Some patients may require 1,000 or more units before there is a drop in the level of glucose in their blood, but Bonnie did not require such a large amount. In the first four hours after she was

---

[35] Drowsiness is defined as a pathological state of sleepiness. Stupor is a state of unconsciousness from which the individual can be aroused. He lapses back into unconsciousness after stimulation ceases. In coma, the patient cannot be aroused. All are different degrees of depression of mental alertness.

admitted to the hospital, she received 330 units of insulin. To ensure a prompt effect, regular insulin was placed in the intravenous fluids as well as injected subcutaneously. Only regular or crystalline insulin is administered in intravenous fluids. Later isophane (N.P.H.), a long-acting insulin, was also prescribed for Bonnie. During the first 24 hours the total amount administered was 400 units. A fall in the level of glucose and the disappearance of ketone bodies from Bonnie's blood and urine indicated that glucose metabolism was sufficient to suppress the excess catabolism of fat. Particularly in patients who are treated aggressively, glucose may be administered by intravenous infusion to prevent or treat iatrogenically induced hypoglycemia. As soon as patients retain fluids taken by mouth, fluids containing glucose, such as orange juice, are often prescribed by the physician.

Simultaneously with the measures instituted to restore carbohydrate metabolism, Bonnie was given intravenous fluids to correct the water and electrolyte deficits. Solutions are usually selected on the basis of the extent of electrolyte deficits and the availability of laboratory facilities to check the level of the electrolytes in the blood plasma. Bonnie received 500 ml of Ringer's lactate solution, 1,000 ml of physiological saline with 5 per cent bicarbonate of soda, and 4,000 ml of physiological saline by intravenous infusion. In addition, she ingested about 2,200 ml of fluids by mouth. Oral fluids consisted of 600 ml of beef broth, 600 ml of orange juice, and approximately 1,000 ml of water. Her total fluid intake was therefore 9,900 ml. Her urine output during the first 24 hours following hospitalization was 1,850 ml. Her relatively small output of urine in relation to the intake of fluid provides a measure of water depletion. Although the 9,900 ml of fluid may appear large, it is probably the average amount required by patients in diabetic acidosis. Patients treated aggressively sometimes receive as much as 10,000 ml over a period of a few hours.

Bonnie was placed on bed rest as soon as she was admitted. Patients with diabetes are usually advised to go to bed immediately when they are unwell. Reduction in activity reduces metabolism and should thereby decrease the catabolism of fat and protein.

To reduce the fluid lost by vomiting and to prevent gastric dilatation, fluids were withheld for two hours after Bonnie was admitted. Gastric lavage, which is frequently performed at the time of the admission of the patient to the hospital, was not performed. Gastric aspiration with or without lavage removes fluids accumulated in the stomach and relieves gastric dilatation. It may shorten the length of time the patient is unable to retain fluids. Usually, fluids

are withheld for one hour after the completion of the gastric aspiration. After fluids were started and until Bonnie received her usual diet, she was given 100 ml each of broth and orange juice. Broth is a good source of sodium and potassium salts as well as of water and is usually well tolerated when served hot. Orange juice is also a good source of potassium as well as of glucose and water. Other fluids, such as ginger ale, serve the same purposes.

The therapeutic plan for Bonnie is similar to that utilized in the medical treatment of most patients in acidosis. Because every patient is an individual, the details of the treatment required by each patient will differ. Physicians differ in their beliefs about how patients should be treated and this will be a modifying factor. Knowledge changes as a result of observation, study, and research. Practices vary because the assumptions on which practice is based vary.

Although all persons who care for the patient have a responsibility for the safety of the patient, perhaps much of the burden for his protection falls on the nurse. During the period when the patient is less than normally responsive, he must be protected from falling and from the effects of pressure. As stated earlier, side rails should be raised or placed on the bed. Bed covering over the lower extremities should be elevated with a cradle. Should the patient be in shock, care should be taken to prevent injury by burning or pressure. If hot-water bottles are used, the temperature should not be greater than 105°F, and the bottle should not rest against the patient. Insofar as possible, patients should be moved and turned regularly unless they are so restless that this is unnecessary. When the patient is restless precautions must be taken to prevent falling or injury from unprotected side rails. He should, of course, also be protected from overheating and chilling. Extra heat should not be applied to patients in a state of shock, as heat increases vasodilatation and intensifies the failure of the circulation. Albeit all patients should be protected from sources of infection, in no patient is this more important.

Nursing Responsibilities and Care of the Patient with Diabetes Mellitus

As emphasized earlier, the response of the patient to therapy and often whether or not he recovers depend on the promptness with which therapy is initiated. Depending on the situation, the nurse may be called on to prepare, administer, and supervise the therapeutic regime prescribed by the physician. In addition, the nurse is responsible for observing the patient and his reaction to therapy. She may be required to modify the therapy in relation to its effects on the patient and report to the physician only when the patient fails to respond in the desired manner to the prescribed therapeutic regime.

As stated earlier, the medical therapy of the patient, including Bonnie, consists of insulin and fluids. The nurse is responsible for administering these promptly and accurately. The nurse usually collects the urine and sometimes tests it for glucose and acetone. Because insulin dosage is usually in relation to the quantity of glucose and acetone in the urine, accurate and regular testing is important. The length of the interval at which testing is performed varies from one-half to two hours. When voided specimens are used, all urine may be checked. In some clinics the collection of urine specimens is facilitated by the introduction of an indwelling catheter. In others this is not done because of the increased possibility of infection of the urinary tract.[36] When urine is used as an index of the level of glucose in the blood at a specific time, a freshly voided specimen must be obtained for testing. The blood may also be tested in place of or to supplement urine testing.

Patients receiving insulin without adequate amounts of glucose may continue to have ketone bodies in their urine in the absence of glycosuria. One patient stands out in the memory of the author. She was a young woman who had an appendectomy in the morning. Because she was a known diabetic, she was given insulin. During the first night after surgery she was found to have ketone bodies but no glucose in her urine. She also had Kussmaul respirations. Her physician was called, and both glucose and insulin were administered. Evidence of developing acidosis was rapidly corrected.

Patients being treated for acidosis may also become hypoglycemic. Although hypoglycemia does not usually occur suddenly, it may. Bonnie developed a mild hypoglycemic reaction after she had been under treatment for acidosis for about six hours.

Any patient who receives a large volume of fluid by intravenous infusion should be carefully observed. Patients may be anuric at the time of admission or may develop anuria later. The reasons for the occurrence of anuria have been presented. Observation of the urine output, including quantity and frequency of voiding, is highly important. As hypovolemia is corrected, urine output should increase. In general, the capacity of the patient to tolerate a large volume of fluid depends on the severity of his hypovolemia, his general health status, and adequacy of his cardiovascular and renal systems.

[36] Diabetics are predisposed to urinary tract infection.

Any patient receiving a large volume of fluid should have the rate of infusion and its general effects closely observed. Depending on the circumstances and available facilities his central venous pressure may be monitored.

Because the recovery of the patient depends on the restoration of homeostasis, the related factors have been emphasized. Although physiological homeostasis is given priority, this does not mean that the patient as a human being should be neglected. Care should be taken to avoid making unwarranted statements in the presence of the patient or talking about other patients in his presence. Conversation should include the patient but should not make unnecessary demands on him. He should be informed about the care he is receiving and the progress he is making. Attention should be paid to his physical comfort. Until the survival of the patient is assured, attention is, however, directed toward three principal objectives: to restore normal carbohydrate metabolism as promptly as possible, to replace the water and electrolyte balance, and to protect the patient from injury. If the recovery of the patient is to be ensured, time is of the essence. Consequently, when a patient is admitted, therapy should be started promptly.

By the evening of the day Bonnie was admitted to the hospital, her hypovolemia had been corrected. Although several days elapsed before her blood glucose became relatively stable, ketonemia had been largely corrected. She was able to eat the food prescribed for her. About 7 o'clock in the evening following her admission, she passed 425 ml of urine and was more alert than she had been. From thence forward, she made rapid progress. A week later she was dismissed from the hospital.

Prevention of Acidosis

Another question that may be raised is why did Bonnie and her parents allow her to become seriously ill before medical attention was sought? Some of the answers sound easy, but in actual practice they may not be. Acidosis ought to be prevented by continuous and conscientious control of diabetes mellitus. All patients, particularly those who have a tendency to ketosis, should go to bed and call a physician at the first indication of an infection. Bonnie has never been a very well-controlled diabetic. Whether the instability of her diabetes is caused by neglect or by an exceptionally severe form of the disease or both is not known. Her mother is a nurse. She assures the physician that his instructions are carefully followed, and they may well be. Treatment was not sought until Bonnie was seriously ill. Why not? Were Bonnie and her family ashamed of their failure, or did they not recognize what was happening? Had other members of the family had a similar illness and recovered promptly? Perhaps neither Bonnie nor her parents really understood the nature of diabetes mellitus. Patients and the members of their families may appear to be more knowledgeable than they really are. Because the answers to the questions about why Bonnie develops acidosis frequently are not known, only guesses can be made about them.

Recently a youngster whose medical history parallels that of Bonnie came to the attention of the author. The child, Bobby, was in and out of the hospital at frequent intervals. On a recent admission to the hospital the nurse who cared for him decided to investigate the reasons for his repeated attacks of acidosis. In this instance, the nurse learned that neither Bobby nor his parents had any real understanding of the nature of diabetes mellitus or why certain procedures were important. The nurse made a detailed teaching plan, checked it with the physician to be sure that what she was planning to present to the patient was not in conflict with his instructions, and proceeded to instruct the patient and family. The mother was delighted. Best of all, six months later Bobby was well and active; he had not missed a day of school nor had he been unwell. This had never happened before. Not all problems in the control of diabetes mellitus are as easily solved as were Bobby's. From his previous history, however, Bobby probably would have continued to be in and out of the hospital if a nurse had not tried to identify the reason for his failure to remain well and initiated an appropriate teaching plan.

In the instance of Bonnie, the answer is not known. Multiple factors including a lack of knowledge, physical and emotional problems of adolescence, and relationship problems with parents, peers, teachers, and others may be involved, as well as the fact that the disease is difficult to control.

Vascular Concomitants

Several abnormalities occur with such great frequency in diabetes mellitus that some authorities refer to them as concomitants of the disease, that is, they are a part of the disease. Although vascular disorders such as atherosclerosis and arteriosclerosis as well as other types of vascular disease occur, the type believed to be characteristic of diabetes is capillary basement membrane thickening.[37] This disorder is

[37] Thomas C. Skillman: "Peripheral Vascular Disease" in *Diabetes Mellitus: Diagnosis and Treatment,* Vol. II, George J. Hamwi and T. S. Danowski, eds. (New York: American Diabetes Association, Inc., 1967), pp. 171–72.

not a complication but a part of the disease. Some go so far as to say small vessel disease initiates diabetes mellitus. The relationship of insulin to vascular disorders is not known. There does not appear to be a relationship between the degree to which diabetes is controlled and the development and progress of small vessel disease.[38]

SMALL VESSEL DISEASE

Retinopathy, nephropathy, and possibly the neuropathy occurring in diabetes are associated with a thickening of the capillary basement membrane. Although these disorders may have their beginning very early in the life of the individual, clinical evidence of their presence becomes increasingly evident with increasing duration of the disease. Despite exceptions most patients who have had diabetes for 20 years or more have evidence of retinopathy and renal disease. Renal disease is now the cause of death in about one half of the young diabetics.

LARGE VESSEL DISEASE

Atherosclerosis occurs in the diabetic at an earlier age than it does in the nondiabetic. The hyperlipemia and hypercholesterolemia that accompany diabetes may be predisposing factors. Among the organs particularly prone to atherosclerosis are those supplying the brain, heart, lower extremities, and kidneys. Recent studies implicate diabetes mellitus as a factor in early coronary artery disease.

With the increase in the life expectancy of patients with diabetes mellitus, chronic disorders involving the vascular and nervous systems and the kidney have become increasingly important. Reference to the patients presented in Table 19-1 shows that four of the six patients have vascular complications; one of the four has a renal disorder as well. Studies indicate that a high percentage of persons who develop diabetes in childhood and live into adult life develop vascular concomitants.

Vascular concomitants also are frequent among persons who are middle-aged or older at the time of onset. They occur earlier and to a more severe degree in diabetics than in nondiabetics. They are more rapidly progressive in young persons who have long-standing diabetes that has been inadequately treated. More than 50 per cent of the deaths in patients who have had diabetes for more than 15 years are caused by vascular lesions. All types of arteriosclerosis occur alone or in combination. The arteries most commonly involved are those supplying the lower extremities, the heart muscle (coro-

[38] *Ibid.,* p. 172.

nary arteries), the brain, the eye, and the kidney.

Vascular disorders are important because they have a high incidence among persons with diabetes. After they are established, they tend to be progressive. They differ from acute complications as they do not cause the diabetes to become more severe. Authorities do not agree about the value of maintaining the level of blood glucose within physiological limits in preventing vascular lesions. Some authorities are questioning whether the present criteria for diabetic control are adequate. The suggestion has been made that periods of *mild* hypoglycemia might be of benefit to the patient.

Complications involving the kidney are very common among persons with long-standing diabetes mellitus. Renal complications include those resulting from nephrosclerosis, intercapillary glomerulosclerosis, and pyelonephritis. All these conditions can and do occur in nondiabetics. They are, however, likely to be more severe and more rapidly progressive in diabetics than in nondiabetics. When they are progressive, they lead to a loss of renal function and with it to azotemia (the accumulation of the waste of protein metabolism in the blood).

Of the renal disorders the one that is most common in diabetes mellitus is pyelonephritis, but the one that is the most characteristic is intercapillary glomerulosclerosis or Kimmelsteil-Wilson's disease. This disorder is frequent and its incidence is rising. Although its diagnosis requires renal biopsy, it is presumed to be present when edema, hypertension, azotemia, and proteinuria are present. In the diabetic other pathology frequently associated with intercapillary sclerosis is diabetic retinopathy and anemia. Although intercapillary sclerosis may remain stable for long periods of time, after severe edema and albuminuria occur the life expectancy of the patient can be measured only in months. The reader may remember that Mr. Benedict has edema and hypertension. Although he is not aware of the seriousness of his condition, his prognosis is guarded. He has had diabetes for 21 years.

Complications arising from the effects of diabetes on the various structures of the eyes are frequent. Arteriosclerosis of the retinal arteries, as well as hemorrhages and exudates into the retina, lead to loss of vision. In three of our patients retinopathy is present. A fourth patient has cataracts. Although the type of cataract occurring most frequently in diabetic patients does not differ from the ordinary senile cataract, they do occur somewhat more frequently among diabetic patients than among nondiabetics. The problems of the patient are those of any individual who is losing or loses his

vision. About 18 per cent of blindness is associated with diabetes mellitus.

Not much is known about the pathological changes responsible for the neurological complications. Neuropathies occur in the peripheral nerves as well as elsewhere in the nervous system. When the spinal cord is involved, the changes in the posterior and lateral columns are identical with those found in pernicious anemia. Patients with peripheral neuritis often suffer numbness, tingling, and pain that is sometimes very severe.

Among the complications involving the skin are furuncles (boils) and carbuncles (multiple boils adjacent to each other). In health, the skin serves as a storehouse for glycogen. In uncontrolled diabetes, the glycogen in the skin is depleted and the glucose content of the skin rises with the hyperglycemia. When diabetes is poorly controlled, the skin is predisposed to infections by the *Staphylococcus aureus*. There is also evidence that function of the polymorphonuclear leukocytes is impaired. Two requirements, that is, control of diabetes and cleanliness of the skin and clothing, are important to the prevention of skin complications.

Vascular, renal, and neurological manifestations usually develop over an extended period of time. Their increasing incidence is related to the fact that diabetics as well as nondiabetics have an improved life expectancy. All these disorders occur earlier and are more rapidly progressive in the diabetic than in the nondiabetic.

Control of Diabetes Mellitus

As stressed earlier, successful control of diabetes mellitus depends on the intelligent cooperation of the patient and his family. Unlike recovery from an acute infectious disease, recovery does not follow a period of acute illness. Diabetes mellitus is permanent. Remissions can and do occur when the disease is discovered early and treated aggressively, but even these patients should not think of themselves as cured. As stated earlier, relapse usually occurs within a few months.

The days and weeks that immediately follow the diagnosis of diabetes mellitus are important in the life of of the patient. During this time he learns what it means to be diabetic and how he can control his disease. The general objectives of his medical therapy include (1) to individualize his regime so that he can live as full and useful a life as is possible within the limitations of his disorder, (2) to correct the underlying metabolic abnormalities in order to restore homeostasis, (3) to attain and maintain ideal body weight, (4) to delay the progression of vascular disorders, and (5) to prevent complications of the disease.

The fundamental methods used in the treatment are insulin or hypoglycemic agents, diet, exercise, and education. In the prevention of complications good hygiene is also important. The continued management and control of diabetes mellitus depends on the patient. Education as to the nature and behavior of his disease is required so that he understands the reasons for what he must do and develops the skills required for it.

Psychological Aspects and Reactions

At the time the patient learns that diabetes is incurable, he should learn that it is controllable. Whether or not it is kept under control depends to a large extent on himself and his family. In the past, physicians have tended to assume the primary responsibility for the regulation of diabetes. The trend is toward placing the responsibility for control on the patient and his family. Doctors and nurses are available and willing to help him assume this responsibility, however. Furthermore, the measures that are required are for his well-being. The patient learns to control his disease because this is the way to good health. He does not take insulin or other medication and regulate his food intake to please the doctor or the nurse or someone else but to promote health. The control of diabetes mellitus is a way of life, but it should not be all of life.

When a person learns that he has diabetes mellitus, even when he has suspected its presence, he experiences disbelief and then grief. The degree of shock will depend on the individual and what the diagnosis and treatment mean to him. Any pre-existing problem can be expected to be intensified. The patient and his family can be expected to react to knowledge of the diagnosis as they do to other crisis situations in life. Authorities frequently emphasize the advantages of diabetes over other chronic disorders. In time the patient may come to a similar conclusion, but at the time the diagnosis is established he is thinking of what he has lost and not of other more serious possibilities. He compares diabetes with health and he prefers health. The nurse can usually be of more help to the patient if she can help him to identify and express his feelings rather than telling him how lucky he is.

When diabetes is diagnosed in a young child, the parents are the ones who experience the negative feelings. Their child is less than perfect. If the disease is to be controlled, the child must have special care and attention. Questions arise. Will other children in the family develop the disease? Is the fact that the child is ill the result of something the parent did or did not do? Of our six patients, Bonnie, at age 4, probably had few, if any, preconceived ideas about diabetes mellitus. Try, however, to imagine the feelings of an 8-year-old boy or a 13-year-old girl who learns that he or she has diabetes. Are they likely to be consoled by the fact that they do not have leukemia?

In addition to the fact of diabetes itself, negative emotions are usually engendered by the measures required in treatment. Although children of five or younger learn to inject their own insulin, older adults find this procedure particularly frightening. Men and women who are employed may be concerned about whether they will be able to continue in their current jobs. Those who are not yet gainfully employed face the possibility that diabetes will limit their choice of vocation as well as their chances of getting and holding a position. Will others know and if they do will the diabetic be accepted? Will he be able to do what his friends do? Will he be able to marry and to have children? Boys who have dreamed of being athletes find their ambitions threatened. Restrictions real and imagined are likely to appear to be insurmountable to the patient and to his family as well.

A danger common to any patient with a disease requiring long-term therapy is that when the person feels well he decides that he is cured and discontinues his regime. Or when he finally realizes that he is not going to get well in the usual interpretation of the term, he may decide to try some quick cure such as a special food or a cure-all. He may also deny that he has diabetes or that anything can be done to change its course. Deviations from the prescribed regime will result in a loss of, at best, the control of his diabetes mellitus and, at worst, his life.

Although much has been accomplished to reduce the cost of insulin, diet, and medical supervision, diabetes mellitus does place an economic burden on families whose incomes are limited. For this reason, patients with diabetes mellitus may be declared medically indigent at a higher level of income than nondiabetics. Enough problems have been raised to suggest that the psychosocial problems arising in relation to a diagnosis of diabetes mellitus are many and highly individualized.

During the period immediately following diagnosis the patient and his family require psychological support. This should start with the patient's admission to the office of the physician, to the clinic, or to the hospital. The type and amount of support will vary with each individual. Both the patient and his family have a right to expect that professional personnel try to understand their feelings and to accept their behavior as having meaning. An important objective in the care of the patient should be to provide a climate in which he feels accepted so that he will feel free to express his feelings and be supported in his attempts to accept his diagnosis and what it entails. The nurse should try to convey to the patient that, while she understands or is trying to understand his feelings, he will be able to learn to do what he must do and will be provided with the necessary assistance.

A second period of stress for the patient occurs when he becomes aware of the fact that he is developing one or more of the chronic manifestations of diabetes. Again he and his family require support while they adjust to the situation. As an example, when Mr. Benedict learned of his kidney disorder, both he and his wife had to adjust not only to a "new disorder" but to the possibility that Mr. Benedict could expect to live only a few months. Not only did he have a wife, but he had two young dependent children. How would this young family manage all the financial and social problems accompanying his illness and following his death?

Accomplishment of Objectives

The objectives of the therapy of diabetes are achieved by diet, insulin, other hypoglycemic agents, exercise, and education. Physicians differ about the degree to which chemical control is necessary. Some advocate strict chemical control so that glycosuria is prevented and the level of glucose in the blood is maintained at normal or nearly normal levels. Both hypo- and hyperglycemia are to be avoided. Those who support strict chemical control state that it reduces the severity of diabetes and lessens the likelihood of degenerative changes developing and that when they develop their rate of progress is slowed. A further argument is that insulin requirements are less when blood glucose is maintained at normal or near-normal levels. For example, at the time Mrs. Keen was admitted, she was taking 35 units of isophane insulin and 24 units of regular insulin each day. At the time she was discharged, she was taking 10 units of Lente insulin daily. For a person on a limited budget, as Mrs. Keen was, the reduction in insulin dosage reduced the cost of treatment, a not unimportant consideration.

Those who disagree with the strict chemical control approach say that this method neglects the individuality of the patient, because the therapy is directed against the disease rather than toward the person. Some physicians believe that hyperglycemia and glycosuria can be disregarded as long as ketosis is avoided and normal weight and strength are maintained. For example, they would not be concerned because Mrs. Keen's blood glucose was elevated most of the time or because she had marked glycosuria more or less continuously. She would be given enough insulin to keep her feeling well and to keep her urine free of ketone bodies. Some physicians who support this approach place few restrictions on the diet. Others encourage the patient to restrict his intake of concentrated carbohydrates, especially those lacking other nutrients. Physicians who favor clinical control believe that the incidence of degenerative disorders is not high enough to warrant the restrictions required to achieve chemical control. Moreover, they say that the patient feels better.

Many physicians and, if the truth were known, patients adopt a regime between the two. The physician tries to prescribe a diet that is acceptable to the patient and takes into account the severity of his disease. Some patients prefer a strict regime, whereas others do better when the approach is more flexible. Since insulin has become available, a nutritious and satisfying diet can usually be achieved.

DIET

Root and Bailey [39] state that diet planned for long-continued use should meet the following criteria:

1. Its caloric content should be sufficient to meet the patient's needs as determined by his age, sex, activity, and growth requirements. For example, because Bonnie is still growing and is presumably more active, she requires a higher caloric intake per unit of body surface than Mrs. Curry. Because Mr. Benedict is a man, he utilizes more calories than women do.

2. The distribution of calories and the proportions of carbohydrate, protein, and fat should remain about the same from day to day. The specific foods eaten may vary greatly. Some authorities make this point by saying that the proportions of the various nutrients as well as the meal schedule should be inflexible. Great flexibility can, however, be exercised in the selection of specific foods.

3. Most diabetic diets contain less carbohydrate than the normal diet. The quantity of protein and fat is usually a little higher. The reduction in carbohydrate is accompanied by the

---

[39] Howard F. Root and C. Cabell Bailey: "Diet in the Treatment of Diabetes Mellitus," *Modern Nutrition in Health and Disease,* 4th ed., Michael G. Wohl and Robert S. Goodhart, eds. (Philadelphia: Lea & Febiger, 1968), p. 786.

elimination of concentrated sweets and pastries.

4. The calories should be planned to support the ideal rather than the actual weight. The obese patient can be expected to lose weight. The underweight person should gain weight.
5. The diet should be planned so that it provides for an adequate intake of all nutrients, including minerals and vitamins.

The physician makes the decision as to the content and distribution of carbohydrates, proteins, and fat in the diet of the patient. The nurse and the dietitian translate the prescription into terms of food and methods of food preparation. In the hospital, the dietitian often is responsible for the formal dietary instruction. In small hospitals and in public health agencies nurses must often assume the responsibility for the basic instruction of the patient. In some public health agencies dietary consultants are available to give guidance and other help to the nurse. Unless the patient receives detailed instruction and the diet is planned to take into account his usual food pattern, he is quite likely to disregard his diet prescription or to unnecessarily restrict his food intake.

Some points to be kept in mind when planning with the patient have already been included and will not be further reviewed. In the achievement of the objective to plan the diet in terms of the individual pattern of living of the patient, the nurse, wherever she is employed, is in a particularly advantageous position to be helpful. The nurse should obtain information about the economic status of the patient, what foods are available to him as well as their cost, his religion, national origin, social status, occupation, idiosyncrasies, misconceptions and beliefs about food, facilities for preparing food, and where and with whom he eats. Unless the family diet is inadequate, the family food pattern is used as a base. One of the objectives is to disrupt the family as little as possible. The diet of the patient is kept as nearly like the rest of the family's as possible. The visiting nurse can often be of great service to the person who prepares the meals for the person with diabetes. For the most part special foods are not required. Water-packed canned fruits and vegetables are now available at most grocery stores. They can be substituted for fresh fruits and vegetables when these are not available or are expensive.

The patient and the person who prepares his meals should learn to identify the carbohydrate, protein, and fat content of foods. They should know why the carbohydrate content is restricted. When a patient is in ketosis, the carbohydrate content may be restricted to 100 g per day, as was done when Bonnie was first admitted. At the time she was dismissed, her diet prescription included 150 g of carbohydrate, which is well within the usual range.

Whether patients are taught to weigh, measure, or approximate the size of servings depends on the views of the physician. Patients with compulsive personalities may be more comfortable when they weigh their food, whereas others may reject the idea entirely. The patient and the person who prepares his food should be well acquainted with food exchange lists and know how to use them.

INSULIN

In many patients, diabetes mellitus cannot be controlled by dietary measures alone. In only two of our six patients was this possible. In young persons and those with moderate or severe diabetes insulin is required. Two general types of insulin, unmodified and modified, are available. Unmodified insulin, commonly known as regular insulin, was the first type to be available. It is promptly absorbed after subcutaneous injection and its effect is begun within one-half hour after it is injected. It reaches its maximum effect in from two to three hours. Because it may be injected intravenously as well as subcutaneously and it acts quickly, it is used in the treatment of diabetic acidosis. It is also used to supplement the effect of the types of insulin with prolonged actions.

Modified insulins differ from regular insulin in that something is added to make the insulin relatively insoluble and thereby delay the rate at which it is absorbed with the result that the period over which the insulin acts is prolonged. Classified according to the length of the period over which they act, modified insulins are of two types: long-acting and intermediate-acting. Protamine zinc insulin, the first of the modified insulins to be developed, has a prolonged action. It was developed by Hagedorn of Denmark, who added a basic protein, protamine—a substance obtained from the sperm of a certain fish—to insulin. Protamine precipitates with insulin and delays the rate at which it is absorbed as the protamine must be broken down before the insulin is released. Because of its prolonged action, hyperglycemia in patients requiring more than 40 units of insulin is difficult to control with protamine zinc insulin. Although the period of maximum action is from 12 to 24 hours, action may continue for from 48 to 72 hours. There is, therefore, an overlapping of dosages, making it difficult to secure a uniform depression of the blood glucose. Hypoglycemic reactions are frequent.

A more nearly physiological effect can be

achieved by administering part of the insulin dosage as unmodified and part as protamine zinc insulin, either as two separate injections or by mixing the two and giving one injection. The success of this method depends on the ability of the patient to assume responsibility for measuring and mixing the two types of insulin. A commercially prepared mixture of protamine zinc insulin and regular insulin is available.

Following the introduction of protamine zinc insulin, other modifications were introduced that more nearly meet all the following criteria. They require only one injection, have a sufficiently rapid onset of action, and are absorbed over an appropriate period of time. The three most successful preparations are isophane or N.P.H. insulin, globin zinc insulin, and Lente insulin. Isophane insulin is a modified protamine zinc insulin. It behaves essentially like a mixture of two parts regular to one part protamine insulin. As the two types are mixed, the problems in administration are simplified. The essential difference between globin and isophane insulin is that globin rather than protamine is used to prolong the period of absorption.

The Lente insulins are the newest preparations. They differ from other slow-acting insulins in that they do not contain a foreign protein. They are made by precipitating insulin with zinc and then resuspending it in an acetate buffer solution. By altering the conditions under which the preparations are made, particles of different sizes can be made. Ultra Lente contains particles of large size and has the duration of action of over 30 hours; its duration of action is similar to that of protamine zinc insulin. Lente insulin contains particles of small size. Insulin is released more rapidly from small than from large particles, and duration of the action of Lente insulin is approximately 24 hours. Semilente insulin is composed of amorphous particles, and the duration of its action is from 12 to 18 hours. The two preparations of insulin in most common use today are isophane and Lente insulin. The types of insulin along with the time of onset and duration of action are summarized in Table 19-2.

The objective of insulin therapy is to enable the individual to utilize sufficient food to meet his nutritional needs and, within limits, his desire for food. For many patients this objective can be achieved by a single injection of protamine zinc insulin or one of the intermediate-acting insulins, either alone or in combination with crystalline insulin. The ideal preparation of insulin would be one in which the insulin is released in response to hyperglycemia. At this time there is no such preparation. A reasonably good approximation can, however, be achieved

TABLE 19-2

Time of Action of Various Insulin Preparations

Type of Insulin	Time of Onset, Hours	Duration of Action
Insulin injection, U.S.P.	½	6
Crystalline zinc insulin	1	8
Globin zinc insulin	2–4	10–24
Isophane insulin injection (N.P.H.)	2	20–30
Protamine zinc injection	6–8	24–36
Lente insulin (insulin zinc suspension)	4–5	20–24

in many patients. This is done by planning the distribution of carbohydrate in the diet of the patient and his pattern of exercise in relation to the duration of action of the type of insulin used. Because individuals differ from each other and the same individual differs from time to time, the details of the therapeutic plan will be different for each person. Persons who require less than 40 units of insulin per day often do very well on a single injection of protamine zinc insulin. Miss Arthur had been able to control her diabetes with 35 units of protamine zinc injected each morning. Those who require more than 40 units of protamine zinc insulin to control their diabetes usually respond better to one of the intermediate insulins either singly or in combination with crystalline insulin. There are some persons whose diabetes is brittle, that is, it is very difficult to control. They have rapid shifts in the level of glucose in their blood, despite attention to the therapeutic regime.

HYPOGLYCEMIA

Although not all patients experience it, hypoglycemia is an ever-present possibility in the patient who takes insulin or one or more oral hypoglycemic agents. Situations that predispose to hypoglycemia, or, as it is commonly called, insulin reaction, include a delay in or omission of a meal, an increase in the amount of exercise taken, or an improvement in the patient's glucose tolerance. An error in the measurement of insulin, resulting in excess dosage, can also be responsible. The manifestations of hypoglycemia have been listed and discussed in Chapter 12. Hypoglycemia, particularly when severe or repeated, is generally regarded as a serious condition.

Because of the importance of hypoglycemia its manifestations will be reviewed here. Signs and symptoms associated with hypoglycemia are caused by its effect on the nervous system. According to Sussman et al.[40] hypoglycemia affects the nervous system in the following order: (1) parasympathetic nervous system, (2) cerebral effects, (3) sympathoadrenal system, and (4) hypoglycemic coma. Parasympathetic effects include hunger, nausea, and bradycardia. Cerebral effects include yawning, lethargy, lassitude, and the inability to carry out a conversation or to count. Although not mentioned by Sussman, some patients may be confused, disoriented, and aphasic. Some patients make inappropriate remarks or develop acute catatonic or manic states. Thus a patient who is receiving insulin should be suspected of developing hypoglycemia when he has a change in mood or personality.

The symptoms most likely to be noted by the patient are those caused by increased sympathoadrenal activity. They include nervousness or anxiety, sweating, and tachycardia. The patient may describe his state by saying that he feels funny or peculiar. Not all patients are aware of their hypoglycemic state and go directly into coma. The patient receiving any hypoglycemic agent may develop coma; those receiving long-acting insulin are most likely to be unaware of developing hypoglycemia.

A marked fall in the blood sugar may be accompanied by unconsciousness. Severe and repeated periods of hypoglycemia may cause permanent damage to the brain. Miss Arthur was unconscious at the time of her admission. She could not explain why she had developed hypoglycemia as she said that she had neither delayed eating nor taken more than her usual amount of exercise. The principal change in her life was that she had taken a new position a week previously. Emotional stress may be reflected in a change in the blood glucose, usually in the direction of an elevation. Possibly Miss Arthur experienced glucosuria and she increased her insulin dosage. She was embarrassed by her condition as she took pride in keeping her diabetes under control; she was also worried lest she lose her new position.

Bonnie had two mild attacks of hypoglycemia as her diabetes was brought under control. She felt nervous and perspired profusely. Both patients recovered promptly following the administration of glucose. Because Miss Arthur was unconscious, she was given 100 ml of 10 per cent glucose by intravenous infusion. Glucagon, 1 mg, given subcutaneously, intramuscularly, or intravenously promptly restores the blood glucose to normal levels. Patients who are unconscious should never be given fluids by mouth. Bonnie was given 2 tsp of corn syrup dissolved in half a glass of water. Suitable substitutes include 100 ml of orange juice or a lump or two of sugar. Patients should be instructed to treat the first indications of hypoglycemia without delay. When patients are hospitalized, they should be encouraged to report suspicious symptoms. There should be no delay in treatment. In some hospitals the method to be used in the treatment of hypoglycemia is included in the standing orders. In others individual physicians leave a prescription or ask to be called. Whatever the practice, there should be no unnecessary delay in instituting effective therapy. Furthermore, should the nurse be in a position where there is some doubt as to whether the patient is hypoglycemic or acidotic, and the physician is not readily available, she should treat the patient for hypoglycemia. Delay in its correction can result in harm to the patient. Five or ten grams of glucose will not affect the course of acidosis appreciably.

The patient who is taking regular insulin is always aware that he is hypoglycemic. He can, therefore, protect himself from a severe reaction. In contrast, the patient who is taking intermediate or long-acting insulin may not have warning and can pass directly into an unconscious state. Generally, intermediate and long-acting insulins lower the blood glucose more gradually than rapidly acting insulin. If he happens to be driving an automobile, or is in a position involving danger, the possible consequences to himself and others are obvious.

The prevention of hypoglycemia is preferable to its cure. Patients should be instructed to maintain an inflexible meal schedule insofar as possible. The distribution of carbohydrate through the day should take into account the time of maximum action of the type of insulin the patient is using. When a meal is delayed, 5 to 10 g of glucose should be taken. This glucose can be subtracted from the next meal. Exercise should be regular rather than sporadic, and when it is increased, the patient may take 5 to 10 g of glucose to prevent hypoglycemia. During a period in which a patient is recovering from an acute illness or his diabetes is being brought under control, as in the instance of Mrs. Keen and Bonnie, nurses should be alert to the possibility that the tolerance of the patient for glucose is likely to be improving and hypoglycemia may occur. Changes in the be-

[40] Karl E. Sussman et al.: "Failure of Warning in Insulin-induced Hypoglycemic Reactions," Diabetes, 12:39 (Jan.–Feb.) 1963.

havior of the patient should be interpreted in this light.

Although the urine may provide information about the level of glucose in the blood, the results may also be misleading. When urine accumulated in the bladder over a period of time is tested, it can contain glucose despite the presence of hypoglycemia at the time. For example, Mr. Rugge, a known diabetic, was admitted to the emergency room of City Hospital in an unconscious state. A catheterized specimen of urine was examined for glucose and produced a maximum color change: it was 4+ for glucose. He was transferred to an inpatient ward, where another sample of urine was obtained and tested for glucose. This time glucose was absent. Mr. Rugge was given 10 g of glucose by intravenous infusion. In a matter of seconds, consciousness returned, and in less time than it takes to tell, he was sitting up in bed demanding, "What happened? Why am I here? I'm hungry. Can't somebody get me something to eat?" Prompt and effective treatment of hypoglycemia quickly restores the individual to well-being. Untreated and severe, it may cause irreparable damage to the brain.

PREVENTION OF HYPOGLYCEMIA

Application of knowledge of the duration of the action of each of the various insulins enables the physician, nurse, or patient to predict when hyperglycemia and hypoglycemia are most likely to occur. The physician prescribes the distribution of carbohydrate in the diet of the patient in relation to the type of insulin used. To protect patients who are receiving protamine zinc insulin from nocturnal hypoglycemia, some of the carbohydrate from the evening meal is saved for a lunch at bedtime. Milk and crackers or toast and butter are satisfactory. Patients taking intermediate-acting insulin are frequently advised to save some of the carbohydrate from their lunch as a mid- or late-afternoon snack. By distribution of the intake of carbohydrate over the time when insulin absorption is at its height, the patient is protected from attacks of hypoglycemia. The importance of the mid-afternoon and prebedtime lunch should be emphasized to the patient. A hypoglycemic reaction may not be too serious when the person is in the protected environment of his home, but a sudden loss of consciousness when out in public can endanger his life. If he is driving a car, not only the person's life but the lives of others are in danger. Some physicians recommend that patients who are planning to drive a car in the later afternoon take 5 to 10 g of glucose before starting out. One-fourth to one-half glass of orange juice or a Life Saver or two contain enough glucose to protect the patient from hypoglycemia. As pointed out earlier, the patient requires less insulin when his diabetes is under control than when he is hyperglycemic. During periods when control is being established, he should, therefore, be observed for signs of hypoglycemia. He should also be asked to report any changes in the way he feels. The patient should learn the common manifestations of hypoglycemia.

Although hypoglycemic attacks may occur at any time, patients on isophane, globin, or Lente insulin are most likely to have them in the late afternoon. Bonnie had an attack of hypoglycemia about 4 o'clock on two successive afternoons. As a result, her physician prescribed that one slice of bread be saved from her lunch and eaten at 3:30 in the afternoon.

EXERCISE

Another factor that predisposes to hypoglycemia is exercise. Exercise is a valuable part of the therapeutic regime, because working muscle does not require insulin to utilize glucose. As a result, the patient with diabetes is encouraged to exercise regularly. The type, amount, and degree of activity should be about the same from day to day. Sudden increases, particularly in the patient who is taking insulin, are to be avoided. The beneficial effect of exercise sometimes creates problems for the patient who has been hospitalized. Hospital space and policy often make it difficult for the patient to duplicate the amount of exercise he takes outside the hospital. After his discharge, he may have a series of hypoglycemic attacks. To prevent this, some physicians encourage patients who are able to leave the hospital for an afternoon, or several afternoons, to try to duplicate their usual activity. When patients must for some reason exercise more than is usual, they should protect themselves by taking 5 to 10 g of glucose (1 to 2 lumps of sugar).

BUYING INSULIN

Because patients have to buy insulin they should know that there are different types but that they should not substitute one type or strength for another without discussing this with their physician. They should also learn that insulin dosage is expressed in units and that a unit has the same power to lower the blood sugar whatever the number per milliliter of solution or the type of insulin. A unit of insulin is determined by its blood sugar-lowering effect when it is injected into a rabbit. Preparations are concentrated so that 1 ml of solution contains 10, 20, 40, 80, or 100 units. Because of the differences in potency, care should be exercised in the identification of the number of units per milliliter. To lessen the chance of error, some hospitals require that two nurses check the label on the bottle against the order and the label against the quantity of insulin in the syringe. Textbooks used in courses of introduction to nursing cover the details of subcutaneous injections, so they will not be repeated here. The physician prescribes the type, dosage, and time insulin is to be administered to the patient as well as when to instruct and who is to be instructed. Ideally, instruction should begin as soon as the diagnosis is established. Joslin says that, when at all possible, the patient should inject his first dose of insulin.[41]

This practice has the advantage of not allowing the patient time to worry about whether or not he will be able to do it. Joslin was of the opinion that delay only increases the difficulty for the patient. Patients should be taught that because insulin is a protein, it is advisable to keep it in a cool place but that it should not be allowed to freeze. With the exception of the Lente insulins, the supply in current use need not be refrigerated. Lente insulins should be refrigerated.

CARE OF EQUIPMENT AND INSULIN

Syringe and needle should be sterilized by boiling before each injection. Boiling is simplified by placing the separated barrel and plunger of the syringe and the needle in a metal strainer. The strainer is placed in a saucepan of cold water and boiled for five minutes. When the syringe is removed from the water, care should be taken not to contaminate any part of the needle or syringe that comes in contact with the insulin or is introduced into the patient. When the syringe and needle are kept in alcohol, the alcohol container should be emptied, washed, and boiled at the time the syringe is sterilized. Before the syringe is filled with insulin, alcohol should be removed from the barrel by moving the plunger in and out of the barrel a number of times. The skin over the site of injection should be clean, and just before the injection is made, it should be cleansed with alcohol.

The hour at which the patient takes his insulin will depend on the type of insulin, the severity of his diabetes, when his blood sugar is highest, and the practices of his physician. The most common time is 20 to 30 minutes before breakfast for patients receiving one injection a day. Modified insulins containing a precipitate should be gently rotated until the sediment is thoroughly mixed with the clear solution. Vigorous shaking should be avoided to prevent bubble formation.

Insulin, though usually called a protein, is a polypeptide and is digested in the alimentary

[41] *Op. cit.,* p. 283.

canal. It must, therefore, be administered parenterally. The usual method is by subcutaneous injection into loose subcutaneous tissues. Because daily, or more frequent, injections are required over the lifetime of the individual, care should be taken to rotate the sites, so that one area is not used more often than once each month. When a patient injects his own insulin, the anterior aspects of the thigh and the abdomen are usually the most convenient sites. For those patients who have automatic syringes, the lateral aspect of the upper arm may also be used.

Local reactions may occur at the site of injection. Local allergic reactions are common when patients are taking protamine zinc insulin and are unusual when other types of insulin are used. The reaction is manifested by redness, swelling, itching, and discomfort at the site of injection. The first symptoms appear in from 2 to 12 hours after the injection and reach their height in from 18 to 24 hours. In from three to four weeks this type of reaction subsides. Fortunately, patients rarely are allergic to the protein of insulin itself. When they are, they are more likely to be allergic to beef or sheep insulins than to pork insulin.

Other local reactions may result from repeated injections of insulin into the same site over a long period of time. In some patients, adipose tissue hypertrophies and causes local areas of swelling. In other patients, adipose tissue atrophies leaving concave depressions in the skin. Children of both sexes and adult females seem to be predisposed to this condition. The cause is not known. The rotation of the sites of injection is encouraged to prevent either hypertrophy or atrophy of adipose tissue. Fat atrophy is also less likely to occur if insulin is administered at room temperature.

A considerable number of persons whose diabetes is rapidly brought under control with insulin develop a temporary presbyopia, a condition in which the individual can see at a distance but has difficulty in accommodating to near vision. Particularly to the young patient, presbyopia may be quite disturbing. He should be reassured that the condition will clear up in from three to four weeks and delay having his eyes examined for glasses as any prescription obtained during this period will not be suitable later.

The patient with diabetes mellitus should carry with him some form of identification that includes not only personal data but the fact that he is diabetic, his insulin dosage, and the name of his physician. Carrying a card is of greatest importance to those who are taking insulin or who are subject to ketosis. A number of types of identification tags and cards are available.

A coin-size tag on a chain or bracelet has the advantage of being less likely to be separated from the individual. Additional information can be placed on a card and carried in a billfold.

When a patient requires insulin, he will usually require at least one injection every day for the remainder of his life. There are exceptions, but this is the general rule. He or a member of his family must learn to measure and to inject the insulin. The instruction of the patient including the injection of his own insulin should be begun immediately. Judgment should be exercised so that the patient is not overwhelmed by too much information offered at one time. Instructions should be repeated as often as necessary.

Besides insulin, what drugs are useful in the control of the level of glucose in the blood?

A landmark in the treatment of diabetes mellitus was the discovery that certain chemical compounds when administered orally have a hypoglycemic effect. Of the compounds developed, two have been most widely used, the sulfonylureas and the biguanides. The sulfonylurea tolbutamide (Orinase) is frequently selected because it is effective and has few toxic effects. It is short acting as its effect lasts about four hours. A second sulfonylurea is chlorpropamide, U.S.P. (Diabinese). The sulfonylureas act on the beta cells to increase the output of insulin. Of the biguanides, phenformin is commonly selected. Unlike tolbutamide, its mechanism of action is unknown. It does not induce hypoglycemia in healthy subjects. One hypothesis is that it increases the anaerobic breakdown of glucose. Similar to tolbutamide it has few toxic effects. It is most frequently used in patients in whom tolbutamide is ineffective, either alone or with it. When the sulfonylureas were found to have a hypoglycemic effect, hope was aroused that an effective oral substitute had been discovered. Subsequent experience with the sulfonylureas has demonstrated that, like other drugs, they have limitations as well as uses. They are effective in newly discovered diabetics who are (1) over 40 years of age, (2) not susceptible to ketosis, (3) not overly obese, but (4) in whom hyperglycemia is not controlled by diet alone. They are not effective in young diabetics or in older diabetics whose disease is severe. For example, tolbutamide, a sulfonylurea, was not successful in controlling hyperglycemia in Mrs. Keen. Patients subject to ketosis or with severe diabetes require insulin. Tolbutamide is sometimes used by patients who require large dosages of insulin to reduce the amount of insulin required. Sulfonylureas may become ineffective, and insulin is then required when diabetes worsens or during an infection or other stress. Tolbutamide is safe and effective; about 35 per cent of patients who are resistant to ketosis respond favorably to it.

Patients receiving oral hypoglycemic agents should know that the drug (1) is effective in many older diabetics but rarely in the young, (2) is not a form of insulin, (3) does not act like insulin, and (4) is not effective during infections or other forms of stress as insulin is required at these times. In some patients the favorable effect of the sulfonylureas lasts only from four to six months. Other measures—diet and exercise—are still important and should not be neglected. The only real change in the regime of the patient is that he can take the drug by mouth rather than taking insulin by subcutaneous injection. When, as is not at all uncommon, the patient is taking several different drugs, some system should be devised that helps him to remember which of these drugs controls his blood sugar and when and how to take each drug.

As repeatedly emphasized, diet, exercise, and, when required, insulin or an oral hypoglycemic agent form the framework in the treatment and control of diabetes mellitus. Because diabetes mellitus is an incurable disease characterized by failure in the homeostasis of glucose, fats, and proteins, good health depends on conforming to the therapeutic regime. As stated earlier, successful control of diabetes mellitus depends on the patient and his family assuming responsibility for the management of his disease. Education has a significant role in therapy.

Unlike many chronic diseases, in diabetes relatively simple methods are available to check the effectiveness of the measures used to control hyperglycemia. The concentration of glucose and of acetone in the blood or urine can be determined by relatively simple tests. Examinations of the urine for glucose and acetone are so simple that laymen easily learn to perform them. Determinations of the level of glucose in the blood are somewhat more complicated. To secure accurate information about the degree to which the homeostasis of glucose is being achieved, food and insulin should be delayed until after the blood has been withdrawn. A newly admitted patient should be instructed about the days when blood is taken to be tested for glucose. He may, sometimes, need to be reminded about why he has not received his breakfast. The nonhospitalized patient who has blood drawn in the office of his physician or in the outpatient clinic should be informed of what is expected of him. He should know whether or not he should omit his breakfast and insulin and whether or not he should bring his insulin and breakfast with him. The latter practice may be encouraged, particularly for patients who have a limited income. In the preparation of the patient for some of the newer screening and diagnostic tests, the patient may be instructed to eat his regular or a special meal.

URINE TESTING

Although the concentration of glucose in the blood of a fasting person provides accurate information about the adequacy of control of diabetes mellitus, the frequency with which the test is performed is limited by the fact that blood must be withdrawn before it can be examined. Under most circumstances, the quantity of glucose in the urine provides a reasonably accurate estimate of the degree to which the homeostasis of glucose is being achieved. Because urine is easily obtained and glucose and acetone are excreted in the urine when the renal threshold is exceeded, and the qualitative test for glucose and acetone are relatively simple, urine is widely used to evaluate the control of diabetes mellitus. Depending on the severity of the diabetes and whether or not the patient takes insulin, as well as the views of the physician, the patient may be instructed to test his urine as frequently as four times a day or as infrequently as once or twice a month. For most individuals who work, two testings a day are a practical maximum. During a period in which a diabetes mellitus is under regulation or is changing, more frequent testing may be desired to determine when hyperglycemia and/or hypoglycemia occurs.

Whereas blood to be tested for glucose is usually taken when the patient is fasting, no simple statement applies to the kinds of samples of urine examined for glucose. All urine may be saved for 24 hours so that the total quantity of glucose excreted per day can be determined. Each and every voiding may be checked as a means of evaluating fluctuations in the blood glucose. The patient may be instructed to void at specific times of the day and the urine is added to previous voidings and mixed. A sample of the mixture is then tested for sugar and acetone. In another method the patient voids and discards the voiding unless a 24-hour specimen is being collected, when the urine is added to previous voidings. He drinks a glass or two of water and then one hour later collects a sample of urine (a fresh specimen) for testing. Because the urine is secreted over a known and relatively short period of time, it more accurately reflects the level of glucose in the blood at the time of testing than is likely to be true of the other methods. Whatever method is used, however, the patient should be instructed in its use. He should have practice not only in performing the method he will use at home but in evaluating the results. If he is to adjust his insulin dosage in relation to the quantity of glucose in his urine, he should also be given explicit written as well as verbal instructions and should practice adjusting his insulin dosage while he is still being instructed.

The standard method for determining the quantity of glucose in the urine is the Benedict test. Benedict's solution is an alkaline solution of cupric hydroxide. When it is heated in the presence of an aldehyde group $H{-}\overset{\overset{\textstyle H}{\textstyle |}}{C}{=}O$, the blue cupric ions are reduced to brick-red cuprous ions. Because the glucose molecule contains an aldehyde group, when urine containing glucose is added to Benedict's solution and the mixture is heated, this reaction occurs. Cuprous hydroxide forms a precipitate that settles out on standing. To perform the test 1 tsp of Benedict's solution is measured and placed in a clean test tube. Eight drops of urine are added. The test tube is placed upright in a pan of boiling water and boiled for five minutes. The color changes vary from the clear blue of cupric hydroxide to the brick red of cuprous hydroxide. Scales for comparison are found in various textbooks. An effective method for teaching nurses and patients to estimate the amount of glucose in the urine is to prepare a series of test tubes containing varying amounts of glucose and then, after heating the solution, to seal the open end of the tube by heating it in an oxhydrogen flame.

Since the introduction of the Benedict test, procedures have been developed that make it possible to test the urine both easily and quickly. These include the following:

1. Clinitest method, a modification of the Benedict test. The reagent tablet is dropped into a measured amount of urine. The results are similar to those of the Benedict test. Because the tablets lose their potency when they are exposed to moisture, bottles containing Clinitest tablets should be tightly stoppered.

2. Galatest. In this test the active agent is bismuth. A drop or two of urine is placed on a small mound of powder. When glucose is present, the bismuth is reduced and the powder changes to gray or black.

3. Glucose oxidase tests. These tests are based on the fact that an enzyme, glucose oxidase, converts glucose to glyconic acid. Unlike other tests for identifying glucose in the urine, these tests are specific for glucose.

    Two commercial tests are available that make use of glucose oxidase reaction. Testape not only identifies the presence of glucose in the urine but gives a rough approximation of the quantity of glucose present. The test is simple to perform, because a strip of impregnated paper is dipped into the urine. Color changes take place in about a minute. When glucose is present, the color changes to varying shades of green or blue.

Clinistik, the second glucose oxidase test, is similar to the testape. A specially prepared tip of a stick is placed in urine. These tests have the advantage of being easy and quick to perform.

When glucose is present in appreciable quantities, the urine is also tested for ketone bodies. To test for diacetic acid, a 10 per cent water solution of ferric chloride is added, drop by drop, to 5 ml of freshly voided urine. A wine-red color indicates the presence of diacetic acid.

Acetest is a simple test for acetone. A drop of freshly voided urine is placed on a tablet that contains aminoacetic acid, disodium phosphate, and sodium nitroprusside. A positive test is indicated by a purple tint, from lavender to a deep purple. The more intense the color, the greater the amount of acetone.

The tests for glucose and for ketone bodies are useful in evaluating the success of the control of diabetes mellitus. The patient should be instructed to seek medical attention immediately when the quantity of glucose in the urine increases over 1+ or 2+ as well as when ketone bodies appear in the urine. An experienced and intelligent diabetic patient may be able to evaluate why glucose appears in his urine and to make the appropriate adjustment. When these adjustments are not successful, he, too, should see his physician.

Diet, insulin, and exercise have as their objective the maintenance of the homeostasis of glucose. Analysis of the blood and urine for glucose and acetone enables the patient and his physician to evaluate success in achieving and maintaining homeostasis. Although not specifically related to the control of diabetes mellitus, certain hygienic habits lessen the danger of skin infections such as boils and also help to protect tissues with a limited blood supply. For convenience, the habits that should be developed by the diabetic are divided into general hygiene, care of special areas, and care of the feet. If the patient is hospitalized, all these measures should be observed in the care of the patient. When the nurse is sufficiently aware of the importance of these measures and encourages the patient to practice what he is taught, the patient is more likely to be impressed with their importance than if they are neglected. Conversely, if the nurse does not carry out the necessary procedures in the care of the patient and does not help the patient to follow them, their importance is likely to be minimized to the patient.

SURGERY AND THE DIABETIC

Because anesthesia and surgery lessen the patient's glucose tolerance, the diabetic who has surgery must be diligently observed for signs of both diabetic ketoacidosis and hypoglycemia. Signs of either should be promptly reported. The patient's fluid intake and output should be promptly and carefully measured and recorded. On the day of surgery and for several days thereafter, all urine voided should be tested for sugar. Orders for parenteral fluids and insulin should be carried out promptly and as ordered. Frequently and regularly turning the patient, encouraging deep-breathing, keeping the patient warm without overheating him, maintaining his fluid intake after food is allowed, and seeing that his diet promptly follows his insulin injection are all important, as is encouraging him to eat all the food on his tray. If he does not, the amount of food left should be reported to the dietitian.

EDUCATION

What should the patient be taught concerning general hygiene?

The diabetic patient should be the cleanest person "on the block." Personal cleanliness, as well as clean clothing, is very important. Diabetic patients are more susceptible to "athlete's foot" and to pyogenic infections of the skin than nondiabetics. Cleanliness reduces the number of bacteria and other microorganisms on the skin. The removal of the secretions from between the toes and from the skin makes conditions less favorable for the growth and multiplication of bacteria.

Instruction must be practical. This means that it should be adapted to the situation of the patient, including his customs, his habits, and his living conditions. For example, although a daily bath is frequently recommended as a desirable practice, some modifications are often necessary. For the patient with very dry skin frequent bathing intensifies the dryness and predisposes to itching. A patient living in a cold-water flat or in a farmhouse where water has to be carried in and out and where only one room is heated may find the effort and lack of privacy great obstacles to seriously considering a daily bath. Habits and customs also differ from one group to another. The elderly man who has always bathed once or twice a week is not likely to take kindly to a daily bath. When frequent bathing is rejected or is impractical, the nurse should stress the daily washing of the feet, the neck, and the pubic region.

In the diabetic patient the care of the feet cannot be overemphasized. Arteriosclerosis develops earlier and progresses more rapidly than it does in the nondiabetic. An injury to the toes that would pass unnoticed in the nondiabetic can, if neglected, lead to gangrene of the toe, foot, and leg. The feet of the diabetic patient require special care.

Today, with increased life expectancy and the availability of insulin for the control of severe diabetes, diabetic patients are living longer than at any other period in history. Diabetic coma, although still a serious complicacation, is no longer responsible for many deaths among young diabetics. Disability and death usually result from vascular pathology: Changes in the walls of large and small vessels result in a lessening of the blood supply to the tissues, which in turn reduces the ability of the tissues to respond favorably to injury. Consequently, when an older diabetic is admitted to the hospital, he should not only receive the care given to the nondiabetic patient but special attention should be given to protect his lower extremities from injury. One of the most common causes of injury to the lower extremities is heat. Diabetics are remarkably sensitive to heat and may be burned by hot-water bottles, electric pads, and hot, moist packs. Therefore, heat in any of these forms should not be applied below the knees. If moist dressings are applied, they should be just warm (37.8 to 40.6°C, 100° to 105°F).

Extremities of the diabetic patient should be protected not only from heat but from the effects of pressure. A cradle placed under the covering at the foot of the bed prevents pressure from above and allows for freedom of movement. If the patient lies in one position more or less continuously, or if his blood supply is especially poor, a soft pillow under the ankle or heel will help lessen the pressure. Nurses caring for diabetic patients cannot exercise too much care in the protection of the patient's feet from injury. Cleanliness, protection of the feet, well-fitting shoes and hose, proper cutting of the nails, and prompt treatment of injuries when they occur are imperative. See Chapter 10 for more detailed instruction.

The diabetic patient should be taught to treat minor infections such as a common cold or an acute gastrointestinal infection by going to bed. He should avoid the use of sweetened cough mixtures and other agents that are sometimes taken during acute respiratory infections. He should test his urine at three-hour intervals during the day and at six-hour intervals during the night. Because any infection in the diabetic patient is an emergency, he should call his doctor and follow his advice.

PREPARATION OF THE PATIENT TO MANAGE HIS DISEASE

The period during which the severity of diabetes is being evaluated and regulation is effected should be utilized to prepare the patient and the members of his family to assume the responsibility for controlling his diabetes. During this period he should learn what he needs to know to understand the nature of his disease and develop the skills needed to maintain his control. The objective should be for him to be the master of diabetes mellitus rather than for it to be his master. The reward of mastery is a more nearly normal life. He should learn to avoid all excesses. Idleness is to be avoided as well as excess strain, tension, anxiety, emotional upsets, and overfatigue. Eight to ten hours' sleep at night and, if convenient, an hour of rest at midday is beneficial.

Some hospitals have well-organized plans for the instruction of patients with diabetes mellitus. Both group and individual instruction are arranged. More recently, some of the content has been programmed and placed on a teaching machine. Each method has its advantages and disadvantages. One of the advantages of group instruction is that the patient may be encouraged when he learns that other people's problems are not unlike his own. Patients may have an opportunity to share experiences and solutions to problems. Individual instruction allows for modification of the plan for the needs and problems of the patient. Programmed instruction permits the patient to progress in learning at his own rate. Theoretically, he does not progress until he has mastered each step. This form of instruction also ensures that each patient receives a minimum of instruction. A well-planned program should cover all aspects required by the patient.

Whether patients are taught in groups or individually, instruction should be carefully planned and adapted to the needs of each individual patient. A variety of factors may interfere with the ability of the patient to learn. Sometimes a patient is of low intellectual level. Other factors are more frequently responsible, however. The fact that the patient is adjusting to a new and anxiety-provoking diagnosis may decrease his learning capacity for the time being because he is unable to give his attention to learning. His ability to learn may be lessened because he is not feeling well. Frequently the time that he is in the hospital is too short to master the necessary knowledge and skill. As soon as he begins to feel well, he is discharged. His ability or willingness to reveal significant factors in his home and work situation may be lacking. He may interpret instructions too literally. For example, Mr. Simon ate hamburgers every day for lunch because his doctor told him to eat what he had been eating in the hospital. This was all he could remember having been served for lunch while he was in the hospital. Also, the patient may not follow through with his prescribed treatment. This may be caused by the stress involved in his adjustment at home or because he fails to understand the importance of continued treatment. Some patients are overly conscientious. They behave as though the disease will go away if they perform each procedure often enough. The nurse should also be aware that the 8- to 12-year-old child may try to mislead his parents and physicians by such maneuvers as testing his friend's urine. The adjustment of the patient and his family is usually facilitated by a visit from a friendly professional nurse. When the patient's instruction has been inadequate, the services of the visiting nurse as a teacher are practically indispensable.

If the patient is to assume the long-term management of diabetes mellitus successfully, he needs to understand its nature and the measures that are used in its control. He also requires practice in a supportive environment until he develops skill and confidence in his ability to carry out the necessary procedures. For the nurse to provide the patient with the assistance that he needs, she should have a body of knowledge and have developed skills in teaching as well as in the performance of necessary procedures. In these programs nurses are usually responsible for certain aspects of the instruction of the patient. They should, therefore, be familiar with the total program. In hospitals and other agencies that do not have an organized instructional plan, the nurse should discuss the content of her plan for teaching with the physician so that the patient is protected from conflicting instructions, as this can be a source of psychological stress to the patient. Furthermore, the nurse may be able to secure the cooperation of the physician and the dietitian in initiating a program of instruction.

If the patient is to be prepared to assume the management of his condition, he should receive the maximum rather than the minimum of instruction. To accomplish this, teaching should begin as soon as the diagnosis is established. When the physician's prescription is required before teaching can be started, it should be sought early. Most of the objections of physicians to nurses teaching patients are based on an experience in which a nurse used poor judgment in what she told a patient. In the experience of the author, these fears usually can be laid to rest by adequate preparation and discussion with the physician before the teaching is started.

Most, though by no means all, patients are motivated to learn. When the patient is unable for one reason or another to learn, members of the family or a neighbor may be enlisted to give the necessary assistance. Mrs. Delft never learned to administer her own insulin. Her son came each morning on his way to work to inject it. Certainly it would have been more convenient had Mrs. Delft learned to administer her own insulin. She refused, however, saying, "I just can't stick myself." Some patients such as Mrs. Curry do not see well enough to measure insulin and to carry out the details of the procedure unless they have a special type of syringe that is available for the use of blind patients.

In addition to making the most of the patient's interest in learning and being sure that he knows what he is to learn, the teaching should provide for thoughtful and understanding learning. Time should be taken to learn what the patient already knows or thinks he knows, as well as what he wants to know about diabetes. In the opinion of the author, there is a tendency to overestimate what persons who have had diabetes for some time know about their disease and its control. Although the average patient may not benefit from knowing the chemical reactions involved in the testing of urine, he is much more likely to test his urine regularly if he understands why he tests it and if he knows how to use the results. Sometimes the physician may ask the patient to keep a record of the results of urine testing. The patient should know that the information will help guide the physician in regulating his diabetes. As in other learning, the program should provide for sufficient repetition to make certain that the patient has had sufficient knowledge and practice to care for himself with confidence. Some of the factors that influence the amount of practice that a given patient needs are the ability of the patient to learn, his interest in learning, and his confidence in himself. A great deal of encouragement is sometimes necessary. Emphasis should be on accomplishment rather than on failure.

As in other types of learning, the situation should provide the patient with an opportunity to perform procedures as nearly as possible as they will be carried out at home. For example, when Bonnie learns to administer her own insulin, she should learn the various parts of the procedure separately, but she should practice the procedure as a whole; that is, she should measure the dosage of insulin, make the injection, and care for the syringe following its use.

Practice periods should be distributed over a

period of time rather than be limited to a single intensive practice. Unless the instruction of the diabetic patient is carefully planned, this factor in learning is likely to be disregarded. Instruction may include little more than a hasty demonstration and inadequate practice. The patient is then dismissed with the vain hope that he has mastered a set of complicated instructions and that he will be able to manage his diabetes. The worried patient goes home hoping for the best. Often, as a result of failure to appreciate the importance of the control of diabetes plus a lack of confidence in his ability to care for himself, the patient lapses into his old habits and sooner or later is readmitted to the hospital where the same procedure is repeated.

It follows that if the instruction of every diabetic patient is to be adequate this instruction must be planned. The plan for the patient's instruction must suit the individual patient and his situation if it is to work. However, whether the instruction of the diabetic patient is given by a special instructor or is shared by a number of people, each person should know what his responsibilities are and every provision should be made to see that these functions are accomplished.

A not unimportant, but frequently little appreciated, part of teaching the patient is the teaching given by the nurse in her care and supervision of the patient. The nurse is in a favorable position to encourage the patient to express and examine his feelings about diabetes mellitus, to learn his misconceptions and doubts, and to answer or obtain answers to his questions. Some instruction she gives directly as instruction. Other teaching is done by example, for if she carries out and supervises his care conscientiously she does much to impress him with its importance. For example, if she collects the urine specimens promptly and correctly, she does much to impress the patient with the importance of regular and frequent testing of the urine. If she uses care in washing his feet and dries them well with a soft cloth, the patient is more certain to follow the example set. If the nurse insists that the patient who starts barefooted for the bathroom stop and put on his slippers, she is not only emphasizing what he has been taught but is giving him actual practice in it. The patient who is provided with a footstool and encouraged to elevate his feet is learning by doing.

Throughout the discussion of the needs of the patient with diabetes mellitus, emphasis has been placed on the importance of preparing the patient to manage himself so that his diabetes is kept under control. Diet, exercise, and, when necessary, insulin or an insulin substitute are the principal measures used in the control of diabetes mellitus. Education is an essential aspect of therapy.

Because the patient and his family must eventually assume the responsibility for the management of the diabetes mellitus, the nurse must not do for the patient what he is able to do for himself. She should, however, interpret her actions so that he understands the reason for encouraging him to care for himself. She should also give recognition to progress made by the patient. The nurse must exercise a high degree of judgment in making the decision that the patient is or is not ready to assume more responsibility for his own care. In some instances, the patient is unable to assume full responsibility for his care and a member of his family must be taught to assist him. Insofar as the patient is able to participate, he should be included in any instruction. Whenever possible, one or more members of the family should also be included in the instructional plan, as family members can be helpful to the patient.

Even when instructions given in the physician's office or in the hospital are well planned and carried out, the patient and/or his family still may have some problems. When a visiting nurse service or public health nurse is available in the community, the patient can be helped to make the adjustment to full responsibility by visits from a nurse. Even when a patient is well taught in the hospital, problems are likely to arise in his adjustment at home or to his work situation. In addition to the usual sources of stress in hospitalized patients, he is adapting to diabetes and all that is entailed in its control.

Two studies of diabetic patients at home indicate that they make many errors in the management of their disease. In the first, made by Watkins and her associates,[42] the patients were rated on the management of insulin, urine tests, diet, foot care, and disease control. Of 60 patients 48 had unacceptable practice in the administration of insulin. In every category from 20 to 80 per cent of the patients made errors. As an example 48 had unacceptable practices in administration of insulin and 31 made errors in dosage. Furthermore, the longer they had the disease, the more insulin errors they made. Those who knew more about diabetes managed better but their disease was more poorly controlled. Only one patient demonstrated acceptable practice in all areas.

In the second study Leifson[43] found that patients made numerous errors in testing urine.

[42] Julia D. Watkins et al.: "A Study of Diabetic Patients at Home," Amer. J. Public Health, 57:452–57 (Mar.) 1967.
[43] June Leifson: "Glycosuria Tests Performed by Diabetics at Home," Public Health Rep., 84:32 (Jan.) 1969.

Eighty-six per cent timed them improperly, 19 per cent used outdated test material, and 67 per cent stored the material improperly.

Both of these studies indicate the need for further study of the kind of help patients need if they are to manage their diabetes. Very likely the kind of assistance patients require changes over time. As an example, as vision fails old methods for measuring insulin may be inadequate. These studies also raise some other questions, such as why should patients who know more about diabetes be in poorer control? Certainly more information is needed if people with chronic conditions are to live productive and healthy lives.

Throughout this text, attention has been given to the problem of enlisting the patient's help in restoring and maintaining his own health.

Mendelsohn [44] challenges some of the current ideas about mass education in public health. To emphasize the point that mass communication efforts of the past have failed despite the expenditure of large sums of money, he cites the ever-rising number of traffic accidents. For educational efforts to be successful, he states [45] that the program must take into account the following:

1. Simple exposure is not enough; interest is a prerequisite.
2. Man is a complex actor-reactor. He functions in dynamic situations that he defines for himself in different ways.
3. Facts are not enough. Time must be spent in altering socially derived perceptions and in helping the patient develop insight into the actual health threat.
4. Two variables are involved in any health

threat, perceived susceptibility (it can or cannot happen to me) and perceived severity.

Tolstoy [46] defined the last when he had Ivan Ilych say "Is it or is it not serious?" He did not care what the diagnosis was. He wanted to know what the implications were.

Although Mendelsohn [47] makes other useful points, one more will be cited. He says that people do not want the facts, nor do they know what to do with them. They must be told what to do in an interesting, explicit, dramatic, and exact manner.

In the practice of nursing, nurses want to help patients with long-term illnesses live as comfortably and usefully as they can. To accomplish this objective we must learn

1. What kinds of help the patient who is newly diagnosed needs and how this help can best be given.
2. What kinds of continuing help and supervision the patient needs and how this help can be given.

Summary

The nurse has two major responsibilities to the diabetic patient. They are the instruction of the patient in the management of his condition and his care during illness. The sick diabetic patient has all the problems of any person who is ill plus special ones that must be recognized and met. The nurse who assists in the care of diabetic patients has the satisfaction of knowing that the diabetic patient who maintains his diabetes under control has a good chance of living almost as long and as well as if he were not a diabetic.

---

[44] Harold Mendelsohn: "Which Shall It Be: Mass Education or Mass Persuasion for Health?" *Amer. J. Public Health,* **58:**131–37 (Jan.) 1968.

[45] *Ibid.,* p. 133.

[46] Leo Tolstoy: "The Death of Ivan Ilyich," *Six Short Masterpieces by Tolstoy* (New York: Dell Publishing Company, 1963), pp. 248–49.

[47] *Op. cit.,* p. 135.

REFERENCES

BOOKS

Beeuwkes, Adelia M. (ed.): *Institute on the Education of the Diabetic and His Family* (Ann Arbor: University of Michigan School of Public Health, 1966).

Duncan, Garfield G.: *A Modern Pilgrim's Progress with Further Revelations for Diabetics,* 2nd ed. (Philadelphia: W. B. Saunders Company, 1967).

Kessler, Edward, Caccamo, Leonard P., and Azneer, J. Leonard: *Diabetic Acidosis: A Pro-*

gramed Text (Philadelphia: F. A. Davis Company, 1967).

Ralli, Elaine P.: *Management of the Diabetic Patient: A Practical Guide* (New York: G. P. Putnam's Sons, 1965).

Report on the Fifty-first Ross Conference on Pediatric Research: *Juvenile Diabetes Mellitus* (Columbus, Ohio: Ross Laboratories, 1965).

Rosenthal, Joseph, and Rosenthal, Helen: *Diabetic Care in Pictures,* 4th ed. (Philadelphia: J. B. Lippincott Company, 1968).

Waife, S. O. (ed.): *Diabetes Mellitus,* 7th ed. (Indianapolis: Eli Lilly Research Laboratories, 1967).

Williams, Robert H.: *Textbook of Endocrinology,* 4th ed. (Philadelphia: W. B. Saunders Company, 1968), pp. 690–92.

PERIODICALS

Current Concepts in Diabetes Mellitus

Anderson, O. Ortved, and Friss, Th.: "The Intravenous Tolbutamide Test in Diagnosing Mild and Latent Diabetes Mellitus," *Acta. Med. Scand.,* 181:535–45 (May) 1967.

Bacon, George E., and Sanbar, Shafeek S.: "Serum Lipids and Lipoproteins in Diabetic Children," *Univ. Mich. Med. Center J.,* 34:84–87 (Mar.–Apr.) 1968.

Berson, Soloman A., and Yalow, Rosalyn S.: "Some Current Controversies in Diabetes Research," *Diabetes,* 14:549–72 (Sept.) 1965.

Bloom, Arnold: "Relation of the Complications of Diabetes to the Clinical State," *Proc. Roy. Soc. Med.,* 60:149–52 (Feb.) 1967.

Bressler, Rubin (guest ed.): "Investigative Issues in Diabetes Mellitus," *Arch. Intern. Med. Symposia,* 123:219–322 (Mar.) 1969.

Brown, Josiah, *et al.:* "Diabetes Mellitus," *Ann. Intern. Med.,* 68:634–61 (Mar.) 1968.

Cahill, George: "Pathophysiology of Diabetes," *Med. Clin. N. Amer.,* 49:881–92 (July) 1965.

Camerini-Davalos, Rafael A.: "Prevention of Diabetes Mellitus," *Med. Clin. N. Amer.,* 49:865–79 (July) 1965.

Colwell, Arthur R.: "Fifty Years of Diabetes in Perspective," *Diabetes,* 17:599–610 (Oct.) 1968.

Davis, Dave M., Shipp, Joseph C., and Pattishall, Evan G.: "Attitudes of Diabetic Boys and Girls Towards Diabetes," *Diabetes,* 14:106–109 (Feb.) 1965.

"The Diagnosis of Diabetes: Programmed Instruction," *GP,* 39:133–49 (Jan.) 1969.

Donaldson, James B.: "Current Concepts in the Treatment of Diabetes Mellitus," *Med. Clin. N. Amer.,* 49:1349–60 (Sept.) 1965.

Eisenstein, Albert B.: "Interrelationship of Nutrition and Endocrinology," *Amer. J. Clin. Nutr.,* 21:467–72 (May) 1968.

Goodner, Charles J.: "Newer Concepts in Diabetes Mellitus, Including Management," *DM,* pp. 2–52 (Sept.) 1965.

Gorman, G. K.: "Hypoglycemia: A Brief Review," *Med. Clin. N. Amer.,* 49:947–59 (July) 1965.

Hodges, Robert E.: "Present Knowledge of Nutrition in Relation to Diabetes Mellitus," *Nutr. Rev.,* 24:257–60 (Sept.) 1966.

Houssay, Bernardo A.: "Hormonal Factors of Diabetic Ketosis," *Diabetes,* 12:481–89 (Nov.–Dec.) 1963.

Klimt, Christian R., *et al.:* "Study of Familial Patterns of Reported Diabetes," *Diabetes,* 16:40–50 (Jan.) 1967.

Krall, Leo P.: "When Is Diabetes?" *Med. Clin. N. Amer.,* 49:893–94 (July) 1965.

Levin, Marvin E., and Recant, Lillian: "Diabetes

and the Environment," *Arch. Environ. Health,* 12:621–30 (May) 1966.

Luft, Rolf: "Some Considerations on the Pathogenesis of Diabetes Mellitus," *New Eng. J. Med.,* 279:1086–92 (Nov. 14) 1968.

Lukens, F. D.: "Diabetes Mellitus—1967," *Perspect. Biol. Med.,* 11:136–52 (Autumn) 1967.

Martin, Marguerite M.: "Diabetes Mellitus: Current Concepts," *Amer. J. Nurs.,* 66:510–14 (Mar.) 1966.

Metz, Robert, *et al.:* "Glucose Tolerance, Plasma Insulin, and Free Fatty Acids in Elderly Subjects," *Ann. Intern. Med.,* 64:1042–48 (May) 1966.

Newill, Vann A.: "The Epidemiology of Diabetes Mellitus," *Med. Sci.,* 14:30–39 (Dec.) 1963.

Osborn, James R., and Goldstein, H. Howard: "Does Diabetes Cause Coronary Disease," *Postgrad. Med.,* 44:137–41 (Sept.) 1968.

Richardson, G. O.: "Endocrine Disorders of the Pancreas," *Practitioner,* 200:494–501 (Apr.) 1968.

Smith, W. Hamilton: "Difficulties in the Management of Diabetes Mellitus," *Med. J. Aust.,* 53:575–77 (Apr. 2) 1966.

Stern, C. B., Jr.: "Diabetes Mellitus; Natural History, Symptoms and Detection," *Amer. Ass. Industr. Nurses J.,* 16:7–9 (Aug.) 1968.

"Taking the Danger out of Diabetes," *Today's Health,* 43:56–57, 82–84 (Apr.) 1965.

Weisenfeld, Shirley, *et al.:* "Adsorption of Insulin to Infusion Bottles and Tubing," *Diabetes,* 17:766–70 (Dec.) 1968.

White, Priscilla: "The Inheritance of Diabetes," *Med. Clin. N. Amer.,* 49:857–63 (July) 1965.

Zuck, David: "Metabolism: The Source of Energy," *Nurs. Times,* 64:1746 (Dec. 27) 1968.

Insulin

Bagdade, J. D.: "Basal Insulin and Obesity," *Lancet,* 2:630–31 (Sept. 14) 1968.

Hernandez, Alfredo, Zorrilla, Eduardo, and Gershberg, Herbert: "Decreased Insulin Production, Elevated Growth Hormone Levels, and Glucose Intolerance in Liver Disease," *J. Lab. Clin. Med.,* 73:25–33 (Jan.) 1969.

"Insulin—How Many Faces," *New Eng. J. Med.,* 277:877–78 (Oct.) 1967.

"Insulin and Pro Insulin," *JAMA,* 207:552 (Jan. 20) 1969.

"Islet-cells and Insulin," *Lancet,* 1:1142–44 (May 27) 1967.

Levine, Rachmiel: "Concerning the Mechanisms of Insulin Action," *Diabetes,* 10:421–31 (Nov.–Dec.) 1961.

Romanoff, Neil E.: "Factors Controlling Release of Insulin from Beta Cell," *New York J. Med.,* 68:385–91 (Feb. 1) 1968.

Seltzer, Holbrooke S., and Allen, E. William: "Hyperglycemia and Inhibition of Insulin Secretion during Administration of Diazoxide and Trichlormethiazide in Man," *Diabetes,* 18:19–28 (Jan.) 1969.

Simpson, Ronald G., *et al,:* "Early Phase Insulin Release," *Diabetes,* 17:684–92 (Nov.) 1968.

Vallance-Owen, J.: "Synalbumin Insulin Antagonism," *Diabetes,* 13:241–46 (May–June) 1964.

Vallance-Owen, J., and Lilley, M. D.: "Insulin Antagonism in the Plasma of Obese Diabetics and Prediabetics," *Lancet,* 1:806–807 (Apr. 15) 1961.

Vallance-Owen, J., Dennes, Elizabeth, and Campbell, P. N.: "Insulin Antagonism in Plasma of Diabetic Patients and Normal Subjects," *Lancet,* 2:336–38 (Aug. 16) 1958.

Wright, Peter H.: "Measurement of Insulin Secretion," *Diabetes,* 17:641–44 (Oct.) 1968.

The Pharmacological Treatment of Diabetes Mellitus

Danowski, T. S.: "Drug Therapy of Diabetes Mellitus," *Postgrad. Med.,* 41:366–72 (Apr.) 1967.

Davidoff, Frank F.: "Oral Hypoglycemic Agents and the Mechanism of Diabetes Mellitus," *New Eng. J. Med.,* 278:148–55 (Jan. 18) 1968.

Devrim, Sevim: "Effects of Tolbutamide and Insulin on Insulin Inhibitory Activity Associated with Plasma Albumin," *Diabetes,* 17:746–51 (Dec.) 1968.

Ferguson, B. Dan: "The Oral Hypoglycemic Compounds," *Med. Clin. N. Amer.,* 49:929–38 (July) 1965.

Hadden, David R., and Weaver, John A.: "Oral Hypoglycaemic Agents," *Practitioner,* 200: 129–36 (Jan.) 1968.

Hadley, William B.: "Insulin Treatment of Diabetes Mellitus," *Med. Clin. N. Amer.,* 49:921–27 (July) 1965.

Keen, H., *et al.:* "The Uses of Biguanides in Diabetes Mellitus," *Postgrad. Med.,* 44:466–71 (June) 1968.

Martin, Marguerite M.: "Insulin Reactions," *Amer. J. Nurs.,* 67:328–31 (Feb.) 1967.

Patient Teaching

Bowen, Rhoda, Rich, Rosemary, and Schlotfeldt, Rozella M.: "Effects of Organized Instruction for Patients with the Diagnosis of Diabetes Mellitus," *Nurs. Res.,* 10:151–59 (Summer) 1961.

Hanchett, Effie S.: "Memory Booster for Drug Taking," *Amer. J. Nurs.,* 69:304 (Feb.) 1969.

Kaufman, Mildred: "A Food Preference Questionnaire for Counseling Patients with Diabetes," *J. Amer. Diet. Ass.,* 49:31–37 (July) 1966.

Leiner, Malvina S., and Rahmer, Ann E.: "The Juvenile Diabetic and the Visiting Nurse," *Amer. J. Nurs.,* 68:106–108 (Jan.) 1968.

Meadows, Dorothy: "Patients Learn About Diabetes from Teaching Machine," *Hospitals,* 39: 77–82 (Dec. 16) 1965.

Mohammed, Mary F. Bucklin: "Patient's Understanding of Written Health Information," *Nurs. Res.,* 13:100–108 (Spring) 1964.

Pond, Helen: "Special Problems of the Diabetic Child," *Practitioner,* 200:527–32 (Apr.) 1968.

Watkins, Julia D., and Moss, Fay T.: "Confusion in the Management of Diabetes," *Amer. J. Nurs.,* 69:521–24 (Mar.) 1969.

BOOKS AND PAMPHLETS FOR PATIENTS WITH DIABETES

ADA Forecast (New York: American Diabetic Association). This magazine is published every other month. Subscription rate is $2.00.

Deaconess, Maud Behrman: *Cookbook for Diabetics* (New York: American Diabetic Association, 1959).

Diabetes (Kalamazoo: Upjohn Company, 1967).

Diabetes in the News (Elkhart, Ind.: Ames Company). This pamphlet is published quarterly and is free upon request.

Diabetic Guidebook (Elkhart, Ind.: Ames Company).

A Guide for the Diabetic (Indianapolis: Eli Lilly Company, 1966).

PART B:

Mr. Allen, A Patient Who Was Burned *

The Patient	Acceptance of the Role as a Sick Person
The Extent of Burn Injury	Physiological Responses
Psychological Responses of the Patient, His Family, and the Staff	Fluid and Electrolyte Disturbances

The Patient

On the evening of January 11, Mr. Marshall Allen left his apartment to attend a public dance against the wishes of his wife. She had planned to go with him, but because she had not been feeling well, she asked him to forego the dance and stay at home to take care of their two infant daughters so that she might rest. Mr. Allen and his wife were married very young, and neither found it easy to accommodate to the responsibilities of parenthood; on the night in question, he was only 20 years old, she was 19, and both were behaving very irresponsibly in the heat of argument. Unwilling to change his plans, Mr. Allen stormed out of the house and attended the dance with friends.

Near midnight, he was standing at the head of the stairs in the dance hall to hear what the commotion was that was going on outside the entrance. Suddenly he felt something cold splash his face, and as he put his hands to his face the cold liquid, which was gasoline from a Molotov cocktail, ignited. The dance hall was soon ablaze, and many were burned. But Mr. Allen remembered very little of what happened at the scene of the fire, despite the fact that he remained conscious. He recalled vaguely being brought to Emergency Hospital in an ambulance and being cared for all that night in the emergency room but could reconstruct no details of the immediate postburn period.

Mr. Allen was in severe pain on admission to the hospital and was given morphine intravenously through a subclavian intracatheter that was inserted immediately to establish a route for fluid therapy.

The Extent of Burn Injury

Mr. Allen had sustained second- and third-degree burns over about 85 per cent of his body; over 50 per cent of them were third-degree. From Figure 19-5 the reader can see that his burns were distributed over all areas except a wedge of his upper anterior chest, the lower portion of his abdomen, the scrotum, buttocks, ankles and feet, and the top of his head. Because he had facial burns, tracheal burns were considered to be a possibility, and a tracheostomy was considered but was determined to be unnecessary as he showed no evidence of respiratory distress. The rule of nines was used by the physician to arrive at the percentage of body surface burned. Figure 19-6 shows the division of the body surface into areas that are each equivalent to approximately 9 per cent, or multiples of 9, of the total body surface.[48]

Physical examination at the time of admission revealed a slender, well-nourished Negro male weighing 140 lb (64 kg), who was 5 ft, 8 in. tall. The history was obtained from the relatives, and revealed the following information:

Age, 20 years; born in Michigan
Married: Wife—living and well, at home
　　　　　Children—two daughters, aged 14 months and 4 months
Father: 43, living and well
Mother: 42, living and well
Siblings: six brothers and sisters, aged 14 to 25
Occupation: employed in automotive industry for the past year
Income: about $120 per week
Health insurance: Group Blue Cross through employment
Living accommodations: apartment in his father's house, which includes heat, electricity, and refrigerator; no telephone

[48] Curtis P. Artz and John A. Moncrief: *The Treatment of Burns,* 2nd ed. (Philadelphia: W. B. Saunders Company, 1969), p. 92.

---

* This part was contributed and revised by Joyce Passos, Associate Professor of Nursing, College of Nursing, Wayne State University, Detroit, Michigan.

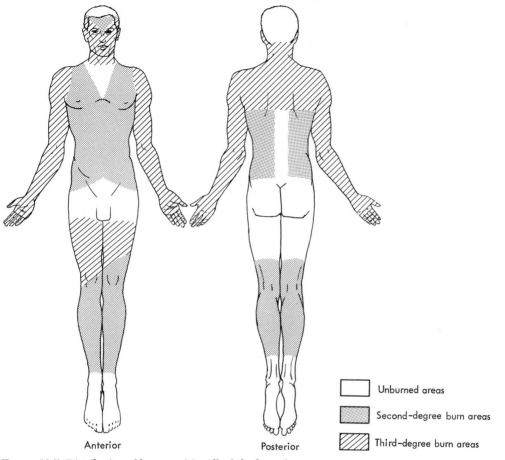

	Unburned areas
	Second-degree burn areas
	Third-degree burn areas

Anterior   Posterior

FIGURE 19-5. Distribution of burns on Mr. Allen's body surface.

Education: high school graduate

Significant persons: two close friends, high school classmates

Religion: Baptist

Past medical history: previously in good health, except for having been hospitalized nine months prior to this admission for treatment of pneumonia; recovery was complete

Personal habits: did not smoke, liked "a few beers" at night

Table 19-3 summarizes and emphasizes the pathophysiological changes that occurred in Mr. Allen because of his burns and specifies the medical therapy instituted and the nursing care required. Because little reference is made in the table to Mr. Allen's behavior, it is necessary to present here a brief description of his psychological response to his injury and subsequent hospitalization. Mr. Allen was admitted to the surgical intensive-care unit the morning after his arrival at Emergency Hospital, and he remained in that unit throughout the 32 post-burn days to which this discussion of his problems and care relate.

Psychological Responses of the Patient, His Family, and the Staff

During the first postburn week, Mr. Allen exhibited an egocentricity and constriction of interest that was graphically illustrative of regressive adaptation; as mentioned previously, he never lost consciousness, and during this first week his overwhelming and single expressed concern was, "What does my face look like?" When he began to realize within two to three days after the fire just how serious his condition was, he began also to ask, "Am I going to live?" As his activity began to be increased by the end of the first week and the beginning of the second week, he expressed to several members of the nursing staff and to his father that he really did not want to live. It is a testimony to his family and to the medical

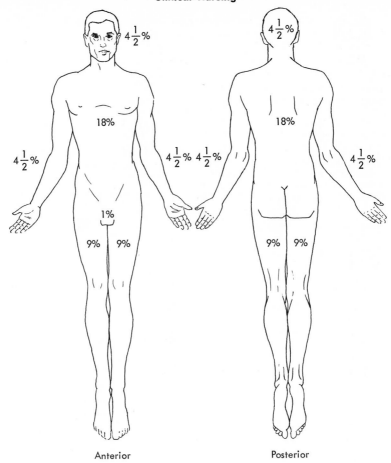

Anterior   Posterior

FIGURE 19-6. Rule of nines. A rapid method of estimating the percentage of body surface involved. (Adapted with permission of W. B. Saunders Company from *The Treatment of Burns*, 2nd ed., 1969, p. 92, by C. P. Artz and J. A. Moncrief.)

and nursing staff that he was helped to feel sufficiently valued and accepted as a whole person during those early postburn weeks that he regained his will to live and even was able to achieve a pseudonormalcy in jesting with staff and in participating with his wife and father in making decisions regarding his own family. A factor that may have exerted a strong influence in helping him to overcome his early feelings of despair was the constant interest and visits of his two close friends; staff and family may be expected to help when one is sick and disfigured, but friends can more easily extricate themselves from the bonds of human relationships. Mr. Allen's trust and confidence in the ability of others to see through his appearance to the person within was by no means generalized to all people. Whenever he met someone for the first time, his eyes were riveted on the newcomer's face to detect any hint of revulsion or rejection. When the time came for plans to

be made for his transfer out of the intensive care unit to a surgical ward, he was very reluctant to go and expressed his apprehension exquisitely: "They'll treat me like a criminal." This transition was eased considerably for him by having the man who would be helping him most with his care on the new ward come in and get acquainted with him for several days prior to the actual transfer.

Throughout his illness, even during the shock phase of his response to his thermal injury, Mr. Allen expressed to those who were closest to him his acute sense of guilt about being in the dance hall the night of the fire. He realized he had behaved irresponsibly toward his wife and children that night and was convinced that his subsequent injuries were punishment for his wrongdoing. He kept pictures of his children on his bedside table and often expressed concern about the welfare of his family and the extent to which his willfulness had jeopardized their welfare. He was grateful that his wife's family were giving her some help with expenses, and he had the satisfaction of knowing that he continued to contribute financially through sickness benefits that continued to come to him through his place of employment. But these factors did not assuage his sense of guilt.

Acceptance of the Role as a Sick Person

In most respects, Mr. Allen fulfilled the role of a patient that is expected in our culture. When he became ill, he was provided with, and accepted, medical treatment. He surrendered his independence and decision-making prerogatives to medical and paramedical personnel. Although he was very ill, he cooperated by making progress toward recovery. As he improved physically, he accepted the care that was necessary. He expressed his appreciation to those who cared for him and followed the instructions (orders) of the professional staff explicitly and without question. As his condition improved, his behavior began to deviate from that expected of the person in the sick role, i.e., despite his verbal assertions that he desired to regain independence and mobility, he frequently whined during treatments and the onset of activity, was easily discouraged and would allow others to do for him things that he had previously been able to manage slowly by himself, and made many requests of personnel. The high tolerance of nurses for deviant behavior of persons in the sick role because of severe burns seems to be a common phenomenon. Davitz and Pendleton found that nurses inferred the greatest degree of suffering in patients who had been burned and consequently might be expected to empathize more with burned patients than with patients having other illnesses.[49] The approval that was accorded Mr. Allen by those responsible for his care may have been caused in part by the fact that his family also behaved as relatives are expected to behave in our culture. His father had not missed a day of visiting him since the night of the fire and served as a strong stabilizing force in helping to maintain Mr. Allen's psychological equilibrium throughout the severe physiological and psychological stress to which he had been subject. His wife came faithfully and even arranged to bring his daughters once when he was beginning to improve physically. Brothers and cousins agreed to help by serving as donors of some of the many homografts required during the endless round of grafting procedures performed on Mr. Allen. All these factors may have contrib-

[49] Jean Davitz and Sydney Harrison Pendleton: "Nurses' Inferences of Suffering," *Nurs. Res.,* **18**:100–107 (Mar.–Apr.) 1969.

uted to the high tolerance of Mr. Allen's prolonged dependency by the nursing staff. The general tenor of their acceptance and empathy was expressed in one succinct entry in the nurses' notes: "Requests are frequent but reasonable."

Physiological Responses

At the time of this writing, Mr. Allen still has a very long way to go to achieve even physiological stability. Formulas developed for predicting survival of burned patients based on age and extent of severe burned body surface predict zero probability of survival for 20-year-olds with 85 per cent of the body surface severely burned.[50] He has already achieved a victory of no small proportions. But his physicians continue to hold a guarded prognosis for him because of the problem of obtaining sufficient grafts, especially autografts, to ensure re-epithelialization. Presently, everyone involved in Mr. Allen's struggle to return to a useful place in society is giving the task all the skill, concern, imagination, and devotion required by the enormity of his problems. If desire, commitment, and energy expended are sufficient to defy statistical probabilities, Mr. Allen will recover.

Fluid and Electrolyte Disturbances

Table 19-3 includes discussion of the fluid and electrolyte disturbances that accompany severe burns; the dangers to which a person is exposed when there is disruption of the integrity of the skin and alterations in the defense mechanisms of the respiratory tract; hazards to a person's convalescence from prolonged immobilization; and alterations in metabolism, especially of proteins, in the immediate and long-term postburn period. In each case the medical therapy instituted for Mr. Allen is presented, and there is elaboration of actions indicated for the nurse. Two illustrations have been developed to graphically represent some of the most significant aspects of Mr. Allen's fluid and electrolyte status during the first 32 days of the postburn period, to assist the reader in applying information presented in Table 19-3 to the condition and treatment of Mr. Allen during the phases of burn shock, reabsorption, and anemia and malnutrition. Figure 19-7 presents a summary of selected serum levels of potassium, calcium, chloride, and sodium; Figure 19-8 presents a summary of his fluid intake, urinary output, and body weights during the same 32 days of the postburn period.

[50] Artz and Moncrief, *op. cit.,* p. 99.

FIGURE 19-7. Serum levels of potassium, calcium, chloride, and sodium for Mr. Allen for 32 days postburn.

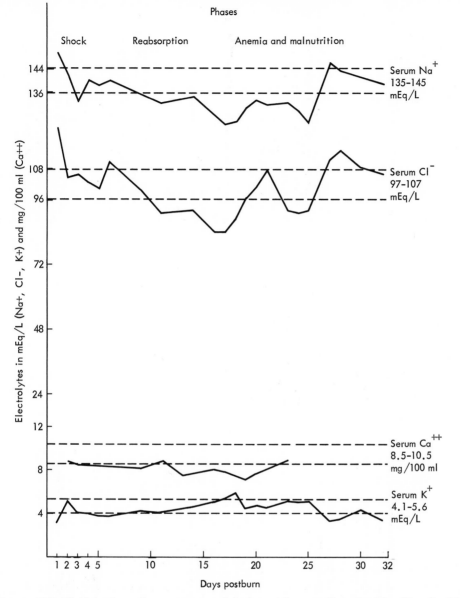

FIGURE 19-8. Fluid intake, urinary output, and body weight recordings for Mr. Allen for 32 days postburn.

TABLE 19-3

Physiological Changes, Medical Prescription and Nursing Responsibilities

Changes	Medical Prescriptions	Nurse Should:
General Description of Physiological Events that Follow Severe Thermal Trauma The end results of the complex, interrelated consequences of thermal trauma are a reduction in plasma and extracellular volume, the development of acidosis, swelling of erythrocytes, elevated hematocrit, microcirculatory stasis, decreased cardiac output, circulatory failure with fall in blood pressure, and decreasing renal blood flow. Medical therapy is aimed at averting, modifying, or correcting these abnormal physiological conditions. Sequence of events is generally as follows: 1. Heat injures cells. 2. Injured cells lose K^+ (as well as Mg^{2+} and PO_4^{2-}) and acquire Na^+. 3. Intracellular enzymes such as proteases, thromboplastin, and various "toxic factors" are released or produced. ATP is converted to ADP and ultimately to inorganic PO_4^{2-} and adenine nucleotides. Histamine is released and its production increased. Damaged cells are anoxic. Tissue perfusion is depressed by blockage of the microcirculation secondary to erythrocyte aggregation by platelet adhesion enhanced by ADP and by formation of microthrombi. Blood viscosity is also increased by these factors plus released tissue thromboplastin and hypercoagulability of the blood. Microcirculatory stasis develops locally and at a distance from the site of trauma, leading to cellular anoxia and resultant metabolic acidosis. Acidosis reduces renal blood flow. If the elevated pCO_2 of respiratory acidosis is superimposed on the reduced bicarbonate concentration of metabolic acidosis, intracellular pH can become dangerously low, leading to rapid and sudden death. 4. The acquisition of Na^+ by injured cells reduces the tonicity of the extracellular fluid; this, together with the increasing H^+ concentration of cells, causes uninjured cells to imbibe water. The intracellular gain in water from hypotonic extracellular fluid has been demonstrated to result in decrease in plasma volume without prior "plasma loss."	Three requirements of an effective burn regimen: 1. Replacement of Na^+ and water gained by the injured tissues. 2. Neutralization of an increased H^+ concentration (metabolic acidosis) and restoration of both bicarbonate and pCO_2 to normal. 3. Reduction in the viscosity and hypercoagulability of the blood.[51]	Acquire operational knowledge of the physiological events that follow severe thermal trauma. Observe for: *Dehydration* Thirst Dry mucosa Decreased turgor of intact skin Decreased salivation Weight loss Decreased urine output Elevated temperature Elevated hematocrit Increased pulse Increased specific gravity of urine Soft tongue *Hyponatremia* Muscle weakness or cramps Apathy Tremors Anorexia Decreased turgor of intact skin Increased pulse Decreased blood pressure and pulse pressure Orthostatic hypotension *Hypokalemia* Anorexia Nausea and vomiting Abdominal distention Paralytic ileus Muscle weakness Absent or weak deep tendon reflexes Depressed sensorium

[51] Charles L. Fox, Jr.: *Management of the Severely Burned Patient, with Special Reference to Fluid Therapy* (North Chicago: Abbott Laboratories, 1968), p. 26.

Metabolic acidosis
Depressed level of consciousness, some degree of disorientation
General malaise
Dull headache
Abdominal pain
Nausea and vomiting
Kussmaul respirations
Elevated pCO_2
Decreased blood pH

5. Plasma constituents, some ions, and some protein molecules accumulate in zones of injury; their transport, via the lymphatics, is greatly increased. Edema represents the influx into the zones of injury of Na^+ and water in isotonic proportions like extracellular fluid; thus the total "loss" of Na^+ in the edema fluid, plus that exchanged for cellular K^+, exceeds the "loss" of edema water into injured tissues. Reduction not only in plasma volume but also in "functioning" extracellular volume follows. The fact is that plasmapheresis (massive removal of plasma protein without salt and water) does not cause shock; plasma protein levels of 1.0g/100ml or lower may prevail with no signs of shock. In marked contrast, removal of Na^+ promptly leads to shock and circulatory collapse. Edema formation is mediated in part by bradykinin produced by the tissue proteases. If blisters are formed, some plasma proteins may be contained therein. Some plasma proteins accumulate in the edema fluid at the site of injury, with cell proteins entering the circulation, but specific "plasma loss" is a minor fraction of the total fluid shift. Actually, the plasma protein concentration is supranormal (8.0–8.5g/100 ml) soon after the burn, before fluid therapy, caused by Na^+ depletion, reflecting the movement of water out of the plasma.[52]

6. A consequence of reduction in extracellular fluid volume is augmentation of aldosterone activity, resulting in Na^+ retention and cellular K^+ loss manifested by urine low in Na^+ but high in K^+. In addition, Cl^- excretion, especially after infusion of NaCl, is relatively suppressed. The resulting metabolic acidosis inhibits the normal vasomotor response to catecholamines, which are produced in supernormal amounts and appear in the urine with bradykinin. Angiotensin II may also be produced, or activated, in small but sufficient amounts to cause intense renal vasoconstriction and stimulate the extrarenal response of increased aldosterone secretion. These factors, as well as metabolic acidosis, all contribute to a decreased renal blood flow. The metabolic acidosis arises from several sources. Following tissue destruction produced by thermal trauma, PO_4^{2-} and other intracellular acidic anions are released. These, together with lactic acid and other acids, which accumulate during intervals of impaired circulation and tissue anoxia, flow into the blood. They cause metabolic acidosis characterized by reduction in plasma HCO_3^-. The blood pH will fall until hyperpnea can ventilate the CO_2 pro-

52 *Ibid.*, pp. 24–25.

887

Table 19-3 (cont.)

Physiological Changes, Medical Prescription and Nursing Responsibilities

Changes	Medical Prescriptions	Nurse Should:
duced, and decrease the pCO_2 below normal, to restore the 20:1 ratio of bicarbonate/carbonic acid.		
7. Frequently the free egress of CO_2 is impeded by actual damage to the airways or by edema of face, nose, and especially the neck, and the pCO_2 becomes elevated above normal. If pCO_2 remains elevated despite assisted ventilation, a normal pH can be obtained only by compensated elevation in bicarbonate. There is a limit to the buffering capacity of the elevated plasma bicarbonate and hence mechanical ventilatory aids and perhaps tracheostomy may be necessary.[53]		
Mr. Allen's admission to Emergency Hospital: Mr. A was considered to be critically burned according to the starred items in the following criteria:		In clear, unexcited, low tones explain to Mr. A— whether or not he asks or seems frightened—that
1. Critical burns.		
*a. Burns complicated by respiratory tract injury.		
*b. Partial-thickness burns of more than 30% of body surface.		
*c. Full-thickness burns of face, hands, feet, genitalia, or more than 10% of body surface.		
d. Burns complicated by fractures or major soft-tissue injury.		
e. Electrical burns.		
2. Moderate burns.		
a. Partial-thickness burns of 15–30% of body surface.		
b. Full-thickness burns less than 10% of body surface, provided the hands, face, or genitalia are not involved.[54]		
3. Minor burns.		
a. Partial-thickness of less than 15% of body surface.		
b. Full-thickness of less than 2% of body surface.[54]		
Extent of Mr. A.'s burn was estimated by the rule of nines (as shown in Figure 19-6). The initial estimate of the type and amount of fluids to be administered to Mr. A in the first 48 hr was calculated by the Brooke formula, according to the severity of the burn:	Intravenous fluids for the first 24 hours:	
1. 0.5 ml of colloid per kg of body weight for each 1% of body surface burned.		

[53] *Ibid.*, p. 25.
[54] Artz and Moncrief, *op. cit.*, p. 95.

2. 1.5 ml of electrolyte (crystalloid) solution per kg of body weight for each 1% of body surface burned.[55]
3. 2000 ml of glucose in water.

Fluid and Electrolytes

Clinical shock is a preventable syndrome, provided adequate therapy can be instituted soon after injury. Patients with burns exceeding 10–15% of body surface receive the fluid equivalent of approximately 10% of body weight, or 100 ml/kg. This is given initially at the rate of at least 500 ml hourly, and more slowly subsequently depending on the status of the patient. A patient weighing 60 kg would thus receive at least 6000 ml of fluid in the first 24 hr. Of this, slightly more than half would be given in the first 12 hr.[56]

Mr. A. arrived at Emergency Hospital 1 hour after he was ignited in the dance hall. To ensure that he would receive uninterrupted fluid and electrolyte therapy essential to the early management of his burns, two percutaneous intracatheters were inserted, one in each of his subclavian veins.

Because changes in body fluids are reflected by changes in body weight, it is of the utmost importance to monitor the patient's weight frequently, regardless of the severity of illness.

Replacement therapy of burn patients cannot be undertaken blindly. The guidelines available from measurements of body weight, blood pH, urine output, and serum and urine electrolytes are of proved value in preventing the patient from being drowned with fluid.[57]

Mr. A was watched closely for signs of renal failure, which fortunately never developed; the lowest urine volume he exhibited during the shock phase was 600 ml/24 hr on the first postburn day.

There are many possible and interrelated causes of renal failure in the burn patient, but the major one is low plasma volume. Others include pigment load from intravascular hemolysis and muscle necrosis, toxins, endotoxemia, and pre-existing renal disease.[58]

Close observation of the pattern of CVP readings must accompany notation of hourly urine outputs, as they are intimately related.

55 *Ibid.*, p. 132.
56 Fox, *op. cit.*, p. 7.
57 *Ibid.*
58 Alfred P. Morgan and Francis D. Moore: "Answers to Questions on Burns," *Hosp. Med.*, **4:**71–89 (Sept.) 1968.

12,000 ml
Colloid: Albumin
Crystalloid: Ringer's Lactate
Water: 5% dextrose in water

Foley to urinometer:
Measure and record every hour.

Vital signs every hour.
Central venous pressure every 2 hr.

Weigh stat. and q.d.

---

he will have
1. Two tubes into his shoulder veins by which to feed him for a while.
2. A tube into his bladder to be sure of how his kidneys are working.
3. Medication to ease the pain and help him relax.

Set up two independent intravenous injection setups with prescribed solutions, placing one on each side of Mr. A.

Prepare a central venous pressure (CVP) set to attach to one of the conduit systems.

Set up a male catheterization tray for physician, or if he is occupied with crucial tasks, obtain a qualified male attendant.

Insert a rectal probe and attach it to the battery-powered box, which registers continuous temperatures.

Take either pedal, femoral, carotid, or supraclavicular pulses, because of the location of Mr. A's burns.

When taking CVP readings, have the bed flat and discontinue the respirator, particularly if it is a pressure-cycle type, provided the patient can tolerate the interruption.

Connect indwelling urinary catheter to sterile drainage set and a sterile, stable, calibrated collecting reservoir. A urinometer that operates automatically every hour is ideal.

Be sure connecting drainage tubing is free of any obstruction that will interfere with free gravity flow and that collecting reservoir is protected against being turned over or broken. (e.g., if a bottle is used, suspend from bed frame.) Be sure measurement is done in a receptacle with calibrations of at least as fine as 5 ml.

Unless otherwise instructed, volumes of less than 30 ml or greater than 50 ml/hour should be reported stat. to the physician.

Measure and record specific gravity every hour or as often as cumulative hourly volumes enable the

TABLE 19-3 (cont.)

Physiological Changes, Medical Prescription and Nursing Responsibilities

Changes	Medical Prescriptions	Nurse Should:

Pulmonary edema with normal CVP is possible but rare. The upper limit of safety varies with the individual patient; 20 cm of water is high (measured from a point 4 cm below the anterior chest wall at the sternal angle) and 30 cm of water is very high. Patients with valvular cardiac disease and invasive gram-negative sepsis appear to tolerate and require a higher CVP than others. Rate of rise is a better guide than absolute level. If an aliquot of 200 ml of plasma given in 30 min causes the venous pressure to increase by 5 cm of water, its absolute value being greater than 10 cm of water, there is probably no immediate need for further volume replacement.[59]
 	
 As the physicians in the emergency room were establishing access for intravenous replacement, they were simultaneously evaluating his respiratory status. They made the decision not to perform a tracheostomy, despite his face and neck burns, but to watch him closely for any signs of obstruction. At no time did Mr. A require either intubation or a tracheostomy, except for purposes of administering anesthesia later in his postburn course when grafting procedures were performed in the operating room, after the third burn day.
 	
 Pulmonary Complications
 Pulmonary complications are replacing burn wound sepsis as the most common cause of death in burn patients, in some burn centers, because of the introduction of topical chemotherapy. Despite the common usage of the term *respiratory burn*, there is little evidence to support the existence of thermal coagulation necrosis of the tracheobronchial tree as a clinical or pathological entity in the absence of inhalation of steam or readily combustible vapors or gases. Reflex closure of the glottis, the cooling effect of the upper airway, and the poor heat-carrying capacity of air all account for the protection of the respiratory tree. Inhalation of irritating combustible products, however, can produce severe respiratory difficulties. Tracheobronchitis may be rapidly progressive and result in necrotizing inflammation in the lower
		urinometer to float. A concentration in excess of 1.020–1.030 may indicate progressive hemoconcentration and should be reported.
		 Note character of the urine for:
		   Deepening amber color
		   Pink tinge (blood ?)
		   Casts, sediment (albumin or cells ?)
		   Odor
		 Observe for signs of pulmonary edema:
		   Increased restlessness
		   Cyanosis of toenail beds, feet, conjunctival sac
		   Increase in moist, labored respirations
		   Complaints of feeling of chest constriction, desire to sit up
		   Marked increase in pulse
		   Alteration (possible decrease) in blood pressure
		   Increased CVP
		   Hemoptysis
		 On admission, observe for:
		   Singed nasal hairs
		   Blackened rim of nares, especially when adjacent skin is not burned
		   Rapid, noisy respirations—as wind passing over a dry reed
		   Dry, wracking cough
		   Cyanosis of unburned skin and toenail beds
		   Rales
		   Black particles and/or blood in sputum
		 Know location and operation of:
		   Oxygen equipment
		   Respirators
		   Laryngoscope
		   Endotracheal tubes
		   Tracheostomy set
		   Aspirator

[59] *Ibid.*, p. 77.

890

respiratory tree with sloughing of the mucosa. In addition, this injury decreases the efficiency with which the ciliated epithelium protects the lower respiratory tree. Mucosal and submucosal swelling results in obstruction of varying degrees. Bronchial wheezing and rales can be heard. Fatal pneumonia is the ultimate result. Burns in the facial area have been suggested as a warning to the physician of this possible complication. However, the extent and depth of burn are of greater significance. Usually the respiratory distress begins 18–36 hr after the injury.[60]

Postmortem pathological findings in the respiratory tree seem to be related to prolonged positive pressure ventilatory assistance with oxygen. Major trauma and shock have been shown to cause decreases in surfacant, with resultant atelectasis causing alterations in diffusion and perfusion. (See Chapter 11.)

If there is doubt as to involvement of the pulmonary tract, fall in pO_2 or a rise in pCO_2 will indicate the need for improving ventilation. In contrast, a falling plasma bicarbonate concentration will indicate need for additional sodium bicarbonate solution rather than the balanced electrolyte solution with which fluid replacement therapy is begun.[61]

Impaired respiratory mechanics and obstruction of the upper airway are the two most critical indications for tracheostomy and/or ventilation. Otherwise, even in the presence of facial and neck burns, singed nasal hairs and a history of smoke inhalation, the decision for tracheostomy should be deferred.[62]

Patients with smoke inhalation may demonstrate immediate or delayed hoarseness or begin expectorating sooty mucus. Humidification is strongly recommended, preferably with ultrasonic nebulizers, which provide very fine water particles less than 5 μ in diameter, which can reach the lower bronchial tree. The hyperventilation of burned patients can quickly desiccate the tracheobronchial mucosa.[63]

Deep-breathing and coughing should be encouraged frequently. Occasionally, instillation of saline through a percutaneous tracheal catheter effectively stimulates the cough reflex. Direct suctioning down the tracheobronchial tree produces considerable truama and irritation of an already inflamed mucosa. Whether through the nasal route or directly through the tracheostomy, suctioning should be performed *gently*. The most important part of the endotracheal aspiration is the stimulation of the cough reflex. As

Cough, deep-breathe frequently. Chest x-ray two times per week.

Measure and record the circumference of the neck q.4.h. (Mr. A's increased 1 in. the first 24 hr; despite this, he was able to breathe adequately unassisted and without tracheostomy.)
Stimulate cough reflex with tip of suction catheter, which should not be passed into the trachea below the larynx or into the bronchi but only to the point of stimulating the patient to cough. Use scrupulous surgical aseptic technique in handling the suction catheter.

Instruct Mr. A to deep-breathe and cough (starred items were not feasible with Mr. A because of the location of his burns):
* 1. Inspire against pressure of nurse's hands on anterolateral surface of thorax.
* 2. Expire forcibly, with assistance of nurse's hands, to compress thorax as completely as possible.
3. After a sequence of exchanges, cough at the onset of the expiratory phase.
4. Have tissue over Mr. A's nose and mouth before he coughs.
5. Instruct, demonstrate, and supervise him in the use of blow bottles.

---

60 Jerry M. Shuck and John A. Moncrief: "The Management of Burns: General Considerations and Sulfamylon Method," *Curr. Probl. Surg.*, p. 7 (Feb.) 1969.
61 Fox, *op. cit.*, p. 14.
62 Shuck and Moncrief, *op. cit.*, p. 12.
63 *Ibid.*, p. 19.

TABLE 19-3 (cont.)

Physiological Changes, Medical Prescription and Nursing Responsibilities

Changes	Medical Prescriptions	Nurse Should:
the patient brings the secretions up high in the trachea, they should then be gently aspirated. Vigorous and deep probing of stiff catheters down the tracheobronchial tree is to be condemned.[64] Progressive activity, especially ambulation when burned surfaces do not include the feet, should begin even during the early postburn period as one of the best means of preventing pulmonary complications.[65] Enthusiasm for the use of intermittent positive pressure breathing must be tempered with caution, as these devices are potential sources of infection.[65] *Skin and Vascular Problems* Although age and general physical condition prior to the thermal injury influence mortality in major burns, the ultimate determining factor in survival is the burn wound itself. Both the depth and extent of the burn are critical. The characteristic pathological lesion caused by thermal injury is coagulation necrosis. Before healing can be complete, this necrotic tissue must be sloughed and replaced by skin. If only a portion of the thickness of skin is involved, then regeneration of skin can take place from remaining epidermal elements. If the full thickness of skin is destroyed, healing of the wound will require the use of skin grafts.[66] As indicated previously, Mr. A had full thickness burns of over 50% of his body surface. Prior to the final healing of the burn wound, the effects of thermal injury on the skin covering of the patient are major factors influencing ultimate survival. The chemical and physical alterations in the skin render this organ incapable of serving its function in the over-all body homeostasis. The vapor barrier capacity of the skin, which preserves the aqueous milieu of the body, is an important quality of normal skin. The keratinized superficial skin layers and the lipids within the skin normally prevent the escape of large volumes of water. A superficial second-degree burn may		Help Mr. A learn how, and how much, to move himself in bed. (More details in relation to mobility problems.) Because Mr. A had no involvement of his feet, he was helped to stand and shift his weight from one foot to the other by the eighth postburn day.

[64] *Ibid.*, p. 20.
[65] *Ibid.*, p. 21.
[66] Shuck and Moncrief, *op. cit.*, pp. 4-5.

Conserve heat loss, and thus energy expenditure, by creating and maintaining environmental temperature and humidity at a level that will allow Mr. A, at rest, to be in a state of thermal neutrality:

1. Collaborate with physicians, hospital engineers and architects, nursing and hospital supervisory personnel, and equipment salesmen to develop means by which to gain more precise control over environmental temperature and humidity.
2. Try to maintain a temperature of 75–80°F and a humidity of 40–70%, being guided to alterations by the response of Mr. A in terms of his report of what feels comfortable, results of frequent measurements of his body temperature, and any objective evidence of shivering.[71]
3. Initiate, request, or offer to participate in multidisciplinary research on the effects of control of environmental temperature and humidity on the duration of the catabolic phase in the postburn period.

destroy the keratinized surface and permit increased water vaporization. Full-thickness coagulation necrosis of the skin destroys not only the keratin but also the lipid-containing portions of the skin. The dry, full-thickness burn has practically no vapor barrier. Although to visual inspection it appears otherwise, evaporation through a dry eschar is much greater than water loss from an equal surface of wet, blistered skin. Not until full, mature epithelium, regrown or grafted, covers the wound does water vaporization return to essentially normal levels.[66]

With a large portion of the body surface burned, loss of water vapor may result in rapid dehydration of a patient. The peak period of vapor loss is between 5 and 10 days postburn. After this time, there is a gradual reduction of water loss, but evaporation continues to be greatly increased until coverage of the burn wound itself by skin is obtained. Because 1 sq m of full-thickness burn can lose up to 3,000 ml of water per hour, an adult with a 50% full-thickness burn can lose over 6 liters of water per day. With each liter of water requiring 560 calories for evaporation, the caloric expense of such a burn may be up to 4,000 calories for evaporation of water alone.[67]

[The total number of calories per hour liberated by an individual is divided by his total body surface area, which, for the average adult, is 1.73 sq m. This means that his basal metabolic rate is 48.3 calories/sq m/hour, or approximately 1965 calories in 24 hr (48.3 calories × 1.73 sq m × 24 hr)].[68] Considering that Mr. A had a 50% full-thickness burn, its caloric expense was more than twice that required by his body surface in the unburned state. Such an enormous expenditure of energy accompanying heat loss usually results in a marked drop in body temperature, resulting in a relative hypothermia. Further energy in the form of muscular activity is then required to maintain the body temperature at anything approaching a normal thermal response. When heat loss exceeds heat production, an absolute hypothermia exists.[69] Clinical data suggest that manipulation of the ambient temperature and water vapor pressure by more precise methods might actually permit the achievement of thermal neutrality in the burned patient.[70]

The flow of blood through vessels of the local area is related to the

67 Ibid., p. 5.
68 Arthur C. Guyton: Textbook of Medical Physiology, 3rd ed. (Philadelphia: W. B. Saunders Company, 1966), pp. 982–83.
69 Shuck and Moncrief, op. cit., p. 5.
70 Ibid., p. 57.
71 William R. Price and MacDonald Wood: "Operating Room Care of Burned Patients Treated with Silver Nitrate," Amer. J. Nurs., 68:1705–1707 (Aug.) 1968.

TABLE 19-3 (cont.)

Physiological Changes, Medical Prescription and Nursing Responsibilities

Changes	Medical Prescriptions	Nurse Should:
vascular alterations from the coagulative thermal injury to the burn tissue. The degree of thrombosis of the blood supply in the wound is in proportion to the intensity and duration of the heat applied. Where the heat injury has been intense, a blood coagulum without fibrin develops in the vessels. In addition, agglutination of red blood cells forms overt thrombi. Within 24 hr, the devitalized tissue at the site of the burn injury shows marked edema, without subcutaneous cellular infiltration. The obstructed circulation around a third-degree burn prevents access of blood-borne inflammatory elements to the site of injury, which is responsible for the minimal inflammatory response in the burn wound, even in the presence of infection of the devitalized tissue. After 1 week, granulation tissue begins to develop and brings with it a new blood supply but is not an effective barrier to infection for 3 weeks.[72] In the absence of infection, the period of avascularity of the partial-thickness burn usually lasts only 24–48 hr, though circulation may be decreased for longer periods. Preservation of the deep epithelial elements from destruction by infection or ischemia prevents the conversion of second-degree burns to third-degree burns.[72]		
One of the most frequent sites of infection is related to the need of the burned patient for intravenous fluids, while his vascular system is ideally suited to the proliferation of microorganisms that may enter via any route. Approximately one fourth of patients who have had a cutdown develop some complication, ranging from mild cellulitis around the cutdown site to frank suppurative thrombophlebitis with septicemia. Although the saphenous venous system is the most common area for suppurative thrombophlebitis, sepsis has occurred from infected veins in the upper extremities as well as the external jugular system.[73] Mr. A showed no evidence of suppurative thrombophlebitis, despite the fact that both subclavian intracatheters were kept in considerably longer, on a continuous basis, than the recommended 72 hr.	Intracatheter 1: Discontinue on postburn day 4. Intracatheter 2: Discontinue on postburn day 16.	Observe for signs and symptoms of (suppurative) thrombophlebitis: 1. Tender vein with a red streak. 2. Pus coming from cutdown site. 3. Abscesses along the course of the vein. 4. Complaint of burning or pain along vein when intracatheter is irrigated to keep it patent. (This is probably the most sensitive and earliest symptom of inflammation of the vein.)[74]

[72] Shuck and Moncrief, op. cit., p. 5.

[73] Ibid., p. 46.

[74] Lucy M. Brand, Assistant Professor, College of Nursing, Wayne State University, Detroit, Michigan: an observation based on her 5 years of experience in caring for the acutely ill surgical patient, including burned patients.

Management of the Burn Wound

Occlusive dressings are no longer recommended for major burns. Patients are frequently febrile and have little control over their temperature-regulating mechanism, and occlusive dressings interfere with heat loss. Dressings must be changed at least every 2–3 days, requiring general anesthetic, which interrupts the patient's oral intake. In addition, the absence of physical therapy, febrile courses, lack of daily inspection of the burn wound, and the requirement of using an operating room all weigh against occlusive dressings as the primary mode of therapy for large areas of burn.[75]

For a short period postburn, the surface of the wound is generally sterile. Within 48 hr, however, bacteria appear to contaminate the surface of the wound and then colonize the depths of the eschar. The source of the contaminating bacteria is not generally agreed on. Studies of the numberous phage types of *Pseudomonas aeruginosa* that may involve the wounds of different patients on the same ward strongly suggest that this microorganism may constitute a part of a given patient's normal flora prior to injury. Thus the role of self-contamination in the pathogenesis of burn wound colonization is presently under serious consideration. Failure to prevent bacterial colonization of wounds under the most aseptic ward precautions may well lie in the problem of self-contamination of wounds by the patient's own cutaneous or fecal flora.[76] The presence of bacteria within the hair follicles may prevent their detection on swab cultures of the skin surface.[77]

All hair should be shaved from the burned area and from adjacent sites of unburned skin and shaved frequently throughout the hospital course to prevent crusting and its attendant proliferating of microorganisms.[78]

Pseudomonas aeruginosa has been recognized with increasing frequency as the most prevalent colonizer and deadly invader of the burn wound. Staphylococci and certainly streptococci no longer occupy the positions of importance that they formerly held in relation to the establishment of fatal infection.[79]

Any successful, objective treatment of patients with extensive burns

Validate with the attending physician whether or not strict medical asepsis, including gown, gloves, and masks, are required before going to the enormous preparation of such a unit. It may be that careful hand washing, careful assignment of the smallest possible number of persons to render care to the patient, and use of pHisoHex for all general hygiene will suffice.

Check with attending physician as to whether or not he wishes the patient to be shaved. If he does, carry out the procedure with sterile technique and pHisoHex solution.

[75] Shuck and Moncrief, *op. cit.*, p. 28.
[76] Artz and Moncrief, *op. cit.*, p. 29.
[77] *Ibid.*, p. 30.
[78] Shuck and Moncrief, *op. cit.*, p. 27.
[79] Artz and Moncrief, *op. cit.*, p. 31.

TABLE 19-3 (cont.)

Physiological Changes, Medical Prescription and Nursing Responsibilities

Changes	Medical Prescriptions	Nurse Should:
must provide for effective wound bacteriostasis, until epithelialization is complete, impede the leak of water vapor through the wound, and permit closure of it with skin or a satisfactory substitute at the earliest possible moment.[80] The ideal topical antiseptic should meet several criteria: 1. Effective clinical bacteriostasis. 2. Nonabsorbability, and therefore lack of systemic toxicity. 3. Absence of direct histotoxicity or of potent allergenicity. One-half per cent aqueous silver nitrate solution reasonably satisfies these criteria, both hypothetically and clinically.[81] Because of the disadvantages of the patient's being constantly wet, and the subsequent added heat and energy loss, silver nitrate cream or ointment base has been developed that has retained all the advantages of the active ingredient, silver nitrate, and has eliminated much of the discomfort for the patient and tediousness of application for the nursing staff of continuous wet dressings. The silver nitrate cream applied to Mr. A was in hydrophilic ointment, which contains the following ingredients:	Apply 0.5% AgNO₃ cream dressings every day to all burned areas and to donor sites. Start immediately on admission from the emergency room (first post-burn day).	Gently remove old dressings. Wash all surfaces with solution of sterile water and pHisoHex. Apply cream to large burn dressings, in advance of uncovering patient by removing his old dressings, to prevent chilling him. Apply dressings to wound, placing them properly the first time, to avoid rubbing dressing across burn surface. Wrap dressings with Kling, flannel, or stockinette. Remove and treat dressings gently to avoid removing grafts.

Stearyl alcohol, 250 g
Methylparaben, 0.25 g
Prophylparaben, 0.15 g
Polyoxyl-40 stearate, 50 g
Propylene glycol, 120 g
Water, 330 g [82]

Silver has practically no allergenic potential and a low systemic toxicity. Because of the minimum absorption of silver that occurs through burn wounds, argyria has not been observed in any patient treated in this way. The silver salts of the biologically important anions (chloride, carbonate, proteinate) are highly insoluble. This is the reason that no significant absorption of silver occurs through wounds. Application of silver nitrate to open burns results in the precipitation of silver salts on the wound. A brown or blue-black keratinous crust of these salts forms over newly healed or epithelializing surfaces and on eschar as well.[83]

80 William A. Monafo: "The Management of Burns: The Silver Nitrate Method," *Curr. Probl. Surg.*, pp. 53–66 (Feb.) 1969.
81 *Ibid.*, p. 54.
82 Contents according to Emergency Hospital Pharmacy.

Because of the insolubility of these silver salts, and because of the hypotonicity of silver nitrate, the dressing causes the leaching from the wounds of significant amounts of the serum minerals and possibly of the water-soluble vitamins and other substances. This loss into the dressing continues until the wounds are epithelialized and, for Na+ and Cl−, is a constant function of the surface area of open wound.[83]

In patients with burns of more than 20% in extent, there are frequently clinically significant deficits of Na+, Cl−, and K+ and less frequently of Ca2+ and Mg2+. Deficits can be induced by the dressing within as little as 6 hr but is most likely to occur within the first few weeks following injury. By this time the patient is usually on oral intake, and so dietary supplement of NaCl, K, and Ca must be adequate and regulated according to the serum and urine concentrations of these minerals and the absence or presence of the clinical signs of their deficits.[84]

NaCl tablets	Observe for:	
Ca gluconate tablets	Hyponatremia	
KCl liquid	Hypochloremia	
Vitamin C tablets	Hypokalemia	
Multivitamin tablets	Hypocalcemia:	
	Tetany	
	Trousseau's sign	
	Chvostek's sign	
	Paresthesias	
	Muscle spasm (especially of facial muscles)	
	Mood changes	

Give vitamin and mineral supplements with feedings or meals to minimize the amount of water required to be taken by Mr. A.

As can be seen in Figure 19-7, Mr. A experienced generalized electrolyte imbalance beginning about the tenth postburn day, which was believed to be caused by the effects of his silver nitrate dressings.

Topical 0.5% silver nitrate is not an escharotic and will not injure regenerating epithelium or other normal tissue. In a series of more than 140 patients treated with topical silver nitrate, not once did a full-thickness wound result at any of the donor sites subsequent to the cutting of split-thickness skin grafts; all donor sites were continuously covered with the silver nitrate dressing. Donor sites treated like this healed regularly within 10–12 days so that the recutting of more skin from them was then routinely possible.[85]

Penicillin and oxacillin are given routinely throughout convalescence as a precaution against streptococcal and staphylococcal lymphangitis.[86]

Aqueous penicillin q.6 h.
Tetracycline q.6 h.
Check temperature q.4 h.
If temperature is over 101°F, get blood culture.
Then give Tylenol p.r.n.

Observe for sensitivity:
Fever with chills
Angioedema
Decreased blood pressure
Increased pulse

83 Monafo, *op. cit.*, p. 55.
84 *Ibid.*
85 *Ibid.*, p. 56.
86 *Ibid.*, p. 57.

TABLE 19-3 (cont.)

Physiological Changes, Medical Prescription and Nursing Responsibilities

Changes	Medical Prescriptions	Nurse Should:
Salt is added to the tub bath to lessen the osmotic gradient and thus to decrease the loss of electrolytes and minimize subsequent dehydration.	Eighth postburn day: Tub bath q.d. for débridement before daily dressings. Add 1½ lb of NaCl to bath water.	Prepare dressings for application before taking Mr. A to tub room. Have tub room as steamy and warm as possible before removing old dressings. Keep water running slowly while Mr. A is in the tub to help maintain temperature of the water. Weigh Mr. A when he gets out of the tub and before applying new dressings.
Homograft skin is placed over the granulating surface for no more than 4–5 days, because its removal becomes progressively difficult. If left longer, at the time of removal bleeding and the retention of dermal homograft remnants in the granulating surface are troublesome.[87]		Be very careful in removing old dressings in tub that homografts are not pulled or washed off. (Mr. A's most severely burned areas were disappointing in their response to homografts. Often the homografts would float to the surface of the bath water soon after Mr. A was immersed.)
Homografts serve many functions in the treatment of the burn wound. Their use tends to clean up untidy wounds, because débridement is effected with each homograft change. They provide a vapor barrier for the granulating surface with resultant decrease in water evaporation and exudation. They also serve as an excellent test of the granulating surface for its acceptability to autograft, which is especially important in large burns in which donor sites are limited and autograft failure can be disastrous. In massive burns, where donor sites must be used more than once, the homograft will preserve granulation tissue until donor sites can be reharvested. After homograft has been applied, the wound becomes immediately and dramatically free of pain.[88]	Discontinue Demerol and Valium (sixteenth postburn day).	
On admission, Mr. A had suffered extensive destruction of his body's first barrier of defense against invasion of microorganisms, and he was covered with charred clothing. He was therefore subject to infection by anaerobic microbes, especially Clostridium tetani.	Tetanus toxoid, 0.5 ml s.c., stat.	Explain that the injection is to protect him against infection. Because this induces active immunity, observe for signs and symptoms of anaphylaxis. (See Chapter 6.)
"Burn wound sepsis" is a pathological entity characterized by the presence of greater than 10^5 organisms per gram of tissue with demonstrable invasion of adjacent unburned tissues.[89] Develop-		Observe for septicemia: Paralytic ileus Increased bleeding tendency

[87] Shuck and Moncrief, op. cit., p. 39.
[88] Ibid.
[89] Ibid.

ment of burn wound sepsis creates a condition that facilitates invasion of the blood stream by colonizing microorganisms. The onset of septicemia may be insidious or acute. A blood culture in any burned patient whose rectal temperature is 103°F or higher is indicated.

Mild jaundice
Elevated body temperature
Increased pulse
Decreased blood pressure
Decreased urine output
Confusion, disorientation

Before leaving discussion of changes in the skin of a burned patient, it is necessary to point out one of the enormous advantages of using topical antiseptics in the treatment of the burn wound; there is absolutely none of the previously characteristic foul smell that promptly identified the presence of a burned patient on any hospital unit. This improvement alone has made the illness and its prolonged treatment more bearable for patients and has helped nursing personnel attack the many nursing problems of the burned patient with greater zeal.

Urinary Bladder

In a two-year study of 88 autopsies on fatally burned individuals at the U.S. Army Surgical Research Unit, 62% were found to have bacteriuria, and 100% of these either still had the indwelling catheter in place or had recently had it removed.[90]

Give scrupulous attention to perineal care, especially around the urethral orifice, while an indwelling catheter is in place.
Urge the physician to endorse removal of the catheter as soon as evidence of Mr. A's fluid status and ability to take oral fluids warrants.

Remove Foley catheter, but continue to measure and record urinary output (seventh postburn day).

Prepare Mr. A's family and visitors for the changes in his appearance, before they go in to visit him, to prevent their shock from being an additional burden on Mr. A's already overstressed psychological status.

Chondritis of the Ear

The pathogenesis of chondritis of the ear in burned patients remains a mystery. The complication usually develops late, during the second and fifth week postburn. Depth of burn is no indication of the ultimate course. *Pseudomonas* and *staphylococcus aureus* are the most frequently cultured organisms from this site, but there are instances of sterile culture and frank necrosis. The incidence is unaffected by the use of topical antiseptic treatment. The patient complains of severe pain, and swelling and redness of the ear become apparent. Spontaneous rupture with drainage of purulent material may occur directly through healed second-degree burn or in areas of complete skin loss. Drainage and total removal of necrotic cartilage are required. When destruction is extensive, it may be necessary to remove all of the cartilage. The end result is a markedly deformed ear.[91] On the twenty-fourth postburn day, Mr. A's right ear and right nostril began to drain green purulent exudate. Within 3 weeks, the entire external ear

90 Artz and Moncrief, *op. cit.*, p. 83.
91 Shuck and Moncrief, *op. cit.*, pp. 48–49.

TABLE 19-3 (cont.)

Physiological Changes, Medical Prescription and Nursing Responsibilities

Changes	Medical Prescriptions	Nurse Should:
had had to be removed, and the distal third of the right side of the nose was also completely excised.		
Eye The problem of burns around the eyes involves primarily the periorbital tissues, especially the lids. Appropriate care involves prevention of secondary injury to the eye from infection or exposure. During the early course of face burns, it is important to irrigate the eyes several times a day with normal saline solution to wash out exudate and debris. After irrigation, an antibiotic ophthalmic ointment or solution should be instilled 3 or 4 times a day.	Bleph gtts. both eyes (o.u.) 5.i.d. Neosporin ophthalmic ointment both eyes at h.s.	
If conjunctiva is exposed because of contraction of eyelids, inflammation and corneal ulceration may develop rapidly. Exposure of the cornea while the patient is sleeping and intractable conjunctivitis are indications for early release of eyelid contractures (by means of tarsorrhaphy).[92]		Speak on entering the room, because Mr. A recognizes voices and can see shapes and colors but is not able to distinguish individuals by their features.
Mr. A developed severe eyelid contractures and by the end of the seventh postburn week had vision limitation because of corneal changes. Treatment was still local, and no surgical procedure had been performed to release the contractures at that time, but it was being considered.		Try to increase amount and frequency of ambulation with someone accompanying him to counteract the increasing sense of isolation that may accompany impairment of this very vital sense. Ask physician if he would approve frequent administration of methyl cellulose eye gtts., to prevent further drying and deterioration of the cornea until such time as the eyelid contractures are released.
Musculoskeletal System One of the most formidable obstacles to maintaining or restoring mobility in the burned patient is the patient's fear of pain or fear of moving a burned extremity because of anticipation of pain. If the patient learns early that he can move his limbs without causing extreme discomfort, he is better able to cooperate with subsequent efforts. After even a few days or a week of absolute	Encourage ambulation (on eighth postburn day). Range-of-motion exercises with dressing changes while in bathtub.	

92 *Ibid.*, p. 50.

immobility following acute burn trauma, the patient will be extremely fearful of and resistant to any passive or active motion.[93] Throughout the period covered by this report of Mr. A's injury and hospitalization, his responses to efforts to move him either passively or actively were consistent with the preceding description; every success in getting him to move either a single joint or his whole body was accomplished only with painstaking persistence, patience, and endless time and reassurance. It is a testimony to his nursing care that within the first 3 weeks postburn Mr. A was able to hold his own glass by cupping both covered hands around the container; was able to get in and out of bed by himself, though it required from 15 to 20 min for each operation; and was able to ambulate around the ward unassisted.

It is significant to note that the extent to which he was willing to make the effort required to accomplish the preceding activities on his own depended largely on who was encouraging or pushing him. It seems evident that, with the severely burned patient perhaps more than with any other type of patient, the nurse must reinforce the will to live and to try by caring enough to continually harass the patient. Perhaps her persistent caring is the best means he has of knowing that, despite his disfigurement and relative helplessness, he is still worthy of being a person with a future.

The goals of physical therapy are relatively simple:
1. Prevention of contracture.
2. Maintenance of joint motion.
3. Maintenance of muscle tone.

Accomplishment of the goals of physical therapy is through the recognized measures of positioning and of active, passive, resistive, and isometric exercise. In positioning, special attention is given to all major joints: ankles, knees, hips, shoulders, elbows, wrists and hands.[94]

Ankles are supported at 90 degrees of dorsiflexion.
Knees are straight but not hyperextended.
Hips are in neutral rotation and symmetrically abducted to 10–15 degrees.
Shoulders are abducted at least 60 degrees and are alternately externally and internally rotated.
Elbows are flexed no more than 30–40 degrees.
Wrists are supported in slight extension.

93 Artz and Moncrief, op. cit., p. 348.
94 Ibid., pp. 348-49.

Alternate flat and elevated headrest to prevent hip flexion deformity.
Apply AgNO$_3$ cream directly to burned surfaces of hands, and then apply white cotton gloves to increase possible range of motion in the hand.
Apply forearm splints during extended rest periods of the day and at h.s.
Teach and remind to do exercises of the facial muscles.

Have Mr. A transferred to a Circo-Electric bed as soon as one is obtained. (This was accomplished for Mr. A at the beginning of the second postburn month.)

Position, turn, and exercise him to provide optimum exposure of all burned areas, redistribution of pressure, and immobilization of arms and head:
1. Head must be in neutral position with sandbags placed to prevent rotation (to protect grafts on neck) when Mr. A is on posterior frame.

TABLE 19-3 (cont.)

Physiological Changes, Medical Prescription and Nursing Responsibilities

Changes	Medical Prescriptions	Nurse Should:
At the metacarpophalangeal joints, fingers are allowed to drop into flexion, and the thumb into an abducted and slightly flexed position. In burns of the neck, the head is positioned so that there is slight extension of the neck but no more than that amount that will allow the patient to close his mouth easily.[95] In each case, the position chosen or prescribed is the one that facilitates the most useful position for subsequent movement of the body. The amount of active motion possible in the burned extremity is determined by whether or not joints are bridged by unburned skin and by whether or not grafts have been applied within the past 48–72 hr.[96] Because of the primary role of the hand in our ability to be self-sufficient, one of the most serious threats to mobility is the development of interphalangeal joint stiffness. This stiffness is not caused by the burn itself, but happens during the period of systemic treatment of the burned patient and results from immobilization, edema, contraction, and fibrous-protein synthesis as the wound begins to heal.[97] Muscle atrophy progresses relentlessly in the catabolic phase following a severe burn; although this cannot be prevented, a degree of muscle tone and muscle awareness can be retained. In the catabolic phase, which in most patients roughly corresponds to that period preceding healthy granulating surfaces or the formation of healthy granulating surfaces, no measures, dietary or otherwise, will bring the patient into nitrogen equilibrium. The nitrogen loss through exudate, but principally through the urine, far exceeds any realistic dietary intake.[98] Evidence does not support the assumption that the routine programmed exercise of the severely burned patient impedes skeletal demineralization. Immobility is only one of the causes of bony atrophy in severe burns, and considered alongside protein deficit		2. On anterior frame, forehead support and body weight promote immobilization. 3. Do not address Mr. A until you are standing directly in his vision. Place bed so he can see those entering his room without having to turn his head. 4. Teach, supervise, and encourage: Quadriceps setting exercises. Gluteal setting exercises. Flexion extension exercises of legs and feet. Wiggling toes and pressing on footboard. (See Chapter 17.) 5. Keep elbow joint as nearly straight as possible, support arms (under elbow to produce extension) with rolled towels, bath blankets, or small pillows to elevate hands just above shoulder (to promote venous return and decrease edema of wrapped hands) when Mr. A is on posterior frame. 6. On anterior frame, support to arms should be placed under wrists with arms extended so that weight of arms will keep elbow joint straight. 7. As soon as facial burns have granulated, Mr. A should be encouraged to chew gum and blow up balloons.

[95] Ibid., pp. 349–50.
[96] Ibid., p. 353.
[97] Erle E. Peacock, Jr., "Burned Hands: And How to Heal Them," Consultant, 9:18–20 (Mar.–Apr.) 1969.
[98] Artz and Moncrief, op. cit., p. 357.

and hyperadrenalism, it could easily be the least important. It is, however, one factor that can be controlled to some extent from the outset. It is safe to assume that exercise affects favorably the degree of local atrophy in burned extremities, whereas its effect on generalized demineralization is probably negligible.[99]

Protein Metabolism

Proteins are the basic components of cellular protoplasm, composed of carbon, hydrogen, oxygen, nitrogen, and often sulfur. With complete hydrolysis, proteins yield various crystalline amino acids, which may be
1. Synthesized into protein.
2. Metabolized to H_2O and CO_2 for energy production.
3. Converted to glucose or fat.

Of the 23 known amino acids, 10 are essential in the diet because they cannot be synthesized in the body; foods containing these are called complete proteins. Incomplete protein can be synthesized from products of glucose and fat metabolism and also occurs in vegetable proteins.

Amino acids absorbed in the intestine go directly to the liver via the portal vein, where some are stored and others are sent on to body tissues.

In the absence of food, protein will be deprived of its nitrogen and converted into glucose to keep up the blood sugar level and to provide the glucose essential to the burning of the body fat for fuel. As much as 58% of protein, by weight, may thus be turned to glucose to be burned along with fat for fuel, or serve as the sole source of fuel when body fat is exhausted. The nitrogen output of the fasting man is thus raised because he uses protein for fuel as well as for building purposes.

To minimize this extravagant use of protein in a patient unable to ingest (or digest) food by the oral route, carbohydrate should be given to supply the glucose necessary to provide energy and spare protein.

The normal adult is in nitrogen equilibrium; intake equals excretion, and the total quantity of protein stores remains essentially

[99] *Ibid.*, p. 358.

Encourage complete proteins:
Milk
Eggs
Cheese and cottage cheese
Fish
Fowl
Liver, kidneys
Veal
Pork
Lamb
Lean meat

Encourage proportional intake of incomplete proteins:
Legumes: 3–4 servings per day
Cereals
Cereal products: whole wheat bread, crackers

Encourage low alkaline ash juices (to minimize renal calculus formation while increasing vitamin, mineral, and fluid intake):
Cranberry juice
Raspberry juice
Plum juice

Assess Mr. A's tolerance for, and encourage:
Cream soups
Eggnogs, flavored if necessary
Meat stock broth
Identify Mr. A's favorite drinks:
Fruit juices
Milk
Beer (This presented some problem to obtain.)

Refrain from forcing more than Mr. A takes willingly.

TABLE 19-3 (cont.)

Physiological Changes, Medical Prescription and Nursing Responsibilities

Changes	Medical Prescriptions	Nurse Should:
stable. Positive nitrogen balance implies that the rate of anabolism exceeds the rate of catabolism. Negative nitrogen balance exists when catabolism exceeds anabolism.		to avoid his developing a strong aversion to food early in his convalescence. Allow 10 to 15 min for offering liquids, as his willingness to drink may be in direct proportion to the relaxation and encouragement of nurse's attitude. Observe closely for: 1. Eructation. 2. Nausea. 3. Abdominal distention. 4. Complaints of cramps, abdominal pain. Discontinue feedings if any of the preceding signs or symptoms develop, and report to physician immediately.
An adult ingesting a normal diet excretes from 10–15 g of urinary nitrogen per day; the same adult, following an extensive burn, may excrete as much as 30 g of urinary nitrogen per day. During the first few days postburn, increased excretion of urinary nitrogen is not evident because of impaired renal function. High excretion becomes evident within 3–5 days postburn, reaching a maximum in the first and second postburn week. Magnitude of urinary nitrogen loss varies with the following factors: 1. There is a rough correlation between the severity of the burn and the amount of nitrogen excreted; the more extensive the burn, the larger the nitrogen excretion. 2. Preburn body weight is positively correlated with nitrogen excretion. 3. Men generally excrete more than women. 4. Usually, increased nitrogen excretion does not occur in patients malnourished before injury.		
Burned patients are usually unable to accept an adequate oral diet during the early postburn period. Starvation, with its disproportionate lean tissue destruction, leads to hypoproteinemia very early. The nitrogen excretion from major thermal injury can approach 40 g/day. Starvation in the uninjured individual is compensated by a decrease in resting metabolism, but the burned patient has a tremendous increase in metabolic activity as reflected by oxygen utilization. The metabolic expenditure during the first postburn week is 200% of normal. In addition, in the burned patient, total metabolic expenditure cannot be lowered, and as catabolism proceeds, there are decreased stores for energy conversion. As open or infected wounds produce exudation, further protein loss occurs. Two to three grams of protein for each percentage of burn is the average loss per 24 hr, and as much		

as 7–8 g of protein for each percentage of body surface burned can be lost from a burn wound in 1 day.[100]

A loss of 30 g of tissue protein represents an accompanying loss of approximately 1 g of total protein per 100 ml of serum; thus early wound closure is of paramount importance. In this same postburn period, a low nitrogen intake contributes further to the negative nitrogen balance.

In the early postburn period, Mr. A was in negative nitrogen balance (excessive catabolism) because of imbalance created by excessive losses in wound exudate and increased excretion of urinary nitrogen, mostly as urea, resulting from hydrolysis of proteins for energy and extensive destruction of tissue protein by burn injury. When amino acids are burned for fuel, they are deprived of their nitrogen and reduced to compounds containing only carbon-hydrogen-oxygen, which burn like sugar and fat. The nitrogen, being of no use as fuel, is converted into a relatively harmless soluble substance, urea, and excreted in the urine.

An energetic nutritional regimen of a high-protein, high-caloric diet, instituted 7–10 days after burning, may reduce substantially the duration of negative nitrogen balance. Unless special efforts are made to achieve ingestion of such a diet, negative nitrogen balance can be expected to last more than a mouth. The well-treated burned patient returns to nitrogen equilibrium, or more likely to positive balance, after a month.

In a high-calorie, high-protein diet, the ratio of calories to nitrogen in the intake is important because protein synthesis will not occur in the absence of adequate caloric intake. The calorie/nitrogen ratio is the ratio of nonprotein calories to protein nitrogen in the diet.
1 g of carbohydrate equals 4 calories.
1 g of fat equals 9 calories.
1 g of protein equals 4 calories.

About 40–50% of the chemical energy of carbohydrate and fat, and 80–85% of the chemical energy of protein, is converted to heat in the process of metabolism. A lack of caloric intake from the first two food sources will result in gradual combustion of body tissue. The burned patient loses weight as he loses muscle

[100] Shuck and Moncrief, op. cit., pp. 8–9.

Weigh dressings when dry, before applying them to Mr. A, and again when they are removed, as a basis for estimating the loss of protein via wound exudate.

4,000-calorie high-protein, high-vitamin, soft (bland) diet, in frequent small feedings (sixth postburn day).

Observe frequency and consistency of bowel movements. (Mr. A was consistently confronted with the added problem of constipation.)
Ask physician for p.r.n. enema order and prevent impaction.

Table 19-3 (cont.)

Physiological Changes, Medical Prescription and Nursing Responsibilities

Changes	Medical Prescriptions	Nurse Should:
mass and fat. His depletion syndrome includes low levels of total body protein, potassium, magnesium, sulfate, and other intracellular ions. Water and extracellular salts tend to remain in excess until the patient approaches nitrogen equilibrium.		
B-complex vitamins, especially thiamine, are essential to the enzyme systems responsible for facilitating use of glucose by the cell.	Multivitamins ii p.o. q.d.	Encourage foods rich in vitamin C. Ask family to contribute some of the following, if not available in quantity from the kitchen: Citrus fruits / Melons / Berries / Tomatoes / Raw vegetables
Ascorbic acid is essential for growth, cell activity, maintenance of strength of blood vessels, and formation of supporting tissues. Plasma ascorbic acid concentration is low after severe burns; ascorbic acid is one of the precursors of the adrenocortical steroids and thus is depleted during the body's response to stress and, in combination with increased tissue demands for vitamin C for healing the extensive areas of injury, requires administration of large doses of ascorbic acid.	Ascorbic acid, 500 mg p.o. t.i.d.	Encourage foods high in iron: Beans / Soybeans / Green leafy vegetables: / Kale / Turnips / Lean meats: liver / Dried fruits: / Prunes / Apricots
Anemia develops rapidly in severely burned patients who survive the initial period of shock. Amount of destruction of red blood cells (RBC's) following thermal injury is variable and in general is a significant problem only with deep burns.		
An additional factor that contributed to the prolonged catabolic phase of Mr. A's postburn period was the development of a Curling's ulcer at the end of the first postburn week, just as he was being given substantial amounts of oral intake.	Give maalox and milk every hour.	Observe for: / * Coffee-ground emesis / Hematemesis / * Poor food tolerance / Melena / Abdominal distention / Epigastric pain / Ileus / Mr. A demonstrated the starred behavior.
The incidence of gastroduodenal ulceration on one series of 88 patients who were fatally burned at the Brooke Army Medical Center was 47%.[101] A remarkable feature of stress ulcers in the study was the frequent lack of inflammatory response. The variation in severity and the inconstancy of the inflammatory response		

101 Artz and Moncrief, op. cit., pp. 73–76.

in these lesions as contrasted to the uniformity of significant leukocytic reactions in peptic ulcer cannot be completely explained.[102]

Mr. A has withstood the onslaught of every one of the insults to which the severely burned patient is subject. A large burn assaults the patient in three overlapping ways: hypovolemic shock, followed by sepsis and starvation, succeeded in turn by a period of limited function and nutritional inadequacy. The response to volume depletion, though doubtless subtle and complex, is at least well enough understood for treatment to be effective. Current understanding of the endocrine and metabolic response to starvation and sepsis in the second phase serves less well as a guide to treatment, and it is here that the majority of patients are lost.[103]

If Mr. A fails to win his battle for life, it will be because he lost the fight against starvation and sepsis.

[102] *Ibid.*
[103] Morgan and Moore, *op. cit.*, p. 81.

REFERENCES

BOOKS AND MONOGRAPHS

Artz, Curtis P., and Moncrief, John A.: *The Treatment of Burns,* 2nd ed. (Philadelphia: W. B. Saunders Company, 1969).

Feller, Irving: *International Bibliography on Burns* (Ann Arbor, Mich.: The American Burn Research Corporation, 1969.)

Fox, Charles L., Jr.: *Management of the Severely Burned Patient: With Special Reference to Fluid Therapy* (North Chicago: Abbott Laboratories, April 1968).

PERIODICALS

"Burns: The Neglected Trauma," *Roche Med. Image,* 10:6–8 (Dec.) 1968.

Craig, Nancy, "Silver Nitrate Stains: How One Hospital Is Meeting the Problem," *Hospitals,* 40:60 (Nov. 1) 1966.

Dominguez, Oscar, Bains, Jerry W., and Lewis, Steven R.: "Treatment of Burns with Silver Nitrate Versus Exposure Method: Analysis of 200 Patients," *Plast. Reconstr. Surg.,* 40:489–93 (Nov.) 1967.

Henley, Nellie L.: "Sulfamylon for Burns," *Amer. J. Nurs.,* 69:2122–23 (Oct.) 1969.

Morgan, Alfred P., and Moore, Francis D.: "Answers to Questions on Burns," *Hosp. Med.,* 4:71–89 (Sept.) 1968.

Peacock, Erle E., Jr.: "Burned Hands: And How to Heal Them," *Consultant,* 9:18–20 (Mar.–Apr.) 1969.

Phares, Richard E., and Paletta, Francis X.: "Silver Nitrate Treatment of Burns Involving Flexor Surfaces of the Body," *Surg. Forum,* 17:473 (Oct.) 1966.

Price, William R., and Wood, MacDonald: "Silver Nitrate Treatment of Burns Controls Infection, Pain, Heat Loss," *Hosp. Top.,* 46:109 (Feb.) 1968.

Price, William R., and Wood, MacDonald: "Operating Room Care of Burned Patients Treated with Silver Nitrate," *Amer. J. Nurs.,* 68:1705–1707 (Aug.) 1968.

Scapicchio, Anthony P., Constable, John D., and Opitz, Betsy F.: "Comparative Effects of Silver Nitrate and Sulfamylon Acetate on Epidermal Regeneration," *Surg. Forum,* 18:510 (Oct.) 1967.

Shuck, Jerry M., Moncrief, John A., and Monafo, William A.: "The Management of Burns," *Curr. Probl. Surg.,* pp. 3–66 (Feb.) 1969.

"Silver Nitrate Cream for Burn Treatment," *Mod. Med.,* 23:66–67 (Dec. 2) 1968.

Wood, MacDonald: "Silver Nitrate and Burns—Caution!" *Arizona Med.,* 22:817 (Oct.) 1965.

PART C:

Assessing the Level of Consciousness of the Patient

Introduction

Definitions

Nursing Responsibilities

Cause of the Disorder

Introduction

THROUGHOUT the book references have been made to conditions altering the level of consciousness of the patient. In the surgical treatment of patients unconsciousness may be induced in order to prevent pain and increase muscular relaxation. A great number of disorders of intrinsic or extrinsic origin may depress or alter cerebral function, such as (1) intracranial pathology—vascular thromboses or hemorrhage, cerebral edema, neoplasm or infection; (2) cranial or skull lesions and injuries; (3) metabolic disorders in which the homeostatic conditions of cells are altered—hypoglycemia, diabetic ketoacidosis, renal failure, liver failure, or iatrogenic disorders in which the levels of electrolytes such as potassium, hydrogen, and calcium are abnormal; (4) respiratory or circulatory disorders, which result in a failure to supply needed materials or to remove products of energy metabolism; and (5) toxic chemicals, including drugs and microbial products that have a depressing effect on the brain. All of the preceding as well as others may be accompanied by some alteration in the patient's state of consciousness.

The level of consciousness is the most important single indicator of cerebral function. The nurse must be able to detect changes as early as possible. According to one estimate, approximately 3 per cent of patients admitted to city hospitals have a disturbance in level of consciousness. Many more develop an alteration after admission. The primary purpose of this section is to present a guide for the assessment of the level of consciousness.

A point that must be emphasized is that the terms *conscious* and *unconscious* are abstractions. They are used differently in general medicine, psychiatry, psychology, and philosophy. The nurse should also know that mental function cannot be divided into clear or distinctive stages between consciousness and unconsciousness.

The nurse observes the patient to gather data to answer two major questions. What is (are) the possible cause(s) of loss of consciousness? What is the direction of change, that is, is the patient improving or getting worse? Descriptions of behavior are more likely to be helpful in answering these questions than naming a stage. As an illustration, Mrs. Beta answers the question "What is your name and where do you live" promptly, slowly, or not at all. In general the level of consciousness is assessed by noting the patient's response to various types of stimuli—verbal, tactile, visual, and painful. As the patient loses consciousness, he goes from alert and purposeful behavior to purposeless behavior. As he improves the reverse is true.

Definitions

Conscious. Alert, awake, aware; responds promptly to visual, auditory, tactile, and painful stimuli. Oriented to time, place, and self. Responds spontaneously to questions. In respect to orientation, awareness of time is first to be lost and awareness of self is last to disappear. Response to simple commands such as "squeeze my hand" is lost following disorientation to self. A point to be kept in mind is that when a person is in a strange environment or his sleeping patterns are disturbed, he may not know the hour of the day or the day of the week. Fully conscious patients may comment about "losing track" of time. On the other hand, gross misjudging of time is usually significant. A patient may appear to be fully alert and reveal some loss of awareness by making an irrelevant remark. As an example, Mrs. Alpha, aged 84, was hospitalized for the treatment of congestive heart failure. She was given digitalis and diuretics. Her serum potassium was 3 mEq/L. The only indication of a disturbance in mentation was a comment to her nurse. She believed that the time was 1913 and that she was in the hospital to have a baby. Her nurse reminded her that it was 1969. The nurse also gave her orange juice to drink and reported and recorded the incident. The patient's judgment may be tested by asking him to interpret a well-known saying such as "The grass is greener on the other side of the fence." The nurse should try to select statements that will have meaning to the patient and remember that the higher the patient's intelligence and level of education, the more difficult it is to test his judgment. Others, such as family members, report failing judgment before a physician or nurse can detect it.

Confusion is used to describe the state of an individual who is unable to recognize and respond to his environment in a normal manner. For example, Mr. Penn thinks that his nurse is his granddaughter. Conversely, some patients believed to be confused are not when all the facts are known.

Lethargy. Drowsiness, somnolence, a dull sluggish state. The patient can be aroused and may be clear mentally, but he is frequently somewhat confused. Answers questions with sentences, but slowly.

Obtundation. Dull, lacks mental acuteness. The patient can be awakened but little more. Uses gestures but few words.

Stupor. The patient can be aroused only by vigorous and continuous stimulation; he may move spontaneously, and he responds to painful, loud noises and bright light. Response is usually by withdrawal, but the patient may be combative. Bowel and bladder control varies. Able to locate site of painful stimulation.

Semicoma. The patient responds only to painful stimuli by mass movement.

Coma. Varies from moderate coma to deep coma. In moderate coma the patient has rudimentary reflex motor responses. In deep coma all psychological and motor responses are lost. The patient is incontinent of feces and urine.

Delirium. A self-limiting state associated with an acute brain syndrome. It is characterized by fluctuating levels of consciousness. The patient is disorientated as to time, place, and person. He may experience anxiety to the point of panic. When his anxiety is severe, he may attempt suicide. He may have hallucinations, especially of the visual type. He may fear that he will be poisoned or harmed in some way.

Sleep. "Commonly looked upon as a periodic temporary cessation, or interruption of the waking state, which is the prevalent mode of existence for the healthy human adult." [102]

[102] Nathaniel Kleitman: *Sleep and Wakefulness* (Chicago: University of Chicago Press, 1963).

Sleep and wakefulness are cyclical states occurring under predictable conditions; a sleeping person can be fully awakened by unusual stimuli. The amount of stimulation required varies with the depth of sleep.

An all too common error is the presumption that any patient admitted in a stuporous or comatose state and who has the odor of alcohol on his breath is intoxicated. He may be, but he may not be. As a result he may be allowed to die from the effects of some treatable disorder such as hypoglycemia or a subdural hematoma.

Nursing Responsibilities

Granted that a disturbance in the level of consciousness is more likely to be associated with some disorders than others, it is a possibility in any seriously ill or toxic individual. The first responsibility of the nurse is to watch over the patient in order to detect any changes in the mental state of the patient. It is well to keep in mind that the patient's mental state may change with great rapidity. He may appear to be alert when seen at one time and five minutes later be stuporous.

When analyzing data, the nurse should be certain that she has enough data to make sound judgments. Care should be taken to validate inferences. Erroneous conclusions may place a patient in jeopardy. For example, Mr. Delta was thought to be confused because he repeatedly told his nurse that the windshield of his car had been damaged a few days before he was admitted to the hospital. Because he was acutely ill from an infectious disease, the inference that he was confused was logical but erroneous. The windshield had in fact been damaged.

Cause of the Disorder

Guide for Assessment of Consciousness

1. Normal sleep.
2. State of consciousness.
   a. Fully alert.
   b. Lethargy.
   c. Obtundation.
   d. Stupor.
   e. Semicoma.
   f. Coma.
   g. Delirium.
3. Other responses.
   a. Skeletal muscle response.
      (1) Ability to move voluntarily on command.

(a) Extremities.
(b) Smile, pucker lips.
(c) Hand grasp.
(d) Eye movements.
(2) Strength of muscle contraction.
b. Reflexes.
(1) Responses to light, noise, pain.
(2) Pupillary responses.
(a) Size.
(b) Reaction to light.
(c) Equality of size.
Note: Fixed dilatation of the pupils is a poor prognostic sign.
c. Swallowing.
d. Continence of urine and feces.
e. As indicated, inspect the condition of the patient's skin, mouth, eyes, and ears.
f. Vital signs.
g. Position.
(1) Assumed by the patient.
(2) Prescribed.

Nursing Actions Depending on or Stemming from Assessment

1. Report and record changes in levels of consciousness in behavioral terms. (Changes indicating improvement are as significant as those indicating deterioration.)
2. Safety precautions.
a. Maintain clear airway. In any patient whose consciousness is depressed, main-tenance of a clear airway takes a high priority. (See Chapters 8 and 17.)
b. Protect the patient who is unable to swallow from his own secretions and test ability to swallow before offering fluids. (See Chapters 8 and 12.)
c. Maintain patient in (prescribed) position.
d. Turn every 1 to 2 hours. (See Chapter 4.)
e. Prevent patient from lying on arm when in the side-lying position. (See Chapters 4 and 17.)
f. Breathing exercises if patient can co-operate.
g. Mouth care. Give particular attention to the area around the uvula in patients who breathe through their mouths for lengthy periods of time. Crusts forming in and around the uvula may break off and be aspirated. (See Chapter 17.)
h. Skin care. (See Chapter 4.)
i. Side rails, padded if necessary.
j. Removal of cigarettes, matches, or other harmful objects if patient is confused or delirious.
3. Maintain fluid and food intake. (See Chapters 9, 11, and 12.)
4. Attention to indwelling urinary catheter. (See Chapter 17.)
5. Protect conjunctiva and cornea from exposure to drying.
a. Remove secretions as indicated.
b. Bandage the eye.

REFERENCES

BOOKS

See medical and physiology texts at beginning of the References in Chapter 4.

Fazekas, Joseph F., and Alman, Ralph W.: *Coma* (Springfield, Ill.: Charles C Thomas, Publisher, 1962).

Plum, Fred, and Posner, J. B.: *The Diagnosis of Stupor and Coma* (Philadelphia: F. A. Davis Company, 1966).

United States Department of Health, Education, and Welfare: *Current Research on Sleep and Dreams* (Washington, D.C.: Superintendent of Documents, U.S. Government Printing Office, 1966).

Webb, Wilse B.: *Sleep: An Experimental Approach* (New York: The Macmillan Company, 1968).

PERIODICALS

Brooks, Helen Louise: "The Golden Rule for the Unconscious Patient," *Nurs. Forum,* 4:12–18 (No. 3) 1965.

Butts, Cl., *et al.:* "The Unresponsive Patient," *Amer. J. Nurs.,* 67:1886–88 (Sept.) 1967.

Gardner, M. Arlene Martin: "Responsiveness as a Measure of Consciousness," *Amer. J. Nurs.,* 68:1035–38 (May) 1968.

Gumnit, R. J.: "The Medical Management of Closed Head Injuries," *Geriatrics,* 22:112–18 (Dec.) 1967.

Luessenhop, Alfred: "Care of the Unconscious Patient," *Nurs. Forum,* 4:6–11 (No. 3) 1965.

Mannarino, E., *et al.:* "Management of Head Injuries," *Surg. Clin. N. Amer.,* 48:723–36 (Aug.) 1968.

Moraczewski, Albert, and Adriani, John: "The Hopelessly Unconscious Patient," *Postgrad. Med.,* 44:126–29 (Dec.) 1968.

INDEX

Abnormalities, 48, 167
Abrasions, defined, 85
Abscesses
  brain, 293
  chronic, 566
  defined, 186
  examples, 187
  obstructive, 248
  spontaneous opening, 186–87
  staphylococcal, 145
Absorption from GI tract, 521
Acalculia, 833
Accidents. *See also* Safety
  death rates, 12, 37
Acetyl coenzyme A, 79, 544, 854–55
Achalasia, 570*t*
Achlorhydria (HCL), cancer of stomach, 638
Acid(s). *See also* specific acids
  buffer systems, 333
  defined, 307
  dilution, 333
  regulation of acid-base equilibrium, 333
  urine, 336, 341–42
Acid-base balance
  equilibrium, 333
  mechanisms for maintaining, 333–37
Acidosis
  bicarbonate anion, 334, 470
  burn patients, 886–88
  diabetes mellitus, 563, 858–62
  fasting, 563
  metabolic
    causes, 337, 470
    signs and symptoms, 291–92, 338, 470
    treatment and nursing care, 338
  from methyl alcohol poisoning, 101
  respiratory
    causes, 260, 338
    prevention, 339
    signs and symptoms, 338–39
    treatment, 226
Acromegaly, 678
ACTH (adrenocorticotrophic hormone), 76*n*
  allergies, 179
  effects, 161, 213, 558, 682
  regulation, 682
  secretion, 198*t,* 677
  testing adrenocortical function, 682
Activity. *See also* Ambulation; Bedrest; Exercise
  daily living, 835–36
  necessary, 76
Adaptation, 42–50, 163–64
  biological, 47–48
  cause of injury, 106, 163
  characteristics, 49–50
  defined, 46

Adaptation (*Cont.*)
  etiology of disease, 54–56
  factors influencing capacity, 48–49
  high altitude, 247
  individual capacity, 55–56, 206
  man to environment, 42–50
  psychological, 48, 206
  syndrome, 163–64
Addiction
  alcohol, 79–80, 422–23
  drugs, 36
Adenohypophysis, relationship to thyroid, 76*n,*
    686–87
Adenosine triphosphate (ATP), 463, 475, 543, 557
Adenoviruses as cause of respiratory disease, 294,
    296
Adiadochokinesia, 721
Adolescence, 741–43
  developmental tasks, 739
  nutrition, 493
Adrenal glands, 679–86. *See also* Injury
  cortex
    adenomas, 685, 686
    atrophy, 76*n,* 682
    hormones, 163–64, 681, 685, 686
    hypersecretion, 685–86
    insufficiency, 682
      nurses' responsibilities, 683
      therapy, 684–85
  medulla
    hormones, 44–45, 679–80
    hyperfunction, 680–81
    relationship to nervous system, 679–80
Adynamic ileus, 527, 788
Aerosol therapy, carrier gas, 281
Agammaglobulinemia, 167
Age
  adaptability, 48–49, 152, 161
  aging process; eight stages in life cycle of man,
    738–40
  healing, 195
  nutrition, 195, 493
  relationship of illness, 118, 152
  response to injury, 152
  senescence
    anemia, 447
    constipation, 526
    emphysema, 265–66
    heart failure, 375
    prolonged sitting, 414
    surgery, 638
Agenesis, 78
Aggression, 229
Agnosia, 725, 834
Agranulocytosis (agranulocytopenia), 182
Agraphia, 833

Neuromuscular irritability, 320, 330, 333
Neurons, 707
Neuropathy, diabetes, 863
Neutrons, defined, 90
Neutrophils, 118
    inflammation, 185
Niacin, deficiency, 567
Nissl bodies, 707
Nitrogen
    balance, 565
    blockage of blood vessels, 245
    blood urea, 341
    component of atmosphere, 244
    emboli, 245
    partial pressure, 244–45
Nitrogen mustards
    administration, 182
    treatment of cancer, 643
Nitroglycerine, angina pectoris, 403–404
Nitrous oxide, 245
Node of Ranvier, 709
Nodular goiter, 691*t*
Nonverbal communication of pain, 805
Norepinephrine (Levarterenol or Levophed), 157,
    406, 423, 429, 680
Normergy, defined, 166
Nose
    cleansing action, 248–49
    mucous membrane, secretion, 249
Nose drops, overuse, 252
Nosocomial infections. *See* Infection
Nuclei, 715*n*, 715, 716, 717
Nucleic acids, antigens, 165, 168. *See* DNA;
    Heredity; and RNA
Nucleotides, 664*n*
Nursing. *See also* specific diseases
    attitudes about patients, 3
    beliefs, 1–2
    case finding, 112, 136
    competencies, 4
    components, 17–18
    contribution to health field, 2
    defined, 2
    diagnosis, 13
    expectations, nurse, 218–19
        patient, 6–10, 217–18
    functions, 46. *See also* specific diseases and con-
        ditions
    hypothesis, 16–17
    objectives, 18
    personalized, 6–8
    practice, culture, 206–19
    process, 14–17
    professional status, 2–3
    relation to social issues, 4, 32–33
    roles, 5–6
        neuromuscular response, 155–56
    scholarly concern, 5
    understanding society, 4–5
    unique skills, 4–5
Nutrition. *See also* Food; Ischemia; Malnutrition;
        specific nutrients
    atrophy, 76
    defined, 482
    effect of neoplasms, 627, 628–29
    elimination diet for allergies, 175

Nutrition (*Cont.*)
    factors affecting, 487–88
        conditioning, 491–92
        cultural, 489–90
        emotional, 490–91
        family, 490
        habits, 472
        psychological, 488
        senses, 487–88
        symbolic value, 491
    feeding physically dependent patient, 730
    health, 482
    immunity, 117
    mental retardation, 485
    requirements, 483–84
    responsibilities of nurse, 483
    surgery
        preoperative evaluation, 757–60
        requirements, 161
    survey of dietary adequacy, 567–68
    value of blood transfusions, 786
Nutritional status, 485. *See also* Malnutrition
    defined, 482
    programs for improvement, 486
    studies, 507–508
    world problems, 486

Obesity
    causes, 547–49
    Cushing's syndrome, 685
    definition, 546
    diabetes mellitus, 547, 847
    Fröhlich's syndrome, 548
    hazards, 547
    heart disease, 390, 401, 547
    heat loss, 596, 596*t*
    hypertension, 434
    hypothyroidism, 692*t*
    mortality rates, 547
    overeating, 547
    predisposition to disease, 547
    prevention, 549
    surgery, 759
    treatment, 549–52
    United States, 546
Observation, nursing process, 15–17
Obstruction. *See also* specific organs and sites
    general effects, 76, 76*n*, 250, 527
Occlusive vascular disease. *See* Circulatory system
Occupational therapy, 230
Old tuberculin (OT), 130
Oliguria. *See* Urine
Oncology, defined, 609
Oncotic pressure, 279
Oral care. *See* Mouth, care
Orthopnea, 279, 290. *See also* Dyspnea
    position, 291, 329, 389
    relief, 379
Oscillometers in peripheral vascular disease, 424
Osmol, 308
Osmolality
    defined, 308
    reduced serum, 326
Osmotic pressure
    colloid, 184, 279
    corrected, 320